BIOACTIVE COMPOUNDS AND CANCER

NUTRITION AND HEALTH

Adrianne Bendich, PhD, FACN, Series Editor

For other titles published in this series, go to
http://www.springer.com/series/7659

BIOACTIVE COMPOUNDS AND CANCER

Edited by

JOHN A. MILNER

National Cancer Institute, Health and Human Services, Rockville, MD

DONATO F. ROMAGNOLO

Department of Nutritional Sciences, The University of Arizona, Tucson, AZ

Forewords by

DAVID S. ALBERTS, MD

Arizona Cancer Center, The University of Arizona, Tucson, AZ

MARIA LLURIA-PREVATT, PhD

Arizona Cancer Center, The University of Arizona, Tucson, AZ

and

SCOTT M. LIPPMAN, MD

Department of Thoracic/Head and Neck Medical Oncology, M. D. Anderson Cancer Center, The University of Texas, Houston, TX

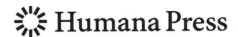 Humana Press

Editors

John A. Milner
Nutritional Science Research Group
Division of Cancer Prevention
National Institutes of Health
Executive Plaza North
Suite 3164
6130 Executive Boulevard
Rockville MD 20892
USA
milnerj@mail.nih.gov

Donato F. Romagnolo
Department of Nutritional Sciences
The University of Arizona
Tucson AZ 85721-0038
Shantz Building
USA
donato@u.arizona.edu

Series Editor

Adrianne Bendich, PhD, FACN
GlaxoSmithKline Consumer Healthcare
Parsippany, NJ
USA

ISBN 978-1-60761-626-9   e-ISBN 978-1-60761-627-6
DOI 10.1007/978-1-60761-627-6
Springer New York Dordrecht Heidelberg London

Library of Congress Control Number: 2010922882

Printed on acid-free paper

Humana Press is part of Springer Science+Business Media (www.springer.com)

Series Editor Introduction

The Nutrition and Health Series of books have, as an overriding mission, to provide health professionals with texts that are considered essential because each includes (1) a synthesis of the state of the science, (2) timely, in-depth reviews by the leading researchers in their respective fields, (3) extensive, up-to-date fully annotated reference lists, (4) a detailed index, (5) relevant tables and figures, (6) identification of paradigm shifts and the consequences, (7) virtually no overlap of information between chapters, but targeted, inter-chapter referrals, (8) suggestions of areas for future research, and (9) balanced, data-driven answers to patient/health professionals questions which are based upon the totality of evidence rather than the findings of any single study.

The Series volumes are developed to provide valuable in-depth information to nutrition health professionals and health providers interested in practical guidelines. Each editor has the potential to examine a chosen area with a broad perspective, both in subject matter and in the choice of chapter authors. The international perspective, especially with regard to public health initiatives, is emphasized where appropriate. The editors, whose trainings are both research and practice oriented, have the opportunity to develop a primary objective for their book; define the scope and focus, and then invite the leading authorities from around the world to be part of their initiative. The authors are encouraged to provide an overview of the field, discuss their own research, and relate the research findings to potential human health consequences. Because each book is developed de novo, the chapters are coordinated so that the resulting volume imparts greater knowledge than the sum of the information contained in the individual chapters.

"Bioactive Compounds and Cancer," edited by John A. Milner, Ph.D., and Donato F. Romagnolo, Ph.D., is a very welcome addition to the Nutrition and Health Series and exemplifies the Series' goals. This volume is especially timely as the number of research papers and meta-analyses in the clinical nutrition arena of cancer research increases every year and clients and patients are very interested in dietary components that have bioactivity and may be able to impact cancer prevention as well as reduce the adverse effects of cancer therapies. The editors have made great efforts to provide health professionals with the most up-to-date and comprehensive volume that highlights the key, nutrition, and cancer information available to date. They have combined their broad backgrounds in research as well as clinical practice to help the reader to better understand the relevant science while providing background information so that the reader can understand and appreciate the importance of the mechanisms of action of the bioactive components in their diets.

Drs. Milner and Romagnolo are internationally recognized leaders in the field of nutrition and cancer biology and have actively investigated the physiological roles of dietary bioactive compounds as modifiers of cancer risk and tumor behavior. The editors are proven excellent communicators and they have worked tirelessly to develop a book that is destined to be the benchmark in the field because of its extensive review of the current state of the science with regard to dietary bioactive compounds and the complex interactions between diet, health, and the development and the progression of cancer. Dr. Milner is the Chief of the Nutritional Science Research Group, Division of Cancer Prevention at the National Institutes of Health's National Cancer Institute (NCI). In this capacity, Dr. Milner is responsible for helping to set the national strategy for cancer research. Prior to joining the NCI, Dr. Milner led the Department of Nutrition at The Pennsylvania State University for over a decade. He also served as the Director of the Division of Nutritional Science at the University of Illinois. Dr. Milner has served as the President of the American Society for Nutrition and as chair of the World Cancer Research Fund/American Institute for Cancer Research Mechanisms Working Group. In 2008, Dr. Milner received the David A. Kritchevsky Career Achievement Award in Nutrition from the American Society for Nutrition. Dr. Romagnolo is Professor of Nutritional and Cancer Biology at the University of Arizona and is a member of the Arizona Cancer Center, BIO5, and the Center for Toxicology. He has served as the chair of the Environmental Gene Expression Group of the Southwest Environmental Health Sciences Center. Thus, both editors are immersed in the discovery and implementation of research to better understand the effects of bioactive molecules from the diet on cancer development and control.

The editors have chosen 76 of the most well-recognized and respected authors from around the world to contribute the 33 informative chapters in the volume. Hallmarks of all of the chapters include complete definitions of terms with the abbreviations fully defined for the reader and consistent use of terms between chapters. Key features of this comprehensive volume include the informative Key Points and key words that are at the beginning of each chapter and suggested readings as well as bibliography at the end of each chapter. The volume contains more than 150 detailed tables and informative figures, an extensive, detailed index and more than 4,300 up-to-date references that provide the reader with excellent sources of worthwhile information about the role of diet, foods, food components, essential nutrients, bioactive phytochemicals, and their potential mechanisms of action in affecting cancer risk.

This comprehensive volume is divided into two major sections beginning with six introductory chapters, followed by the section on bioactive molecules divided into three logical subsections – eight chapters on dietary macro-constituents; eight chapters covering carotenoids, vitamins, and minerals; and the final section including 10 chapters on the most researched of the myriad of non-nutritionally essential bioactive components in the diet. The final chapter examines the challenges of communicating food and cancer relationships to consumers, clients, and patients. The volume begins with an introductory chapter that examines the overall cancer rates in the United States, the major cancer types, and the populations most affected by cancer. We learn that about 1.5 million new cancers will be diagnosed each year and over half a million persons will die from this disease annually. For both men and women, lung and bronchus cancers are the leading cause of cancer deaths even though most individuals think that breast and prostate cancers are the major cancer killers. There is an extensive discussion of the Surveillance, Epidemiology and End Results (SEER) Program from the NCI, and the numerous tables and figures provide examples of the cancer statistics for incidence and survival rates in the US population. The next chapter reminds us that only about 5% of cancer cases are genetically inherited, whereas 95% are linked to environmental factors including diet. There is a clear explanation of the developmental phases of cancer and the potential for bioactive molecules in the diet to affect the early stages of initiation and promotion. As an example, the interactions between nutritional factors and genes, defined as nutrigenomics, are carefully examined so that the reader is provided with the basics of this new area of research. An excellent explanation concerning the newest research tools including high-throughput proteomic and metabolomic approaches are placed in perspective to better understand their value in nutrition and cancer research. Examples of bioactive compounds found in foods include essential nutrients such as vitamins and minerals and essential lipids; plant polyphenols, carotenoids, xenobiotics, and numerous other molecular entities. The complex interactions between the bioactive molecules and genetic components including histones, DNA methylation, transcription factors, cell cycle regulators, and other factors are introduced and explanations are provided so that the reader can better understand the importance of these interactions.

Cancer begins with changes in the cell's DNA and the next chapter comprehensively reviews the major changes that result is cellular malignancy and examines the data suggesting that certain dietary factors can interfere with the progression of cells through the steps resulting in a cancerous cell. The reader is alerted that dietary factors that affect cells in cell culture may not be effective in vivo. Dietary substances that are briefly discussed include resveratrol, sulforaphane, apigenin (a flavonoid found in many fruits and vegetables), curcumin, EGCG and quercetin, and several other examples that are examined in greater depth in subsequent individual chapters. Within the cell, changes in single nucleotides (single nucleotide polymorphisms or SNPs) can result in changes to the structure, function, and/or the cellular content of a specific protein. If the SNP is located in genes involved in the metabolism of bioactive dietary factors, then this genetic change can result in alterations in cellular responses to potential carcinogens as one example. The next chapter, on nutrigenetics, closely examines nutrient–gene interactions. The epidemiological associations between antioxidants, folates, and dietary phytoestrogens, and reduced risk as well as the associations between meats and the compounds generated during cooking and increased cancer risk are reviewed with the aid of informative figures. Epigenetic processes that can alter the regulation of genes is the logical topic of the next chapter and it concentrates on the importance of dietary sources of methyl donors including folate, choline, and methionine. The final chapter in the introductory section examines the role of transcription factors that can initiate changes in the DNA in cells and the potential for dietary factors to modulate the actions of these transcription factors. The information contained within the first six chapters provides the reader with a firm grounding in the complexities of the cellular events that ultimately can lead to cancer and informs the reader of the newest research to identify key components in the diet that may be able to reduce the risk of forming cancerous cells.

The second section begins with the subsection on macro-constituents and the first chapter concerns the macronutrients, obesity, and the potential for calorie restriction (using diets that provide the full measure of essential nutrients in a calorie restricted matrix) and physical activity to reduce cancer risk by altering the synthesis of endogenous hormones and growth factors that are stimulated by caloric intakes. In addition to macronutrients, diets contain fiber that is defined as the plant parts that are resistant to hydrolysis by human gastrointestinal (GI) enzymes. The importance of fiber (prebiotics) as well as metabolic products of the probiotic microbes that reside in the human alimentary tract and their role in the development of cancer – especially in the GI tract, is the topic of the next chapter. The following chapter explores the importance of the gut microbiota in greater detail and provides discussions of specific microbes in the gut and their influence on not only cancer risk but also potentially precancerous inflammatory responses in the colon and other organ systems as well.

Flame-cooked red meats and processed meat consumption is consistently associated with increased risk of cancers in the GI tract. The mechanisms by which these meats can increase cancer risk are clearly explained and strategies to reduce risk are included in the next chapter. Meats contain a higher proportion of saturated to unsaturated fats and the next chapter reviews the evidence linking higher intakes of most saturated fats with increased risk of cancer. The following chapter examines the early evidence from in vitro and animal studies that certain isomers of one fatty acid found in meat and dairy products, conjugated linoleic acid (CLA), may reduce the risk of certain cancers; the chapter includes almost a dozen relevant figures that help the reader to better understand the complexity of the findings with CLA. In contrast to most of the fats in meats, the polyunsaturated fats, primarily long-chain n−3 fatty acids from fish or other sources (discussed in a separate chapter), have been associated with a decreased risk of cancer possibly by affecting translational regulation of genes and thereby reducing cell proliferation. The next chapter, containing over 200 references and two detailed tables of the relevant clinical studies, reviews the data linking higher intakes of n-6 unsaturated fatty acids with increased risk of cancer that may be due to the increased cell proliferation and inflammation associated with n-6 fatty acid metabolites. These five chapters highlight the complexity of making generalizations about all fats; nevertheless, the authors, who are recognized leaders in this area of research, clearly present compelling arguments for maintaining overall fat intake at about 30% of calories/day, keeping saturated fat intake to 10% of calories, and maintaining a 1–2:1 ratio of n-6 to n-3 fatty acids in the daily diet.

In the section entitled carotenoids, vitamins, and minerals, there are individual chapters on carotenoids, vitamin A, vitamin D, folate, selenium, calcium, iron, and zinc contributed by the major researchers of these nutrients. The chapter on carotenoids highlights the consistent association between fruit and vegetable intakes with decreased cancer risks and examines in detail two individual carotenoids found in the human diet: β-carotene and lycopene. The authors remind the reader that even though the immediate headlines from the ATBC study published in 1994 suggested that Finnish smokers who were in the β-carotene arm had increased rates of lung cancer, data published 6 years later no longer found this association; four other β-carotene intervention studies found no increased risk of lung cancer in smokers although the number of smokers in these studies was not as great as in the ATBC and CARET studies. The entire literature concerning lycopene in major in vitro and all in vivo studies is tabulated for the reader. The authors conclude with a recommendation for individuals to eat five servings of fruits and vegetables/day and make five of those choices lycopene-containing tomato products each week. Certain carotenoids can be metabolized to vitamin A (retinol), which is an essential nutrient critical for controlling cell growth and differentiation into normal cells in contrast to cancerous cells. Retinoic acid (RA), a metabolite of retinol, is a direct activator of genetic functions and has been examined as a chemopreventive drug over many years. Many RA derivatives have been synthesized and tested as cancer treatments. This chapter points out the difficulties found in moving from positive in vitro and animal studies to human studies of both chemoprevention and chemotherapy with vitamin A as well as the retinoids. With regard to vitamin D, discussed in the next chapter, its role in cancer development and potential in treatment is a very new area of research associated with the capability of non-renal tissues to locally synthesize the active form of the vitamin whereas cancerous tissue appears to lose this function. The epidemiology and the mechanism of action studies are carefully reviewed and a recommendation is made for increased intake of vitamin D. Synthesis of DNA as well as the methylation of this molecule and others within the body requires folate, an essential water-soluble B vitamin. Epidemiological data point to the inverse association between folate intake and risk of cancers of the colon and esophagus. However, intervention studies with folic-acid supplementation have not shown reduction in precancerous colon polyps. It may be that unrecognized genetic polymorphisms in the enzymes controlling folate and other B vitamin metabolism have reduced the potential to see the beneficial effects of folate and/or may even increase the risk of carcinogenesis. Given that many nations have implemented a folic-acid fortification program to reduce the occurrence of neural tube birth defects, it is critical to better understand the timing and dose of folate needed to reduce and not enhance cancer development and/or progression.

Selenium is the first essential mineral reviewed and as has been seen with many of the nutrients, there are several bioactive forms in the food supply as well as in the body. Likewise, selenium has a number of functions within the body as it is a component of an antioxidant enzyme and many other selenoproteins involved in cellular metabolism. In vitro, animal and epidemiological data support a chemopreventive role for selenium. However, the two clinical trials have provided inconsistent results for prostate cancer that may be due to many factors not the least of which could be the baseline selenium status of the cohort. Calcium, the mineral discussed in the next chapter, has been shown to significantly reduce the rate of colon polyp recurrence. Moreover, recent data from a large cohort suggests that supplemental intakes of calcium are associated with reduced risk of total cancers in post-menopausal women. The data for prostate cancer associations are inconsistent. Iron, another essential element, is required for the synthesis of energy in the form of ATP. There are no data suggesting that increased iron intake reduces the risk of cancers, rather in individuals with the homozygous genetic defect that causes iron overload, there is an increased risk of liver cancer and in heterozygotes there are increases in risks of several cancers. Other genes and proteins associated with iron metabolism and cancer risk are tabulated in this chapter. Epidemiological data show inconsistent associations between high iron intakes and cancer risks that may reflect red meat consumption (mentioned in the chapter on meat and cancer as well). The final chapter in this section looks at the role of zinc in cancer development and prevention. Zinc is an essential component of over 300 human enzymes and is thus involved in virtually all aspects of cellular function. Yet, the research on zinc and cancer is in its infancy. In vitro cell culture studies have shown important effects of zinc and studies in zinc-deficient animal models find increased cancer development. There are consistent epidemiological associations of low zinc status and increased risk of oral and esophageal cancers, but no intervention studies of zinc alone have been initiated.

Non-nutritive bioactive molecules found in foods, spices, and herbs and their potential role in cancer prevention and/or treatment is an exciting and very active area of research. Drs. Milner and Romagnolo have chosen ten of the most well-studied bioactives and have also enlisted the investigators who have done the most work on these compounds to provide informative chapters. As the research on the effects of the bioactive compounds is at the early states of investigation, many have not been used in clinical intervention studies. Cruciferous vegetables contain isothiocyanates and indoles; these compounds have been shown to affect tumor cell cycles, gene expressions, apoptosis, inflammatory responses, and other factors associated with lowering the risk of initiation and growth of malignant cells. Broccoli is the most commonly consumed cruciferous vegetable in US diets at about once/week, and cooking inactivates some of the bioactive compounds. Genotypes likely affect the cancer preventive potential of these compounds. There are no full-scale clinical studies; the epidemiological studies are tabulated. Garlic and the bioactive sulfur compounds isolated from garlic have been shown to reduce cell proliferation and enhance DNA repair and in laboratory animal studies, garlic decreased cancer formation following exposure to carcinogens. However, epidemiological and clinical data are not available, so this is a new area for clinical investigation.

Two polyphenol compounds are reviewed in the next chapter that examines the anticarcinogenic potential of resveratrol and genistein in animal models and cell culture studies. In rodent models of breast or prostate cancer, the two compounds individually and in combination appeared to reduce the size and progression of these tumors. Tea catechins, fruit and vegetable flavonols, and procyandins have also been shown to be of benefit against tumor development in animal models. The epidemiological evidence for tea consumption and reduced cancer risk is tabulated; results from small intervention studies are reviewed. The next chapter provides an in depth review of the isoflavones genistein and daidzein from soy (more than 200 cited references) and concludes that these compounds have anti-carcinogenic effects in animal models and a number of mechanisms of action. Because of their estrogenic activity, clinical investigations may concentrate on non-estrogen responsive cancers. Many culinary herbs and spices including rosemary, oregano, basil, chilies, turmeric, ginger, and cloves have demonstrated antioxidant and anti-inflammatory activities in cell culture and some have been tested in animal models of cancer. Emphasis in this chapter is placed on the data concerning curcumin from turmeric where there have been some small clinical investigations in cancer patients looking at biomarkers of activity. Berries, such as strawberries, blueberries, cranberries, and raspberries, have been consumed by humans throughout history. These fruits contain essential nutrients as well as other bioactive phytochemicals including phenolic acids and flavonoids. The anthocyanins are one of the most abundant flavonoids in berries. Extracts can reduce cellular carcinogenesis in culture and in certain animal models. Pilot intervention studies have shown that berry concentrates can modulate biomarkers of cancer development. Pomegranates have also been consumed by humans for centuries and there is interest in the phytochemicals in the rind and juice produced from the whole fruit that contains a tannin, punicalagin. A pilot intervention study with pomegranate juice in men with prostate cancer found an increase in the time with no rise in prostate-specific antigen.

Alcohol use has been consistently associated with an increased risk of breast cancer in women and with cancers of the aerodigestive tract. Cell studies and animal models document that ethanol is the carcinogen in alcohol and the cancer risk is related directly to dose. The alcohol–cancer relationship can be modified by many factors including dietary status, concomitant smoking or other environmental toxins, gender, age, and by genetics. Over 200 references are included in this chapter. The other major classes of compounds that can increase the risk of cancer are the xenobiotics from the environment including polycyclic aromatic hydrocarbons and dioxins. The mechanisms of cancer formation and the potential to reduce the effects of exposure with the consumption of foods that contain beneficial bioactive molecules is the topic of the next chapter. Flavonols that can activate detoxifying enzymes may reduce the risk of cancer formation by lowering the body burden of these environmental toxins.

The final chapter of the volume is of great practical relevance and unique to this volume. The chapter examines the opportunities and challenges of communicating to consumers about foods and cancer risk. Effective communication is critically important as we do not appear to be able to stem the obesity epidemic; and obesity is a significant risk factor for many cancers. Consumer research from the 2008 International Food Information Council (IFIC) Food and Health Survey into attitudes and awareness of the role of dietary components in their health is reviewed. It is important to determine how clients, patients, and colleagues interpret the health messages that the media develop from research studies such as those presented in this volume.

In conclusion, "Bioactive Compounds and Cancer" edited by John A. Milner, Ph.D., and Donato F. Romagnolo, Ph.D., provides health professionals in many areas of research and practice with the most up-to-date, well-referenced volume on the importance of diet and its effects on cancer risk. This volume will serve the reader as the benchmark in this complex area of interrelationships between food, dietary intakes, and body weight, the myriad of mechanisms by which bioactive components in our diet can reduce the risk of initiation, promotion, and progression of malignancies. Moreover, the interactions between environmental and genetic factors are clearly delineated so that practitioners can better understand the complexities of these interactions. The editors are applauded for their efforts to develop this volume which now stands as the benchmark in the field of nutrition and cancer. This excellent text is a very welcome addition to the Nutrition and Health Series.

Adrianne Bendich, PhD, FACN

Foreword by David S. Alberts, MD, and Maria Lluria-Prevatt, PhD

While we have begun to see documented decline of both the incidence and death rates from all cancers combined in both men and women *(1)*, cancer still accounts for more deaths than heart disease in persons younger than 85 years of age. Our Western lifestyle literally is killing us! In order to extend the success in reducing cancer incidence and death, our knowledge of the effects of nutrition and physical activity in cancer causation, prevention, and intervention are essential. After all, there is a growing consensus that we must "get off the couch and out to the refrigerator" if we are to survive.

There is an expected more than 1.5 million new cases of invasive cancer and 560,000 cancer deaths in the United States in 2009 *(2)*. Alarmingly, with our present rate of increase in obesity, it is estimated that the current patterns of overweight and obesity in the United States could account for 14% of all deaths from cancer in men and 20% of those in women *(3)*. The vast majority of these cancer cases are preventable.

The multistage model of carcinogenesis demonstrates the stages of initiation, promotion, and progression as a multiyear process. If we understand that for most common cancer types there may be an estimated lag time of 20–30 years from the first initiated (i.e., DNA damaged) cancer cell to death from metastatic cancer, then there are between 11 million and 17 million people in the United States who currently have some phase of premalignant disease who, ultimately, will die from cancer. There is a wide window of opportunity within this long lag period or premalignant phase in which enhanced physical activity and nutritionally targeted cancer prevention can effectively influence the course of this disease process (Fig. 1).

The editors, Drs. John A. Milner and Donato F. Romagnolo, of "Bioactive Compounds and Cancer" have brought together 76 world renowned authors to provide the most up-to-date, comprehensive volume discussing numerous dietary components that have demonstrated an impact on cancer risk and prevention in preclinical models and/or clinically. This text provides health professionals the most relevant science-based knowledge with regard to dietary bioactive compounds and their effects on the progression of cancer.

There have been a large number of observational studies showing a reduction in the risk of several types of epithelial malignancies among populations with higher intakes of fruits and vegetables *(5)* or reduction in fat intake *(6)*. While a primary prevention strategy might involve the promotion of a high fruit and vegetable and/or low-fat diet to reduce the frequency of initiated cells or to repair damage manifested by initiated cells, the authors of this text have taken the process a step further by identifying the actual dietary component that specifically demonstrates bioactivity in a wide variety of cancers in preclinical and/or clinical settings. These authors provide scientific data of the mechanisms of action of these compounds and in many cases have been able to identify

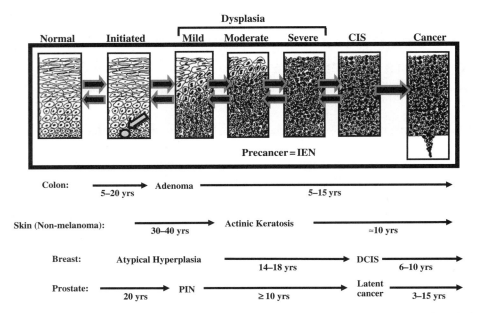

Fig. 1. Progression of precancer to cancer in humans is a multiyear process. Adapted from O'Shaughnessy et al. *(4)*.

specific cancer genes, signaling proteins, transcription factors, or epigenetic events that the bioactive components are able to regulate.

The initial section of this text gives an introduction to the potential influence of nutrition on cancer risk and prevention strategies and how investigators have begun to document the roles of bioactive compounds. One strategy to understand nutritional effects in cancer is nutrigenomics. Nutrigenomics is the study of the effects of food and food constituents on gene expression. This allows for the identification of bioactive food compounds, which affect specific targets that influence the carcinogenesis process. The identification of these bioactive compounds and the key molecular targets is attained through the use of high-throughput proteomics and metabolomic approaches. Here, the authors describe the potential interactions between bioactive molecules and genetic components such as histones, DNA methylation, transcription factors, and cell cycle regulators. The bioactive compounds found in food include essential nutrients such as vitamins and minerals and essential lipids, plant polyphenols, carotenoids, xenobiotics and numerous, other molecular entities. One specific transcription factor, AP-1, has been identified as a potential target for regulation and chemoprevention by nutrients, including epigallocatechin gallate (EGCG) *(7)*, theaflavins, caffeine *(8)*, [6]-gingerol *(9)*, resveratrol *(10)*, and flavonols such a as kaempherol, quercetin *(10)*, and myricetin *(11)*. This transcription factor appears to play a role in proliferation, differentiation, apoptosis, and angiogenesis *(12)*. In the case of DNA methylation, nutrients can supply the methyl groups in the formation of *S*-adenosylmethionine (SAM) and modify the utilization of methyl groups by DNA methyltransferases. In addition, nutrients may play a role in DNA demethylation activity and DNA methylation may influence the specific response to a nutrient. Understanding the complexities of the cellular events in carcinogenesis has paved the road to identify the key components in the diet that may be able to reduce the risk of cancer development.

A comprehensive discussion of macronutrients, obesity, and the potential for calorie restriction and physical activity to reduce cancer risk are discussed in Chapters 7–14. These authors have pulled together much of the current knowledge, including their own extensive research to discuss the effect of dietary balance involving calorie restriction and specific dietary components involved in cancer risk and prevention. The authors in this section present data concerning the use of compounds such as bifidobacteria, lactobacilli, and *Clostridium butyricum* to modulate gut microbiota and the intake of fiber for colon cancer prevention. In addition to a discussion of the recommended reduction in red meat intake and the resulting exposure to their carcinogenic chemical compounds, polycyclic aromatic hydrocarbons (PAH) formed in grilled meat, these authors have extensively explained the bioactivity of two polyunsaturated fatty acids (PUFA): n-6 PUFA and n-3 PUFA. N-6 PUFA metabolites are associated with increased cell proliferation and inflammation providing a potential mechanism in the extensive clinical studies linking increased cancer risk with intake of high levels of this PUFA. In contrast, n-3 PUFA are often found in fish and other food sources and have been associated with a decrease risk of cancer by affecting translational regulation of genes and subsequently reducing cellular proliferation. Recent data have identified a family of isomers, conjugated linoleic acid (CLA), that are found in meat and dairy products. In vitro studies demonstrated CLA inhibited growth of several cancer cell lines and induced expression of apoptotic genes. A reduction in tumors by CLA was also seen in rodent models. However, there can be no recommendation for CLA consumption for prevention or therapy until more extensive preclinical and clinical studies can be undertaken. This section of the book brings forth the evidence needed for the recommended reduction of overall fat intake, discussing the specific compounds found in fat that are associated with increased cancer risk, and providing evidence of the mechanism by which they act to increase cancer risk.

Many patients today use alternative therapies to manage their health. It is difficult for the health-care professionals to keep up with the evolving field. With a large selection of combination of vitamins and supplements available to the individual and the frequent mention of the positive impact to health from the lay media, health professionals are undoubtedly left to answer the patient's request of vitamin and nutrient supplement selection. From a scientific perspective, the authors of Chapter 15–22 discuss the most recent studies of carotenoids, vitamin A, vitamin D, folate, selenium, calcium, iron, and zinc. Both the carotenoids, β-carotene and lycopene, are highlighted in this section. Lycopene found in tomato food sources has been associated with the reduction in prostate cancer risk potentially through a mechanism of decreasing the expression of androgen-producing enzymes. β-carotene levels have been used as a biomarker for fruit and vegetable intake which is associated with reduced cancer risk. Controversial studies of high doses β-carotene and increased lung cancer risk in heavy, current smokers are addressed. The authors of this chapter recommend the five-a-day servings of fruit and vegetables and suggest that five of those in a week be lycopene-containing tomato products.

Vitamin A (retinol) is an essential nutrient involved in controlling cell growth and differentiation into normal cells; however, its use in cancer prevention has been limited to non-melanoma skin cancer chemoprevention due to the side effects associated with it. The authors do not present evidence that warrants a change in recommendations for dietary vitamin A for the purpose of cancer prevention. The discussions concerning vitamin D and its preventive cancer effects are quite limited; however, there is evidence that the ability to produce vitamin D3 is often lost as cancer develops. This leaves open the possibility that with restoration of this synthesis mechanism, there could be modulation of the carcinogenesis process.

Unfortunately, the role of folate in cancer prevention has been contradictory, especially since the mid-1990s when folic-acid supplementation of the US food supply was initiated. Essentially, too much of a "good thing" may not be so "good." The chapters on the minerals, selenium, and calcium provide well-documented preclinical and clinical data of their potential to prevent cancer. The putative mechanisms for cancer prevention are described for both. Selenium has been connected to antioxidant protection and anti-inflammatory effects while calcium provides protection by decreasing cell proliferation and stimulating cell differentiation in numerous types of cells. In contrast, excess iron accumulation can lead to increased risk of cancer and diseases associated with iron overload, but iron is required for many normal cell functions and therefore poses a dilemma with respect to long-term supplementation.

Currently, there has been an increased interest in zinc consumption because of its activity in boosting immune function and "fighting" the common cold. There is preclinical evidence to support that zinc has a potential role in cancer prevention. This concept has been formulated primarily because dietary zinc deficiency has been associated with increased tumors in epidemiological, clinical, and animal model studies. Esophageal cancer translational research efforts demonstrated an effect on NF-kB-COX-2 signaling pathway regulation by zinc that might contribute to prevention of this and other types of cancer.

Chapters 23–30 provide a large amount of reference supported research on specific compounds in different food components. One such compound is sulforaphane found in cruciferous vegetables and noted to block inflammatory responses. Cruciferous vegetable intake may reduce the risk of several cancers, including the hematologic malignancies, multiple myeloma, and non-Hodgkins lymphoma. Cruciferous vegetables contain isothiocyanates and indoles that have demonstrated advantageous cancer prevention effects on tumor cell cycles, gene expression, apoptosis, inflammatory responses, and other mechanisms associated with lowering of cancer risk. The bioactive sulfur compounds of garlic also have been shown to reduce cell proliferation and enhance DNA repair in animal models. Garlic decreased cancer formation subsequent to carcinogen exposure.

The polyphenols, resveratrol and genistein, individually and in combination reduced the size and progression of breast and prostate tumors in animal models. The benefits of tea intake are discussed and accompanied by a complete table of the epidemiological studies of tea consumption and the associated reduction in cancer risk. Another set of bioactive compounds extensively reviewed in this text are the isoflavones, genistein, and diadzein from soy. These compounds demonstrate a multitude of mechanisms contributing to their anti-carcinogenic effects. Also the phytochemicals of berries and pomegranates are introduced. In berries, the most active compounds are the anthocyanins. Berries inhibit carcinogenesis by inhibiting growth of cells, inhibiting angiogenesis and inflammation, and stimulating apoptosis, cell differentiation, and cell adhesion. Topical ointments containing berry extract have been associated with a reduction in histological grade and restoration of loss of heterozygosity in oral dysplastic lesions. The authors go so far as to advise the daily consumption of several grams of berry powder to elicit protection from cancer development.

Pomegranate ellagitannins metabolize into urolithins by the gut flora, which have demonstrated bioactivity in inhibiting prostate cancer cell growth, NFκ-B, and HIF-1α-dependent activation of VEGF. The consumption of pomegranate juice appears to cause a decrease in the rate of PSA after radiation or surgery in prostate cancer treatment. The second to last chapter in this text brings forth the biological data on alcohol consumption and its contribution to the development of many types of cancers of the aerodigestive tract. Discussed in the final chapter is the aryl hydrocarbon receptor (AhR). When activated by agonists, the AhR leads to a decreased expression of the tumor suppressor genes p16 and BRCA-1 and may be a risk factor in various types of cancer. Under current investigations are the potential benefits of using natural modulators of the AhR, including resveratrol and other indole compounds to work as cancer chemoprevention drugs.

The authors of many of these chapters rightfully address the difficulties in moving positive in vitro and animal studies of these bioactive compounds to human studies of chemoprevention (13). The suggested evidence necessary for a compound to qualify as a chemopreventive agent that could be developed naturally is shown in Fig. 2.

In an era where either the patients are asking "how and why" to prevent cancer or patients circumstances require the motivation for healthier living, "Bioactive Compound and Nutrition" provides the health-care professionals the concrete research behind calorie restriction, increased physical activity, reduction of intake of certain foods, including the moderation of vitamin and supplement consumption, and the increased intake of

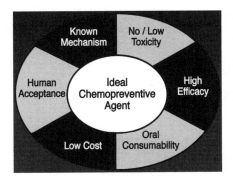

Fig. 2. Qualities of an ideal chemopreventive agent.

other healthful nutrients. With the identification of the actual bioactive compounds in the diet and understanding the molecular interactions that occur with these compounds, there will be greater confidence that effective chemoprevention agents can be developed from these dietary components.

David S. Alberts, MD
Maria Lluria-Prevatt, PhD

REFERENCES

1. Jemal, A., Thun, M.J., Ries, L.A., Howe, H.L., Weir, H.K., Center, M.M. et al. (2008) Annual report to the nation on the status of cancer, 1975–2005, featuring trends in lung cancer, tobacco use, and tobacco control. *J Natl Cancer Inst* **100**(23), 1672–94.
2. Jemal, A., Siegel, R., Ward, E., Hao, Y., Xu, J., Thun, M.J. et al. (2009) Cancer statistics, 2009. *CA Cancer J Clin* **59**(4), 225–49.
3. Calle, E.E., Rodriguez, C., Walker-Thurmond, K., Thun, M.J., Calle, E.E., Rodriguez, C. et al. (2003) Overweight, obesity, and mortality from cancer in a prospectively studied cohort of U.S. adults.[see comment]. *New Engl J Med* **348**(17), 1625–38.
4. O'Shaughnessy, J.A., Kelloff, G.J., Gordon, G.B., Dannenberg, A.J., Hong, W.K., Fabian, C.J. et al. (2002) Treatment and prevention of intraepithelial neoplasia: an important target for accelerated new agent development.[see comment]. *Clin Cancer Res* **8**(2), 314–46.
5. Alberts, D.S. (1999) A unifying vision of cancer therapy for the 21st century. *J Clin Oncol* **17**(11 Suppl), 13–21.
6. Prentice, R.L., Thomson, C.A., Caan, B., Hubbell, F.A., Anderson, G.L., Beresford, S.A. et al. (2007) Low-fat dietary pattern and cancer incidence in the Women's Health Initiative Dietary Modification Randomized Controlled Trial.[see comment]. *J Natl Cancer Inst* **99**(20), 1534–43.
7. Chen, W., Dong, Z., Valcic, S., Timmermann, B.N., and Bowden, G.T. (1999) Inhibition of ultraviolet B–induced c-fos gene expression and p38 mitogen-activated protein kinase activation by (-)-epigallocatechin gallate in a human keratinocyte cell line. *Mol Carcinog* **24**(2), 79–84.
8. Nomura, M., Ma, W.Y., Huang, C., Yang, C.S., Bowden, G.T., Miyamoto, K. et al. (2000) Inhibition of ultraviolet B-induced AP-1 activation by theaflavins from black tea. *Mol Carcinog* **28**(3), 148–55.
9. Bode, A.M., Ma, W.Y., Surh, Y.J., and Dong, Z. (2001) Inhibition of epidermal growth factor-induced cell transformation and activator protein 1 activation by [6]-gingerol. *Cancer Res* **61**(3), 850–53.
10. Lee, K.W., Kang, N.J., Heo, Y.S., Rogozin, E.A., Pugliese, A., Hwang, M.K. et al. (2008) Raf and MEK protein kinases are direct molecular targets for the chemopreventive effect of quercetin, a major flavonol in red wine. *Cancer Res* **68**(3), 946–55.
11. Jung, S.K., Lee, K.W., Byun, S., Kang, N.J., Lim, S.H., Heo, Y.S. et al. (2008) Myricetin suppresses UVB-induced skin cancer by targeting Fyn. *Cancer Res* **68**(14), 6021–29.
12. Cooper, S.J., and Bowden, G.T. (2007) Ultraviolet B regulation of transcription factor families: roles of nuclear factor-kappa B (NF-kappaB) and activator protein-1 (AP-1) in UVB-induced skin carcinogenesis. *Curr Cancer Drug Targets* **7**(4), 325–34.
13. Alberts, D.S. (2002) Reducing the risk of colorectal cancer by intervening in the process of carcinogenesis: a status report. *Cancer J* **8**(3), 208–21.

Foreword by Scott M. Lippman, MD

Natural agents have a long, exciting history in cancer prevention that extends back to 1925, when Wolbach and Howe reported early animal studies of vitamin A, foreshadowing the founding of the field of modern cancer chemoprevention by pioneers such as Lee Wattenberg, Michael B. Sporn, and Waun Ki Hong in the 1960s, 1970s, and 1980s. In the wake of several negative, some even harmful, major trials of natural agents for chemoprevention, however, a recent editorial stated that the prospects for cancer prevention through natural agents "have never looked worse" *(1)*. Although this observation is perfectly understandable, no one should rush to count natural bioactive compounds out, as the chapters of this book, *Bioactive Compounds and Cancer*, make abundantly clear.

This comprehensive textbook is an excellent research source of in-depth reviews in every chapter, illustrating the complexity of the field and useful both for research and for clinical practice. Every major area of natural-agent research is covered. Wide-ranging chapters on biology, technology, and mechanisms include one chapter each on nutrigenomics and nutrigenetics and a chapter on diet and epigenetics. Research varying from whole foods to extracts to specific compounds is presented in a clear, useable format. There are individual chapters on a host of bioactive compounds including folate, selenium, vitamin D, zinc, iron, garlic, isoflavones, berries and anthocyanines, herbs and spices, pomegranates, and many more. The book's broad scope is illustrated further by chapters on caloric restriction/energy balance, gut microbiotica, aryl hydrocarbon receptor-mediated carcinogenesis, carcinogenic effects of meat and alcohol, and (in four chapters) the double-edged sword of fatty acids.

Although illuminated in this book, much of the leading-edge methodology of natural-agent research did not enter into the backgrounds and rationales of the large randomized controlled trials (RCTs) beginning in the mid-1990s that led to the gloomy outlook quoted above. Beta-carotene and vitamin A analogues (retinoids) increased lung cancer incidence and mortality in smokers. Folic acid increased the risk of advanced colorectal adenomas and prostate cancer. Vitamin E (α-tocopherol) marginally increased prostate cancer in the largest cancer prevention RCT ever conducted (the Selenium and Vitamin E Cancer Prevention Trial [SELECT]), in addition to increasing mortality in meta-analyses of clinical trials. The only positive micronutrient RCT involved is calcium, which produced a significant, albeit modest, reduction in colorectal adenomas. RCTs of many other natural compounds, including complex combinations of vitamins and minerals, have yielded negative-neutral results. Many complex aspects of these results remain unresolved, including the apparent non-linear dose–response of many of the natural agents, potential effects in nutrient-deficient (not replete) populations, and pharmacogenomic considerations such as have been reported recently for selenium.

The primary basis of most of these RCTs was epidemiologic data, which can be confounded by many factors. The enormous SELECT went further, basing its rationale largely on compelling secondary RCT data, which did not lead to positive results. In view of these trials' somewhat limited rationales and preponderantly negative results, cancer prevention experts have proposed a new model of natural agent development, a model that develops consistent cross-discipline preliminary data from preclinical models, epidemiology, pharmacogenetics, risk-modeling, and early-phase clinical trials prior to the launch of large, expensive, and time-consuming RCTs. Strong efforts are needed in the step of early-phase clinical trials, including presurgical studies within intraepithelial neoplasia or cancer and important correlative assessments such as of molecular profiles of efficacy.

The editorial mentioned in the opening paragraph also aptly said, "The primary lesson from our experience in the nutritional prevention of cancer is that it is not simple." Nevertheless, the complexity of feasible, desired early evidence will lead, at last, to the most-promising areas for registration or definitive RCTs of natural agents. These RCTs will represent the distillation of large, heterogeneous populations of somewhat-increased – risk individuals down into cohorts of highest-risk, pharmacogenomically appropriate individuals, who will receive formulations, doses, and durations of single or combined natural agents with the highest activity and safety profiles in preclinical and early-stage clinical studies. This proposed agent-development scheme applies not only to the natural agents described by world leaders in this remarkable book, but as well to the development of molecular-targeted or other synthetic agents for cancer prevention. Movement toward achieving the goal of fully stepped natural-agent development includes efforts of the new American Association for Cancer Research (AACR) journal *Cancer Prevention Research*, which is the leading home for preclinical (in vitro and in vivo), pharmacogenomic, molecular risk assessment, and early-phase clinical studies relevant to natural bioactive compounds.

In sum, the prospects for prevention through natural agents have never looked better, thanks to the growing impetus for effective drug development reflected in the extraordinary body of work represented in *Bioactive Compounds and Cancer*.

Scott M. Lippman, MD

REFERENCE

1. Kristal, A.R., and Lippman, S.M. (2009 Mar 18) Nutritional prevention of cancer: new directions for an increasingly complex challenge. *J Natl Cancer Inst* **101**(6), 432–35.

Preface

Cancer is a global issue. While cancer risk may vary depending on location there is mounting evidence that the incidence and associated morbidity and mortality will continue to mount. This increase is in part due to an aging society, but also to the escalating incidence of obesity throughout the world. Only a small percentage of cancers are familial suggesting that environmental factors including dietary intakes are critical for determining risk and tumor behavior. The impetus to developing this volume stems from the wealth of evidence pointing to specific dietary bioactive components as modifiers of cancer-related processes. Thirty-three chapters have been assembled from world renowned experts who have conducted a systematic review of the relevant literature and provided an assessment of cancer prevention opportunities using bioactive food compounds. The tone of this text is to establish a "proof-of-principle" about the importance of nutrition and cancer prevention while realizing that space limitations may not have allowed for all areas to be adequately addressed. The text has been divided into several sections to aid in the assimilation of the materials provided. *Part I: Understanding the Role of Nutrition in Health* addresses the cancer response to bioactive food components, how "omics" approaches have been used to investigate individual variability due to genetic and epigenetic nutrient regulation of signaling proteins and associated small-molecular-weight compounds. This section defines the cellular cancer processes and molecular targets for food components and identifies those individuals who are likely to benefit by assessing the relevance of selected polymorphisms. Part II: *Role of Dietary Bioactive Components in Cancer Prevention and/or Treatment* was developed realizing that cancer risk is influenced by dietary behavior and interactions among dietary *Macro-constituents* including dietary energy balance, protein, fats, and microflora. Moreover, the effects of certain macronutrients on the cancer process may be modified by synergies with other bioactive components including *Carotenoids, Vitamins, and Minerals*, and many *Bioactive Food Components* found in fruits and vegetables, which in concert may alter the susceptibility to cancer risk. Attention was given to the fact diet may also be a vehicle for cancer-promoting substances including *Alcohol* and to the biological basis of prevention by natural bioactive compounds against certain *Dietary Xenobiotics* with cancer-promoting effects. Finally, this volume provides a forum to discuss opportunities and challenges for communicating food and health relationships to *Consumers*.

In preparing this text, efforts were directed to presenting epidemiological, clinical, and preclinical experimental evidence supporting the role of selected bioactive food components in cancer prevention or causation. Because bioactive food components are promiscuous and influence a multitude of molecular and cellular targets, particular attention was given to discussion of the mechanisms of action, review of experimental data supporting tissue-specific cancer preventative effects, and whenever available, to the totality of evidence supporting the use of specific bioactive food components for the prevention or management of specific types of neoplasms. Areas for future nutrition and cancer research are also highlighted throughout. When possible, global recommendations are provided as general guides for use by those committed to reducing cancer burden.

ACKNOWLEDGMENTS

Special thanks are due to Adrianne Bendich, Series Editor for her support through thought-full comments, suggestions, and encouragements. The editors acknowledge the editorial assistance of Amanda Rutherford of the Undergraduate Program in Nutritional Sciences and Theresa Spicer of the Department of Nutritional Sciences, at The University of Arizona; the grant support to Donato F. Romagnolo from the Susan G. Komen for the Cure and the Arizona Biomedical Research Commission, Phoenix, AZ. The editors would like to offer special accolades for the efforts of the multiple authors who have contributed to the development of this state-of-the-science text.

MEMORIAL

Professor Sheila Bingham, coauthor of Chapter 10 on Meats, Protein, and Cancer, was an international leader in nutritional epidemiology. She investigated the biological mechanisms underlying the effects of nutrition on health and chronic diseases, including cancer. Sadly, we acknowledge her death on 16th June 16, 2009.

Contents

Contributors

B.H. AKTAS, PHD, DVM • *Laboratory for Translational Research, Brigham and Women's Hospital and Harvard Medical School, Cambridge, MA*

SEAN F. ALTEKRUSE, DVM, PHD • *Surveillance Research Program, National Cancer Institute (NCI), Bethesda, MD*

CHRISTINE B. AMBROSONE, PHD • *Department of Cancer Prevention and Control, Roswell Park Cancer Institute, Buffalo, NY*

LYSSA BALICK, MS, CNS • *Information Specialist, McCormick Science Institute, 18, Loveton Circle, Sparks, MD*

STEPHEN BARNES, PHD • *Department of Pharmacology and Toxicology, Center for Nutrient-Gene Interaction, University of Alabama at Birmingham, Birmingham, AL; Purdue University-University of Alabama at Birmingham Botanicals Center for Age-Related Disease, University of Alabama at Birmingham, Birmingham, AL*

SHEILA A. BINGHAM, PHD • *Medical Research Council, Dunn Human Nutrition Unit, Cambridge, UK*

ANN M. BODE, PHD • *The Hormel Institute, University of Minnesota, Austin, MN*

ALEXANDER D. BOROWSKY MD • *Department of Pathology, School of Medicine, Center for Comparative Medicine, University of California, Davis, CA*

SUSAN BORRA, RD • *Formally with International Food Information Council (IFIC) and the Foundation, Washington, DC*

G. TIM BOWDEN, PHD • *Department of Cell Biology and Anatomy, The Arizona Cancer Center, The University of Arizona, Tucson, AZ*

JIA CHEN, SCD • *Mount Sinai School of Medicine, New York, NY*

M. CHOREV, PHD • *Laboratory for Translational Research, Brigham and Women's Hospital and Harvard Medical School, Cambridge, MA*

JAMES R. CONNOR, PHD • *Department of Neurosurgery, Penn State Hershey Cancer Institute, The Pennsylvania State University College of Medicine & M.S. Hershey Medical Center, Hershey, PA*

LEAH M. COOK, MS • *Department of Pharmacology and Toxicology, University of Alabama at Birmingham, Birmingham, AL*

PATRIZIA DAMONTE, PHD • *Department of Pathology, School of Medicine, Center for Comparative Medicine, University of California, Davis, CA*

CINDY D. DAVIS, PHD • *Nutritional Science Research Group, Division of Cancer Prevention, National Cancer Institute, Rockville, MD*

REBECCA DEANGEL, MPH • *Department of Nutritional Sciences, University of Texas, Austin, TX*

STEPHANIE C. DEGNER, PHD • *Department of Nutritional Sciences, The University of Arizona, Tucson, AZ; Department of Veterinary Science and Microbiology, The University of Arizona, Tucson, AZ*

SALLY DICKINSON, PHD • *Arizona Cancer Center, The University of Arizona, Tucson, AZ*

ZIGANG DONG, MD, DR. PHD • *The Hormel Institute, University of Minnesota, Austin, MN*

BRENDA K. EDWARDS, PHD • *Surveillance Research Program, National Cancer Institute (NCI), Bethesda, MD*

JOHN W. ERDMAN JR., PHD • *Division of Nutritional Sciences, Department of Food Science and Human Nutrition, University of Illinois at Urbana-Champaign, IL*

KENT L. ERICKSON, PHD • *Department of Cell Biology and Human Anatomy, School of Medicine, University of California, Davis, CA*

JAMES C. FLEET, PHD • *Department of Foods and Nutrition, Purdue University, West Lafayette, IN*

LOUISE Y.Y. FONG, PHD • *Department of Pharmacology and Experimental Therapeutics, Kimmel Cancer Center, Thomas Jefferson University, Pennsylvania, PA, USA*

MICHELE R. FORMAN, PHD • *Department of Epidemiology, MD Anderson Cancer Center, Houston TX*

GLENN R. GIBSON, PHD • *Food Microbial Sciences Unit, Department of Food Biosciences, The University of Reading, Reading, UK*

J.A. HALPERIN, MD • *Laboratory for Translational Research, Brigham and Women's Hospital and Harvard Medical School, Cambridge, MA*

CURT E. HARPER, PHD • *Department of Pharmacology and Toxicology, University of Alabama at Birmingham, Birmingham, AL*

DAVID HEBER MD, PHD • *Department of Medicine, David Geffen School of Medicine at UCLA, UCLA Center for Human Nutrition, Los Angeles, CA*

STEPHEN S. HECHT, PHD • *Masonic Cancer Center, University of Minnesota, Minneapolis, MN*

LEENA HILAKIVI-CLARKE, PHD • *Lombardi Comprehensive Cancer Center, Georgetown University, Washington, DC*

NADIA HOWLADER, MS • *Surveillance Research Program, National Cancer Institute (NCI), Bethesda, MD*

NEIL E. HUBBARD, PHD • *Department of Cell Biology and Human Anatomy, School of Medicine, University of California, Davis, CA*

STEPHEN D. HURSTING, PHD, MPH • *Department of Nutritional Sciences, University of Texas, Austin, TX; Department of Carcinogenesis, University of Texas-MD Anderson Cancer Center, Smithville, TX*

GUY H. JOHNSON, PHD • *McCormick Science Institute, 18, Loveton Circle, Sparks, MD*

WENDY REINHARDT KAPSAK, MS, RD • *International Food Information Council (IFIC) and the Foundation, Washington, DC*

GUNTER G.C. KUHNLE, PHD • *Medical Research Council, Dunn Human Nutrition Unit, Cambridge, UK*

CORAL A. LAMARTINIERE, PHD • *Department of Pharmacology and Toxicology, University of Alabama at Birmingham, Birmingham, AL; UAB Comprehensive Cancer Center, University of Alabama at Birmingham, Birmingham, AL*

JOSHUA D. LAMBERT, PHD • *Department of Chemical Biology, Ernest Mario School of Pharmacy, Rutgers, The State University of New Jersey, Piscataway, NJ*

JOAN M. LAPPE, PHD, RN, FAAN • *Creighton University, Omaha, NE*

LAURA LASHINGER, PHD • *Department of Nutritional Sciences, University of Texas, Austin, TX; Department of Carcinogenesis, University of Texas-MD, Anderson Cancer Center, Smithville, TX*

SANG Y. LEE, PHD • *Department of Neurosurgery, Penn State Hershey Cancer Institute, The Pennsylvania State University College of Medicine & M.S. Hershey Medical Center, Hershey, PA*

BRIAN L. LINDSHIELD PHD • *Department of Human Nutrition, Kansas State University Manhattan, KS*

AMY LIU, MPH • *Fred Hutchinson Cancer Research Center, Cancer Prevention Research Program, Seattle, WA*

MARIE LOF, PHD, MSC • *Department of Medical Epidemiology and Biostatistics, Karolinska Institute, Stockholm, Sweden*

SOMDAT MAHABIR, PHD, MPH • *Department of Epidemiology, MD Anderson Cancer Center, Houston TX*

SUSAN R. MALLERY, DDS, PHD • *Division of Oral Surgery, Pathology and Anesthesiology, College of Dentistry, The Ohio State University, Columbus, OH*

SUSAN E. MCCANN, PHD, RD • *Department of Cancer Prevention and Control, Roswell Park Cancer Institute, Buffalo, NY*

JOHN A. MILNER, PHD • *Nutritional Science Research Group, Division of Cancer Prevention, National Cancer Institute, Rockville, MD*

LETICIA NOGUEIRA, BS • *Department of Nutritional Sciences, University of Texas, Austin, TX*

SUSAN OLIVO-MARSTEN, PHD, MPH • *Cancer Prevention Fellowship Program, Office of Preventive Oncology, Division of Cancer Prevention National Cancer Institute, NIH, Bethesda, MD*

BRIJESH B. PATEL, MS • *Department of Pharmacology and Toxicology, University of Alabama at Birmingham, Birmingham, AL*

SUSAN N. PERKINS, PHD • *Department of Nutritional Sciences, University of Texas, Austin, TX*

MARY E. PLATEK, PHD • *Department of Cancer Prevention and Control, Roswell Park Cancer Institute, Buffalo, NY*

ELIZABETH RAHAVI, RD • *International Food Information Council (IFIC) and the Foundation, Washington, DC*

MARGARET P. RAYMAN DPHIL, RPHNUTR • *Nutritional Sciences Division, Faculty of Health and Medical Sciences, University of Surrey, Guildford, UK*

MICHELLE R. ROBERTS, MA • *Department of Cancer Prevention and Control, Roswell Park Cancer Institute, Buffalo, NY*

DONATO F. ROMAGNOLO, PHD, MS • *Department of Nutritional Sciences, The University of Arizona, Tucson, AZ*

A. CATHARINE ROSS, PHD • *Department of Nutritional Sciences, Pennsylvania State University, University Park, PA; Huck Institute for the Life Sciences, Pennsylvania State University, University Park, PA*

SHARON A. ROSS, PHD • *Nutritional Science Research Group, Division of Cancer Prevention, National Cancer Institute, National Institutes of Health, Department of Health and Human Services, Bethesda, MD*

CHRISTINE SARDO, MPH, RD • *Comprehensive Cancer Center, The Ohio State University College of Medicine, Columbus, OH*

ORNELLA SELMIN, PHD • *Department of Nutritional Sciences, The University of Arizona, Tucson, AZ*

KEITH SINGLETARY, PHD • *Department of Food Science and Human Nutrition, University of Illinois, Urbana, IL*

JOANNE L. SLAVIN, PHD, RD • *Department of Food Science and Nutrition, University of Minnesota, St. Paul, MN*

SARAH M. SMITH, PHD • *Department of Nutritional Sciences, University of Texas, Austin, TX; Department of Carcinogenesis, University of Texas-MD Anderson Cancer Center, Smithville, TX*

MARIA L. STEWART, MS • *Department of Food Science and Nutrition, University of Minnesota, St. Paul, MN*

GARY D. STONER, PHD • *Division of Hematology and Oncology, Department of Internal Medicine, Innovation Centre, The Ohio State University College of Medicine, Columbus, OH; Comprehensive Cancer Center, The Ohio State University College of Medicine, Columbus, OH*

CYNTHIA A. THOMSON, PHD, RD • *Department of Nutritional Sciences, The University of Arizona, Tucson, AZ*

CORNELIA M. ULRICH, PHD • *Fred Hutchinson Cancer Research Center, Cancer Prevention Research Program, Seattle, Washington, WA; NCT Division of Preventive Oncology, German Cancer Research Center, Heidelberg, Germany*

GEMMA E. WALTON, PHD • *Food Microbial Sciences Unit, Department of Food Biosciences, The University of Reading, Reading, UK*

JUN WANG, MD • *Department of Pharmacology and Toxicology, University of Alabama at Birmingham, Birmingham, AL*

TIMOTHY G. WHITSETT JR., PHD • *Department of Pharmacology and Toxicology, University of Alabama at Birmingham, Birmingham, AL*

LI-SHU WANG, PHD • *Comprehensive Cancer Center, The Ohio State University College of Medicine, Columbus, OH*

CHUNG S. YANG, PHD • *Department of Chemical Biology, Ernest Mario School of Pharmacy, Rutgers, The State University of New Jersey, Piscataway, NJ*

XINRAN XU, PHD • *Mount Sinai School of Medicine, New York, NY*

NANCY ZIKRI, PHD • *Department of Cardiovascular Medicine, The Ohio State University College of Medicine, Columbus, OH*

I Understanding the Role of Nutrition in Health

1 Monitoring the Burden of Cancer in the United States

Nadia Howlader, Sean F. Altekruse, and Brenda K. Edwards

Key Points

1. The American Cancer Society estimates that approximately 1,437,180 new cancer cases will be diagnosed in 2008, and approximately 565,650 individuals are expected to die as a result of cancer.
2. The prevalence of invasive cancer in the United States appears to be increasing, in part due to aging of the US population. However, a larger proportion of cases are diagnosed at earlier stages and prognoses improve with more effective therapies. On January 1, 2005, the number of persons in the United States diagnosed with invasive cancer was estimated at 11,098,450.
3. Each year, cancer cases are reported by registries that participate in the SEER Program. A cancer's stage describes the extent or spread of disease at the time of diagnosis. Several staging systems are available.
4. The three leading cancer sites for men (prostate, lung and bronchus, and colon and rectum) accounted for one-half of male cancer deaths. Cancer of the lung and bronchus was responsible for 2.5 times more deaths than prostate cancer, the most common cancer site among men.
5. The three leading cancer sites among women (breast, lung and bronchus, and colon and rectum) caused ~50% of female cancer deaths. Cancer of the lung and bronchus caused 1.5 times more deaths than breast cancer, the leading incident cancer site for women.
6. After decades of steady increases in cancer incidence and death rates, overall rates appear to be declining. In particular, the incidence and death rates for cancers of the breast, prostate, and colon and rectum are declining.

Key Words: Cancer; burden; surveillance; incidence; mortality; survival; prevalence

1. INTRODUCTION

Cancer represents a major public health concern. The American Cancer Society estimates that approximately 1,437,180 new cancer cases will be diagnosed in 2008, and approximately 565,650 individuals are expected to die as a result of cancer *(1)*. In recognition of the significant burden of cancer in the United States, the National Cancer Act was enacted into law in 1971. As part of this Act, Congress provided funding to the

From: *Nutrition and Health: Bioactive Compounds and Cancer*
Edited by: J.A. Milner, D.F. Romagnolo, DOI 10.1007/978-1-60761-627-6_1,
© Springer Science+Business Media, LLC 2010

National Cancer Institute (NCI) for the Surveillance, Epidemiology, and End Results (SEER) Program. The SEER Program now collects, analyzes, and disseminates cancer statistics from population-based cancer registries that cover 26% of the US population.

During the past 30 years, statistics from the SEER Program have informed many cancer control efforts. The SEER Program is the principal source of cancer incidence and survival information in the United States. This database is used widely by scientists, decision makers, and the public. The SEER Program provides cancer statistics and data regarding trends such as the number of new cancer cases, cancer-related deaths, and how long people survive after being diagnosed with cancer. The purpose of this chapter is to provide a brief overview of the burden of cancer on the general population using data collected by the SEER registries and data on US cancer deaths compiled by the Center for Disease Control and Prevention's (CDC) National Center for Health Statistics (NCHS). Data are presented on cancer incidence, mortality, survival, and prevalence for the overall population by gender, race and ethnicity, and age. A primary source of these statistics is the annual Cancer Statistics Review (CSR) published by the SEER Program on its web site (http://seer.cancer.gov). Additional cancer statistics are available on the SEER web site, including the Fast Stats and Cancer Query systems and public use files.

1.1. Collection of Cancer Data

Cancer cases are identified through records from hospitals, private laboratories, radiotherapy units, nursing homes, and other health service units in a registry's defined geographic area. In addition, each registry collects data on patient demographics, primary tumor site and extent of disease, and first course of treatment. The original nine registries in the SEER Program, denoted as SEER-9, consist of Atlanta, Connecticut, Detroit, Hawaii, Iowa, New Mexico, San Francisco–Oakland, Seattle–Puget Sound, and Utah. Data are available for patients diagnosed since 1973 with the exception of Seattle–Puget Sound (1974) and Atlanta (1975). Reports on long-term incidence cancer trends are based on SEER-9, which represents 10% of the US population. The SEER-13 registries consist of SEER-9 plus Los Angeles, San Jose–Monterey, Rural Georgia, and the Alaska Native Tumor Registry. Data are available for cases diagnosed since 1992. The SEER-17 registries consist of the SEER-13 as described above, plus Greater California, Kentucky, Louisiana, and New Jersey and data are available for all cases diagnosed starting in 2000. These registries report data based on race (Native American, Asian Pacific islanders) and include information on more than five million cancer cases. This chapter is based on cases diagnosed from 1975 through 2005.

1.2. Case Definition

Site and extent of cancer cases in SEER registries are coded according to the International Classification of Diseases for Oncology, Third edition (ICD-O-3) (2). Cases collected before 2001 were machine converted to ICD-O-3 codes. Each year, cancer cases are reported by registries that participate in the SEER Program. A cancer's stage describes the extent or spread of disease at the time of diagnosis. Several staging systems are available. The SEER historic stage is used for descriptive and statistical analysis of tumor registry data and comprises four categories: in situ, localized, regional, and distant (3).

1.3. Incidence and Death Rates

In all 50 states and the District of Columbia, deaths by cancer site are reported on a yearly basis to the NCHS *(4)* as a component of the state vital health reporting systems. This data source is used to generate age-adjusted death rates for this chapter. Population estimates that are used to calculate incidence and death rates are obtained from the US Census Bureau *(5)*, which provides data organized by 5-year age group, gender, county, and race ethnicity enabling estimates of age-adjusted incidence and death rates by gender for four racial groups (White, Black, Asian and Pacific Islander, and American Indian/Alaska Native) and one ethnic group (Hispanic).

Incidence and death rates presented in this chapter are expressed as the number of new primary cancers and deaths per 100,000 persons. For cancer sites that pertain to one sex only, the population at risk is the sex-specific population (e.g., prostate cancer). Incidence and death rates are age adjusted according to the 2000 US standard population based on 5-year age groups *(6)*. Age adjustment minimizes the effect due to differences in age distributions when comparing rates.

1.4. Delay Adjustment and Trend Analysis

When cancer cases in SEER registries are reported to NCI in November of each year, data are ~98% complete for all cancer sites combined. Cancer registries continuously update their databases, and SEER uses statistical modeling to adjust data for underestimation due to reporting delays estimated from the receipt of data files in subsequent years *(7)*. The delay-adjustment factor increases the age-adjusted incidence rates in the more current reporting years.

Trends over a given time interval are summarized by annual percent change (APC) *(8)*. The APC is obtained by fitting a regression line through the logarithms of the rates for the given time period using weighted least squares. The slope of the line is tested for significant increases or decreases. In addition, the joinpoint regression model *(8)* is used to characterize changes in cancer rates over time. Each joinpoint denotes a statistically significant change in trend (p-value ≤ 0.05) and a maximum of four joinpoints and five line segments are allowed. For this chapter, we present final segment APCs to capture recent changes in incidence and mortality trends for selected cancer sites.

1.5. Survival and Prevalence

Cancer survival is estimated in different ways, depending on the intended purpose. Relative survival is calculated by comparing observed survival with expected survival from a set of people with the same characteristics as the patient cohort with respect to age, race, sex, and calendar period *(9)*. Relative survival estimates present the effect of the cancer being considered on survival in the absence of other causes of death. Complete prevalence is the number of people in a population who are alive on a certain date and have been diagnosed with cancer at any time in their lives *(10, 11)*. It differs from incidence in that it considers both newly diagnosed and previously diagnosed cases. Prevalence is a function of both the incidence of the disease and survival.

Prevalence is estimated for all races by applying the completeness index method to limited-duration prevalence (http://seer.cancer.gov/csr/1975_2005/index.html). The US cancer prevalence counts at January 1, 2005, were estimated by multiplying the SEER age- and race-specific prevalence proportions by the corresponding US population esti-mates based on the average of 2004 and 2005 population estimates from the US Bureau of the Census. US cancer prevalence counts for all races were estimated by combining US estimated counts for White/unknown, Black, and other races.

1.6. All Malignant Cancers Combined

The incidence rate for all malignant cancers combined in SEER-9 registries during the period 2001–2005 was 471.1 cases per 100,000 people (Table 1). Based on a joinpoint analysis of incidence rates from 1975 through 2005, a statistically significant decrease in APC was observed in the most recent joinpoint segment, 1999–2005 (APC=−1.2%, $P \leq 0.05$; Table 1).

Annual incidence rates for all malignant cancers in SEER-9 registries from 1975 to 2005 are represented by unfilled triangles (Fig. 1). Rates generally rose from 1975 through 1992, with the increase in APC from 1989 through 1992 indicated by the rising slope of the solid line segment (joinpoint model). Cancer incidence rates varied between 1992 and 2005, with two decreasing and one increasing joinpoint segments.

Although cancer incidence rates from 2001 to 2005 were higher among males (551.9 per 100,000) than females (415.2 per 100,000), the magnitude of the decline in APC for the recent joinpoint segment was larger for men (−2.3%) than for women (−0.8%; Table 1). The annual death rate for all malignant cancers combined in the United States for the years 2001–2005 was 189.8 cases per 100,000 people (Table 1). Based on a joinpoint analysis of death rates from 1975 through 2005, a statistically signif-icant decrease in APC was seen in the most recent joinpoint segment, 2002–2005 (APC=−1.8, $P \leq 0.05$; Table 1).

Annual death rates for all malignant cancers in the United States from 1975 to 2005 are depicted by solid triangles in Fig. 1. Rates generally rose from 1975 through 1992 and have declined thereafter. Joinpoint segments from 1975 to 1992 showed increas-ing APCs, whereas joinpoint segments from 1992 to 2005 showed decreasing APCs ($P \leq 0.05$, data not shown; Fig. 1). Cancer death rates from 2001 to 2005 were higher among males (234.4 per 100,000) than females (159.9 per 100,000). However, the mag-nitude of the decline in APC for men from 2001 to 2005 was slightly larger (−2.0%) than the decline in APC for women from 2002 to 2005 (−1.6%; Table 1).

1.7. Top Three Cancer Sites for Men and Women

Between 2001 and 2005, three cancer sites accounted for more than half of all new malignant cancers in men in the order of prostate, lung and bronchus, and colon and rectum (Table 1). Similarly, three cancer sites accounted for more than one-half of all new malignant cancers in women in the order of breast, lung and bronchus, and colon and rectum. With the exception of cancer of the lung and bronchus in women, incidence rates for the top three cancer sites in both sexes decreased significantly during the most recent joinpoint segment time period (Table 1). Significant declines in the rate of cancer

Table 1

Age-adjusted Cancer Incidence and Death Rates for All Malignant Cancers, the Top Three Cancer Sites of Men and Women, and Two Sites with Increasing Incidence and Death Rates, 2001–2005, Annual Percentage Changes for Last Joinpoint Segment, SEER-9*

		Incidence			Death		
		Rate	Most recent joinpoint segment		Rate	Most recent joinpoint segment	
Gender	Cancer site	2001–2005	Time period	APC	2001–2005	Time period	APC
Both sexes	All malignant cancers	471.1	1999–2005	-1.2[a]	189.8	2002–2005	-1.8[a]
Males	All malignant cancers	551.9	2001–2005	-2.3[a]	234.4	2001–2005	-2.0[a]
	Top three cancer sites						
	Prostate	168.2	2001–2005	-4.9[a]	26.7	1994–2005	-4.1[a]
	Lung and bronchus	77.7	1991–2005	-1.9[a]	72.0	1993–2005	-1.9[a]
	Colon and rectum	58.5	1998–2005	-3.0[a]	22.7	2002–2005	-4.3[a]
	Selected sites (increasing)						
	Liver/intrahepatic bile duct	9.2	1996–2005	2.4[a]	7.3	1999–2005	2.6[a]
	Esophagus	8.2	1975–2005	0.7[a]	7.8	1994–2005	0.4[a]
Females	All malignant cancers	415.2	1998–2005	-0.8[a]	159.9	2002–2005	-1.6[a]
	Top three cancer sites						
	Breast	129.1	1999–2005	-2.4[a]	25.0	1990–2005	-2.2[a]
	Lung and bronchus	51.9	1998–2005	-0.2	41.0	1995–2005	0.1
	Colon and rectum	43.8	1998–2005	-2.4[a]	15.9	2002–2005	-4.4[a]

Table 1
(Continued)

Gender	Cancer site	Incidence				Death			
		Rate 2001–2005	Most recent joinpoint segment		Rate 2001–2005	Most recent joinpoint segment			
			Time period	APC		Time period	APC		
	Selected sites (increasing)								
	Liver/intrahepatic bile duct	3.3	1975–2005	2.9[a]	3.1	2001–2005	2.1[a]		
	Esophagus	2.0	1975–2005	−0.3[a]	1.7	2000–2005	−1.5[a]		

APC, Annual Percent Change. Rates per 100,000 population.
[a]Slope of joinpoint regression line not equal to zero, $P \leq 0.05$, best fitting model selected, up to four joinpoint segments allowed.
Source: Cancer Statistics Review http://seer.cancer.gov/csr/1975_2005/index.html

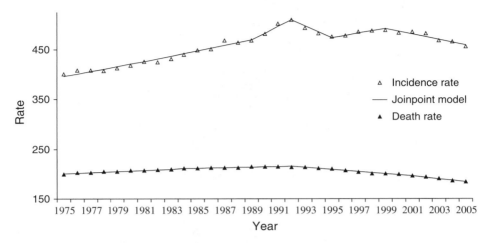

Fig. 1. Annual incidence (SEER-9 registries*) and death rates (United States) for all malignant cancers combined, 1975–2005, with best fitting joinpoint models.

of the lung and bronchus were observed among men between 1982 and 2005 (Fig. 2). Incidence rates of colorectal cancer declined for both men and women since the mid-1980s. Furthermore, female breast cancer and prostate cancer have declined since the beginning of the twenty-first century (Fig. 3). Stable incidence rates for cancer of the lung and bronchus in women from 1998 to 2005 (Table 1) reflect an inversion from an uptrend observed up to 1998.

The three leading cancer sites for men (prostate, lung and bronchus, and colon and rectum) accounted for one-half of male cancer deaths. Cancer of the lung and bronchus was responsible for 2.5 times more deaths than prostate cancer, the most common cancer site among men (Table 1). Similarly, the three leading cancer sites among women (breast, lung and bronchus, and colon and rectum) caused ~50% of female cancer deaths. Cancer of the lung and bronchus caused 1.5 times more deaths than breast cancer, the leading incident cancer site for women (Table 1). Only the APC for cancer mortality of the lung and bronchus in women did not decrease in the most recent joinpoint segment time period.

Although overall trends show progress in reducing cancer burden, the incidence and death rates for cancers of the liver and intrahepatic bile duct have increased in both men and women (Table 1). In addition, incidence and death rates for esophageal cancer have increased among men. Cancers of these sites carry a poor prognosis; 1-year survival rates from time of diagnosis is less than 50% (data not shown).

1.8. Tumor Histology: The Example of Esophageal Cancer

Cancer is a general term for a broad group of diseases, each with its own etiologic risk factors. Thus, in addition to determining the anatomic site of tumors, information on tumor histology is important in cancer surveillance programs. For example, in SEER-9 registries, overall incidence rates of esophageal cancer increased from 1975 to 2005 (Fig. 4). The modest, but steady increase occurred even as overall cancer incidence rates

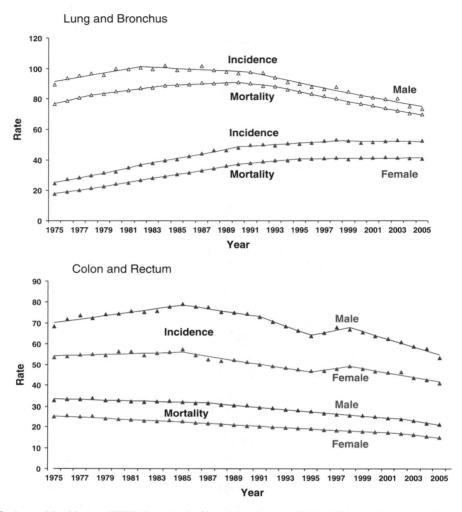

Fig. 2. Annual incidence (SEER-9 registries*) and death rates (United States) for cancer of the lung and bronchus and colon and rectum by gender, 1975–2005, with best fit joinpoint model.

began to decline in the 1990s. However, the incidence rates of squamous cell carcinomas markedly declined from 1975 to 2005, with an acceleration of the downtrend starting in 1986 (Fig. 3). Conversely, a marked increase in adenocarcinoma contributed to the overall increase in esophageal cancer.

Although smoking and low fruit and vegetable consumption are risk factors for both esophageal cancer histologies, alcohol consumption and low body mass are risk factors for esophageal squamous cell carcinoma, which disproportionately affects black males. Conversely, overweight and gastroesophageal reflux are risk factors for esophageal adenocarcinomas. Incidence rates of this cancer are increasing most pronouncedly among white males *(12)*. This example illustrates that information about tumor histology is

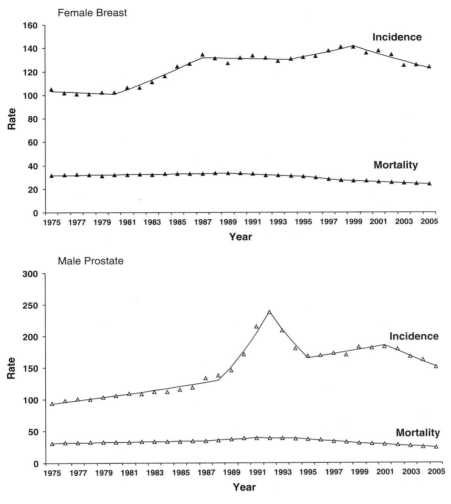

Fig. 3. Annual incidence (SEER-9 registries*) and death rates (United States) for cancer of the breast (female) and prostate (male), 1975–2005, with best fit joinpoint model.

important in defining risk factors for specific cancers and developing effective control programs and tumor-specific treatments. Tumor classification is by no means a static discipline. The study of molecular biomarkers is likely to lead to further improvement of tumor classification and herald an era of personalized oncology.

1.9. Incidence and Death Rates by Race and Ethnicity

In SEER-13 registries from 2001 to 2005, black populations had the highest total cancer incidence rate among racial and ethnic subgroups. Black men had the highest rate among men, and white women had the highest rate among women (Table 2). Regardless of racial group, prostate cancer incidence rates were higher than those for lung

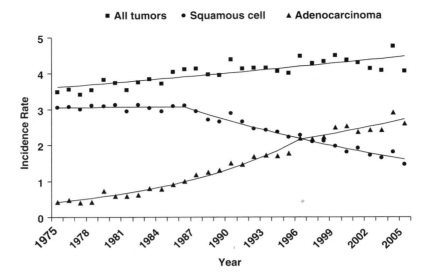

| Histology | Segments | Years | Incidence | | Annual Percent |
			Start	End	Change (APC)
All	1	1975–2005	3.5	4.1	0.7*
Squamous	2	1975–1986	3.1	1.5	0.04
cell		1986–2005	3.1	4.9	−3.4*
Adeno-	1	1975–1996	0.4	2.2	8.1*
carcinoma		1996–2005	2.2	2.6	2.6*

Fig. 4. Annual incidence rates (SEER-9 registries*) for all cancers of the esophagus and for the primary esophageal cancer histologies (squamous cell and adenocarcinoma), 1975–2005, with best fit joinpoint model.

and colorectal cancer. Among Hispanics, men had higher incidence of colorectal cancer compared with cancer of the lung and bronchus. Among women, breast cancer incidence rates were higher than any other cancer regardless of racial and ethnic group, followed by cancers of the lung and bronchus among blacks and whites, and cancer of the colon and rectum among American Indians/Alaskan Natives, Asian/Pacific Islanders, and women of Hispanic ethnicity.

US death rates for all cancers combined (2001–2005) were highest for blacks and lowest for Asians and Pacific Islanders (Table 3). Cancers of the lung, prostate, and colon and rectum were in the order of the three leading causes of cancer death among men for all racial and ethnic subgroups, except for Asian and Pacific Islander men, for whom cancer of the liver ranked second after cancer of the lung and bronchus. The leading causes of death for women were cancer of the lung and bronchus, breast, colon and rectum, except among Hispanic women, for whom breast and lung and bronchus cancer contributed equally.

Table 2

Age-adjusted Cancer Incidence Rates, All Malignant Cancers and Selected Cancer Sites by Gender and Race/Ethnicity, SEER 13 Registries, 2001–2005

Gender	Cancer site	Race/ethnicity				
		White	Black	AI/AN	API	Hispanic[a]
Both sexes	All malignant cancers	469.6	498.9	266.4	327.8	350.2
Male	All malignant cancers	543.4	646.4	287.5	370.8	412.3
	Top three cancer sites					
	Prostate	161.0	248.9	61.9	98.7	137.0
	Lung and bronchus	72.3	104.7	46.5	56.7	42.5
	Colon and rectum	56.5	70.3	39.4	51.6	45.7
	Selected sites (increasing)					
	Liver/intrahepatic bile duct	8.0	13.8	11.5	21.9	15.5
	Esophagus	7.9	9.2	6.7	4.5	5.5
Female	All malignant cancers	419.8	399.1	253.0	300.5	312.0
	Top three cancer sites					
	Breast	131.8	118.0	66.6	94.2	88.7
	Lung and bronchus	50.8	55.3	33.1	29.3	23.4
	Colon and rectum	42.0	53.9	34.3	37.7	31.7
	Selected sites (increasing)					
	Liver/intrahepatic bile duct	2.9	4.3	6.1	8.5	5.9
	Esophagus	1.9	3.2	1.9	1.2	1.0

AI/AN, American Indian/Alaska Native; API, Asians and Pacific Islander.
[a]Hispanic ethnicity is not mutually exclusive of race.
Source: Cancer Statistics Review http://seer.cancer.gov/csr/1975_2005/index.html

Table 3
Age-adjusted Death Rates, All Malignant Cancers and Selected Sites by Gender and Race/Ethnicity, United States, 2001–2005

Gender	Cancer site	White	Black	AI/AN	API	Hispanic[a]
Both sexes	All malignant cancers	188.0	234.4	128.5	114.1	136.6
Males	All malignant cancers	231.0	313.9	152.1	139.2	172.3
	Top three cancer sites					
	Prostate	24.6	59.7	17.9	11.0	23.1
	Lung and bronchus	71.4	93.3	42.7	37.6	39.5
	Colon and rectum	22.1	31.9	15.7	14.5	17.9
	Selected sites (increasing)					
	Liver/intrahepatic bile duct	6.7	10.3	8.1	15.2	10.2
	Esophagus	7.8	9.8	5.3	3.1	4.6
Females	All malignant cancers	159.1	186.9	112.1	96.1	112.7
	Top three cancer sites					
	Breast	24.4	33.6	14.3	12.6	16.7
	Lung and bronchus	42.0	40.0	28.9	18.5	16.7
	Colon and rectum	15.3	22.4	10.6	10.2	12.1
	Selected sites (increasing)					
	Liver/intrahepatic bile duct	2.9	3.9	4.7	6.6	4.6
	Esophagus	1.6	2.8	1.4	0.8	1.0

AI/AN, American Indian/Alaska Native; API, Asians and Pacific Islander.
[a]Hispanic ethnicity is not mutually exclusive of race.
Sources: Centers for Disease Control and Prevention, National Center for Health Statistics. Mortality rates for Hispanic ethnicity exclude Minnesota data for 2002, North Dakota data for 2001–2003. Cancer Statistics Review http://seer.cancer.gov/csr/1975_2005/index.html

1.10. Five-Year Relative Survival Rates by Stage Distribution

In the SEER-9 areas, patients diagnosed at an earlier stage of disease generally had higher 5-year survival rates than those diagnosed at more advanced stages (Table 4). For cancers that are readily detected by screening, such as breast, prostate, and colon and rectum, most cases were diagnosed with localized-stage disease. In contrast, the majority of lung and bronchus cancer cases were diagnosed with distant-stage disease. The 5-year relative survival rate for all sites combined was higher for females (92.8%) than males (83.9%) suggesting a higher proportion of women were diagnosed with localized and regional cancer.

The 5-year relative survival for selected sites is shown by stage at diagnosis, sex, and race in Table 5. For prostate cancer, the relative 5-year survival for the localized stage was 100.0% suggesting this cohort survives longer than other cancer populations. In contrast, the 5-year survival rate for cases diagnosed with distant prostate cancer was only 31.5%. Similarly, the overall 5-year relative survival rate for female breast cancer was 89.3%, with a much better prognosis for localized-stage breast cancer (∼98.3%) and a far worse prognosis for cases with distant stage (∼28.3%) at the time of diagnosis.

The overall 5-year survival rate for colon and rectal cancer in men and women was ∼65.0%, with a steady decline in the 5-year survival rate for progressively higher stage cancer from localized, to regional, and distant stage at diagnosis, respectively (Table 5). Among the top three cancers for men and women, cancers of the lung and bronchus had the worst prognosis, reflecting the high proportion of cases with distant-stage disease at the time of diagnosis (Table 4). Relative survival rates were higher for white than black patients regardless of type of tumor and gender. For example, there was a 10-percentage-point difference between 5-year survival rates for all white and black cases (both male and female) diagnosed with colon and rectum cancer, where lower survival rates in blacks generally seen based on stage at diagnosis. In addition, the 5-year relative survival rate for female breast cancer for all stages combined was 90.5% in white women vs. 77.8% in black women. An even greater racial difference was seen for distant-stage (metastatic) breast cancer (29.9% for whites vs. 19.6% for blacks). Overall, 5-year survival rates for cancers of the prostate and lung and bronchus (both sexes) were approximately 3%–4% higher in whites than in blacks. The NCI survival monograph provides more detailed histology and race/ethnicity data *(13)*.

1.11. Prevalence of People Living in the US with a History of Invasive Cancer

On January 1, 2005, the number of persons in the United States diagnosed with invasive cancer was estimated at 11,098,450 (Table 6). The history of invasive cancer increased with age. At least one episode of invasive cancer was estimated for ∼100,000 children from 0 to 19 years of age and for 500,000 young adults from 20 to 39 years of age who were alive on January 1, 2005. About 70% of the more than 11 million individuals with prevalent invasive cancer who were alive on January 1, 2005 were 60 or more years of age. Compared with January 1, 2004, the 2005 prevalence estimate increased by 336,236 cases *(14)*. The increase in cancer prevalence in the US population is attributed to a number of factors including increased incidence, improvement in survival, and the aging population of US.

Table 4

Five-Year Relative Survival Rates by Stage, All Cancer Sites Combined and Top Three Cancer Sites[a] of Men and Women, 1996–2004 (SEER-9)[b]

Gender	Cancer site(s)	Five-year relative survival rate (%)					Stage distribution (%)				
		All stages (%)	Localized (%)	Regional (%)	Distant (%)	Unstaged (%)	All stages (N)	Localized (%)	Regional (%)	Distant (%)	Unstaged (%)
Both sexes	All malignant cancers	66.3	89.9	58.2	18.2	46.3	906,914	32.1	19.4	19.7	12.9
Male	All malignant cancers	66.0	83.9	46.4	17.4	46.9	469,927	51.8	15.2	19.6	13.4
	Top three cancer sites										
	Prostate[c]	98.9	100.0	–	31.5	80.3	155,194	92.2	–	4.6	3.2
	Lung and bronchus	13.5	45.3	19.6	2.4	8.1	62,563	14.7	26.3	52.7	6.3
	Colon and rectum	65.4	90.0	68.9	10.7	42.5	48,678	40.7	36.3	19.3	3.8
Female	All malignant cancers	66.6	92.8	66.0	19.1	45.7	436,987	43.7	23.9	19.9	12.4
	Top three cancer sites										
	Breast	89.3	98.3	83.8	28.3	56.8	140,739	62.6	29.8	5.7	1.9
	Lung and bronchus	18.2	54.7	23.5	3.4	9.5	50,447	18.0	24.8	50.3	6.9
	Colon and rectum	65.3	90.2	69.2	10.8	37.6	47,634	39.0	37.5	18.6	4.9

[a]The top three cancer sites among men and women account for more than 50% of new cancer cases (SEER-9) and US cancer deaths.
[b]Acturial method. No adjustment for heterogeneity.
[c]Localized/regional stages are combined for prostate cases and reported under "localized" heading for prostate and for all sites (male).
Source: Cancer Statistics Review http://seer.cancer.gov/csr/1975_2005/index.html

Table 5
Five-Year Relative Survival Rate by Stage for the Top Three[a] Cancer Sites of Men and Women, by Race, 1996–2004 (SEER-9)[b].

Gender	Cancer site	Race	All stages (%)	5-Year survival (%)			
				Localized (%)	Regional (%)	Distant (%)	Unstaged (%)
Male	Prostate[c]	All races	98.9	100.0	–	31.5	80.3
		White	99.4	100.0	–	31.1	80.7
		Black	95.9	100.0	–	28.2	71.8
	Colon and rectum	All races	65.4	90.0	68.9	10.7	42.5
		White	66.4	90.6	70.1	10.7	42.3
		Black	56.1	84.4	61.8	10.2	41.5
	Lung and bronchus	All races	13.5	45.3	19.6	2.4	8.1
		White	13.7	46.1	19.7	2.3	7.3
		Black	11.0	38.4	16.0	2.4	11.4
Female	Breast	All races	89.3	98.3	83.8	28.2	56.9
		White	90.5	98.8	85.2	29.9	57.7
		Black	77.8	93.4	71.6	19.6	49.5
	Colon and rectum	All races	65.2	90.5	69.4	10.9	33.3
		White	66.2	91.0	70.3	11.1	31.6
		Black	55.9	84.6	61.6	8.4	40.0
	Lung and bronchus	All races	18.2	54.7	23.5	3.4	9.5
		White	18.4	55.0	23.5	3.3	9.2
		Black	15.1	46.0	21.9	3.3	10.1

[a]The top three cancer sites among men and women account for more than 50% of new cancer cases (SEER-9) and US cancer deaths.
[b]Actuarial method. No adjustment for heterogeneity.
[c]Localized/regional stages are combined for prostate cases and reported under "localized" heading for prostate.
Source: Cancer Statistics Review http://seer.cancer.gov/csr/1975_2005/index.html

Table 6

Complete Prevalence Counts, All Invasive Cancers Combined and the Top Three Sites of Men and Women as of January 1, 2005, by Age at Prevalence, United States[a]

Cancer site	Sex	All ages[b]	Age at prevalence (Years)							
			0–9	10–19	20–29	30–39	40–49	50–59	60–69	70+
All sites	Both sexes	11,098,450	30,547	72,038	150,370	357,602	917,205	1,768,647	2,454,249	5,347,792
	Males	5,017,159	16,399	39,131	72,187	144,424	325,302	684,471	1,158,366	2,576,879
	Females	6,081,291	14,148	32,907	78,183	213,178	591,903	1,084,176	1,295,883	2,770,913
Colon and rectum	Both sexes	1,095,283	11	150	1,929	9,738	41,408	121,209	212,781	708,059
	Males	531,875	11	58	908	4,952	21,683	65,986	117,180	321,098
	Females	563,408	0	92	1,021	4,786	19,725	55,223	95,601	386,961
Lung and bronchus	Both sexes	360,081	22	132	627	2,617	15,157	48,564	100,554	192,408
	Males	172,426	22	88	267	1,144	6,635	23,556	50,032	90,682
	Females	187,655	0	44	360	1,473	8,522	25,008	50,522	101,726
Breast (female)	Females	2,477,847	0	70	2,367	35,542	205,803	485,718	597,083	1,151,266
Prostate	Males	2,106,499	22	69	93	286	16,233	179,722	532,480	1,377,594

APC, annual percent change.

[a]US 2005 cancer prevalence counts are based on 2005 cancer prevalence proportions from the SEER-9 registries. Cases diagnosed more than 30 years ago were estimated using the completeness index method (10).

[b]Due to rounding, the sum of age-specific estimates may not equal the all-ages estimate.

Source: Cancer Statistics Review http://seer.cancer.gov/csr/1975_2005/index.html

1.12. Goal of Surveillance and Factors Influencing Major Cancer Trends

The primary goal of the NCI-SEER Program is to collect complete and accurate data on all cancers diagnosed among residents of geographic areas covered by SEER cancer registries, currently comprising 26% of the US population, with demographic and educational attributes comparable to the general US population. The SEER Program provides clinicians and researchers with the longitudinal data to monitor cancer trends and identify changing patterns of cancer burden across diverse US population subgroups. The cancer statistics presented in this chapter were organized by gender, race, ethnicity, stage of disease, and 5-year age group. These detailed population-based statistics are a valuable public health resource that helps to define at-risk populations, monitor temporal trends, and evaluate the effectiveness of cancer control efforts.

After decades of steady increases in cancer incidence and death rates, overall rates appear to be declining (Fig. 1). In particular, the incidence and death rates for cancers of the breast, prostate, and colon and rectum are declining (Fig. 2). Modeling of breast cancer mortality data suggests that both screening mammography and treatment have helped to reduce the rate of death in the United States *(15)*. Modeling of incidence and death data for prostate cancer suggests that screening for prostate-specific antigen (PSA) likely assisted in reducing mortality in the United States *(16)*. In addition, it is estimated that 45%–70% of the recently observed decline in prostate cancer mortality could be attributed to stage shift associated with PSA screening. We observed a sustained decrease in lung cancer death rates among men and a plateauing of lung cancer death rates among women *(17)*.

Substantial changes in prostate cancer incidence trends (Fig. 2) were seen after the introduction of the PSA blood test. This test was first approved by the US Food and Drug Administration (FDA) in 1986 as a method to monitor prostate cancer progression. Changes in PSA levels were quickly and widely adopted as an early prostate cancer marker. As a result, prostate cancer incidence rates increased sharply, reaching a peak in 1993 *(18)*. This uptrend was followed by a steep decline through 1995 and stabilization to background level in subsequent years *(19)*.

Results of the Women's Health Initiative (WHI) trial results published in 2002 suggested that hormone replacement therapy (HRT) increased the risk of breast cancer in postmenopausal women *(20)*. The subsequent abrupt decline in the use of HRT was partially responsible for the dramatic drop in breast cancer rates observed in SEER registries during years 2002 and 2003. Breast cancer rates began to level off in 2004 *(21)*.

Dietary folate is thought to decrease the risk of certain epithelial cancers of the uterine cervix, stomach, esophagus, lung, and colon and rectum *(22)*. However, there is concern that provision of folate could increase tumorigenesis among individuals with existing preneoplastic lesions of the colon and rectum. It has been hypothesized that a temporal relationship between folic acid fortification of foods in the 1980s and the increase in cancer of the colon and rectum incidence rates observed in the 1990s (Fig. 2) may be related to the promoting effects of folate on tumor growth *(23)*.

Important gender differences in lung cancer incidence are illustrated in Fig. 2. Compared to men, there has been a delayed increase and decrease of lung and bronchus cancer incidence among women *(24)*. These temporal differences reflect the fact that women who began cigarette smoking typically did so during and after World War II, while men began to adopt the habit in the early twentieth century, beginning in World War I *(25)*.

Age-adjusted incidence and mortality rates from 2001 to 2005 (Tables 2 and 3) indicate that black men and women experience elevated overall cancer incidence and death rates compared to other racial ethnic groups. The underlying patterns vary by cancer site. For example, black men and women had the highest incidence and death rates for cancer of the lung and bronchus and cancer of the colon and rectum. In contrast, white women had the highest breast cancer incidence rates. Despite lower incidence rates of breast cancer among black women, death rates were higher among black women compared with white women. This increased death rate among black women was attributed in part to cancer diagnosis at later stages *(26)*.

1.13. Impact of Race and Ethnicity

Asian and Pacific Islander men had the highest liver and intrahepatic bile duct cancer incidence and death rates, followed by Hispanic and black men. This racial distribution is attributed to the elevated occurrence of chronic Hepatitis B infection among Asians and Pacific Islanders *(27)*. An epidemic of Hepatitis C affecting Hispanics, blacks, and whites in the United States during the 1960s and 1970s and a successful global immunization campaign against Hepatitis B are expected to alter the racial distribution of liver cancer in the United States during the first half of the twenty-first century.

The highest rates of esophageal adenocarcinoma are seen in white males *(28)*. The incidence of this highly fatal cancer is increasing as the incidence of esophageal squamous cell carcinoma declines (Fig. 3). The increased occurrence of esophageal adenocarcinoma is partially attributed to obesity and low fruit and vegetable consumption *(12)*. Increased body mass and gastroesophageal acid reflux disease contribute to Barrett's disease, a lesion that precedes esophageal adenocarcinoma. The differential contribution of esophageal adenocarcinoma and squamous cell carcinoma to esophageal cancers would be unapparent without data collection by registries on esophageal tumor histology.

Rates for Asians and Pacific Islanders, American Indians and Alaska Natives, and Hispanics may be slightly biased because of delay in reporting adjustments for these racial/ethnic groups. Also, determination of the cancer burden among these populations has been difficult due to lack of systematic data collection, and underestimation of cancer cases and size of populations *(29, 30)*. Agencies and nonprofit organizations that contribute to cancer surveillance are committed to improving the quality of data collection related to race and ethnicity.

1.14. Prognosis

Survival statistics, a measure of prognosis, vary considerably by age and stage at diagnosis, gender, race/ethnicity, and initial treatment (Tables 4 and 5). Survival statistics have some limitations for estimating net survival due to cancer. For example, valid life tables are required to produce reliable estimates of relative survival. However, life tables do not exist for racial groups other than whites and blacks *(31)*. Thus, survival estimates cannot be accurately calculated for Asians and Pacific Islanders, American Indians and

Alaska Natives, and Hispanics. At present, cause-specific survival rates are available for these groups. This estimate of survival requires reliably coded information on cause of death. Even when cause of death information is available to the cancer registry via death certificate, the clear, underlying cause of death may not be available. Therefore, caution must be exercised when interpreting cause-specific survival estimates.

1.15. Conclusions and the Future of Cancer Surveillance

Cancer surveillance is improving in the United States as more registries contribute cancer data to SEER and CDC's National Program of Cancer Registries (NPCR). Combined programs for 49 states, six metropolitan areas, and the District of Columbia cover approximately 98% of the US population (32). As the post-World War II birth cohort (baby boomers) ages, an increase in cancer incidence is anticipated. Patients are expected to live longer after cancer diagnosis because of early detection and better treatments. An increasingly aging population combined with better survival rates contribute to increasing prevalence of people living with a history of invasive cancer, estimated to be approaching 12 million as of January 1, 2005. The increasing prevalence of cancer and comorbid conditions in the cohort of more than 70 million aging baby boomers will have a profound effect on cancer prevention and treatment (33). The SEER Program is an important source of information to monitor trends in burden of cancer in an ever changing US population (34).

REFERENCES

1. American Cancer Society. (2008) Cancer Facts and Figures 2008. Atlanta: American Cancer Society.
2. Fritz, A., Percy, C., Jack, A. et al. (2000) International Classification of Diseases for Oncology. 3rd ed. Geneva: World Health Organization.
3. Johnson C.H., Adamo M., eds (2007) SEER Program Coding and Staging Manual 2007. Bethesda, MD: National Cancer Institute, NIH Pub. 07-5581.
4. Centers for Disease Control and Prevention/National Center for Health Statistics. Available at: http://www.cdc.gov/nchs/Default.htm . Accessed November 15, 2006
5. United States Department of Health and Human Services. Population Estimates Used in NCI's SEER*Stat Software. Bethesda, MD: National Cancer Institute. Accessed on August, 2008
6. Ries, L.A., Harkins, D., Krapcho, M. et al. (2006) SEER Cancer Statistics Review, 1975–2003. Bethesda, MD: National Cancer Institute
7. Clegg, L.X., Feuer, E.J., Midthune, D.N. et al. (2002) Impact of reporting delay and reporting error on cancer incidence rates and trends. *J Natl Cancer Inst* **94**, 1537–45.
8. Kim, H.J., Fay, M.P., Feuer, E.J. et al. (2001) Permutation tests for join point regression with applications to cancer rates. *Stat Med* **19**, 335–51.
9. Ederer, F., Axtell, L.M., and Cutler, S.J. (1961) The relative survival rate: A statistical methodology. *J Natl Cancer Inst Monogr* **6**, 101–21.
10. Merrill, R.M., Capocaccia, R., Feuer, E.J., and Mariotto, A. (2000) Cancer prevalence estimates based on tumour registry data in the Surveillance, Epidemiology, and End Results (SEER) Program. *Int J Epidemiol* **29**, 197–207.
11. Gigli, A., Mariotto, A., Clegg, L.X., Tavilla, A., Corazziari, I., Capocaccia, R., Hachey, M., and Scoppa, S. (2006) Estimating the variance of cancer prevalence from population-based registries. *Stat Methods Med Res* **15**, 235–53.

12. Engel, L.S., Chow, W.H., Vaughan, T.L., Gammon, M.D., Risch, H.A., Stanford, J.L., Schoenberg, J.B., Mayne, S.T., Dubrow, R., Rotterdam, H., West, A.B., Blaser, M., Blot, W.J., Gail, M.H., and Fraumeni, J.F., Jr. (2003) Population attributable risks of esophageal and gastric cancers. *J Natl Cancer Inst* **95**, 1404–13.

13. Ries L.A.G., Melbert D., Krapcho M., Mariotto A., Miller B.A., Feuer E.J., Clegg L., Horner M.J., Howlader N., Eisner M.P., Reichman M., Edwards B.K., eds (2008) Cancer Statistics Review, 1975–2005. Bethesda, MD: National Cancer Institute, http://seer.cancer.gov/csr/19752005

14. Ries L.A.G., Young J.L., Keel G.E., Eisner M.P., Lin Y.D., Horner M.-J. eds (2007) SEER Survival Monograph: Cancer Survival Among Adults: U.S. SEER Program, 1988–2001, Patient and Tumor Characteristics. Bethesda, MD: National Cancer Institute, SEER Program: NIH Pub. 07-6215.

15. Berry, D.A., Cronin, K.A., Plevritis, S.K. et al. (2005) Effect of screening and adjuvant therapy on mortality from breast cancer. *N Engl J Med* **353**, 1784–92.

16. Etzioni, R., Tsodikov, A., Mariotto, A., Szabo, A., Falcon, S., Wegelin, J., Ditommaso, D., Karnaofski, K., Gulati, R., Penson, D.F., and Feuer, E.J. (2008) Quantifying the role of PSA screening in the US prostate cancer mortality decline. *Cancer Causes Control* **19**, 175–81.

17. Jemal, A., Thun, M., Ries, L.A.G. et al. (2008) Annual report to the nation on the status of cancer, 1975–2005, featuring trends in lung cancer, tobacco use, and tobacco control. *J Natl Cancer Inst* **100**, 1672–94.

18. Potosky, A.L., Miller, B.A., Albertsen, P.C., and Kramer, B.S. (1995) The role of increasing detection in the rising incidence of prostate cancer. *JAMA* **273**, 548–52.

19. Feuer, E.J., and Wun, L.-M. (1992) How much of the recent rise in breast cancer incidence can be explained by increases in mammography utilization? A dynamic population model approach. *Am J Epidemiol* **136**, 1423–36.

20. Rossouw, J.E., Anderson, G.L., Prentice, R.L.,, LaCroix, A.Z., Kooperberg, C., Stefanick, M.L., Jackson, R.D., Beresford, S.A., Howard, B.V., Johnson, K.C., Kotchen, J.M., and Ockene, J. (2002) Risks and benefits of estrogen plus progestin in healthy postmenopausal women: Principal results from the Women's Health Initiative randomized controlled trial. *JAMA* **288**, 321–33.

21. Ravdin, P.M., Cronin, K.A., Howlader, N. et al. (2007) The decrease in breast-cancer incidence in 2003 in the United States. *N Engl J Med* **356**, 1670–74.

22. Ulrich, C.M., and Potter, J.D. (2007) Folate and cancer—timing is everything. *JAMA* **297**, 2408–9.

23. Mason, J.B., Dickstein, A., Jacques, P.F. et al. (2007) A temporal association between folic acid fortification and an increase in colorectal cancer rates may be illuminating important biological principles: A hypothesis. *Cancer Epidemiol Biomarkers Prev* **16**, 1325–29.

24. Devesa, S.S., Blot, W.J., and Fraumeni, J.F., Jr. (1989) Declining lung cancer rates among young men and women in the United States: A cohort analysis. *J Natl Cancer Inst* **81**, 1568–71.

25. Jemal, A., Chu, K.C., and Tarone, R.E. (2001) Recent trends in lung cancer mortality in the United States. *J Natl Cancer Inst* **93**, 277–83.

26. Morris, G.J., and Mitchell, E.P. (2008) Higher incidence of aggressive breast cancers in African-American women: A review. *J Natl Med Assoc* **100**, 698–702.

27. El-Serag, H.B., Davila, J.A., Petersen, N.J., and McGlynn, K.A. (2003) The continuing increase in the incidence of hepatocellular carcinoma in the United States: An update. *Ann Intern Med* **139**, 817–23.

28. Devesa, S.S., Blot, W.J., and Fraumeni, J.F., Jr. (1998) Changing patterns of the incidence of esophageal and gastric carcinoma in the United States. *Cancer* **83**, 2049–53.

29. Swan, J., and Edwards, B.K. (2003) Cancer rates among American Indians and Alaska Natives: Is there a national perspective? *Cancer* **98**, 1262–72.

30. Miller, B.A., Chu, K.C., Hankey, B.F., and Ries, L.A. (2008) Cancer incidence and mortality patterns among specific Asian and Pacific Islander populations in the U.S. *Cancer Causes Control* **19**, 227–56.

31. Rosenberg, H.M., Maurer, J.D., Sorlie, P.D. et al. (1999) Quality of death rates by race and Hispanic origin: A summary of current research, 1999. *Vital Health Stat 2* **128**, 1–13.

32. U.S. Cancer Statistics Working Group. (2007) United States Cancer Statistics: 2004 Incidence and Mortality Data. Atlanta: US Department of Health and Human Services, Centers for Disease Control and Prevention and National Cancer Institute.

33. Mariotto, A.B., Rowland, J.H., Ries, L.A., Scoppa, S., and Feuer, E.J. (2007) Multiple cancer prevalence: A growing challenge in long-term survivorship. *Cancer Epidemiol Biomarkers Prev* **16**, 566–71.
34. Hayat, M.J., Howlader, N., Reichman, M.E., and Edwards, B.K. (2007) Cancer statistics, trends, and multiple primary cancer analyses from the Surveillance, Epidemiology, and End Results (SEER) Program. *Oncologist* **12**, 20–37.

2 Cancer Biology and Nutrigenomics

John A. Milner and Donato F. Romagnolo

Key Points

1. Current cancer models comprise those that are inherited through the germline and represent only ∼5% of total cases of human cancers. These tumors originate because of mutational events. The remaining ∼95% originate as sporadic events and evolve as a result of exposure to the environment, which includes exposure to both environmental contaminants and dietary agents.

2. The multistage model of carcinogenesis identifies various phases, initiation, promotion, and progression, which determine the evolution of normal somatic cells to heterogeneous populations with cancer potential. This process appears to be influenced by tissue microenvironment and organization. Significant opportunities in nutrition and cancer prevention exist in the early stages of initiation and promotion prior to clonal expansion of heterogeneous populations. Targeting initiators, cocarcinogens, and promoters may provide the best opportunity in cancer prevention since the majority of advanced solid tumors are resistant to therapy.

3. Nutrigenomics represents a strategy that can be applied to the study and prevention of many diseases including cancer. It has been defined as a pyramidal approach that encompasses the study of molecular relationships between nutrients and genes (nutrigenetics), how these interactions influence changes in the profile of transcripts (transcriptomics), proteins (proteomics), and metabolites (metabolomics). DNA methylation and histone modifications are epigenetic events that mediate heritable changes in gene expression and chromatin organization in the absence of changes in the DNA sequence. The age-increased susceptibility to cancer may derive from accumulation of epigenetic changes and represents a potential target for therapies with bioactive compounds.

4. Factors that mediate the response to dietary factors include nuclear receptors and transcription factors, which function as sensors to dietary components and determine changes in the profile of transcripts.

5. Integration of high-throughput proteomic and metabolomic approaches with computational techniques is necessary to understand the complexity of the biological response to specific bioactive compounds or associations of nutrients and identify key molecular targets in cancer prevention and treatment.

Key Words: Nutrigenomics; cancer biology; multistage carcinogenesis; bioactive compounds; molecular targets; prevention

From: *Nutrition and Health: Bioactive Compounds and Cancer*
Edited by: J.A. Milner, D.F. Romagnolo, DOI 10.1007/978-1-60761-627-6_2,
© Springer Science+Business Media, LLC 2010

1. INTRODUCTION

1.1. Multistage Carcinogenesis

Cancer statistics indicate that only 5% of known cancers are linked to heredity, whereas the remaining 95% are sporadic, i.e., tumors originate in the absence of family history and are caused by a variety of factors. The classical model of multistage carcinogenesis identifies three phases: initiation, promotion, and progression. The first phase, initiation, is characterized by induction of unchecked replication, which may result from one or more events including exposure to DNA damaging agents, loss of DNA repair functions, fixation of mutations in tumor suppressor genes, or activation of protooncogenes *(1)*. A likely consequence of initiation is that selected cells may gain a resistant phenotype to certain carcinogens, DNA damaging agents, or escape programmed cell death. However, at this stage the presence of initiated cells is not necessarily associated with clonal growth. The second stage, promotion, is believed to be a quantitative phase during which initiated cells increase in number under the influence of selective, non-DNA reactive, pressures and in the context of a specific tissue microenvironment (e.g., stroma) *(2)*. Therefore, specific proliferative stimuli (e.g., estrogens) or chronic inflammation may have a central role as cocarcinogens and promote proliferation of existing focal lesions *(3)*. This process is essentially quantitative and facilitates growth of cancer foci under the influence of the tissue microenvironment (e.g., influence of paracrine factors) *(4)*. The net effect of events that occur during promotion may be the selective proliferation of initiated cells. The third phase, progression, has been characterized as a qualitative process during which cell heterogeneity arises and divergent cell populations grow inside focal lesions. The clonal evolution of specific cell subsets during progression contributes to the heterogeneity of tumors and is influenced by the tissue microenvironment or organization, which regulates the rate of cancer progression and metastasis *(1)*.

Key questions in cancer prevention pertain to identifying the timing in life of exposure to initiators; predicting the latency between time of exposure and cancer manifestation; and dissecting the molecular and biochemical mechanisms responsible for neoplastic growth. If these conditions were known, then they might be targeted with preventive naturally occurring dietary compounds or dietary patterns. For example, the importance of timing of nutrient exposure in cancer prevention is highlighted by experimental evidence showing that supplementation with the isoflavone genistein during the prepubertal or prepubertal plus adult periods protected against mammary carcinogenesis *(5)*. Similarly, epidemiological studies in Chinese women reported an inverse association between intake of soy during adolescence and the risk of breast cancer in adult life *(6)*. The risk of certain cancers (e.g., breast cancer) increases in association with Western diets compared to Mediterranean or native Mexican diets. Therefore, nutrition strategies need to be developed to prevent the effects of carcinogenic agents; target and eliminate premalignant lesions at early stages; and antagonize (i.e., induce apoptosis) the proliferation of clonal neoplastic populations *(7)*.

Based on the multistage model of carcinogenesis, multiple time points of intervention may exist. However, previous decades of experience in cancer therapeutics suggest that significant opportunities in nutrition and cancer prevention exist in the early stages of initiation and promotion prior to clonal expansion of heterogeneous populations. As cancer cells diverge from progenitor cells, they may acquire differences in nutrient requirements, gain proliferative advantages, or become refractory to therapeutic bioactive food components and drugs. Targeting initiators, cocarcinogens, and promoters may provide the best opportunity in cancer prevention since the majority of advanced solid tumors is resistant to therapy *(8)*. Therefore, ideally bioactive components (e.g., *Symphytum officinale*) should not contribute to cancer risk per se *(9)* and halt or eliminate premalignant lesions. An interesting example is provided by polyphenols, which in combination with transition metals (e.g., copper) increase at higher levels in cancer cells the production of reactive oxygen species and cause DNA damage. Therefore, interactions between nutrients may be exploited in therapies specifically targeted to cancer cells *(10)*.

An important area of study is whether high doses of certain bioactive compounds or associations of bioactives could become co-carcinogens. An example of this potential risk is provided by folate, which may function as a cancer promoter of colonic lesions *(11)*. Similarly, exposure to indol-3-carbinol, an indole contained in cruciferous vegetables, increased in a rat model the incidence of uterine lesions including atypical hyperplasia and adenocarcinomas *(12)*. Therefore, studies are needed to determine the upper limits or thresholds of supplementation.

The main goal of nutrigenomics is to profile global changes induced by nutrients and develop dietary-intervention strategies to maintain homeostasis and prevent diseases including cancer *(13)*. The main challenge is that of integrating information pertaining to expression of more than 30,000 genes, for most of which the function is not known, and computing changes in expression for more than 100,000 proteins and several thousand metabolites *(14)*. A major drawback in developing prevention strategies comes from differences in approach between preclinical and clinical research. Most, if not all, preclinical studies with in vitro and animal models tend to focus on single bioactive food components without considerations of the complex interactions that occur among bioactive food components present in the human diet. This problem is addressed in part by epidemiological studies that focus on the average anticarcinogenic or procarcinogenic effects of specific groups of bioactive compounds (e.g., n-3 fatty acids) in the context of dietary exposure (e.g., Western vs. Asian diet). Nevertheless, results of population studies may not find statistical differences or be biased if the analysis comprises individuals with mutations in tumor suppressor genes or carrying specific polymorphisms. For example, individuals with the TT polymorpshism at nucleotide 677 for methylenetetrahydrofolate reductase (MTHFR) ($\sim$5–20% population worldwide) appear to be at decreased risk for colorectal adenomas in the presence of high plasma levels of folate *(15)*. Therefore, the interaction between levels of exposure to certain bioactive food components and genetics (nutrigenetics) may influence the risk of cancer in certain subpopulations and is an important component of nutrigenomic studies.

Whereas it is recognized that cancer requires multiple molecular changes, it is also known that certain genetic alterations play a hierarchical role in cancer development in certain tissues. For example, loss of BRCA-1 expression through epigenetic silencing may confer a high probability of breast cancer *(16)*. Loss of DNA repair functions controlled by BRCA-1 may lead to subsequent genetic alterations in genes that control proliferation and apoptosis. During the last two decades a tremendous amount of information has been gathered concerning the role of signaling pathways in cancer development. Nutrigenomic strategies are an important tool to decode pyramidal effects and establish the minimum requirements for cancer development and prevention.

1.2. Gene × Diet Interactions

Analysis of worldwide occurrence of cancer suggests that certain geographical areas have higher incidence for specific types of tumors. For example, historically Japan was a region with relatively low incidence of colon cancer, yet Japanese populations that relocated to the United States experience an increase in the incidence of colon cancers and a reduction in the incidence of stomach cancers. Similarly, increased incidence for breast and prostate cancer has been reported for migrant populations (17–19). These observations suggest that heredity alone does not explain the susceptibility to these and other tumor types, and point to environmental and dietary factors as potential causative agents (20). A second but very important factor that should be considered is that the overall occurrence of cancer increases with age. The age-increased susceptibility to cancer may derive from accumulation of epigenetics changes and represents a potential target for prevention with bioactive compounds.

If one excludes mutations in cancer susceptibility genes or occupational exposure to chemical carcinogens, diet alone likely represents the most significant risk factor in the etiology of sporadic tumors. In support of this notion, the 2007 AICR/WCRF Second Expert Report on Food, Nutrition, Physical Activity, and the Prevention of Cancer suggested that about one-third of all cancer deaths may be attributable to dietary factors (21). The ability of dietary compounds to influence the risk of cancer may result from tissue-specific influences on cellular processes including inflammation, carcinogen metabolism, hormone regulation, cell differentiation, DNA repair, apoptosis, and cell growth cycle. Whereas about 30% of all cancer cases may relate to dietary habits, the impact of diet on these processes is influenced by the specific foods consumed, the specific type of cancer, and interactions among compounds, which may act additively or synergistically when combined in the human diet.

Modern approaches in cancer prevention should address the issue of tissue specificity and identify nutrients that in animal and cell culture models prevent tumors of the same type as those associated with human exposure (8). An obvious challenge is the establishment of a cause–effect relationship between exposure to specific bioactive compounds and tissue-specific cancer prevention.

1.3. Nutrigenomics

Conceptually, nutrigenomics represents a strategy that can be applied to the study and prevention of many diseases. It provides a pyramidal approach that encompasses the study of molecular relationships between nutrients and genes (nutrigenetics), how these interactions influence changes in the profile of transcripts (transcriptomics), proteins (proteomics), and metabolites (metabolomics) (22). The underpinning concept is that thousands of bioactive compounds function as signals and influence the organism's response (23). The opportunity of targeting nutrients–gene interactions to influence the cancer process is modulated by genetic variations in human populations, epigenetic modifications that selectively and permanently alter gene expression, by complex interactions/associations among dietary components, and heterogeneity of cells within a certain tumor. Therefore, integration of information about gene polymorphisms, identification of gene targets that regulate cell and tissue-specific pathways, and development of diagnostic strategies to control for clinical heterogeneity are important to understand how nutrigenomics may be used in cancer prevention *(24)*. Other chapters in this volume will discuss specifically how nutrigenetics, epigenetics, transcriptomics, and metabolomics may help to assess the effects of specific nutrients on the cancer process. Here, we will highlight examples of how integration of nutrigenomic data may be useful to understand the correlation between consumption of specific bioactive compounds and protection toward specific tumor types.

A key point that should be made is that changes in gene or protein expression do not necessarily translate into changes in metabolic profiles. Conversely, changes in promoter activities and transcript profiles do not necessarily lead to changes in protein expression and functions. Therefore, integration and the parallel use of all components of nutrigenomics through high-throughput and computational techniques are necessary to understand the complexity of the biological response to specific bioactive compounds or associations of nutrients and identify key molecular targets *(25, 26)*. The ultimate goal of nutrigenomics is that of developing genomics-based biomarkers that help in the early detection and prevention of diet-related diseases, including cancer. To reach this goal it is important to develop tissue-specific dietary responses that can be used as signatures or fingerprints to estimate risk *(27)*. The availability of nutritional biomarkers at early stages (e.g., initiation) may be used as prognostic tools. A complicating factor is that diet contains a large number of compounds and that each nutrient has different gene targets and affinities. An example is the cross talk of estrogens and isoflavones with estrogen receptors and how this interaction may affect the development and prevention of breast cancer *(28)*.

One of the mechanisms through which nutrients influence cellular responses is through interactions with members of the nuclear receptor superfamily of transcription factors, which integrate genomic and nongenomic effects. This family comprises many members that bind with various affinities to hormones, nutrients, and metabolites *(29)*. In essence, these receptors function as sensors and transmit signals to specific molecular targets to induce an adaptive response and changes in transcript levels. Receptors are binding proteins that translocate from the cytoplasm to the nucleus. Examples of these nuclear receptors are the glucocorticoid (GR), estrogen (ERα and β), retinoic acid (RARα, β, and γ), vitamin D (VDR), peroxisome proliferators activated receptor (PPARa, β/δ, and γ), and retinoid-X (RXRα, β, and γ) receptor. The RXR participates in the formation of heterodimers with many nuclear receptors including ER, VDR, and PPAR *(30)*. The formation of heterodimers and the presence of isoforms for receptors increase the number of potential complexes that can bind to specific DNA consensus sequence, thus amplifying the diversity of biological actions induced by receptor ligands. Numerous members of the nuclear receptor family are orphan since no apparent endogenous ligands have been found. Orphan receptors may function as activator or repressors. For example, the AhR activates the transcription of P450 genes, while repressing transcription of estrogen-inducible promoters *(31)*.

Consensus sequences for nuclear receptor complexes are harbored within or in close proximity to promoter regions and influence the chromatin organization and transcription of target genes. Nuclear receptors may act at as homodimers at inverted repeats (Class I), heterodimers at direct repeats (Class II), homodimers at direct repeats (Class III), and monomers at core sites (Class IV). The spatial arrangement and organization of these responsive elements is important to understand the responsiveness of certain genes to receptor ligands and cooperativity among multiple *cis*-regulatory elements. Receptors that are known to mediate responses to nutrients include members of the PPAR subfamily, which binds fatty acids and eicosanoid metabolites. In turn, the activated PPAR regulates the expression of genes involved in lipid metabolism *(32)*. A thorough overview of the application of transcriptomics to study PPAR-dependent gene regulation can be found in Bunger et al. *(33)*. The ER is known to bind to natural phytoestrogens (e.g., genistein) found in soy products *(34)* and the phytoalexin resveratrol. The AhR binds a vast number of compounds including tea catechins and indoles (indol-3-carbinol (I3C)) and 3,3′diindolyilmethane (DIM) (more details in Chapter 32).

The molecular structure and concentration of ligands influences the ability to activate specific receptors and the direction and intensity of the response. Likely, the exposure to many dietary ligands occurs in the context of chronic exposure at concentrations (μM–mM) higher than those known for classical nuclear receptor ligands (nM) *(32)*. Therefore, the action of dietary ligands (e.g., isoflavones or resveratrol) for nuclear receptors (e.g., ER) may antagonize that of endogenous ligands (e.g., estrogen) and offer opportunities to prevent the growth of cancer lesions.

Transcription factors that have been shown to exert an important role in cancer include NFkB and the activator protein-1 (AP-1). Both factors play a key role in chronic inflammation, which is associated with cancer development. The transcription factor AP-1 is required for activation of NFkB and mediates the effects of tumor promoters including epidermal growth factor (EGF) and UV. Therefore, both AP-1 and NFkB have been identified as promising molecular targets for cancer prevention *(35–37)*. The activation of NFkB, e.g., by prostaglandins or bile acids *(38)* promotes cell proliferation and has been identified in solid tumors (breast, colon), leukemia, and lymphoma. NFkB is a homodimer and heterodimer of the Rel/NFkB family of proteins. In its inactive form, NFkB is sequestered to the cytosol bound to the cofactor IkB. The phosphorylation of IkB by the kinase Ikk leads to dissociation of IkB and translocation of NFkB to the nucleus where it targets promoter regions at specific binding sites. Dietary compounds found to inhibit the activity of NFkB include dimeric procyanidin B2 (B2), which prevents binding of NFkB to target DNA sequences. Procyanidins are oligomers formed from flavan-3-ols found in flavonoid-rich foods including cocoa, grapes, cranberries, red wine, and apples *(39)*. Other anti-NFkB bioactives include curcumin, a natural component of the rizhome of *Curcuma longa*, carnosol (rosemary and sage), benzyl-isothiocyanates and sulforaphane (cruciferous vegetables), and kaempferol *(40)*.

AP-1 comprises protein homodimers (jun-jun) and heterodimers (jun-fos, jun-ATF). It belongs to the class of basic leucine zipper (bZIP) transcription factors and binds promoters at sequence-specific sites, thus transactivating or repressing transcription. Bioactive compounds that inhibit AP-1 include rosmarinic acid *(41)*, isoliquiritigenin (a licorice flavonoid), luteolin *(42)*, conjugated linoleic acid *(43)*, eicosapentaenoic acid *(44)*, and sulforaphane.

A wealth of studies utilized DNA microarrays to understand cancer and identify transcriptional targets for bioactive food compounds. In general, investigations have attempted to classify clusters of genes based on their functional food categories. Epidemiological studies have suggested that high fish intake is associated with a decreased risk of colorectal cancer. This protective effect has been attributed to the high content of n-3 polyunsaturated fatty acids (PUFAs), eicosapentaenoic acids (EPA), and docosahexaenoic acid (DHA) in some fish. cDNA array studies suggested that the protective effects of n-3 PUFA were associated with upregulation of phase II enzymes (GSTT2) and Bax, and downregulation of pro-inflammatory genes (COX-2) *(45)*

Genome-wide analysis of gene expression in response to dietary fats has been used as a paradigm to study the nutrigenomics of PPARs. The PPAR receptor system is of interest primarily as a sensor to dietary lipids. However, most of the genome-wide analyses of PPAR functions have utilized pharmacological agonists *(33)*. Dietary fat-induced changes in gene expression have been examined before and during puberty in rodent models. Recent gene microarray analyses documented that expression of PPARγ was increased in the mammary gland of 50-day-old rats prepubertally fed low-fat n-3 PUFA. The reduction in mammary tumorigenesis was associated with increased expression of antioxidant genes and lower expression of genes that stimulate cell proliferation *(46)*. Combination of laser capture microdissection of mammary ductal epithelial cells and measurements of genes expression revealed fatty acid-enriched diets significantly stimulated proliferation and activation of cell cycle genes during puberty *(47)*. Oligonucleotide microarray analyses have been used to identify genes involved in enhanced growth of human prostate cancer. These studies revealed upregulation of IGF-1 receptor expression in prostate cancer xenografts under high-fat diets *(48)*. Increased expression of IGF-II and plasminogen activator inhibitor-1 (PAI-1) protein was detected in HepG2 cells following in vitro treatment with low (50 μM) levels of palmitate *(49)*. Both IGF-II and PAI-1 are involved in metabolic syndrome. The latter study combined mRNA expression profiling with in silico promoter analysis (Genomatix Gene2Promotor, Matinspector and Biobase Transfac programs) to identify common transcription factor binding sites in the promoter regions of palmitate-regulated genes. Genes were divided into groups of downregulated and upregulated genes. Recognition elements for the transcription factors AhR, EKLF, MAZF, MTF, NRSF, PAX5, and ZBPF were identified within the promoter regions of five downregulated metallothionein genes. The SREBP-1 binding element was found in the regulatory regions of the genes MT1E, MT1F, and MT2A. In the promoter regions of the upregulated genes, common recognition elements for the transcription factors EKLF, GREF, MZF, and ZBPF were identified. cDNA microarrays have also been used to detect changes in transcript expression of ~5,700 genes in radical prostatectomies in men after 6 weeks of low-fat/low-glycemic diets *(50)*.

Genomic-wide analyses based on ChIP and DNA microarrays illustrated that global features of estrogen-regulated genes included occupancy by ERα and histone acetylation *(51)*. The ER influences the expression of many genes by either binding as a homodimer to estrogen response elements (ERE), or by forming complexes with AP-1or specificity protein (Sp). These genes may be targeted by soy isoflavones because of their ability to act on the ER. Whole-genome microarray hybridization with 25,000 oligonucleotides has been used to investigate the impact of ER status (MCF-7=ER+ vs.

MDA-MB-231=ER−) and differences between normal (MCF-10A) and cancerous cells after lycopene exposure. These studies revealed that lycopene, which may have preventive roles in breast cancer, affected genes involved in apoptosis and cell cycle *(52)*. Differential expression studies in breast cancer cells documented that the phytoalexin resveratrol was more active in ER+ (MCF-7) than ER− (MDA-MB-231) breast cancer cells *(53)*. The specificity of resveratrol for ER+ breast cancer cells may provide the mechanistic basis for the development of prevention therapies against ER+ breast cancers.

Epigenetic events including DNA methylation and histone modifications can alter chromatin organization and modulate gene transcription in a site-specific and cooperative manner *(54)*. Octamers of core histones (two each of H2A, H2B, H3, and H4) are wrapped by ∼146 bp of DNA to form the nucleosome, considered to be the minimum and basic structure of chromatin. Histone tails provide binding sites for regulatory proteins and are subject to dynamic posttranslational modifications including methylation, acetylation, phosphorylation, ADP-ribosylation, ubiquitination, and sumoylation *(55)*. DNA methylation of cytosines by DNA methyltransferases (DMNTs) results in chromatin reorganization governed by the methyl-binding proteins (MBPs). In addition, DNA methylation inhibits the binding of transcription factors and produces binding sites for chromatin modifying complexes such as the histone deacetylase complexes (HDACs). The removal of acetyl groups from amino-terminal lysine residues of histones by HDACs permits the subsequent methylation of histone H3 on lysine 9 (H3-K9) by the histone methyltransferases (HMTases), SUV39H1 and SUV39H2 *(56)*. The methylation of histone H3 lysine 9 allows for the recruitment of the HP-1 protein and also interferes with phosphorylation of histone H3 at serine-10 *(57)*. In contrast to histone deacetylation by HDACs, histone acetylation is generally associated with transcriptional activity *(55)*. Cofactors that contain histone acetyltransferase activity (HAT) include CBP/p300, p/CAF, and SRC-1 *(58)*.

Besides genetic changes, epigenetic alterations have been proposed to play a key role in the onset of a variety of tumors by inducing stable, heritable changes in gene expression that are propagated over cell generations *(59)*. Patterns and levels of DNA methylation and histone acetylation are reported to be profoundly altered in human pathologies including inflammation and cancer *(60)*. However, it is not clear how the cross talk between histone modifications and DNA methylation influences gene expression, and how the hierarchical order of these changes leads to silencing during tumor development.

It remains to be clearly established whether histone modifications need to occur before changes in DNA methylation or DNA methylation changes guide histone modifications. Answering this question has paramount implications in identifying the initiating events involved in cancer development and guide in the development of strategy for cancer prevention and treatment. Acetylations of histone H3Lys9 and Lys18 and deacetylation of Lys14 were associated with PI3K-dependent activation of PTEN through antioxidant-responsive element (ARE) *(61)*. Loss of histone H4K20 trimethylation was reported in early precursor lung cancer lesions *(62)*. Methylation of CpG islands in promoter regions has been reported for tumor suppressor genes, hormone receptors, and other genes involved in detoxification and DNA repair *(63)*. ERα and

BRCA-1 promoter methylation have been reported in subsets of sporadic breast cancers *(16)*. The CpG island methylator phenotype in colorectal cancer is frequently characterized by hypermethylation of promoter regions in tumor suppressor genes. This methylation event increases with age. Specific promoters found to be methylated in patients with CpG island methylator phenotype tumors include p16 and TIMP3. Methylation of these genes increased with age *(64)*.

Epigenetic changes can occur randomly or in response to the environment (diet). However, unlike genetic mutations, epigenetic events may be reversible *(65)* and represent viable targets for dietary intervention. For example, (–)-epigallocatechin-3-gallate (EGCG), the major polyphenol from green tea, and genistein, the major isoflavone present in soy, have been used to restore the expression of methylation-silenced genes including RARβ, p16, and O^6-methylguanine methyltransferase (MGMT) *(66, 67)*. The reversal effects of EGCG and genistein were attributed primarily to inhibition of DNA methyltransferase, although the effect of genistein was weaker than that of EGCG. The reactivation of p16 by genistein was associated with inhibition of cell growth and weak inhibition of HDAC activity. The combination of genistein plus sulforaphane, a HDAC inhibitor present in broccoli, augmented the reactivation of expression of RARβ, p16, and MGMT by genistein. In human cancer cells, sulforaphane, butyrate, and metabolites of garlic organosulfur compounds (allyl mercaptan, AM) inhibited HDAC activity *(68, 69)*. The depression in HDAC activity by AM was associated with increased histone acetylation, binding of Sp3 to the promoter region of p21, and cell cycle arrest. These results documented that combination of agents that target DNA methyltransferase and HDAC activity may be effective in epigenetic therapies targeted to reactivation of tumor suppressor and receptor genes and halt proliferation of cancer cells. In theory, one potential drawback of using bioactive compounds in cancer therapies is the lack of specificity. For example, a depression in DNA methyltransferase activity may lead to global hypomethylation leading to chromosomal instability and tumors *(70)*. Furthermore, HATs and HDACs and their inhibitors modify acetylation of nonhistone proteins, such as transcription factors. Ideally, these potential problems might be addressed using combinations of (weak) HDAC and DNMT inhibitors and concentrations sufficient to induce synergistic and tissue-specific effects.

The use of specific biomarker profiles that function as sentinel indicators may assist in the detection of changes in gene expression linked to nuclear receptors, transcription factors, signaling pathways, and metabolites *(71)*. Nevertheless, this approach is complicated by the multitude of compounds that affect multiple target genes, which in turn can exert polygenic effects and influence a large number of downstream targets. Moreover, more than 350 oncogenes and tumor suppressor genes have been implicated in the etiology of cancer *(1)*. Furthermore, intake of a particular bioactive food component or precursor does not equate to exposure at the tissue or cell levels *(72)*. The complexity of this system requires the development of genome-based tissue-specific signatures to correlate phenotypic responses to nutrition.

A specific target for nutrigenomic strategies is endocrine cancers, including breast, ovarian, endometrial, and prostate cancers. The vast majority of breast cancers is estrogen receptor (ER)-positive and occurs in postmenopausal women. Because breast tissues undergo complex programs of growth and development that are under the influence of ovarian steroids, studies have considered nutrition factors that alter or interfere with estrogen and progesterone-dependent regulation.

The interest on isoflavones in breast cancer prevention derives from the fact breast cancer risk for women residing in geographical areas of high consumption of soy products during puberty is lower compared to that of women living in Western countries or Asian women who had a low soy intake *(73)*. However, clinical trials reported small *(74)* or no effect of supplementation with isoflavones on breast cancer risk *(75–78)*, and administration of isoflavones elicited in some cases an estrogen-like effect. Other studies indicated that the reduction in breast cancer risk due to soy intake was limited to Asian populations *(79)*. A case–control study conducted in Southeast China in 2004–2005 reported that premenopausal and postmenopausal women in the highest quartile of total isoflavone intake had a reduced risk for all receptor (ER/PR) status of breast cancer with a dose–response relationship. The protective effect was more pronounced for women with ER+/PR+ and ER–/PR– breast tumors *(80)*.

Several factors may be responsible for the inconsistent effects of soy-related diets on cancer outcome (Table 1). These include age, reproductive history, genetic background, dose and timing of exposure, and dietary patterns. For example, because of their binding affinity for the ER, isoflavones may function as agonists or antagonists depending on the concentration. The differential binding of isoflavones to the ER may interfere with or activate the genomic actions of the ER. Moreover, the agonist/competing effects of isoflavones for the ER may be modified by interactions with polymorphisms for the ER *(81)*. For example, polymorphisms in the ERβ have been shown to modify the association between isoflavone intake and breast cancer risk *(82)*. Given the role of cross talk between ER and isoflavones in breast cancer risk, genome-wide studies are required to examine the effects of isoflavones and exposure levels on promoter sequences that are targeted by the ER. DNA microarray technologies have been used to monitor genome-wide effects by isoflavones. For example, studies measured patterns of gene expression in the developing uterus and ovaries of Sprague-Dawley rats on GD 20, exposed to graded dosages of 17alpha-ethynyl estradiol (EE), genistein, or bisphenol A (BPA) from GD 11 to GD 20. Analysis of the transcript profile of these tissues was used to determine the estrogenicity of different compounds *(83)*. Studies that examined the impact of isoflavones on the epigenetic process reported that elevation of histone acetylation and coactivator activity of ER may reduce the risk of estrogen-related diseases *(84)*,

Nutrigenetics takes into account how the cellular response to specific nutrients is influenced by interindividual genetic variations including single nucleotide polymorphisms (SNPs). The cell response to isoflavones may also be influenced by the presence of mutations in specific tumor suppressor genes. For example, the growth of *BRCA1* mutant cells (SUM1315MO2) carrying the 185delAG *BRCA1* mutation was strongly inhibited by genistein, whereas this isoflavone only had a weak effect in cells expressing wild-type BRCA1 protein. The responsiveness of BRCA1 mutant cells was linked to higher expression of ERβ gene. These data suggested that genistein may be an efficient inhibitor of cancer development in *BRCA1* mutant breast cancer cells *(85)*. With respect to BRCA-1 status in ovarian cancers, genistein induced apoptosis in both wild-type and mutated BRCA-1 ovarian cancer (BG-1) cells. However, this effect was mediated by different pathways since genistein inhibited ERα in BRCA-1 deficient cells, whereas it activated ERβ when BRCA-1 was present *(86)*.

Table 1
Isoflavones and Nutrigenomic Approaches in Female Cancers

Experimental model	Dietary bioactive compounds	References
Transcriptomics		
Human MCF-7 breast cancer cells	Natural estrogens (17beta-estradiol, estriol, estrone, genistein)	Terasaka et al. *(91)*
Human MCF-7 breast cancer cells	Isoflavones (genistein, daidzein, glycitein, biochanin A and ipriflavone), flavones (chrysin, luteolin, and apigenin), flavonols (kaempferol and quercetin), and a coumestan, a flavanone and a chalcone (coumestrol, naringenin, and phloretin, respectively)	Ise et al. *(92)*
Uterus and ovaries of Sprague-Dawley rats	Genistein	Naciff et al. *(83)*
Human Ishikawa endometrial cancer cells	Genistein	Konstantakopoulos et al. *(93)*
Human MCF-7 breast cancer cells	Genistein	Shioda et al. *(94)*
Human MCF-7, T47D breast cancer cells	Genistein	Buterin et al. *(95)*
FVB female mice	Isoflavones, of which 66.5% was genistein, 32.3% daidzein, and 1.2% glycitein	Thomsen et al. *(96)*
Epigenetics		
ER-mediated core histone acetylation, Chromatin preparations from *Drosophila*	Equol, genistein, daidzein	Hong et al. *(84)*
Proteomics		
Rat mammary gland	Genistein	Rowell et al. *(97)*
Metabolomics		
Premenopausal women	Soy or miso consumption	Solanky et al. *(98)*
Postmenopausal women	Soy milk	Pino et al. *(99)*
Postmenopausal female monkeys	Soy protein isolate	Wood et al. *(100)*
Premenopausal women	Soy (40 mg genistein/day)	Kumar et al. *(101)*

Isoflavones may also alter gene expression by inducing chromatin modifications at target promoters. For example, genistein was shown to suppress DNA-cytosine methyltransferase-1 (DNMT) and reverse DNA hypermethylation in mammary cancer cells in vitro *(87)*. Therefore, epigenetic changes such as alterations in DNA methylation could account for the preventive effects of genestein and other soy isoflavones. A recent study reported that intake of soy isoflavones had an antiestrogenic effect and altered mammary promoter hypermethylation in healthy premenopausal women *(88)*. Low circulating levels of genistein were associated with decreased methylation of RARβ2 and CCND2, whereas promoter methylation of these genes increased with high circulating levels. Hypermethylation of both RARβ and CCND2 is correlated with breast carcinogenesis. The fact that the circulating levels of genestein may influence the direction and methylation levels represents important evidence of potential for epigenetic regulation by isoflavones in breast tissue.

The effects of isoflavones in mammary tissue have been related to either stimulation or repression of a number of processes. Pathways and processes that are stimulated by isoflavones include cell cycle arrest, apoptosis, cyclin-dependent inhibitors (p21 and p27), BRCA-1 and BRCA-2, PPARγ, MAPK signaling (p38 phosphorylation and JNK), and IGF-1 plasma levels. Conversely, isoflavones have been reported to downregulate cdc2 activity, Akt1, NFκB, AP-1, phosphorylation of ERK1/2, levels of VEGF and cell migration, xenobiotic metabolism, and enzymatic activities of estrogen sulfotransferases (SULT) *(73)*. The SULT enzymes regulate in endocrine tissue such as breast and endometrium the sulfonation of various substrates including estrogens and phenols *(89)*.

The chemical reactivity of isoflavones compared to that of estrogens may influence their preventative role in breast cancer. For example, genistein is metabolized to quinones with a short half-life, and it is subsequently hydrated to generate a catechol genistein which has estrogen-like properties, but low reactivity with DNA. Conversely, catechol estrogen quinones have a longer half-life and can damage DNA via depurination reactions *(90)*. Therefore, competition for quinone formation by genistein may reduce the formation of genotoxic quinone metabolites.

2. CONCLUSIONS

From the data discussed in this chapter it is apparent that clarifications of the mechanisms of action of bioactive compounds are complex (Table 2) and require simultaneous examination of changes in gene expression (transcriptomics), study of molecular relationships between nutrients and genes (nutrigenetics), how these interactions influence changes in the profile of proteins (proteomics), study of multiple signaling and metabolic pathways (metabolomics), and how associations of different compounds exert synergistic, additive, or opposing effects. DNA methylation and histone modifications are epigenetic events that mediate heritable changes in gene expression and chromatin organization in the absence of changes in the DNA sequence. Examples of large-scale analyses include microarray studies of estrogen-responsive genes in response to natural and industrial chemicals *(91)* and phytoestrogens *(92)*. Based on these studies, it emerges that nutritional strategies targeted to the prevention of endocrine tumors should consider multiple signaling pathways.

Table 2
Factors Affecting Nutrigenomics Research

Approach	Definition and factors
Transcriptomics	*Identification of transcription factors that respond to nutrients and gene targets* RNA amplification procedure (quantity, quality, replicates, real-time PCR, high-density analysis) Quantity of starting tissue/cell material Fold change in expression Intraindividual and interindividual variations in healthy and diseased subjects Heterogeneity of cell populations and single-cell gene expression profiling Combination of gene variants (SNPs) Data processing and interpretation
Epigenetics	*Characterization of chromatin modifications that influence gene expression and impact of nutrients* Histone modifications DNA methylation Nucleosome organization Order, interdependence and intradependence, and reversibility of histone modifications Cross talk and mutual dependency between histone modifications, DNA methylation, and methyl-binding proteins
Proteomics	*Linking gene expression studies with protein functions* Protein structure Tissue and cellular localization Plasma levels Expression level Posttranslational modifications Protein–protein interactions Cellular function Bioinformatics and data processing
Metabolomics	*Linking exposure to biological effects induced by metabolites* Interindividual differences in metabolism and disposition Measurement of metabolites in specimens (urine, plasma) Recovery methods from tissue/plasma Metabolic origin and overlapping pathways Handling of metabolic data

REFERENCES

1. Sonnenschein, C., and Soto, A.M. (2008 Oct) Theories of carcinogenesis: An emerging perspective. *Semin Cancer Biol* **18**(5), 372–77.
2. Philip, M., Rowley, D.A., and Schreiber, H. (2004 Dec) Inflammation as a tumor promoter in cancer induction. *Semin Cancer Biol* **14**(6), 433–39.
3. Iannaccone, P.M., Weinberg, W.C., and Deamant, F.D. (1987 Jun 15) On the clonal origin of tumors: A review of experimental models. *Int J Cancer* **39**(6), 778–84.
4. Laconi, E., Doratiotto, S., and Vineis, P. (2008 Oct) The microenvironments of multistage carcinogenesis. *Semin Cancer Biol* **18**(5), 322–29.
5. Lamartiniere, C.A., Cotroneo, M.S., Fritz, W.A., Wang, J., Mentor-Marcel, R., and Elgavish, A. (2002 Mar) Genistein chemoprevention: Timing and mechanisms of action in murine mammary and prostate. *J Nutr* **132**(3), 552S–558S.
6. Boyapati, S.M., Shu, X.O., Ruan, Z.X., Dai, Q., Cai, Q., Gao, Y.T., and Zheng, W. (2005 Jul) Soyfood intake and breast cancer survival: A followup of the Shanghai Breast Cancer Study. *Breast Cancer Res Treat* **92**(1), 11–17.
7. Martin, K.R. (2007 Aug) Using nutrigenomics to evaluate apoptosis as a preemptive target in cancer prevention. *Curr Cancer Drug Targets* **7**(5), 438–46.
8. Carbone, M., and Pass, H.I. (2004 Dec) Multistep and multifactorial carcinogenesis: When does a contributing factor become a carcinogen? *Semin Cancer Biol* **14**(6), 399–405.
9. Mei, N., Guo, L., Zhang, L., Shi, L., Sun, Y.A., Fung, C., Moland, C.L., Dial, S.L., Fuscoe, J.C., and Chen, T. (2006 Sep 26) Analysis of gene expression changes in relation to toxicity and tumorigenesis in the livers of Big Blue transgenic rats fed comfrey (Symphytum officinale). *BMC Bioinformatics* **7**(Suppl 2), S16.
10. Hadi, S.M., Bhat, S.H., Azmi, A.S., Hanif, S., Shamim, U., and Ullah, M.F. (2007 Oct) Oxidative breakage of cellular DNA by plant polyphenols: A putative mechanism for anticancer properties. *Semin Cancer Biol* **17**(5), 370–76.
11. Yang, K., Kurihara, N., Fan, K., Newmark, H., Rigas, B., Bancroft, L., Corner, G., Livote, E., Lesser, M., Edelmann, W., Velcich, A., Lipkin, M., and Augenlicht, L. (2008 Oct 1) Dietary induction of colonic tumors in a mouse model of sporadic colon cancer. *Cancer Res* **68**(19), 7803–10.
12. Yoshida, M., Katashima, S., Ando, J., Tanaka, T., Uematsu, F., Nakae, D., and Maekawa, A. (2004 Nov) Dietary indole-3-carbinol promotes endometrial adenocarcinoma development in rats initiated with N-ethyl-N'-nitro-N-nitrosoguanidine, with induction of cytochrome P450s in the liver and consequent modulation of estrogen metabolism. *Carcinogenesis* **25**(11), 2257–64.
13. D'Ambrosio, S.M. (2007 Oct) Phytonutrients: A more natural approach toward cancer prevention. *Semin Cancer Biol* **17**(5), 345–46.
14. Müller, M., and Kersten, S. (2003 Apr) Nutrigenomics: Goals and strategies. *Nat Rev Genet* **4**(4), 315–22.
15. Marugame, T., Tsuji, E., Kiyohara, C., Eguchi, H., Oda, T., Shinchi, K., and Kono, S. (2003 Feb) Relation of plasma folate and methylenetetrahydrofolate reductase C677T polymorphism to colorectal adenomas. *Int J Epidemiol* **32**(1), 64–66.
16. Wei, M., Xu, J., Dignam, J., Nanda, R., Sveen, L., Fackenthal, J., Grushko, T.A., and Olopade, O.I. (2008 Sep) Estrogen receptor alpha, BRCA1, and FANCF promoter methylation occur in distinct subsets of sporadic breast cancers. *Breast Cancer Res Treat* **111**(1), 113–20.
17. Hsing, A.W., Tsao, L., and Devesa, S.S. (2000 Jan 1) International trends and patterns of prostate cancer incidence and mortality. *Int J Cancer* **85**(1), 60–67.
18. Shimizu, H., Ross, R.K., Bernstein, L., Yatani, R., Henderson, B.E., and Mack, T.M. (1991 Jun) Cancers of the prostate and breast among Japanese and white immigrants in Los Angeles County. *Br J Cancer* **63**(6), 963–66.
19. Cook, L.S., Goldoft, M., Schwartz, S.M., and Weiss, N.S. (1999 Jan) Incidence of adenocarcinoma of the prostate in Asian immigrants to the United States and their descendants. *J Urol* **161**(1), 152–55.
20. Imai, K., Suga, K., and Nakachi, K. (1997 Nov–Dec) Cancer-preventive effects of drinking green tea among a Japanese population. *Prev Med* **26**(6), 769–75.

21. AICR/WCRF. (2007) Second Expert Report on Food, Nutrition, Physical Activity, and the Prevention of Cancer. Washington, DC: AICR/WCRF.

22. Davis, C.D., and Milner, J. (2004 Jul 13) Frontiers in nutrigenomics, proteomics, metabolomics and cancer prevention. *Mutat Res* **551**(1–2), 51–64, Review. Erratum in: *Mutat Res* (2005 Mar) 1;570(2), 305.

23. Kaput, J. (2005 Dec) Decoding the pyramid: A systems-biological approach to nutrigenomics. *Ann N Y Acad Sci* **1055**, 64–79.

24. Ross, S.A. (2007 Dec) Nutritional genomic approaches to cancer prevention research. *Exp Oncol* **29**(4), 250–56.

25. Gaj, S., Eijssen, L., Mensink, R.P., and Evelo, C.T. (2008 Dec) Validating nutrient-related gene expression changes from microarrays using RT(2) PCR-arrays. *Genes Nutr* **3**(3–4), 153–57.

26. Gaj, S., van Erk, A., van Haaften, R.I., and Evelo, C.T. (2007 Sep) Linking microarray reporters with protein functions. *BMC Bioinformatics* **26**(8), 360.

27. Afman, L., and Müller, M. (2006 Apr) Nutrigenomics: From molecular nutrition to prevention of disease. *J Am Diet Assoc* **106**(4), 569–76.

28. Magee, P.J., and Rowland, I.R. (2004 Apr) Phyto-oestrogens, their mechanism of action: Current evidence for a role in breast and prostate cancer. *Br J Nutr* **91**(4), 513–31.

29. Mangelsdorf, D.J., Thummel, C., Beato, M., Herrlich, P., Schutz, G., Umesono, K., Blumberg, B., Kastner, P., Mark, M., Chambon, P., and Evans, R.M. (1995) The nuclear receptor superfamily: The second decade. *Cell* **83**(6), 835–39.

30. Wang, K., Chen, S., Xie, W., and Wan, Y.J. (2008 Jun 1) Retinoids induce cytochrome P450 3A4 through RXR/VDR-mediated pathway. *Biochem Pharmacol* **75**(11), 2204–13.

31. Khan, S., Barhoumi, R., Burghardt, R., Liu, S., Kim, K., and Safe, S. (2006 Sep) Molecular mechanism of inhibitory aryl hydrocarbon receptor-estrogen receptor/Sp1 cross talk in breast cancer cells. *Mol Endocrinol* **20**(9), 2199–214.

32. Francis, G.A., Fayard, E., Picard, F., and Auwerx, J. (2003) Nuclear receptors and the control of metabolism. *Annu Rev Physiol* **65**, 261–311.

33. Bünger, M., Hooiveld, G.J., Kersten, S., and Müller, M. (2007 Aug) Exploration of PPAR functions by microarray technology–a paradigm for nutrigenomics. *Biochim Biophys Acta* **1771**(8), 1046–64, E-pub 2007 Jun 2.

34. Kuiper, G.G., Carlsson, B., Grandien, K., Enmark, E., Häggblad, J., Nilsson, S., and Gustafsson, J.A. (1997 Mar) Comparison of the ligand binding specificity and transcript tissue distribution of estrogen receptors alpha and beta. *Endocrinology* **138**(3), 863–70.

35. Young, M.R., Yang, H.S., and Colburn, N.H. (2003 Jan) Promising molecular targets for cancer prevention: AP-1, NF-kappa B and Pdcd4. *Trends Mol Med* **9**(1), 36–41.

36. Maeda, S., and Karin, M. (2003 Feb) Oncogene at last–c-Jun promotes liver cancer in mice. *Cancer Cell* **3**(2), 102–4.

37. Eferl, R., and Wagner, E.F. (2003 Nov) AP-1: A double-edged sword in tumorigenesis. *Nat Rev Cancer* **3**(11), 859–68.

38. Glinghammar, B., Inoue, H., and Rafter, J.J. (2002 May) Deoxycholic acid causes DNA damage in colonic cells with subsequent induction of caspases, COX-2 promoter activity and the transcription factors NF-kB and AP-1. *Carcinogenesis* **23**(5), 839–45.

39. Mackenzie, G.G., Adamo, A.M., Decker, N.P., and Oteiza, P.I. (2008 Apr 1) Dimeric procyanidin B2 inhibits constitutively active NF-kappaB in Hodgkin's lymphoma cells independently of the presence of IkappaB mutations. *Biochem Pharmacol* **75**(7), 1461–71.

40. Pan, M.-H., and Ho, C.-T. (2008 Nov) Chemopreventive effects of natural dietary compounds on cancer development. *Chem Soc Rev* **37**(11), 2558–74, E-pub 2008 Sep 24.

41. Scheckel, K.A., Degner, S.C., and Romagnolo, D.F. (2008 Nov) Rosmarinic acid antagonizes activator protein-1-dependent activation of cyclooxygenase-2 expression in human cancer and nonmalignant cell lines. *J Nutr* **138**(11), 2098–105.

42. Jang, S., Kelley, K.W., and Johnson, R.W. (2008 May 27) Luteolin reduces IL-6 production in microglia by inhibiting JNK phosphorylation and activation of AP-1. *Proc Natl Acad Sci USA* **105**(21), 7534–39.

43. Degner, S.C., Kemp, M.Q., Bowden, G.T., and Romagnolo, D.F. (2006 Feb) Conjugated linoleic acid attenuates cyclooxygenase-2 transcriptional activity via an anti-AP-1 mechanism in MCF-7 breast cancer cells. *J Nutr* **136**(2), 421–27.

44. Zhao, Y., and Chen, L.H. (2005 Feb) Eicosapentaenoic acid prevents lipopolysaccharide-stimulated DNA binding of activator protein-1 and c-Jun N-terminal kinase activity. *J Nutr Biochem* **16**(2), 78–84.

45. Habermann, N., Lund, E.K., Pool-Zobel, B.L., and Glei, M. (2009 Mar) Modulation of gene expression in eicosapentaenoic acid and docosahexaenoic acid treated human colon adenoma cells. *Genes Nutr* **4**(1), 73–76.

46. Olivo-Marston, S.E., Zhu, Y., Lee, R.Y., Cabanes, A., Khan, G., Zwart, A., Wang, Y., Clarke, R., and Hilakivi-Clarke, L. (2008 Dec) Gene signaling pathways mediating the opposite effects of prepubertal low-fat and high-fat n-3 polyunsaturated fatty acid diets on mammary cancer risk. *Cancer Prev Res (Phila PA)* **1**(7), 532–45.

47. Medvedovic, M., Gear, R., Freudenberg, J.M., Schneider, J., Bornschein, R., Yan, M., Mistry, M.J., Hendrix, H., Karyala, S., Halbleib, D., Heffelfinger, S., Clegg, D.J., and Anderson, M.W. (2009 Apr 7) Influence of fatty acid diets on gene expression in rat mammary epithelial cells. *Physiol Genomics.* [Epub ahead of print] PubMed PMID: 19351911.

48. Narita, S., Tsuchiya, N., Saito, M., Inoue, T., Kumazawa, T., Yuasa, T., Nakamura, A., and Habuchi, T. (2008 Feb 15) Candidate genes involved in enhanced growth of human prostate cancer under high fat feeding identified by microarray analysis. *Prostate* **68**(3), 321–35.

49. Vock, C., Gleissner, M., Klapper, M., and Döring, F. (2007 Sep) Identification of palmitate-regulated genes in HepG2 cells by applying microarray analysis. *Biochim Biophys Acta* **1770**(9), 1283–88, E-pub 2007 Jul 10.

50. Lin, D.W., Neuhouser, M.L., Schenk, J.M., Coleman, I.M., Hawley, S., Gifford, D., Hung, H., Knudsen, B.S., Nelson, P.S., and Kristal, A.R. (2007 Oct) Low-fat, low-glycemic load diet and gene expression in human prostate epithelium: A feasibility study of using cDNA microarrays to assess the response to dietary intervention in target tissues. *Cancer Epidemiol Biomarkers Prev* **16**(10), 2150–54.

51. Kininis, M., Chen, B.S., Diehl, A.G., Isaacs, G.D., Zhang, T., Siepel, A.C., Clark, A.G., and Kraus, W.L. (2007 Jul) Genomic analyses of transcription factor binding, histone acetylation, and gene expression reveal mechanistically distinct classes of estrogen-regulated promoters. *Mol Cell Biol* **27**(14), 5090–104.

52. Chalabi, N., Satih, S., Delort, L., Bignon, Y.J., and Bernard-Gallon, D.J. (2007 Feb) Expression profiling by whole-genome microarray hybridization reveals differential gene expression in breast cancer cell lines after lycopene exposure. *Biochim Biophys Acta* **1769**(2), 124–30.

53. Le Corre, L., Chalabi, N., Delort, L., Bignon, Y.J., and Bernard-Gallon, D.J. (2006) Differential expression of genes induced by resveratrol in human breast cancer cell lines. *Nutr Cancer* **56**(2), 193–203.

54. Kishimoto, M., Fujiki, R., Takezawa, S., Sasaki, Y., Nakamura, T., Yamaoka, K., Kitagawa, H., and Kato, S. (2006 Apr) Nuclear receptor mediated gene regulation through chromatin remodeling and histone modifications. *Endocr J* **53**(2), 157–72.

55. Schreiber, S.L., and Bernstein, B.E. (2002 Dec 13) Signaling network model of chromatin. *Cell* **111**(6), 771–78.

56. Rea, S., Eisenhaber, F., O'Carroll, D., Strahl, B.D., Sun, Z.W., Schmid, M., Opravil, S., Mechtler, K., Ponting, C.P., Allis, C.D., and Jenuwein, T. (2000 Aug 10) Regulation of chromatin structure by site-specific histone H3 methyltransferases. *Nature* **406**(6796), 593–99.

57. Shilatifard, A. (2006) Chromatin modifications by methylation and ubiquitination: Implications in the regulation of gene expression. *Annu Rev Biochem* **75**, 243–69.

58. Jenuwein, T., and Allis, C.D. (2001 Aug 10) Translating the histone code. *Science* **293**(5532), 1074–80.

59. Herman, J.G., and Baylin, S.B. (2003 Nov 20) Gene silencing in cancer in association with promoter hypermethylation. *N Engl J Med* **349**(21), 2042–54.

60. Vaissière, T., Sawan, C., and Herceg, Z. (2008 Jul–Aug) Epigenetic interplay between histone modifications and DNA methylation in gene silencing. *Mutat Res* **659**(1–2), 40–48.

61. Sakamoto, K., Iwasaki, K., Sugiyama, H., and Tsuji, Y. (2009 Mar) Role of the tumor suppressor PTEN in antioxidant responsive element-mediated transcription and associated histone modifications. *Mol Biol Cell* **20**(6), 1606–17.

62. Van Den Broeck, A., Brambilla, E., Moro-Sibilot, D., Lantuejoul, S., Brambilla, C., Eymin, B., Khochbin, S., and Gazzeri, S. (2008 Nov 15) Loss of histone H4K20 trimethylation occurs in pre-neoplasia and influences prognosis of non-small cell lung cancer. *Clin Cancer Res* **14**(22), 7237–45.

63. Egger, G., Liang, G., Aparicio, A., and Jones, P.A. (2004 May 27) Epigenetics in human disease and prospects for epigenetic therapy. *Nature* **429**(6990), 457–63.

64. Kawakami, K., Ruszkiewicz, A., Bennett, G., Moore, J., Grieu, F., Watanabe, G., and Iacopetta, B. (2006 Feb 27) DNA hypermethylation in the normal colonic mucosa of patients with colorectal cancer. *Br J Cancer* **94**(4), 593–98.

65. Lyko, F., and Brown, R. (2005 Oct 19) DNA methyltransferase inhibitors and the development of epigenetic cancer therapies. *J Natl Cancer Inst* **97**(20), 1498–506.

66. Fang, M.Z., Wang, Y., Ai, N., Hou, Z., Sun, Y., Lu, H., Welsh, W., and Yang, C.S. (2003 Nov 15) Tea polyphenol(–)-epigallocatechin-3-gallate inhibits DNA methyltransferase and reactivates methylation-silenced genes in cancer cell lines. *Cancer Res* **63**(22), 7563–70.

67. Fang, M.Z., Chen, D., Sun, Y., Jin, Z., Christman, J.K., and Yang, C.S. (2005 Oct 1) Reversal of hypermethylation and reactivation of p16INK4a, RARbeta, and MGMT genes by genistein and other isoflavones from soy. *Clin Cancer Res* **11**(19 Pt 1), 7033–41.

68. Myzak, M.C., and Dashwood, R.H. (2006 Apr) Histone deacetylases as targets for dietary cancer preventive agents: Lessons learned with butyrate, diallyl disulfide, and sulforaphane. *Curr Drug Targets* **7**(4), 443–52.

69. Nian, H., Delage, B., Ho, E., and Dashwood, R.H. (2009 Apr) Modulation of histone deacetylase activity by dietary isothiocyanates and allyl sulfides: Studies with sulforaphane and garlic organosulfur compounds. *Environ Mol Mutagen* **50**(3), 213–21.

70. Eden, A., Gaudet, F., Waghmare, A., and Jaenisch, R. (2003 Apr 18) Chromosomal instability and tumors promoted by DNA hypomethylation. *Science* **300**(5618), 455.

71. Davis, C.D., and Milner, J.A. (2007 Sep) Biomarkers for diet and cancer prevention research: Potentials and challenges. *Acta Pharmacol Sin* **28**(9), 1262–73.

72. Lampe, J.W., and Chang, J.L. (2007 Oct) Interindividual differences in phytochemical metabolism and disposition. *Semin Cancer Biol* **17**(5), 347–53.

73. Steiner, C., Arnould, S., Scalbert, A., and Manach, C. (2008 May) Isoflavones and the prevention of breast and prostate cancer: New perspectives opened by nutrigenomics. *Br J Nutr* **99E**(Suppl 1), ES78–ES108.

74. Trock, B.J., Hilakivi-Clarke, L., and Clarke, R. (2006 Apr 5) Meta-analysis of soy intake and breast cancer risk. *J Natl Cancer Inst* **98**(7), 459–71.

75. Messina, M., McCaskill-Stevens, W., and Lampe, J.W. (2006 Sep 20) Addressing the soy and breast cancer relationship: Review, commentary, and workshop proceedings. *J Natl Cancer Inst* **98**(18), 1275–84.

76. Maskarinec, G., Williams, A.E., and Carlin, L. (2003 Apr) Mammographic densities in a one-year isoflavone intervention. *Eur J Cancer Prev* **12**(2), 165–69.

77. Maskarinec, G., Takata, Y., Franke, A.A., Williams, A.E., and Murphy, S.P.A. (2004 Nov) 2-year soy intervention in premenopausal women does not change mammographic densities. *J Nutr* **134**(11), 3089–94.

78. Atkinson, C., Warren, R.M., Sala, E., Dowsett, M., Dunning, A.M., Healey, C.S., Runswick, S., Day, N.E., and Bingham, S.A. (2004) Red-clover-derived isoflavones and mammographic breast density: A double-blind, randomized, placebo-controlled trial. *Breast Cancer Res* **6**(3), R170-R79, E-pub 2004 Feb 24.

79. Wu, A.H., Yu, M.C., Tseng, C.C., and Pike, M.C. (2008 Jan 15) Epidemiology of soy exposures and breast cancer risk. *Br J Cancer* **98**(1), 9–14.

80. Zhang, M., Yang, H., and Holman, C.D. (2009 Feb 28) Dietary intake of isoflavones and breast cancer risk by estrogen and progesterone receptor status. *Breast Cancer Res Treat*. [E-pub ahead of print] PubMed PMID: 19252980.

81. Low, Y.L., Taylor, J.I., Grace, P.B., Dowsett, M., Scollen, S., Dunning, A.M., Mulligan, A.A., Welch, A.A., Luben, R.N., Khaw, K.T., Day, N.E., Wareham, N.J., and Bingham, S.A. (2005 Jan) Phytoestrogen exposure correlation with plasma estradiol in postmenopausal women in European Prospective Investigation of Cancer and Nutrition-Norfolk may involve diet-gene interactions. *Cancer Epidemiol Biomarkers Prev* **14**(1), 213–20.

82. Iwasaki, M., Hamada, G.S., Nishimoto, I.N., Netto, M.M., Motola, J., Jr, Laginha, F.M., Kasuga, Y., Yokoyama, S., Onuma, H., Nishimura, H., Kusama, R., Kobayashi, M., Ishihara, J., Yamamoto, S., Hanaoka, T., and Tsugane, S. (2009 May) Isoflavone, polymorphisms in estrogen receptor genes and breast cancer risk in case-control studies in Japanese, Japanese Brazilians and non-Japanese Brazilians. *Cancer Sci* **100**(5), 927–33.

83. Naciff, J.M., Jump, M.L., Torontali, S.M., Carr, G.J., Tiesman, J.P., Overmann, G.J., and Daston, G.P. (2002 Jul) Gene expression profile induced by 17alpha-ethynyl estradiol, bisphenol A, and genistein in the developing female reproductive system of the rat. *Toxicol Sci* **68**(1), 184–99.

84. Hong, T., Nakagawa, T., Pan, W., Kim, M.Y., Kraus, W.L., Ikehara, T., Yasui, K., Aihara, H., Takebe, M., Muramatsu, M., and Ito, T. (2004 Apr 23) Isoflavones stimulate estrogen receptor-mediated core histone acetylation. *Biochem Biophys Res Commun* **317**(1), 259–64.

85. Privat, M., Aubel, C., Arnould, S., Communal, Y., Ferrara, M., and Bignon, Y.J. (2009 Feb 13) Breast cancer cell response to genistein is conditioned by BRCA1 mutations. *Biochem Biophys Res Commun* **379**(3), 785–89, E-pub 2009 Jan 4.

86. Thasni, K.A., Rojini, G., Rakesh, S.N., Ratheeshkumar, T., Babu, M.S., Srinivas, G., Banerji, A., and Srinivas, P. (2008 Jul 7) Genistein induces apoptosis in ovarian cancer cells via different molecular pathways depending on Breast Cancer Susceptibility gene-1 (BRCA1) status. *Eur J Pharmacol* **588**(2–3), 158–64.

87. Fang, M., Chen, D., and Yang, C.S. (2007 Jan) Dietary polyphenols may affect DNA methylation. *J Nutr* **137**(1 Suppl), 223S–228S.

88. Qin, W., Zhu, W., Shi, H., Hewett, J.E., Ruhlen, R.L., MacDonald, R.S., Rottinghaus, G.E., Chen, Y.C., and Sauter, E.R. (2009) Soy isoflavones have an antiestrogenic effect and alter mammary promoter hypermethylation in healthy premenopausal women. *Nutr Cancer* **61**(2), 238–44.

89. Pasqualini, J.R. (2009 Feb) Estrogen sulfotransferases in breast and endometrial cancers. *Ann N Y Acad Sci* **1155**, 88–98.

90. Zhang, Q., Tu, T., d'Avignon, D.A., and Gross, M.L. (2009 Jan 28) Balance of beneficial and deleterious health effects of quinones: A case study of the chemical properties of genistein and estrone quinones. *J Am Chem Soc* **131**(3), 1067–76.

91. Terasaka, S., Aita, Y., Inoue, A., Hayashi, S., Nishigaki, M., Aoyagi, K., Sasaki, H., Wada-Kiyama, Y., Sakuma, Y., Akaba, S., Tanaka, J., Sone, H., Yonemoto, J., Tanji, M., and Kiyama, R. (2004 May) Using a customized DNA microarray for expression profiling of the estrogen-responsive genes to evaluate estrogen activity among natural estrogens and industrial chemicals. *Environ Health Perspect* **112**(7), 773–81.

92. Ise, R., Han, D., Takahashi, Y., Terasaka, S., Inoue, A., Tanji, M., and Kiyama, R. (2005 Mar 14) Expression profiling of the estrogen responsive genes in response to phytoestrogens using a customized DNA microarray. *FEBS Lett* **579**(7), 1732–40.

93. Konstantakopoulos, N., Montgomery, K.G., Chamberlain, N., Quinn, M.A., Baker, M.S., Rice, G.E., Georgiou, H.M., and Campbell, I.G. (2006 Oct) Changes in gene expressions elicited by physiological concentrations of genistein on human endometrial cancer cells. *Mol Carcinog* **45**(10), 752–63.

94. Shioda, T., Chesnes, J., Coser, K.R., Zou, L., Hur, J., Dean, K.L., Sonnenschein, C., Soto, A.M., and Isselbacher, K.J. (2006 Aug 8) Importance of dosage standardization for interpreting transcriptomal signature profiles: Evidence from studies of xenoestrogens. *Proc Natl Acad Sci USA* **103**(32), 12033–38, E-pub 2006 Aug 1.

95. Buterin, T., Koch, C., and Naegeli, H. (2006 Aug) Convergent transcriptional profiles induced by endogenous estrogen and distinct xenoestrogens in breast cancer cells. *Carcinogenesis* **27**(8), 1567–78, E-pub 2006 Feb 10.

96. Thomsen, A.R., Almstrup, K., Nielsen, J.E., Sørensen, I.K., Petersen, O.W., Leffers, H., and Breinholt, V.M. (2006 Oct) Estrogenic effect of soy isoflavones on mammary gland morphogenesis and gene expression profile. *Toxicol Sci* **93**(2), 357–68.

97. Rowell, C., Carpenter, D.M., and Lamartiniere, C.A. (2005 Dec) Chemoprevention of breast cancer, proteomic discovery of genistein action in the rat mammary gland. *J Nutr* **135**(12 Suppl), 2953S–2959S.

98. Solanky, K.S., Bailey, N.J., Beckwith-Hall, B.M., Bingham, S., Davis, A., Holmes, E., Nicholson, J.K., and Cassidy, A. (2005 Apr) Biofluid 1H NMR-based metabonomic techniques in nutrition research – metabolic effects of dietary isoflavones in humans. *J Nutr Biochem* **16**(4), 236–44.

99. Pino, A.M., Valladares, L.E., Palma, M.A., Mancilla, A.M., Yáñez, M., and Albala, C. (2000 Aug) Dietary isoflavones affect sex hormone-binding globulin levels in postmenopausal women. *J Clin Endocrinol Metab* **85**(8), 2797–800.

100. Wood, C.E., Register, T.C., and Cline, J.M. (2007 Apr) Soy isoflavonoid effects on endogenous estrogen metabolism in postmenopausal female monkeys. *Carcinogenesis* **28**(4), 801–8.

101. Kumar, N.B., Cantor, A., Allen, K., Riccardi, D., and Cox, C.E. (2002 Feb 15) The specific role of isoflavones on estrogen metabolism in premenopausal women. *Cancer* **94**(4), 1166–74.

3 Cellular Cancer Processes and Their Molecular Targets for Nutritional Preemption of Cancer

Cindy D. Davis

Key Points

1. Malignant cells are characterized by numerous alterations in multiple signaling pathways that promote proliferation, inhibit apoptosis, promote angiogenesis in the case of solid tumors and enable cancer cells to invade and migrate through tissues.
2. Bioactive dietary components have been shown to modify all of the major signaling pathways which are deregulated in cancer. Estimates suggest that 30–70% of all cancer cases might be preventable by diet, depending on the dietary components and the specific type of cancer.
3. A better understanding of the bioactive components present in food, the mechanism(s) of action of these dietary components toward cancer prevention, the critical intake of dietary components, duration and when they should be provided to optimize the desired physiological response is needed. The response can be complex since the effects of dietary components can depend on the cell type examined and these components typically influence more than one cancer process.
4. One of the greatest challenges is the identification of which process(es), either singly or in combination, is/are most important in bringing about a phenotypic change. Unfortunately, most of the mechanistic information has been obtained in cell culture studies, often with unachievable concentrations.
5. When interpreting the results from in vitro studies, care must be taken to consider dose, cell type, culture conditions and treatment time, as each of these can affect the biological outcome.

Key Words: Cell proliferation; apoptosis; inflammation; immunity; angiogenesis

1. INTRODUCTION

Evidence continues to mount that altering dietary habits is an effective and cost-efficient approach for both reducing cancer risk and for modifying the biological behavior of tumors. The World Cancer Research Fund/American Institute of Cancer Research has estimated that cancer is 30–40% preventable by appropriate food and nutrition, regular physical activity, and avoidance of obesity *(1)*. On a global scale, they have estimated

From: *Nutrition and Health: Bioactive Compounds and Cancer*
Edited by: J.A. Milner, D.F. Romagnolo, DOI 10.1007/978-1-60761-627-6_3,
© Springer Science+Business Media, LLC 2010

that this represents over 3–4 million cases of cancer that can be prevented in these ways, every year *(1)*.

While optimizing the intake of specific foods and/or their bioactive components seems a practical, noninvasive, and cost-effective strategy for reducing the cancer burden, this is far from a simple process *(2)*. The magnitude of the problem in identifying critical dietary components is evident by the literally thousands of compounds consumed each day *(2, 3)*. Furthermore, the dearth of quantitative information about some food constituents limits the ability to unravel which are most important. While it is estimated that humans consume >5,000 individual flavonoids, only a few have been examined for their cancer protective effects *(2)*. Unfortunately many bioactive food components remain largely uncharacterized and thus can lead to confusion about the true role of diet in determining health. Interactions, both synergistic and antagonistic, between the different components within a food may explain why isolated components do not always result in similar biological outcomes to the intact food *(4)*. Likewise, interactions among foods and their constituents may contribute to the overall relationship between eating behaviors and cancer *(4)*.

In addition to identifying bioactive dietary components, it is critical to define the amount of the specific bioactive component that is needed to achieve concentrations in target tissues that will lead to a phenotypic change. The response can be complex since the effects of dietary components can depend on the cell type examined and the likelihood that food components will have multiple sites of action. Thus, one of the greatest challenges is the identification of which process(es), either singly or in combination, is/are most important in bringing about a phenotypic change. Unfortunately, most of the mechanistic information has been obtained in cell culture studies, often with unachievable concentrations. Thus, the extrapolation of these data to humans is difficult, if not impossible *(5)*. The interpretation of observations from preclinical studies involving cells or experimental models must be viewed cautiously and consider dose, cell type, culture conditions, and exposure duration, as each of these factors can affect the biological response.

All of the major signaling pathways, which are deregulated in cancer and have been examined as targets for cancer prevention, can be modified by one or more dietary components. These include, but are not limited to, carcinogen metabolism, DNA repair, cell proliferation, apoptosis, inflammation, immunity, differentiation, and angiogenesis. Since multiple responses may occur simultaneously, it is difficult to determine which is most important in dictating the overall biological response. Furthermore, the ability of several nutrients to influence the same or multiple biological processes raises issues about possible synergy, as well as antagonistic interactions, that may occur within and among foods *(4, 6)*.

2. CELL PROLIFERATION

Generally, the growth rate of preneoplastic or neoplastic cells outpaces that of normal cells because of malfunctioning or dysregulation of their cell-growth and cell-death machineries. Proteins involved in cell cycle regulation include cyclins, cyclin-dependent kinases (CDKs), CDK inhibitors (CDKIs), regulatory proteins (retinoblastoma [Rb] and p53), and the E2F transcription factor. These proteins guide the cell through distinct and sequential replicative phases from quiescence (G0 phase) through the first "gap" or gap1 (G1 phase), DNA synthesis (S phase), the second gap (G2 phase), during which the cell prepares itself for division, and finally mitosis (M phase), during which the chromosomes separate and the cell divides. Pivotal to progression through the cell cycle at G1, S, and G2 phases is the release of the transcription factor E2F from the Rb protein when Rb is phosphorylated by the CDKs. Therefore, specific molecular features for each phase of the cell cycle control Rb phosphorylation and thereby regulate cell cycle progression at the G1 and G2 checkpoints (Fig. 1).

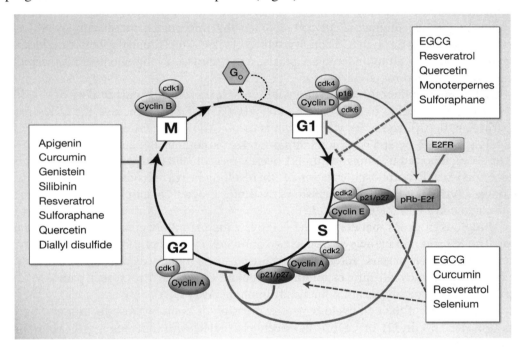

Fig. 1. The various phases of the cell cycle (G1, S, G2, and M), and the different cyclins and their cyclin-dependent kinases (CDKs) that control progression through the cell cycle. Different dietary components act at different cell cycle checkpoints and some act on multiple checkpoints or targets. *Arrows* indicate activation and *blocked lines* indicate inhibitory effects.

The progression from one phase of the cell cycle to the next is regulated by sequential activation and inactivation of many "check points" that monitor the status of the cell *(7)*. These "check points" are mechanisms whereby the cell actively halts progression through the cell cycle until it can ensure that an earlier process, such as DNA replication or mitosis, is complete. In response to DNA damage, checkpoints can also trigger the induction of necessary repair genes or cause cells to undergo programmed cell death or apoptosis. The DNA damage checkpoint arrests cells in the G1, S, or G2 phase depending upon the cell cycle status of the cell at the time damage was incurred *(8)*.

The D cyclins (cyclin D1, D2, and D3) are expressed during G1 and are required for the cell to traverse the G1 checkpoint and transverse to S phase. Cyclins function by forming complexes with specific catalytic partners among the family of CDKs. Cyclin D1 assembles with Cdk-4 and/or Cdk-6. These CDKs cause cell cycle progression by phosphorylating, and thereby activating, the Rb tumor suppressor protein, releasing E2F from negative regulators, and facilitating transcription of E2F-responsive genes including cyclins E and A *(9)*. Progression through S phase appears to be dependent on CDK2–cyclin E complexes and cyclin A which bind and activate both CDK2 and CDK1 (during S phase and in G2, respectively). Early in the S phase, before cellular DNA synthesis and replication, cyclins D and E are degraded. Cyclin A levels increase leading to the activation of CDK2 and enable the initiation of DNA and histone biosynthesis. If DNA replication is successful, cyclin A/CDK2 levels are reduced, cells enter into G2, and cyclin B/CDK1 accumulates. The cell regulates this important protein complex at many levels, particularly through p53 activity, which blocks M phase entry when DNA is damaged, causing the cell to undergo apoptosis. After mitosis, cyclin B is degraded rapidly to prevent a second round of division.

CDKIs interact directly with cyclin/CDK complexes to block their activity by directly competing for binding to Cdk4 and Cdk6 *(10)*. CDKI families include the INK4 family (p15, p16, p18, and p19), which inhibits the G1 CDKs specifically and the CIP/KIP family (p21, p27, and p57), which inhibits CDKs throughout all phases of the cell cycle. It has been reported that both cyclin D1 overexpression and p16 protein alterations produce persistent hyperphosphorylation of Rb, resulting in evasion of cell cycle arrest *(11)*. Conversely, loss of cyclin D expression constitutes a signal for exit from the mitotic cell cycle and entry into the G0 state *(12)*.

Mutations in genes that control the cell cycle are extremely common in human cancer. The Rb and p53 pathways are the two main cell cycle control pathways frequently targeted in tumorigenesis. Alterations occurring in each pathway depend on the tumor type *(13)*. Virtually all human tumors deregulate either the Rb or p53 pathway, and oftentimes both pathways are influenced simultaneously *(13)*.

Deregulation of the cell cycle by overexpression of kinases involved in growth promotion (i.e., cyclin D1 or CDKs) has been associated with carcinogenesis. Many different bioactive dietary components have been shown to inhibit different phases of the cell cycle (Fig. 1). Nevertheless, the effects on cell cycle arrest can either be direct or indirect *(14)*. EGCG has been shown to directly inhibit CDKs in various cancer cells (prostate, lung, and skin) *(7)*, or indirectly by inducing the expression of p21 and p27 genes and inhibiting the expression of cyclin D1 and Rb phosphorylation in a dose and time-dependent manner *(15, 16)*.

Some dietary components have been shown to have multiple molecular targets that can affect different phases of the cell cycle. Moreover, the specific molecular targets may depend on the specific type of cell being treated. Several studies indicate that resveratrol, a polyphenol found at high concentrations in red wine and grapes, inhibits cell cycle progression at different stages of the cell cycle in cancer cells *(17, 18)*. Treatment of LNCaP and PC-3 prostate cancer cells with resveratrol (19–150 μmol/l) reduced the expression of cyclin D1, E, and CDK4. The reduction in cyclin D1/CDK4 kinase activity resulted in G1/S phase cell cycle arrest *(17)*. However, animal and human studies consistently indicate plasma resveratrol concentrations of 1–2 μmol/l *(19)*. In contrast, in HL-60 cells, resveratrol arrested cells at the S/G2 phase via an overexpression of cyclins

A and E without modification of p21 expression *(18)*. Sulforaphane is another dietary component that can modulate different phases of the cell cycle. In DU-145 prostate cancer cells, sulforaphane induces a G0/G1 block via downregulation of the expression of cyclin D1 and CDK4 *(20)*. Sulforaphane also induces cell cycle arrest at the G2/M phase by increasing expression of cyclin B1 in human colon and breast cells *(21)*. In HT-29 cells, this G2/M phase arrest was a consequence of maintaining the cdc2 kinase in its active dephosphorylated form and was associated with phosphorylation/activation of Rb *(22)*. In contrast, sulforaphane treatment of either prostate PC-3 cells or bladder UM-UC-3 cells reduced the expression of cyclin B1 *(23, 24)*. Sulforaphane treatment of UM-UC-3 cells also resulted in S phase arrest via reduced expression of cyclin A *(24)*. These results demonstrate that the molecular targets for bioactive dietary components will depend on the specific cell of interest.

Although cell culture models are useful in obtaining mechanistic insights, experimental observations obtained with in vitro models need to be verified in vivo in animal models at physiologically relevant concentrations. The dietary flavonoid apigenin is widely distributed in many fruits and vegetables, including onions, parsley, celery, and oranges. In vitro studies with prostate cancer cells demonstrated that apigenin caused a G0/G1 cell cycle arrest by reducing total and phosphorylated Rb protein and decreased the expression of cyclin D1, D2, and E as well as their regulatory partners CDK2, CDK4, and CDK6 *(25)*. Similarly, studies in mice have shown that apigenin reduced in a dose-dependent fashion the growth of prostate cancer cell xenografts. This antiproliferative effect was associated with decreased phosphorylation of RB and reduced protein expression of cyclins D1, D2 and E, and CDK2, CDK4, and CDK6 *(26)*. These effects were observed at intakes of 20 µg/mouse/day, which is similar to the median intake of 40–50 mg/day apigenin measured in humans *(27)*.

Curcumin is another dietary component for which in vitro molecular targets have been verified in vivo. Bioavailability data suggest that in vitro studies with curcumin at concentration of 10 µmol/l or lower are physiologically relevant to humans *(19)*. The treatment of either LNCaP or PC-3 prostate cancer cells with 10 µmol/l curcumin inhibited cyclin D1, cyclin E and induced the CDK inhibitors p16, p21, and p27 *(28)*. In rats, a gavage administration of curcumin (200 or 600 mg/kg) inhibited diethylnitrosamine-induced hepatic hyperplasia by increasing p21 expression, while decreasing the expression of cyclin E and cdc2 *(29)*.

It is also important to realize that combinations of dietary compounds may be more efficacious than individual components. For example, in an in vitro model of oral cancer, EGCG blocked cells in the G0/G1 phase, while curcumin blocked cells in the G2/M phase of the cell cycle. The combination of EGCG plus curcumin showed synergistic interactions in growth inhibition *(30)*. While tea or curcumin individually decreased the number and volume of dimethylbenzanthracene-induced oral tumors in hamster, only the combination decreased the proliferation index of squamous cell carcinoma *(31)*.

Human supplementation studies have demonstrated that dietary components, such as calcium or low-fat dairy foods *(32, 33)* or dietary fiber *(34)* can inhibit colonic or rectal epithelial cell proliferation in vivo. However, these studies did not investigate the molecular targets for the dietary components. Moreover, it is difficult to critically evaluate the effect of dietary components on cell proliferation in humans because of the difficulty in obtaining human tissues noninvasively.

3. APOPTOSIS

Apoptosis, interchangeably referred to as programmed cell death, is a key pathway for regulating homeostasis. It helps to establish a natural balance between cell death and cell renewal by destroying excess, damaged, or abnormal cells. Apoptosis is one of the most potent defenses against cancer since this process eliminates potentially dele-terious, damaged cells. Factors that trigger apoptosis include DNA damage, disruption of the cell cycle, hypoxia, detachment of cells from their surrounding tissue, and loss of trophic signaling (35). It is characterized by cell shrinkage, chromatin condensa-tion, and fragmentation of the cell into compact membrane-enclosed structures, called "apoptotic-bodies" that are engulfed by macrophages and removed from the tissue in a controlled manner (36). These morphological changes are a result of characteristic molecular and biochemical events, most notably the activation of proteolytic enzymes. Proteolytic cleavage of procaspases is an important step leading to caspase activation, which in turn is amplified by the cleavage and activation of other downstream caspases in the apoptosis cascade. Caspases are a family of cysteinyl aspartate-specific proteases involved in apoptosis and subdivided into initiation (8, 9, and 10) and executioner (3, 6, and 7) caspases (37). Apoptosis occurs through two pathways, the extrinsic (death receptor pathway) or intrinsic pathway (mitochondrial pathway), which are activated, respectively, by caspase-8 and caspase-9 (Fig. 2). A critical element to both pathways is the involvement of caspase-3, which results in cleavage and inactivation of key cellu-lar proteins including the DNA repair enzyme poly(-ADP-ribose) polymerase (PARP). In addition, mitogenic and stress responsive pathways are involved in the regulation of apoptotic signaling.

The extrinsic apoptotic pathway is activated at the cell surface when a specific lig-and binds to its corresponding cell-surface death receptor. Death receptors belong to the tumor necrosis factor (TNF)-related superfamily and include TNF, TNF-related apoptosis-inducing ligand (TRAIL) receptor, and Fas (38). These proteins recruit adapter proteins including Fas-associated death domain protein (FADD) to cytoso-lic death domains, resulting in the binding of procaspase-8 and procaspase-10 to a supramolecular complex called the death-inducing signaling complex (38). Activated caspase-8 directly cleaves and activates caspase-3, which in turn cleaves other caspases (39). Caspase-8 can also activate Bcl-2 interacting domain (Bid), a proapoptotic member of the Bcl-2 family, by converting it to its truncated form (39).

The intrinsic or mitochondrial pathway of apoptosis occurs when there is permeabi-lization of the outer membrane and subsequent release of mitochondrial proteins into the cyctosol as a consequence of cellular stress. The first protein to be released following permeabilization is cytochrome c, which binds to apoptotic protease-activating factor 1 (Apaf-1). Other mitochondrial proteins include secondary mitochondrial-derived activa-tor of caspase (Smac) and DIABLO. These proteins can bind and activate the apoptotic protease-activating factor-1 (Apaf-1) promoting binding and activation of procaspase-9, followed by the subsequent activation of caspase-3, caspase-6, and caspase-7 (40).

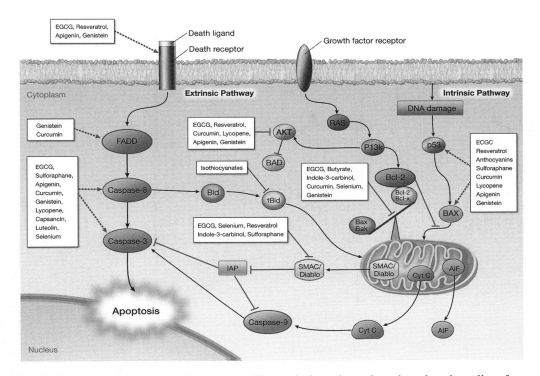

Fig. 2. The two main pathways of apoptosis. The extrinsic pathway is activated at the cell surface when a specific ligand binds to its corresponding cell-surface death receptor and activates caspase-8. The intrinsic or mitochondrial pathway occurs when there is release of mitochondrial proteins leading to the activation of caspase-9. Both pathways converge in the activation of caspase-3. Different dietary components can affect different molecular targets associated with apoptosis. Some dietary components can act on multiple molecular targets. *Arrows* indicate activation and *blocked lines* indicate inhibitory effects.

Moreover, the mitochondrial pathway is regulated by the Bcl-2 family of proteins, including the anti-apoptotic proteins Bcl-2 and Bcl-X$_L$, and the proapoptotic proteins Bad, Bid, Bax, and Bak *(41)*.

Compelling evidence of in vitro studies suggests that bioactive dietary components may trigger apoptosis though numerous intracellular molecular targets in both apoptotic pathways (Fig. 2, Tables 1 and 2). Distinct from the apoptotic events in the normal physiological process, which are mediated mainly by the interaction between death receptors and their relevant ligands *(58)*, many bioactive dietary components appear to induce apoptosis through the mitochondria-mediated pathway. Dietary compounds generally induce oxidative stress, which downregulates anti-apoptotic molecules such as Bcl-2 or Bcl-x and upregulates proapoptotic molecules such as Bax or Bak *(59)*. Furthermore, many of these dietary agents appear to exhibit some degree of specificity for neoplastic cells while sparing normal cells. For example, β-carotene induces apoptosis in various tumor cells from human prostate, colon, breast, and leukemia, whereas normal cells are largely resistant to the induction of apoptosis by β-carotene *(60)*.

Table 1

Examples of Bioactive Dietary Components that Induce the Extrinsic/Death Receptor Pathway of Apoptosis

Dietary agent	Molecular target/mechanism	Cell line(s)/concentration	References
Lupeol	Increased Fas receptor and FADD protein expression	LNCaP, CRW22Rv1 1–30 μmol/l	Saleem et al. (42)
Sulforaphane	Increased Fas ligand and cleavage of caspase-8 and caspase-3	MDA-MB-231 15–25 μmol/l	Pledgie-Tracy et al. (43)
Curcumin	Increased TRAIL-induced apoptosis via inhibition of NF-6B	LNCaP, PC-3 10–30 μmol/l	Deeb et al. (44)
Diindolylmethane	Increased TRAIL-induced apoptosis via downregulation of c-FLIP; increased caspase-8 cleavage	HepG2, HT-29 20 μmol/l	Zhang et al. (45)
EGC or EGCG	Caspase-8 activation and proteolytic cleavage of Bid	SH-SY5Y 50 μmol/l	Das et al. (46)
Genistein	Decreased expression of TNF ligand and receptor family	SPC-A-A 20 μmol/l	Zou et al. (47)

Please note that this table just contains selected examples.

Table 2

Examples of Bioactive Dietary Components that Induce the Intrinsic/Mitochondrial Pathway of Apoptosis

Dietary agent	Molecular target/mechanism	Cell line(s)/concentration	References
Curcumin	Mitochondrial swelling and collapse of the mitochondrial membrane potential	HepG2 0–40 μg/ml	Cao et al. (48)
Sulforaphane	Collapse of mitochondrial membrane potential, activation of caspase-3, downregulation of Bcl-2	U937 0–4 μmol/l	Choi et al. (49)

Table 2
(Continued)

β-Carotene	Loss of mitochondrial membrane potential, increased cytochrome c release, activation of caspase-9	HL-60, HT-29, SK-MEL-2 0–20 μmol/l	Palozza et al. (50)
Genistein	Decreased Bcl-2 and increased Bax mRNA and protein expression	SG7901 cells injected into nude mice 0.5–1.5 mg/kg diet	Zhou et al. (51)
EGCG	Decreased Bcl-2 and PARP cleavage and increased Bax protein expression	MDA-MB-231 50 μg/ml	Thangapazham et al. (52)
Apigenin	Increased cytochrome c release and activation of caspase-3 and caspase-9; decreased Bcl-2 and increased Bax protein	22Rv1 10–80 μmol/l	Shukla and Gupta (53)
Luteolin	Activation of caspase-3 and caspase-9 and PARP cleavage	SCC-4 0–100 μmol/l	Yang et al. (54)
Diallyl disulfide	Decreased mitochondrial membrane potential, cytochrome c, and Smac into the cytosol, decreased Bcl-2 and some BIRC proteins, activation of caspase-9 and caspase-3	T98G and U87MG 100 μmol/l	Das et al. (55)
Selenium	Decreased mitochondrial membrane potential, release of cytochrome c into the cytosol, activation of caspase-9 and caspase-3	LNCaP 2.5 μmol/l	Xiang et al. (56)
Resveratrol	Cleavage of immature caspase-3 into active fragments (p12, p17, and p20), increased caspase-3 activity, and PARP cleavage	MD-MB-231 50 μmol/l	Alkhalaf et al. (57)

Please note that this table just contains selected examples.

It is important to consider whether the concentrations used in cell culture models are nutritional or pharmacological. For example, the concentrations of EGCG needed to significantly downregulate anti-apoptotic proteins and induce programmed cell death in vitro (20 μmol/l) are much higher than the physiological concentrations that could be obtained in humans by typical tea consumption *(19)*. Consumption of 6–7 cups of green tea/day (~30 mg/kg/day EGCG) would generate a plasma EGCG concentration of about 1 μmol/l *(61)*. Therefore, to achieve higher plasma concentrations, EGCG supplements are needed *(62)*. In contrast, human consumption of onions and applesauce with peel resulted in peak plasma concentrations of quercetin of 225 ± 43 and 331 ± 7 μmol/l, respectively *(63)*, which are significantly higher than concentrations shown to induce apoptosis in vitro (30–100 μmol/l) *(64)*. These data suggest that for quercetin, the effects observed in cell culture are nutritionally relevant.

Another important consideration is that dietary components have been shown to exert additive and synergistic effects on apoptosis induction. Resveratrol and quercetin additively activated caspase-3 and cytochrome c release in a human pancreatic cell line *(65)*. Quercetin and ellagic acid, respectively, at concentrations of 5 and 10 μmol/l also synergistically induced apoptosis in human leukemia MOLT-4 cells *(66)*. Selenium and vitamin E have been shown to exert synergistic effects on apoptosis induction in human prostate cancer cells *(67)*. This synergy was accounted for primarily by selenium and vitamin E modifying distinct signaling pathways of caspase activation. Selenium activated caspase-1 and caspase-12, whereas vitamin E activated caspase-9. Thus, the combination of selenium and vitamin E may activate multiple molecular targets for apoptosis induction, the endoplasmic reticulum stress/cytokine signaling pathway and mitochondrial pathway, respectively. The combinatorial effects of selenium and vitamin E may target the entire battery of initiator caspases and "switch on the full force of the apoptotic machinery" *(67)*. These studies suggest that combinations of bioactive compounds that target different mechanisms of action can likely achieve synergistic effects in cancer prevention.

Studies in human subjects have demonstrated that dietary compounds can influence apoptosis. Thirty-two patients diagnosed by biopsy with prostate cancer were given tomato sauce pasta entries (30 mg lycopene/day) for 3 weeks before prostatectomy *(68)*. Tomato sauce consumption resulted in a significant increase in the percentage of apoptotic cells in benign prostatic hyperplasia (from 0.66 ± 0.13% to 1.38 ± 0.31%) and in carcinomas (0.84 ± 0.13% to 2.76 ± 0.58%). This increase was associated with decreased Bax expression in the carcinomas *(68)*. Similarly, 18 men with prostate cancer who consumed 160 mg/day of red clover-derived isoflavones, containing a mixture of genistein, daidzen, formononectin, and biochanin A, prior to prostatectomy had significantly higher percentage of apoptotic cells (1.14%) in the radical prostatectomy samples compared to the control group (0.24%) *(69)*. While these data are encouraging, additional human studies are needed to determine whether other dietary components, at physiologically relevant concentrations, can modulate specific molecular targets associated with apoptosis.

4. INFLAMMATION

Inflammation represents a physiological response to invading microorganisms, trauma, chemical irritation, or foreign tissues. The inflammatory response is a complex tightly regulated process to prevent extensive damage to the host. However, uncontrolled and persistent inflammation is detrimental to the host and can increase cancer risk. Evidence for this comes from epidemiologic data showing an association between chronic inflammatory conditions and subsequent malignant transformation in the inflamed tissue. Clinical trials showed decreased cancer risk with the use of anti-inflammatory drugs. Animal studies showed increased cancer incidence with genetically (transgenic/knockout animals) or chemically induced chronic inflammation *(70)*. Experimental evidence indicates that there are multiple mechanisms linking inflammation to cancer and that there are multiple targets for cancer prevention by bioactive dietary compounds (Fig. 3, Table 3).

Chronic inflammation promotes carcinogenesis by inducing gene mutations, inhibiting apoptosis, and stimulating cell proliferation and angiogenesis. At the molecular level, free radicals and aldehydes produced during chronic inflammation can induce gene mutations and posttranslational modifications of key cancer-related proteins *(74)*.

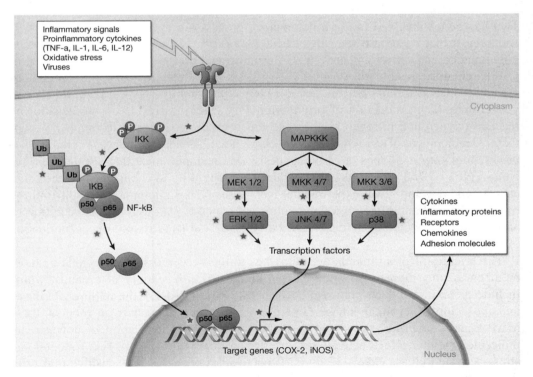

Fig. 3. The inflammatory cascade. The binding of proinflammatory cytokines to their receptors activates the mitogen-activated protein kinase family of proteins which activate NF-kB and induce expression of target genes such as COX-2 and iNOS. *Stars* indicate potential molecular targets for bioactive dietary components.

Table 3
Molecular Targets for Representative Dietary Bioactive Components that Influence Inflammation (71–73)

Molecular target	Dietary components
Inhibit NF-κB activation	Curcumin, resveratrol, gingerol, indole-3-carbinol, ellagic acid, green tea polyphenols, S-allyl-cysteine, lycopene, caffeic acid phenethyl ester, capsaicin, gingerol, ginseng
Inhibit mitogen-activated protein kinases (MAPK)	Curcumin, indole-3-carbinol, resveratrol, green tea polyphenols, capsaicin, gingerol, ginseng
Inhibit COX-2 activity	Luteolin, apigenin, genistein, green tea polyphenol, curcumin, resveratrol, kaempferol, quercetin, vitamin D, capsaicin, gingerol, ginseng, genistein
Inhibit iNOS activity	Curcumin, gingerol, EGCG, resveratrol, indole-3-carbinol, ginseng, genistein

Two key genes involved in the inflammatory process are cyclooxygenase-2 (COX-2) and nuclear factor-kappa B (NF-κB). These factors provide a mechanistic link between inflammation and cancer and are targets for nutritional prevention of cancer.

Inflammatory insults result in the synthesis and secretion of proinflammatory cytokines such as tumor necrosis factor- (TNF-), interleukin-1 (IL-1), IL-6, IL-12, and γ-interferon. The production of proinflammatory cytokines results in an elevation in reactive oxygen and nitrogen species and has been directly linked to tumor development. Development of cytokine gene knockout mice has demonstrated the vital role of proinflammatory cytokines in carcinogenesis. For example, mice that are deficient for either TNFα or TNFα receptors have reduced susceptibility to chemically induced skin cancers and develop fewer experimental metastases (75). Inflammation is self-limiting because the production of proinflammatory cytokines is followed by the secretion of anti-inflammatory cytokines (e.g., IL-4, IL-10, and TGF-β) to reduce the accumulation of reactive species.

The binding of proinflammatory cytokines to their receptors activates one or more members of the mitogen-activated protein kinase (MAPK) family of proteins, which include the extracellular signal-regulated protein kinase (ERK), the p38 MAP kinase, and the c-Jun N-terminal kinase (JNK). The improper activation of each of these MAP kinases amplifies the signal cascades through phosphorylation of downstream molecules including IκB, activating transcription factor–2 (ATF–2), Elk, mitogen and stress-activated kinase (Msk), leading to coactivation of two redox-sensitive transcription factors, namely, NFκ and c–Jun. The latter is a member of the activator protein–1 (AP–1) transcription factor. In resting cells, NF-κB resides in the cytoplasm as an inactive complex with the inhibitory protein IκB, which undergoes rapid phosphorylation, ubiquitination, and subsequent proteasomal degradation in response to a variety of stimuli, such as mitogens, proinflammatory cytokines, ultraviolet (UV) radiation, viral proteins, and bacterial toxins *(76)*. Dissociation of IκB from NF-κB allows the activated free dimer to translocate to the nucleus, where it binds to a κB element located in the promoter region of target genes, controlling their expression *(77)*. In normal cells, NF-κB is tightly regulated, whereas in tumor cells NF-κB becomes constitutively activated leading to deregulated expression of its target genes *(78)*.

NFκ and AP-1 activate the expression of over 400 genes including cytokines, chemokines, adhesion molecules, acute phase protein, growth factors, as well as specific enzymes such as inducible nitric oxide synthase (iNOS) and COX-2 *(79)*. In turn, these enzymes directly influence the levels of reactive oxygen species (ROS), reactive nitrogen species (RNS), and eicosanoids. ROS profoundly affect numerous critical cellular functions, and the absence of efficient cellular detoxification mechanisms that remove these radicals can increase cancer risk *(80)*. ROS and RNS are potentially damaging to cellular macromolecules such as DNA, proteins, and lipids. ROS can also specifically activate certain intracellular signaling cascades and thus contribute to tumor development and metastasis through the regulation of cellular phenotypes such as proliferation, death, and motility *(80)*.

The enzyme COX-2 catalyzes the first two steps in the biosynthesis of prostaglandins from arachidonic acid. Inappropriate upregulation of COX-2 has been implicated in the pathogenesis of various types of malignancies including colorectal, breast, and pancreatic cancers and well as cancers of the head and neck *(81)*. Transgenic mice overexpressing COX-2 had higher cancer incidence compared to COX-2 knockout animals *(82, 83)*. There is abundant evidence that a number of dietary components are COX-2 enzyme inhibitors (Table 3). For example, COX-2 transcription is inhibited in vitro not only by quercetin aglycone, but also by the quercetin conjugates that are found in human plasma (e.g., quercetin 3-glucoronide, quercetin 3′-sulfate, and 3′-methylquercetin 3′-glucoronide). Both quercetin and quercetin 3′-sulfate also inhibit COX-2 enzyme activity *(84)*. Additionally, the biologically active form of vitamin D [1,25 $(OH)_2D$] or calcitriol regulates multiple genes involved in the prostaglandin pathway *(85)*. These effects include calcitriol's action to decrease COX-2 synthesis, to increase COX-2 catabolism, and to inhibit expression of prostaglandin receptors. In combination, these three mechanisms reduce prostaglandin levels and signaling thereby attenuating the growth stimulatory effects of prostaglandins.

Nitric oxide is a short-lived radical that diffuses freely within cells and acts as an important intracellular and intercellular signaling molecule in almost every tissue in the body. Nitric oxide is synthesized from L-arginine by members of the nitric oxide synthase family including iNOS. Whereas low concentrations of nitric oxide may act as antioxidants and alter the transcriptional activity of NF-κB and AP-1, excess production of nitric oxide by iNOS may damage DNA, thereby enhancing the risk of cancer *(86)*. Thus, the control of iNOS expression is an important mechanism for cancer prevention. A variety of flavonoids, including apigenin, luteolin, kaempferol, myricetin, and genistein downregulate nitric oxide production and/or iNOS protein expression and activity in RAW 264.7 macrophage cells *(87)*.

In humans, evidence of efficacy for many bioactive food components is lacking. However, there is evidence that 1.5 g of eicosapentaenoic acid compared to placebo significantly reduces COX-2 protein expression in the esophageal mucosa of Barrett's esophagus patients. Moreover, the change in COX-2 expression was inversely related to a change in eicosapentaenoic concentrations (88). There is also evidence from a double-blind, placebo-controlled trial that consumption of a tomato-based drink (Lyc-o-Mato, containing 5.7 mg lycopene, 3.7 mg phytoene, 2.7 mg phytofluene, 1 mg β-carotene, and 1.8 mg -tocopherol) for 26 days reduced TNF- production by 34.4% compared to a placebo drink (same test and flavor but void of active compounds) (89). While these studies support the results obtained with in vitro models, additional studies in humans are warranted.

5. IMMUNITY

The main function of the immune system is to monitor tissue homeostasis, to protect against invading or infectious pathogens, and to eliminate damaged cells (90). The immune system may have the ability to eliminate nascent transformed cells (cancer immunosurveillance). Cancer immunosurveillance involves adaptive immune responses specific for antigens on malignant cells, as well as innate immune responses to non-self status or stress-induced ligands of transformed or malignant cells (91). The innate immune response provides a first line of defense and requires no previous exposure to a pathogen. The innate immune response involves recognition of common pathogen-associated molecules by cell-surface receptors, followed by infiltration of natural killer (NK) cells, macrophages, neutrophils, basophils, eosinophils, and mast cells at the site of infection that function to engulf and digest the pathogen. In contrast, the adaptive immune response represents a learned response to a previous exposure. Molecular changes that consistently occur during the carcinogenic process that might be recognized as "flags" on tumor cells could include: (1) products of oncogenes or tumor suppressor genes that are often mutated in cancer cells; (2) normal cellular proteins that are either overexpressed or aberrantly expressed in cancer cells; (3) oncogenic virus products; and/or (4) overexpression of stress-inducible proteins (91).

The adaptive immune system is comprised of B-lymphocytes and T-lymphocytes. B-lymphocytes recognize and engulf specific circulating antigens, triggering their clonal expansion and maturation into antibody secreting plasma cells. These antibodies bind to and mark pathogens for phagocytosis by cells of the innate immune system (92). Adaptive immunity involves the recognition of tumor antigens that are expressed in conjunction with HLA molecules by tumor-specific cytotoxic T-lymphocytes. These cells secrete tumoricidal molecules (such as perforin) or produce cytokines (such as IFN-γ and TNF-α) that can either directly inhibit tumor cell growth or potentiate the antitumor activity of other lymphoid effectors. However, although cancer cells typically express recognizable surface antigens, some tumor cells can escape detection and survive when the mutated gene products in question are not presented as MHC/peptide complexes (93). Mechanisms for immune escape are considered a hallmark of tumor progression (94).

DNA damage transcriptionally induces the expression of the mRNA for ligands of the immune receptor NKG2D (95). NK2GD is a cell-surface receptor that is expressed by many cell types in the immune system, including natural killer cells, $\gamma\delta$ T cells, CD8$^+$

T cells, and some activated CD4$^+$ cells *(96)*. In NK cells, NK2GD triggers cytotoxic activity and cytokine production *(97)*. These data suggest that DNA damage, in addition to stimulating cell cycle arrest and enhancing DNA repair activity or triggering apoptosis, may also participate in alerting the immune system to the presence of potentially cancerous cells.

The immune system not only plays a crucial role in preventing tumor growth, but it can also facilitate cancer progression, at least in part, by selecting tumors with lower immunogenicity *(98)*. Specifically, tumors derived from immunodeficient mice, such as recombination-activating gene-2 (RAG2)$^{-/-}$, Jα18$^{-/-}$ (NKT deficient), perforin$^{-/-}$, nude, or Scid mice are more immunogenic and less tumorigenic as a group, compared to the tumors derived from mice with an intact immune system (*reviewed in 98*). In addition, an abundance of infiltrating innate immune cells can contribute to cancer development. Tumor-infiltrating leukocytes can facilitate tumor progression by secreting growth factors, reactive oxygen and nitrogen species, proteases, prostaglandins, and angiogenic growth factors. ROS and RNS may directly promote tumor progression by inducing DNA damage and, therefore, the acquisition of additional mutations.

Because improved systemic immune function correlates with a reduction in tumor growth in several transplantable tumor models *(99, 100)*, as well as a reduced intestinal polyp number and increased survival in a spontaneous tumor model *(101)*, dietary components that increase immune function offer promise for nutritional preemption of cancer. For example, in mice fed a diet supplemented with probiotics in the form of yogurt, there was a correlation between enhanced mucosal cytokine production and a reduction in chemically induced colon carcinogenesis in the mice that consumed yogurt *(102)*. Fish oil consumption has also been linked to decreased cancer risk in a number of animal models and these effects may be modulated by alterations in the immune system. Fish oil consumption has been shown to improve macrophage function in Walker 256 tumor-bearing rats *(103)* and alter the balance between CD4$^+$ T-helper (TH1 and Th2) subsets by directly suppressing Th1 cell development *(104)*. This is noteworthy because Th2 cells mediate resistance to extracellular pathogens.

Both energy restriction and increased physical activity have also been associated with decreased cancer risk. When mice were fed either an energy restricted diet (30% reduction compared to control energy intake) and/or exercise (voluntary wheel reduction), there were alterations in both systemic and mucosal immune function *(105)*. Although energy restriction significantly enhanced NK cell function, it significantly impaired splenic and intestinal T-cell proliferation and had an inhibitory effect on cytokine production by intestinal lymphocytes. In contrast to energy restriction, exercise enhanced both mucosal T-cell proliferation and cytokine productions, as well as IFN-γ production in the spleen *(105)*. Therefore, exercise and energy restriction are working via different biological mechanisms to regulate NK and T-cell function.

Selenium is another nutrient, whose status has been linked with cancer risk. In preclinical models, selenium deficiency decreases antibody production by B-cells and decreases neutrophil chemotaxis and activity, while selenium supplementation enhances T-cell response by upregulation of the T-cell IL-2 receptor and increased antibody synthesis *(106)*. Moreover, selenium supplementation has been shown to enhance the immune system in humans. In a double-blind placebo-controlled study, 50 or 100 μg of selenium/day for 15 weeks augmented the cellular immune response through an increased production of IFN-γ and other cytokines, an earlier peak T-cell proliferation and an increase in T helper cells *(107)*. Selenium-supplemented subjects also showed more rapid clearance of poliovirus and the reverse transcriptase-polymerase chain reaction products recovered from the feces of the supplemented subjects contained a lower number of mutations *(107)*.

Many different dietary components have been shown to enhance γδ T-cell function and may play a role in cancer prevention *(108)*. These include vitamin E, mistletoe extract, nucleotides, n-3 fatty acids, conjugated linoleic acids, tea, and fruit and vegetable juice concentrate *(108)*. For example, in a randomized, double-blind, placebo-controlled trial, the γδ T cells from subjects who consumed a green tea capsule for 3 months proliferated 28% more and secreted 26% more IFN-γ in response to γδ T-cell antigens, as compared to the γδ T cells from subjects taking placebo *(109)*. Human consumption of a fruit and vegetable juice concentrate has also been associated with increased circulating γδ T cells *(110)*. Although it is logical to assume that a change in tumoricidal cell activity will coincide with cancer prevention, direct evidence for this is lacking, and thus firm conclusions regarding the impact of these alterations on cancer risk cannot be made.

6. ANGIOGENESIS

Tumor angiogenesis is the proliferation of a network of blood vessels that penetrates into cancerous growths, supplying nutrients and oxygen and removing waste products. Tumor angiogenesis is a complex process that involves the tight interplay of tumor cells, endothelial cells, phagocytes and their secreted factors, which act as promoters or inhibitors of angiogenesis. Neoplastic cells have an inherent propensity to produce angiogenic molecules to initiate neoangiogenesis by paracrine regulation of endothelial cells. Endothelial cells are stimulated and attracted to the site where the new blood supply is needed by various growth factors such as vascular endothelial growth factor (VEGF), fibroblast growth factor (FGF), and insulin-like growth factor-1 (IGF-1), and inflammatory molecules including IL-8, COX-2, and iNOS (Fig. 4) *(111, 112)*. Chemotactic migration along this gradient is, however, possible only through the degradation of extracellular matrix components *(113)*. This is accomplished via matrix metalloproteinases (MMPs) *(114, 115)*. MMPs include collagenases (MMP-1, MMP-8, and MMP-13), gelatinases (MMP-2 and MMP-9), stromelysins (MMP-3, MMP-10, and MMP-7), and elastase (MMP-12) *(116)*.

The expression of matrix metalloproteinases is regulated by the AP-1 transcription complex, which can be activated by several mechanisms involving growth factors, cell–cell interactions, and interactions among cells and matrix *(117)*. In addition, natural MMP inhibitors (tissue inhibitors of metalloproteinases, TIMPs) are also involved in regulating the activation and activity of these enzymes. MMPs are involved in many physiological processes involving matrix remodeling and appear to be essential in angiogenesis, tumor cell invasion, and metastasis. In addition to removing physical barriers to migration through degradation of the extracellular matrix, MMPs can modulate cell

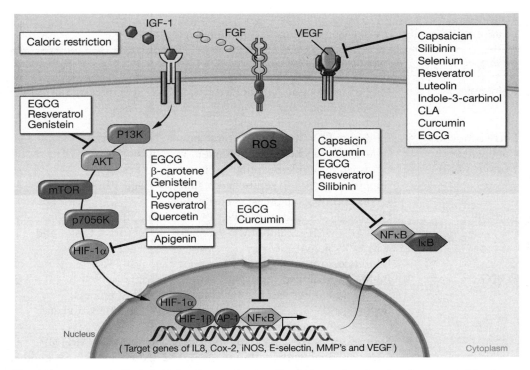

Fig. 4. Angiogenesis. Endothelial cells are stimulated and attracted to the site where a new blood supply is needed by various growth factors. Different dietary components can affect different molecular targets associated with angiogenesis. Some dietary components can act on multiple molecular targets. *Arrows* indicate activation and *blocked lines* indicate inhibitory effects.

adhesion and generate extracellular matrix degradation products that are chemotactic for endothelial cells.

Inhibition of angiogenesis serves two purposes. First, it limits tumor size by restricting oxygen and nutrients. Second, it decreases the opportunities for metastatic cells to enter the circulatory system. Several dietary components have surfaced as inhibitors of angiogenesis in various animal and cell culture models (Table 4). In addition, experimental findings suggest that energy restriction suppresses tumor angiogenesis in prostate cancer, human gliomas, and intracerebral growth of malignant tumors *(121, 122)*. A recent study in rats implanted with prostate cancer cells demonstrated that a 40% caloric restriction reduced serum concentrations of IGF-1 by 35%, VEGF mRNA by 30%, and secreted VEGF protein by 33% compared to control animals *(123)*. Moreover, in vitro studies with the prostate cancer cells demonstrated dose- and time-dependent stimulation of VEGF expression by IGF-1. These results suggest that dietary restriction reduces endocrine and prostate tumor autocine/paracrine IGF-1 expression, which contributes to reduced VEGF expression and signaling, to inhibit tumor angiogenesis associated with prostate tumorigenesis *(123)*.

Table 4
Examples of Bioactive Dietary Components that Inhibit Angiogenesis[a]

Dietary agent	Effect on angiogenesis
Apigenin	Inhibits hypoxia-inducible factor 1- and VEGF expression in human ovarian cancer cells Inhibits in vitro angiogenesis
	Inhibits in vitro angiogenesis
Berry extracts	Inhibition of VEGF expression in human keratinocytes
Conjugated linoleic acid	Inhibits angiogenesis in vitro and in vivo by suppression of formation of microcapillary networks
	Suppression of both serum and mammary gland VEGF concentrations in breast cancer model
Curcumin	Downregulates transcript levels of VEGF and bFGF and suppresses VEGF, MMP-2, and MMP-9 expression, NF-6B, COX-2, and MAPKs activity
	Inhibits microvessels density in tumor xenografts
EGCG	Inhibits growth and survival of endothelial cells
	Suppresses tumor vasculature in tumor xenograft models
	Suppresses ERK1/2 activity and inhibits VEGF expression and secretion in cancer cells
	Suppresses MMP-2/9 expression and activation in the TRAMP model, along with inhibition of COX-2, iNOS, and NF-6B in other tumor models
Genistein	Downregulates MMP-9 and upregulates TIMP-1
	Suppresses endothelial cell proliferation, migration, and invasion
	Inhibits VEGF and COX-2 expression and suppresses VEGF-induced tyrosine phosphorylation of receptor kinases
Grape seed procyanidins	Inhibits growth, survival, migration, and matrigel invasion of HUVEC
	Decreases VEGF expression and microvessel density in tumor xenograft model
Indole-3-carbinol	Decreases VEGF and Flk-1 expression in endothelial cells
	Inhibits growth of HUVEC and inhibits in vitro angiogenesis in matrigel
	Decreases iNOS expression
Inositol hexaphosphate	Decreases VEGF expression and microvessel density in tumor xenograft model
	Inhibits growth, survival, migration, and matrigel invasion of HUVEC
Luteolin	Inhibition of VEGF-induced proliferation of HUVEC
Phenylethyl isothiocyanate	Inhibits VEGF secretion and lowers VEGF-R expression
	Lowers survival rate of HUVEC cells, inhibits capillary-like tube formation and migration of HUVEC cells
Quercetin	Inhibits MMP-2 and MMP-9 secretion from tumor cells and suppresses endothelial cell proliferation, migration, and tube formation

Table 4
(Continued)

Dietary agent	Effect on angiogenesis
Resveratrol	Inhibits capillary-like tube formation by HUVEC and capillary diffentiation and VEGF binding to HUVEC
	Decreases iNOS and VEGF expression
Retinoic acid	Inhibits responsiveness of endothelial cells to angiogenic growth factors
Selenium	Suppresses VEGF expression, lowers microvessel density, and inhibits genolytic activity of MMP-2 in rat mammary carcinoma
	Initiates apoptotic death in HUVEC cells
Silibinin	Inhibits growth and survival of endothelial cells via disrupting VEGF and IGF-1 signaling
	Inhibits MMP-2 expression and tube formation in HUVEC
	Inhibits VEGF secretion from human cancer cells
	Decreases iNOS and VEGF expression and microvessel density in mouse lung tumors

[a]Additional information can be obtained from recent reviews on dietary modification of angiogenesis *(118–120)*.

While angiogenesis may be inhibited by many dietary components, this process also serves many important physiological functions such as the healing of wounds, acute injury, and chronic damages of the gastrointestinal mucosa.

A better understanding of the differential effects of dietary components on tumor versus physiological angiogenesis is needed.

7. CONCLUSIONS

Dietary behavior is one of the most important modifiable determinants of cancer risk and tumor behavior. Overwhelming evidence demonstrates that a variety of dietary components can influence a number of key intracellular targets that are associated with the cancer process. Unraveling the role of bioactive food components is complicated by the multiple steps in the cancer process, which can be modified simultaneously, including sites such as drug metabolism, DNA repair, cell proliferation, apoptosis, inflammation, immunity, differentiation, and angiogenesis. Bioactive food components typically influence more than one process. The dose dependency of these changes needs to be examined in much more detail as they relate to phenotypic differences in tumor incidence and/or tumor behavior. There is a growing body of evidence to suggest that even if single agents are inactive at low concentrations, combinations of two or more components might be more efficacious *(4)*. Additionally, the timing and duration of exposure needed to bring about a response deserves greater attention.

A fundamental action of several bioactive food components is that they serve as regulators of gene expression and/or modulate gene products. Transcriptomic or microarray analysis can provide clues about the mechanisms that underlie the beneficial or adverse effects of dietary components. Such analysis can identify important genes and related events that are altered in the predisease state, and may, therefore, serve as molecular biomarkers and/or assist in identifying and characterizing the basic molecular pathways influenced by food components.

Typically, increasing the intensity and duration of exposure to dietary components increases the number of genes whose expressions are modified *(124, 125)*. Thus, dose and duration of exposure become fundamental considerations in interpreting findings from microarray studies. Additionally, while most studies are simple snapshots of genomic expression changes that can help identify important possible targets, they must be interpreted cautiously because of inherent biological variability *(126)*. Determining which one of the targets is most important in altering tumor growth will not be a simple task. Likewise, unraveling the multitude of interactions among nutrients with these key events makes the challenge even more daunting. Finally, interindividual differences, probably reflecting genetic polymorphisms, can mask the response to a nutrient and thereby complicate this undertaking to an even greater extent. Nevertheless, deciphering the role of diet is fundamental to optimizing health and preventing disease. Access to this information should help resolve the inconsistencies within the literature and provide clues to strategies that may be developed to assist individuals in preventing cancer.

REFERENCES

1. World Cancer Research Fund/American Institute for Cancer Research Food. (2007) Nutrition, Physical Activity and the Prevention of Cancer: A Global Perspective. Washington, DC: AICR.
2. Milner, J.A. (2004) Molecular targets for bioactive food components. *J Nutr* **134**, 2492S–98S.
3. Liu, R.H. (2003) Health benefits of fruit and vegetables are from additive and synergistic combinations of phytochemicals. *Am J Clin Nutr* **78**, 517S–20S.
4. Davis, C.D. (2007) Nutritional interactions: Credentialing of molecular targets for cancer prevention. *Exp Biol Med* **232**, 176–83.
5. Liu, R.H. (2003) Health benefits of fruit and vegetables are from additive and synergistic combinations of phytochemicals. *Am J Clin Nutr* **78**, 517s–20s.
6. Sarkar, F.H., and Li, Y. (2007) Targeting multiple signal pathways by chemopreventive agents for cancer prevention and therapy. *Acta Pharmacol Sin* **28**, 1305–15.
7. Meeran, S.M., and Katiyar, S.K. (2008) Cell cycle control as a basis for cancer chemoprevention through dietary agents. *Frontiers Biosci* **13**, 2191–202.
8. Mailand, N., Falck, J., Lukas, C., Syljuasen, R.G., Welcker, M., Barteck, J., and Lukas, J. (2000) Rapid destruction of human Cdc25A in response to DNA damage. *Science* **288**, 1425–29.
9. Sherr, C.J. (2000) The Pezcoller lecture: Cancer cell cycles revisited. *Cancer Res* **60**, 3689–95.
10. Santamaria, D., and Ortega, S. (2006) Cyclins and CDKS in development and cancer: Lessons from genetically modified mice. *Front Biosci* **11**, 1164–88.
11. Beasley, M.B., Lantuojoul, S., Abbondanzo, S., Chu, W.S., Hasleton, P.S., Travis, W.D., and Brambilla, E. (2003) The P16/cyclin D1/Rb pathway in neuroendocrine tumors of the lung. *Hum Pathol* **34**, 136–42.
12. Belleti, B., Nicoloso, M.S., Schiappacassi, M., Chimienti, E., Berton, S., Lovat, F., Colombatti, A., and Baldassare, G. (2005) p27(kip1) functional regulation in human cancer: A potential target for therapeutic designs. *Med Chem* **12**, 1589–605.
13. Macaluso, M., Montanari, M., Cinti, C., and Giordano, A. (2005) Modulation of cell cycle components by epigenetic and genetic events. *Semin Oncol* **32**, 452–57.
14 Fresco, P., Borges, F., Diniz, C., and Marques, M.P. (2006) New insights on the anticancer properties of dietary polyphenols. *Med Res Rev* **26**, 747–66.

15. Semczuk, A., and Jakowicki, J.A. (2004) Alterations of pRB1-cyclin D1-cdk4/6-p16(INK4A) pathway in endometrial carcinogenesis. *Cancer Lett* **203**, 1–12.

16. Shankar, S., Suthakar, G., and Srivastava, R.K. (2007) Epigallocatchin-3-gallate inhibits cell cycle and induces apoptosis in pancreatic cancer. *Front Biosci* **12**, 5039–51.

17. Benitz, D.A., Pozo-Guisado, E., Alvarez-Barrientos, A., Fernandez-Salguero, P.M., and Castellon, E.A. (2007) Mechanisms involved in resveratrol-induced apoptosis and cell cycle arrest in prostate cancer derived cell lines. *J Androl* **28**, 282–93.

18. Suh, N., Luyengi, L., Fong, H.H., Kinghorn, A.D., and Pezzuto, J.M. (1995) Discovery of natural product chemopreventive agents using HL-60 cell differentiation as a model. *Anticancer Res* **15**, 233–39.

19. Howell, L.M., Moiseeva, E.P., Neal, C.P., Foreman, B.E., Andreadi, C.K., Sun, Y., Hudson, E.A., and Manson, M.M. (2007) Predicting the physiological relevance of in vitro cancer preventive activities of phytochemicals. *Acta Pharmacol Sin* **28**, 1274–304.

20. Wang, L., Liu, D., Ahmed, T., Chung, F.L., Conaway, C., and Chiao, J.W. (2004) Targeting cell cycle machinery as a molecular mechanism of sulforaphane in prostate cancer prevention. *Int J Oncol* **24**, 187–92.

21. Jackson, S.J., and Singletary, K.W. (2004) Sulforaphane inhibits human MCF-7 mammary cancer cell mitotic progression and tubulin polymerization. *J Nutr* **134**, 2229–36.

22. Parnaud, G., Li, P., Cassar, G., Rouimi, P., Tulliez, J., Combaret, L., and Gamet-Payrastre, L. (2004) Mechanism of sulforaphane-induced cell cycle arrest and apoptosis in human colon cancer cells. *Nutr Cancer* **48**, 198–206.

23. Singh, S.V., Herman-Antosiewicz, A., Singh, A.V., Lew, K.L., Srivastava, S.K., Kamath, R., Brown, K.D., Zhang, L., and Baskaran, R. (2004) Sulforaphane-induced G2/M phase cell cycle arrest involves checkpoint kinase 2-mediated phosphorylation of cell division cycle 25C. *J Biol Chem* **279**, 25813–22.

24. Tang, L., and Zhang, Y. (2005) Mitochondria are the primary target in isothiocyanate-induced apoptosis in human bladder cancer cells. *Mol Cancer Ther* **4**, 1250–59.

25. Shukla, S., and Gupta, S. (2007) Apigenin-induced cell cycle arrest is mediated by modulation of MAPK, P13K-Akt, and loss of cyclin D1 associated retinoblastoma dephosphorylation in human prostate cancer cells. *Cell Cycle* **6**, 1102–14.

26. Shukla, S., and Gupta, S. (2006) Molecular targets for apigenin-induced cell cycle arrest and apoptosis in prostate cancer cell xenograft. *Mol Cancer Ther* **4**, 843–52.

27. Hollman, P.C., and Katan, M.B. (1999) Health effects and bioavailability of dietary flavanols. *Free Radic Res* **1**, 75–80.

28. Srivastava, R.K., Chen, Q., Siddiqui, I., Sarva, K., and Shankar, S. (2007) Linkage of curcumin-induced cell cycle arrest and apoptosis by cyclin-dependent kinase inhibitor p21$^{/WAF1/CIP1}$. *Cell Cycle* **6**, 2953–61.

29. Chuang, S.E., Cheng, A.L., Lin, J.K., and Kuo, M.L. (2000) Inhibition by curcumin of diethylnitrosamine-induced hepatic hyperplasia, inflammation, cellular gene products and cell-cycle-related proteins in rats. *Food Chem Toxicol* **38**, 991–95.

30. Khafif, A., Schantz, S.P., Chou, T.L.C., Edelstein, D., and Sacks, P.G. (1998) Quantitation of chemopreventive synergism between (–)-epigallocatechin-3-gallate and curcumin in normal, premalignant and malignant human oral epithelial cells. *Carcinogenesis* **19**, 419–24.

31. Lin, N., Chen, X., Liao, J., Yang, G., Wang, S., Josephson, Y., Han, C., Huang, M.T., and Yang, C.S. (2002) Inhibition of 7,12-dimethylbenz{a}antrhracene (DMBA)-induced oral carcinogenesis in hamsters by tea and curcumin. *Carcinogenesis* **23**, 1307–13.

32. Holt, P.R., Wolper, C., Moss, S.F., Yang, K., and Lipkin, M. (2001) Comparison of low-fat dairy foods on epithelial cell proliferation and differentiation. *Nutr Cancer* **41**, 150–55.

33. Rozen, P., Lubin, F., Papo, N., Knaani, J., Farbstein, H., Farbstein, M., and Zajicek, G. (2001) Calcium supplements interact significantly with long-term diet while suppressing rectal epithelial proliferation of adenoma patients. *Cancer* **91**, 833–40.

34. Weerasooriya, V., Rennie, M.J., Anant, S., Alpers, D.H., Patterson, B.W., and Klein, S. (2006) Dietary fiber decreases colonic epithelial cell proliferation and protein synthetic rates in human subjects. *Am J Physiol Endocrinol Metab* **290**, E1104–E08.

35. Sun, S.Y., Hail, N., and Lotan, R. (2004) Apoptosis as a novel target for cancer chemoprevention. *J Natl Cancer Inst* **96**, 662–72.

36. Rodriguez, M., and Schaper, J. (2005) Apoptosis: Measurement and technical issues. *J Mol Cell Cardiol* **38**, 15–20.

37. Fischer, U., and Schulze-Ostoff, K. (2005) Apoptosis-based therapies and drug targets. *Cell Death Differ* **12**, 942–61.

38. Khan, N., Afaq, F., and Mukhtar, H. (2007) Apoptosis by dietary factors: The suicide solution for delaying cancer growth. *Carcinogenesis* **28**, 233–39.

39. Cho, S.G., and Choi, E.J. (2002) Apoptotic signaling pathways: Caspases and stress-activated protein kinases. *J Biochem Mol Biol* **35**, 24–27.

40. Watson, R.W., and Fitzpatrick, J.M. (2005) Targeting apoptosis in prostate cancer: Focus on caspases and inhibitors of apoptosis proteins. *BJI Int* **96**, 30–34.

41. Li, P., Nijhawan, D., and Wang, X. (2004) Mitochondrial activation of apoptosis. *Cell* **116**, S57–S9.

42. Saleem, M., Kweon, M.H., Yun, J.M., Adhami, M., Khan, N., Syed, D.N., and Mukhtar, H. (2005) A novel dietary triterpene leueol induces fas-mediated apoptotic death of androgen-sensitive prostate cancer cells and inhibits tumor growth in a xenograft model. *Cancer Res* **65**, 11203–13.

43. Pledgie-Tracy, A., Sobolewski, M.D., and Davidson, N.E. (2007) Sulforaphane induces cell type-specific apoptosis in human breast cancer cell lines. *Mol Cancer Ther* **6**, 1013–21.

44. Deeb, D., Jiang, H., Gao, X., Al-Holou, S., Danyluk, A.L., Dulchavsky, S.A., and Gautam, S.C. (2007) Curcumin [1,7-Bis(4-hydroxy-3-methoxyphenyl)-1-6-heptadine-3,5-dione] sensitizes human prostate cancer cells to tumor necrosis factor-related apoptosis-inducing ligand/Apo2L-induced apoptosis by suppressing nuclear factor-6B via inhibition of the prosurvival Akt signaling pathway. *J Pharmacol Exp Ther* **321**, 616–25.

45. Zhang, S., Shen, H.M., and Ong, C.N. (2005) Down-regulation of c-FLIP contributes to the sensitization effect of 3,3′-diindolylmethane on TRAIL-induced apoptosis in cancer cells. *Mol Cancer Ther* **4**, 1972–81.

46. Das, A., Banik, N.L., and Ray, S.K. (2006) Mechanism of apoptosis with the involvement of calpain and caspase cascades in human malignant neuroblastoma SH-SY5Y cells exposed to flavonoids. *Int J Cancer* **119**, 2575–85.

47. Zou, H., Zhan, S., and Cao, K. (2008) Apoptotic activity of genistein on human lung adenocarcinoma SPC-A-1 cells and preliminary exploration of its mechanisms using microarray. *Biomed Pharmacother* (E-pub).

48. Cao, J., Liu, Y., Zhou, H.M., Kong, Y., Yang, G., Jiang, L.P., Li, Q.J., and Zhong, L.F. (2007) Curcumin induces apoptosis through mitochondrial hyperpolization and mtDNA damage in human hepatoma G2 cells. *Free Rad Med Biol* **43**, 968–75.

49. Choi, W.Y., Choi, B.T., Lee, W.H., and Choi, Y.H. (2008) Sulforaphane generates reactive oxygen species leading to mitochondrial perturbation for apoptosis in human leukemia U937 cells. *Biomed Pharmacother* (E-pub).

50. Palozza, P., Serini, S., Torsello, A., Di Nicuolo, F., Maggiano, N., Ranelletti, F.O., Wolf, C.I., and Calviello, G. (2003) Mechanisms of activation of caspase cascade during beta-carotene-induced apoptosis in human tumor cells. *Nutr Cancer* **47**, 76–87.

51. Zhou, H.B., Chen, J.M., Cai, J.T., Du, Q., and Wu, C.N. (2008) Anticancer activity of genistein on implanted tumor of human SG7901 cells in nude mice. *World J Gastroenterol* **14**, 627–31.

52. Thangapazham, R.L., Passi, N., and Maheshwair, R.K. (2007) Green tea polyphenol and epigallocatechin gallate induce apoptosis and inhibit invasion in human breast cancer cells. *Cancer Biol Ther* **6**, 1938–43.

53. Shukla, S., and Gupta, S. (2008) Apigenin-induced prostate cancer cell death is initiated by reactive oxygen species and p53 activation. *Free Radic Biol Med* **44**, 1833–45.

54. Yang, S.F., Yang, W.E., Chang, H.R., Chu, S.C., and Hsieh, Y.S. (2008) Luteolin induces apoptosis in oral squamous cancer cells. *J Dent Res* **87**, 401–06.

55. Das, A., Banik, N.L., and Ray, S.K. (2007) Garlic compounds generate reactive oxygen species leading to activation of stress kinases and cysteine proteases for apoptosis in human glioblastoma T98G and U87MG cells. *Cancer* **110**, 1083–94.

56. Xiang, N., Zhao, R., and Zhong, W. (2008) Sodium selenite induces apoptosis by generation of super-oxide via the mitochondrial-dependent pathway in human prostate cancer cells. *Cancer Chemother Pharmacol* (E-pub).

57. Alkhalaf, M., El-Mowafy, A., Renno, W., Rachid, O., Ali, A., and Al-Attyiah, R. (2008) Resveratrol-induced apoptosis in human breast cancer cells is mediated primarily through the caspase-3-dependent pathway. *Arch Med Res* **39**, 162–68.

58. Krammer, P.H. (2000) CD95's deadly mission in the immune system. *Nature* **407**, 789–95.

59. Chen, C., and Kong, A.N. (2005) Dietary cancer-chemopreventive compounds: From signaling and gene expression to pharmacological effects. *Trends Pharmacol Sci* **26**, 318–26.

60. Palooza, P. (2005) Can beta-carotene regulate cell growth by a redox mechanism? An answer from cultured cells. *Biochim Biophys Acta* **740**, 215–21.

61. Yang, C.S., Chen, L., Lee, M.J., Balentine, D., Kuo, M.C., and Schantz, S.P. (1998) Blood and urine levels of tea catechins after ingestion of different amounts of green tea by human volunteers. *Cancer Epidemiol Biomarkers Prev* **7**, 351–54.

62. Chow, H.H., Cai, Y., Alberts, D.S., Hamkin, I., Dorr, R., Shahi, F., Crowell, J.A., Yang, C.S., and Hara, Y. (2001) Phase 1 pharmacokinetic study of tea polyphenols following single-dose administration of epigallocatechin gallate and polyphenon E. *Cancer Epidemiol Biomarkers Prev* **10**, 53–58.

63. Nemeth, K., and Piskula, M.K. (2007) Food content, processing, absorption and metabolism of onion flavonoids. *Critical Rev Food Sci Nutr* **47**, 397–409.

64. Kim, Y.H., Lee, D.H., Jeong, J.H., Guo, Z.S., and Lee, Y.J. (2008) Quercetin augments TRAIL-induced apoptotic death: Involvement of the ERK signal transduction pathway. *Biochem Pharmacol* **75**, 1946–58.

65. Mouria, M., Gukovskaya, A.S., Jung, Y., Buechler, P., Hines, O.J., Reber, H.A., and Pandol, S.J. (2002) Food-derived polyphenols inhibit pancreatic cancer growth through mitochondrial cytochrome C release and apoptosis. *Int J Cancer* **98**, 761–69.

66. Mertens-Talcott, S.U., and Percival, S.S. (2005) Ellagic acid and quercetin interact synergistically with resveratrol in the induction of apoptosis and cause transient cell cycle arrest in human leukemia cells. *Cancer Lett* **218**, 141–51.

67. Zu, K., and Ip, C. (2003) Synergy between selenium and vitamin E in apoptosis induction is associated with activation of distinctive initiator caspases in human prostate cancer cells. *Cancer Res* **63**, 6988–95.

68. Kim, H.S., Bowen, P., Chen, L., Duncan, C., Ghosh, L., Sharifi, R., and Christov, K. (2003) Effects of tomato sauce consumption on apoptotic cell death in prostate benign hyperplasia and carcinoma. *Nutr Cancer* **47**, 40–47.

69. Jarred, R.A., Keikha, M., Dowling, C., McPherson, S.J., Clare, A.M., Husband, A.J., Pedersen, J.S., Frydenberg, M., and Risbridger, G.P. (2002) Induction of apoptosis in low to moderate-grade human prostate carcinoma by red clover-derived dietary isoflavones. *Cancer Epidemiol Biomarkers Prev* **11**, 1689–96.

70. Hofseth, L.J., and Ying, L. (2006) Identifying and defusing weapons of mass inflammation in carcinogenesis. *Biochim Biophys Acta* **1765**, 74–84.

71. Ichikawa, H., Nakamura, Y., Kashiwada, Y., and Aggarwal, B.B. (2007) Anticancer drugs designed by mother nature: Ancient drugs by modern targets. *Curr Pharm Des* **13**, 3400–16.

72. Surh, Y.J., and Kundu, J.K. (2007) Cancer preventive phytochemicals as speed breakers in inflammatory signaling involved in aberrant COX-2 expression. *Current Cancer Drug Targets* **7**, 447–58.

73. Murakami, A., and Ohigashi, H. (2007) Targeting NOX, iNOS, and COX-2 in inflammatory cells: Chemoprevention using food phytochemicals. *Int J Cancer* **121**, 2357–63.

74. Hussain, S.P., Hofseth, L.J., and Harris, C.C. (2003) Radical causes of cancer *Nat. Rev. Cancer* **3**, 276–85.

75. Moore, R.J., Owens, D.M., Stamp, G., Arnott, C., Burke, F., East, N., Holdsworth, H., Turner, L., Rollins, B., Pasparakis, M., Kollias, G., and Balkwill, F. (1999) Mice deficient in tumor necrosis factor-alpha are resistant to skin carcinogenesis. *Nat Med* **5**, 828–31.

76. Naugler, W.E., and Karin, M. (2008) NF-kappaB and cancer-identifying targets and mechanisms. *Curr Opin Genet Dev* (E-pub).

77. Greten, F.R., and Karin, M. (2004) The IKK/NF-kappaB activation pathway-a target for prevention and treatment of cancer. *Cancer Lett* **206**, 193–99.
78. Dolcet, X., Llobet, D., Pallares, J., and Matias-Guiu, X. (2005) NF-6B in development and progression of human cancer. *Virchows Arch* **446**, 475–82.
79. Nam, N.H. (2006) Naturally occurring NF-kappaB inhibitors. *Mini Rev Med Chem* **6**, 945–51.
80. Storz, P. (2005) Reactive oxygen species in tumor progression *Front. Bioscience* **10**, 1881–96.
81. Harris, R.E. (2007) Cyclooxygenase-2 (cox-2) and the inflammogenesis of cancer. *Subcell Biochem* **42**, 93–126.
82. Oshima, H., Oshima, M., Inaba, K., and Taketo, M.M. (2004) Hyperplastic gastric tumors induced by activated macrophages in COX-2/mPGES-1 transgenic mice. *EMBO J* **23**, 1669–78.
83. Oshima, M., Dinchuk, J.E., Kargman, S.L., Oshima, H., Hancock, B., Kwong, E., Trzaskos, J.M., Evans, J.F., and Taketo, M.M. (1996) Suppression of intestinal polyposis in Apc delta716 knockout mice by inhibition of cyclooxygenase 2 (COX-2). *Cell* **87**, 803–09.
84. O'Leary, K.A., de Pascual-Tereasa, S., Needs, P.W., Bao, Y.P., O'Brien, N.M., and Williamson, G. (2004) Effect of flavonoids and vitamin E on cyclooxygenase-2 (COX-2) transcription. *Mutat Res* **551**, 245–54.
85. Feldman, D., Krishnan, A., Moreno, J., Swami, S., Peehl, D.M., and Srinivas, S. (2007) Vitamin D inhibition of the prostaglandin pathway as therapy for prostate cancer. *Nutr Rev* **65**, S113–S15.
86. Hofseth, L.J., Saito, S., Hussain, S.P., Espey, M.G., Miranda, K.M., Araki, Y., Jhappan, C., Higashimoto, Y., He, P., Linke, S.P., Quezado, M.M., Zurer, I., Rotter, V., Wink, D.A., Appella, E., and Harris, C.C. (2003) Nitric oxide-induced cellular stress and p53 activation in chronic inflammation. *Proc Natl Acad Sci U S A* **100**, 143–48.
87. Kim, H.K., Cheon, B.S., Kim, Y.H., Kim, S.Y., and Kim, H.P. (1999) Effect of naturally occurring flavonoids on nitric oxide production in the macrophage cell line RAW 264.7 and their structural-activity relationships. *Biochem Pharmacol* **58**, 759–65.
88. Mehta, S.P., Boddy, A.P., Cook, J., Sams, V., Lund, E.K., Johnson, I.T., and Rhodes, M. (2008) Effect of n-3 polyunsaturated fatty acids on Barrett's epithelium in the human lower esophagus. *Am J Clin Nutr* **87**, 949–56.
89. Riso, P., Visioli, F., Grande, S., Guarnieri, S., Gardana, C., Simonetti, P., and Porrini, M. (2006) Effect of tomato-based drink on markers of inflammation, immunomodulation and oxidative stress. *J Agric Food Chem* **54**, 2563–66.
90. de Visser, K.E., Eichten, A., and Coussens, L.M. (2006) Paradoxical roles of the immune system during cancer development. *Nat Rev Cancer* **6**, 24–37.
91. Nakachi, K., Hayashi, T., Imai, K., and Kusunoki, Y. (2004) Perspectives on cancer immuno-epidemiology. *Cancer Sci* **95**, 921–29.
92. Philpot, M., and Ferguson, L.R. (2004) Immunonutrition and cancer. *Mutat Res* **551**, 29–42.
93. Wu, J., and Lainer, L.L. (2003) Natural killer cells and cancer. *Adv Cancer Res* **90**, 127–56.
94. Marincola, F.M., Jaffee, E.M., Hicklin, D.J., and Ferrone, S. (2000) Escape of human solid tumors from T-cell recognition: Molecular mechanisms and functional significance. *Adv Immunol* **74**, 181–273.
95. Gasser, S., Orsulic, S., Brown, E.J., and Raulet, D.H. (2005) The DNA damage pathway regulates innate immune system ligands of the NKG2D receptor. *Nature* **436**, 1186–90.
96. Raulet, D.H. (2003) Roles of the NKG2D immunoreceptor and its ligands. *Nat Rev Immunol* **3**, 781–90.
97. Billadeau, D.D., Upshaw, J.L., Schoon, R.A., Dick, C.J., and Leibson, P.J. (2003) NKG2D-DAP10 triggers human NK cell-mediated killing via a Syk-independent regulatory pathway. *Nat Immunol* **4**, 557–64.
98. Ikeda, T., Chamoto, K., Tsuji, T., Suzuki, Y., Wakita, D., Takeshima, T., and Nishimura, T. (2004) The critical role of type-1 innate and acquired immunity in tumor immunotherapy. *Cancer Sci* **95**, 697–803.
99. Palena, C., Abrams, S.I., Schlom, J., and Hodge, J.W. (2006) Cancer vaccines: Preclinical studies and novel strategies. *Adv Cancer Res* **95**, 115–45.

100. Jones, E., Golgher, D., Simon, A.K., Dahm-Vicker, M., Screaton, G.L., Elliot, T., and Gallimore, A. (2004) The influence of CD25+ cells on the generation of immunity to tumour cell lines in mice. *Novartis Found Symp* **256**, 149–52.

101. Revaz, V., and Nardelli-Haefliger, D. (2005) The importance of mucosal immunity in defense against epithelial cancers. *Curr Opin Immunol* **17**, 175–79.

102. Rachid, M.M., Gobbato, N.M., Valdez, J.C., Vitalone, H.H., and Perdigon, G. (2002) Effect of yogurt on the inhibition of an intestinal carcinoma by increasing cellular apoptosis. *Int J Immunopathol Pharmacol* **15**, 209–16.

103. Pizato, N., Bonatto, S., Piconcelli, M., de Souza, L.M., Sassaki, G.L., Naliwaiko, K., Nunes, E.A., Curi, R., Calder, P.C., and Fernandes, L.C. (2006) Fish oil alters T-lymphocyte proliferation and macrophage responses in Walker 256 tumor-bearing rats. *Nutrition* **22**, 425–32.

104. Chapkin, R.S., Davidson, L.A., Ly, L., Weeks, B.R., Lupton, J.R., and McMurray, D.N. (2007) Immunomodulatory effects of (n-3) fatty acids: Putative link to inflammation and colon cancer. *J Nutr* **137**, 200S–4S.

105. Rogers, C.J., Berrigan, D., Zaharoff, D.A., Hance, K.W., Patel, A.C., Perkins, S.N., Schlom, J., Greiner, J.W., and Hursting, S.D. (2008) Energy restriction and exercise differentially enhance components of systemic and mucosal immunity in mice. *J Nutr* **138**, 115–22.

106. Arthur, J.R., McKenzie, R.C., and Beckett, G.J. (2003) Selenium in the immune system. *J Nutr* **133**, 1457s–59s.

107. Broome, C.S., McArdle, F., Kyle, J.A.M., Andrews, F., Lowe, N.M., Hart, C.A., Arthur, J.R., and Jackson, M.J. (2004) An increase in selenium intake improves immune function and poliovirus handling in adults with marginal selenium status. *Am J Clin Nutr* **80**, 154–62.

108. Percival, S.S., Bukowski, J.F., and Milner, J. (2008) Bioactive food components that enhance $\gamma\delta$T cell function may play a role in cancer prevention. *J Nutr* **138**, 1–4.

109. Nantz, M.P., Rowe, C.A., Nieves, C., and Percival, S.S. (2006) Immunity and antioxidant capacity in humans is enhanced by consumption of a dried, encapsulated fruit and vegetable juice concentrate. *J Nutr* **136**, 2606–10.

110. Rowe, C.A., Nantz, M.P., Bukowski, J.F., and Percival, S.S. (2007) Specific formulation of *Camellia sinensis* prevents cold and flu symptoms and enhances $\gamma\delta$T cell function: A randomized, double-blind, placebo-controlled study. *Am Coll Nutr* **26**, 445–52.

111. Presta, M., Dell'Era, P., Mitola, S., Moroni, E., Ronca, R., and Rusnati, M. (2005) Fibroblast growth factor/fibroblast growth factor receptor system in angiogenesis. *Cytokine Growth Factor Rev* **16**, 159–78.

112. Albini, A., Tosetti, F., Benelli, R., and Noonan, D.M. (2005) Tumor inflammatory angiogenesis and chemoprevention. *Cancer Res* **65**, 10637–41.

113. Pfeffer, U., Ferrari, N., Morini, M., Benelli, R., Noonan, D.M., and Albini, A. (2003) Antioangiogenic activity of chemopreventive drugs. *Int J Biol Markers* **18**, 70–74.

114. Cockett, M.I., Murphy, G., Birch, M.L., O'Connell, J.P., Crabbe, T., Millican, A.T., Hart, I.R., and Docherty, A.J. (1998) Matrix metalloproteinases and metastatic cancer. *Biochem Soc Symp* **63**, 295–313.

115. Ii, M., Yamamoto, H., Adachi, Y., Maruyama, Y., and Shinomura, Y. (2006) Role of matrix metalloproteinase-7 (matrilysin) in human cancer invasion, apoptosis, growth and angiogenesis. *Exp Biol Med* **231**, 20–27.

116. Bisacchi, D., Benelli, R., Vanzetto, C., Ferrari, N., Tosetti, F., and Albini, A. (2003) Antiangiogenesis and angioprevention: Mechanisms, problems and perspectives. *Cancer Detect Prev* **27**, 229–38.

117. Westermarck, J., and Kahari, V.M. (1999) Regulation of matrix metalloproteinase expression in tumor invasion. *FASEB J* **13**, 781–92.

118. Singh, R.P., and Agarwal, R. (2007) Inducible nitric oxide synthase-vascular endothelial growth factor axis: A potential target to inhibit tumor angiogenesis by dietary agents. *Curr Cancer Drug Targets* **7**, 475–83.

119. Bhat, T.A., and Singh, R.P. (2008) Tumor angiogenesis – a potential target in cancer chemoprevention. *Food Chem Toxicol* **46**, 1334–45.

120. Dulak, J. (2005) Nutraceuticals as anti-angiogenic agents: Hopes and reality. *J Physiol Pharmacol* **56**, 51–69.

121. Mukherjee, P., Sotnikov, A.V., Mangian, H.J., Zhou, J.R., Visek, W.J., and Clinton, S.K. (1999) Energy intake and prostate tumor growth, angiogeneis, and vascular endothelial growth factor expression. *J Natl Cancer Inst* **91**, 512–23.

122. Mukherjee, P., Al-Abbadi, M.M., Kasperzyk, J.L., Ranes, M.K., and Seyfried, T.N. (2002) Dietary restriction reduces angiogenesis and growth in an orthotopic mouse brain tumour model. *Br J Cancer* **86**, 1615–21.

123. Powolny, A.A., Wang, S., Carlton, P.S., Hoot, D.R., and Clinton, S.K. (2008) Interrelationships between dietary restriction, the IGF-1 axis, and the expression of vascular endothelial growth factor by prostate adenocarcinoma in rats. *Mol Carcinog* **47**, 458–65.

124. El-Bayoumy, K., and Sinha, R. (2005) Molecular chemoprevention by selenium: A genomic approach. *Mutat Res* **591**, 224–36.

125. Prima, V., Tennant, M., Gorbatyuk, O.S., Muzyczka, N., Scarpace, P.J., and Zolotkhin, S. (2004) Differential modulation of energy balance by leptin, ciliary neurotrophic factor, and leukemia inhibitory factor gene delivery: Microarray deoxyribonucleic acid-chip analysis of gene expression. *Endocrinology* **145**, 2035–45.

126. Zakharkin, S.O., Kim, K., Mehta, T., Chen, L., Barnes, S., and Scheirer, K.E. (2005) Sources of variation in Affymetrix microarray experiments. *BMC Bioinformatics* **6**, 214.

4 Nutrigenetics: The Relevance of Polymorphisms

Susan E. McCann, Michelle R. Roberts, Mary E. Platek, and Christine B. Ambrosone

Key Points

1. Nutrigenetics has been defined as "an integrated framework that simultaneously examines genetics and associated polymorphisms with diet-related diseases" and may lead to a better understanding of how diet may influence cancer risk.
2. Nutrigenetics enables us to better understand mechanisms of action of numerous food components in relation to cancer risk, and to better clarify risk relationships by focusing on those most likely to be impacted based upon genetics.
3. Single nucleotide polymorphisms (SNP) can change the structure, function, and cellular content of a specific protein. If the SNPs are harbored in genes involved in the metabolism of drugs, environmental agents, or dietary components, then they may greatly affect how an individual responds to specific exposures.
4. Fruits and vegetables are sources of many bioactive food components that possess anticarcinogenic properties, and the intake of specific bioactive components found in fruits and vegetables modulate the relationship between genetic variants and cancer risk.
5. Individuals with defective endogenous protection from oxidative stress may benefit from dietary antioxidants. Conversely, the intake of fruits and vegetables may have little impact on cancer risk in subjects with higher endogenous antioxidant potential.
6. It should be noted that regardless of one's genotype a balanced diet high in fruits, vegetables, and whole grains and low in meat and fats may be beneficial for overall health and well-being and prevention of numerous diseases other than cancer.

Key Words: Nutrigenetics; polymorphisms; oxidative stress; diet; prevention

1. INTRODUCTION

Although experimental studies provide insights into how specific macronutrients and micronutrients may affect the carcinogenic process, it is through epidemiologic studies that associations between dietary components and specific cancers may be inferred, and risk estimates calculated. Following strong leads from epidemiologic studies, clinical

From: *Nutrition and Health: Bioactive Compounds and Cancer*
Edited by: J.A. Milner, D.F. Romagnolo, DOI 10.1007/978-1-60761-627-6_4,
© Springer Science+Business Media, LLC 2010

prevention trials may be conducted to determine if specific food components do, in fact, reduce risk of cancer or surrogate endpoints, such as polyps as a precursor of colorectal cancer. However, despite work in the last decades to better understand associations between diet and cancer risk, results for many cancers remain inconsistent, and findings from association studies are often not validated in intervention studies.

Difficulties in clearly defining risk relationships, if they exist, between bioactive compounds and cancer risk are often attributed to methodological issues. There is likely a good degree of misclassification of dietary intake with the use of Food Frequency Questionnaires (FFQs), which are most often used in epidemiologic studies to ascertain usual patterns of consumption. It is also possible that assessment of current or recent diet does not capture the most important, relevant periods in life, which may be earlier in the carcinogenic process in cancers with a long latency period. Other study considerations likely play a role, including bias in selection of cases and controls, differences in time periods between dietary assessment and cancer in cohort studies, and most importantly, sample size and statistical power.

Inconsistencies in results, however, may also occur because of the heterogeneity of study populations, in that not all individuals respond in the same way to similar exposures or to foods consumed. In the pharmaceutical field, it is known that some individuals may have "allergies" to certain drugs, which is actually a reaction due to metabolic differences in drug activation and detoxification. This field of pharmacogenetics has led the FDA to include label warnings for specific drugs, indicating that dose should be adjusted based on the genetic makeup of the patient. This field was later extended to studying interactions between the environment and genetics, "ecogenetics," and more recently to understanding how genetics influence the interaction between dietary intake and cancer risk. Nutrigenetics has been defined as "an integrated framework that simultaneously examines genetics and associated polymorphisms with diet-related diseases" *(1)* and may lead to a better understanding of how diet may influence cancer risk. In this chapter, we will first review the concept of genetic variability, and then discuss how it influences the response to specific dietary components, including fruits and vegetables, meats, and phytoestrogens.

1.1. One Size Does Not Fit All

Except for monozygotic twins, no two individuals look exactly the same, and the majority of this heterogeneity is due to genetic makeup. Similarly, there are common differences between biologic and biochemical processes in individuals due to variations in DNA coding. The human genome is comprised of millions of base pairs of nucleotides in various reading frames of four basic nucleotides: adenine, cytosine, guanine, and thymine (Fig. 1). The order in which these nucleotides occur determines which proteins will be synthesized and, more importantly, the level of expression and protein stability. Inherited single nucleotide substitutionsin a part of the gene that encodes a protein, such as a cytosine instead of a guanine (Fig. 2), are called single nucleotide polymorphisms (SNPs), and can change the structure, function, or amount of the protein that is made.

The discovery of numerous commonly occurring SNPs in most genes has led to investigations of how these genetic variants may affect cancer risk. If the SNPs are in genes

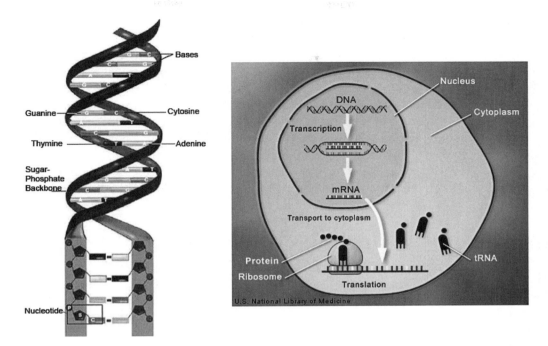

Fig. 1. DNA structure, and translation into proteins.

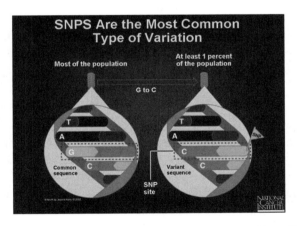

Fig. 2. A G to C substitution single nucleotide polymorphism (SNP).

that are important in the metabolism of drugs, environmental agents, or dietary components, then they may greatly affect how an individual responds to specific exposures, putting some groups at greater risk than others. For example, certain populations may consist of individuals whose genetic makeup requires different levels of antioxidants, as well as those whose endogenous antioxidant capabilities are high. Blending these groups of heterogeneous individuals may mask potential relationships between consumption of fruits and vegetables and cancer risk. Similarly, certain populations may be particularly susceptible to potential carcinogens formed during cooking of meats at high temperatures, based upon how they metabolize those carcinogens or how well their DNA repair capabilities function to compensate for DNA-damaging agents. However, the association between meat consumption and cancer risk may not be detectable if these individuals are clustered within groups whose genetic background does not put them at risk. The field of nutrigenetics may be useful for separating out those groups that are most susceptible or can most benefit from intake of specific food components and allow for better estimation of risk among strata of the entire population. If associations between cancer and bioactive compounds are examined based on genotypic differences, it may become clear whether intake of a specific nutrient increases or decreases cancer risk for certain subgroups. Below we apply this concept to a number of food components and nutrients.

2. FRUIT AND VEGETABLE CONSUMPTION AND CANCER RISK

Consumption of fruits and vegetables has been proposed to reduce the risk of a number of cancers. However, for many tumor types results are not consistent. A recent publication by the World Cancer Research Fund and the American Institute for Cancer Research (2) reported there is no "convincing" evidence that the intake of fruits and vegetables decreases cancer risk. The same report noted that there is "probable" evidence that foods containing lycopene and selenium reduce risk of prostate cancer; that non-starchy vegetables reduces the risk of cancers of the mouth, pharynx, larynx, esophagus, and stomach; and that intake of fruits reduces the risk of cancers of the mouth, pharynx, larynx, esophagus, lung, and stomach. Fruits and vegetables are sources of many bioactive food components likely to possess anticarcinogenic properties. In this section, we discuss how intake of specific components of fruits and vegetables modulates the potential relationships between diet, genetic variants, and cancer risk.

2.1. Cruciferous Vegetables, SNPs in Metabolic Enzymes, and Cancer Risk

Based upon experimental data supporting a role in carcinogenesis for compounds found in cruciferous vegetables, such as precursors of isothiocyanates (ITCs), potential associations have been evaluated in relation to a number of cancer sites. Because ITC metabolites are excreted in the urine, thus exposing urinary bladder cells to their effects in urine, cruciferous vegetable intake has been evaluated in two cohort studies of bladder cancer. In the Health Professionals Follow-up Study (HPFS) (3), cruciferae were the only vegetable group associated with decreased risk of bladder cancer, with the strongest associations noted for broccoli and cabbage. However, in the ATBC study (4), an intervention trial among male smokers, no associations were reported between risk and intake of cruciferous vegetables. We recently showed that consumption of cruciferous vegetables decreased risk of bladder cancer, with strongest relationships detected among higher consumers of raw vegetables (5). This association is biologically plausible since the strength of isothiocyanates is reduced when cruciferous vegetables are heated.

Somewhat consistent findings have been noted for prostate cancer. In one cohort and three case–control studies, including our own analysis in the Western New York Diet

Study *(6)*, associations were noted between higher intake of cruciferous vegetables and decreased risk *(7–9)*, although other studies observed no effect *(10, 11)*. In the HPFS *(12)* a weak, non-significant inverse association between intake of cruciferous vegetable and prostate cancer risk was observed. However, the inverse association was strengthened when analyses were restricted to men who received PSA screening tests.

In the EPIC study, no associations were noted between intake of cruciferous vegetables and risk of breast cancer *(13)*. Conversely, the Pooling Project *(14)* reported inverse, non-significant associations between risk of breast cancer and high intake of broccoli and Brussels sprouts. These findings were replicated in a large case–control study in Sweden *(15)*. We also found that consumption of cruciferous vegetables, particularly broccoli, was marginally inversely associated with breast cancer risk in premenopausal women *(16)*. In the Shanghai Breast Cancer Study *(17)*, urinary levels of ITCs were inversely associated with breast cancer risk among both premenopausal and postmenopausal women.

Genetic variability in metabolic pathways may explain some of the inconsistencies in relationships between cruciferous vegetable consumption and cancer risk. The metabolism of ITCs involves four polymorphic genes in the mercapturic acid pathway: glutathione transferase (GST), γ-glutamyltranspeptidase (γ-GT), cysteinylglycinase (CG), and *N*-acetyltransferase (NAT). The bioavailability of ITCs depends upon their clearance by these metabolic enzymes. Furthermore, ITCs are potent inhibitors of phase I and inducers of phase II enzymes, such as glutathione S-transferases (GSTs). The induction of phase II enzymes could lead to more efficient excretion of reactive intermediates of phase I metabolism.

Most of the research that examined the associations between intake of cruciferous vegetables, genetic polymorphisms, and cancer risk have focused on the role of GSTs. Lin et al. *(18)* reported an inverse association between broccoli consumption and risk of colorectal adenomas. This was attributed to genotypes null for *GST*M1. In a colon cancer study *(19)*, high consumers with GSTM1 null genotypes had a two-thirds reduction in risk, while GSTM1 present genotypes were associated with reduced risk regardless of diet. In a Chinese study, risk of colorectal cancer was also lowest among those individuals with *GSTM1* and *GSTT1* null genotypes and high dietary ITCs *(20)*.

The detoxifying effects of GSTs may play an important role in the risk of lung cancer, where carcinogen exposure is a known risk factor. London and colleagues *(21)* found that individuals with detectable urinary ITCs were at decreased risk of lung cancer. The risk was lowest among those individuals who carried deletions in *GSTM1* and *GSTT1*. These associations were also observed in a large case–control study in Europe *(22)*. Conversely, a study by Spitz et al. *(23)* found that the risk was *greatest* among those individuals who were null for GST and consumed low levels of ITCs. Among higher consumers of ITCs, risk was greater for GST null individuals than those with GST present genotypes. Similarly, in a large case–control study *(24)*, higher cruciferous vegetable intake reduced lung cancer risk only among those with *GSTM1* present genotypes. Among non-smoking women in China, however, the strongest inverse association between intake of ITC and lung cancer risk was seen in individuals with *GSTM1* and *GSTT1* null genotypes *(25)*.

There are also inconsistencies in the breast cancer literature. In the Western New York Diet Study, an inverse relationship was observed between cruciferous vegetable intake and risk of breast cancer, but polymorphisms in *GSTM1* and *GSTT1* did not modify risk relationships *(16)*. However, in the Long Island Breast Cancer Study Project (LIBCSP), women who had *GSTA1* genotypes related to lower activity and who consumed lower levels of cruciferous vegetables were at significantly increased risk *(26)*. Similar relationships were noted in the Shanghai Breast Cancer Study for the *GSTP1* genotype *(27)*. In contrast, no associations were observed in the LIBCSP study between breast cancer risk, intake of cruciferous vegetables, and *GSTM1, GSTT1*, and *GSTP1* polymorphisms *(28)*.

The impact of polymorphisms in other genes in ITC metabolic pathways have yet to be extensively examined in relation to cruciferous vegetable intake and cancer risk. In one study of bladder cancer, Zhao and colleagues *(29)* found that inverse relationships between intake of cruciferous vegetables and bladder cancer risk were not modified by polymorphisms in *GSTM1, GSTT1*, or *NAT2*.

Inconsistencies between these molecular epidemiologic studies could be attributed to study design issues or to chance. However, GST genotypes encode for enzymes that are highly inducible by numerous exposures and processes and participate in extremely complex pathways. Thus, associations for one cancer site may vary from those for another, and other exposures that are also substrates for GSTs may impact risk relationships. This biochemical complexity in studying the effects of genetic variants in metabolic pathways cannot be oversimplified. Epidemiologic research needs to develop approaches to comprehensively account for phenotypic effects of genetic polymorphisms. Nonetheless, it can be concluded from the majority of these analyses that cruciferous vegetables are likely to play an important role in cancer prevention, the strength of which may be dependent to some extent upon exposure to other carcinogens and genotypes for GSTs, as well as other metabolic enzymes.

2.2. Dietary Antioxidants, Genetics of Oxidative Stress, and DNA Repair

Experimental evidence from in vitro and in vivo studies indicates that dietary antioxidants are likely to play a role in the prevention of breast cancer. However, epidemiological studies have not consistently found inverse associations between risk of several cancers and fruit and vegetable consumption, or specific dietary antioxidants. It is possible that variability in endogenous antioxidant capabilities, resulting from genetic variants in enzymes that generate or neutralize reactive oxygen species (ROS), may alter the needs of individuals for dietary antioxidants. For example, individuals with less endogenous protection from oxidative stress may require greater protection from dietary antioxidants. Conversely, the intake of fruits and vegetables may have little impact on cancer risk in individuals with higher endogenous antioxidant capabilities.

Our group has been investigating this hypothesis for the last several years, with focused attention on the pathway of reduction of superoxide radicals. As shown in Fig. 3, superoxide radicals can be reduced through superoxide dismutase (SOD), resulting in production of hydrogen peroxide (H_2O_2), a weak ROS. The enzyme catalase (CAT) breaks down H_2O_2 into H_2O and oxygen gas (O_2). Gluthathione peroxide (GPX)

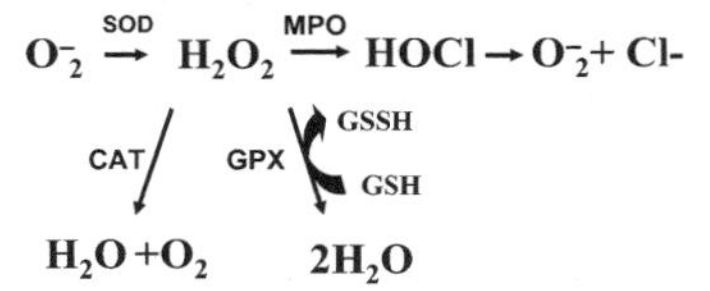

$$O_2^- \xrightarrow{\text{SOD}} H_2O_2 \xrightarrow{\text{MPO}} HOCl \rightarrow O_2^- + Cl-$$

$$H_2O + O_2 \qquad 2H_2O$$

Fig. 3. Illustration of conversion of superoxide to either greater reactive species through myeloperoxidase, or reduced by catalase or glutathione peroxidase.

performs a similar function. However, H_2O_2 is also a substrate for myeloperoxidase (MPO), which in the presence of chloride anion (Cl^-) generates the cytotoxic hypochlorous acid (HOCl). It is likely that genetic variants in any of these enzymes will alter the ultimate levels of ROS, which in turn may affect the endogenous antioxidant potential and needs for dietary antioxidants.

Manganese superoxide dismutase (MnSOD) is synthesized in the cytosol and post-transcriptionally modified for transport into the mitochondria. There is a structural mutation in the gene, a T to C substitution in the mitochondrial targeting sequence, which changes an amino acid in the signal peptide resulting in better transport of MnSOD into mitochondria. We first showed that women with CC genotypes were at significantly higher risk of breast cancer than those with A alleles, but the risk associated with the CC genotypes was greatly reduced by higher consumption of dietary fruits and vegetables *(30)*. A number of groups subsequently investigated this hypothesis in relation to breast cancer, with many noting associations between MnSOD variants particularly in relation to a low antioxidant environment. Results of the Nurses' Health Study suggested that C alleles were associated with increased risk only in women who were smokers at the time of enrollment into the cohort *(31)*. The same study reported that *MnSOD* variants increased risk among women who also had low-activity genotypes for *GPx (32)*. In the Shanghai Breast Cancer Study, C alleles were associated with a slight increase in risk, which was strongest among women who were low consumers of fruits and vegetables *(33)*, consistent with our earlier findings. In a large German study of breast cancer, there were no main effects for *MnSOD* polymorphisms, nor was there significant modification by diet or smoking. However, women with C alleles who were higher consumers of alcohol had greater risk than those with T alleles who did not drink *(34)*. In the Carolina Breast Cancer Study, there were greater than additive effects for *MnSOD* genotypes and smoking and radiation to the chest, with a reduction in risk with the use of non-steroidal anti-inflammatory drugs (NSAIDs) *(35)*. However, no associations were reported between breast cancer risk and *MnSOD* genotypes in relation to antioxidant or prooxidant exposure in the LIBCSP *(36)*.

Relationships between *MnSOD* genotypes and oxidative stress-related exposures have also been examined in relation to prostate cancer. In the ATBC Study, C alleles for *MnSOD* were associated with increased risk of high-grade tumors, but there was no modification by α-tocopherol supplementation *(37)*. The Physicians' Health Study reported a lower risk of prostate cancer among men with A alleles and high selenium, lycopene, and α-tocopherol levels *(38)*, similar to our findings for breast cancer. Similar associations were also noted in the HPFS *(39)*, the Prostate, Lung, Colorectal, and

Ovarian Cancer Screening Trial *(40)*, and the CARET study *(41)*. These results confirm the important role of genetics in modifying relationships between diet and cancer risk.

Myeloperoxidase (MPO), an antibacterial agent released by neutrophils, is found in breast tissue and milk. There is a G to A polymorphism in the 5′ upstream region of the MPO gene causing greater transcription in the G allele carriers due to disruption of the binding site. In the LIBCSP, we found that the low activity A alleles were associated with more than a 2.0-fold reduction in risk of premenopausal breast cancer. Importantly, the reduction in risk was confined to those individuals who were higher consumers of fruits and vegetables *(42)*. These results were replicated in the Nurses' Health Study, which reported reduced risk with *MPO* A alleles only among higher consumers of fruits and vegetables and those individuals with the highest level of plasma carotenoids, a good surrogate marker for fruit and vegetable consumption *(43)*. We recently evaluated MPO genotypes and breast cancer risk in the context of oxidant and antioxidant exposures in the American Cancer Society cohort and noted similar, but nonsignificant findings *(44)*.

An alternate pathway for H_2O_2 conversion is through reduction by CAT or GPX. A few studies have evaluated polymorphisms in CAT and GPX as potential modifiers of relationships between diet and cancer risk. We assessed the role of both genes in the LIBCSP. We found no associations between *GPX1* and risk, nor any significant modification by dietary intake of fruits and vegetables *(45)*. In the same study, we noted a slight reduction of breast cancer risk for women with low-activity CAT genotypes *(46)*. Importantly, there was notable modification of relationships by dietary intake of fruits and vegetables, with significant risk reduction limited to those with high dietary consumption. To our knowledge, this was the first published study that examined the impact of dietary habits and variants in *GPX1* or *CAT* on risk of breast cancer.

One factor involved in repair of oxidative DNA damage is XRCC1 *(47)*. In a small case–control study of prostate cancer in North Carolina, the intake of lycopene significantly reduced risk only among men with Arg/Arg polymorphisms in XRCC1, with no effects among men with Gln alleles. Similar associations were seen for plasma levels of α-tocopherol and β-carotene *(48)*. Similar relationships were noted for XRCC1 codon 194 Arg to Trp polymorphisms and dietary antioxidants and breast cancer risk in the LIBCSP *(49)*. In the Nurses' Health Study, this polymorphism was also associated with decreased risk of breast cancer, with a significant interaction with plasma carotene levels *(50)*. XRCC1 gene polymorphisms were also evaluated in relation to lung cancer risk, and individuals with the Arg194Trp allele were at lower risk, particularly if they had higher serum levels of α-tocopherol and retinol *(51)*. These studies clearly illustrate the complex interactions between endogenous and exogenous antioxidants and polymorphisms in DNA repair genes. Importantly, they demonstrate that genetic heterogeneity dilutes relationships between dietary antioxidants and cancer risk when all populations are taken together, regardless of relevant genotypes.

2.3. Folate and Folate Metabolism

Folate refers to compounds that have nutritional properties similar to those of folic acid and are found naturally in foods and biological tissues *(52)*. Folic acid is a water-soluble B vitamin rarely found in nature. It is the most common synthetic form of the vitamin, more bioavailable than natural folates, and is the form used in fortified food products, supplements, and drugs *(52)*. The bioavailability of natural folate in food varies greatly as biochemically reduced forms of folate are labile and easily oxidized *(52)*. It is estimated that folate bioavailability from a mixed diet is only about 50% *(52)*. High-quality food sources of folate include fresh green vegetables such as spinach, Brussels sprouts, broccoli, asparagus, and turnip greens. Additionally, legumes, lentils, and fruits (especially strawberries and oranges) are good sources of folate *(52)*.

Folate-dependent intermediary metabolism, also referred to as one-carbon metabolism, is a series of biochemical reactions necessary for the synthesis of purines and pyrimidines, the compounds that are the backbone of nucleic acids. These reactions are also required for the formation of S-adenosylmethionine (SAM), important for the methylation of substrates including RNA, protein, and DNA *(53)*. Other nutrients such as choline, methionine, and vitamin B12 can supply or transport methyl groups, but only folate is capable of de novo generation of one-carbon groups *(54)*.

A consistent body of epidemiologic evidence supports the preventive role of adequate folate status to sustain nucleotide synthesis and decrease mutations in replicating tissues *(55)*. Epidemiological studies have reported inverse associations for colorectal cancer among those with high folate intake *(56)*. Accordingly, inadequate folate status was associated with increased risk for cancer of the cervix, brain, pancreas, lung, prostate, breast, esophagus, and blood *(57–60)*. It is important to note here that folate is considered a "double-edged sword" in that supraphysiological levels of folate due to extreme folate supplementation at different times during the carcinogenic process may negatively affect risk for cancer or survival. Here, we focus on inadequate or adequate body folate status based on median values of control populations for either dietary and/or supplemental intake, blood levels, or plasma and/or red blood cell folate levels, for which normal physiological levels have been defined for the United States population.

Alcohol consumption may affect folate status by altering the absorption, activation, and storage of folate, as well as affecting dietary intake of folate-rich foods. Alcohol directly affects internal folate metabolism and results in a reduction of serum folate levels and tissue supply *(61)*. Furthermore, high levels of acetaldehyde, a by-product of alcohol metabolism, induce cleavage of folate at the C9–N10 bond *(62)*. Epidemiological studies provide evidence that low folate status due to high alcohol intake increases the risk of breast cancer *(55)*.

Folate metabolism is complex and numerous genes are involved in one-carbon metabolism. Polymorphisms of genes involved in folate metabolism may influence cancer risk (Fig. 4). Several gene variants have been evaluated in epidemiologic studies, but the best-studied folate related gene is the rate limiting enzyme methylenetetrahydrofolate reductase (MTHFR). *MTHFR* is a ubiquitous cytosolic enzyme that catalyzes the irreversible reduction of 5, 10-methylenetetrahydrofolate (CH2-THF) to 5-methyltetrahydrofolate (CH3-THF) *(63)*. CH3-THF is the most abundant form of circulating folate. Therefore, *MTHFR* is important for the maintenance of adequate intracellular levels of folate *(63)*. *MTHFR*'s substrate, CH2-THF, is found primarily within cells and is important for de novo purine synthesis and maintenance of the deoxynucleotide pool required for DNA synthesis *(63, 64)*. *MTHFR* plays a key role in

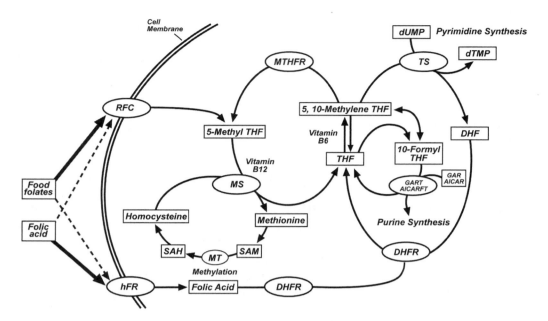

Fig. 4. Schematic drawing of one-carbon metabolism TTCC *(179).*

one-carbon metabolism by redirecting one-carbon moieties from nucleic acid synthesis to production of methionine and methylation reactions *(63, 64).*

A well-studied polymorphism of the MTHFR gene (677 C to T) causes an amino acid change from alanine to valine. The 677 variant heterozygotes (CT) and homozygotes (TT) have, respectively, 65 and 30% enzyme activity compared with the common variant (CC) *(65).* In a cross-sectional examination of folate intake within the Nurses' Health Study, plasma folate and homocysteine concentrations were investigated by *MTHFR* genotype status. An inverse association between plasma folate and homocysteine was modified by the *MTHFR*677 genotype (p for interaction = 0.05) *(66).*

To date, there are a number of research studies reporting on the interaction of folate and *MTHFR* 677 in relation to colorectal cancer risk. Chen et al. from the HPFS reported that folate, as part of the dietary methyl supply, was critical for those with the TT variant genotype of MTHFR 677 *(67).* In the Physicians' Health Study, Ma et al. reported that men with the TT variant of MTHFR 677 and adequate folate levels had a decreased risk for colorectal cancer (OR=0.32, CI=0.15–0.68) compared to those individuals with wild-type (CC) or heterozygote (CT) genotype. At a decreased level of folate, this change in risk was diminished *(68).* Studies examining colon cancer outcomes have shown that those with the TT variant and higher intakes of folate had a decreased risk of either adenomatous polyps or carcinoma. However, those with the variant genotype and a lower intake of folate had an increased risk of adenomas *(19, 69–72).*

There have been several other epidemiological investigations of the potential association of the MTHFR C677T genetic polymorphism, diet and risk for other cancers. Chen et al. examined the *MTHFR* C677T polymorphism within the LIBCSP and found that the 677TT genotype was associated with an increased risk (OR=1.37;

CI=1.06–1.78), which was most pronounced in women with the lowest intake of dietary folate *(73)*. Lin et al. reported a 3.0-fold increase in risk of bladder cancer among those with the *MTHFR* 677CT or TT genotypes and low dietary folate intake compared to those with the CC genotypes and high dietary intake of folate *(74)*. Additionally, Goodman et al. demonstrated that women with the *MTFHR* 677CT or TT genotype and lower folate intake had an increased risk for cervical cancer that was 2.0- to 3.0-fold higher than women with the CC genotypes and folate intake above the median *(75)*.

Folate is an excellent example of a bioactive nutrient and a well-known genetic polymorphism that together impact cancer risk, with the combined effects altering risk estimates beyond that which would be expected. The influence of this interaction on cancer risk estimates may differ depending on the type of cancer, the variance in dietary intake, the use of folic acid supplements (amount and recent or lifetime use), and the amount of alcohol consumption (amount and recent or lifetime use). Furthermore, risk estimates can differ based on the limitations of the epidemiological study design. Nonetheless, the *MTHFR* C677T polymorphism and folate intake interaction is biochemically plausible and shows a fairly reliable relationship with cancer that is supported by animal and in vitro studies.

3. PHYTOESTROGENS AND HORMONE METABOLISM PATHWAYS

Phytoestrogens are naturally occurring polyphenolic compounds ubiquitous in plant foods *(76)*. Although a number of polyphenols have been shown to have phytoestrogenic activities, phytoestrogens are generally grouped into three main classes: isoflavones, coumestans, and lignans. Isoflavones include genistein and daidzein, among others, and are found predominantly in soybeans and soy products. Non-soy legumes also contribute isoflavones. Coumestans are found in bean sprouts, refried beans, and pinto beans. The richest source of lignans is flaxseed; additional sources include other seeds, whole grains, vegetables, and fruits.

Because of the structural similarities of phytoestrogens to estradiol, early research focused on the hormonal aspects of these compounds in cancer etiology *(76)*. In addition to antioxidant, antiangiogenic, and antiproliferative effects, phytoestrogens have been shown to have estrogenic activities in vitro and in vivo. However, phytoestrogens may also act as antiestrogens either through competition for the estrogen receptor or through modification of steroid hormone metabolism.

Several phytoestrogens have been shown to be metabolized by, as well as to modify, the activity of enzymes in the CYP450 family *(77)*. In experimental studies, genistein, quercetin, and resveratrol (polyphenols) have been shown to decrease both transcription and activity of CYP1A1 and CYP1B1, two enzymes involved in the metabolism and clearance of estrogens *(78)*. Catechol-*O*-methyl transferase, which catalyzes the *O*-methylation of estrogens to catechol estrogens, is inhibited by quercetin *(79)* and most likely by other flavonoids. Probably the best known inhibitory target of phytoestrogens is CYP19 (aromatase), which catalyzes the conversion of androgens to estradiol *(80)*. Another important enzyme in estrogen biosynthesis, 17β-hydroxysteroid dehydrogenase, is inhibited by isoflavones, flavones, coumestrol, and lignans *(81–83)*.

Steroid sulfatase, an enzyme that hydrolyzes estrone sulfate to estradiol and dehy-droepiandrosterone sulfate to DHEA, can be inhibited by several flavonoids includ-ing quercetin and daidzein. Isoflavones inhibit sulfotransferases (SULT1E1, SULT1A1) *(84, 85)*.

Of relevance to breast cancer and possibly prostate and colon cancer, several phytoe-strogens have been shown to affect the expression of estrogen receptor-α (ERα) and estrogen receptor-β (ERβ) *(80)*. Although the binding affinity of phytoestrogens for the ER is weak relative to that of estradiol, individuals consuming large amounts of phytoestrogens (e.g., vegetarians, herbal supplement users) could conceivably achieve pharmacologic levels that compete with endogenous estrogens for the ER. The relative expression of ERalpha and ERbeta may be modified by differences in concentration of available substrate.

Epidemiologic studies investigating the role of phytoestrogens in the etiology of cancers of the breast *(86)*, prostate *(87)*, and colon/rectum *(88)* have often produced inconsistent findings. Some of these inconsistencies may be due to interactions between genetic variations and exposure to phytoestrogens.

3.1. Genetic Variation in Hormone Metabolizing Genes and Response to Phytoestrogen Exposure

Circulating levels of endogenous steroid hormones and other cancer-related biomark-ers can be affected by genetic variation in genes responsible for their metabolism. Given the accumulating evidence establishing that many of these genes can be either inhibited or upregulated by dietary phytoestrogens, it is becoming increasingly recognized that these exposures might have differential effects depending upon an individual's genetic makeup.

Several observational as well as experimental studies have investigated phytoestrogen–gene interactions. A randomized, double-blind, placebo-controlled, crossover dietary intervention trial with 117 healthy postmenopausal women investi-gated the effect of soy isoflavones on several parameters including plasma total, HDL, and LDL cholesterol, triglycerides, lipoprotein(a), glucose, insulin, and the homeostasis model of insulin resistance. These measurements and other related biomarkers were assessed in conjunction with SNPs in several related genes including ERα (*Xba*I and *Pvu*II), ERβ (*Alu*I), ERβ(cx), endothelial nitric oxide synthase (eNOS), apolipoprotein E (*Apo E2, E3*, and *E4*), cholesteryl ester transfer protein (CETP) (*Taq*IB), and leptin receptor *(17)*. The impact of equol producer status on these relationships was also investigated. Although the intervention had no impact on any of the biomarkers examined in the study, there was a statistically significant difference in response to isoflavones supplementation for HDL cholesterol among women who had the ERβ(cx) *Tsp*509I AA genotype, but not GG or GA.

In a separate study, 205 women ranging from 49 to 65 years of age and with high breast density were randomly assigned to either an isoflavones supplement or placebo for 1 year *(89)*. The goal of this study was to assess the effect of the isoflavones sup-plementation on changes in breast density, serum estradiol, follicle stimulating hor-mone (FSH), luteinizing hormone (LH), menopausal symptoms, and lymphocyte tyrosine kinase activity. Results of this study showed no difference between supplement and placebo for changes in breast density overall but did observe a significant interaction between the supplementation group and the ER *PvuII* polymorphism for change in breast density. Although both the placebo and the supplementation groups had reduced density from baseline to postintervention, isoflavone-supplemented women with the TT genotype tended to show very little decrease over time, whereas all other groups and genotypes showed decreases averaging from 3 to 10%. No interactions were observed for polymorphisms in *CYP17* or *CYP19*. A borderline significant interaction between *CYP19* polymorphism and FSH was observed across treatment groups, with decreases in FSH for all groups except for the isoflavone-supplemented women carrying the *CYP19* GG allele.

In a moderate-sized clinical trial among 132 postmenopausal women consuming 10 g/day ground flaxseed (a rich source of phytoestrogen lignans) for 7 days, urinary hydroxyestrone metabolism was shown to vary by polymorphisms in *CYP1B1* (Leu432Val) and *COMT* (Val158Met) *(90)*. Whereas there was little effect of genotype on hydroxyestrone metabolism at baseline, in the supplementation group with flaxseed the 2-hydroxyestrone:16α-hydroxyestrone ratio increased with increasing numbers of variant alleles for *COMT*, and especially for *CYP1B1*. These findings provide support that many hormone-related genes may modify the effect of dietary phytoestrogen on estrogen metabolism.

A number of cross-sectional investigations have been conducted using data and samples from the European Prospective Investigation of Cancer and Nutrition (EPIC). Studies by Low et al. *(91)* with 125 women participating in EPIC and Nutrition-Norfolk documented that urinary excretion of isoflavones was negatively correlated with plasma estradiol, especially among postmenopausal women with the CC genotype for the ESR1 *PvuII* polymorphism *(91)*. In 2006, these investigators extended their studies to include 1,988 healthy postmenopausal women participating in EPIC-Norfolk. Results of these investigations revealed that SHBG levels were positively associated with urinary isoflavones excretion, especially among women with the N variant of the SHBG D356N polymorphism *(92)*. Finally, Low et al. *(93)* reported that urinary excretion of lignans was positively associated with plasma SHBG and negatively associated with plasma testosterone. They also reported that equol, a metabolite of soy isoflavones, was negatively associated with plasma estradiol. Importantly, significant interactions were observed between polymorphisms in the estrogen receptor 1 (ESR-1) and lignans, whereas women with the GG or GA, but not AA, genotypes had lower estrone levels in association with higher excretion of lignans. Also reported was an interaction between isoflavones excretion and NR1I2-6 (*nuclear receptor subfamily 1, group I, member 2 gene*) polymorphism. For women with the AA genotype there was a positive association between isoflavones excretion and estrone levels, whereas for women with the GG genotype this study revealed a positive association between isoflavones excretion and estradiol levels.

Similarly, Low et al. *(94)* demonstrated that among 267 men in EPIC-Norfolk polymorphisms in *CYP19* modified the associations between serum and urinary phytoestrogens and plasma androgens. Both urinary and serum equol were associated with plasma testosterone among men with the TT genotype, but not the CC or CT genotypes, for the CYP19 3′untranslated region (UTR) T-C polymorphism. Similar associations were shown for urinary and serum enterolactone associations with testosterone.

3.2. Genetic Variation, Phytoestrogen Exposure, and Disease Risk

Only a few studies have investigated the combined effect of genetic variation and intake of phytoestrogens on cancer outcome. Two case–control studies have demonstrated a modifying effect of *CYP17* polymorphism on the association between dietary lignan intakes and breast cancer *(95, 96)*. Among 207 women with breast cancer and 188 controls in Western New York, breast cancer risk was greatly reduced for premenopausal women with at least one *CYP17* A2 allele in the highest tertile of dietary lignan intake *(95)*. Piller et al. reported a similar interaction in a larger study of 267 premenopausal women with breast cancer and 573 age-matched population controls. In this study, lignan exposure was expressed as levels of plasma enterolactone and dietary intake. Only in A2A2 carriers, both plasma enterolactone and dietary intake were inversely related to breast cancer risk *(96)*.

Interactions between genes and phytoestrogens have been investigated for prostate cancer as well. In a nested case–control study among participants in EPIC-Norfolk, prospectively collected biomarkers and dietary data were examined to study the association between genetic variations in a number of steroid hormone metabolizing genes and risk of prostate cancer *(97)*. The relatively small study included 89 men who had developed prostate cancer after enrollment into EPIC and 178 men without prostate cancer. Isoflavones and lignans were measured in spot urine and serum samples, and dietary intake calculated from food diaries and a food frequency questionnaire. Prostate cancer risk was elevated for men with the CC vs. TT genotype for the estrogen receptor I *Pvu*II polymorphism, but no association was observed for prostate cancer risk and phytoestrogen exposure, nor were there interactions between genotype and phytoestrogens.

On the other hand, a much larger case–control study involving 1,314 prostate cancer patients and 782 controls reported an interaction between dietary phytoestrogens and genetic variation in association with risk of prostate cancer *(98)*. In this population-based case–control study conducted in Sweden, carriers of the variant allele of a promoter SNP in the ERβ gene (ESR2) had strongly reduced prostate cancer risks with increasing intakes of total phytoestrogens, isoflavonoids, and coumestrol, but these associations were not observed in men with the common alleles. These findings are not necessarily contradictory to those of Low et al. ERβ is highly expressed in the prostate, and phytoestrogens tend to bind more strongly to ERβ compared to ERα. Additional studies are necessary to fully delineate how these interactions modulate the risk of prostate cancer.

Finally, two studies have investigated phytoestrogen–gene interactions in endometrial cancer. In the Shanghai Endometrial Cancer Study, 1,204 endometrial cancer cases and 1,212 community controls provided blood samples and information on dietary intakes of usual soy food intake *(99)*. Daily intakes of soy protein and soy isoflavones were calculated from the food frequency questionnaire, and genotyping for two polymorphisms (rs2676530 and rs605059) in *17β-HSD1* was performed using Taq-Man assays. *17β-HSD1*, which is inhibited by isoflavones, is an enzyme that catalyzes the conversion of estrone to estradiol. No associations with endometrial cancer were observed for the rs2676530 polymorphism, but women with at least one A allele of the rs605059 polymorphism had a 20% lower risk of endometrial cancer compared to those with the GG genotype. Furthermore, among premenopausal carriers of at least one A allele of rs605059, those women in the highest tertile of soy intake had a 60% reduction in endometrial cancer risk compared with women in the lowest tertile of intake. No interactions between genotype and isoflavones intake were observed among postmenopausal women.

In a separate study, several polymorphisms in *CYP19A1* were examined in association with soy food and tea consumption in the Shangai Endometrial Cancer Study *(100)*. In this study, higher intakes of soy foods and tea were both inversely associated with endometrial cancer risk. There was no interaction between soy intake and SNPs in any of the *CYP19A1* polymorphisms examined, but several SNPs modified the association between endometrial cancer and tea consumption. Tea contains high levels of polyphenols which have been shown to inhibit aromatase activity *(101)*.

4. MEAT CONSUMPTION, GENETICS, AND CANCER RISK

Conflicting epidemiological evidence exists between meat consumption and risk of colon, breast, and prostate cancers. Consumption of processed meat products has been associated with an increased risk of developing colorectal cancer in prospective studies *(102–104)*, but the role of red meat intake in cancer etiology is less well known, with studies reporting both positive *(102, 105)* and no associations *(103)*. Two meta-analyses concluded that greater consumption of meat was associated with increased risk of breast cancer (OR=1.17, 95% CI 1.06–1.29; OR=1.18 95% CI 1.06–1.32) *(106, 107)*. While case–control studies have yielded conflicting results *(108, 109)*, prospective studies have generally found no associations between meat consumption and breast cancer risk *(110–112)*, except for one study in which meat consumption was associated with increased risk of ER-positive breast cancer *(113)*. Red and processed meat consumption has also been positively associated with risk of prostate cancer in prospective and case–control studies *(105, 114–118)*. Reasons for the inconsistencies observed in these studies include variations in study design, sample size, measurement of dietary exposures, biases relating to exposure recall or participant selection, and genetic variability in xenobiotic metabolizing enzymes.

Cooking of meats such as chicken, beef, pork, and fish results in the formation of several mutagens and carcinogens including heterocyclic amines (HCAs), nitrosamines (NAs), and polycyclic aromatic hydrocarbons (PAHs). The most prevalent HCA found in meats is 2-amino-1-methyl-6-phenylimidazo[4,5-b]-pyridine (PhIP). Following metabolic activation, PhIP, along with other HCAs, causes the production of DNA adducts and is carcinogenic in rat colon, mammary, and prostate tissues *(119–121)*. In rodents and cell lines, PhIP has been shown to stimulate signaling pathways resulting in increased cellular proliferation *(119, 120, 122, 123)*.

4.1. Heterocyclic Amines, Genetics, and Cancer Risk

Heterocyclic amines are metabolized through an oxidation reaction catalyzed by cytochrome p450 enzymes including CYP1A2, and to a lesser extent, by CYP1A1, 1B1, and 3A4 *(124, 125)*. The oxidized molecules are then acetylated by the two isozymes of N(O)-acetyltransferase, NAT1 and NAT2, or sulfated by sulfotransferases (SULT) *(126)*. The acetylated products can undergo spontaneous hydrolysis to form arylnitrenium ions, which can covalently bind DNA to form DNA adducts that may increase the risk of mutagenesis and subsequent development of cancer *(126–132)*. Genetic polymorphisms exist for cytochrome p450, NAT, and SULT *(133)*. Therefore, cancer risk related to metabolism of HCA may differ based on genotype.

Because meat consumption is an accepted risk factor for colorectal cancer, a number of studies have evaluated the role of HCAs in the etiology of this type of tumor. One prospective study of *NAT* genotype, red meat intake, and colorectal cancer risk in men found that neither *NAT1* nor *NAT2* genotype was independently related to risk of colorectal cancer. However, there was an association between red meat intake and colorectal cancer among men who were rapid acetylators at either the *NAT1* or *NAT2* locus *(134)*. Three case–control studies have demonstrated an increased risk of colorectal cancer among those individuals with the *NAT2* rapid acetylator genotypes who consume well-done meat *(122, 135, 136)*. In one study, this association was limited to ever-smokers *(136)*. A recent study revealed positive associations between colorectal cancer and *NAT1*, but not *NAT2*, genotype for increased consumption of HCAs, estimated using an exposure index that accounted for frequency of consumption, cooking method, and level of doneness of meat *(137)*. This finding is consistent with an earlier study that found a 6.0-fold increase in risk of colorectal adenoma among *NAT1* rapid acetylators (OR=6.50; 95% CI 2.16–19.6) with daily consumption of greater than 27 ng of one type of HCA, 2-amino-3,8-dimethylimidazo[4,5-f]quinoxaline (MeIQx) *(138)*. Two case–control studies have demonstrated an increased risk of colorectal cancer among those subjects with the CYP1A2 rapid metabolizing phenotype who consume meat cooked well done *(122, 136)*. Additionally, an analysis of six single nucleotide polymorphisms in the *CYP1A2, CYP2E1, CYP1B1*, and *CYP2C9* genes found that three allelic variant combinations were associated with increased risk of colorectal cancer with higher red meat consumption *(137)*.

Case–control studies have yielded conflicting results concerning the relationships between *NAT1* genotype, HCA consumption, and breast cancer risk. Two studies found an increased risk of breast cancer among carriers of the *NAT1* rapid acetylator genotype who consumed high levels of red meat or meat cooked well done *(140, 141)*. Conversely, two separate studies failed to find similar relationships *(108, 109)*. Likewise, results of case–control studies examining *NAT2* genotype have been equivocal. Four studies have revealed no associations between *NAT2* genotype, risk of breast cancer, and meat intake or meat doneness *(109, 142–144)*. Two case–control studies, however, found an increased risk of breast cancer among women with the *NAT2* rapid or intermediate acetylator genotype who consumed higher levels of red meat or meat cooked well done *(108, 145)*.

Human prostate tissue has been demonstrated to metabolically activate heterocyclic amines formed when meat is cooked *(146)*. In rats, PhIP has been shown to produce PhIP-DNA adducts and prostate tumors *(147)*. Consumption of grilled red meats has been associated with higher levels of PhIP-DNA adduct levels *(148)*. One prospective study linked data from a meat-cooking preferences questionnaire to a database estimating intake of benzo[a]pyrene, MeIQx, 2-amino-3,4,8-trimethylimidazo[4,5-f]quinoxaline (DiMeIQx), and PhIP. An intake of greater than 10 g/day of very well-done meat was associated with increased risk of prostate cancer. The highest quintile of PhIP intake was also associated with increased risk, although intake of MeIQx or DiMeIQx was not *(149)*. While *NAT1* and *NAT2* genotypes have been associated with increased risk of prostate cancer *(150)*, a case–control study examining intake of MeIQx and PhIP found no association between prostate cancer and either *NAT1* or *NAT2* acetylator genotypes *(151)*. In humans, mutagenicity testing of HCAs has indicated that N-hydroxy-PhIP is activated specifically by SULT1A1 *(152)*. Transcripts of SULT1A1 have been found in prostate tissue *(153)*. A polymorphism in *SULT1A1* has been associated with increased *N*-hydroxy-PhIP DNA adduct catalytic activity *(154)*. This polymorphism was not associated with prostate cancer in a small population *(155)*, but a larger study found that both *SULT1A1* genotype and enzymatic activity increased the risk of prostate cancer *(156)*.

4.2. Nitrosamines and Colorectal Cancer

Nitrosamines are activated by cytochrome p450 enzymes. CYP2E1 catalyzes the α-hydroxylation of many types of nitrosamines to activate and allow them to bind to DNA *(157)*. The intake of processed meats, an important source of nitrosamines, has been associated with an increased risk of colorectal cancer *(158)*. Polymorphisms in *CYP2E1* have been associated with increased risk of colorectal cancer *(159, 160)*. Conversely, a case–control study reported no evidence of an association between *CYP2E1* genotype, red or processed meat consumption, and risk of colorectal cancer. However, there was an increased risk of rectal cancer for those individuals with high intake of red or processed meat and the high-activity *CYP2E1* genotype *(161)*. The enzyme CYP2A6 has also been shown to metabolize nitrosamines and is overexpressed in colorectal cancers *(162)*. Nevertheless, to date, there have been no studies that investigated potential interactions of CYP2A6 with meat consumption and risk of colorectal cancer.

4.3. Polycyclic Aromatic Hydrocarbons and Breast Cancer

PAHs are known carcinogens in humans, have been shown to cause mammary tumors in rodents *(163)*, and form PAH-DNA adducts in human breast cells *(164)*. Exposure to these compounds has been linked to development of postmenopausal breast cancer *(165)*, and levels of PAH-DNA adducts have been associated with risk of breast cancer *(166–168)*. PAHs are metabolized by cytochrome p450 and GST enzymes (GSTM-1 and GSTT-1) *(169, 170)*. Studies have generally concluded there is no association between polymorphisms in these GST genes and risk of breast cancer *(171–175)*, although one study found that the GSTM1 null genotype was predictive of PAH-DNA adduct levels in breast tissue *(176)*. While one case–control study concluded there was no relationship between GSTM1 or GSTT1 null genotypes, meat consumption, and risk of breast cancer *(109)*, another study found an increased risk among women with either null genotype who consumed meats consistently well or very well done *(177)*.

5. CONCLUSIONS

The above examples illustrate the complex relationships between dietary factors and cancer risk, and the importance of consideration of genetic makeup in assessing risk relationships in epidemiologic studies. Nutrigenetics enables us to better understand mechanisms of action of numerous food components in relation to cancer risk, and to better clarify risk relationships by focusing on those most likely to be impacted based upon genetics. However, we do not believe that nutrigenetics is a doorway to individualized genotyping for risk assessment and dietary counseling. First, the biochemistry underlying gene–diet interactions is complex. For example, we measured the activity of catalase in red blood cells in several hundred healthy controls and noted clear dose–response relationships between phenotype and genotype of the CAT promoter polymorphism *(178)*. However, these relationships between phenotype and genotype varied based on fruits and vegetables consumption. As shown in Fig. 5, for those with *CAT* genotypes that confer higher enzyme activity (CC), geometric means for CAT activity in units/mg hemoglobin in each tertile of consumption were very similar (118.9, 117.0, 115.0 for tertiles 1, 2, and 3, respectively). However, among those with low-activity genotypes (CT and TT), CAT levels were highest among those with low consumption, with decreasing levels with increasing tertiles of fruit and vegetable consumption (93.0, 78.0, and 74.7 for tertiles 1, 2, and 3, respectively). These data indicate that there are feedback mechanisms involved and that, in a high endogenous antioxidant environment, the effects of dietary antioxidants on oxidative balance may be minimal. However, if there is lower consumption of dietary antioxidants, there may be compensation through activation of endogenous enzyme systems. Therefore, genotyping may reveal only part of an intricate picture. Furthermore, because so little is known about relation-

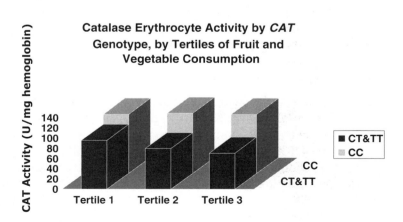

Fig. 5. Tertiles of fruit and vegetable consumption.

ships between SNPs, diet, and cancer risk, extrapolation of research data to individual risk assessment remains difficult.

Finally, it should be noted that regardless of one's genotype a balanced diet high in fruits, vegetables, and whole grains and low in meat and fats may be beneficial for over-all health and well-being and prevention of numerous diseases in addition to cancer. Thus, although applying genetics to studies of diet and cancer will help us to refine relationships and understand mechanisms and may, in the future, identify those individuals whose needs are greater for specific nutrients or food components, the public health message of consumption of a healthy diet should not be influenced by knowledge of one's genetic makeup.

REFERENCES

1. Davis, C.D., and Milner, J. (2004) Frontiers in nutrigenomics, proteomics, metabolomics and cancer prevention. *Mutat Res* **551**, 51–64.
2. American Institute for Cancer Research. (2007) World Cancer Research Fund. Food, Nutrition, Physical Activity, and the Prevention of Cancer: A Global Perspective. Washington, DC: American Institute for Cancer Research.
3. Michaud, D.S., Spiegelman, D., Clinton, S.K., Rimm, E.B., Willett, W.C., and Giovannucci, E.L. (1999) Fruit and vegetable intake and incidence of bladder cancer in a male prospective cohort. *J Natl Cancer Inst* **91**, 605–13.
4. Michaud, D.S., Pietinen, P., Taylor, P.R., Virtanen, M., Virtamo, J., and Albanes, D. (2002) Intakes of fruits and vegetables, carotenoids and vitamins A, E, C in relation to the risk of bladder cancer in the ATBC cohort study. *Br J Cancer* **87**, 960–65.
5. Tang, L., Zirpoli, G.R., Guru, K., Moysich, K.B., Zhang, Y., Ambrosone, C.B., and McCann, S.E. (2008) Consumption of raw cruciferous vegetables is inversely associated with bladder cancer risk. *Cancer Epidemiol Biomarkers Prev* **17**, 938–44.
6. Joseph, M.A., Moysich, K.B., Freudenheim, J.L., Shields, P.G., Bowman, E.D., Zhang, Y., Marshall, J.M., and Ambrosone, C.B. (2004) Cruciferous vegetables, genetic polymorphisms in glutathione S-transferases M1 and T1, and prostate cancer risk. *Nutr Canc* **50**, 206–13.
7. Cohen, J.H., Kristal, A.R., and Stanford, J.L. (2000) Fruit and vegetable intakes and prostate cancer risk. *J Natl Cancer Inst* **92**, 61–68.
8. Jain, M.G., Hislop, G.T., Howe, G.R., and Ghadirian, P. (1999) Plant foods, antioxidants, and prostate cancer risk: Findings from case, control studies in Canada. *Nutr Canc* **34**, 173–84.
9. Schuurman, A.G., Goldbohm, R.A., Dorant, E., and Van Den Brandt, P.A. (1998) Vegetable and fruit consumption and prostate cancer risk: A cohort study in the Netherlands. *Cancer Epidemiol Biomarkers Prev* **7**, 673–80.
10. Le Marchand, L., Hankin, J.H., Kolonel, L.N., and Wilkens, L.R. (1991) Vegetable and fruit consumption in relation to prostate cancer risk in Hawaii: A reevaluation of the effect of dietary beta-carotene. *Am J Epidemiol* **133**, 215–19.
11. Villeneuve, P.J., Johnson, K.C., Kreiger, N., Mao, Y., Paulse, B., Dewar, R., Dryer, D., Whittaker, H., Robson, D., Fincham, S., and Le, N. (1999) Risk factors for prostate cancer: Results from the Canadian National Enhanced Cancer Surveillance System. *Cancer Causes Control* **10**, 355–67.
12. Giovannucci, E., Rimm, E.B., Liu, Y., Stampfer, M.J., and Willett, W.C. (2003) A prospective study of cruciferous vegetables and prostate cancer. *Cancer Epidemiol Biomarkers Prev* **12**, 1403–09.
13. Van Gils, C.H., Peeters, P.H.M., Bueno-de-Mesquita, H.B., Boshuizen, H.C., Lahmann, P.H., Clavel-Chapelon, F., Thiébaut, A., Kesse, E., Sieri, S., Palli, D., Tumino, R., Panico, S., Vineis, P., Gonzalez, C.A., Ardanaz, E., Sánchez, M.-J., Amiano, P., Navarro, C., Quirós, J.R., Key, T.J., Allen, N., Khaw, K.-T., Bingham, S.A., Psaltopoulou, T., Koliva, M., Trichopoulou, A., Nagel, G., Linseisen, J.,

Boeing, H., Berglund, G., Wirfält, E., Hallmans, G., Lenner, P., Overvad, K., Tjønneland, A., Olsen, A., Lund, E., Engeset, D., Alsaker, E., Norat, T., Kaaks, R., Slimani, N., and Riboli, E. (2005) Consumption of vegetables and fruits and risk of breast cancer. *J Am Med Assoc* **293**, 183–93.

14. Smith-Warner, S.A., Spiegelman, D., Yaun, S.-S., Adami, H.-O., Beeson, W.L., Van Den Brandt, P.A., Folsom, A.R., Fraser, G.E., Freudenheim, J.L., Goldbohm, R.A., Graham, S., Miller, A.B., Potter, J.D., Rohan, T.E., Speizer, F.E., Toniolo, P., Willett, W.C., Wolk, A., Zeleniuch-Jacquotte, A., and Hunter, D.J. (2001) Intake of fruits and vegetables and risk of breast cancer: A pooled analysis of cohort studies. *J Am Med Assoc* **285**, 769–76.

15. Terry, P., Wolk, A., Persson, I., Magnusson, C., Smith-Warner, S.A., Willett, W.C., Spiegelman, D., and Hunter, D. (2001) Brassica vegetables and breast cancer risk [3]. *J Am Med Assoc* **285**, 2975–77.

16. Ambrosone, C.B., McCann, S.E., Freudenheim, J.L., Marshall, J.R., Zhang, Y., and Shields, P.G. (2004) Breast Cancer Risk in Premenopausal Women Is Inversely Associated with Consumption of Broccoli, a Source of Isothiocyanates, but Is Not Modified by GST Genotype. *J Nutr* **134**, 1134–38.

17. Hall, W.L., Vafeiadou, K., Hallund, J., Bugel, S., Reimann, M., Koebnick, C., Zunft, H.-F., Ferrari, M., Branca, F., Dadd, T., Talbot, D., Powell, J., Minihane, A.-M., Cassidy, A., Nilsson, M., Dahlman-Wright, K., Gustafsson, J.-Å., and Williams, C.M. (2006) Soy-isoflavone-enriched foods and markers of lipid and glucose metabolism in postmenopausal women: Interactions with genotype and equol production. *Am J Clin Nutr* **83**, 592–600.

18. Lin, H.J., Probst-Hensch, N.M., Louie, A.D., Kau, I.H., Witte, J.S., Ingles, S.A., Frankl, H.D., Lee, E.R., and Haile, R.W. (1998) Glutathione transferase null genotype, broccoli, and lower prevalence of colorectal adenomas. *Cancer Epidemiol Biomarkers Prev* **7**, 647–52.

19. Slattery, M.L., Kampman, E., Samowitz, W., Caan, B.J., and Potter, J.D. (2000) Interplay between dietary inducers of GST and the GSTM-1 genotype in colon cancer. *Int J Cancer* **87**, 728–33.

20. Seow, A., Yuan, J.-M., Sun, C.-L., Van Den Berg, D., Lee, H.-P., and Yu, M.C. (2002) Dietary isothiocyanates, glutathione S-transferase polymorphisms and colorectal cancer risk in the Singapore Chinese Health Study. *Carcinogenesis* **23**, 2055–61.

21. London, S.J., Yuan, J.-M., Chung, F.-L., Gao, Y.-T., Coetzee, G.A., Ross, R.K., and Yu, M.C. (2000) Isothiocyanates, glutathione S-transferase M1 and T1 polymorphisms, and lung-cancer risk: A prospective study of men in Shanghai, China. *Lancet* **356**, 724–29.

22. Brennan, P., Hsu, C.C., Moullan, N., Szeszenia-Dabrowska, N., Lissowska, J., Zaridze, D., Rudnai, P., Fabianova, E., Mates, D., Bencko, V., Foretova, L., Janout, V., Gemignani, F., Chabrier, A., Hall, J., Hung, R.J., Boffetta, P., and Canzian, F. (2005) Effect of cruciferous vegetables on lung cancer in patients stratified by genetic status: A mendelian randomisation approach. *Lancet* **366**, 1558–60.

23. Spitz, M.R., Duphorne, C.M., Detry, M.A., Pillow, P.C., Amos, C.I., Lei, L., De Andrade, M., Gu, X., Hong, W.K., and Wu, X. (2000) Dietary intake of isothiocyanates: Evidence of a joint effect with glutathione S-transferase polymorphisms in lung cancer risk. *Cancer Epidemiol Biomarkers Prev* **9**, 1017–20.

24. Wang, L.I., Giovannucci, E.L., Hunter, D., Neuberg, D., Su, L., and Christiani, D.C. (2004) Dietary intake of Cruciferous vegetables, Glutathione S-transferase (GST) polymorphisms and lung cancer risk in a Caucasian population. *Cancer Causes Control* **15**, 977–85.

25. Zhao, B., Seow, A., Lee, E.J.D., Poh, W.-T., Teh, M., Eng, P., Wang, Y.-T., Tan, W.-C., Yu, M.C., and Lee, H.-P. (2001) Dietary isothiocyanates, glutathione S-transferase -M1, -T1 polymorphisms and lung cancer risk among Chinese women in Singapore. *Cancer Epidemiol Biomarkers Prev* **10**, 1063–67.

26. Ahn, J., Gammon, M.D., Santella, R.M., Gaudet, M.M., Britton, J.A., Teitelbaum, S.L., Terry, M.B., Neugut, A.I., Eng, S.M., Zhang, Y., Garza, C., and Ambrosone, C.B. (2006) Effects of glutathione S-transferase A1 (GSTA1) genotype and potential modifiers on breast cancer risk. *Carcinogenesis* **27**, 1876–82.

27. Lee, S.-A., Fowke, J.H., Lu, W., Ye, C., Zheng, Y., Cai, Q., Gu, K., Gao, Y.-T., Shu, X.-O., and Zheng, W. (2008) Cruciferous vegetables, the GSTP1 Ile105Val genetic polymorphism, and breast cancer risk. *Am J Clin Nutr* **87**, 753–60.

28. Steck, S.E., Gaudet, M.M., Britton, J.A., Teitelbaum, S.L., Terry, M.B., Neugut, A.I., Santella, R.M., and Gammon, M.D. (2007) Interactions among GSTM1, GSTT1 and GSTP1 polymorphisms, cruciferous vegetable intake and breast cancer risk. *Carcinogenesis* **28**, 1954–59.

29. Zhao, H., Lin, J., Grossman, H.B., Hernandez, L.M., Dinney, C.P., and Wu, X. (2007) Dietary isothiocyanates, GSTM1, GSTT1, NAT2 polymorphisms and bladder cancer risk. *Int J Cancer* **120**, 2208–13.

30. Ambrosone, C.B., Freudenheim, J.L., Thompson, P.A., Bowman, E., Vena, J.E., Marshall, J.R., Graham, S., Laughlin, R., Nemoto, T., and Shields, P.G. (1999) Manganese superoxide dismutase (MnSOD) genetic polymorphisms, dietary antioxidants, and risk of breast cancer. *Cancer Res* **59**, 602–06.

31. Tamimi, R.M., Hankinson, S.E., Spiegelman, D., Colditz, G.A., and Hunter, D.J. (2004) Manganese superoxide dismutase polymorphism, plasma antioxidants, cigarette smoking, and risk of breast cancer. *Cancer Epidemiol Biomarkers Prev* **13**, 989–96.

32. Cox, D.G., Tamimi, R.M., and Hunter, D.J. (2006) Gene x Gene interaction between MnSOD and GPX-1 and breast cancer risk: A nested case-control study. *BMC Cancer* **6**, 217.

33. Cai, Q., Shu, X.O., Wen, W., Cheng, J.R., Dai, Q., Gao, Y.T., and Zheng, W. (2004) Genetic polymorphism in the manganese superoxide dismutase gene, antioxidant intake, and breast cancer risk: Results from the Shanghai Breast Cancer Study. *BCR* **6**, R647–R55.

34. Slanger, T.E., Chang-Claude, J., and Wang-Gohrke, S. (2006) Manganese superoxide dismutase Ala-9Val polymorphism, environmental modifiers, and risk of breast cancer in a German population. *Cancer Causes Control* **17**, 1025–31.

35. Millikan, R.C., Player, J., de Cotret, A.R., Moorman, P., Pittman, G., Vannappagari, V., Tse, C.K., and Keku, T. (2004) Manganese superoxide dismutase Ala-9Val polymorphism and risk of breast cancer in a population-based case-control study of African Americans and whites. *BCR* **6**, R264–R74.

36. Gaudet, M.M., Gammon, M.D., Santella, R.M., Britton, J.A., Teitelbaum, S.L., Eng, S.M., Terry, M.B., Bensen, J.T., Schroeder, J., Olshan, A.F., Neugut, A.I., and Ambrosone, C.B. (2005) MnSOD Val-9Ala genotype, pro- and anti-oxidant environmental modifiers, and breast cancer among women on Long Island, New York. *Cancer Causes Control* **16**, 1225–34.

37. Woodson, K., Tangrea, J.A., Lehman, T.A., Modali, R., Taylor, K.M., Snyder, K., Taylor, P.R., Virtamo, J., and Albanes, D. (2003) Manganese superoxide dismutase (MnSOD) polymorphism, α-tocopherol supplementation and prostate cancer risk in the Alpha-Tocopherol, Beta-Carotene Cancer Prevention Study (Finland). *Cancer Causes Control* **14**, 513–18.

38. Li, H., Kantoff, P.W., Giovannucci, E., Leitzmann, M.F., Gaziano, J.M., Stampfer, M.J., and Ma, J. (2005) Manganese superoxide dismutase polymorphism, prediagnostic antioxidant status, and risk of clinical significant prostate cancer. *Cancer Res* **65**, 2498–504.

39. Mikhak, B., Hunter, D.J., Spiegelman, D., Platz, E.A., Wu, K., Erdman, J.W., Jr, and Giovannucci, E. (2008) Manganese superoxide dismutase (MnSOD) gene polymorphism, interactions with carotenoid levels, and prostate cancer risk. *Carcinogenesis* **29**(12), 2335–40.

40. Kang, D., Lee, K.-M., Sue, K.P., Berndt, S.I., Peters, U., Reding, D., Chatterjee, N., Welch, R., Chanock, S., Huang, W.-Y., and Hayes, R.B. (2007) Functional variant of manganese superoxide dismutase (SOD2 V16A) polymorphism is associated with prostate cancer risk in the prostate, lung, colorectal, and ovarian cancer study. *Cancer Epidemiol Biomarkers Prev* **16**, 1581–86.

41. Choi, J.-Y., Neuhouser, M.L., Barnett, M.J., Hong, C.-C., Kristal, A.R., Thornquist, M.D., King, I.B., Goodman, G.E., and Ambrosone, C.B. (2008) Iron intake, oxidative stress-related genes (MnSOD and MPO) and prostate cancer risk in CARET cohort. *Carcinogenesis* **29**, 964–70.

42. Ahn, J., Gammon, M.D., Santella, R.M., Gaudet, M.M., Britton, J.A., Teitelbaum, S.L., Terry, M.B., Neugut, A.I., Josephy, P.D., and Ambrosone, C.B. (2004) Myeloperoxidase genotype, fruit and vegetable consumption, and breast cancer risk. *Cancer Res* **64**, 7634–39.

43. He, C., Tamimi, R.M., Hankinson, S.E., Hunter, D.J., and Han, J. (2008) A prospective study of genetic polymorphism in MPO, antioxidant status, and breast cancer risk. *Breast Canc Res Treat* 1–10.

44. Li, Y., Hong, C.-C., McCullough, M.J., Ahn, J., Stevens, V.L., Thun, M.J., and Ambrosone, C.B. Oxidative stress-related genotypes, fruit and vegetable consumption and breast cancer risk. In review.

45. Ahn, J., Gammon, M.D., Santella, R.M., Gaudet, M.M., Britton, J.A., Teitelbaum, S.L., Terry, M.B., Neugut, A.I., and Ambrosone, C.B. (2005) No association between glutathione peroxidase Pro198Leu polymorphism and breast cancer risk. *Cancer Epidemiol Biomarkers Prev* **14**, 2459–61.

46. Ahn, J., Gammon, M.D., Santella, R.M., Gaudet, M.M., Britton, J.A., Teitelbaum, S.L., Terry, M.B., Nowell, S., Davis, W., Garza, C., Neugut, A.I., and Ambrosone, C.B. (2005) Associations between breast cancer risk and the catalase genotype, fruit and vegetable consumption, and supplement use. *Am J Epidemiol* **162**, 943–52.

47. Vodicka, P., Kumar, R., Stetina, R., Sanyal, S., Soucek, P., Haufroid, V., Dusinska, M., Kuricova, M., Zamecnikova, M., Musak, L., Buchancova, J., Norppa, H., Hirvonen, A., Vodickova, L., Naccarti, A., Matousu, Z., and Hemminki, K. (2004) Genetic polymorphisms in DNA repair genes and possible links with DNA repair rates, chromosomal aberrations and single-strand breaks in DNA. *Carcinogenesis* **25**, 757–63.

48. Goodman, M., Bostick, R.M., Ward, K.C., Terry, P.D., Van Gils, C.H., Taylor, J.A., and Mandel, J.S. (2006) Lycopene intake and prostate cancer risk: Effect modification by plasma antioxidants and the XRCC1 genotype. *Nutr Canc* **55**, 13–20.

49. Shen, J., Gammon, M.D., Terry, M.B., Wang, L., Wang, Q., Zhang, F., Teitelbaum, S.L., Eng, S.M., Sagiv, S.K., Gaudet, M.M., Neugut, A.I., and Santella, R.M. (2005) Polymorphisms in XRCC1 modify the association between polycyclic aromatic hydrocarbon-DNA adducts, cigarette smoking, dietary antioxidants, and breast cancer risk. *Cancer Epidemiol Biomarkers Prev* **14**, 336–42.

50. Han, J., Hankinson, S.E., De Vivo, I., Spiegelman, D., Tamimi, R.M., Mohrenweiser, H.W., Colditz, G.A., and Hunter, D.J. (2003) A Prospective Study of XRCC1 Haplotypes and Their Interaction with Plasma Carotenoids on Breast Cancer Risk. *Cancer Res* **63**, 8536–41.

51. Ratnasinghe, D.L., Yao, S.X., Forman, M., Qiao, Y.L., Andersen, M.R., Giffen, C.A., Erozan, Y., Tockman, M.S., and Taylor, P.R. (2003) Gene-environment interactions between the codon 194 polymorphism of XRCC1 and antioxidants influence lung cancer risk. *Anticancer Res* **23**, 627–32.

52. Groff, J., Gropper, S., and Smith, D. (2009) Advanced Nutrition and Human Metabolism. Belmont: Wadsworth.

53. Bailey, L., and Gregory, J. (1999) Folate metabolism and requirements. *J Nutr* **129**, 779–82.

54. Jacob, R. (2000) Folate, DNA methylation, and gene expression: Factors of nature and nurture. *Am J Clin Nutr* **72**, 903–4.

55. Ulrich, C. (2007) Folate and cancer prevention: A closer look at a complex picture. *Am J Clin Nutr* **86**, 271–73.

56. Sanjoaquin, M., Allen, N., Cuoto, E., Roddam, A., and Key, T. (2005) Folate intake and colorectal cancer risk: A meta-analytical approach. *Int J Cancer* **113**(5), 825–28.

57. Kim, Y. (1999) Folate and carcinogenesis: Evidence, mechanisms and implications. *J Nutr Biochem* **10**, 66–88.

58. Heijmans, B., Boer, J., Suchiman, H., Cornelisse, C. et al. (2003) A common variant of the methylenetetrahydrofolate reductase gene (1p36) is associated with an increased risk of cancer. *Cancer Res* **63**, 1249.

59. Zhang, S., Willett, W., Selhub, J., Hunter, D., Giovannucci, E., Holmes, M., Colditz, G., and Hankinson, S. (2003) Plasma folate, vitamin B6, vitamin B12, homocysteine, and risk of breast cancer. *J Natl Cancer Inst* **95**, 373–80.

60. Ziegler, R., Weinstein, S., and Fears, T. (2002) Nutritional and genetic inefficiencies in one-carbon metabolism and cervical cancer risk. *J Nutr* **132**, 2345S.

61. Steinberg, S., Campbell, C., and Hillman, R. (1980) The toxic effects of alcohol on folate metabolism. *Clin Toxicol* **17**, 407–11.

62. Shaw, S., Jayatileke, E., Herbert, V., and Colman, N. (1989) Cleavage of folates during ethanol metabolism: Role of acetaldehyde/xanthine oxidase-generated superoxide. *Biochem J* **257**, 277–80.

63. Bailey, L., and Gregory, J. (1999) Polymorphisms of methylenetetrahydrofolate reductase and other enzymes: Metabolic significance, risks and impact on folate requirement. *J Nutr* **129**, 919–22.

64. Schwahn, B., and Rozen, R. (2001) Polymorphisms in the methylenetetrahydrofolate reductase gene. *Am J Pharmacogenomics* **1**, 189–201.

65. Rozen, R. (1997) Genetic predisposition to hyperhomocysteinemia:deficiency of methylenetetrahydrofolate reductase (MTHFR). *Thromb Haemost* **78**, 523–26.

66. Chiuve, S.E., Giovannucci, E.L., Hankinson, S.E., Hunter, D.J., Stampfer, M.J., Willett, W.C., and Rimm, E.B. (2005) Alcohol intake and methylenetetrahydrofolate reductase polymorphism

modify the relation of folate intake to plasma homocysteine. *Am J Clin Nutr* **82**, 155–62.

67. Chen, J., Giovannucci, E., Kelsey, K., Rimm, E., Stampfer, M., Colditz, G. et al. (1996) A methylenetetrahydrofolate reductase polymorphism and the risk of colorectal carcinoma. *Cancer Res* **56**, 4862.

68. Ma, J., Stampfer, M., Giovannucci, E. et al. (1997) Methylenetetrahydrofolate reductase polymorphism, dietary interactions and risk of colorectal cancer. *Cancer Res* **57**, 1098.

69. Ulrich, C., Kampman, E., Bigler, J. et al. (1999) Colorectal adenomas and the C677T MTHFR polymorphism: Evidence for gene-environment interaction? *Cancer Epidemiol Biomarkers Prev* **8**, 659–68.

70. Levine, A., Siegmund, K., Ervin, C. et al. (2000) The methylenetetrahydrofolate reductase C677T polymorphism and distal colorectal adenoma risk. *Cancer Epidemiol Biomarkers Prev* **9**, 657–63.

71. Ulvik, A., Evensen, E., Lien, E. et al. (2001) Smoking, folate and methylenetetrahydrofolate reductase status as interactive determinants of adenomatous and hyperplastic polyps of colorectum. *AmJ Med Genet* **101**, 246–54.

72. Le Marchand, L., Donlon, T., Hankan, J. et al. (2002) B-vitamin intake, metabolic genes and colorectal cancer risk (United States). *Cancer Causes Control* **13**, 239–48.

73. Chen, J., Gammon, M., Chan, W., Palomeque, C., Wetmur, J., Kabat, G., Teitelbaum, S., Britton, J., Terry, M., Neugut, A., and Santella, R. (2005) One-carbon metabolism, MTHFR polymorphisms, and risk of breast cancer. *Cancer Res* **65**, 1606–14.

74. Lin, J., Spitz, M., Wang, Y., Schabath, M. et al. (2004) Polymorphisms of folate metabolic genes and susceptibility to bladder cancer: A case-control study. *Carcinogenesis* **25**, 1639.

75. Goodman, M.T., McDuffie, K., Hernandez, B., Wilkens, L.R. et al. (2001) Association of methylenetetrahydrofolate reductase polymorphism C677T and dietary folate with the risk of cervical dysplasia. *Cancer Epidemio Biomarkers Prev* **10**, 1275.

76. Humfrey, C.D. (1998) Phytoestrogens and human health effects: Weighing up the current evidence. *Nat Toxins* **6**, 51–59.

77. Mense, S.M., Hei, T.K., Ganju, R.K., and Bhat, H.K. (2008) Phytoestrogens and breast cancer prevention: Possible mechanisms of action. *Environ Health Perspect* **116**, 426–33.

78. Moon, Y.J., Wang, X., and Morris, M.E. (2006) Dietary flavonoids: Effects on xenobiotic and carcinogen metabolism. *Toxicol In Vitro* **20**, 187–210.

79. Zhu, B.T., Ezell, E.L., and Liehr, J.G. (1994) Catechol-O-methyltransferase-catalyzed rapid O-methylation of mutagenic flavonoids. Metabolic inactivation as a possible reason for their lack of carcinogenicity in vivo. *J Biol Chem* **269**, 292–99.

80. Rice, S., and Whitehead, S.A. (2008) Phytoestrogens oestrogen synthesis and breast cancer. *J Steroid Biochem Mol Biol* **108**, 186–95.

81. Sanderson, J.T., Hordijk, J., Denison, M.S., Springsteel, M.F., Nantz, M.H., and van den, B.M. (2004) Induction and inhibition of aromatase (CYP19) activity by natural and synthetic flavonoid compounds in H295R human adrenocortical carcinoma cells. *Toxicol Sci* **82**, 70–79.

82. Brooks, J.D., and Thompson, L.U. (2005) Mammalian lignans and genistein decrease the activities of aromatase and 17beta-hydroxysteroid dehydrogenase in MCF-7 cells. *J Steroid Biochem Mol Biol* **94**, 461–67.

83. Makela, S., Poutanen, M., Lehtimaki, J., Kostian, M.L., Santti, R., and Vihko, R. (1995) Estrogen-specific 17 beta-hydroxysteroid oxidoreductase type 1 (E.C. 1.1.1.62) as a possible target for the action of phytoestrogens. *Proc Soc Exp Biol Med* **208**, 51–59.

84. Huang, Z., Fasco, M.J., and Kaminsky, L.S. (1997) Inhibition of estrone sulfatase in human liver microsomes by quercetin and other flavonoids. *J Steroid Biochem Mol Biol* **63**, 9–15.

85. Mesia-Vela, S., and Kauffman, F.C. (2003) Inhibition of rat liver sulfotransferases SULT1A1 and SULT2A1 and glucuronosyltransferase by dietary flavonoids. *Xenobiotica* **33**, 1211–20.

86. Peeters, P.H., Keinan-Boker, L., van der Schouw, Y.T., and Grobbee, D.E. (2003) Phytoestrogens and breast cancer risk. Review of the epidemiological evidence. *Breast Cancer Res Treat* **77**, 171–83.

87. Ganry, O. (2005) Phytoestrogens and prostate cancer risk. *Prev Med* **41**, 1–6.

88. Lechner, D., Kallay, E., and Cross, H.S. (2005) Phytoestrogens and colorectal cancer prevention. *Vitam Horm* **70**, 169–98.

89. Atkinson, C., Warren, R.M., Sala, E., Dowsett, M., Dunning, A.M., Healey, C.S., Runswick, S., Day, N.E., and Bingham, S.A. (2004) Red-clover-derived isoflavones and mammographic breast density: A double-blind, randomized, placebo-controlled trial [ISRCTN42940165]. *BCR* **6**, R170–R79.

90. McCann, S.E., Wactawski-Wende, J., Kufel, K., Olson, J., Ovando, B., Kadlubar, S.N., Davis, W., Carter, L., Muti, P., Shields, P.G., and Freudenheim, J.L. (2007) Changes in 2-hydroxyestrone and 16α-hydroxyestrone metabolism with flaxseed consumption: Modification by COMT and CYP1B1 genotype. *Cancer Epidemiol Biomarkers Prev* **16**, 256–62.

91. Low, Y.-L., Taylor, J.I., Grace, P.B., Dowsett, M., Scollen, S., Dunning, A.M., Mulligan, A.A., Welch, A.A., Luben, R.N., Khaw, K.-T., Day, N.E., Wareham, N.J., and Bingham, S.A. (2005) Phytoestrogen exposure correlation with plasma estradiol in postmenopausal women in European Prospective Investigation of Cancer and Nutrition-Norfolk may involve diet-gene interactions. *Cancer Epidemiol Biomarkers Prev* **14**, 213–20.

92. Low, Y.-L., Dunning, A.M., Dowsett, M., Luben, R.N., Khaw, K.-T., Wareham, N.J., and Bingham, S.A. (2006) Implications of gene-environment interaction in studies of gene variants in breast cancer: An example of dietary isoflavones and the D356N polymorphism in the sex hormone-binding globulin gene. *Cancer Res* **66**, 8980–83.

93. Low, Y.-L., Dunning, A.M., Dowsett, M., Folkerd, E., Doody, D., Taylor, J., Bhaniani, A., Luben, R., Khaw, K.-T., Wareham, N.J., and Bingham, S.A. (2007) Phytoestrogen exposure is associated with circulating sex hormone levels in postmenopausal women and interact with ESR1 and NR1I2 gene variants. *Cancer Epidemiol Biomarkers Prev* **16**, 1009–16.

94. Low, Y.-L., Taylor, J.I., Grace, P.B., Dowsett, M., Folkerd, E., Doody, D., Dunning, A.M., Scollen, S., Mulligan, A.A., Welch, A.A., Luben, R.N., Khaw, K.-T., Day, N.E., Wareham, N.J., and Bingham, S.A. (2005) Polymorphisms in the CYP19 gene may affect the positive correlations between serum and urine phytoestrogen metabolites and plasma androgen concentrations in men. *J Nutr* **135**, 2680–86.

95. McCann, S.E., Moysich, K.B., Freudenheim, J.L., Ambrosone, C.B., and Shields, P.G. (2002) The risk of breast cancer associated with dietary lignans differs by CYP17 genotype in women. *J Nutr* **132**, 3036–41.

96. Piller, R., Verla-Tebit, E., Wang-Gohrke, S., Linseisen, J., and Chang-Claude, J. (2006) CYP17 genotype modifies the association between lignan supply and premenopausal breast cancer risk in humans. *J Nutr* **136**, 1596–603.

97. Low, Y.-L., Taylor, J.I., Grace, P.B., Mulligan, A.A., Welch, A., Scollen, S., Dunning, A.M., Luben, R.N., Khaw, K.-T., Day, N.E., Wareham, N.J., and Bingham, S.A. (2006) Phytoestrogen exposure, polymorphisms in COMT, CYP19, ESR1, and SHBG genes, and their associations with prostate cancer risk. *Nutr Canc* **56**, 31–39.

98. Hedelin, M., Bälter, K.A., Chang, E.T., Bellocco, R., Klint, A., Johansson, J.-E., Wiklund, F., Thellenberg-Karlsson, C., Adami, H.-O., and Grönberg, H. (2006) Dietary intake of phytoestrogens, estrogen receptor-beta polymorphisms and the risk of prostate cancer. *Prostate* **66**, 1512–20.

99. Dai, Q., Xu, W.-H., Long, J.-R., Courtney, R., Xiang, Y.-B., Cai, Q., Cheng, J., Zheng, W., and Shu, X.-Q. (2007) Interaction of soy and 17β-HSD1 gene polymorphisms in the risk of endometrial cancer. *Pharmacogenetics Genom* **17**, 161–67.

100. Xu, W.H., Dai, Q., Xiang, Y.B., Long, J.R., Ruan, Z.X., Cheng, J.R., Zheng, W., and Shu, X.O. (2007) Interaction of soy food and tea consumption with CYP19A1 genetic polymorphisms in the development of endometrial cancer. *Am J Epidemiol* **166**, 1420–30.

101. Way, T.-D., Lee, H.-H., Kao, M.-C., and Lin, J.-K. (2004) Black tea polyphenol theaflavins inhibit aromatase activity and attenuate tamoxifen resistance in HER2/neu-transfected human breast cancer cells through tyrosine kinase suppression. *Eur J Cancer* **40**, 2165–74.

102. Giovannucci, E., Rimm, E.B., Stampfer, M.J., Colditz, G.A., Ascherio, A., and Willett, W.C. (1994) Intake of fat, meat, and fiber in relation to risk of colon cancer in men. *Cancer Res* **54**, 2390–97.

103. Goldbohm, R.A., van den Brandt, P.A., van't Veer, P., Brants, H.A., Dorant, E., Sturmans, F., and Hermus, R.J. (1994) A prospective cohort study on the relation between meat consumption and the risk of colon cancer. *Cancer Res* **54**, 718–23.

104. Gonzalez, C.A., and Riboli, E. (2006) Diet and cancer prevention: Where we are, where we are going. *Nutr Cancer* **56**, 225–31.

105. Hu, J., La Vecchia, C., DesMeules, M., Negri, E., Mery, L., and Canadian Cancer Registries Epidemiology Research Group (2008) Meat and fish consumption and cancer in Canada. *Nutr Cancer* **60**, 313–24.

106. Boyd, N.F., Martin, L.J., Noffel, M., Lockwood, G.A., and Trichler, D.L. (1993) A meta-analysis of studies of dietary fat and breast cancer risk. *Br J Cancer* **68**, 627–36.

107. Boyd, N.F., Stone, J., Vogt, K.N., Connelly, B.S., Martin, L.J., and Minkin, S. (2003) Dietary fat and breast cancer risk revisited: A meta-analysis of the published literature. *Br J Cancer* **89**, 1672–85.

108. Egeberg, R., Olsen, A., Autrup, H., Christensen, J., Stripp, C., Tetens, I., Overvad, K., and Tjonneland, A. (2008) Meat consumption, N-acetyl transferase 1 and 2 polymorphism and risk of breast cancer in Danish postmenopausal women. *Eur J Cancer Prev* **17**, 39–47.

109. van der Hel, O.L., Peeters, P.H., Hein, D.W., Doll, M.A., Grobbee, D.E., Ocke, M., and Bueno de Mesquita, H.B. (2004) GSTM1 null genotype, red meat consumption and breast cancer risk (The Netherlands). *Cancer Causes Control* **15**, 295–303.

110. Holmes, M.D., Colditz, G.A., Hunter, D.J., Hankinson, S.E., Rosner, B., Speizer, F.E., and Willett, W.C. (2003) Meat, fish and egg intake and risk of breast cancer. *Int J Cancer* **104**, 221–27.

111. Missmer, S.A., Smith-Warner, S.A., Spiegelman, D., Yaun, S.S., Adami, H.O., Beeson, W.L., van den Brandt, P.A., Fraser, G.E., Freudenheim, J.L., Goldbohm, R.A., Graham, S., Kushi, L.H., Miller, A.B., Potter, J.D., Rohan, T.E., Speizer, F.E., Toniolo, P., Willett, W.C., Wolk, A., Zeleniuch-Jacquotte, A., and Hunter, D.J. (2002) Meat and dairy food consumption and breast cancer: A pooled analysis of cohort studies. *Int J Epidemiol* **31**, 78–85.

112. Voorrips, L.E., Brants, H.A., Kardinaal, A.F., Hiddink, G.J., van den Brandt, P.A., and Goldbohm, R.A. (2002) Intake of conjugated linoleic acid, fat, and other fatty acids in relation to postmenopausal breast cancer: The Netherlands Cohort Study on Diet and Cancer. *Am J Clin Nutr* **76**, 873–82.

113. Cho, E., Chen, W.Y., Hunter, D.J., Stampfer, M.J., Colditz, G.A., Hankinson, S.E., and Willett, W.C. (2006) Red meat intake and risk of breast cancer among premenopausal women. *Arch Intern Med* **166**, 2253–59.

114. Kolonel, L.N. (1996) Nutrition and prostate cancer. *Cancer Causes Control* **7**, 83–44.

115. Kolonel, L.N. (2001) Fat, meat, and prostate cancer. *Epidemiol Rev* **23**, 72–81.

116. Rodriguez, C., McCullough, M.L., Mondul, A.M., Jacobs, E.J., Chao, A., Patel, A.V., Thun, M.J., and Calle, E.E. (2006) Meat consumption among Black and White men and risk of prostate cancer in the Cancer Prevention Study II Nutrition Cohort. *Cancer Epidemiol Biomarkers Prev* **15**, 211–16.

117. Rohrmann, S., Platz, E.A., Kavanaugh, C.J., Thuita, L., Hoffman, S.C., and Helzlsouer, K.J. (2007) Meat and dairy consumption and subsequent risk of prostate cancer in a US cohort study. *Cancer Causes Control* **18**, 41–50.

118. Ross, R.K. (1996) Epidemiology of prostate cancer and bladder cancer: An overview. *Cancer Treat Res* **88**, 1–11.

119. Creton, S.K., Zhu, H., and Gooderham, N.J. (2007) The cooked meat carcinogen 2-amino-1-methyl-6-phenylimidazo[4,5-b]pyridine activates the extracellular signal regulated kinase mitogen-activated protein kinase pathway. *Cancer Res* **67**, 11455–62.

120. Gooderham, N.J., Zhu, H., Lauber, S., Boyce, A., and Creton, S. (2002) Molecular and genetic toxicology of 2-amino-1-methyl-6-phenylimidazo[4,5-b]pyridine (PhIP). *Mutat Res* **506–507**, 91–99.

121. Snyderwine, E.G. (1994) Some perspectives on the nutritional aspects of breast cancer research. Food-derived heterocyclic amines as etiologic agents in human mammary cancer. *Cancer* **74**, 1070–77.

122. Lang, N.P., Butler, M.A., Massengill, J., Lawson, M., Stotts, R.C., Hauer-Jensen, M., and Kadlubar, F.F. (1994) Rapid metabolic phenotypes for acetyltransferase and cytochrome P4501A2 and putative exposure to food-borne heterocyclic amines increase the risk for colorectal cancer or polyps. *Cancer Epidemiol Biomarkers Prev* **3**, 675–82.

123. Lauber, S.N., Ali, S., and Gooderham, N.J. (2004) The cooked food derived carcinogen 2-amino-1-methyl-6-phenylimidazo[4,5-b] pyridine is a potent oestrogen: A mechanistic basis for its tissue-specific carcinogenicity. *Carcinogenesis* **25**, 2509–17.

124. Hammons, G.J., Milton, D., Stepps, K., Guengerich, F.P., Tukey, R.H., and Kadlubar, F.F. (1997) Metabolism of carcinogenic heterocyclic and aromatic amines by recombinant human cytochrome P450 enzymes. *Carcinogenesis* **18**, 851–54.

125. Yamazoe, Y., Shimada, M., Kamataki, T., and Kato, R. (1983) Microsomal activation of 2-amino-3-methylimidazo[4,5-f]quinoline, a pyrolysate of sardine and beef extracts, to a mutagenic intermediate. *Cancer Res* **43**, 5768–74.

126. Chou, H.C., Lang, N.P., and Kadlubar, F.F. (1995) Metabolic activation of N-hydroxy arylamines and N-hydroxy heterocyclic amines by human sulfotransferase(s). *Cancer Res* **55**, 525–29.

127. Buonarati, M.H., and Felton, J.S. (1990) Activation of 2-amino-1-methyl-6-phenylimidazo[4,5-b]pyridine (PhIP) to mutagenic metabolites. *Carcinogenesis* **11**, 1133–38.

128. Buonarati, M.H., Turteltaub, K.W., Shen, N.H., and Felton, J.S. (1990) Role of sulfation and acetylation in the activation of 2-hydroxyamino-1-methyl-6-phenylimidazo[4,5-b]pyridine to intermediates which bind DNA. *Mutat Res* **245**, 185–90.

129. Kato, R., Kamataki, T., and Yamazoe, Y. (1983) N-hydroxylation of carcinogenic and mutagenic aromatic amines. *Environ Health Perspect* **49**, 21–25.

130. Kato, R., and Yamazoe, Y. (1987) Metabolic activation and covalent binding to nucleic acids of carcinogenic heterocyclic amines from cooked foods and amino acid pyrolysates. *Jpn J Cancer Res* **78**, 297–311.

131. Minchin, R.F., Reeves, P.T., Teitel, C.H., McManus, M.E., Mojarrabi, B., Ilett, K.F., and Kadlubar, F.F. (1992) N-and O-acetylation of aromatic and heterocyclic amine carcinogens by human monomorphic and polymorphic acetyltransferases expressed in COS-1 cells. *Biochem Biophys Res Commun* **185**, 839–44.

132. Wallin, H., Mikalsen, A., Guengerich, F.P., Ingelman-Sundberg, M., Solberg, K.E., Rossland, O.J., and Alexander, J. (1990) Differential rates of metabolic activation and detoxication of the food mutagen 2-amino-1-methyl-6-phenylimidazo[4,5-b]pyridine by different cytochrome P450 enzymes. *Carcinogenesis* **11**, 489–92.

133. Glatt, H., Boeing, H., Engelke, C.E., Ma, L., Kuhlow, A., Pabel, U., Pomplun, D., Teubner, W., and Meinl, W. (2001) Human cytosolic sulphotransferases: Genetics, characteristics, toxicological aspects. *Mutat Res* **482**, 27–40.

134. Chen, J., Stampfer, M.J., Hough, H.L., Garcia-Closas, M., Willett, W.C., Hennekens, C.H., Kelsey, K.T., and Hunter, D.J. (1998) A prospective study of N-acetyltransferase genotype, red meat intake, and risk of colorectal cancer. *Cancer Res* **58**, 3307–11.

135. Chan, A.T., Tranah, G.J., Giovannucci, E.L., Willett, W.C., Hunter, D.J., and Fuchs, C.S. (2005) Prospective study of N-acetyltransferase-2 genotypes, meat intake, smoking and risk of colorectal cancer. *Int J Cancer* **115**, 648–52.

136. Le Marchand, L., Hankin, J.H., Wilkens, L.R., Pierce, L.M., Franke, A., Kolonel, L.N., Seifried, A., Custer, L.J., Chang, W., Lum-Jones, A., and Donlon, T. (2001) Combined effects of well-done red meat, smoking, and rapid N-acetyltransferase 2 and CYP1A2 phenotypes in increasing colorectal cancer risk. *Cancer Epidemiol Biomarkers Prev* **10**, 1259–66.

137. Butler, L.M., Millikan, R.C., Sinha, R., Keku, T.O., Winkel, S., Harlan, B., Eaton, A., Gammon, M.D., and Sandler, R.S. (2008) Modification by N-acetyltransferase 1 genotype on the association between dietary heterocyclic amines and colon cancer in a multiethnic study. *Mutat Res* **638**, 162–74.

138. Ishibe, N., Sinha, R., Hein, D.W., Kulldorff, M., Strickland, P., Fretland, A.J., Chow, W.H., Kadlubar, F.F., Lang, N.P., and Rothman, N. (2002) Genetic polymorphisms in heterocyclic amine metabolism and risk of colorectal adenomas. *Pharmacogenetics* **12**, 145–50.

139. Kury, S., Buecher, B., Robiou-du-Pont, S., Scoul, C., Sebille, V., Colman, H., Le Houerou, C., Le Neel, T., Bourdon, J., Faroux, R., Ollivry, J., Lafraise, B., Chupin, L.D., and Bezieau, S. (2007) Combinations of cytochrome P450 gene polymorphisms enhancing the risk for sporadic colorectal cancer related to red meat consumption. *Cancer Epidemiol Biomarkers Prev* **16**, 1460–67.

140. Krajinovic, M., Ghadirian, P., Richer, C., Sinnett, H., Gandini, S., Perret, C., Lacroix, A., Labuda, D., and Sinnett, D. (2001) Genetic susceptibility to breast cancer in French-Canadians: Role of carcinogen-metabolizing enzymes and gene-environment interactions. *Int J Cancer* **92**, 220–25.

141. Zheng, W., Deitz, A.C., Campbell, D.R., Wen, W.Q., Cerhan, J.R., Sellers, T.A., Folsom, A.R., and Hein, D.W. (1999) N-acetyltransferase 1 genetic polymorphism, cigarette smoking, well-done meat intake, and breast cancer risk. *Cancer Epidemiol Biomarkers Prev* **8**, 233–39.

142. Ambrosone, C.B., Freudenheim, J.L., Sinha, R., Graham, S., Marshall, J.R., Vena, J.E., Laughlin, R., Nemoto, T., and Shields, P.G. (1998) Breast cancer risk, meat consumption and N-acetyltransferase (NAT2) genetic polymorphisms. *Int J Cancer* **75**, 825–30.

143. Delfino, R.J., Sinha, R., Smith, C., West, J., White, E., Lin, H.J., Liao, S.Y., Gim, J.S., Ma, H.L., Butler, J., and Anton-Culver, H. (2000) Breast cancer, heterocyclic aromatic amines from meat and N-acetyltransferase 2 genotype. *Carcinogenesis* **21**, 607–15.

144. Gertig, D.M., Hankinson, S.E., Hough, H., Spiegelman, D., Colditz, G.A., Willett, W.C., Kelsey, K.T., and Hunter, D.J. (1999) N-acetyl transferase 2 genotypes, meat intake and breast cancer risk. *Int J Cancer* **80**, 13–17.

145. Deitz, A.C., Zheng, W., Leff, M.A., Gross, M., Wen, W.Q., Doll, M.A., Xiao, G.H., Folsom, A.R., and Hein, D.W. (2000) N-Acetyltransferase-2 genetic polymorphism, well-done meat intake, and breast cancer risk among postmenopausal women. *Cancer Epidemiol Biomarkers Prev* **9**, 905–10.

146. Williams, J.A., Martin, F.L., Muir, G.H., Hewer, A., Grover, P.L., and Phillips, D.H. (2000) Metabolic activation of carcinogens and expression of various cytochromes P450 in human prostate tissue. *Carcinogenesis* **21**, 1683–89.

147. Shirai, T., Sano, M., Tamano, S., Takahashi, S., Hirose, M., Futakuchi, M., Hasegawa, R., Imaida, K., Matsumoto, K., Wakabayashi, K., Sugimura, T., and Ito, N. (1997) The prostate: A target for carcinogenicity of 2-amino-1-methyl-6-phenylimidazo[4,5-b]pyridine (PhIP) derived from cooked foods. *Cancer Res* **57**, 195–98.

148. Tang, D., Liu, J.J., Rundle, A., Neslund-Dudas, C., Savera, A.T., Bock, C.H., Nock, N.L., Yang, J.J., and Rybicki, B.A. (2007) Grilled meat consumption and PhIP-DNA adducts in prostate carcinogenesis. *Cancer Epidemiol Biomarkers Prev* **16**, 803–08.

149. Cross, A.J., Peters, U., Kirsh, V.A., Andriole, G.L., Reding, D., Hayes, R.B., and Sinha, R. (2005) A prospective study of meat and meat mutagens and prostate cancer risk. *Cancer Res* **65**, 11779–84.

150. Hein, D.W., Leff, M.A., Ishibe, N., Sinha, R., Frazier, H.A., Doll, M.A., Xiao, G.H., Weinrich, M.C., and Caporaso, N.E. (2002) Association of prostate cancer with rapid N-acetyltransferase 1 (NAT1*10) in combination with slow N-acetyltransferase 2 acetylator genotypes in a pilot case-control study. *Environ Mol Mutagen* **40**, 161–67.

151. Rovito, P.M., Jr., Morse, P.D., Spinek, K., Newman, N., Jones, R.F., Wang, C.Y., and Haas, G.P. (2005) Heterocyclic amines and genotype of N-acetyltransferases as risk factors for prostate cancer. *Prostate Cancer Prostatic Dis* **8**, 69–74.

152. Muckel, E., Frandsen, H., and Glatt, H.R. (2002) Heterologous expression of human N-acetyltransferases 1 and 2 and sulfotransferase 1A1 in Salmonella typhimurium for mutagenicity testing of heterocyclic amines. *Food Chem Toxicol* **40**, 1063–68.

153. Dooley, T.P., Haldeman-Cahill, R., Joiner, J., and Wilborn, T.W. (2000) Expression profiling of human sulfotransferase and sulfatase gene superfamilies in epithelial tissues and cultured cells. *Biochem Biophys Res Commun* **277**, 236–45.

154. Nowell, S., Ambrosone, C.B., Ozawa, S., MacLeod, S.L., Mrackova, G., Williams, S., Plaxco, J., Kadlubar, F.F., and Lang, N.P. (2000) Relationship of phenol sulfotransferase activity (SULT1A1) genotype to sulfotransferase phenotype in platelet cytosol. *Pharmacogenetics* **10**, 789–97.

155. Steiner, M., Bastian, M., Schulz, W.A., Pulte, T., Franke, K.H., Rohring, A., Wolff, J.M., Seiter, H., and Schuff-Werner, P. (2000) Phenol sulphotransferase SULT1A1 polymorphism in prostate cancer: Lack of association. *Arch Toxicol* **74**, 222–25.

156. Nowell, S., Ratnasinghe, D.L., Ambrosone, C.B., Williams, S., Teague-Ross, T., Trimble, L., Runnels, G., Carrol, A., Green, B., Stone, A., Johnson, D., Greene, G., Kadlubar, F.F., and Lang, N.P. (2004) Association of SULT1A1 phenotype and genotype with prostate cancer risk in African-Americans and Caucasians. *Cancer Epidemiol Biomarkers Prev* **13**, 270–76.

157. Yang, C.S., Yoo, J.S., Ishizaki, H., and Hong, J.Y. (1990) Cytochrome P450IIE1: Roles in nitrosamine metabolism and mechanisms of regulation. *Drug Metab Rev* **22**, 147–59.

158. Knekt, P., Jarvinen, R., Dich, J., and Hakulinen, T. (1999) Risk of colorectal and other gastro-intestinal cancers after exposure to nitrate, nitrite and N-nitroso compounds: A follow-up study. *Int J Cancer* **80**, 852–56.

159. Kiss, I., Sandor, J., Pajkos, G., Bogner, B., Hegedus, G., and Ember, I. (2000) Colorectal cancer risk in relation to genetic polymorphism of cytochrome P450 1A1, 2E1, and glutathione-S-transferase M1 enzymes. *Anticancer Res* **20**, 519–22.

160. Morita, M., Tabata, S., Tajima, O., Yin, G., Abe, H., and Kono, S. (2008) Genetic Polymorphisms of CYP2E1 and Risk of Colorectal Adenomas in the Self Defense Forces Health Study. *Cancer Epidemiol Biomarkers Prev* **17**, 1800–07.

161. Le Marchand, L., Donlon, T., Seifried, A., and Wilkens, L.R. (2002) Red meat intake, CYP2E1 genetic polymorphisms, and colorectal cancer risk. *Cancer Epidemiol Biomarkers Prev* **11**, 1019–24.

162. Matsuda, Y., Saoo, K., Yamakawa, K., Yokohira, M., Suzuki, S., Kuno, T., Kamataki, T., and Imaida, K. (2007) Overexpression of CYP2A6 in human colorectal tumors. *Cancer Sci* **98**, 1582–85.

163. el-Bayoumy, K., Chae, Y.H., Upadhyaya, P., Rivenson, A., Kurtzke, C., Reddy, B., and Hecht, S.S. (1995) Comparative tumorigenicity of benzo[a]pyrene, 1-nitropyrene and 2-amino-1-methyl-6-phenylimidazo[4,5-b]pyridine administered by gavage to female CD rats. *Carcinogenesis* **16**, 431–34.

164. Stampfer, M.R., Bartholomew, J.C., Smith, H.S., and Bartley, J.C. (1981) Metabolism of benzo[a]pyrene by human mammary epithelial cells: Toxicity and DNA adduct formation. *Proc Natl Acad Sci U S A* **78**, 6251–55.

165. Bonner, M.R., Han, D., Nie, J., Rogerson, P., Vena, J.E., Muti, P., Trevisan, M., Edge, S.B., and Freudenheim, J.L. (2005) Breast cancer risk and exposure in early life to polycyclic aromatic hydro-carbons using total suspended particulates as a proxy measure. *Cancer Epidemiol Biomarkers Prev* **14**, 53–60.

166. Gammon, M.D., Santella, R.M., Neugut, A.I., Eng, S.M., Teitelbaum, S.L., Paykin, A., Levin, B., Terry, M.B., Young, T.L., Wang, L.W., Wang, Q., Britton, J.A., Wolff, M.S., Stellman, S.D., Hatch, M., Kabat, G.C., Senie, R., Garbowski, G., Maffeo, C., Montalvan, P., Berkowitz, G., Kemeny, M., Citron, M., Schnabel, F., Schuss, A., Hajdu, S., and Vinceguerra, V. (2002) Environmental toxins and breast cancer on Long Island. I. Polycyclic aromatic hydrocarbon DNA adducts. *Cancer Epidemiol Biomarkers Prev* **11**, 677–85.

167. Gammon, M.D., Sagiv, S.K., Eng, S.M., Shantakumar, S., Gaudet, M.M., Teitelbaum, S.L., Britton, J.A., Terry, M.B., Wang, L.W., Wang, Q., Stellman, S.D., Beyea, J., Hatch, M., Kabat, G.C., Wolff, M.S., Levin, B., Neugut, A.I., and Santella, R.M. (2004) Polycyclic aromatic hydrocarbon-DNA adducts and breast cancer: A pooled analysis. *Arch Environ Health* **59**, 640–49.

168. Rundle, A., Tang, D., Hibshoosh, H., Estabrook, A., Schnabel, F., Cao, W., Grumet, S., and Per-era, F.P. (2000) The relationship between genetic damage from polycyclic aromatic hydrocarbons in breast tissue and breast cancer. *Carcinogenesis* **21**, 1281–89.

169. Rebbeck, T.R. (1997) Molecular epidemiology of the human glutathione S-transferase genotypes GSTM1 and GSTT1 in cancer susceptibility. *Cancer Epidemiol Biomarkers Prev* **6**, 733–43.

170. Strange, R.C., Spiteri, M.A., Ramachandran, S., and Fryer, A.A. (2001) Glutathione-S-transferase family of enzymes. *Mutat Res* **482**, 21–26.

171. Ambrosone, C.B., Freudenheim, J.L., Graham, S., Marshall, J.R., Vena, J.E., Brasure, J.R., Laughlin, R., Nemoto, T., Michalek, A.M., and Harrington, A. (1995) Cytochrome P4501A1 and glutathione S-transferase (M1) genetic polymorphisms and postmenopausal breast cancer risk. *Cancer Res* **55**, 3483–85.

172. Bailey, L.R., Roodi, N., Verrier, C.S., Yee, C.J., Dupont, W.D., and Parl, F.F. (1998) Breast cancer and CYPIA1, GSTM1, and GSTT1 polymorphisms: Evidence of a lack of association in Caucasians and African Americans. *Cancer Res* **58**, 65–70.

173. Egan, K.M., Cai, Q., Shu, X.O., Jin, F., Zhu, T.L., Dai, Q., Gao, Y.T., and Zheng, W. (2004) Genetic polymorphisms in GSTM1, GSTP1, and GSTT1 and the risk for breast cancer: Results from the Shanghai Breast Cancer Study and meta-analysis. *Cancer Epidemiol Biomarkers Prev* **13**, 197–204.

174. Helzlsouer, K.J., Selmin, O., Huang, H.Y., Strickland, P.T., Hoffman, S., Alberg, A.J., Watson, M., Comstock, G.W., and Bell, D. (1998) Association between glutathione S-transferase M1, P1, and T1 genetic polymorphisms and development of breast cancer. *J Natl Cancer Inst* **90**, 512–18.

175. Vogl, F.D., Taioli, E., Maugard, C., Zheng, W., Pinto, L.F., Ambrosone, C., Parl, F.F., Nedelcheva-Kristensen, V., Rebbeck, T.R., Brennan, P., and Boffetta, P. (2004) Glutathione S-transferases M1, T1, and P1 and breast cancer: A pooled analysis. *Cancer Epidemiol Biomarkers Prev* **13**, 1473–79.

176. Rundle, A., Tang, D., Zhou, J., Cho, S., and Perera, F. (2000) The association between glutathione S-transferase M1 genotype and polycyclic aromatic hydrocarbon-DNA adducts in breast tissue. *Cancer Epidemiol Biomarkers Prev* **9**, 1079–85.

177. Zheng, W., Wen, W.Q., Gustafson, D.R., Gross, M., Cerhan, J.R., and Folsom, A.R. (2002) GSTM1 and GSTT1 polymorphisms and postmenopausal breast cancer risk. *Breast Cancer Res Treat* **74**, 9–16.

178. Ahn, J., Nowell, S., McCann, S.E., Yu, J., Carter, L., Lang, N.P., Kadlubar, F.F., Ratnasinghe, L.D., and Ambrosone, C.B. (2006) Associations between catalase phenotype and genotype: Modification by epidemiologic factors. *Cancer Epidemiol Biomarkers Prev* **15**, 1217–22.

179. Ulrich, C. M. et al. *Cancer Epidemiol Biomarkers Prev* 2006;**15**, 189–93.

5 Diet and Epigenetics

Sharon A. Ross

Key Points

1. Diet and dietary factors are important contributing factors to health and disease. Since an inappropriate diet may contribute significantly to the causation of chronic disease, including cancer, it is important to uncover the molecular mechanisms of dietary bioactive factors in health and disease in order to determine the best strategies for intervention.
2. Evidence suggests that diet and other environmental factors may be significant regulators of epigenetic events, including DNA methylation, histone posttranslational modification, noncoding RNAs, and factors/proteins that regulate chromatin structure and dynamics.
3. At least four ways in which nutrients may be interrelated with DNA methylation have been found. First, nutrients may influence the supply of methyl groups for the formation of S-adenosylmethionine (SAM). Second, nutrients may modify the utilization of methyl groups by DNA methyltransferases. A third possible mechanism may relate to DNA demethylation activity. Fourth, the DNA methylation patterns may influence the response to a nutrient.
4. One example of the influence of diet in DNA methylation and cancer is the finding that dietary methyl deficiency (of folate, choline, or methionine) has been shown to alter hepatic DNA methylation patterns and induce hepatocarcinogenesis in the absence of a carcinogen in Fisher 344 rats.
5. Although the cancer epigenetic field has advanced in the last decade, much remains to be revealed especially with respect to potential modification by bioactive dietary components. Research needs to address the quantity of dietary components needed to bring about a biological effect, the effects of timing of exposure, and how chemical form and duration of exposure influence the cancer process.

Key Words: Bioactive food components; diet; DNA methylation; histone; polycomb repressive complex; microRNA; epigenetics

1. INTRODUCTION

Several lines of evidence, including epidemiological and preclinical studies, suggest that the increased intake of certain bioactive food components (BFCs) including folate, choline, zinc, genistein, epigallocatechin gallate, diallyl disulfide, and sulforaphane may modulate cancer risk. However, the specific molecular mechanisms for these observations about BFCs and the quantities needed (as well as issues of frequency, duration, and timing of exposure in the life span) to bring about the anticancer effect remain largely

From: *Nutrition and Health: Bioactive Compounds and Cancer*
Edited by: J.A. Milner, D.F. Romagnolo, DOI 10.1007/978-1-60761-627-6_5,
© Springer Science+Business Media, LLC 2010

unresolved. It has also been known that these dietary constituents influence the cellular milieu by modulating several cellular processes, including DNA repair, hormonal regulation, differentiation, inflammation, apoptosis, cell cycle control/proliferation, carcinogen metabolism, and angiogenesis, among others. Cancer has been hypothesized to develop from cells that have escaped normal regulation of these processes along with disordered intercellular relationships. These functional abnormalities are thought to arise from deregulated expression of key genes, resulting in altered cellular phenotype *(1)*. Such anomalous gene expression may result from genetic disruption, i.e., mutation, or from epigenetic modulation by silencing genes that should be active or activating genes that should be silent. Diet and bioactive food factors may directly influence both processes.

Many studies provide intriguing evidence that part of the anticancer properties attributed to several BFCs may relate to modulation of epigenetic processes, including DNA methylation of the cytosine phosphate guanine dinucleotide (CpG) islands in promoters and other regions of the genome, chromatin remodeling and higher order chromatin structural alterations, posttranslational ATP-dependent modifications which include methylation, acetylation, ubiquitination, and phosphorylation of histone tail domains, as well as gene regulation through noncoding RNAs (Fig. 1). We have previously delineated *(2)* at least four ways in which nutrients may be interrelated with DNA methylation. The first is that nutrients may influence the supply of methyl groups for the formation of S-adenosylmethionine (SAM). The second mechanism is that nutrients may modify utilization of methyl groups by processes including altered DNA methyltransferase activity. The third possible mechanism may relate to DNA demethylation activity. Finally, the DNA methylation patterns may influence the response to a nutrient. Intriguingly, such interactions may apply similarly to the way in which diet

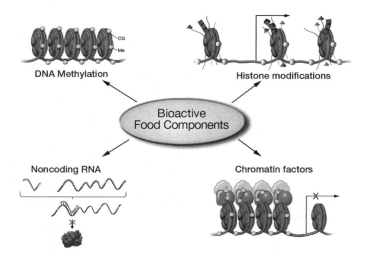

Fig. 1. Evidence suggests that bioactive food components can modify several epigenetic mechanisms, including DNA methylation, histone modifications, noncoding RNA, and chromatin factors such as the polycomb repressive complex 1.

impacts histone methylation marks and processes. The interrelationship between nutrients, epigenetics, and cancer will be further explored in this review by providing additional examples and highlighting areas for further research.

2. EPIGENETICS AND CANCER

The cellular epigenetic apparatus consists of chromatin, which contains a histone protein-based structure around which DNA is wrapped, histone posttranslational modifications, and covalent modifications of a methyl group to cytosines residing at the dinucleotide sequence CG in DNA (3). These modifications determine the accessibility of the transcriptional machinery to the genome. Recently, small noncoding RNAs have also been hypothesized to provide an additional level of epigenetic regulation in the nucleus (4).

The most widely studied epigenetic modification in humans is cytosine methylation of DNA within the dinucleotide CpG (5). DNA methylation does not act in isolation, but interacts with histone modifications and chromatin-remodeling complexes to inform chromatin structure and gene regulation (6). One-carbon metabolism provides the methyl group for all biologic methylation reactions, which are dependent on methyl donors and cofactors (e.g., methionine, choline, folic acid, vitamin B12, and pyridoxal phosphate) to synthesize the universal methyl donor SAM. DNA methyltransferases (DNMTs) catalyze the transfer of a methyl group from SAM onto the 5′ position of the cytosine ring at the dinucleotide sequence CG. Three DNMTs – DNMT1, DNMT3A and DNMT3B – have been extensively studied in developmental processes and in cancer. DNMT1, known as a "maintenance" methyltransferase, has a preference for a hemimethylated substrate and is involved in copying DNA methylation patterns during cellular replication (7). DNMT3A and DNMT3B are responsible for "de novo" methylation. Emerging evidence suggests that DNMT targeting to DNA is more complicated in that these enzymes appear to target specific genes with the assistance of sequence-specific factors (8). DNA methylation is thought to be removed passively by blocking methylation of newly synthesized DNA during DNA replication (9). However, the presence of an active DNA demethylase has long been speculated in mammalian cells and recent experimental findings suggest that the methyl DNA binding protein MBD2 and de novo DNA methyltransferases DNMT3A and DNMT3B possess DNA demethylase activity in mammalian cells (9, 10). These findings need to be replicated and further explored to determine whether active mammalian demethylation plays a role in the regulation of DNA methylation.

Regions rich in CpG dinucleotides, termed CpG islands, span the 5′ end region (promoter, untranslated region, and exon 1) of many genes and are usually unmethylated in normal cells (11). This unmethylated status is associated with the ability of CpG island-containing genes to be transcribed in the presence of the necessary transcriptional activators. Conversely, methylation at these critical sites inhibits the binding of transcription factors to their recognition elements and recruits methylated DNA binding proteins such as MeCP2 to the gene and chromatin modification enzymes such as histone deacetylases (HDACs) which in turn introduce histone modifications, resulting in the silencing of chromatin *(12)*. In cancer cells, the transcriptional silencing of tumor suppressor genes by CpG island-promoter hypermethylation is thought to be an early response in the tumorigenic process *(13)*. In addition to region-specific hypermethylation, widespread global DNA hypomethylation *(14)* and increased DNA methyltransferase *(15)* activity are common characteristics of tumor cells. Importantly, DNA methylation changes are thought to be inherited mitotically in somatic cells, providing a potential mechanism by which environmental effects, including dietary exposures, on the epigenome can have long-term effects on gene expression *(16)*.

The secondary structure of chromatin is arranged as a chain of nucleosomes consisting of an octamer of histone proteins inclusive of the H3–H4 histone protein tetramer flanked on either side with a H2A–H2B histone protein dimer and 147 base pairs of double-stranded DNA twisted around this protein complex *(17)*. Arrangement in this multinucleosomal order is important for organization and stablization of DNA, as well as for regulation of transcription of genetic information, DNA replication, and repair processes. The N-terminal tails of the histone proteins are extensively modified by methylation *(18)*, phosphorylation *(19)*, acetylation *(20)*, sumoylation *(21)* ubiquitination *(22)*, and biotinylation *(23)*. These modifications confer functional attributes, for example, histone acetylation typically facilitates the decondensation of the chromatin, relaxing nucleosomal connections between DNA and histones, and thereby promoting the transcription process, whereas deacetylation and condensation generally suppress transcription *(24)*. The specific pattern of histone modifications has been proposed to form a "histone code," which explains, in part, the sections of the genome to be expressed at a given point in time in a given cell type *(25)*. It has been hypothesized that similar to a genetic mutation, a change in the posttranslational modification of histone tails around a regulatory region of a gene can silence an active gene, resulting in "loss of function," or activate a silent gene, leading to "gain of function." Such modifications may also enhance or impair levels of gene expression in the absence of complete gene silencing or activation. In fact, aberrant histone posttranslational modifications have been associated with cancer. For example, a common hallmark of human tumor cells is the loss of monoacetylation and trimethylation of histone H4 *(26)*.

Histone acetylation is regulated by several enzymatic activities with the capacity to either transfer acetyl groups or to induce histone deacetylation, which is associated with gene silencing. A common observation in cancer cells is an imbalance of histone acetyltransferase (HAT) and HDAC activities *(27)*. It is interesting to note that aberrant targeting of HDACs has been associated with transcriptional silencing of tumor suppressor genes, including *p21* – which encodes a cyclin-dependent kinase inhibitor that blocks cell cycle progression from G_1 into S phase *(28)*. The expression of p21 has been found to be diminished in many different tumors, permitting uncontrolled cell division. Interestingly, HDAC inhibitors have been shown to reactivate p21 expression, thereby preventing tumor cell proliferation *(28)*. Furthermore, the HDAC inhibitor-induced expression of p21 has been found to correlate with an increase in the acetylation of histones associated with the p21 promoter region. These discoveries have led to the development of HDAC inhibitors as chemotherapeutic agents in clinical trials *(27)*. Recent studies implicating histone posttranslational modifications with cell identity, including stem cell identity and characteristics such as pluripotency, suggest that HATs and histone acetylation in concert with other chromatin modifications may regulate stem cell pluripotency, and deregulation of such histone marking may lead to tumorigenesis (24).

Several proteins or protein complexes have recently been identified that regulate chromatin structure and dynamics. For example, ATP-dependent chromatin-remodeling factors alter the position of nucleosomes around the transcription start site and define accessibility to the transcription machinery (29). The SWItch/Sucrose NonFermentable (Swi/SNF) complex is a chromatin-remodeling complex that uses the energy of ATP hydrolysis to modify chromatin structure and regulate gene expression; recent observations link an aberrant SWI/SNF complex to cancer (30). Evidence is emerging that both gene activation complexes and gene repressive complexes contain chromatin-remodeling activities (31). A DNA helicase/ATPase-containing complex termed nucleosome remodeling and deacetylase corepressor complex (or NuRD), which represses transcription through chromatin remodeling (31), has recently been found to direct aberrant gene repression and transmission of epigenetic repressive marks in acute promyelocytic leukemia (32).

The polycomb group (PcG) proteins, which function as transcriptional repressors that silence specific sets of genes through chromatin modification, may also contribute to the pathogenesis of cancer (33). At least two distinct complexes, PcG complex 1 and 2, are thought to be involved in chromatin modification. PcG complex 2, composed of several factors/proteins including histone methylase activity, is first recruited to silence chromatin with concomitant methylation of histone H3 at lysine 27 (K27me3). This is followed by recruitment of the PcG complex 1 through recognition of this histone mark, which thereby triggers ubiquitination of histone H2A and/or inhibits chromatin remodeling to maintain the silenced state of the locus (34). PcG-deficient mice have provided biological evidence that these chromatin repressive complexes are essential for sustaining stem cell activity. Furthermore, enrichment of polycomb repressive complexes is correlated with cancer progression and prognosis and is also associated with cancer stem cell activity. How and in what context these and other epigenetic mechanisms and regulatory factors may interact to regulate chromatin structure, dynamics, and gene expression in cancer development and prevention is an active area of research.

The role of small noncoding RNA molecules in the regulation of gene expression is an emerging area of research. Noncoding RNAs (e.g., microRNA) have been shown to modulate posttranscriptional silencing (i.e., the targeted degradation of mRNAs) and there is much interest in studying deregulation of these small RNAs in various diseases, including cancer (35). It has been recently reported that microRNAs (miRNAs) may also transcriptionally silence gene expression in the nucleus (36). In this study, investigators performed a bioinformatic search for miRNA target sites proximal to known gene transcription start sites in the human genome. One conserved miRNA, *miR-320*, that was identified is encoded within the promoter region of the cell cycle gene POLR3D in the antisense orientation. Evidence for a *cis*-regulatory role for *miR-320* in transcriptional silencing of POLR3D expression was provided. Interestingly, using chromatin immunoprecipitation (ChIP) assays, *miR-320* was suggested to direct the association of RNA interference (RNAi) protein Argonaute-1 (AGO1), polycomb group component EZH2, and trimethylation of histone H3 lysine 27 (H3K27me3) to the POLR3D promoter. These results support the existence of an epigenetic mechanism for miRNA-directed transcriptional gene silencing (TGS) in mammalian cells. These investigators hypothesized that misregulation of endogenous miRNAs that target gene promoters may potentially play a role in the aberrant epigenetic silencing of cancer-related genes. Moreover, epigenetic modifications have recently been found to be induced and directed by other small RNA molecules in human cells (37). These small RNAs are thought to act like the exogenous small inhibitory RNAs (siRNAs) in gene inactivation. In fact, this endogenous small RNA-mediated transcriptional gene silencing was shown to be correlated with changes in chromatin structure (including modulation of histone marks and DNA methylation) at specific sites in promoter regions (37). The impact of this epigenetic mechanism in cancer development is currently being explored.

Evidence for interactions between dietary components and each of the epigenetic mechanism described above – DNA methylation, histone posttranslational modification, chromatin remodeling and other chromatin factors, as well as noncoding RNAs – and their impact on cancer development and prevention are highlighted in the sections that follow. Ultimately, it will be important to understand how these and other newly identified epigenetic components work interactively and simultaneously to impose gene regulatory information.

3. DIET AND DNA METHYLATION: TIMING OF EXPOSURE

Recent preclinical evidence suggests that prenatal and early postnatal diet may alter DNA methylation marks and processes which may impact the risk of developing disease later in life (38–43). It has also been suggested that diet-induced epigenetic alterations might also be inherited transgenerationally, thereby potentially affecting the health of future generations. In this regard, it was recently shown that individuals who were prenatally exposed to famine during the Dutch Hunger Winter in 1944–1945 had, 6 decades later, less DNA methylation of the imprinted *insulin-like growth factor II* (IGF2) gene compared with their unexposed, same-sex siblings (44). The results of these studies support the fetal basis or developmental origins of the adult-onset disease hypothesis. This intriguing hypothesis implies that an organism can adapt to environmental signals in early life, but that these adaptations may also increase the risk of developing chronic diseases, including cancer, later in life when there is a disparity between the perceived environment and that which is encountered in adulthood.

Some of the best evidence for the impact of diet on DNA methylation comes from studies examining the yellow agouti (A^{vy}) mouse model. In this model, an endogenous retrovirus-like transposon sequence is inserted close to the gene coding for the agouti protein (45). Normally, a cryptic promoter within the retrotransposon is silenced by methylation allowing normal tissue-specific and regulated agouti expression. However, if this site is undermethylated the promoter is active and drives constitutive ectopic expression of the agouti gene, leading to yellow coat color and obesity (as well as increased susceptibility to other chronic diseases, including cancer). Dietary supplementation of folic acid, vitamin B12, choline, betaine, and zinc to yellow agouti dams in utero has been shown to lead to changes in DNA methylation as well as profound effects on phenotype of the offspring (38–41, 46). In initial experiments this supplementation regime to maternal diets was associated with a change in coat color from a yellow to an agouti or pseudo-agouti coat in the offspring *(38)*. This phenotype change is typically associated with a lower risk of cancer, diabetes, obesity, and prolonged life in this model *(38, 46)*. Furthermore, representative yellow mice displayed more hypomethylated long terminal repeats 5′ of the *agouti* gene and the representative agouti coat mice were found to have a greater degree of hypermethylation in the long terminal repeat 5′ of the *agouti* gene *(46)*.

Another group of investigators verified these findings (supplementing with folic acid, vitamin B12, choline and betaine, but not zinc) and also compared the shift in the distribution of coat color to changes in CpG methylation of the *agouti* locus in methyl-supplemented vs. non-supplemented animals *(39)*. They found that changes in pigmentation of the mouse pup coat, ranging from yellow to brown, were significantly associated with supplementation status of the mother's diet during pregnancy. Furthermore, these coat color changes were directly associated with alterations in DNA methylation and there was a distribution shift toward increased CpG methylation at the A^{vy} locus with methyl supplementation. Moreover, the coat color phenotype and A^{vy} methylation relationship persisted into adulthood as evidenced by a comparison of tail DNA at 21 days and liver DNA at 100 days. These studies clearly demonstrate that maternal methyl donor supplementation during gestation can alter offspring phenotype by methylating the epigenome. It is not yet evident, however, which of the dietary constituents are necessary or sufficient for the DNA methylation and phenotypic change.

Similar alterations in coat color and DNA methylation were induced in offspring through maternal dietary supplementation of genistein, the major phytoestrogen in soy, at amounts comparable to those a human might receive through a high soy diet (250 mg/kg diet) *(41)*. Furthermore, the offspring exposed to genistein in utero with DNA hypermethylation at the A^{vy} locus appeared to be protected against obesity in adulthood, indicating that maternal dietary supplementation is associated with not only altered fetal methylation patterns but also methylation-dependent susceptibility to disease. The mechanism of how genistein effects methylation and epigenetic pathways has yet to be determined as these investigators did not find an association between genistein supplementation and the one-carbon metabolism. Changes in other epigenetic marks or regulation of specific nuclear transcription factors are potential sites of action of genistein to explore in future research.

The agouti mouse has also been utilized as an environmental biosensor to evaluate the effects of maternal dietary exposure to a xenobiotic chemical on the fetal epigenome *(47)*. In utero or neonatal exposure to bisphenol A (BPA), a high-production volume chemical used in the manufacture of polycarbonate plastic, is associated with higher body weight, increased breast and prostate cancer, and altered reproductive function. Maternal exposure to this endocrine active compound (50 mg of BPA/kg) shifted the coat color distribution of A^{vy} mouse offspring toward yellow by decreasing CpG methylation in an intracisternal-A particle (IAP) retrotransposon upstream of the *agouti* gene. It is fascinating that maternal nutritional supplementation with either methyl donors or the phytoestrogen genistein rescued the BPA exposed animals by shifting the coat color distribution toward the control animal as well as by negating the DNA hypomethylating effect of BPA. These studies present convincing evidence that early developmental exposure to a xenobiotic chemical such as BPA can change offspring phenotype by stably altering the epigenome, an effect that can be counteracted by maternal dietary supplements.

The agouti model has also recently been utilized to examine whether diet influences phenotype transgenerationally. Interestingly, passing the A^{vy} allele through three maternal generations resulted in amplification of obesity in the offspring of the mice fed a NIH-31 control (or unsupplemented group) diet in each successive generation (48). By the third generation in the methyl-supplemented offspring, however, there was a significant decrease in body weight relative to the unsupplemented group, thereby suggesting a preventive effect on transgenerational amplification of obesity in adulthood. This is an interesting study because it examines the effect of maternal obesity among three generations of genetically identical mice which had an inclination to overeat due to the A^{vy} allele. Furthermore, the authors hypothesize that the methyl supplements affected body weight by interfering with the area of the brain that regulates appetite.

Studies using another murine metastable epiallele, *axin fused* (*Axin*^{Fu}), found similar epigenetic plasticity to maternal diet as the agouti mouse model (42). *Axin*^{Fu} is a mutation in mice which causes kinked, fused tails and other developmental abnormalities including axial duplications. The *Axin* gene is located proximally on chromosome 17 and encodes a component of the Wnt signaling pathway, an important regulator of embryonic axis formation in mammals. The mutant *Axin*^{Fu} allele results from insertion of an IAP, a murine retrotransposon, into intron 6 of the *Axin* gene. This mutant allele is able to produce wild-type transcript, as well as mutant transcripts, arising from either alternative splicing or initiation of transcription from a cryptic promoter. It has been suggested that the mutant gene leads to the fused phenotype through a gain-of-function effect. Female mice supplemented with methyl donors and factors (including choline, betaine, folic acid, vitamin B12, methionine, and zinc) before and during pregnancy were found to have offspring with an increase in DNA methylation at the *Axin*^{Fu} locus and reduced incidence of tail kinking (42). The hypermethylation was tail specific, suggesting a mid-gestation effect. The investigators speculate that the results indicate a stochastic establishment of an epigenotype at metastable epialleles, which is labile to methyl donor nutrition and such influences are likely not limited to early embryonic development.

It is important to clarify how observations in the agouti and *Axin Fused* models may relate to human phenotype and disease. Although the A^{vy} locus and *Axin*^{Fu} locus – retrovirus-like transposon sequences – are not found in the human genome, there is the possibility that metastable epialleles ("metastable" refers to the labile nature of the epigenetic state of these alleles; "epiallele" defines their potential to maintain epigenetic marks transgenerationally (49)) associated with other transposable elements could similarly be influenced by methylation or another epigenetic regulating process via in utero exposure to dietary factors. It has been intriguingly proposed that transposable elements in the mammalian genome may cause considerable phenotypic variability, making each individual mammal a "compound epigenetic mosaic" (50). Whether such an epigenetic mosaic can be modulated by early diet and how such phenotypes alter susceptibility to chronic disease, including cancer, in adulthood requires further study. In addition, other regions of the genome which may be susceptible to epigenetic variation need to be identified and characterized in human tissues. There is also a need to further our understanding of the interaction between diet, epigenetics, and crucial times of exposure during development and throughout the entire life span.

In this regard, another group has hypothesized that epigenetics in early infancy, childhood, and puberty might also be susceptible to effects of one of the involved methyl donor nutrients described above, namely dietary folate *(51)*. These investigators examined the effects of timing and duration of dietary folate intervention provided during the postweaning period on genomic DNA methylation of adult Sprague Dawley rat liver. Folate deficiency beginning at weaning and continued through puberty followed by control diet in adulthood until 30 weeks of age (when animals were sacrificed) induced a significant 34–49% increase in genomic DNA methylation in adult rat liver compared with control- and folate-supplemented diets provided in the same manner. The authors hypothesized that a compensatory upregulation of DNMT and of choline and betaine-dependent transmethylation pathways occurred in response to folate deficiency during the postweaning period. This was thought to result in genomic DNA hypermethylation in the liver and this pattern was maintained in the presence of adequate folate when the animals were fed the control diet at puberty through adulthood. In contrast, dietary folate deficiency or supplementation continually imposed from weaning to adulthood or from puberty to adulthood did not significantly affect genomic DNA methylation in adult rat liver. These data suggest that early folate nutrition during postnatal development can impact epigenetic programming that can have a permanent effect in adulthood. More studies on the long-term functional consequences of such dietary epigenetic programming are encouraged.

Folate supplementation may also bring about epigenetic changes in adult humans as demonstrated by an interesting study in dialysis patients with uremia and hyperhomocysteinemia *(52)*. In this study, global DNA methylation was reduced in patients with uremia and hyperhomocysteinemia, but both DNA hypomethylation and hyperhomocysteinemia were reversed by administration of folate (15 mg oral methyltetrahydrofolate a day for 8 weeks). Furthermore, the DNA hypomethylation was linked to defects in the expression of genes regulated by methylation. To study this gene regulation, the pattern of allelic expression for the normally imprinted *H19* gene in peripheral mononuclear cells in seven of the dialysis patients that were heterozygous for *H19* RsaI restriction fragment length polymorphisms (RFLP) was examined. The RFLP analysis showed a shift from monoallelic to biallelic expression of *H19* (expression of both *H19* T and H19 C alleles in the heterozygotes could be identified) when plasma total homocysteine concentration was between 39 and 62 μmol/L. Interestingly, in the three patients with high total homocysteine concentrations (<62 μmol/L) reverse transcriptase-PCR analysis showed a shift back to monoallelic expression of *H19* after folate treatment. These data suggest that treatment of hyperhomocysteinemia with folate in these patients corrects DNA hypomethylation and provides a mechanism for the relevant changes of gene expression. This intriguing study needs replication and follow-up for other affected genes and conditions.

In addition to silencing inappropriately activated genes (e.g., imprinted genes) by DNA methylation, dietary components have been shown to reactivate inappropriately silenced genes (e.g., tumor suppressor genes) by demethylation in cell culture systems. The prevention or reversal of hypermethylation-induced inactivation of key tumor suppression or DNA repair genes, for example, in cancer cells could be an effective approach for cancer prevention. As examples, epigallocatechin 3-gallate (EGCG) (5–50 μM) from green tea and genistein (2–20 μmol/L) from soybean have been found to restore methylation patterns and gene expression of tumor suppressor genes in neoplastic cells in culture *(53–55)*. Both dietary factors have been shown to inhibit DNA methyltransferase activity which was associated with demethylation of CpG islands in the gene promoters and the reactivation of methylation-silenced genes such as *p16INK4a, retinoic acid receptor beta, O6-methylguanine methyltransferase, human mutL homolog 1*, and *glutathione S-transferase-pi (53–55)*. These modifications have been observed in human esophageal, colon, prostate, and mammary cancer cell lines and were also associated with cell growth inhibition.

The Annurca apple, a variety of southern Italy, is rich in polyphenols that are associated with anticancer properties. For example, populations in southern Italy have lower incidences of colorectal cancer than elsewhere in the Western world. Recently, investigators evaluated the anticancer effects of Annurca polyphenol extract (APE) using RKO, SW48, and SW480 human colorectal cancer cells in culture *(56)*. Because some sporadic colorectal cancers display the CpG island methylator (CIMP) phenotype, DNA methylation of selected tumor suppressor genes were also evaluated in these cells after treatment with APE and compared with the synthetic demethylating agent 5-aza-2′deoxycytidine (5-aza-2dC). APE treatment (polyphenol dose comparable to that from dietary consumption of 1 apple) decreased cell viability and enhanced apoptosis in the RKO and SW48 cell lines, both in vitro models for CIMP. A similar dose of APE reduced DNA methylation in the promoters of *hMLH1, p14(ARF)*, and *p16(INK4a)* genes with consequent restoration of normal mRNA expression in RKO cells. These effects were qualitatively comparable with those obtained with 5-aza-2dC. A significant reduction in expression of DNMT-1 and DNMT-3b proteins after treatment without changes in messenger RNA was also observed. Thus, APE, like EGCG and genistein, appears to have demethylating activity through the inhibition of DNMT proteins.

Because of the relatively low bioavailability of most polyphenolic compounds, the exact effect dietary polyphenols would have on DNA methylation in humans is not clear *(53)*. The effect of normal dietary consumption of a single polyphenolic compound is not likely to affect healthy individuals. However, the combinational and additive effects of polyphenols with various epigenetic activities might produce biological consequences. On the other hand, the consumption of excessive amounts of polyphenols from dietary supplements would seem to be more likely to affect DNA methylation status and perhaps other epigenetic processes as well, but such possibilities remain to be examined. Although polyphenols are thought to selectively induce apoptosis or reduce proliferation in cancer cells but not in normal cells, additional research is also warranted to determine beneficial vs. deleterious responses to these BFCs during vulnerable periods of the life span.

The putative mechanism of action for selenium in cancer prevention has been an active research emphasis since the start of the Selenium and Vitamin E Cancer Prevention Trial (SELECT) *(57)*. Recently, selenium has been shown to induce promoter DNA demethylation and gene reexpression in LNCaP prostate cancer cells, suggesting that epigenetic modifications may be a possible mechanism for cancer prevention *(58)*. In particular, selenite treatment (at physiologically achievable levels) caused partial promoter DNA demethylation and reexpression of the *pi-class glutathione-S-transferase* (*GSTP1*) in a dose- and time-dependent manner. Selenite treatment decreased mRNA levels of DNMTs 1 and 3A and protein levels of DNMT1. Additionally, selenite treatment caused partial promoter demethylation and reexpression of the tumor suppressor adenomatous polyposis coli and cellular stress response 1. Both of these genes have been shown to be hypermethylated in human prostate cancer cells. Interestingly, selenite also decreased histone deacetylase activity and increased levels of acetylated lysine 9 on histone H3 (H3K9), but decreased levels of methylated H3K9. More specifically, selenite treatment influenced epigenetic marks associated with the *GSTP1* promoter, including reduced levels of DNMT1 and methylated H3K9, but increased levels of acetylated H3K9. These epigenetic marks are correlated with gene activation. The relationship between particular histone modifications and DNA methylation in gene reactivation may be gene specific and requires additional study, preferably in an in vivo setting.

Although the interactions between bioactive food components and DNA methylation are among the earliest studies of the relationship between diet and epigenetics in cancer prevention, there continues to be a growing body of literature encompassing more and more dietary factors that may impact DNA methylation at various times of vulnerability, including during cancer development and prevention. How these single observations will be united to reflect the complexity of human dietary patterns as well as how the many epigenetic mechanisms and marks will be integrated to provide an understanding of specific and global gene regulation are the hopeful outcomes of future endeavors.

4. HISTONE MODIFICATION BY BIOACTIVE FOOD COMPONENTS AND DIET COMPOSITION

Several dietary factors, including butyrate (formed in the colon from the fermentation of dietary fiber), diallyl disulfide (present in garlic and other *Allium* vegetables), and sulforaphane (found in cruciferous vegetables) have been found to inhibit HDAC enzymes *(59, 60)*. These bioactive food components have also been shown to enhance histone acetylation *(60)* and possibly alter additional histone posttranslational modifications that modify chromatin structure in specific regions as the model in Fig. 2 depicts. Butyrate, diallyl disulfide, and sulforaphane have all been associated with cancer prevention in various preclinical and clinical studies. It is certainly possible that the inhibition of HDAC activity and concomitant enhanced histone acetylation is directly linked with the cancer protective effects of these dietary components. It is interesting to note that butyrate, diallyl disulfide, and sulforaphane have all been shown to inhibit cell proliferation and stimulate apoptosis in a manner analogous to other nondietary HDAC inhibitors.

Butyrate has been reported to inhibit HDAC activity and increase histone acetylation in a number of cell lines *(60)*. These butyrate-induced alterations in histone enzymes and marks have been associated with several processes, including cellular differentiation, cell cycle arrest, apoptosis and inhibition of invasion and metastasis. Butyrate has also been found to alter transcriptional regulation in a manner comparable to other

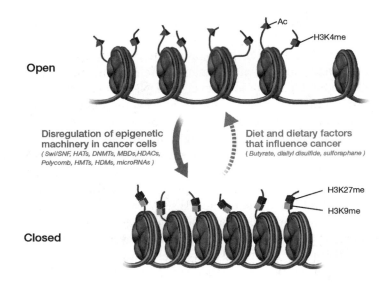

Fig. 2. A model depicting dysregulation of epigenetic machinery in cancer cells and the putative reversal actions of dietary factors. Butyrate, diallyl disulfide, and sulforaphane have been shown to inhibit histone deacetylase activity and increase acetylation on histone proteins *(59, 60)*. Ac, acetylation; H3K4me, histone 3 lysine 4 methylation; H3K27me, histone 3 lysine 27 methylation; H3k9me, histone 3 lysine 9 methylation; Swi/SNF, SWItch/Sucrose NonFermentable complex; HATs, histone acetyltransferases; DNMTs, DNA methyltransferases; MBDs, methyl-CpG binding domain proteins; HDACs, histone deacetylases; HMTs, histone methyltransferases; HDMs, histone demethylases.

HDAC inhibitors, such as trichostatin A *(61)*. As was observed for trichostatin A, butyrate caused down-regulation of c-myc mRNA expression which likely accounts for its effect on reducing cell proliferation *(62)*. Furthermore, both trichostatin A and butyrate increased histone H3 and H4 acetylation within the *CDKN1A* promoter (using ChIP experiments), which regulates the p21 protein, in colorectal cancer cells in culture *(63)*. Because only 2% of genes are thought to be regulated by butyrate, specificity of HDAC inhibition and consequent transcriptional regulation may be due to sequences such as butyrate response elements in the promoter region of certain genes *(64)*. Epigenome-wide analysis of both genetic sequence and epigenetic marks could assist in uncovering this specificity.

The active garlic constituent diallyl disulfide (DADS) has been shown to induce cell cycle arrest in the G_2/M phase in both HT-29 and Caco-2 human colon cancer cell lines. These antiproliferative effects were correlated with increased CDKN1A mRNA and p21 protein levels, as well as increased H4 and/or H3 acetylation within the *CDKN1A* promoter *(65, 66)*. The findings suggest that histone hyperacetylation of the promoter region may account for the cell cycle arrest induced by DADS. Histone acetylation changes have been observed in rat liver and transplanted Morris hepatoma 7,777 cells with DADS treatment (200 mg/kg body weight), demonstrating that altered acetylated histone status is achievable in vivo *(67)*. Furthermore, using a nontumorigenic animal model, investigators found that DADS (200 mg/kg) treatment increased histone H4 and H3 acetylation in isolated colonocytes *(68)*. More research that compares the effects of garlic constituents on normal and cancer cells is advocated in order to decipher the biological effects. Physiologic concentrations (low micromolar range) of S-allyl-mercaptocysteine, another organosulfur compound found in garlic, has also been reported to induce growth arrest in various cell lines and increase the levels of acetylated histones H3 and H4 *(69)*. Much of the work on these epigenetic modulations utilized a very large dose of garlic constituent (i.e., 200 μM), consequently there is a need to perform dose–response experiments to delineate the physiological vs. pharmacological effects that may provide indications for either prevention or therapy.

Sulforaphane (SFN) (3–15 μM) has been shown to inhibit HDAC activity and in parallel increase acetylated histones in several cell systems, including human embryonic kidney 293 cells, HCT116 human colorectal cancer cells, and various prostate epithelial cell lines (BPH-1, LnCaP, and PC-3) *(60)*. This increased histone acetylation induced by sulforaphane was linked with increased apoptosis and a greater number of cells in G_2/M cell cycle arrest than control treated cells *(60)*. Moreover, these observations were associated with increased acetylated histone H4 in the *p21* promoter and concomitant increased p21 protein expression *(70)*. Furthermore, sulforaphane dose-dependently increased the amount of acetylated histone H4 associated with the *p21* promoter *(71)*. Using the Apc^{min} mouse model, sulforaphane (443 mg/kg diet) suppressed tumor development and increased acetylated histones in gastrointestinal polyps, including acetylated histones specifically associated with the promoter region of the *p21* and *bax* genes *(72)*. Most remarkable is the finding that in healthy human subjects ($N=3$), a single ingestion of 68 g (1 cup) of broccoli sprouts rich in SFN inhibited HDAC activity in circulating peripheral blood mononuclear cells 3–6 h after consumption, with simultaneous induction of histone H3 and H4 acetylation *(73)*. The biological consequences of reduced HDAC activity and enhanced histone acetylation in normal compared to cancer cells require further study. Although SFN has been shown to selectively induce apoptosis and growth inhibition in cancer cells but not in normal cells, additional research is warranted to determine beneficial vs. harmful responses to BFCs during vulnerable periods. Another isothiocyanate present in cruciferous vegetables, namely phenethyl isothiocyanate (1 μM), was also found to inhibit the level and activity of HDACs in prostate cancer cells, induce selective histone acetylation and methylation for chromatin unfolding *(74)*. These results demonstrate that isothiocyanates can inhibit HDAC activity in vitro and in vivo and suggest that this inhibition might contribute to the cancer preventive effects of cruciferous vegetables.

A recent report revealed that genistein (at both 10 and 25 μmol/l) induced the expression of the tumor suppressor genes *p21* and *p16* (INK4a) with a concomitant decrease in cyclins in prostate cancer cells *(75)*. These investigators found that genistein increased acetylation of histones H3, H4, and H3 lysine 4 (H3K4) at the *p21* and *p16* transcription start sites with concomitant increased expression of histone acetyltransferases. Interestingly, DNA methylation analysis revealed the absence of *p21* promoter methylation prior to genistein exposure. Furthermore, these same investigators found that genistein (50 μM) activated expression of several aberrantly silenced tumor suppressor genes that have unmethylated promoters such as PTEN, CYLD, p53, and FOXO3a in prostate cancer cells *(76)*. Instead of turning on tumor suppressor genes through promoter demethylation, these investigators found that genistein influenced remodeling of the heterochromatic domains at promoters by reducing/modulating histone H3 lysine 9 (H3K9) methylation and deacetylation. These findings suggest that genistein may be protective against cancers with various epigenetic profiles. Furthermore, the relationship between genistein, histone, and DNA methylation modifications in gene reactivation, which may be gene specific, is not entirely clear and requires further study.

The story is further complicated for soy consumption because of the activity of other constituents found in soy that may modify chromatin in a somewhat opposing fashion. In fact, lunasin, a unique 43-amino acid soybean peptide that has cancer prevention capability, has been found to inhibit acetylation of core histones in mammalian cells and selectively kills cells that are in the process of transformation (e.g., E1A-transfected mouse fibroblast NIH 3T3 cells), but does not affect the growth rate of normal and established cancer cell lines at 10 μM concentrations *(77)*. An epigenetic mechanism of action has been proposed whereby lunasin selectively kills cells being transformed or newly transformed cells by binding to deacetylated core histones exposed by the transformation event, thereby disrupting the dynamics of histone acetylation and deacetylation. These results point to the importance of understanding the timing of cellular vulnerability to epigenetic modulation. Recently, investigators observed the histone H3 and H4 acetylation inhibitory properties of lunasin from different Korean soybean varieties used for various food purposes *(78)*. They found that various amounts of lunasin are found in the soybean varieties (4.40–70.49 ng of lunasin per μg of protein) and that the amount was correlated with the extent of inhibition of core histone acetylation. Furthermore, the blood from rats fed lunasin-enriched soy protein, but not the blood from control fed rats, was found to inhibit histone acetylation activity. Delineating the epigenetic activity of various soy constituents and products in different cellular contexts is potential area for future research.

Recently, the maternal diet has been shown to alter histone acetylation and gene expression profiles in the developing primate offspring *(79)*. In this study, chronic consumption of a maternal high-fat diet (35% fat vs. 13% fat for control animals) resulted in a threefold increase in fetal liver triglycerides and histologic correlates of fatty liver disease, which was accompanied by hyperacetylation of fetal hepatic tissue at histone 3 lysine 14 (H3K14) and decreased HDAC1 mRNA, protein, and activity. Gene expression changes were also observed, including increased glutamic pyruvate transaminase (alanine aminotransferase) 2 (*GPT2*), *DNAJA2* (a heat shock protein 70 co-chaperone), and *Rdh12* (an all *trans* and 9-*cis* retinol dehydrogenase responsive to oxidative stress) in fetal hepatic tissue from maternal caloric-dense diet animals when compared with control. Furthermore, the gene *Npas2*, a peripheral circadian regulator, was significantly down-modulated in the offspring of high-fat diet animals. Definitive conclusions regarding the role of H3K14 acetylation with respect to the observed altered gene expression requires additional study. These results, however, suggest that a caloric-dense maternal diet leading to obesity epigenetically alters fetal chromatin structure in primates via covalent modifications of histones and hence offers a molecular basis to the fetal origins of adult-onset disease hypothesis.

The majority of the evidence for dietary-induced histone posttranslational modifications concerns the effects of dietary HDAC inhibitors and the effects of diet on histone acetylation, much of which is described above. Additional histone posttranslational modifications and their enzymatic partners have been shown to be influenced by dietary factors that have also been implicated in cancer prevention pathways. These include interactions between a methyl-deficient diet and histone methylation in early hepatocellular carcinogenesis *(80)* and the nutrient biotin and histone biotinylation in repression of transposable elements in cancer cells *(81)*. These reports provide evidence for the impact of dietary factors on histone modification and in determining chromatin structures, including whether the chromatin is in the open (active) or closed (inactive) state. Research on the identification and characterization of dietary triggers of histone modifications and associated affects such as gene silencing or activation is emergent. Some of these efforts will likely examine specificity of bioactive food factors for particular histone modifying enzymes and perhaps will utilize epigenome approaches to map the numerous histone posttranslational marks in normal and cancer cells following dietary exposure(s).

5. DIETARY MODULATION OF POLYCOMB REPRESSIVE COMPLEXES

Histone modifications triggered by polycomb repressive complex signaling are thought to be important during embryonic stem (ES) cell differentiation. For example, PcG complex 2 binding mediates trimethylation of lysine 27 (K27me3) on histone H3, but this histone mark is lost on developmental genes that are transcriptionally induced during ES cell differentiation. The active vitamin A constituent retinoic acid (RA) is involved in differentiation of ES cells as well as differentiation of various cancer cells in culture. Interestingly, a decrease in the H3K27me3 mark was recently observed in as little as 3 days after differentiation of mouse ES cells induced by RA (1 μM) treatment *(82)*. The enzyme histone K27 methyltransferase EZH2, which mediates the K27me3 mark, also decreased with RA treatment. A loss of EZH2 binding and H3K27me3 was observed locally on PcG complex 2 target genes induced after 3 days of RA, including the gene *nestin*. In contrast, direct RA-responsive genes that are rapidly induced, such as *Hoxa1*, showed a loss of EZH2 binding and K27me3 within only a few hours of RA treatment. These observations suggest that there are likely temporal stages of derepression of polycomb complex target genes during early differentiation and also emphasize the complexity of the histone code in regulating gene transcription as increased histone acetylation was found to override this H3K27me3 repressive mark to induce gene transcription in some genes.

After the PcG complex 2 binds and increases H3K27me3 in a specific gene region, the second polycomb repressive complex 1 (PcG complex 1), which contains the protein Bmi-1, binds to the K27me3 in histone H3 and catalyzes the ubiquitinylation of histone H2A. This cooperation between the two PcG complexes is what leads to silencing of gene expression. PcG complex 1, including Bmi-1, appears to remain attached to the chromatin after these events are completed. Bmi-1 is overexpressed in some human cancers, including colorectal cancer *(83)* and human non-small cell lung cancer *(84)*, as well as markedly elevated in epidermal squamous cell carcinoma cells *(85)*.

The polyphenol EGCG reduces skin cancer cell survival. Thus, the impact of EGCG on the PcG complex 1 chromatin factor in cultured squamous cell carcinoma cells was recently examined to determine the involvement of Bmi-1 in the activity of EGCG *(86)*.

EGCG (40 μM) was found to suppress Bmi-1 levels and reduce Bmi-1 phosphorylation, resulting in displacement of the Bmi-1 polycomb protein complex from chromatin and reducing survival of transformed cells. These observations provide additional evidence for the role of dietary components in reducing cancer cell survival by altering epigenetic control of gene expression. The importance of the polycomb repressive complexes in the development of cancer is currently an active research enterprise. An important area for future research will be to clarify the role of dietary regulation of PcGs (primarily focusing on cancer stem cells and perhaps adult stem cells) during cancer prevention as well as cancer progression and during other periods of vulnerability.

6. SMALL, NONCODING RNA, EPIGENETICS, AND DIETARY FACTORS

The methyl-deficient model of endogenous hepatocarcinogenesis (HCC) in rodents is unique in that dietary insufficiency rather than the addition of chemical carcinogens or viral agents can lead to tumor formation (87). Specifically, deficiency of the major dietary sources of methyl groups and cofactors – methionine, choline, folic acid, and vitamin B12 – is sufficient to induce liver tumor formation in male rats and certain mouse strains (88–91). The methyl deficiency induced in these animals has been associated with several defects, including increased genome-wide and gene-specific hypomethylation (91–94). Recent studies examining the early stages of hepatocarcinogenesis induced by methyl deficiency in rats found significant alterations in other aspects of the epigenetic machinery, including aberrant expression of DNA methyltransferases and methyl CpG binding proteins (95), defects in histone methyltransferase protein expression and histone posttranslational modifications (80), and changes in the expression of microRNAs (miRNA) (96, 97). The aberrant epigenetic alterations imposed by this diet have been hypothesized to be the primary mechanism responsible for malignant transformation of rat liver cells (80, 91, 92, 94, 98), but which of the epigenetic defects is initially responsible for transformation has not been determined. In this regard, development of methyl-deficient induced HCC was shown to be characterized by prominent early changes in the expression of miRNA genes that are involved in the regulation of apoptosis, cell proliferation, cell-to-cell connection, and epithelial–mesenchymal transition (97). Specifically, inhibition of expression of *miR-34a*, *miR-127*, *miR-200b*, and *miR-16a* with corresponding changes in the levels of E2F3, NOTCH1, BCL6, ZFHX1B, and BCL2, proteins that are targeted by these miRNAs, was observed. The significance of the disruption of miRNAs expression in HCC was confirmed by the persistence of these miRNA alterations in the livers of methyl-deficient rats refed a methyl-adequate diet. These investigators hypothesized that the early occurrence of alterations in miRNA expression and their persistence during the entire process of hepatocarcinogenesis indicated that the dysregulation of microRNA expression is likely to be an important contributing factor in the development of HCC. Whether the inhibition of expression of these specific miRNAs in this HCC model are the earliest trigger(s) toward fixing the neoplastic state requires further study. It is interesting to note that the sequence of pathological and molecular events in the methyl-deficient model of liver carcinogenesis is remarkably similar to the development of human hepatocellular carcinoma associated with viral hepatitis B and C infections, alcohol exposure, and metabolic liver diseases *(99)*, thus advocating this model for further study.

Curcumin, derived from the rhizome of *Curcuma longa*, is a naturally occurring flavanoid with apoptotic activity and has recently been shown to alter the expression profiles of miRNA in human BxPC-3 pancreatic cancer cells *(100)*. In this study, 11 miRNAs were significantly upregulated and 18 miRNAs were significantly downregulated after 72 h of treatment with 10 μmol/L curcumin in these cells. For example, curcumin upregulated miRNA-22 and downregulated miRNA-199a*, and these findings were confirmed by real-time PCR analysis. Furthermore, the expression of two computationally predicted targets for miRNA-22 (because miRNA-22 function is unknown), SP1 transcription factor (SP1) and estrogen receptor 1 (ESR1), was investigated in the pancreatic cancer cells. Upregulation of miRNA-22 expression by either treatment with 10 μmol/L curcumin or transfections with synthetic miRNA-22 mimics reduced the expression of its target genes SP1 and ESR1, while experiments using miRNA-22 antisense enhanced SP1 and ESR1 expression. These findings suggest that alterations of miRNA expression by curcumin may be an important mediator of its anticancer effects in pancreatic cancer cells.

The above evidence suggests that nutrient deficiency as well as bioactive food component supplementation may modulate the expression of microRNA and that this modulation has consequences in cancer pathways of progression and/or prevention. Whether the affected miRNA is acting in an epigenetic fashion through miRNA-directed transcriptional gene silencing *(36)* as well as by modulating posttranscriptional silencing (i.e., the targeted degradation of mRNAs) has not been delineated. In fact, the role that microRNAs themselves can have as chromatin modifiers is only beginning to be understood *(101)*. Recent evidence suggests that this regulation can involve a direct or indirect repression of DNA and histone modifying enzymes, as well as chromatin-remodeling factors. It is also interesting to note that microRNA genes are also epigenetically modified in cancer cells *(101)*. Evidence suggests that miRNA genes are subject to hypermethylation and hypomethylation in a tumor- and tissue-specific manner. Further characterization of the downstream mRNA targets for these miRNAs will shed light on the functional consequences of their altered epigenetic regulation and how this contributes to human tumorigenesis. Whether dietary factors also influence DNA methylation near or within miRNA genes is another research topic for consideration. In addition to miRNA, other noncoding RNA will likely to be impacted by dietary modulation as well as have activity in epigenetic pathways and in cancer. Investigators have only begun to understand how small noncoding RNAs act in gene regulation and disease.

7. CONCLUSIONS

Recent evidence suggests that dietary components – as diverse as selenium, retinoids, and sulforaphane – exert cancer protective effects through modulation of epigenetic mechanisms, such as DNA methylation of CpG islands in promoters and other regions of the genome, chromatin silencing complexes, posttranslational modifications of histone tail domains, and regulation of noncoding RNAs. Diet and bioactive food components may alter several cellular processes that participate in cancer risk and prevention, including DNA repair, hormonal regulation, differentiation, inflammation, apoptosis, cell cycle control/proliferation, carcinogen metabolism, and angiogenesis, among others. Accumulating data suggest that dietary factors may alter these cancer processes through modifications of epigenetic mechanisms.

In the near future, epigenomic approaches are likely to assist in characterizing genome-wide epigenetic marks that are targets for dietary regulation. The ability to characterize reference epigenomes (be it profiles of DNA methylation or histone modifications) will greatly impact the ability to determine, on a global level, how diet impacts differential epigenetic effects on normal vs. cancer tissue, elucidate epigenetic changes resulting from dietary exposures during critical periods of prenatal and postnatal development, adolescence, and senescence, as well as investigate the potential impact of diet on transgenerational transmission of epigenetic changes. Research also indicates that links between genetics and epigenetics may provide additional insights about transcriptional regulation in cancer risk and prevention. How dietary factors participate in these interactions will likely need to be unraveled. Moreover, the identification and characterization of novel epigenetic marks and mechanisms with the capacity to differentially silence and activate gene expression are likely to surface over the next few years. Understanding how diet and dietary factors influence these evolving mechanisms will provide additional research opportunities.

Although the cancer epigenetic field has advanced in the last decade, much remains to be revealed especially with respect to potential modification by bioactive dietary components. Issues remain about the quantity of dietary components needed to bring about a biological effect, the timing of exposure and other variables (chemical form, duration of exposure) that can influence the response. Importantly, for the future of nutrigenomics and personalized nutrition, epigenetic marks may be useful as biomarkers of cancer prevention, early disease, or nutritional status, as well as function as potential molecular targets that are modulated by dietary interventions.

REFERENCES

1. Wiseman, M. (2008) The Second World Cancer Research Fund/American Institute for Cancer Research Expert Report. Food, nutrition, physical activity, and the prevention of cancer: A global perspective. *Proc Nutr Soc* **67**, 253–56.
2. Ross, S.A. (2003) Diet and DNA methylation interactions in cancer prevention. *Ann NY Acad Sci* **983**, 197–207.
3. McGowan, P.O., Meaney, M.J., and Szyf, M. (2008) Diet and the epigenetic (re)programming of phenotypic differences in behavior. *Brain Res* **1237**, 12–24.
4. Kim, D.H., Saetrom, P., Snøve, O., Jr., and Rossi, J.J. (2008) MicroRNA-directed transcriptional gene silencing in mammalian cells. *Proc Natl Acad Sci USA* **105**, 16230–35.
5. Esteller, M. (2005) Aberrant DNA methylation as a cancer-inducing mechanism. *Annu Rev Pharmacol Toxicol* **45**, 629–56.
6. Tost, J. (2009) DNA methylation: An introduction to the biology and the disease-associated changes of a promising biomarker. *Methods Mol Biol* **507**, 3–20.
7. Razin, A., and Riggs, A.D. (1980) DNA methylation and gene function. *Science* **210** , 604–10.
8. Brenner, C., Deplus, R., Didelot, C., Loriot, A., Viré, E., De Smet, C., Gutierrez, A., Danovi, D., Bernard, D., Boon, T., Pelicci, P.G., Amati, B., Kouzarides, T., de Launoit, Y., Di Croce, L., and Fuks, F. (2005) Myc represses transcription through recruitment of DNA methyltransferase corepressor. *EMBO J* **24** , 336–46.

9. Ooi, S.K., and Bestor, T.H. (2008) The colorful history of active DNA demethylation. *Cell* **133**, 1145–48.

10. Kim, J.K., Samaranayake, M., and Pradhan, S. (2008) Epigenetic mechanisms in mammals. *Cell Mol Life Sci* Nov 3. [Epub ahead of print].

11. Esteller, M. (2007) Cancer epigenomics: DNA methylomes and histone-modification maps. *Nat Rev Genet* **8**, 286–98.

12. Li, E. (2002) Chromatin modification and epigenetic reprogramming in mammalian development. *Nat Rev Genet* **3**, 662–73.

13. Belinsky, S.A. (2005) Silencing of genes by promoter hypermethylation: Key event in rodent and human lung cancer. *Carcinogenesis* **26**, 1481–87.

14. Ehrlich, M. (2002) DNA methylation in cancer: Too much, but also too little. *Oncogene* **21**, 5400–13.

15. Kautiainen, T.L., and Jones, P.A. (1986) DNA methyltransferase levels in tumorigenic and nontumorigenic cells in culture. *J Biol Chem* **261**, 1594–98.

16. Wolffe, A.P. (1994) Inheritance of chromatin states. *Dev Genet* **15**, 463–70.

17. Kornberg, R.D., and Lorch, Y. (1999) Twenty-five years of the nucleosome, fundamental particle of the eukaryote chromosome. *Cell* **98**, 285–94.

18. Jenuwein, T. (2001) Re-SET-ting heterochromatin by histone methyltransferases. *Trends Cell Biol* **11**, 266–73.

19. Oki, M., Aihara, H., and Ito, T. (2007) Role of histone phosphorylation in chromatin dynamics and its implications in diseases. *Subcell Biochem* **41**, 319–36.

20. Wade, P.A., Pruss, D., and Wolffe, A.P. (1997) Histone acetylation: Chromatin in action. *Trends Biochem Sci* **22**, 128–32.

21. Shiio, Y., and Eisenman, R.N. (2003) Histone sumoylation is associated with transcriptional repression. *Proc Natl Acad Sci USA* **100**, 13225–30.

22. Shilatifard, A. (2006) Chromatin modifications by methylation and ubiquitination: Implications in the regulation of gene expression. *Annu Rev Biochem* **75**, 243–69.

23. Kothapalli, N., Camporeale, G., Kueh, A., Chew, Y.C., Oommen, A.M., Griffin, J.B., and Zempleni, J. (2005) Biological functions of biotinylated histones. *J Nutr Biochem* **16**, 446–48.

24. Shukla, V., Vaissière, T., and Herceg, Z. (2008) Histone acetylation and chromatin signature in stem cell identity and cancer. *Mutat Res* **637**, 1–15.

25. Jenuwein, T., and Allis, C.D. (2001) Translating the histone. *Code Sci* **293**, 1074–80.

26. Fraga, M.F., Ballestar, E., Villar-Garea, A., Boix-Chornet, M., Espada, J., Schotta, G., Bonaldi, T., Haydon, C., Ropero, S., Petrie, K., Iyer, N.G., Pérez-Rosado, A., Calvo, E., Lopez, J.A., Cano, A., Calasanz, M.J., Colomer, D., Piris, M.A., Ahn, N., Imhof, A., Caldas, C., Jenuwein, T., and Esteller, M. (2005) Loss of acetylation at Lys16 and trimethylation at Lys20 of histone H4 is a common hallmark of human cancer. *Nat Genet* **37**, 391–400.

27. Rosato, R.R., and Grant, S. (2003) Histone deacetylase inhibitors in cancer therapy. *Cancer Biol Ther* **2**, 30–37.

28. Gibbons, R.J. (2005) Histone modifying and chromatin remodeling enzymes in cancer and dysplastic syndromes. *Hum Mol Genet* **14**, R85–R92.

29. Varga-Weisz, P.D., and Becker, P.B. (2006) Regulation of higher-order chromatin structures by nucleosome-remodelling factors. *Curr Opin Genet Dev* **16**, 151–56.

30. Medina, P.P., and Cespedes, M.S. (2008) Involvement of the chromatin-remodeling factor BRG1/SMARCA4 in human cancer. *Epigenetics* **3**, 64–68.

31. Xue, Y., Wong, J., Moreno, G.T., Young, M.K., Côté, J., and Wang, W. (1998) NURD, a novel complex with both ATP-dependent chromatin-remodeling and histone deacetylase activities. *Mol Cell* **2**, 851–61.

32. Morey, L., Brenner, C., Fazi, F., Villa, R., Gutierrez, A., Buschbeck, M., Nervi, C., Minucci, S., Fuks, F., and Di Croce, L. (2008) MBD3, a component of the NuRD complex, facilitates chromatin alteration and deposition of epigenetic marks. *Mol Cell Biol* **28**, 5912–23.

33. Sparmann, A., and van Lohuizen, M. (2006) Polycomb silencers control cell fate, development and cancer. *Nat Rev Cancer* **6**, 846–56.

34. Takihara, Y. (2008) Role of polycomb-group genes in sustaining activities of normal and malignant stem cells. *Int J Hematol* **87**, 25–34.
35. Fabbri, M., Croce, C.M., and Calin, G.A. (2008) MicroRNAs. *Cancer J* **14**, 1–6.
36. Kim, D.H., Saetrom, P., Snøve, O., Jr., and Rossi, J.J. (2008) MicroRNA-directed transcriptional gene silencing in mammalian cells. *Proc Natl Acad Sci USA* **105**, 16230–35.
37. Hawkins, P.G., and Morris, K.V. (2008) RNA and transcriptional modulation of gene expression. *Cell Cycle* **7**, 602–07.
38. Wolff, G.L., Kodell, R.L., Moore, S.R., and Cooney, C.A. (1998) Maternal epigenetics and methyl supplements affect agouti gene expression in Avy/a mice. *FASEB J* **12**, 949–57.
39. Waterland, R.A., and Jirtle, R.L. (2003) Transposable elements: Targets for early nutritional effects on epigenetic gene regulation. *Mol Cell Biol* **23**, 5293–300.
40. Cropley, J.E., Suter, C.M., Beckman, K.B., and Martin, D.I. (2006) Germ-line epigenetic modification of the murine A vy allele by nutritional supplementation. *Proc Natl Acad Sci USA* **103**, 17308–12.
41. Dolinoy, D.C., Weidman, J.R., Waterland, R.A., and Jirtle, R.L. (2006) Maternal genistein alters coat color and protects A^{vy} mouse offspring from obesity by modifying the fetal epigenome. *Environ Health Perspect* **114**, 567–72.
42. Waterland, R.A., Dolinoy, D.C., Lin, J.R., Smith, C.A., Shi, X., and Tahiliani, K.G. (2006) Maternal methyl supplements increase offspring DNA methylation at Axin Fused. *Genesis* **44**, 401–06.
43. Waterland, R.A., Lin, J.R., Smith, C.A., and Jirtle, R.L. (2006) Post-weaning diet affects genomic imprinting at the insulin-like growth factor 2 (*IGF2*) locus. *Hum Mol Genet* **15**, 705–16.
44. Heijmans, B.T., Tobi, E.W., Stein, A.D., Putter, H., Blauw, G.J., Susser, E.S., Slagboom, P.E., and Lumey, L.H. (2008) Persistent epigenetic differences associated with prenatal exposure to famine in humans. *Proc Natl Acad Sci USA* **105**, 17046–49.
45. Duhl, D.M., Vrieling, H., Miller, K.A., Wolff, G.L., and Barsh, G.S. (1994) Neomorphic agouti mutations in obese yellow mice. *Nat Genet* **8**, 59–65.
46. Cooney, C.A., Dave, A.A., and Wolff, G.L. (2002) Maternal methyl supplements in mice affect epigenetic variation and DNA methylation of offspring. *J Nutr* **132**, 2393S–400S.
47. Dolinoy, D.C., Huang, D., and Jirtle, R.L. (2007) Maternal nutrient supplementation counteracts bisphenol A-induced DNA hypomethylation in early development. *Proc Natl Acad Sci USA* **104**, 13056–61.
48. Waterland, R.A., Travisano, M., Tahiliani, K.G., Rached, M.T., and Mirza, S. (2008) Methyl donor supplementation prevents transgenerational amplification of obesity. *Int J Obes (Lond)* **32**, 1373–79.
49. Rakyan, V.K., Blewitt, M.E., Druker, R., Preis, J.I., and Whitelaw, E. (2002) Metastable epialleles in mammals. *Trends Genet* **18**, 348–51.
50. Whitelaw, E., and Martin, D.I. (2001) Retrotransposons as epigenetic mediators of phenotypic variation in mammals. *Nat Genet* **27**, 361–65.
51. Kotsopoulos, J., Sohn, K.J., and Kim, Y.I. (2008) Postweaning dietary folate deficiency provided through childhood to puberty permanently increases genomic DNA methylation in adult rat liver. *J Nutr* **138**, 703–09.
52. Ingrosso, D., Cimmino, A., Perna, A.F., Masella, L., De Santo, N.G., De Bonis, M.L., Vacca, M., D'Esposito, M., D'Urso, M., Galletti, P., and Zappia, V. (2003) Folate treatment and unbalanced methylation and changes of allelic expression by hyperhomocysteinaemia in patients with uraemia. *Lancet* **61**, 1693–99.
53. Fang, M., Chen, D., and Yang, C.S. (2007) Dietary polyphenols may affect DNA methylation. *J Nutr* **137**, 223S–8S.
54. Fang, M.Z., Wang, Y., Ai, N., Hou, Z., Sun, Y., Lu, H., Welsh, W., and Yang, C.S. (2003) Tea polyphenol (-)-epigallocatechin-3-gallate inhibits DNA methyltransferase and reactivates methylation-silenced genes in cancer cell lines. *Cancer Res* **63**, 7563–70.
55. Fang, M.Z., Chen, D., Sun, Y., Jin, Z., Christman, J.K., and Yang, C.S. (2005) Reversal of hyper-methylation and reactivation of p16INK4a, RARbeta, and MGMT genes by genistein and other isoflavones from soy. *Clin Cancer Res* **11**, 7033–41.
56. Fini, L., Selgrad, M., Fogliano, V., Graziani, G., Romano, M., Hotchkiss, E., Daoud, Y.A., De Vol, E.B., Boland, C.R., and Ricciardiello, L. (2007) Annurca apple polyphenols have potent

demethylating activity and can reactivate silenced tumor suppressor genes in colorectal cancer cells. *J Nutr* **137**, 2622–28.

57. Klein, E.A., Thompson, I.M., Lippman, S.M., Goodman, P.J., Albanes, D., Taylor, P.R., and Coltman, C. (2000) SELECT: The selenium and vitamin E cancer prevention trial: Rationale and design. *Prostate Cancer Prostatic Dis* **3**, 145–51.

58. Xiang, N., Zhao, R., Song, G., and Zhong, W. (2008) Selenite reactivates silenced genes by modifying DNA methylation and histones in prostate cancer cells. *Carcinogenesis* **29**, 2175–81.

59. Garfinkel, M.D., and Ruden, D.M. (2004) Chromatin effects in nutrition, cancer and obesity. *Nutrition* **20**, 56–62.

60. Myzak, M.C., and Dashwood, R.H. (2006) Histone deacetylases as targets for dietary cancer preventive agents: Lessons learned with butyrate, diallyl disulfide and sulforaphane. *Curr Drug Targets* **7**, 443–52.

61. Mariadason, J.M., Corner, G.A., and Augenlicht, L.H. (2000) Genetic reprogramming in pathways of colonic cell maturation induced by short chain fatty acids: Comparison with trichostatin A, sulindac, and curcumin and implications for chemoprevention of colon cancer. *Cancer Res* **60**, 4561–72.

62. Bernhard, D., Ausserlechner, M.J., Tonko, M., Löffler, M., Hartmann, B.L., Csordas, A., and Kofler, R. (1999) Apoptosis induced by the histone deacetylase inhibitor sodium butyrate in human leukemic lymphoblasts. *FASEB J* **13**, 1991–2001.

63. Fang, Y.J., Chen, Y.X., Lu, J., Lu, R., Yang, L., Zhu, H.Y., Gu, W.Q., and Lu, L.G. (2004) Epigenetic modification regulates both expression of tumor-associated genes and cell cycle progressing in human colon cancer cell lines: Colo-320 and SW1116. *Cell Res* **14**, 217–26.

64. Davie, J.R. (2003) Inhibition of histone deacetylase activity by butyrate. *J Nutr* **133**, 2485S–93S.

65. Druesne, N., Pagniez, A., Mayeur, C., Thomas, M., Cherbuy, C., Duée, P.H., Martel, P., and Chaumontet, C. (2004) Diallyl disulfide (DADS) increases histone acetylation and p21[waf1/cip1] expression in human colon tumor cell lines. *Carcinogenesis* **25**, 1227–36.

66. Druesne-Pecollo, N., Pagniez, A., Thomas, A., Cherbuy, C., Duée, P.H., Martel, P., and Chaumontet, C. (2006) Diallyl disulfide increases CDKN1A promoter-associated histone acetylation in human colon tumor cell lines. *J Agric Food Chem* **54**, 7503–07.

67. Lea, M.A., and Randolph, V.M. (2001) Induction of histone acetylation in rat liver and hepatoma by organosulfur compounds including diallyl disulfide. *Anticancer Res* **21**, 2841–46.

68. Druesne-Pecollo, N., Chaumontet, C., Pagniez, A., Vaugelade, P., Bruneau, A., Thomas, M., Cherbuy, C., Duée, P.H., and Martel, P. (2007) In vivo treatment by diallyl disulfide increases histone acetylation in rat colonocytes. *Biochem Biophys Res Commun* **354**, 140–47.

69. Lea, M.A., Rasheed, M., Randolph, V.M., Khan, F., Shareef, A., and desBordes, C. (2002) Induction of histone acetylation and inhibition of growth of mouse erythroleukemia cells by S-allylmercaptocysteine. *Nutr Cancer* **43**, 90–102.

70. Myzak, M.C., Karplus, A., Chung, F.-L., and Dashwood, R.H. (2004) A novel mechanism of chemoprotection by sulforaphane: Inhibition of histone deactylase. *Cancer Res* **64**, 5767–74.

71. Myzak, M.C., Hardin, K., Wang, R., Dashwood, R.H., and Ho, E. (2006) Sulforaphane inhibits histone deacetylase activity in BPH-1, LnCaP and PC-3 prostate epithelial cells. *Carcinogenesis* **27**, 811–19.

72. Myzak, M.C., Dashwood, W.M., Orner, G.A., Ho, E., and Dashwood, R.H. (2006) Sulforaphane inhibits histone deacetylase in vivo and suppresses tumorigenesi in *APC* [min] mice. *FASEB J* **20**, 506–08.

73. Myzak, M.C., Tong, P., Dashwood, W.M., Dashwood, R.H., and Ho, E. (2007) Sulforaphane retards the growth of human PC-3 xenografts and inhibits HDAC activity in human subjects. *Exp Biol Med (Maywood)* **232**, 227–34.

74. Wang, L.G., Belkemisheva, A., Liu, X.M., Ferrari, A.C., Feng, J., and Chiao, J.W. (2007) Dual action on promoter demethylation and chromatin by an isothiocyanate restored GSTP1 silenced in prostate cancer. *Mol Carcinog* **46**, 24–31.

75. Majid, S., Kikuno, N., Nelles, J., Noonan, E., Tanaka, Y., Kawamoto, K., Hirata, H., Li, L.C., Zhao, H., Okino, S.T., Place, R.F., Pookot, D., and Dahiya, R. (2008) Genistein induces the p21WAF1/CIP1

and p16INK4a tumor suppressor genes in prostate cancer cells by epigenetic mechanisms involving active chromatin modification. *Cancer Res* **68**, 2736–44.

76. Kikuno, N., Shiina, H., Urakami, S., Kawamoto, K., Hirata, H., Tanaka, Y., Majid, S., Igawa, M., and Dahiya, R. (2008) Genistein mediated histone acetylation and demethylation activates tumor suppressor genes in prostate cancer cells. *Int J Cancer* **123**, 552–60.

77. Lam, Y., Galvez, A., and de Lumen, B.O. (2003) Lunasin suppresses E1A-mediated transformation of mammalian cells but does not inhibit growth of immortalized and established cancer cell lines. *Nutr Cancer* **47**, 88–94.

78. Jeong, H.J., Jeong, J.B., Kim, D.S., and de Lumen, B.O. (2007) Inhibition of core histone acetylation by the cancer preventive peptide lunasin *J Agri Food Chem* **55**, 632–37.

79. Aagaard-Tillery, K.M., Grove, K., Bishop, J., Ke, X., Fu, Q., McKnight, R., and Lane, R.H. (2008) Developmental origins of disease and determinants of chromatin structure: Maternal diet modifies the primate fetal epigenome. *J Mol Endocrinol* **41**, 91–102.

80. Pogribny, I.P., Ross, S.A., Tryndyak, V.P., Pogribna, M., Poirier, L.A., and Karpinets, T.V. (2006) Histone H3 lysine 9 and H4 lysine 20 trimethylation and the expression of Suv-20h2 and Suv-39h1 histone methyltransferases in hepatocarcinogenesis induced by methyl deficiency in rats. *Carcinogenesis* **27**, 1180–86.

81. Chew, Y.C., West, J.T., Kratzer, S.J., Ilvarsonn, A.M., Eissenberg, J.C., Dave, B.J., Klinkebiel, D., Christman, J.K., and Zempleni, J. (2008) Biotinylation of histones represses transposable elements in human and mouse cells and cell lines and in Drosophila melanogaster. *J Nutr* **138**, 2316–22.

82. Lee, E.R., Murdoch, F.E., and Fritsch, M.K. (2007) High histone acetylation and decreased polycomb repressive complex 2 member levels regulate gene specific transcriptional changes during early embryonic stem cell differentiation induced by retinoic acid. *Stem Cells* **25**, 2191–99.

83. Kim, J.H., Yoon, S.Y., Kim, C.N., Joo, J.H., Moon, S.K., Choe, I.S., Choe, Y.K., and Kim, J.W. (2004) The Bmi-1 oncoprotein is overexpressed in human colorectal cancer and correlates with the reduced p16INK4a/p14ARF proteins. *Cancer Lett* **203**, 217–24.

84. Vonlanthen, S., Heighway, J., Altermatt, H.J., Gugger, M., Kappeler, A., Borner, M.M., van Lohuizen, M., and Betticher, D.C. (2001) The bmi-1 oncoprotein is differentially expressed in non-small cell lung cancer and correlates with INK4A-ARF locus expression. *Br J Cancer* **84**, 1372–76.

85. Lee, K., Adhikary, G., Balasubramanian, S., Gopalakrishna, R., McCormick, T., Dimri, G.P., Eckert, R.L., and Rorke, E.A. (2008) Expression of Bmi-1 in epidermis enhances cell survival by altering cell cycle regulatory protein expression and inhibiting apoptosis. *J Invest Dermatol* **128**, 9–17.

86. Balasubramanian, S., Lee, K., Adhikary, G., Gopalakrishnan, R., Rorke, E.A., and Eckert, R.L. (2008) The Bmi-1 polycomb group gene in skin cancer – Regulation of function by (-)-Epigallocatechin-3-gallate (EGCG). *Nutr Rev* **66**, S65–S68.

87. Pogribny, I.P., Tryndyak, V.P., Muskhelishvili, L., Rusyn, I., and Ross, S.A. (2007) Methyl deficiency, alterations in global histone modifications, and carcinogenesis. *J Nutr* **137**, 216S–22S.

88. Newberne, P.M. (1986) Lipotropic factors and oncogenesis. *Adv Exp Med Biol* **206**, 223–51.

89. Poirier, L.A. (1994) Methyl group deficiency in hepatocarcinogenesis. *Drug Metab Rev* **26**, 185–99.

90. Denda, A., Kitayama, W., Kishida, H., Murata, N., Tsutsumi, M., Tsujiuchi, T., Nakae, D., and Konishi, Y. (2002) Development of hepatocellular adenomas and carcinomas associated with fibrosis in C57BL/6 J male mice given a choline-deficient, L-amino acid-defined diet. *Jpn J Cancer Res* **93**, 125–32.

91. Christman, J.K. (2003) Diet, DNA methylation and cancer. In: Daniel, H., and Zempleni, J. eds.. *Molecular Nutrition*. Oxon: CABI Publishing, 237–65.

92. Wainfan, E., and Poirier, L.A. (1992) Methyl groups in carcinogenesis: Effects on DNA methylation and gene expression. *Cancer Res* **52**, 2071S–7S.

93. Christman, J.K., Sheikhnejad, G., Dizik, M., Abileah, S., and Wainfan, E. (1993) Reversibility of changes in nucleic acid methylation and gene expression in rat liver by severe dietary methyl deficiency. *Carcinogenesis* **14**, 551–57.

94. Pogribny, I.P., James, S.J., Jernigan, S., and Pogribna, M. (2004) Genomic hypomethylation is specific for preneoplastic liver in folate/methyl deficient rats and does not occur in non-target tissues. *Mutat Res* **548**, 53–59.

95. Ghoshal, K., Li, X., Datta, J., Bai, S., Pogribny, I., Pogribny, M., Huang, Y., Young, D., and Jacob, S.T. (2006) A folate- and methyl-deficient diet alters the expression of DNA methyltransferases and methyl CpG binding proteins involved in epigenetic gene silencing in livers of F344 rats. *J Nutr* **136**, 1522–27.

96. Kutay, H., Bai, S., Datta, J., Motiwala, T., Pogribny, I., Frankel, W., Jacob, S.T., and Ghoshal, K. (2006) Downregulation of miR-122 in the rodent and human hepatocellular carcinomas. *J Cell Biochem* **99**, 671–78.

97. Tryndyak, V.P., Ross, S.A., Beland, F.A., and Pogribny, I.P. (2008) Down-regulation of the microRNAs miR-34a, miR-127, and miR-200b in rat liver during hepatocarcinogenesis induced by a methyl-deficient diet. *Mol Carcinog* Oct 21 [Epub ahead of print].

98. Pogribny, I.P., Ross, S.A., Wise, C., Pogribna, M., Jones, E.A., Tryndyak, V.P., James, S.J., Dragan, Y.P., and Poirier, L.A. (2006) Irreversible global DNA hypomethylation as a key step in hepatocarcinogenesis induced by dietary methyl deficiency. *Mutat Res* **593**, 80–87.

99. Powel, C.L., Kosyk, O., Bradford, B.U., Parker, J.S., Lobenhofer, E.K., Denda, A., Uematsu, F., Nakae, D., and Rusyn, I. (2005) Temporal correlation of pathology and DNA damage with gene expression in a choline-deficient model of rat liver injury. *Hepatology* **42**, 1137–47.

100. Sun, M., Estrov, Z., Ji, Y., Coombes, K.R., Harris, D.H., and Kurzrock, R. (2008) Curcumin (diferuloylmethane) alters the expression profiles of microRNAs in human pancreatic cancer cells. *Mol Cancer Ther* **7**, 464–73.

101. Guil, S., and Esteller, M. (2009) DNA methylomes, histone codes and miRNAs: Tying it all together. *Int J Biochem Cell Biol* **41**, 87–95.

6 Nutrient Signaling – Protein Kinase to Transcriptional Activation

Ann M. Bode and Zigang Dong

Key Points

1. The widespread opinion today is that cancer may be prevented or treated by targeting specific cancer genes, signaling proteins, and transcription factors. Transcriptions factors are comprised of one or more proteins that bind to a specific DNA gene sequence and act to initiate transcription.
2. The molecular mechanisms explaining how normal cells undergo transformation to cancer cells induced by tumor promoters have been the subject of intense investigation. These studies have revealed that the mitogen-activated protein (MAP) kinase signaling pathways are activated differentially by various tumor promoters.
3. The activation of transcription factors including AP-1, NF-κB, p53, NFAT, and CREB protein results in transcription of genes whose proteins regulate a multitude of cellular responses including apoptosis, proliferation, inflammation, differentiation, and development.
4. Nutrients and dietary factors have attracted a great deal of interest because of their perceived ability to act as highly effective chemopreventive agents by targeting protein kinases and/or transcription factors, with very few adverse side effects.
5. The AP-1 transcription factor is a potential target mediated by upstream kinase cascades for regulation and chemoprevention by specific nutrients, including epigallocatechin gallate (EGCG), theaflavins, caffeine, [6]-gingerol, resveratrol, and various flavonols such as kaempferol, quercetin, and myricetin.

Key Words: Activator protein-1; transcriptome; signal transduction; transcriptomics; MAP kinase; tumor promotion; [6]-gingerol; EGCG; theaflavin; flavonol; resveratrol

1. INTRODUCTION

Experimental evidence clearly shows that the process of carcinogenesis involves changes in expression of many genes and proteins that are crucial in the regulation of all cellular functions. The transcriptome is the set of all messenger RNA (mRNA) molecules, or "transcripts," produced in a population of cells. Environmental factors, including nutrition, can have a strong influence on the transcriptome because unlike the genome, which is generally established for a particular cell type, the transcriptome

From: *Nutrition and Health: Bioactive Compounds and Cancer*
Edited by: J.A. Milner, D.F. Romagnolo, DOI 10.1007/978-1-60761-627-6_6,
© Springer Science+Business Media, LLC 2010

varies under the influence of external and internal factors. The expanding science of transcriptomics examines the expression level of mRNAs in a specific cell population and is key in identifying the molecular and cellular mechanisms involved in cancer development. In the cell, the transcriptome is regulated by the activity of transcription factors. A transcription factor is comprised of one or more proteins that bind to a specific gene DNA sequence and act either to initiate or repress transcription leading to increased or decreased mRNA production. DNA binding is commonly induced by protein kinases and transcription factors that act downstream of these signaling cascades are heavily involved in cellular functions that include survival, development, proliferation, apoptosis, cell cycle regulation, inflammation, and differentiation (Fig. 1). Signal transduction is the process by which information from a stimulus outside the cell is transmitted through the cell membrane (e.g., through a protein receptor) into the cell and along an intracellular chain of signaling proteins (e.g., protein kinases) to cause a response (Fig. 1). Dysfunctional transduction of external and/or internal signals can lead to diseases such as cancer. Protein kinase signaling, resulting in the induction of transcriptional activation of specific transcription factors, plays a critical role in carcinogenesis. A protein kinase catalyzes a reaction called phosphorylation, in which one or more phosphate groups are added to a target protein (i.e., substrate). Phosphorylation causes a change in the function of a target protein substrate that can include enhanced or reduced activity, alterations in cellular localization, or changes in

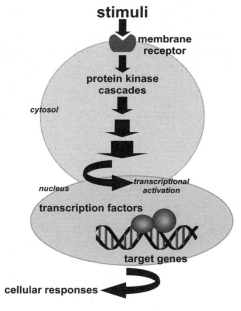

Fig. 1. General scheme of signal transduction from membrane receptor to transcription factor(s) via protein kinase cascades. Membrane receptors respond to external (or internal) stimuli. The response (signal) is transmitted from the membrane and amplified through protein kinase cascades to the nucleus where it results in the binding of transcription factors to DNA response elements modulating transcription of the target gene.

association with other proteins. Kinases phosphorylate both serine and threonine residues and some act on tyrosine, whereas a few have dual specificity and act on all three residues. Approximately 500 protein kinases are known to control most cellular pathways including critical signal transduction pathways that regulate proliferation and cell death and, therefore, their activity is normally very tightly regulated. Aberrant regulation of kinase activity and associated transcriptional activation is closely associated with carcinogenesis and thus these molecules might be ideal targets for cancer prevention and/or therapy *(1)*. One of the most important outcomes in cancer research has been the clarification of signal transduction pathways induced by tumor promoters, including phorbol esters, growth factors, and ultraviolet (UV) irradiation in cancer development. It is widely accepted that cancer may be prevented or treated by targeting specific cancer genes, signaling proteins, and transcription factors. Cancer is believed to be a multistage process that includes an initiation stage, which can be relatively short and irreversible, and a promotion stage, which is a long-term process that requires chronic exposure to a tumor promoter. Promotion is often considered as rate limiting to the overall process of cancer development. Therefore, understanding the molecular mechanisms of promotion is crucial for the development of effective anticancer agents.

Dietary factors have attracted a great deal of interest because of their potential ability to act as effective chemopreventive agents by preventing or reversing premalignant lesions and/or reducing tumor incidence *(2)*. A wealth of experimental evidence suggests that many nutrients might be used alone or in combination with traditional chemotherapeutic agents to prevent or treat cancer. Therefore, identifying the specific signal transduction pathways, gene, protein, and transcription factor targets, and mechanisms explaining the purported anticancer activity of specific dietary factors might provide effective alternatives or additions to traditional methods of cancer prevention (i.e., chemoprevention) or cancer treatment (i.e., chemotherapy).

The molecular mechanisms explaining how normal cells undergo transformation to cancer cells induced by tumor promoters have been the subject of intense investigation. These studies have revealed the mitogen-activated protein (MAP) kinase signaling pathways (Fig. 2) are activated differentially by various tumor promoters (reviewed in *(3–11)*). Various environmental stimuli also activate MAP kinase cascades, which regulate many cellular responses that result in the transcriptional activation of immediate-early-response genes (IEG) *(12)*. The rapid induction of IEG by external stimuli is associated with the delivery of intracellular signals to transcription factors and cofactors at regulatory elements as well as nucleosomes present both at the promoter and within the transcribed region of genes *(13)*. In particular, the Ras/extracellular signal-regulated kinase (Ras/ERK) pathway (Fig. 2) plays a critical role in regulating cell proliferation, survival, growth and motility *(14, 15)*, and tumorigenesis *(16)*.

MAP kinases are activated by translocation to the nucleus, where they phosphorylate a variety of target transcription factors that are important in tumor development. The MAP kinases include the extracellular-signal-regulated protein kinases (ERK), c-Jun N-terminal kinases/stress-activated protein kinases (JNK/SAPK), and the

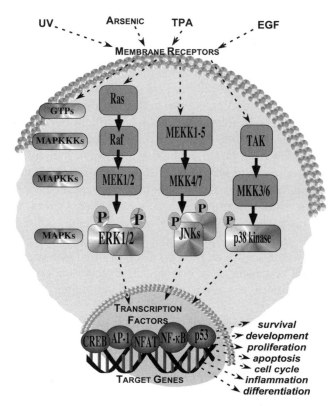

Fig. 2. The mitogen-activated protein kinase cascades. Tumor promoters such as UV, TPA, EGF, or arsenic stimulate membrane receptors that activate various MAP kinase cascades. Although not mutually exclusive, ERK generally transduces signals initiated by tumor promoters such as TPA, EGF, and PDGF. The JNKs/SAPKs and p38 kinases are strongly stimulated by UV and arsenic. MAP kinase cascades regulate transcription factors with a proven role in carcinogenesis including AP-1, NF-κB, p53, NFAT, and CREB. Cellular responses may be survival, development, proliferation, apoptosis, regulation of cell cycle, inflammation, and differentiation.

p38 kinases. ERK generally transmit signals initiated by tumor promoters such as 12-*O*-tetradecanoylphorbol-13-acetate (TPA), epidermal growth factor (EGF), and platelet-derived growth factor (PDGF) *(17)*. The JNK/SAPK and p38 kinases are strongly stimulated by stresses such as UV irradiation *(18)* and arsenic *(19–21)*. MAP kinase cascades (Fig. 2) regulate transcription factors with a proven role in carcinogenesis including AP-1 and NF-κB *(5, 22)*, p53 *(4)*, NFAT *(23, 24)*, and CREB *(25)*. The activation of these signaling cascades can result in transcriptional activation of genes whose protein products regulate a multitude of cellular responses including apoptosis, proliferation, inflammation, differentiation, and development. This chapter will focus on AP-1 as a target transcription factor of upstream kinase cascades and regulation by specific nutrients including EGCG, theaflavins, caffeine, [6]-gingerol, the isoflavandiol equol, resveratrol (and analogues), and various flavonols such as kaempferol, quercetin, and myricetin.

2. NUTRIENTS AND AP-1 ACTIVATION

AP-1 is a very well-characterized transcription factor composed of homodimers and/or heterodimers of the Jun, Fos, ATF (activating transcription factor), and MAF (musculoaponeurotic fibrosarcoma) protein families (26, 27). The Jun protein family comprises c-Jun, JunB, and JunD whereas the Fos family consists of c-Fos, FosB, Fra-1, and Fra-2. The activation and subsequent binding of AP-1 protein dimers to specific gene sequences results in stimulation of cell proliferation and survival functions (Fig. 3). AP-1 plays a major role in cell transformation and is crucial in tumor promotion, progression, and metastasis (28–33). Notably, neoplastic transformation and TPA-induced cancer progression are blocked by inhibiting tumor promoter-induced AP-1 activity (29, 34–37). Constitutive elevation of AP-1 levels has been observed in malignant but not in benign mouse epidermal cells (38). -(-) Epigallocatechin gallate (EGCG) (reviewed in (22, 39–46)), theaflavins (7), caffeine (47), [6]-gingerol (48, 49), equol (50), resveratrol or analogues (51–57), kaempferol, quercetin (58), and myricetin (59) were shown to markedly inhibit cell transformation and carcinogenesis mediated by AP-1 (60).

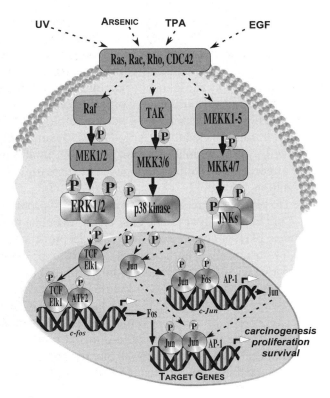

Fig. 3. Activation of signaling cascades and AP-1 in tumor promotion. Tumor promoters, including TPA, EGF, arsenic, and UV irradiation, induce signaling cascades leading to AP-1 activation, which may result in tumor formation, proliferation, and survival. Three MAP kinase pathways (ERK, p38, JNK) and their target molecules lead to AP-1 activation.

2.1. AP-1 Transcriptional Activation Is Suppressed by EGCG

EGCG, a polyphenolic compound, accounts for ~50–80% of the total catechins found in green tea *(7, 45, 46, 61–63)*. Research data suggest that EGCG suppresses carcinogenesis in a variety of tissues through inhibition of MAP kinases, growth factor-related cell signaling, activation of NF-κB, topoisomerase I, and matrix metalloproteinases (reviewed in *(7, 39, 43, 44, 46, 61)*). However, EGCG appears to exert many of its anticancer effects through suppression of AP-1-mediated activation of transcription. EGCG was reported to inhibit tumor promoter-induced MAP kinase and AP-1 activation and cell transformation in JB6 *(64, 65)*, A172, and NIH3T3 *(66)* cell lines. UVB exposure of mouse skin epidermis or cultured skin cells caused a major increase in AP-1 activation that was substantially suppressed by treatment with EGCG or theaflavins *(67, 68)*. Suppression of UVB-induced AP-1 activation may very likely be related to EGCG-dependent inhibition of UVB-induced transcriptional activation of the *c-fos* gene and accumulation of the c-Fos protein *(69)*, an important component of the AP-1 protein complex.

Activation of Fyn, a nonreceptor tyrosine kinase and member of the Src family, plays a critical role in the development of skin cancer *(70, 71)*. Interactions of Fyn with various signaling molecules regulate diverse biological functions important in the progression of carcinogenesis *(72, 73)*. Activated Fyn promotes oral cancer progression via ERK and integrin β6 signaling *(74)*. The Fyn tyrosine kinase is a downstream mediator of Rho/PKR2 function in keratinocyte cell–cell adhesion *(75)*. Recently, He et al. *(76)* reported that EGCG suppressed EGF-induced cell transformation in JB6 cells mediated through Fyn kinase activation and phosphorylation. EGCG directly bound to the Fyn-SH2 domain, but not the Fyn-SH3 domain. Compared with control JB6 Cl41 cells, EGF-induced phosphorylation and DNA-binding activity of ATF-2 (Thr71) and signal transducer and activator of transcription-1 (STAT1) (Thr727) were decreased by siRNA against Fyn and inhibited by EGCG in JB6 cells. Therefore, inhibition of Fyn kinase activity is a novel and important mechanism that may contribute to EGCG-induced inhibition of cell transformation *(76)*.

EGCG was reported to directly target and inhibit a number of proteins associated with the MAP kinase/AP-1 signaling pathway. The zeta chain-associated protein of 70 kDa (ZAP-70) tyrosine kinase plays a critical role in T-cell receptor-mediated signal transduction and the immune response. A high level of ZAP-70 expression is observed in leukemia. ZAP-70 and EGCG displayed high binding affinity ($K_d = 0.6207$ μmol/l) and EGCG effectively suppressed ZAP-70, MAP kinase kinase activities, and the activation of AP-1 and interleukin-2 induced by CD3 *(77)*. Notably, EGCG induced caspase-mediated apoptosis in ZAP-70 expressing leukemia cells, but not in ZAP-70 deficient cells. Molecular docking studies, supported by site-directed mutagenesis experiments, showed that EGCG could form a series of intermolecular hydrogen bonds and hydrophobic interactions within the ATP-binding domain contribute to the stability of the ZAP-70/EGCG heterocomplex *(77)*.

The *Ras* pathway is critical in the activation of AP-1. Mutations of the *Ras* gene occur frequently in many cancers and are associated with uncontrolled growth. Chung et al. *(78)* reported that the H-*Ras*-activated AP-1 pathway is a growth stimulant in transformed mutant *H-ras* JB6 cells. Treatment of JB6 cells with green or black tea polyphenols strongly suppressed cell growth and phosphorylation of ERK, c-Jun, Fra-1, and also decreased AP-1 activity *(78)*. In intestinal epithelial cells (RIE-1), EGCG was reported to inhibit Ras-induced cell proliferation, perhaps through suppression of cyclin D1 expression, leading to G1 arrest *(79)*. Notably, the inhibitory effects of EGCG were more pronounced in transformed cells than in non-transformed cells *(79)*. Similarly, EGCG was shown to have no effect on normal human fetal colon cells. Nevertheless, it inhibited growth of a variety of colon cancer cell lines including Caco2, HCT116, HT29, SW480, and SW837 *(80)*. One marked difference between normal and cancer cell lines used in these studies was the overexpression and constitutive activation of the EGF receptor (EGFR) and HER2 proteins in the colon cancer cell lines *(80)*. Decreased phosphorylation of EGFR, HER2, ERKs, and Akt proteins and an induction of G1 arrest and apoptosis were also observed following treatment with EGCG. These effects appeared to be mediated through a suppression of AP-1, c-Fos, NF-κB, and cyclin D1 activities *(80)*. These findings strongly support the idea that EGCG prevents malignant transformation by suppressing MAP kinase-dependent activation of AP-1.

2.2. Black Tea Theaflavins Inhibit AP-1 Transactivation

Theaflavins are formed from catechins during enzymatic oxidation and confer black tea its characteristic color and taste. Polyphenols included in this group are theaflavin (TF), theaflavin-3-gallate (TF-2a), theaflavin-3′-gallate (TF-2b), and theaflavin-3,3′-digallate (TF-3) *(81)*. Research data suggest that theaflavins might act through different mechanisms and have a more potent anticancer activity compared to EGCG. Both EGCG and TF-3 were reported to inhibit phosphorylation of c-Jun and ERKs, but only TF-3 inhibited p38 *(78)*. Further studies *(82)* confirmed that either EGCG or TF-3 decreased phosphorylation of ERK and MEK, but TF-3 acted at earlier time points (15 min) whereas the effects of EGCG were not apparent until 60 min post-treatment. Furthermore, TF-3 decreased Raf-1 protein levels, whereas EGCG decreased the association of Raf-1 with MEK1 *(82)*. Theaflavins were stronger inhibitors of UVB-induced AP-1 activation compared to EGCG *(68)*. Theaflavins were shown to inhibit UVB-induced phosphorylation of JNK at very low concentrations (0.5 μM) *(83)*. Recently, theaflavins (20 μM) and TF-3 were reported to induce EGFR down-regulation in JB6 Cl41 mouse epidermal and A431 human EGFR-overexpressing epidermoid carcinoma cells *(84)*. Furthermore, TF-3 suppressed EGFR-induced phosphorylation and downstream signaling to ERK and AP-1 resulting in inhibition of EGF-induced cell transformation *(84)*. Therefore, theaflavins appeared to act on AP-1 mainly through EGFR/MAP kinase signaling.

2.3. Xanthine 70, a Caffeine Analogue, but Not Caffeine, Inhibits AP-1 Activation

Caffeine (1,3,7-trimethylxanthine) is a natural compound present in cocoa, cola nuts, coffee, and tea *(47)*. Various analogues of caffeine, referred to as 1,3,7-trialkylxanthines or xanthines, have been examined for their anticancer activity. Mechanistically, caffeine has been reported to primarily affect cell cycle function, induce programmed cell death or apoptosis, and perturb key regulatory proteins including the tumor suppressor protein, p53 *(85, 86)*. Although the effects of caffeine have been vastly investigated, much of the research data regarding caffeine's effects on cell cycle and proliferation are somewhat inconclusive. A potential explanation is that the effects of caffeine have been investigated in a wide range of experimental conditions, using different cell types, and a wide range of concentrations (μM to high mM). In humans, achieving a 2 mM blood level of caffeine would require the simultaneous consumption of over 100 cups of coffee *(87)*, suggesting mM concentrations used in certain studies are largely supraphysiological.

Previous studies revealed that caffeine inhibited chemically induced tumors of the skin *(88)*, lung *(89)*, stomach *(90)*, and liver *(91)*. The oral administration of caffeine was also reported to substantially inhibit UVB-induced skin carcinogenesis in SKH-1 mice *(92)*. Caffeine suppressed the proliferation of various cancer and transformed cell lines including human neuroblastoma cells, human pancreatic adenocarcinoma cells, and human A549 lung adenocarcinoma cells *(85, 93, 94)*. Proliferation *(95)* and tumor promoter-induced neoplastic transformation *(96)* of JB6 cells were also inhibited by caffeine treatment. The compounds 1,3-dimethylxanthine (theophylline) and 1-methyl-3-propyl-7-butylxanthine (xanthine 77) were proposed to be potential anticancer drugs especially in combination with other chemotherapeutic drugs *(97–100)*. Xanthine analogues containing methyl groups were also reported to enhance the killing of p53-deficient cells *(101)*. A recent study investigated the potential chemopreventive activities of 50 different 1,3,7-trialkylxanthines, which resemble caffeine in their structures, but differ in the length of the alkyl side chains *(102)*. Interestingly, xanthine 70, but not caffeine, potently inhibited EGF-induced AP-1 activation and TPA- or H-Ras-induced neoplastic transformation. Overall, results indicated that the number of carbons at R1 or R3 was important for the antitumor-promoting activity of trialkylxanthines and that xanthine 70 might be a potential anticancer agent *(102)*. However, the specific target for xanthine remains to be identified.

2.4. [6]-Gingerol Modulates AP-1 Activation

One of the most popular and highly consumed dietary substances in the world is derived from plants of the ginger (*Zingiber officinale* Roscoe, Zingiberaceae) family *(103)*. The oleoresin or oil from ginger root contains [6]-gingerol (1-[4'-hydroxy-3'-methoxyphenyl]-5-hydroxy-3-decanone), which is the major pharmacologically active component, and a variety of other gingerols, gingerdiols, paradols, and zingerones. The medicinal, chemical, and pharmacological properties of ginger have been extensively reviewed *(49, 104–106)*. Numerous research studies have reported that specific components of ginger suppress cancer cell growth *(107–110)*. Various reports proposed indirect mechanisms by which ginger compounds exert their antitumorigenic effects, which have been extensively reviewed *(48, 49, 59, 111)*. Ginger appears to exert chemopreventive activity through a combination of antioxidant and pro-apoptotic activities. Although cyclooxygenase-2 (COX-2) and NF-κB are clearly affected by various components of ginger, specific molecular targets have not been clearly identified. The effect of two structurally related compounds of the ginger family,

[6]-gingerol and [6]-paradol, on EGF-induced cell transformation and AP-1 activation were investigated *(107)*. Results of these studies indicated that both compounds blocked EGF-induced cell transformation and although [6]-gingerol, but not paradol, inhibited AP-1 activation, both could induce apoptosis *(107)*. Independent studies showed that [6]-paradol and structurally related derivatives, [10]-paradol, [3]-dehydroparadol, [6]-dehydroparadol, and [10]-dehydroparadol inhibited proliferation and induced apoptosis in KB oral squamous carcinoma cells *(112)*. These cumulative results suggest that components of ginger may be effective anticancer agents, but additional studies are needed to determine the specific mechanism of action and their molecular targets.

2.5. Resveratrol and AP-1

Resveratrol is a member of the phytoalexin family of compounds that are produced in plants during times of environmental stress or in response to pathogenic attack *(113)*. Studies that have investigated the anticarcinogenic effects of resveratrol (for review see *52–57*) did not identify AP-1 as the primary molecular target. However, an analogue of resveratrol, RSVL2, was shown to inhibit AP-1 transactivation, *c-fos* activation, and cell transformation through suppression of MEK. RSVL2, but not resveratrol, inhibited TPA-induced phosphorylation of ERK and p90RSK *(114)*. The constitutive activation of MEK1 results in cellular transformation. Both MEK1 and MEK2 have a unique inhibitor-binding pocket adjacent to the MgATP-binding site. MEK1-selective small molecule inhibitors (i.e., PD318088, PD184352, PD098059, U0126) may share a common or overlapping binding site for MEK1 and lock MEK1 into a closed inactive species *(115–117)*. Notably, RSVL2 was also shown to directly bind to MEK1, suggesting the mechanism of MEK inactivation by RSVL2 may be similar to that of MEK1 inhibitors. In addition, although both resveratrol and RSVL2 were reported to bind to and inhibit COX-2 activation, RSVL2 was a stronger inhibitor *(118)*. Importantly, blocking ERK activity using a dominant negative ERK2 or the MEK1 inhibitor, PD098059, blocked TPA- or EGF-induced AP-1 and cell transformation *(119)*. MEK1 and MEK2 share 79% amino acid identity and are equally effective at phosphorylating ERK substrates *(120)*. Evidence suggests that MEK plays a key role in the transformation of cells and development of tumors because small molecular inhibitors of MEK suppressed transformation and tumor growth in both cell culture and mouse models *(17, 121)*. These data indicate that more potent anticancer agents can be derived from the parent compound resveratrol leading to the development of more effective anticancer strategies based on the combined use of resveratrol and its synthetic analogues.

2.6. The Flavonol Compounds, Kaempferol, Quercetin, and Myricetin, Effectively Suppress AP-1 Activation

Flavonols such as myricetin, quercetin, and kaempferol are found in edible plants. The highest total flavonol content is found in onion leaves (quercetin at 1,497.5 mg/kg and kaempferol at 832.0 mg/kg) *(122)*. Kaempferol has been shown to inhibit RSK2 activity *(123, 124)*, which leads to cell proliferation and anchorage-independent cell transformation. RSK2 is a key regulator for tumor promoter-induced cell transformation and ectopic expression of RSK2 in JB6 Cl41 cells caused increased proliferation as well as anchorage-independent transformation *(125)*. Furthermore, knockdown of RSK2 by siRNA almost totally blocked foci formation in NIH3T3 cells. These results demonstrated that RSK2 was a key regulator of cell transformation induced by the tumor promoters EGF or TPA, and kaempferol suppressed cell proliferation and EGF-induced transformation in JB6 Cl41 cells *(125)*.

Experimental evidence suggests that Raf and/or Ras is constitutively activated in several tumor cell lines, and that the transforming actions of several oncogenes are dependent on the activation of the MEK/ERK/AP-1 pathway *(78, 82, 126)*. No substrates for MEK1 have been identified other than ERK1 and ERK2, and activated MEK1 catalyzes the phosphorylation of ERK at Thr183 and Tyr185 *(120)*. This selectivity, coupled with a unique ability to phosphorylate both tyrosine and threonine residues, indicates that MEK is essential for integrating signals into the MAP kinase pathway. MEK plays a critical role in signal cascades initiated by the tumor promoters TPA, EGF, and PDGF *(5, 17)*. Additionally, a mutant *H-ras* gene perpetually activates the MEK/ERK signaling pathway and predisposes transition to anchorage-independent growth *(78, 82, 126)*. Because the abnormal activation of the ERK pathway has been reported to be pivotal in various human tumors *(127, 128)*, targeted inhibition of the ERK pathway by small molecules is a main goal of current chemopreventative strategies.

Compared to resveratrol, the flavonol content of red wine is about 30 times higher. The two major flavonols found in red wine are 3,3,4,5,5,7-hexahydroxyflavone (myricetin) and 3,3,4,5,7-pentahydroxyflavone (quercetin) *(129)*. These compounds represent ~20–50% of the total flavonol content found in red wine *(129)*. Quercetin exerted protective effects in 9,10-dimethyl-1,2-benzanthracene (DMBA)-initiated and TPA-promoted two-stage mouse skin cancer models *(130)*. Quercetin directly binds to and strongly inhibits MEK1 and Raf1 activities *(131)*. The inhibition of MEK1 by quercetin suppressed downstream ERK phosphorylation and activation of AP-1 and NF-κB, which subsequently inhibited EGF- or H-Ras-induced neoplastic transformation. Quercetin was more effective than PD098059 in inhibiting MEK1 activity *(131)*. In addition, quercetin was reported to induce apoptosis of human osteosarcoma cells. Inhibition of JNK using the inhibitor SP600125 or siRNA against JNK sensitized tumor cells to quercitin-induced apoptosis through down-regulation of JunD *(132)*. Quercetin also reduced the protein expression levels of MMP-9 and MMP-2 and AP-1 reporter activation in human fibrosarcoma cells *(133)*.

Myricetin (3,3′,4′,5,5′,7-hexahydroxyflavone) is a major flavonol found in onions, berries, grapes, and red wine *(134, 135)*. Research data have shown that myricetin exerts antioxidant, antitumor, and anti-inflammatory effects *(136–138)*, but like many natural compounds, it also can act as a prooxidant *(139)*. Reports indicate that myricetin does not cause tumor formation in mice and attenuates the number of diol-epoxide-induced pulmonary tumors per mouse *(140)*. It inhibited PAH metabolism and subsequent PAH-DNA adduct formation in mouse epidermis and lung *(141)*. Myricetin exerted protective effects against two-stage skin tumorigenesis *(142)* and inhibited the growth of A549 lung cancer cells by suppressing thioredoxin reductase activity *(143)*. Myricetin has been shown to suppress invasion and both protein expression and enzyme activity of MMP-2 in colorectal carcinoma cells *(144)*. These cumulative data provide evidence that myricetin is an effective chemopreventive agent. Lee et al. *(145)* demonstrated that myricetin is a powerful inhibitor of MEK1 kinase activity leading to inhibition of AP-1 transactivation, *c-fos* activation, and EGF- or TPA-induced cell transformation. Jung et al. *(146)* also reported that myricetin directly bound to Fyn and was an ATP-competitive inhibitor leading to suppression of UVB-induced COX-2 expression in JB6 P+ mouse skin epidermal cells and in mouse dorsal skin. In a mouse skin tumorigenesis model, myricetin strongly reduced the incidence of UVB-induced mouse skin tumors *(146)*.

Equol (4′,7-isoflavandiol) is a nonsteroidal estrogen isoflavandiol originating from metabolism of the isoflavone daidzein by intestinal bacteria. In many cell types, equol is a more potent antioxidant than daidzein *(147)*. For example, equol at concentrations that approximated physiological levels was protective against hydrogen peroxide-mediated DNA damage in human lymphocytes *(148)* and UV-induced DNA damage in hairless mice *(149)*. Moreover, equol was shown to protect against UV-induced skin cancer in the hairless mouse model *(150)*. The UV-induced activation of ornithine decarboxylase, a biomarker of skin tumor promotion, was attenuated by equol treatment. These data indicated that the anticancer activity of equol may be attributed to inhibition of the tumor promotion phase of carcinogenesis *(150)*. Studies have compared the effects of equol and daidzein on TPA-induced AP-1 activity and cell transformation in JB6 P+ cells. Results indicated that equol, but not daidzein, was a potent inhibitor of MEK activity preventing *c-fos* activation, AP-1 transactivation, and cell transformation *(151)*. Equol specifically bound to MEK noncompetitively with ATP to inhibit MEK activity *(151)*. Taken together, these data indicate that flavonoids are effective anticancer agents that act primarily by targeting MEK.

3. CONCLUSIONS

A great deal of scientific data have accumulated to help elucidate the molecular mechanisms involved in the etiology of cancer and the action of anticancer agents. This research has provided the basis for understanding the carcinogenic process caused by environmental agents and molecular targets for cancer prevention. These discoveries have identified key molecular targets that can be used for screening novel natural anticancer drugs with fewer side effects. Dietary factors may be effective preventive agents by inhibiting or reversing premalignant lesions and/or reducing tumor incidence. Many dietary compounds appear to target multiple cellular pathways. Compounds that show promise as therapeutic agents include EGCG, theaflavins, caffeine, ginger, and flavonoids. Rigorous investigations are necessary to determine the molecular actions, long-term effectiveness, and safety of these agents. Large-scale preclinical studies are needed to address the bioavailability, toxicity, molecular target, signal transduction pathways, and side effects of bioactive food components. Clinical trials based on clear mechanistic approaches are also needed to assess in humans the effectiveness of dietary factors as preventive and therapeutic agents.

ACKNOWLEDGMENTS

This work is supported by The Hormel Foundation, the Rochester Eagle's Telethon, Hormel Foods, Pediatric Pharmaceuticals, University of Minnesota Office Vice President of Research, and grants from the American Institute for Cancer Research and NIH grants CA027502, CA081064, CA077646, CA088961, CA111356, CA074916, CA111536, CA120388, ES016548, and CA077451.

REFERENCES

1. Darnell, J.E., Jr. (2002) Transcription factors as targets for cancer therapy. *Nat Rev Cancer* **2**, 740–49.
2. Hong, W.K. (2003) General keynote: The impact of cancer chemoprevention. *Gynecol Oncol* **88**, S56–S58.
3. Bode, A.M., and Dong, Z. (2003) Mitogen-Activated Protein Kinase Activation in UV-Induced Signal Transduction. *Sci STKE* **2003**, re2.
4. Bode, A.M., and Dong, Z. (2004) Post-translational modification of p53 in tumorigenesis. *Nat Rev Cancer* **4**, 793–805.
5. Bode, A.M., and Dong, Z. (2005) Signal transduction pathways in cancer development and as targets for cancer prevention. *Prog Nucleic Acid Res Mol Biol* **79**, 237–97.
6. Bode, A.M., and Dong, Z. (2005) Inducible covalent posttranslational modification of histone H3. *Sci STKE* **2005**, re4.
7. Bode, A.M., and Dong, Z. (2006) Molecular and cellular targets. *Mol Carcinog* **45**, 422–30.
8. Bode, A.M., and Dong, Z. (2007) The functional contrariety of JNK. *Mol Carcinog* **46**, 591–98.
9. Wu, W.S., Wu, J.R., and Hu, C.T. (2008) Signal cross talks for sustained MAPK activation and cell migration: The potential role of reactive oxygen species. *Cancer Metastasis Rev* **27**, 303–14.
10. Friday, B.B., and Adjei, A.A. (2008) Advances in targeting the Ras/Raf/MEK/Erk mitogen-activated protein kinase cascade with MEK inhibitors for cancer therapy. *Clin Cancer Res* **14**, 342–46.
11. Fecher, L.A., Amaravadi, R.K., and Flaherty, K.T. (2008) The MAPK pathway in melanoma. *Current Opin Oncol* **20**, 183–89.
12. Treisman, R. (1996) Regulation of transcription by MAP kinase cascades. *Curr Opin Cell Biol* **8**, 205–15.
13. Hazzalin, C.A., and Mahadevan, L.C. (2002) MAPK-regulated transcription: A continuously variable gene switch? *Nat Rev Mol Cell Biol* **3**, 30–40.
14. Pearson, G., Robinson, F., Beers Gibson, T., Xu, B.E., Karandikar, M., Berman, K., and Cobb, M.H. (2001) Mitogen-activated protein (MAP) kinase pathways: Regulation and physiological functions. *Endocr Rev* **22**, 153–83.
15. Schaeffer, H.J., and Weber, M.J. (1999) Mitogen-activated protein kinases: Specific messages from ubiquitous messengers. *Mol Cell Biol* **19**, 2435–44.
16. Cho, Y.Y., Bode, A.M., Mizuno, H., Choi, B.Y., Choi, H.S., and Dong, Z. (2004) A novel role for mixed-lineage kinase-like mitogen-activated protein triple kinase alpha in neoplastic cell transformation and tumor development. *Cancer Res* **64**, 3855–64.
17. Cowley, S., Paterson, H., Kemp, P., and Marshall, C.J. (1994) Activation of MAP kinase kinase is necessary and sufficient for PC12 differentiation and for transformation of NIH 3T3 cells. *Cell* **77**, 841–52.
18. Kallunki, T., Su, B., Tsigelny, I., Sluss, H.K., Derijard, B., Moore, G., Davis, R., and Karin, M. (1994) JNK2 contains a specificity-determining region responsible for efficient c-Jun binding and phosphorylation. *Genes Dev* **8**, 2996–3007.
19. Huang, C., Ma, W.Y., Li, J., and Dong, Z. (1999) Arsenic induces apoptosis through a c-Jun NH2-terminal kinase-dependent, p53-independent pathway. *Cancer Res* **59**, 3053–58.
20. Bode, A.M., and Dong, Z. (2000) Apoptosis induction by arsenic: Mechanisms of actions and possible clinical applications for treating therapy-resistant cancers. *Drug Resist Updat* **3**, 21–29.

21. Bode, A.M., and Dong, Z. (2002) The paradox of arsenic: Molecular mechanisms of cell transformation and chemotherapeutic effects. *Crit Rev Oncol Hematol* **42**, 5–24.
22. Bode, A.M., and Dong, Z. (2004) Targeting signal transduction pathways by chemopreventive agents. *Mutat Res* **555**, 33–51.
23. Lu, H., and Huan, C. (2007) Transcription factor NFAT, its role in cancer development, and as a potential target for chemoprevention. *Curr Cancer Drug Targets* **7**, 343–53.
24. Medyouf, H., and Ghysdael, J. (2008) The calcineurin/NFAT signaling pathway: A novel therapeutic target in leukemia and solid tumors. *Cell Cycle* **7**, 297–303.
25. Siu, Y.T., and Jin, D.Y. (2007) CREB–a real culprit in oncogenesis. *FEBS J* **274**, 3224–32.
26. Angel, P., and Karin, M. (1991) The role of Jun, Fos and the AP-1 complex in cell-proliferation and transformation. *Biochim Biophys Acta* **1072**, 129–57.
27. Eferl, R., and Wagner, E.F. (2003) AP-1: A double-edged sword in tumorigenesis. *Nat Rev Cancer* **3**, 859–68.
28. Barthelman, M., Chen, W., Gensler, H.L., Huang, C., Dong, Z., and Bowden, G.T. (1998) Inhibitory effects of perillyl alcohol on UVB-induced murine skin cancer and AP-1 transactivation. *Cancer Res* **58**, 711–16.
29. Dong, Z., Birrer, M.J., Watts, R.G., Matrisian, L.M., and Colburn, N.H. (1994) Blocking of tumor promoter-induced AP-1 activity inhibits induced transformation in JB6 mouse epidermal cells. *Proc Natl Acad Sci U S A* **91**, 609–13.
30. Dong, Z., Watts, S.G., Sun, Y., and Colburn, N.H. (1995) Progressive elevation of AP-1 activity during preneoplastic-to neoplastic progression as modeled in mouse JB6 cell variants. *Int J Oncol* **7**, 359–64.
31. Matthews, C.P., Colburn, N.H., and Young, M.R. (2007) AP-1 a target for cancer prevention. *Curr Cancer Drug Targets* **7**, 317–24.
32. Ozanne, B.W., Spence, H.J., McGarry, L.C., and Hennigan, R.F. (2007) Transcription factors control invasion: AP-1 the first among equals. *Oncogene* **26**, 1–10.
33. Verde, P., Casalino, L., Talotta, F., Yaniv, M., and Weitzman, J.B. (2007) Deciphering AP-1 function in tumorigenesis: Fra-ternizing on target promoters. *Cell Cycle* **6**, 2633–39.
34. Dong, Z., Crawford, H.C., Lavrovsky, V., Taub, D., Watts, R., Matrisian, L.M., and Colburn, N.H. (1997) A dominant negative mutant of jun blocking 12-O-tetradecanoylphorbol-13- acetate-induced invasion in mouse keratinocytes. *Mol Carcinog* **19**, 204–12.
35. Huang, C., Ma, W.-Y., and Dong, Z. (1996) Inhibitory effects of ascorbic acid on AP-1 activity and transformation of JB6 cells. *Int J Oncol* **8**, 389–93.
36. Huang, C., Ma, W.Y., Dawson, M.I., Rincon, M., Flavell, R.A., and Dong, Z. (1997) Blocking activator protein-1 activity, but not activating retinoic acid response element, is required for the antitumor promotion effect of retinoic acid. *Proc Natl Acad Sci U S A* **94**, 5826–30.
37. Li, J.J., Dong, Z., Dawson, M.I., and Colburn, N.H. (1996) Inhibition of tumor promoter-induced transformation by retinoids that transrepress AP-1 without transactivating retinoic acid response element. *Cancer Res* **56**, 483–89.
38. Domann, F.E., Jr., Levy, J.P., Finch, J.S., and Bowden, G.T. (1994) Constitutive AP-1 DNA binding and transactivating ability of malignant but not benign mouse epidermal cells. *Mol Carcinog* **9**, 61–66.
39. Chen, D., Milacic, V., Chen, M.S., Wan, S.B., Lam, W.H., Huo, C., Landis-Piwowar, K.R., Cui, Q.C., Wali, A., Chan, T.H., and Dou, Q.P. (2008) Tea polyphenols, their biological effects and potential molecular targets. *Histol Histopathol* **23**, 487–96.
40. Ikeda, I. (2008) Multifunctional effects of green tea catechins on prevention of the metabolic syndrome. *Asia Pacific J Clini Nutr* **17**(Suppl 1), 273–4.
41. Kim, J.A. (2008) Mechanisms underlying beneficial health effects of tea catechins to improve insulin resistance and endothelial dysfunction. *Endocrine Metab Immune Disord Drug Targets* **8**, 82–88.
42. Na, H.K., and Surh, Y.J. (2008) Modulation of Nrf2-mediated antioxidant and detoxifying enzyme induction by the green tea polyphenol EGCG. *Food Chem Toxicol* **46**, 1271–78.
43. Shankar, S., Ganapathy, S., and Srivastava, R.K. (2007) Green tea polyphenols: Biology and therapeutic implications in cancer. *Front Biosci* **12**, 4881–99.

44. Chen, L., and Zhang, H.Y. (2007) Cancer preventive mechanisms of the green tea polyphenol (-)-epigallocatechin-3-gallate. *Molecules* **12**, 946–57.

45. Ju, J., Lu, G., Lambert, J.D., and Yang, C.S. (2007) Inhibition of carcinogenesis by tea constituents. *Semin Cancer Biol* **17**, 395–402.

46. Yang, C.S., Lambert, J.D., Ju, J., Lu, G., and Sang, S. (2007) Tea and cancer prevention: Molecular mechanisms and human relevance. *Toxicol Appl Pharmacol* **224**, 265–73.

47. Bode, A.M., and Dong, Z. (2007) The enigmatic effects of caffeine in cell cycle and cancer. *Cancer Lett* **247**, 26–39.

48. Aggarwal, B.B., Kunnumakkara, A.B., Harikumar, K.B., Tharakan, S.T., Sung, B., and Anand, P. (2008) Potential of Spice-Derived Phytochemicals for Cancer Prevention. *Planta Medica* **74**(13), 1560–69.

49. Bode, A.M., and Dong, Z., eds. (2004) Ginger. New York: Marcel Dekker.

50. Zhao, L., and Brinton, R.D. (2007) WHI and WHIMS follow-up and human studies of soy isoflavones on cognition. *Expert Rev Neurother* **7**, 1549–64.

51. Bode, A.M., and Dong, Z. (2004) Beneficial effects of resveratrol. In: Bao Y., Fenwick R., eds. Phytochemicals in Health and Disease. New York: Marcel Dekker, Inc, 257–84.

52. Gatz, S.A., and Wiesmuller, L. (2008) Take a break–resveratrol in action on DNA. *Carcinogenesis* **29**, 321–32.

53. Harikumar, K.B., and Aggarwal, B.B. (2008) Resveratrol: A multitargeted agent for age-associated chronic diseases. *Cell Cycle* **7**, 1020–35.

54. Kundu, J.K., and Surh, Y.J. (2008) Cancer chemopreventive and therapeutic potential of resveratrol: Mechanistic perspectives. *Cancer Lett* **269**(2), 243–61.

55. Pirola, L., and Frojdo, S. (2008) Resveratrol: One molecule, many targets. *IUBMB Life* **60**, 323–32.

56. Reagan-Shaw, S., Mukhtar, H., and Ahmad, N. (2008) Resveratrol imparts photoprotection of normal cells and enhances the efficacy of radiation therapy in cancer cells. *Photochem Photobiol* **84**, 415–21.

57. Saiko, P., Szakmary, A., Jaeger, W., and Szekeres, T. (2008) Resveratrol and its analogs: Defense against cancer, coronary disease and neurodegenerative maladies or just a fad? *Mutat Res* **658**, 68–94.

58. Boots, A.W., Haenen, G.R., and Bast, A. (2008) Health effects of quercetin: From antioxidant to nutraceutical. *Eur J Pharmacol* **585**, 325–37.

59. Aggarwal, B.B., and Shishodia, S. (2006) Molecular targets of dietary agents for prevention and therapy of cancer. *Biochem Pharmacol* **71**, 1397–421.

60. Ichimatsu, D., Nomura, M., Nakamura, S., Moritani, S., Yokogawa, K., Kobayashi, S., Nishioka, T., and Miyamoto, K. (2007) Structure-activity relationship of flavonoids for inhibition of epidermal growth factor-induced transformation of JB6 Cl 41 cells. *Mol Carcinog* **46**, 436–45.

61. Bode, A.M., and Dong, Z. (2003) Signal transduction pathways: Targets for green and black tea polyphenols. *J Biochem Mol Biol* **36**, 66–77.

62. Graham, H.N. (1992) Green tea composition, consumption, and polyphenol chemistry. *Prev Med* **21**, 334–50.

63. Yang, C.S., and Wang, Z.Y. (1993) Tea and cancer. *J Natl Cancer Inst* **85**, 1038–49.

64. Chen, N.Y., Ma, W.Y., Yang, C.S., and Dong, Z. (2000) Inhibition of arsenite-induced apoptosis and AP-1 activity by epigallocatechin-3-gallate and theaflavins. *J Environ Pathol Toxicol Oncol* **19**, 287–95.

65. Dong, Z., Ma, W., Huang, C., and Yang, C.S. (1997) Inhibition of tumor promoter-induced activator protein 1 activation and cell transformation by tea polyphenols, (-)-epigallocatechin gallate, and theaflavins. *Cancer Res* **57**, 4414–19.

66. Ahn, H.Y., Hadizadeh, K.R., Seul, C., Yun, Y.P., Vetter, H., and Sachinidis, A. (1999) Epigallocathechin-3 gallate selectively inhibits the PDGF-BB-induced intracellular signaling transduction pathway in vascular smooth muscle cells and inhibits transformation of sis-transfected NIH 3T3 fibroblasts and human glioblastoma cells (A172). *Mol Biol Cell* **10**, 1093–104.

67. Barthelman, M., Bair, W.B., III, Stickland, K.K., Chen, W., Timmermann, B.N., Valcic, S., Dong, Z., and Bowden, G.T. (1998) (-)-Epigallocatechin-3-gallate inhibition of ultraviolet B-induced AP-1 activity. *Carcinogenesis* **19**, 2201–04.

68. Nomura, M., Ma, W.Y., Huang, C., Yang, C.S., Bowden, G.T., Miyamoto, K., and Dong, Z. (2000) Inhibition of ultraviolet B-induced AP-1 activation by theaflavins from black Tea. *Mol Carcinog* **28**, 148–55.
69. Chen, W., Dong, Z., Valcic, S., Timmermann, B.N., and Bowden, G.T. (1999) Inhibition of ultraviolet B–induced c-fos gene expression and p38 mitogen-activated protein kinase activation by (-)-epigallocatechin gallate in a human keratinocyte cell line. *Mol Carcinog* **24**, 79–84.
70. Calautti, E., Missero, C., Stein, P.L., Ezzell, R.M., and Dotto, G.P. (1995) Fyn tyrosine kinase is involved in keratinocyte differentiation control. *Genes Dev* **9**, 2279–91.
71. Matsumoto, T., Jiang, J., Kiguchi, K., Ruffino, L., Carbajal, S., Beltran, L., Bol, D.K., Rosenberg, M.P., and DiGiovanni, J. (2003) Targeted expression of c-Src in epidermal basal cells leads to enhanced skin tumor promotion, malignant progression, and metastasis. *Cancer Res* **63**, 4819–28.
72. Matsumoto, T., Jiang, J., Kiguchi, K., Carbajal, S., Rho, O., Gimenez-Conti, I., Beltran, L., and DiGiovanni, J. (2002) Overexpression of a constitutively active form of c-src in skin epidermis increases sensitivity to tumor promotion by 12-O-tetradecanoylphorbol-13-acetate. *Mol Carcinog* **33**, 146–55.
73. Resh, M.D. (1998) Fyn, a Src family tyrosine kinase. *The Int J Biochem Cell Biol* **30**, 1159–62.
74. Li, X., Yang, Y., Hu, Y., Dang, D., Regezi, J., Schmidt, B.L., Atakilit, A., Chen, B., Ellis, D., and Ramos, D.M. (2003) Alphavbeta6-Fyn signaling promotes oral cancer progression. *J Biol Chem* **278**, 41646–53.
75. Calautti, E., Grossi, M., Mammucari, C., Aoyama, Y., Pirro, M., Ono, Y., Li, J., and Dotto, G.P. (2002) Fyn tyrosine kinase is a downstream mediator of Rho/PRK2 function in keratinocyte cell-cell adhesion. *J Cell Biol* **156**, 137–48.
76. He, Z., Tang, F., Ermakova, S., Li, M., Zhao, Q., Cho, Y.Y., Ma, W.Y., Choi, H.S., Bode, A.M., Yang, C.S., and Dong, Z. (2008) Fyn is a novel target of (-)-epigallocatechin gallate in the inhibition of JB6 Cl41 cell transformation. *Mol Carcinog* **47**, 172–83.
77. Shim, J.H., Choi, H.S., Pugliese, A., Lee, S.Y., Chae, J.I., Choi, B.Y., Bode, A.M., and Dong, Z. (2008) (-)-Epigallocatechin gallate regulates CD3-mediated T-cell receptor signaling in leukemia through the inhibition of ZAP-70 kinase. *J Biol Chem* **283**(42), 28370–79.
78. Chung, J.Y., Huang, C., Meng, X., Dong, Z., and Yang, C.S. (1999) Inhibition of activator protein 1 activity and cell growth by purified green tea and black tea polyphenols in H-ras-transformed cells: Structure-activity relationship and mechanisms involved. *Cancer Res* **59**, 4610–17.
79. Peng, G., Wargovich, M.J., and Dixon, D.A. (2006) Anti-proliferative effects of green tea polyphenol EGCG on Ha-Ras-induced transformation of intestinal epithelial cells. *Cancer Lett* **238**, 260–70.
80. Shimizu, M., Deguchi, A., Lim, J.T., Moriwaki, H., Kopelovich, L., and Weinstein, I.B. (2005) (-)-Epigallocatechin gallate and polyphenon E inhibit growth and activation of the epidermal growth factor receptor and human epidermal growth factor receptor-2 signaling pathways in human colon cancer cells. *Clin Cancer Res* **11**, 2735–46.
81. Yang, C.S., Chung, J.Y., Yang, G., Chhabra, S.K., and Lee, M.J. (2000) Tea and tea polyphenols in cancer prevention. *J Nutr* **130**, 472S–8S.
82. Chung, J.Y., Park, J.O., Phyu, H., Dong, Z., and Yang, C.S. (2001) Mechanisms of inhibition of the Ras-MAP kinase signaling pathway in 30.7b Ras 12 cells by tea polyphenols (-)-epigallocatechin-3-gallate and theaflavin-3,3′-digallate. *FASEB J* **15**, 2022–24.
83. Zykova, T.A., Zhang, Y., Zhu, F., Bode, A.M., and Dong, Z. (2005) The signal transduction networks required for phosphorylation of STAT1 at Ser727 in mouse epidermal JB6 cells in the UVB response and inhibitory mechanisms of tea polyphenols. *Carcinogenesis* **26**, 331–42.
84. Mizuno, H., Cho, Y.Y., Zhu, F., Ma, W.Y., Bode, A.M., Yang, C.S., Ho, C.T., and Dong, Z. (2006) Theaflavin-3, 3′-digallate induces epidermal growth factor receptor downregulation. *Mol Carcinog* **45**, 204–12.
85. He, Z., Ma, W.Y., Hashimoto, T., Bode, A.M., Yang, C.S., and Dong, Z. (2003) Induction of apoptosis by caffeine is mediated by the p53, Bax, and caspase 3 pathways. *Cancer Res* **63**, 4396–401.
86. Ito, K., Nakazato, T., Miyakawa, Y., Yamato, K., Ikeda, Y., and Kizaki, M. (2003) Caffeine induces G2/M arrest and apoptosis via a novel p53-dependent pathway in NB4 promyelocytic leukemia cells. *J Cell Physiol* **196**, 276–83.

87. Lelo, A., Miners, J.O., Robson, R., and Birkett, D.J. (1986) Assessment of caffeine exposure: Caffeine content of beverages, caffeine intake, and plasma concentrations of methylxanthines. *Clin Pharmacol Ther* **39**, 54–59.

88. Huang, M.T., Xie, J.G., Wang, Z.Y., Ho, C.T., Lou, Y.R., Wang, C.X., Hard, G.C., and Conney, A.H. (1997) Effects of tea, decaffeinated tea, and caffeine on UVB light-induced complete carcinogenesis in SKH-1 mice: Demonstration of caffeine as a biologically important constituent of tea. *Cancer Res* **57**, 2623–29.

89. Lu, G., Liao, J., Yang, G., Reuhl, K.R., Hao, X., and Yang, C.S. (2006) Inhibition of adenoma progression to adenocarcinoma in a 4-(methylnitrosamino)-1-(3-pyridyl)-1-butanone-induced lung tumorigenesis model in A/J mice by tea polyphenols and caffeine. *Cancer Res* **66**, 11494–501.

90. Nishikawa, A., Furukawa, F., Imazawa, T., Ikezaki, S., Hasegawa, T., and Takahashi, M. (1995) Effects of caffeine on glandular stomach carcinogenesis induced in rats by N-methyl-N'-nitro-N-nitrosoguanidine and sodium chloride. *Food Chem Toxicol* **33**, 21–26.

91. Hosaka, S., Nagayama, H., and Hirono, I. (1984) Suppressive effect of caffeine on the development of hepatic tumors induced by 2-acetylaminofluorene in ACI rats. *Gann* **75**, 1058–61.

92. Lou, Y.R., Lu, Y.P., Xie, J.G., Huang, M.T., and Conney, A.H. (1999) Effects of oral administration of tea, decaffeinated tea, and caffeine on the formation and growth of tumors in high-risk SKH-1 mice previously treated with ultraviolet B light. *Nutr Canc* **33**, 146–53.

93. Jang, M.H., Shin, M.C., Kang, I.S., Baik, H.H., Cho, Y.H., Chu, J.P., Kim, E.H., and Kim, C.J. (2002) Caffeine induces apoptosis in human neuroblastoma cell line SK-N-MC. *J Korean Med Sci* **17**, 674–78.

94. Qi, W., Qiao, D., and Martinez, J.D. (2002) Caffeine induces TP53-independent G(1)-phase arrest and apoptosis in human lung tumor cells in a dose-dependent manner. *Radiat Res* **157**, 166–74.

95. Hashimoto, T., He, Z., Ma, W.Y., Schmid, P.C., Bode, A.M., Yang, C.S., and Dong, Z. (2004) Caffeine Inhibits Cell Proliferation by G(0)/G(1) Phase Arrest in JB6 Cells. *Cancer Res* **64**, 3344–49.

96. Nomura, M., Ichimatsu, D., Moritani, S., Koyama, I., Dong, Z., Yokogawa, K., and Miyamoto, K. (2005) Inhibition of epidermal growth factor-induced cell transformation and Akt activation by caffeine. *Mol Carcinog* **44**, 67–76.

97. Hirsh, L., Dantes, A., Suh, B.S., Yoshida, Y., Hosokawa, K., Tajima, K., Kotsuji, F., Merimsky, O., and Amsterdam, A. (2004) Phosphodiesterase inhibitors as anti-cancer drugs. *Biochem Pharmacol* **68**, 981–88.

98. Sadzuka, Y., Egawa, Y., Sugiyama, T., Sawanishi, H., Miyamoto, K., and Sonobe, T. (2000) Effects of 1-methyl-3-propyl-7-butylxanthine (MPBX) on idarubicin-induced antitumor activity and bone marrow suppression. *Jpn J Cancer Res* **91**, 651–57.

99. Sadzuka, Y., Iwazaki, A., Sugiyama, T., Sawanishi, T., and Miyamoto, K. (1998) 1-Methyl-3-propyl-7-butylxanthine, a novel biochemical modulator, enhances therapeutic efficacy of adriamycin. *Jpn J Cancer Res* **89**, 228–33.

100. Yoshida, Y., Hosokawa, K., Dantes, A., Tajima, K., Kotsuji, F., and Amsterdam, A. (2000) Theophylline and cisplatin synergize in down regulation of BCL-2 induction of apoptosis in human granulosa cells transformed by a mutated p53 (p53 val135) and Ha-ras oncogene. *Int J Oncol* **17**, 227–35.

101. Jiang, X., Lim, L.Y., Daly, J.W., Li, A.H., Jacobson, K.A., and Roberge, M. (2000) Structure-activity relationships for G2 checkpoint inhibition by caffeine analogs. *Int J Oncol* **16**, 971–78.

102. Rogozin, E.A., Lee, K.W., Kang, N.J., Yu, H., Nomura, M., Miyamoto, K., Conney, A.H., Bode, A.M., and Dong, Z. (2008) Inhibitory effects of caffeine analogues on neoplastic transformation: Structure-activity relationship. *Carcinogenesis* **29**, 1228–34.

103. Surh, Y.J., Chun, K.S., Cha, H.H., Han, S.S., Keum, Y.S., Park, K.K., and Lee, S.S. (2001) Molecular mechanisms underlying chemopreventive activities of anti-inflammatory phytochemicals: Downregulation of COX-2 and iNOS through suppression of NF-kappa B activation. *Mutat Res* **480–481**, 243–68.

104. Afzal, M., Al-Hadidi, D., Menon, M., Pesek, J., and Dhami, M.S. (2001) Ginger: An ethnomedical, chemical and pharmacological review. *Drug Metabol Drug Interact* **18**, 159–90.

105. Grant, K.L., and Lutz, R.B. (2000) Ginger. *Am J Health Syst Pharm* **57**, 945–47.

106. Langner, E., Greifenberg, S., and Gruenwald, J. (1998) Ginger: History and use. *Adv Ther* **15**, 25–44.

107. Bode, A.M., Ma, W.Y., Surh, Y.J., and Dong, Z. (2001) Inhibition of epidermal growth factor-induced cell transformation and activator protein 1 activation by [6]-gingerol. *Cancer Res* **61**, 850–53.

108. Lee, E., Park, K.K., Lee, J.M., Chun, K.S., Kang, J.Y., Lee, S.S., and Surh, Y.J. (1998) Suppression of mouse skin tumor promotion and induction of apoptosis in HL-60 cells by Alpinia oxyphylla Miquel (Zingiberaceae). *Carcinogenesis* **19**, 1377–81.

109. Lee, E., and Surh, Y.J. (1998) Induction of apoptosis in HL-60 cells by pungent vanilloids, [6]-gingerol and [6]-paradol. *Cancer Lett* **134**, 163–68.

110. Surh, Y.J., Lee, E., and Lee, J.M. (1998) Chemoprotective properties of some pungent ingredients present in red pepper and ginger. *Mutat Res* **402**, 259–67.

111. Surh, Y.J. (2002) Anti-tumor promoting potential of selected spice ingredients with antioxidative and anti-inflammatory activities: A short review. *Food Chem Toxicol* **40**, 1091–97.

112. Keum, Y.S., Kim, J., Lee, K.H., Park, K.K., Surh, Y.J., Lee, J.M., Lee, S.S., Yoon, J.H., Joo, S.Y., Cha, I.H., and Yook, J.I. (2002) Induction of apoptosis and caspase-3 activation by chemopreventive [6]-paradol and structurally related compounds in KB cells. *Cancer Lett* **177**, 41–47.

113. Dercks, W., and Creasy, L.L. (1989) The significance of stilbene phytoalexins in the Plasmopara viticola-grapevine interaction. *Physiol Mol Plant Path* **34**, 189–202.

114. Lee, K.W., Kang, N.J., Rogozin, E.A., Oh, S.M., Heo, Y.S., Pugliese, A., Bode, A.M., Lee, H.J., and Dong, Z. (2008) The resveratrol analogue 3,5,3′,4′,5′-pentahydroxy-trans-stilbene inhibits cell transformation via MEK. *Int J Cancer* **123**, 2487–96.

115. Alessi, D.R., Cuenda, A., Cohen, P., Dudley, D.T., and Saltiel, A.R. (1995) PD 098059 is a specific inhibitor of the activation of mitogen-activated protein kinase kinase in vitro and in vivo. *J Biol Chem* **270**, 27489–94.

116. Favata, M.F., Horiuchi, K.Y., Manos, E.J., Daulerio, A.J., Stradley, D.A., Feeser, W.S., Dyk, D.E.V., Pitts, W.J., Earl, R.A., Hobbs, F., Copeland, R.A., Magolda, R.L., Scherle, P.A., and Trzaskos, J.M. (1998) Identification of a novel inhibitor of mitogen-activated protein kinase kinase. *J Biol Chem* **273**, 18623–32.

117. Ohren, J.F., Chen, H., Pavlovsky, A., Whitehead, C., Zhang, E., Kuffa, P., Yan, C., McConnell, P., Spessard, C., Banotai, C., Mueller, W.T., Delaney, A., Omer, C., Sebolt-Leopold, J., Dudley, D.T., Leung, I.K., Flamme, C., Warmus, J., Kaufman, M., Barrett, S., Tecle, H., and Hasemann, C.A. (2004) Structures of human MAP kinase kinase 1 (MEK1) and MEK2 describe novel noncompetitive kinase inhibition. *Nat Struct Mol Biol* **11**, 1192–97.

118. Zykova, T.A., Zhu, F., Zhai, X., Ma, W.Y., Ermakova, S.P., Lee, K.W., Bode, A.M., and Dong, Z. (2008) Resveratrol directly targets COX-2 to inhibit carcinogenesis. *Mol Carcinog* **47**(10), 797–805.

119. Watts, R.G., Huang, C., Young, M.R., Li, J.J., Dong, Z., Pennie, W.D., and Colburn, N.H. (1998) Expression of dominant negative Erk2 inhibits AP-1 transactivation and neoplastic transformation. *Oncogene* **17**, 3493–98.

120. Anderson, N.G., Maller, J.L., Tonks, N.K., and Sturgill, T.W. (1990) Requirement for integration of signals from two distinct phosphorylation pathways for activation of MAP kinase. *Nature* **343**, 651–53.

121. Sebolt-Leopold, J.S., Dudley, D.T., Herrera, R., Becelaere, K., Wiland, A., Gowan, R.C., Tecle, H., Barrett, S.D., Bridges, A., Przybranowski, S., Leopold, W.R., and Saltiel, A.R. (1999) Blockade of the MAP kinase pathway suppresses growth of colon tumors in vivo. *Nat Med* **5**, 810–16.

122. Miean, K.H., and Mohamed, S. (2001) Flavonoid (myricetin, quercetin, kaempferol, luteolin, and apigenin) content of edible tropical plants. *J Agr Food Chem* **49**, 3106–12.

123. Cohen, M.S., Zhang, C., Shokat, K.M., and Taunton, J. (2005) Structural bioinformatics-based design of selective, irreversible kinase inhibitors. *Science* **308**, 1318–21.

124. Smith, J.A., Poteet-Smith, C.E., Xu, Y., Errington, T.M., Hecht, S.M., and Lannigan, D.A. (2005) Identification of the first specific inhibitor of p90 ribosomal S6 kinase (RSK) reveals an unexpected role for RSK in cancer cell proliferation. *Cancer Res* **65**, 1027–34.

125. Cho, Y.Y., Yao, K., Kim, H.G., Kang, B.S., Zheng, D., Bode, A.M., and Dong, Z. (2007) Ribosomal S6 kinase 2 is a key regulator in tumor promoter induced cell transformation. *Cancer Res* **67**, 8104–12.

126. Shapiro, P. (2002) Ras-MAP kinase signaling pathways and control of cell proliferation: Relevance to cancer therapy. *Crit Rev Clin Lab Sci* **39**, 285–330.

127. Gioeli, D., Mandell, J.W., Petroni, G.R., Frierson, H.F., Jr., and Weber, M.J. (1999) Activation of mitogen-activated protein kinase associated with prostate cancer progression. *Cancer Res* **59**, 279–84.

128. Oka, H., Chatani, Y., Hoshino, R., Ogawa, O., Kakehi, Y., Terachi, T., Okada, Y., Kawaichi, M., Kohno, M., and Yoshida, O. (1995) Constitutive activation of mitogen-activated protein (MAP) kinases in human renal cell carcinoma. *Cancer Res* **55**, 4182–87.

129. Waterhouse, A.L. (2002) Wine phenolics. *Ann N Y Acad Sci* **957**, 21–36.

130. Soleas, G.J., Grass, L., Josephy, P.D., Goldberg, D.M., and Diamandis, E.P. (2006) A comparison of the anticarcinogenic properties of four red wine polyphenols. *Clin Biochem* **39**, 492–97.

131. Lee, K.W., Kang, N.J., Heo, Y.S., Rogozin, E.A., Pugliese, A., Hwang, M.K., Bowden, G.T., Bode, A.M., Lee, H.J., and Dong, Z. (2008) Raf and MEK protein kinases are direct molecular targets for the chemopreventive effect of quercetin, a major flavonol in red wine. *Cancer Res* **68**, 946–55.

132. Kook, S.H., Son, Y.O., Jang, Y.S., Lee, K.Y., Lee, S.A., Kim, B.S., Lee, H.J., and Lee, J.C. (2008) Inhibition of c-Jun N-terminal kinase sensitizes tumor cells to flavonoid-induced apoptosis through down-regulation of JunD. *Toxicol Appl Pharmacol* **227**, 468–76.

133. Kong, C.S., Kim, Y.A., Kim, M.M., Park, J.S., Kim, J.A., Kim, S.K., Lee, B.J., Nam, T.J., and Seo, Y. (2008) Flavonoid glycosides isolated from Salicornia herbacea inhibit matrix metalloproteinase in HT1080 cells. *Toxicol In Vitro* **22**(7), 1742–48.

134. German, J.B., and Walzem, R.L. (2000) The health benefits of wine. *Annu Rev Nutr* **20**, 561–93.

135. Hakkinen, S.H., Karenlampi, S.O., Heinonen, I.M., Mykkanen, H.M., and Torronen, A.R. (1999) Content of the flavonols quercetin, myricetin, and kaempferol in 25 edible berries. *J Agr Food Chem* **47**, 2274–79.

136. Ribeiro de Lima, M.T., Waffo-Teguo, P., Teissedre, P.L., Pujolas, A., Vercauteren, J., Cabanis, J.C., and Merillon, J.M. (1999) Determination of stilbenes (trans-astringin, cis- and trans-piceid, and cis- and trans-resveratrol) in Portuguese wines. *J Agr Food Chem* **47**, 2666–70.

137. Sellappan, S., and Akoh, C.C. (2002) Flavonoids and antioxidant capacity of Georgia-grown Vidalia onions. *J Agr Food Chem* **50**, 5338–42.

138. Aherne, S.A., and O'Brien, N.M. (1999) Protection by the flavonoids myricetin, quercetin, and rutin against hydrogen peroxide-induced DNA damage in Caco-2 and Hep G2 cells. *Nutr Cancer* **34**, 160–66.

139. Echeverry, C., Blasina, F., Arredondo, F., Ferreira, M., Abin-Carriquiry, J.A., Vasquez, L., Aspillaga, A.A., Diez, M.S., Leighton, F., and Dajas, F. (2004) Cytoprotection by neutral fraction of tannat red wine against oxidative stress-induced cell death. *J Agric Food Chem* **52**, 7395–99.

140. Chang, R.L., Huang, M.T., Wood, A.W., Wong, C.Q., Newmark, H.L., Yagi, H., Sayer, J.M., Jerina, D.M., and Conney, A.H. (1985) Effect of ellagic acid and hydroxylated flavonoids on the tumorigenicity of benzo[a]pyrene and (+/–)-7 beta, 8 alpha-dihydroxy-9 alpha, 10 alpha-epoxy-7,8,9,10-tetrahydrobenzo[a]pyrene on mouse skin and in the newborn mouse. *Carcinogenesis* **6**, 1127–33.

141. Das, M., Khan, W.A., Asokan, P., Bickers, D.R., and Mukhtar, H. (1987) Inhibition of polycyclic aromatic hydrocarbon-DNA adduct formation in epidermis and lungs of SENCAR mice by naturally occurring plant phenols. *Cancer Res* **47**, 767–73.

142. Mukhtar, H., Das, M., Khan, W.A., Wang, Z.Y., Bik, D.P., and Bickers, D.R. (1988) Exceptional activity of tannic acid among naturally occurring plant phenols in protecting against 7,12-dimethylbenz(a)anthracene-, benzo(a)pyrene-, 3-methylcholanthrene-, and N-methyl-N-nitrosourea-induced skin tumorigenesis in mice. *Cancer Res* **48**, 2361–65.

143. Lu, J., Papp, L.V., Fang, J., Rodriguez-Nieto, S., Zhivotovsky, B., and Holmgren, A. (2006) Inhibition of Mammalian thioredoxin reductase by some flavonoids: Implications for myricetin and quercetin anticancer activity. *Cancer Res* **66**, 4410–18.

144. Ko, C.H., Shen, S.C., Lee, T.J., and Chen, Y.C. (2005) Myricetin inhibits matrix metalloproteinase 2 protein expression and enzyme activity in colorectal carcinoma cells. *Mol Cancer Ther* **4**, 281–90.

145. Lee, K.W., Kang, N.J., Rogozin, E.A., Kim, H.G., Cho, Y.Y., Bode, A.M., Lee, H.J., Surh, Y.J., Bowden, G.T., and Dong, Z. (2007) Myricetin is a novel natural inhibitor of neoplastic cell transformation and MEK1. *Carcinogenesis* **28**, 1918–27.

146. Jung, S.K., Lee, K.W., Byun, S., Kang, N.J., Lim, S.H., Heo, Y.S., Bode, A.M., Bowden, G.T., Lee, H.J., and Dong, Z. (2008) Myricetin suppresses UVB-induced skin cancer by targeting Fyn. *Cancer Res* **68**, 6021–29.

147. Arora, A., Nair, M.G., and Strasburg, G.M. (1998) Antioxidant activities of isoflavones and their biological metabolites in a liposomal system. *Arch Biochem Biophys* **356**, 133–41.

148. Sierens, J., Hartley, J.A., Campbell, M.J., Leathem, A.J., and Woodside, J.V. (2001) Effect of phytoestrogen and antioxidant supplementation on oxidative DNA damage assessed using the comet assay. *Mutat Res* **485**, 169–76.

149. Widyarini, S. (2006) Protective effect of the isoflavone equol against DNA damage induced by ultraviolet radiation to hairless mouse skin. *J Vet Sci (Suwon-si, Korea)* **7**, 217–23.

150. Widyarini, S., Husband, A.J., and Reeve, V.E. (2005) Protective effect of the isoflavonoid equol against hairless mouse skin carcinogenesis induced by UV radiation alone or with a chemical cocarcinogen. *Photochem Photobiol* **81**, 32–37.

151. Kang, N.J., Lee, K.W., Rogozin, E.A., Cho, Y.Y., Heo, Y.S., Bode, A.M., Lee, H.J., and Dong, Z. (2007) Equol, a metabolite of the soybean isoflavone daidzein, inhibits neoplastic cell transformation by targeting the MEK/ERK/p90RSK/activator protein-1 pathway. *J Biol Chem* **282**, 32856–66.

II ROLE OF DIETARY BIOACTIVE COMPONENTS IN CANCER PREVENTION AND/OR TREATMENT: MACROCONSTITUENTS

7 Dietary Energy Balance, Calorie Restriction, and Cancer Prevention

Stephen D. Hursting, Sarah M. Smith, Leticia Nogueira, Rebecca DeAngel, Laura Lashinger, and Susan N. Perkins

Key Points

1. The prevalence of obesity, an established epidemiologic risk factor for many cancers, has risen steadily in the past several decades in the United States. Particularly alarming are the increasing rates of obesity among children, indicative of further increases in obesity-related cancers for many years to come unless new prevention strategies can be developed.

2. Estimates from an American Cancer Society (ACS) study, the largest prospective analysis to date of the weight/cancer relationship, suggest 14% of all cancer deaths in men and 20% of all cancer deaths in women from a range of cancer types are attributable to overweight and obesity.

3. Calorie restriction (CR), long known to be the most effective and reproducible intervention for increasing life span in a variety of animal species, is also the most potent, broadly acting cancer prevention regimen in experimental carcinogenesis models.

4. The typical CR dietary regimen provides essential nutrients and vitamins but limits the total energy intake of the animal. CR is often incorrectly equated with starvation; however, adequate nutriture is designed into CR regimens to avoid the confounding effects of malnutrition. Modest calorie decreases of 15–30% relative to an ad libitum (AL) diet can be equated to a normal, healthy level of intake. In fact, CR animals are almost always healthier, sleeker, and more active than their AL counterparts, which are invariably overweight and tend to develop obesity in mid-life.

5. Several hormones and growth factors serve as intermediate and long-term communicators of nutritional state and have been implicated in both energy balance and carcinogenesis. These hormones include IGF-1, insulin, adiponectin, and leptin, as well as several factors associated with inflammation and oxidative stress.

Key Words: Obesity; cancer; caloric restriction; energy; hormones; inflammation; oxidative stress

1. INTRODUCTION

Energy balance refers to the state at which the number of calories taken in equals the number of calories used. This term integrates the effects of diet (particularly energy derived from food and drink), physical activity, and genetics on growth, metabolism,

From: *Nutrition and Health: Bioactive Compounds and Cancer*
Edited by: J.A. Milner, D.F. Romagnolo, DOI 10.1007/978-1-60761-627-6_7,
© Springer Science+Business Media, LLC 2010

and body weight. Lucretius (~50 BC) and Lord Francis Bacon (1561–1626) have been credited with early statements on the role of overindulgence with food in premature aging and in the etiology of degenerative diseases, such as cancer *(1, 2)*. Today, the emerging obesity epidemic in the United States and throughout the world has increased the importance of understanding the effects of energy balance on the development and progression of cancer and in cancer patients' quality of life during and after treatment *(3)*. The prevalence of obesity has increased dramatically in the last two decades in the United States *(4)*. As defined by the Body Mass Index (BMI), among adults aged ≥20 years in 1999–2002, 65.7% were overweight (BMI = 25.0–29.9), 30.6% were obese (BMI ≥ 30.0), and 5.1% were extremely obese (BMI > 40). Between the early 1960s and 2002 mean BMI increased approximately 3 BMI units in both men and women *(5)*. On average, this translates to an increase of more than 20 pounds, while during the same time period mean height increased by approximately one inch *(5)*. Of particular concern is that these same trends have also appeared in children *(4)*.

In a large cohort study conducted by the American Cancer Society (ACS), obesity in adult men and women was associated with increased mortality from cancers of the colon, breast (in postmenopausal women), endometrium, kidney (renal cell), esophagus (adenocarcinoma), gastric cardia, pancreas, prostate, gallbladder, and liver *(6)*. Estimates from this ACS study, the largest prospective analysis to date of the weight/cancer relationship, suggest 14% of all cancer deaths in men and 20% of all cancer deaths in women from a range of cancer types are attributable to overweight and obesity *(6)*. The International Agency for Research on Cancer (IARC) Working Group on the Evaluation of Weight Control and Physical Activity (2002) also concluded that there is consistent epidemiologic evidence for a protective effect of physical activity for many cancers. However, the report stated that the relationship between energy balance and cancer is poorly understood. Furthermore, a gap was identified in the existing literature regarding the mechanisms mediating the anti-cancer effects of CR or physical activity, the major lifestyle-based strategies for reducing/maintaining weight *(7)*.

The first tests in animal models of the link between calorie intake and cancer were reported in 1909 by Moreschi and confirmed by Rous in 1914; both investigators demonstrated that calorie restriction (CR), an experimental mode in which test animals receive a lower-calorie diet than ad libitum (AL)-fed controls, inhibited the growth of transplanted tumors in mice *(8)*. Intense interest in the comparison of AL versus CR animals developed in the 1930s, when McCay et al. showed that a reduced food intake increased life span in rodents *(9)*. This work was extended by Tannenbaum and colleagues, who consistently showed that the incidence of tumors in mice decreased when food intake was reduced *(10, 11)*. To date, CR has been the most widely studied and most effective experimental strategy for increasing the survival of mammals *(12)* and is also the most potent, broadly acting dietary intervention known for preventing carcinogenesis in experimental models *(13)*.

The typical CR dietary regimen provides essential nutrients and vitamins but limits the total energy intake of the animal (usually by 15–40% relative to AL controls). Unfortunately, CR is often incorrectly equated with starvation and this misconception has, at least to some degree, limited the translation of important findings from CR research into human disease prevention strategies. In actuality, adequate nutriture is designed into CR regimens to avoid the confounding effects of malnutrition, and modest calorie decreases of 15–30% relative to an AL diet can be equated to a normal, healthy level of intake. In fact, CR animals are almost always healthier, sleeker, and more active than their AL counterparts, which are invariably overweight (based on adiposity levels) and tend to develop obesity in mid-life. CR regimens administered throughout life, beginning within a few weeks of weaning, are generally more protective than adult-onset CR *(12, 14)*. However, both modalities prevent adult-onset obesity, significantly extend life span, and suppress tumorigenesis, prompting many investigators to suggest that obesity prevention may be a key underlying factor in the anti-aging and anti-cancer effects of CR *(13, 15, 16)*.

In light of the obesity epidemic and the epidemiologic associations between obesity and many cancers, the development of intervention strategies that break the obesity-cancer link have become increasingly urgent. Unfortunately, the effects and mechanistic targets of interventions that modulate energy balance, such as reduced calorie diets and physical activity, on the carcinogenesis process have not been well characterized. The purpose of this chapter is to provide a strong foundation for the translation of mechanism-based research in this area by describing key animal and human studies of energy balance modulations involving diet or physical activity and by focusing on the interrelated pathways affected by alterations in energy balance. Particular attention is placed on signaling through critical energy-dependent growth factor (particularly the insulin and insulin-like growth factor (IGF)-1 receptor) pathways and nutrient-sensing pathways. These include components of the Akt, AMP-kinase, mammalian target of rapamycin (mTOR), and sirtuin signaling pathways downstream of these growth factor receptors and nutrient-sensing components. These pathways have emerged as potential targets for disrupting the obesity–cancer link. The ultimate goal of this work is to provide the missing mechanistic information necessary to identify targets for the prevention and control of cancers related to or caused by excess body weight.

2. CALORIE RESTRICTION AND CANCER IN EXPERIMENTAL MODELS

CR is the only established intervention that extends lifetime survival (including mean and maximal life span) in mammals *(12, 17)*. The anti-aging effects of CR have been observed in diverse organisms, including protozoa, yeast (*Saccharomyces cerevisiae*), nematode (*Caenorhabditis elegans*), several insect species including fruitfly (*Drosophila melanogaster*), mouse, rat, hamster, guinea pig, dog, cow, and apparently in several non-human primate species *(12, 17–20)*. Thus, the mechanism(s) underlying the survival extension in response to CR, imposed using a variety of dietary compositions, feeding strategies, and levels of restriction, appears to be evolutionarily conserved. This suggests that a better understanding of these mechanisms will reveal important clues about the biology of aging.

The effect of CR on cancer has been best studied in rodent models, and we have recently reviewed this literature *(3, 21)*. In brief, CR inhibits a variety of spontaneous neoplasia in experimental cancer model systems, including tumors arising in several knockout and transgenic mouse models, such as p53-deficient mice and Wnt-1 transgenic mice *(22)*. In rodents, CR also suppresses the carcinogenic action of several classes of chemicals including polycyclic hydrocarbons, e.g., benzo(a)pyrene *(11, 23)* and DMBA *(24, 25)*; alkylating and methylating agents, e.g., diethylnitrosamine *(26)*; and aromatic amines, e.g., *p*-cresidine *(27)*. In addition, CR inhibits several forms of radiation-induced cancers *(28, 29)*. Thus, the inhibitory action of CR on carcinogenesis is effective in several species, for a variety of tumor types, and for both spontaneous tumors and chemically induced neoplasia.

2.1. CR in Humans and Non-human Primates

Observational studies suggest that CR has beneficial effects on longevity in humans. These studies include natural experiments, such as a study of Spanish nursing home residents suggesting that reduced caloric intake reduces morbidity and mortality *(30)*. Moreover, physiological changes analogous to those observed in CR monkeys, including HDL cholesterol increases, are reported in Muslims who fast during the daylight hours of the holy month of Ramadan *(31)*. In addition, inhabitants of Okinawa, Japan, who until recently consumed fewer calories than residents of the main Japanese islands, displayed lower death rates from cancer and vascular diseases *(32)*. The relationship between reduced calories and reduced mortality in Okinawa, relative to the rest of Japan, could be confounded by other factors such as genetic or other dietary differences, but these observations are intriguing. Data from certain historical events, such as the Dutch famine during World War II, are also suggestive of decreased mortality from cancer and other age-related diseases following extended reductions in calorie intake. However, these observations are difficult to interpret because of confounding factors such as malnutrition *(33)*.

In humans, more controlled demonstrations of the metabolic effects of CR include the Biosphere 2 and the ongoing Netherlands Toxicology and Nutrition Institute study. Biosphere 2, which took place in a closed ecosystem in Arizona from 1991 to 1993, involved four men and four women who experienced, on average, a 30% calorie restriction relative to their usual energy intake. Although this sample was too small and uncontrolled to allow clear conclusions, many of the physiological parameters associated with the anti-aging and anti-cancer effects of CR in rodents and non-human primates were observed in these subjects *(34)*. The Netherlands study was more controlled, with 8 control subjects and 16 subjects on a 20% CR (relative to their usual calorie intake) regimen. As in Biosphere 2, the Netherlands study subjects on the CR regimen displayed decreased fat mass and lowered blood pressure relative to the controls *(35)*.

In the past decade, four longevity studies involving long-term CR versus AL consumption have been initiated in several non-human primate species *(30, 36)*. It remains to be seen whether the extension of life span and/or reduction in tumor development demonstrated consistently in rodents will be replicated in non-human primates. However, preliminary reports on chronic disease-associated markers and initial tumor incidence and mortality data suggest that monkeys on CR regimens are less likely to develop diabetes, cardiovascular disease, obesity, autoimmune diseases, and cancer than their AL counterparts *(30, 36)*. In addition, the National Institute of Aging has invested in a randomized, controlled clinical trial to assess the effects of CR in humans.

The Comprehensive Assessment of Long-Term Effects of Reducing Intake of Energy (CALERIE) study involves three sites and is following 250 healthy volunteers assigned to a 25% CR or control intervention for 2 years (from 2007 to 2009). Endpoints of this study are markers of glucose metabolism, oxidative stress, muscle function, cognitive function, and other outcomes.

2.2. *Physical Activity and Cancer in Humans and Animals*

The International Agency for Research on Cancer (IARC) Working Group on the Evaluation of Weight Control and Physical Activity (2003), as well as the recent World Cancer Research Fund/American Institute for Cancer Research Expert Report (2007) concluded that there is consistent epidemiologic evidence for a protective effect of physical activity against many cancers *(37)*. Many of the studies have identified some form of protective effect of either voluntary or involuntary exercise on carcinogenesis *(37)*. To the detriment of the field, the number of studies has not increased dramatically over the years and, perhaps more importantly, few studies have focused on plausible biological mechanisms that might explain the effect of exercise on cancer prevention. Mechanisms most commonly cited as potential mediators include enhanced antioxidant defense mechanisms, altered growth factor milieu (i.e., changes in insulin, insulin-like growth factor-1, IGF-binding proteins), decreases in reproductive hormone levels, enhanced anti-tumor immunity, and a reduction in chronic inflammation *(37)*. There are also site-specific mechanisms for various cancers such as a decreased colonic transit time in relation to colon cancer. Many of the mechanisms that have received more attention in human studies, such as alterations in estrogen and IGF-1 levels, have not received much focus in animal models of exercise, and vice versa (e.g., exercise and immune function has been well studied in animal models but not in humans).

3. MECHANISTIC TARGETS OF CALORIE RESTRICTION

3.1. *Energy Balance-Related Hormones and Growth Factors*

Several hormones and growth factors serve as intermediate and long-term communicators of nutritional state throughout the body and have been implicated in both energy balance and carcinogenesis. These hormones include IGF-1, insulin, adiponectin, and leptin, as well as several factors associated with inflammation and oxidative stress, and will be the focus of the following mechanistic discussion.

IGF-1 is a central component of a complex network of molecules that controls long bone growth and energy metabolism *(38)*. Its involvement in cancer was first suspected when in vitro studies consistently showed that IGF-1 enhances the growth of a variety of cancer cell lines *(39–42)*. There is now abundant epidemiological evidence supporting the hypothesis that IGF-1 is involved in several types of human cancer. IGF-1 acts either directly on cells via the IGF-1 receptor (IGF-1R), which is overexpressed in many tumors, or indirectly through its action with other cancer-related molecules, such as the p53 tumor suppressor protein *(43, 44)*. The circulating level of IGF-1 is mainly determined by hepatic synthesis, which is regulated by growth hormone and influenced by nutrient intake, particularly intake of energy and protein *(45)*. Regulation of IGF-1 in extrahepatic tissues is more complex, involving pituitary-derived growth hormone, other hormones and growth factors, and IGF-binding proteins (IGFBPs), of which there are at least six isoforms that determine the systemic half-life and local availability of IGF-1 *(38)*.

IGF-1 has been identified as a cell cycle progression factor based on its ability in many normal and cancer cell types to stimulate progression through the cell cycle from G1 to S phase, purportedly by activating the phosphatidylinositol 3-kinase (PI3K)/Akt signal transduction pathway and modulating cyclin-dependent kinases. IGF-1 can also suppress apoptosis in a variety of cell types, and cells overexpressing IGF-1R show decreased apoptosis *(46, 47)*.

Mounting experimental evidence suggests that IGF-1 mediates at least some of the anti-proliferative, pro-apoptotic, and anti-cancer effects of CR through its role in an evolutionarily conserved regulatory pathway that is responsive to energy availability *(21, 48)*. This conclusion does not exclude other mediators, which may be regulated by IGF-1 or function independently of IGF-1. The role of IGF-1 in the anti-cancer effects of exercise is less clear, with the findings to date consistent with little or no long-term effects of exercise on circulating IGF-1 levels *(49–51)*. However, IGFBP activity may increase with physical activity, and thus overall IGF-1 bioavailability and activity may decrease with exercise *(52)*.

Insulin, particularly under conditions of chronic hyperinsulinemia and insulin resistance, increases risk for cancer at several sites *(53)*, although it is unclear if the tumor-enhancing effects of insulin are due to direct effects via the insulin receptor on preneoplastic cells or indirect effects via stimulation of IGF-1, estrogens, or other hormones. Certainly, high circulating levels of insulin promote the hepatic synthesis of IGF-1 and decrease the production of IGFBP-1, thus increasing the biologic activity of IGF-1 *(53)*. Furthermore, both insulin and IGF-1 act in vitro as growth factors to promote cancer cell proliferation and decrease apoptosis *(54)*. Insulin resistance, a state of reduced responsiveness of tissues to the physiological actions of insulin, results in a compensatory rise in plasma insulin levels and is affected by both adiposity and physical activity. Intra-abdominal obesity is associated with insulin resistance *(55)*, whereas physical activity improves insulin sensitivity *(56)*. A growing body of epidemiologic evidence suggests that type 2 diabetes, which is usually characterized by hyperinsulinemia and insulin resistance for long periods, is associated with increased risks of endometrial, colon, pancreas, kidney, and postmenopausal breast cancers *(53)*.

Downstream targets of IGF-1 receptor and insulin receptor comprise a signaling network that regulates cellular growth and metabolism predominately through induction of the PI3K/Akt pathway, recently reviewed in *(57)*. The importance of this signaling cascade in human cancers has recently been highlighted by the observation that it is one of the most commonly altered pathways in human epithelial tumors *(58–61)*. Engagement of the PI3K/Akt pathway allows both intracellular and environmental cues, such as energy availability and growth factor supply, to affect cell growth, proliferation, survival, and metabolism.

Activation of receptor tyrosine kinases (RTKs) and/or the Ras proto-oncogene stimulates PI3K to produce the lipid second messenger, phosphatidyl-inositol-3,4,5-

trisphosphate (PIP3). PIP3 recruits and anchors Akt to the cell membrane where it can be further phosphorylated and activated *(58, 60, 61)*. Akt is a cAMP-dependent, cGMP-dependent protein kinase that when constitutively active is sufficient for cellular transformation by stimulating cell cycle progression and cell survival as well as inhibiting apoptosis *(62, 63)*. Frequently associated with the aberrant Akt signaling commonly seen in human cancers is an elevation in mTOR (mammalian target of rapamycin) signaling. mTOR is a highly conserved serine/threonine protein kinase which is activated by Akt and also inhibited by an opposing signal from AMP-activated kinase (AMPK). At the interface of the Akt and AMPK pathways, mTOR dictates translational control of new proteins in response to both growth factor signals and nutrient availability through phosphorylation of its downstream mediators, S6K and 4EBP-1 *(64–66)*. Ultimately, activation of mTOR results in cell growth, cell proliferation, and resistance to apoptosis.

An important convergent point for these signaling cascades is the tumor suppressor, tuberous sclerosis complex (TSC), reviewed in *(67–69)*. Briefly, the TSC binds to and sequesters Rheb, a G-protein required for mTOR activation, thus inhibiting mTOR and downstream targets. However, phosphorylation of the TSC elicits inactivation and Rheb is released, allowing for direct interaction with ATP and subsequent activation of mTOR *(70, 71)*. Alternatively, when the TSC is inhibited, Rheb is able to phosphorylate and activate mTOR.

Energy balance can influence both the Akt and AMPK pathways of mTOR activation. For example, overweight and obese conditions are positively associated, as previously mentioned, with high serum levels of IGF-1. We and others have found that obesity is associated with enhanced induction of the PI3K/Akt pathway *(72, 73)*. However, nutrient deprivation, by way of calorie restriction, is congruent with reduced PI3K/Akt signaling as a result of decreased circulating levels of IGF-1 *(72, 73)*. Furthermore, genetic reduction of circulating IGF-1 mimics the effects of CR on tumor development and PI3K/Akt signaling *(74)*. Additionally, recent literature suggests that elevated cellular amino acid, glucose, and ATP concentrations, as are present during high-energy conditions, signal for mTOR activation *(75)*. Conversely, low glucose availability, high AMP/ATP ratios, and decreased amino acids, such as those achieved during calorie restriction, can lead to growth arrest, apoptosis, and autophagy through an AMPK-induced repression of mTOR *(76)*. These coordinated pathways not only function to reduce cellular energy expenditure, but they also protect against stress-induced apoptosis. Although nutrient and growth factor availability directly regulates mTOR, no causal associations have been made between mTOR activation or repression, energy balance, and tumorigenesis.

Leptin is a peptide hormone secreted from adipocytes that is involved with appetite control and energy metabolism through its hypothalamic influence. In the non-obese state, rising leptin levels result in decreased appetite through a series of neuroendocrine changes. The obese state is associated with high circulating levels of leptin *(70, 71, 75, 76)*, suggesting that the obese may develop leptin resistance. This resistance appears to explain much of the inability of exogenous leptin administration to prevent weight gain and may result in a higher "set-point" for body weight *(77)*. The limited number of studies to date are suggestive of an association between circulating leptin levels and cancer risk, with the most consistent findings thus far for colon *(78)* and prostate cancer (particularly progression of prostate cancer, as suggested by Chang *(79)* and Saglam *(80)*). In vitro, leptin stimulates proliferation of multiple types of preneoplastic and neoplastic cells (but not "normal" cells, as reported by Fenton *(42)*) and in animal models appears to promote angiogenesis and tumor invasion *(81)*.

The primary physiologic role of leptin may be the regulation of energy homeostasis by providing a signal to the central nervous system regarding the size of fat stores, as circulating leptin levels correlate strongly with adipose tissue levels in animals and humans *(82)*. The canonical pathway transducing leptin's signal from its receptor (OB-R) is the Janus kinase 2/signal transducer and activator of transcription 3 (JAK2/STAT3) pathway. Leptin may also exert its metabolic effects, at least in part, by activating AMPK in muscle and liver, thus decreasing several anabolic pathways (including glucose-regulated transcription and fatty acid and triglyceride synthesis) and increasing several ATP-producing catabolic pathways *(83)*. In addition, there is emerging evidence of crosstalk between the JAK/STAT family of transcription factors, the insulin/IGF-1/Akt pathway, and AMPK *(84)*. Furthermore, leptin plays a role in regulating the hypothalamus/pituitary/adrenal axis and thus influences IGF-1 synthesis *(83)*. Finally, leptin functions as an inflammatory cytokine and appears to influence immune function, possibly by triggering release of interleukin (IL)-6 and other obesity-related cytokines *(42, 85)*. Thus, although not well studied to date, leptin is certainly positioned as a central player in the energy balance and cancer association.

Adiponectin is a 28-kDa peptide hormone produced exclusively by adipocytes and intimately involved in the regulation of insulin sensitivity and carbohydrate and lipid metabolism. The link between adiponectin and cancer risk is not well characterized, although there is a report that adiponectin infusion inhibits endothelial proliferation and transplanted fibrosarcoma growth *(86)*. Plasma levels of adiponectin, in contrast with other adipokines, are decreased in response to several metabolic impairments, including type 2 diabetes, dyslipidemia, and extreme obesity. This obesity-related decrease can be partially reversed by weight loss, although recent reports suggest these changes are relatively small unless there are drastic weight changes due to severe calorie restriction or surgical intervention *(87, 88)*. Recent findings suggest leptin and adiponectin interact antagonistically to influence carcinogenesis *(89, 90)*, although this interaction has not been well established.

Steroid hormones, including estrogens, androgens, progesterone, and adrenal steroids, reportedly play a role in the relationship between energy balance and certain types of cancer. Adipose tissue is the main site of estrogen synthesis in men and postmenopausal (or otherwise ovarian hormone-deficient) women, through the ability of aromatase (a P450 enzyme present in adipose tissue) to convert androgenic precursors produced in the adrenals and gonads to estrogens *(53)*. In addition, adipose tissue is the second major source of circulating IGF-1, after liver. The increased insulin and bioactive IGF-1 levels that typically accompany increased adiposity can feed back to reduce levels of sex hormone-binding globulin (SHBG), resulting in an increased fraction of bioavailable estradiol in both men and women *(53)*. The epidemiologic literature clearly suggests that the increased bioavailability of sex steroids that accompanies increased adiposity is strongly associated with risk of endometrial and postmenopausal breast cancers *(91)* and may impact colon and other cancers as well. Adrenal glucocorticoid hormones may play a role in the anti-cancer effects of CR, especially at restriction levels above 30% CR, which markedly increase corticosterone levels in rodents *(92–94)*. Glucocorticoid hormones have long been known to inhibit tumor promotion *(95)*. In addition to the anti-inflammatory effects of corticosterone, it can induce p27 and thus influence cell cycle machinery *(93)*. Birt and colleagues have shown that the CR induction of corticosterone can inhibit protein kinase C and MAP kinase signaling, including reduced ERK-1 and -2 signaling and AP1:DNA binding *(92)*.

3.2. The Role of Inflammation in the Link Between Energy Balance and Cancer

The association between chronic inflammation and cancer is widely accepted *(96)*. To date, the effect of exercise on inflammatory processes has been better characterized than the effects of obesity, CR, or other energy balance perturbations. However, obesity is clearly associated with increased inflammation, while we and others have shown that CR and physical activity, alone and in combination, decrease certain inflammatory markers *(21, 97)*.

In general, acute inflammation is a process that is beneficial to the host by providing protection from invading pathogens and initiating wound healing. In the acute phase response, the pro-inflammatory cytokines tumor necrosis factor-alpha (TNF-α) and interleukin-1-beta (IL-β) are produced locally at the site of infection by macrophages. They stimulate the release of IL-6, which has been shown to have both pro-inflammatory and anti-inflammatory effects *(98)*, and the secretion of C-reactive protein (CRP) by the liver into the blood. Following clearance of the infection, the production of IL-1β and TNF-α is dampened by the production and release of IL-1 receptor antagonist (IL-1Ra) and soluble TNF-α receptors (sTNF-R), respectively, by altering signal transduction via these receptors *(99)*. Additionally, IL-10, an anti-inflammatory cytokine that works by deactivating macrophages, is produced by T lymphocytes and is important in controlling the inflammatory response *(100, 101)*.

Chronic (low-grade) systemic inflammation, which typically accompanies obesity, has been described as a condition in which there is a two to threefold increase in the circulating levels of TNF-α, IL-1β, IL-6, IL-1Ra, sTNF-R, and CRP. The origin of the cytokine cascade is not believed to be due to the presence of a foreign pathogen. However, the initial stimuli and the cause of this elevation in cytokines with chronic systemic inflammation are not understood. The source of TNF-α production in chronic systemic inflammation may be adipose tissue itself *(102, 103)* or macrophages that reside in the adipose tissue of obese, but not lean, animals and humans *(104, 105)*. Additional studies are needed to determine the initiating stimuli and the source of inflammatory cytokines in chronic low-grade systemic inflammation. Chronic low-grade systemic inflammation is observed as part of the aging process *(106–110)* and in several chronic diseases, including type 2 diabetes *(111–114)*, atherosclerosis *(108, 115, 116)*, and some cancers *(117, 118)*. Furthermore, numerous cross-sectional epidemiologic studies have shown an association between physical inactivity and systemic inflammation *(119–126)*. One mechanism by which physical activity may reduce cancer risk is via a reduction in chronic inflammation. In particular, the exercise-induced increase in systemic IL-6 may result in reduced pro-inflammatory mediators and elevated anti-inflammatory factors.

3.3. Sirtuins

Sirtuins are a family of proteins that have been implicated in the regulation of aging (127), transcription (128), endocrine signaling (129), stress-induced apoptosis (130), and most recently in metabolic changes associated with obesity (reviewed in (131)). Sirtuins were originally studied in the budding yeast *S. cerevisiae* (132, 133) and nematode *C. elegans* (134), where CR was shown to increase life span as well as increase the levels and activity of the Sir2 protein. In mammals, it has been shown that the levels of SIRT1, a mammalian homologue of Sir2, also rise during CR and promote long-term survival of cells. SIRT1 is an NAD^+-dependent deacetylase that acts on Ku70, which in turn sequesters the proapoptotic factor Bax from the mitochondria, thus inhibiting stress-induced apoptotic cell death (130). Additionally, SIRT1 has been shown to repress PPAR-γ (peroxisome proliferators-activated receptor-γ) by docking with its cofactors and thereby repressing PPAR-γ responsive genes. Therefore, conditions of CR and SIRT1 upregulation result in mobilization of fatty acids from white adipose tissue, lipolysis, and loss of fat (135). Decreases in sirtuin levels during obesity, specifically SIRT1 levels, have been shown to regulate many other metabolic alterations linked to obesity. SIRT1 has been shown to play a role in regulation of adiponectin (136, 137), insulin secretion (138), plasma glucose levels and insulin sensitivity (139), and regulation of oxygen consumption and mitochondrial capacity (140, 141). Another yeast Sir2 homologue, mammalian SIRT3, has been shown to be selectively downregulated at both the gene and protein levels in a mouse model of type 2 diabetes, but not in a model of insulin deficiency without diabetes. These studies documented that insulin-deficient mice lacked muscle insulin receptor (MIRKO mice), but maintained normal levels of insulin, glucose, and insulin-regulated genes. The same MIRKO mice with streptozotocin (STZ)-induced diabetes, however, modeled the metabolic changes associated with type 2 diabetes, including downregulation of Sirt1 (142). These findings further suggested sirtuins may be involved in the control of important downstream transcriptional regulatory mechanisms involved in glucose metabolism.

While CR has long been shown to have a dramatic effect on life span and tumor suppression in almost every tumor type tested, the specific role of sirtuins in cancer development/progression has yet to be elucidated (143). Studies have shown conflicting data as to whether SIRT1 can act as a tumor suppressor gene or an oncogene. SIRT1 is upregulated in several tumor types and can inhibit apoptosis and downregulate the expression of tumor suppressor genes to extend the longevity of epithelial cancer cells (144). SIRT1 is upregulated in tumors and cancer cells lacking the tumor suppressor gene, HIC1 (145) and upregulated in mouse and human prostate cancers (146). In addition, DBC1 (deleted in breast cancer 1)-mediated repression of SIRT1 was shown to increase p53 function (147, 148). However, there is also evidence that SIRT1 can act to suppress polyp formation in the APC^{min} intestinal tumor model (149). Additionally, preclinical studies of resveratrol, a CR mimetic shown to activate sirtuins, have suggested that the activation of SIRT1 may be viable target in cancer prevention or therapy (150).

4. CONCLUSIONS AND FUTURE DIRECTIONS

The findings described above with resveratrol reinforce the notion that the identification and development of natural or synthetic agents that mimic some of the protective effects of CR may constitute a new strategy for cancer prevention. Numerous studies have used microarray analyses to profile the molecular targets responding to CR and other changes in dietary energy balance *(151–156)*. Most of these studies were focused on understanding CR effects related to aging, and they revealed that the extent to which CR modulates the transcriptome is species-specific, tissue-specific, and dependent on the duration and intensity of CR. Nonetheless, some patterns from these studies have emerged suggesting that transcripts involved in inflammation, growth factor signaling (particularly related to the insulin and IGF-1 pathways), oxidative stress, and nutrient metabolism are commonly altered by CR *(21)*. Application of the emerging field of metabolomics to this question should accelerate the identification of additional targets.

As described above, the IGF-1 and Akt/mTOR pathways have emerged as potential key mediators of CR's anti-cancer and anti-aging effects and are initial targets for possible CR mimetics. Agents or interventions that reduce IGF-1 without requiring drastic dietary changes may provide an effective physiological or pharmacological mimetic of those effects, which could be readily adopted by a large proportion of the population, particularly those at high risk for cancer or other chronic diseases associated with high IGF-1 levels. Small-molecule inhibitors of IGF-1 *(157)* or IGF/IGFBP *(158)*, as well as antisense IGF-1 inhibitor approaches *(159)* and anti-IGF-1 antibody therapies *(160)*, are under development. In addition, a wide variety of agents with demonstrated cancer chemopreventive or chemotherapeutic activity have recently been reported to inhibit the IGF-1 pathway *(161–164)*, including retinoids (e.g., fenretinide and all-*trans* retinoic acid), soy isoflavones (e.g., genistein and daidzein), flavonoids (e.g., quercetin and kaempferol), somatostatin analogues (e.g., octreotide), and selective estrogen receptor modulators (e.g., tamoxifen). Physical activity may also affect IGF-1, although the limited findings to date have been mixed *(165–167)*. More evidence is needed regarding the role of IGF-1 in the cancer-preventive effects of these agents or interventions, but current data suggest that targeting IGF-1 or downstream components of the IGF-1 pathway (such as mTOR) with CR, phytonutrients, pharmacological agents, or other means may constitute a plausible cancer prevention strategy.

Although the epidemiologic associations between overweight/obesity and several cancers are becoming well defined, the causal relationships between energy balance, hormones, and cancer risk are not well established. For example, key unanswered questions include the following: (a) Which, if any, of the hormonal changes (i.e., IGF-1, insulin, leptin, sex steroids) or other physiological changes (i.e., weight, adiposity, insulin resistance, inflammation, alterations in energy metabolism) accompanying energy imbalance are causally linked to carcinogenesis? (b) Does reversal of obesity through diet, exercise, or pharmacologic regimens decrease cancer risk or impact existing cancers? (c) Are there important differences between anti-obesity regimens (caloric restriction, exercise, drugs) in terms of the pathways targeted and anti-cancer effects, or is weight reduction/maintenance the key irrespective of the means? (d) Can specific activators of the sirtuin pathway or inhibitors of the IGF/insulin/Akt signaling pathway (such as iGF-1R inhibitors or rapamycin and its newer derivatives), of the leptin/JAK/STAT pathway (such as STAT3 inhibitors), or of the inflammatory cascade disrupt the link between obesity and cancer in the absence of weight loss, which for many individuals is very difficult? (e) What is the impact of different energy balance states and their associated effects on physiology (i.e., lean versus obese; insulin resistant versus insulin sensitive; high versus low postmenopausal estrogen levels) on the response to cancer prevention or cancer therapy regimens? Progress in this area will require a multidisciplinary approach, and these and other key questions will only be answered through well-designed studies in both animals and humans that incorporate molecular, genetic, and metabolic/nutritional tools and expertise.

REFERENCES

1. Kritchevsky, D. (1993) Colorectal cancer: The role of dietary fat and caloric restriction. *Mutat Res* **290**(1), 63–70.
2. McCay, C.M., and Crowell, M.F. (1934) Prolonging the life span. *Sci Mon* **39**, 405–14.
3. Hursting, S.D. et al. (2007) Energy balance and carcinogenesis: Underlying pathways and targets for intervention. *Curr Cancer Drug Targets* **7**(5), 484–91.
4. Hedley, A.A. et al. (2004) Prevalence of overweight and obesity among US children, adolescents, and adults, 1999–2002. *J Am Med Assoc* **291**(23), 2847–50.
5. Ogden, C.L., Advance Data from Vital Health Statistics. 2004, CDC.
6. Calle, E.E. et al. (2003) Overweight, obesity, and mortality from cancer in a prospectively studied cohort of U.S. adults. *N Engl J Med* **348**(17), 1625–38.
7. IARC. (2002) IARC Handbooks of Cancer Prevention: Weight Control and Physical Activity. Vol. 6, Lyon: IARC Press.
8. Kritchevsky, D. (1993) Undernutrition and chronic disease: Cancer. *Proc Nutr Soc* **52**(1), 39–47.
9. McCay, C.M., Crowell, M.F., and Maynard, L.A. (1935) The effect of retarded growth upon the length of life span and upon the ultimate body size. *J Nutr* **10**, 63–79.
10. Tannenbaum, A. (1944) The dependence of the genesis of induced skin tumors on the caloric intake during different stages of carcinogenesis. *Cancer Res* **4**, 673–79.
11. Tannenbaum, A. (1940) The initiation and growth of tumors. I. Introduction. Effects of underfeeding. *Am J Cancer* **38**, 335–50.
12. Weindruch, R., and Walford, R. (1988) The Retardation of Aging and Disease by Dietary Restriction. Springfield, IL: Charles C Thomas.
13. Hursting, S.D., and Kari, F.W. (1999) The anti-carcinogenic effects of dietary restriction: Mechanisms and future directions. *Mutat Res* **443**(1–2), 235–49.
14. Berrigan, D. et al. (2002) Adult-onset calorie restriction and fasting delay spontaneous tumorigenesis in p53-deficient mice. *Carcinogenesis* **23**(5), 817–22.
15. Kritchevsky, D. (1999) Caloric restriction and experimental carcinogenesis. *Toxicol Sci* **52**(2 Suppl), 13–16.
16. Thompson, H.J., Zhu, Z., and Jiang, W. (2002) Protection against cancer by energy restriction: All experimental approaches are not equal. *J Nutr* **132**(5), 1047–49.
17. Roth, G.S., Ingram, D.K., and Lane, M.A. (2001) Caloric restriction in primates and relevance to humans. *Ann N Y Acad Sci* **928**, 305–15.
18. Pinney, D.O., Stephens, D.F., and Pope, L.S. (1972) Lifetime effects of winter supplemental feed level and age at first parturition on range beef cows. *J Anim Sci* **34**(6), 1067–74.
19. Defossez, P.A., Lin, S.J., and McNabb, D.S. (2001) Sound silencing: The Sir2 protein and cellular senescence. *Bioessays* **23**(4), 327–32.
20. Kealy, R.D. et al. (2002) Effects of diet restriction on life span and age-related changes in dogs. *J Am Vet Med Assoc* **220**(9), 1315–20.

21. Hursting, S.D. et al. (2003) Calorie restriction, aging, and cancer prevention: Mechanisms of action and applicability to humans. *Annu Rev Med* **54**, 131–52.

22. Hursting, S.D., and Lubet, R.A. (2002) The utility of transgenic mouse models for cancer prevention research. In: Tumor Models and Cancer Research. Totowa: Humana, 263–74.

23. Tannenbaum, A. (1942) The genesis and growth of tumors. II. Effects of caloric restriction per se. *Cancer Res* **2**, 460–64.

24. Andreou, K.K., and Morgan, P.R. (1981) Effect of dietary restriction on induced hamster cheek pouch carcinogenesis. *Arch Oral Biol* **26**(6), 525–31.

25. Boissonneault, G.A., Elson, C.E., and Pariza, M.W. (1986) Net energy effects of dietary fat on chemically induced mammary carcinogenesis in F344 rats. *J Natl Cancer Inst* **76**(2), 335–38.

26. Lagopoulos, L., and Stalder, R. (1987) The influence of food intake on the development of diethylnitrosamine-induced liver tumours in mice. *Carcinogenesis* **8**(1), 33–37.

27. Dunn, S.E. et al. (1997) Dietary restriction reduces insulin-like growth factor I levels, which modulates apoptosis, cell proliferation, and tumor progression in p53-deficient mice. *Cancer Res* **57**(21), 4667–72.

28. Gross, L., and Dreyfuss, Y. (1990) Prevention of spontaneous and radiation-induced tumors in rats by reduction of food intake. *Proc Natl Acad Sci U S A* **87**(17), 6795–97.

29. Gross, L., and Dreyfuss, Y. (1984) Reduction in the incidence of radiation-induced tumors in rats after restriction of food intake. *Proc Natl Acad Sci U S A* **81**(23), 7596–98.

30. Roth, G.S., Ingram, D.K., and Lane, M.A. (1999) Calorie restriction in primates: Will it work and how will we know? *J Am Geriatr Soc* **47**(7), 896–903.

31. Temizhan, A. et al. (2000) The effects of Ramadan fasting on blood lipid levels. *Am J Med* **109**(4), 341–2.

32. Kagawa, Y. (1978) Impact of Westernization on the nutrition of Japanese: Changes in physique, cancer, longevity and centenarians. *Prev Med* **7**(2), 205–17.

33. van Noord, P.A., and Kaaks, R. (1991) The effect of wartime conditions and the 1944–45 'Dutch famine' on recalled menarcheal age in participants of the DOM breast cancer screening project. *Ann Hum Biol* **18**(1), 57–70.

34. Walford, R.L., Harris, S.B., and Gunion, M.W. (1992) The calorically restricted low-fat nutrient-dense diet in Biosphere 2 significantly lowers blood glucose, total leukocyte count, cholesterol, and blood pressure in humans. *Proc Natl Acad Sci U S A* **89**(23), 11533–37.

35. Velthuis-te Wierik, E.J. et al. (1994) Energy restriction, a useful intervention to retard human ageing? Results of a feasibility study. *Eur J Clin Nutr* **48**(2), 138–48.

36. Lane, M.A. et al. (2001) Caloric restriction in primates. *Ann N Y Acad Sci* **928**, 287–95.

37. Rogers, C.J. et al. (2008) Physical activity and cancer prevention: Pathways and targets for intervention. *Sports Med* **38**(4), 271–96.

38. Le Roith, D. et al. (2001) The somatomedin hypothesis: 2001. *Endocr Rev* **22**(1), 53–74.

39. Macaulay, V.M. (1992) Insulin-like growth factors and cancer. *Br J Cancer* **65**(3), 311–20.

40. LeRoith, D. et al. (1995) Insulin-like growth factors and cancer. *Ann Intern Med* **122**(1), 54–59.

41. Singh, P. et al. (1996) Proliferation and differentiation of a human colon cancer cell line (CaCo2) is associated with significant changes in the expression and secretion of insulin-like growth factor (IGF) IGF-II and IGF binding protein-4: Role of IGF-II. *Endocrinology* **137**(5), 1764–74.

42. Fenton, J.I. et al. (2005) Leptin, insulin-like growth factor-1, and insulin-like growth factor-2 are mitogens in Apc[Min/+] but not Apc[+/+] colonic epithelial cell lines. *Cancer Epidemiol Biomarkers Prev* **14**(7), 1646–52.

43. Buckbinder, L. et al. (1995) Induction of the growth inhibitor IGF-binding protein 3 by p53. *Nature* **377**(6550), 646–49.

44. Takahashi, K., and Suzuki, K. (1993) Association of insulin-like growth-factor-I-induced DNA synthesis with phosphorylation and nuclear exclusion of p53 in human breast cancer MCF-7 cells. *Int J Cancer* **55**(3), 453–58.

45. Hursting, S.D. et al. (1993) The growth hormone: Insulin-like growth factor 1 axis is a mediator of diet restriction-induced inhibition of mononuclear cell leukemia in Fischer rats. *Cancer Res* **53**(12), 2750–57.

46. Resnicoff, M. et al. (1995) The insulin-like growth factor I receptor protects tumor cells from apoptosis in vivo. *Cancer Res* **55**(11), 2463–69.

47. Dunn, S.E. et al. (1998) A dominant negative mutant of the insulin-like growth factor-I receptor inhibits the adhesion, invasion, and metastasis of breast cancer. *Cancer Res* **58**(15), 3353–61.

48. Gems, D., and Partridge, L. (2001) Insulin/IGF signalling and ageing: Seeing the bigger picture. *Curr Opin Genet Dev* **11**(3), 287–92.

49. Atkinson, C. et al. (2004) Effects of a moderate intensity exercise intervention on estrogen metabolism in postmenopausal women. *Cancer Epidemiol Biomarkers Prev* **13**(5), 868–74.

50. Schmitz, K.H., Ahmed, R.L., and Yee, D. (2002) Effects of a 9-month strength training intervention on insulin, insulin-like growth factor (IGF)-I, IGF-binding protein (IGFBP)-1, and IGFBP-3 in 30–50-year-old women. *Cancer Epidemiol Biomarkers Prev* **11**(12), 1597–604.

51. Colbert, L.H. et al. (2003) Exercise and intestinal polyp development in APCMin mice. *Med Sci Sports Exerc* **35**(10), 1662–69.

52. Yu, H., and Rohan, T. (2000) Role of the insulin-like growth factor family in cancer development and progression. *J Natl Cancer Inst* **92**(18), 1472–89.

53. Calle, E.E., and Kaaks, R. (2004) Overweight, obesity and cancer: Epidemiological evidence and proposed mechanisms. *Nat Rev Cancer* **4**(8), 579–91.

54. Yakar, S., Leroith, D., and Brodt, P. (2005) The role of the growth hormone/insulin-like growth factor axis in tumor growth and progression: Lessons from animal models. *Cytokine Growth Factor Rev* **16**(4–5), 407–20.

55. Abate, N. (1996) Insulin resistance and obesity. The role of fat distribution pattern. *Diabetes Care* **19**(3), 292–94.

56. Grimm, J.J. (1999) Interaction of physical activity and diet: Implications for insulin-glucose dynamics. *Public Health Nutr* **2**(3A), 363–68.

57. Carling, D. (2004) The AMP-activated protein kinase cascade–a unifying system for energy control. *Trends Biochem Sci* **29**(1), 18–24.

58. Hardie, D.G., Carling, D., and Carlson, M. (1998) The AMP-activated/SNF1 protein kinase subfamily: Metabolic sensors of the eukaryotic cell? *Annu Rev Biochem* **67**, 821–55.

59. Johnson, L.N., Noble, M.E., and Owen, D.J. (1996) Active and inactive protein kinases: Structural basis for regulation. *Cell* **85**(2), 149–58.

60. Hawley, S.A. et al. (2003) Complexes between the LKB1 tumor suppressor, STRAD alpha/beta and MO25 alpha/beta are upstream kinases in the AMP-activated protein kinase cascade. *J Biol* **2**(4), 28.

61. Woods, A. et al. (2003) LKB1 is the upstream kinase in the AMP-activated protein kinase cascade. *Curr Biol* **13**(22), 2004–08.

62. Brazil, D.P., Yang, Z.Z., and Hemmings, B.A. (2004) Advances in protein kinase B signalling: AKTion on multiple fronts. *Trends Biochm Sci* **29**, 233–42.

63. Guertin, D.A., and Sabatini, D.M. (2005) An expanding role for mTOR in cancer. *Trends Mol Med* **11**(8), 353–61.

64. Shaw, R.J. et al. (2004) The LKB1 tumor suppressor negatively regulates mTOR signaling. *Cancer Cell* **6**(1), 91–99.

65. Corradetti, M.N. et al. (2004) Regulation of the TSC pathway by LKB1: Evidence of a molecular link between tuberous sclerosis complex and Peutz-Jeghers syndrome. *Genes Dev* **18**(13), 1533–38.

66. Shaw, R.J. et al. (2004) The tumor suppressor LKB1 kinase directly activates AMP-activated kinase and regulates apoptosis in response to energy stress. *Proc Natl Acad Sci U S A* **101**(10), 3329–35.

67. Inoki, K., Corradetti, M.N., and Guan, K.L. (2005) Dysregulation of the TSC-mTOR pathway in human disease. *Nat Genet* **37**(1), 19–24.

68. Tee, A.R., and Blenis, J. (2005) mTOR, translational control and human disease. *Semin Cell Dev Biol* **16**(1), 29–37.

69. Eng, C. (2003) PTEN: One gene, many syndromes. *Hum Mutat* **22**, 183–98.

70. Woods, S.C. et al. (1998) Signals that regulate food intake and energy homeostasis. *Science* **280**(5368), 1378–83.

71. Zhang, Y., and Leibel, R. (1998) Molecular physiology of leptin and its receptor. *Growth Genet Horm* **14**, 17–35.

72. Jiang, W., Zhu, Z., and Thompson, H. (2008) Dietary energy restriction modulates the activity of AMP-activated protein kinase, Akt, and mammalian target of rapamycin in mammary carcinomas, mammary gland, and liver. *Cancer Res* **68**, 5492–99.

73. Moore, T., Beltran, L., Carbijal, S., Strom, S., Traag, J., Hursting, S.D., and DiGiovanni, J. (2008) Dietary energy balance modulates signaling through the Akt/mTOR pathway in multiple tissues. *Cancer Prev Res* **1**, 65–76.

74. Moore, T., Carbijal, S., Beltran, L., Perkins, S.N., Hursting, S.D., and DiGiovanni, J. (2008) Reduced susceptibility to two-stage skin carcinogenesis in mice with low circulating IGF-1 levels. *Cancer Res* **68**, 3680–88.

75. Lonnqvist, F., Wennlund, A., and Arner, P. (1997) Relationship between circulating leptin and peripheral fat distribution in obese subjects. *Int J Obes Relat Metab Disord* **21**(4), 255–60.

76. Montague, C.T. et al. (1997) Depot- and sex-specific differences in human leptin mRNA expression: Implications for the control of regional fat distribution. *Diabetes* **46**(3), 342–47.

77. Wilding, J., Widdowson, P., and Williams, G. (1997) Neurobiology. *Br Med Bull* **53**(2), 286–306.

78. Stattin, P. et al. (2004) Obesity and colon cancer: Does leptin provide a link? *Int J Cancer* **109**(1), 149–52.

79. Chang, S. et al. (2001) Leptin and prostate cancer. *Prostate* **46**(1), 62–67.

80. Saglam, K. et al. (2003) Leptin influences cellular differentiation and progression in prostate cancer. *J Urol* **169**(4), 1308–11.

81. Bouloumie, A. et al. (1998) Leptin, the product of Ob gene, promotes angiogenesis. *Circ Res* **83**(10), 1059–66.

82. Ostlund, R.E., Jr. et al. (1996) Relation between plasma leptin concentration and body fat, gender, diet, age, and metabolic covariates. *J Clin Endocrinol Metab* **81**(11), 3909–13.

83. Rajala, M.W., and Scherer, P.E. (2003) Minireview: The adipocyte – at the crossroads of energy homeostasis, inflammation, and atherosclerosis. *Endocrinology* **144**(9), 3765–73.

84. Gonzalez, R.R. et al. (2006) Leptin signaling promotes the growth of mammary tumors and increases the expression of vascular endothelial growth factor (VEGF) and its receptor type two (VEGF-R2). *J Biol Chem* **281**(36), 26320–28.

85. Loffreda, S. et al. (1998) Leptin regulates proinflammatory immune responses. *FASEB J* **12**(1), 57–65.

86. Bråkenhielm, E. et al. (2004) Adiponectin-induced antiangiogenesis and antitumor activity involve caspase-mediated endothelial cell apoptosis. *PNAS* **101**, 2476–81.

87. Diker, D. et al. (2006) mpact of gastric banding on plasma adiponectin levels. *Obes Surg* **9**, 1057–61.

88. Ryan, A. et al. (2003) Adiponectin levels do not change with moderate dietary induced weight loss and exercise in obese postmenopausal women. *Int J Obes* **27**, 1066–71.

89. Amitabha, R., Katai, N., and Cleary, M. (2007) Effects of leptin on human breast cancer cell lines in relationship to estrogen receptor and HER2 status. *Int J Oncol* **6**, 1499–509.

90. Grossmann, M. et al. (2008) Effects of adiponectin on breast cancer cell growth and signaling. *Br J Cancer* **98**, 370–79.

91. Kaaks, R., Lukanova, A., and Kurzer, M.S. (2002) Obesity, endogenous hormones, and endometrial cancer risk: A synthetic review. *Cancer Epidemiol Biomarkers Prev* **11**(12), 1531–43.

92. Birt, D.F. et al. (2004) Identification of molecular targets for dietary energy restriction prevention of skin carcinogenesis: An idea cultivated by Edward Bresnick. *J Cell Biochem* **91**(2), 258–64.

93. Jiang, W. et al. (2002) Mechanisms of energy restriction: Effects of corticosterone on cell growth, cell cycle machinery, and apoptosis. *Cancer Res* **62**(18), 5280–87.

94. Pashko, L.L., and Schwartz, A.G. (1992) Reversal of food restriction-induced inhibition of mouse skin tumor promotion by adrenalectomy. *Carcinogenesis* **13**(10), 1925–28.

95. Boutwell, R.K. (1964) Some biological aspects of skin carcinogenisis. *Prog Exp Tumor Res* **19**, 207–50.

96. Coussens, L.M., and Werb, Z. (2002) Inflammation and cancer. *Nature* **420**(6917), 860–67.

97. Sohal, R.S., and Weindruch, R. (1996) Oxidative stress, caloric restriction, and aging. *Science* **273**(5271), 59–63.

98. Tilg, H., Dinarello, C.A., and Mier, J.W. (1997) IL-6 and APPs: Anti-inflammatory and immunosuppressive mediators. *Immunol Today* **18**(9), 428–32.

99. Dinarello, C.A. (2000) The role of the interleukin-1-receptor antagonist in blocking inflammation mediated by interleukin-1. *N Engl J Med* **343**(10), 732–34.

100. Moore, K.W. et al. (1993) Interleukin-10. *Annu Rev Immunol* **11**, 165–90.

101. Pretolani, M. (1999) Interleukin-10: An anti-inflammatory cytokine with therapeutic potential. *Clin Exp Allergy* **29**(9), 1164–71.

102. Coppack, S.W. (2001) Pro-inflammatory cytokines and adipose tissue. *Proc Nutr Soc* **60**(3), 349–56.

103. Dandona, P., Aljada, A., and Bandyopadhyay, A. (2004) Inflammation: The link between insulin resistance, obesity and diabetes. *Trends Immunol* **25**(1), 4–7.

104. Weisberg, S.P. et al. (2003) Obesity is associated with macrophage accumulation in adipose tissue. *J Clin Invest* **112**(12), 1796–808.

105. Xu, H. et al. (2003) Chronic inflammation in fat plays a crucial role in the development of obesity-related insulin resistance. *J Clin Invest* **112**(12), 1821–30.

106. Ballou, S.P. et al. (1996) Quantitative and qualitative alterations of acute-phase proteins in healthy elderly persons. *Age Ageing* **25**(3), 224–30.

107. Paolisso, G. et al. (1998) Advancing age and insulin resistance: Role of plasma tumor necrosis factor-alpha. *Am J Physiol* **275**(2 Pt 1), E294-E99.

108. Bruunsgaard, H. et al. (1999) Exercise induces recruitment of lymphocytes with an activated phenotype and short telomeres in young and elderly humans. *Life Sci* **65**(24), 2623–33.

109. Bruunsgaard, H. et al. (2000) Ageing, tumour necrosis factor-alpha (TNF-alpha) and atherosclerosis. *Clin Exp Immunol* **121**(2), 255–60.

110. Bruunsgaard, H. et al. (2004) The IL-6-174G>C polymorphism is associated with cardiovascular diseases and mortality in 80-year-old humans. *Exp Gerontol* **39**(2), 255–61.

111. Vgontzas, A.N. et al. (2000) Sleep apnea and daytime sleepiness and fatigue: Relation to visceral obesity, insulin resistance, and hypercytokinemia. *J Clin Endocrinol Metab* **85**(3), 1151–58.

112. Feingold, K.R., and Grunfeld, C. (1992) Role of cytokines in inducing hyperlipidemia. *Diabetes* **41**(Suppl 2), 97–101.

113. Winkler, G. et al. (1998) Elevated serum tumor necrosis factor-alpha concentrations and bioactivity in Type 2 diabetics and patients with android type obesity. *Diabetes Res Clin Pract* **42**(3), 169–74.

114. Mishima, Y. et al. (2001) Relationship between serum tumor necrosis factor-alpha and insulin resistance in obese men with Type 2 diabetes mellitus. *Diabetes Res Clin Pract* **52**(2), 119–23.

115. Harris, T.B. et al. (1997) Carrying the burden of cardiovascular risk in old age: Associations of weight and weight change with prevalent cardiovascular disease, risk factors, and health status in the Cardiovascular Health Study. *Am J Clin Nutr* **66**(4), 837–44.

116. Volpato, S. et al. (2001) Cardiovascular disease, interleukin-6, and risk of mortality in older women: The women's health and aging study. *Circulation* **103**(7), 947–53.

117. Erlinger, T.P. et al. (2004) C-reactive protein and the risk of incident colorectal cancer. *J Am Med Assoc* **291**(5), 585–90.

118. Lehrer, S. et al. (2005) C-reactive protein is significantly associated with prostate-specific antigen and metastatic disease in prostate cancer. *BJU Int* **95**(7), 961–2.

119. King, D.E. et al. (2003) Inflammatory markers and exercise: Differences related to exercise type. *Med Sci Sports Exerc* **35**(4), 575–81.

120. Wannamethee, S.G. et al. (2002) Physical activity and hemostatic and inflammatory variables in elderly men. *Circulation* **105**(15), 1785–90.

121. Abramson, J.L., and Vaccarino, V. (2002) Relationship between physical activity and inflammation among apparently healthy middle-aged and older US adults. *Arch Intern Med* **162**(11), 1286–92.

122. Geffken, D.F. et al. (2001) Association between physical activity and markers of inflammation in a healthy elderly population. *Am J Epidemiol* **153**(3), 242–50.

123. Smith, J.K. et al. (1999) Long-term exercise and atherogenic activity of blood mononuclear cells in persons at risk of developing ischemic heart disease. *J Am Med Assoc* **281**(18), 1722–27.

124. Mattusch, F. et al. (2000) Reduction of the plasma concentration of C-reactive protein following nine months of endurance training. *Int J Sports Med* **21**(1), 21–24.

125. Taaffe, D.R. et al. (2000) Cross-sectional and prospective relationships of interleukin-6 and C-reactive protein with physical performance in elderly persons: MacArthur studies of successful aging. *J Gerontol A Biol Sci Med Sci* **55**(12), M709–M15.

126. Fallon, K.E., Fallon, S.K., and Boston, T. (2001) The acute phase response and exercise: Court and field sports. *Br J Sports Med* **35**(3), 170–73.

127. Longo, V.D., and Kennedy, B.K. (2006) Sirtuins in aging and age-related disease. *Cell* **126**(2), 257–68.

128. Anastasiou, D., and Krek, W. (2006) SIRT1: Linking adaptive cellular responses to aging-associated changes in organismal physiology. *Physiology (Bethesda)* **21**, 404–10.

129. Yang, T. et al. (2006) SIRT1 and endocrine signaling. *Trends Endocrinol Metab* **17**(5), 186–91.

130. Cohen, H.Y. et al. (2004) Calorie restriction promotes mammalian cell survival by inducing the SIRT1 deacetylase. *Science* **305**(5682), 390–92.

131. Metoyer, C.F., and Pruitt, K. (2008) The role of sirtuin proteins in obesity. *Pathophysiology* **15**(2), 103–08.

132. Lin, S.J., Defossez, P.A., and Guarente, L. (2000) Requirement of NAD and SIR2 for life-span extension by calorie restriction in Saccharomyces cerevisiae. *Science* **289**(5487), 2126–28.

133. Anderson, R.M. et al. (2003) Nicotinamide and PNC1 govern lifespan extension by calorie restriction in Saccharomyces cerevisiae. *Nature* **423**(6936), 181–85.

134. Tissenbaum, H.A., and Guarente, L. (2001) Increased dosage of a sir-2 gene extends lifespan in Caenorhabditis elegans. *Nature* **410**(6825), 227–30.

135. Picard, F. et al. (2004) Sirt1 promotes fat mobilization in white adipocytes by repressing PPAR-gamma. *Nature* **429**(6993), 771–76.

136. Qiang, L., Wang, H., and Farmer, S.R. (2007) Adiponectin secretion is regulated by SIRT1 and the endoplasmic reticulum oxidoreductase Ero1-L alpha. *Mol Cell Biol* **27**(13), 4698–707.

137. Qiao, L., and Shao, J. (2006) SIRT1 regulates adiponectin gene expression through Foxo1-C/enhancer-binding protein alpha transcriptional complex. *J Biol Chem* **281**(52), 39915–24.

138. Bordone, L. et al. (2007) SIRT1 transgenic mice show phenotypes resembling calorie restriction. *Aging Cell* **6**(6), 759–67.

139. Ramsey, K.M. et al. (2008) Age-associated loss of Sirt1-mediated enhancement of glucose-stimulated insulin secretion in beta cell-specific Sirt1-overexpressing (BESTO) mice. *Aging Cell* **7**(1), 78–88.

140. Nemoto, S., Fergusson, M.M., and Finkel, T. (2005) SIRT1 functionally interacts with the metabolic regulator and transcriptional coactivator PGC-1{alpha}. *J Biol Chem* **280**(16), 16456–60.

141. Nisoli, E. et al. (2005) Calorie restriction promotes mitochondrial biogenesis by inducing the expression of eNOS. *Science* **310**(5746), 314–17.

142. Yechoor, V.K. et al. (2004) Distinct pathways of insulin-regulated versus diabetes-regulated gene expression: An in vivo analysis in MIRKO mice. *Proc Natl Acad Sci U S A* **101**(47), 16525–30.

143. Lim, C.S. (2006) SIRT1: Tumor promoter or tumor suppressor? *Med Hypotheses* **67**(2), 341–44.

144. Ford, J., Jiang, M., and Milner, J. (2005) Cancer-specific functions of SIRT1 enable human epithelial cancer cell growth and survival. *Cancer Res* **65**(22), 10457–63.

145. Chen, W.Y. et al. (2005) Tumor suppressor HIC1 directly regulates SIRT1 to modulate p53-dependent DNA-damage responses. *Cell* **123**(3), 437–48.

146. Huffman, D.M. et al. (2007) SIRT1 is significantly elevated in mouse and human prostate cancer. *Cancer Res* **67**(14), 6612–18.

147. Kim, J.E., Chen, J., and Lou, Z. (2008) DBC1 is a negative regulator of SIRT1. *Nature* **451**(7178), 583–86.

148. Zhao, W. et al. (2008) Negative regulation of the deacetylase SIRT1 by DBC1. *Nature* **451**(7178), 587–90.

149. Firestein, R. et al. (2008) The SIRT1 deacetylase suppresses intestinal tumorigenesis and colon cancer growth. *PLoS One* **3**(4), e2020.

150. Baur, J.A., and Sinclair, D.A. (2006) Therapeutic potential of resveratrol: The in vivo evidence. *Nat Rev Drug Discov* **5**(6), 493–506.

151. Lee, C.K. et al. (1999) Gene expression profile of aging and its retardation by caloric restriction. *Science* **285**(5432), 1390–93.

152. Lee, C.K., Weindruch, R., and Prolla, T.A. (2000) Gene-expression profile of the ageing brain in mice. *Nat Genet* **25**(3), 294–97.

153. Weindruch, R. et al. (2002) Gene expression profiling of aging using DNA microarrays. *Mech Ageing Dev* **123**(2–3), 177–93.

154. Pletcher, S.D. et al. (2002) Genome-wide transcript profiles in aging and calorically restricted Drosophila melanogaster. *Curr Biol* **12**(9), 712–23.

155. Cao, S.X. et al. (2001) Genomic profiling of short- and long-term caloric restriction effects in the liver of aging mice. *Proc Natl Acad Sci U S A* **98**(19), 10630–35.

156. Kayo, T. et al. (2001) Influences of aging and caloric restriction on the transcriptional profile of skeletal muscle from rhesus monkeys. *Proc Natl Acad Sci U S A* **98**(9), 5093–98.

157. Vogt, A. et al. (1998) Disruption of insulin-like growth factor-1 signaling and down-regulation of cdc2 by SC-alphaalphadelta9, a novel small molecule antisignaling agent identified in a targeted array library. *J Pharmacol Exp Ther* **287**(2), 806–13.

158. Chen, C. et al. (2001) Discovery of a series of nonpeptide small molecules that inhibit the binding of insulin-like growth factor (IGF) to IGF-binding proteins. *J Med Chem* **44**(23), 4001–10.

159. Scotlandi, K. et al. (2002) Effectiveness of insulin-like growth factor I receptor antisense strategy against Ewing's sarcoma cells. *Cancer Gene Ther* **9**(3), 296–307.

160. Granerus, M., and Engstrom, W. (2001) Effects of insulin-like growth factor-binding protein 2 and an IGF-type I receptor-blocking antibody on apoptosis in human teratocarcinoma cells in vitro. *Cell Biol Int* **25**(8), 825–28.

161. Friedl, A., Jordan, V.C., and Pollak, M. (1993) Suppression of serum insulin-like growth factor-1 levels in breast cancer patients during adjuvant tamoxifen therapy. *Eur J Cancer* **29A**(10), 1368–72.

162. Shojamanesh, H. et al. (2002) Prospective study of the antitumor efficacy of long-term octreotide treatment in patients with progressive metastatic gastrinoma. *Cancer* **94**(2), 331–43.

163. Decensi, A. et al. (2001) Long-term effects of fenretinide, a retinoic acid derivative, on the insulin-like growth factor system in women with early breast cancer. *Cancer Epidemiol Biomarkers Prev* **10**(10), 1047–53.

164. Zujewski, J. (2002) Selective estrogen receptor modulators (SERMs) and retinoids in breast cancer chemoprevention. *Environ Mol Mutagen* **39**(2–3), 264–70.

165. Nicklas, B.J. et al. (1995) Testosterone, growth hormone and IGF-I responses to acute and chronic resistive exercise in men aged 55–70 years. *Int J Sports Med* **16**(7), 445–50.

166. Eliakim, A. et al. (1996) Physical fitness, endurance training, and the growth hormone-insulin-like growth factor I system in adolescent females. *J Clin Endocrinol Metab* **81**(11), 3986–92.

167. Smith, A.T. et al. (1987) The effect of exercise on plasma somatomedin-C/insulinlike growth factor I concentrations. *Metabolism* **36**(6), 533–37.

8 Fiber and Microbially Generated Active Components

Joanne L. Slavin and Maria L. Stewart

Key Points

1. Dietary fiber is a heterogeneous group of compounds consisting of the remnants of plant cells resistant to hydrolysis by human alimentary enzymes.
2. Dietary fiber has effects throughout the digestive tract, although its effects in the colon are of greatest interest in cancer prevention.
3. Dietary fiber reduces transit time, dilutes potential carcinogens, stimulates bacterial anaerobic fermentation, and leads to the production of short chain fatty acids that have favorable effects on cell growth regulation.
4. Populations that consume more dietary fiber have less chronic disease, including many forms of cancer. Results of epidemiologic studies of dietary fiber and cancer prevention are inconsistent, although typical intakes of dietary fiber in Western countries are low and studies find protection with dietary fiber when intakes are greater than 35 g/day.
5. Clinical studies find that intake of dietary fiber has beneficial effects on risk factors for developing cancers, including higher stool weights, lowered fecal pH, and increased production of short chain fatty acids. Additionally, high-fiber diets are low in energy density, another dietary attribute linked to cancer protection.
6. Typical Western diseases include diabetes, hypercholesterolemia, heart disease, diverticular disease, and cancer. This may be due to the usual dietary fiber intake at only 15 g/day, about half of recommended levels.

Key Words: Dietary fiber; cancer; short chain fatty acids; microflora

1. INTRODUCTION

1.1. What Is Fiber?

The term *dietary fiber* was not coined until 1953, but the anti-constipating effects of high-fiber foods have been long appreciated. In 430 BC, Hippocrates compared the superior laxative effects of coarse wheat and refined wheat *(1)*. Graham (of graham cracker fame) denounced the harmful effects of refined carbohydrate foods during the nineteenth century, and the first Kellogg's and Post cereals were formulated in response

From: *Nutrition and Health: Bioactive Compounds and Cancer*
Edited by: J.A. Milner, D.F. Romagnolo, DOI 10.1007/978-1-60761-627-6_8,
© Springer Science+Business Media, LLC 2010

to increasing interest in dietary fiber. In the 1920s, J.H. Kellogg published extensively on the attributes of bran, claiming it increased stool weight, promoted laxation, and prevented disease. Dietary fiber was studied throughout the 1930s and then forgotten.

Denis Burkitt is usually credited with popularizing the contemporary idea that dietary fiber may protect against the development of Western diseases, including diabetes, hypercholesterolemia, heart disease, diverticular disease, and cancer (2). Whether isolated dietary fiber has the same physiologic properties as the dietary fiber found naturally in grains, fruits, and vegetables with associated substances is unknown and difficult to study.

Interest in dietary fiber has been limited by our inability to agree on definitions for dietary fiber and recommended intake levels. In 2002, the Food and Nutrition Board of the National Academy of Sciences published a new set of definitions for dietary fiber (3). Whereas the new definition suggested that the term dietary fiber would describe the nondigestible carbohydrates and lignin that are intrinsic and intact in plants, functional fiber consists of the isolated nondigestible carbohydrates that have beneficial physiological effects in humans. Total fiber would then be the sum of dietary fiber plus functional fiber. Nondigestible means not digested and absorbed in the human small intestine. Fibers can be fermented in the large intestine or can pass through the digestive tract unfermented.

There is no biochemical assay that reflects dietary fiber or functional fiber nutritional status, e.g., blood fiber levels cannot be measured because fiber is not absorbed. No data are available to determine an estimated average requirement (EAR) and thus calculate a recommended dietary allowance (RDA) for total fiber, so an adequate intake (AI) was instead developed. The AI for fiber is based on the median fiber intake level observed to achieve the lowest risk of coronary heart disease (CHD). A tolerable upper intake level (UL) was not set for dietary fiber or functional fiber.

Dietary fiber is part of a plant matrix which is largely intact. Nondigestible plant carbohydrates in foods are usually a mixture of polysaccharides that are integral components of the plant cell wall or intercellular structure. This definition recognizes that the three-dimensional plant matrix is responsible for some of the physicochemical properties attributed to dietary fiber. In addition, dietary fiber contains other nutrients normally found in foods that may have health effects. Cereal brans, which are obtained by grinding, are anatomical layers of the grain consisting of intact cells and substantial amounts of starch and protein; they are categorized as dietary fiber sources.

According to the DRI panel, the relationship of fiber intake to colon cancer is the subject on ongoing investigation. The DRI panel suggested the recommended intakes of total fiber may ameliorate constipation and diverticular disease, provide fuel for colonic cells, reduce blood glucose and lipid levels, and provide a source of nutrient-rich, low-energy-dense foods that could contribute to satiety, although these benefits were not used as the basis for the AI.

Dietary fiber intake continues to be less than recommended in the United States averaging only 15 g/day (3). Many popular American foods contain little dietary fiber. Servings of commonly consumed grains, fruits, and vegetables contain only 1–3 g of dietary fiber (4). Major sources of dietary fiber in the US food supply include grains and vegetables (5). White flour and white potatoes provide the most fiber to the diet, about 16 and

9%, respectively, not because they are concentrated fiber sources, but because they are widely consumed. Legumes are very rich in dietary fiber, but because of low consumption they only provide about 6% of the fiber in the US diet. Fruits provide only 10% of the fiber in the overall US diet, because of low fruit consumption and the low amount of fiber in fruits, except for dried fruits.

A variety of definitions of dietary fiber exist (6). Some are based primarily on analytical methods used to isolate and quantify dietary fiber whereas others are physiologically based. Dietary fiber is primarily the storage and cell wall polysaccharides of plants that cannot be hydrolyzed by human digestive enzymes. Lignin, which is a complex molecule of polyphenylpropane units and present only in small amounts in the human diet, is also usually included as a component of dietary fiber. In labels of food products within the United States, dietary fiber is defined as the material isolated by analytical methods approved by the Association of Official Analytical Chemists, generally AOAC Method 985.29 (6). A variety of low-molecular carbohydrates such as resistant starch, polydextrose, and nondigestible oligosaccharides including fructo- and galacto-oligosaccharidies are being developed and increasingly used in food processing. Generally, these compounds are not captured by AOAC Method 985.29. Other AOAC accepted methods to measure the fiber content of these novel fibers have been developed or are currently in development (6).

Although the IOM report recommended that the terms soluble and insoluble fibers not be used (3), food labels still may include soluble and insoluble fiber data. Water-soluble fiber is precipitated in a mixture of enzymes and ethanol. Dietary fiber was divided into soluble and insoluble fibers in an attempt to assign physiological effects to chemical types of fiber. Oat bran, barley bran, and psyllium, mostly soluble fiber, have health claims for their ability to lower blood lipids. Wheat bran and other more insoluble fibers are typically linked to improved laxation and colon cancer prevention. Yet, scientific support that soluble fibers lower blood cholesterol, while insoluble fibers increase stool size, is inconsistent at best.

Resistant starch (the sum of starch and starch-degradation products not digested in the small intestine) (7) reaches the large intestine and would function as dietary fiber. Legumes are a primary source of resistant starch, with as much as 35% of legume starch escaping digestion (8). Small amounts of resistant starch are produced by processing and baking of cereal and grain products. Many new functional fibers increasingly being added to processed foods are resistant starches. Murphy et al. (9) estimated resistant starch intakes in the United States. A database of resistant starch concentrations in foods was developed from published values. These values were linked to foods reported in 24-h dietary recalls from participants in the 1999–2002 National Health and Nutrition Examination Surveys to estimate resistant starch intakes. Americans aged 1 year and older were estimated to consume approximately 4.9 g/day of resistant starch (range 2.8–7.9 g/day).

Dietary fiber includes plant nonstarch polysaccharides (e.g., cellulose, pectin, gums, hemicellulose, β-glucans, and fiber contained in oat and wheat bran), plant carbohydrates that are not recovered by alcohol precipitation (e.g., inulin, oligosaccharides, and fructans), lignin, and some resistant starch. Potential functional fibers include isolated, nondigestible plant (e.g., resistant starch, pectin, and gums), animal (e.g., chitin and chitosan), or commercially produced (e.g., resistant starch, polydextrose, inulin, and indigestible dextrins) carbohydrates *(3)*. Additionally, dietary fiber is a marker of a plant-based diet and associated with a wide range of phytochemicals that also have potential roles in cancer prevention. Also, high-fiber diets are generally low-fat diets, so the protective properties of high-fiber diets may be confounded by low-fat intakes.

2. CANCER BACKGROUND

Cancers of the gastrointestinal tract represent the second most common cancer in the United States and are second only to cancer of the respiratory tract as a cause of cancer-related mortality. The development of colon cancer involves a complex interplay between environmental and genetic factors. As the colorectal epithelium progresses from normal histology to one that is hyperproliferative, adenomatous, and finally malignant, multiple molecular alterations, including the activation of proto-oncogenes, the inactivation of tumor-suppressor genes, and mutations in mismatch repair genes, occur *(10)*. Environmental factors may also contribute to cancer, but unlike genetic factors, they may be modifiable and targeted by prevention strategies. Estimates suggest that 35% of all cancers are attributable to diet and that up to 90% of colorectal cancers in the United States could be avoidable through dietary intervention *(11)*. However, establishing a cause-and-effect relationship between diet and colorectal cancer is a difficult task.

Investigations that examine the impact of diet on cancer incidence include epidemiological studies where dietary variables are compared across populations. Case–control studies examine differences in diet between people who have colon cancer compared to those who do not. A serious limitation of retrospective studies is the accuracy with which intakes of dietary factors can be estimated. It is difficult to recall dietary intakes in former years and disease tends to alter dietary habits. A stronger epidemiological design is the cohort study in which subjects exposed to a particular agent are followed over time and their cancer incidence is compared with those who have not been exposed. These studies are costly and require a large number of subjects. Intervention studies allow investigators to make a dietary change and then follow the course of a disease. Intervention studies are limited by the slow progressive nature of the cancer process and the large number of subjects needed to reach adequate statistical power.

Strategies to avoid these problems include studying individuals who are at high risk for developing cancer to determine whether a chemopreventive agent can prevent the development of cancer. Second, studies use intermediate biomarkers of the cancer process as end points rather than waiting for the cancer to occur. Chemoprevention trials in high-risk individuals use intermediate biomarkers to determine the role of dietary ingredients on colon cancer causation.

Many studies use animal models to investigate the relationship between dietary fiber and colon cancer. Animal studies offer the advantage of greater control of experimental variables, allow for a broader range of interventions, and are generally less expensive than human studies. However, animal models may generate species-related results, which for dietary fiber may be difficult to interpret. For example, the gastrointestinal tract of the rat varies significantly from that of humans. Therefore, extrapolation of data obtained in rodents to humans may not be accurate. Very often, cancer research related to fiber is conducted in cell culture using cancer cell lines. Also, mechanistic studies that investigate the role of dietary fiber in colon cancer prevention utilize healthy human subjects.

The translational significance of studies that examine the impact of dietary fiber on the cancer process may be hampered by problems in defining, measuring, and quantitating dietary fiber. This difficulty is exacerbated by lack of a standard chemical method to assess dietary fiber. Epidemiological studies generally rely on food frequency instruments that estimate dietary fiber. These estimates are largely inadequate when estimating fermentable carbohydrates that reach the colon. Earlier studies by Hill *(12)* suggested that we return to foods for epidemiologic studies rather than attempting to measure dietary fiber, which obviously is problematic.

3. RATIONALE WHY FIBER AND ITS FERMENTATION PRODUCTS PROTECT AGAINST CANCER

Dietary fiber exerts physiological effects throughout the gastrointestinal tract that may explain its protectiveness against cancer. Although we generally think of dietary fiber as most active in the large intestine, it is known that fiber alters hormone functions in the upper digestive tract. These changes may alter satiety, slow digestion, and aid in weight maintenance. Potential mechanisms for the protective effects of dietary fiber against colon cancer are listed in Table 1. The fermentation of carbohydrates in the colon produces short chain fatty acids (SCFA) that help maintain the integrity of the gut *(13)*. More than 75% of dietary fiber in an average diet is broken down in the large intestine resulting in the production of carbon dioxide, hydrogen, methane, and SCFA

Table 1
Mechanisms by Which Fiber Can Protect Against the Development of Cancer

Increased stool bulk
  Decreased transit time
  Dilution of carcinogens
Binds with bile acids or other potential carcinogens
Lower fecal pH
  Inhibits bacterial degradation of normal food constituents to potential carcinogens
Changes in microflora
Fermentation by fecal flora to short chain fatty acids
  Decrease in colonic pH
  Inhibition of carcinogens
Increase in lumenal antioxidants
Peptide growth factors
Alteration of sex hormone status
Change in satiety resulting in lowered body weight
Alterations in insulin sensitivity and/or glucose metabolism

including butyrate, propionate, and acetate. Propionate and acetate are metabolized in colonic epithelial cells or peripheral tissue. Butyrate regulates colonic cell proliferation and serves as an energy source. Propionate is transported to the liver where it may suppress cholesterol synthesis. This may provide a potential explanation for how soluble dietary fiber lowers serum cholesterol.

According to calculations by Cummings and McFarlane (14), fermentation of ~20 g/day of fiber in the colon generates ~200 mM of SCFA (62% acetate, 25% propionate,16% butyrate). Colonic absorption of SCFA is concentration-dependent with no evidence of a saturable process. The mechanism by which SCFA crosses the colonic mucosa is thought to be passive diffusion of the unionized acid into the mucosa cell. SCFAs are respiratory fuels for the colonic mucosa. In isolated human colonocytes, butyrate is actively metabolized to CO_2 and ketone bodies, which account for about 80% of the oxygen consumption by colonocytes.

Butyrate exerts trophic effects on normal colonocytes in vitro and in vivo. In contrast, butyrate arrests the growth of neoplastic colonocytes and inhibits the preneoplastic hyperproliferation induced by some tumor promoters in vitro (15). Butyrate induces differentiation of colon cancer cell lines and regulates the expression of factors involved in colonocyte growth and adhesion.

The effects of butyrate on colonic tumor cell lines in vitro seem to contradict what has been shown in vivo (16). Butyrate appears to have two contrasting effects. It serves as the primary energy source for normal colonic epithelium and stimulates growth of colonic mucosa, yet in colonic tumor cell lines it inhibits growth and induces differentiation and apoptosis. Since SCFAs are volatile, they are quickly absorbed from the lumen. SCFAs acidify the gut, which may affect development of colon cancer because changes in gut pH will affect solubility of metabolites and activities of bacterial enzymes (17).

Hamer et al. (18) reviewed the role of butyrate on colonic function and agreed that butyrate is an important energy source for intestinal epithelial cells and plays a role in the maintenance of colonic homeostasis. Butyrate inhibits inflammation and carcinogenesis. Two important mechanisms include the inhibition of nuclear factor-κB activation and histone deacetylation. Human data for the role of butyrate in cancer prevention are limited and in vitro data depend heavily on concentration of butyrate used and the model system.

Bordonaro et al. (19) suggested that the effects of fiber and butyrate on colon cancer risk may be mediated through Wnt signaling, a pathway that is constitutively activated in most colorectal cancers. Analyses of 10 human colorectal cancer cell lines exposed to butyrate found the levels of apoptosis in these cells were dependent on the fold induction of the canonical Wnt transcriptional activity. The same authors proposed that the existence of colorectal cancer subtypes, individual- and population-specific variations in butyrate-producing colonic microflora, and the timing colorectal lesions are exposed to fiber/butyrate are all factors that may influence the protective role of fiber against colorectal cancer.

Reddy et al. (20) reported that in healthy subjects receiving equal amounts of fiber, the concentration of fecal secondary bile acids and mutagenic activity were significantly lower following supplementation with wheat bran compared to supplementation with oat bran or control diets. Other studies have examined fiber's ability to increase fecal bulk and speed intestinal transit. Dietary fibers differ in their ability to hold water and their resistance to bacterial degradation in the gut. Pectin is effective in holding water, but is quickly fermented in the gut and cannot be found in feces. Conversely, wheat bran has consistently been found to have the most effect on stool bulk, probably because it is slowly fermented and survives transit through the gut. Milling of wheat bran may affect the laxative properties of the bran, with larger particle sizes causing larger increases in fecal weight.

Dietary fiber sources such as wheat bran are complex matrices and attempts have been made to isolate the effects of specific components of wheat bran. In an animal study, rats were fed wheat bran, dephytinized wheat bran, and phytic acid alone and aberrant crypt foci were measured after treatment with azoxymethane *(21)*. Dephytinized wheat bran was less protective than intact wheat bran, suggesting that the protective effects of wheat bran may be due to fiber and phytic acid. Certain components of dietary fiber are more protective than others against colorectal cancer. Insoluble fibers have consistently been found to decrease cell proliferation, whereas soluble fibers may even increase cell proliferation. Lu et al. *(22)* found that lignin, a component of insoluble dietary fiber, acted as a free radical scavenger. These authors suggested that the ability of dietary fiber to protect against colorectal cancer may be determined by the amount of lignin as well as the free radical scavenging ability of lignin.

A common criticism of animal studies is the use of large amounts of dietary fiber. For example, dietary fibers have been fed at levels of 30% of the diet or more. These levels of fiber intake have no bearing on typical or recommended intakes in humans.

4. EFFECT OF DIETARY FIBER ON STOOL CHEMISTRY

Many fiber sources, including cereal brans, psyllium seed husk, methylcellulose, and a mixed high-fiber diet increase stool weight thereby promoting normal laxation. Stool weight parallels fiber intake increases *(23)*, but the added fiber tends to normalize defecation frequency to one bowel movement daily and gastrointestinal transit time to 2–4 days. The increase in stool weight is caused by the fiber mass, the water-holding capacity of fiber, and bacterial mass fermenting the fiber. If the fiber is fully and rapidly fermented in the large bowel, as are most soluble fiber sources, there is no increase in stool weight *(24)*. It is a common but erroneous belief that the increased stool weight is due primarily to water. The moisture content of human stool is 70–75% and this does not change when more fiber is consumed. Fiber in the colon is no more effective at holding water in the lumen than the other components of stool. The one known exception is psyllium seed husk, which does increase the concentration of stool water to ~80%. As fiber consumption increases, stool weight increases. Therefore, increased fluid consumption should be recommended to account for the increased loss of fecal water.

Unlike blood, fecal samples have not been collected and evaluated for a large cohort of healthy subjects. Cummings et al. *(24)* conducted a meta-analysis of 11 studies in which daily fecal weight was measured accurately in 26 groups of people ($n = 206$) on controlled diets of known fiber content. Fiber intakes were significantly related to stool weight ($r = 0.84$). Stool weight varied greatly among subjects from different countries, ranging from 72 to 470 g/day. Stool weight was inversely related to colon cancer risk in this study. Spiller *(25)* suggested that there is a critical fecal weight of 160–200 g/day for adults, below which colon function becomes unpredictable and risk of colon cancer increases. Stool weights in healthy UK adults averaged only 106 g/day. It is likely that average stool weights in the United States are also low as Cummings et al. *(24)* reported that stool weights in Westernized populations ranged from 80 to 120 g/day.

Studies have reported that dietary fibers have differential effects on fecal weight. For example, fecal weight increased 5.4 g/g of wheat bran fiber (mostly insoluble), 4.9 g/g fruits and vegetables (soluble and insoluble), 3 g/g isolated cellulose (insoluble), and 1.3 g/g isolated pectin (soluble) *(24)*. When subjects were fed 15, 30, or 42 g/day diet fiber from a mixed diet, there was a significant increase in stool weight on all diets. Most of the increased stool weight was from undigested dietary fiber, although the mid-range of fiber intake was also associated with an increase in bacterial mass *(26)*.

In addition to fiber, other food components determine stool weight. Slavin et al. *(27)* fed liquid diets containing 0, 30, and 60 g of soy fiber and compared stool weights to those of subjects consuming their habitual diets. Daily fecal weight averaged 145 g/day on the habitual diets. On the liquid diets with added fiber stool weight averaged, respectively, 67, 100, and 150 g/day. Estimated fiber intake on the habitual diet was less than 20 g/day, supporting the conclusion that other factors in solid foods besides dietary fiber increase stool weight.

Besides food intake, other factors also affect stool size. These are often noted in studies, but are not well studied in research trials. For example, stress associated with exams or competition can increase intestinal transit. Exercise may stimulate intestinal transit *(28)*, although data on this effect remain conflicting. Bingham and Cummings *(29)* found that on a controlled dietary intake, transit time increased in nine subjects and decreased in five subjects when a 9-week exercise program was introduced. Other measures of bowel function, including stool weight or fecal frequency, were not changed by the exercise program.

Even on rigidly controlled diets of the same composition, there is a large variation in daily stool weight among subjects. Gender is known to alter colonic functions *(30)*. Tucker et al. *(31)* examined the predictors of stool weight when completely controlled diets were fed to normal volunteers. These investigators found that personality was a better predictor of stool weight than dietary fiber intake, with outgoing subjects more likely to produce higher stool weights.

5. EFFECT OF DIETARY FIBER ON METHANE AND SULFUR GASES

It is estimated that for every 10 g of carbohydrates that reach the large intestine, 100 mmol SCFA, 100 ml hydrogen gas, and 3 g bacterial mass are produced *(14)*. Hydrogen gas accumulation can adversely affect metabolism, so it must be disposed of efficiently. The primary means of hydrogen disposal include methane and hydrogen sulfide (H_2S) production and excretion via breath and flatus *(32)*.

Methane is produced by bacteria (methanogens) such as *Methanobrevibacter smithii* that reside in approximately 30% of the population. Methane production is beneficial for two reasons: (1) methane is nontoxic and (2) for every mole of methane generated, 4 mol of hydrogen gas are removed from the colonic lumen *(32)*. Sulfate reducing bacteria (SRB) compete with methanogens for hydrogen gas when sufficient sulfate is available due to the thermodynamic favorability of H_2S production *(32, 33)*. Dietary sulfate is the primary source of colonic sulfate, but mucins, sulfated glycoproteins, and sulfated polysaccharides also contribute to the colonic sulfate pool *(32)*. H_2S-impaired oxidation of SCFA is a major component of inflammatory bowel disease (IBD), but the role of SRB in the development of IBD is still under debate *(34)*. IBD is associated with an increased risk of colorectal cancer *(35)*. H_2S has not been shown to act as a direct carcinogen, but several studies supported the role of H_2S in epithelial dysregulation and altered signal transduction *(36)*.

6. CANCER

6.1. Large Bowel Cancer

Extensive epidemiological evidence supports the theory that dietary fiber may protect against large bowel cancer. Studies that compared colorectal cancer incidence or mortality rates in various nations with relative estimates of dietary fiber consumption suggested that dietary fiber may protect against colon cancer. Data collected from 20 populations in 12 countries showed that average stool weight varied from 72 to 470 g/day and was inversely related to colon cancer risk *(37)*. When results of 13 case–control studies of colorectal cancer rates and dietary practices were pooled, the authors concluded that the results provided substantive evidence that consumption of fiber-rich foods is inversely related to risks of both colon and rectal cancers *(38)*. The latter study estimated that the risk of colorectal cancer in the US population could be reduced by about 31% with an average increase in fiber intake of about 13 g/day from food sources.

Park et al. *(39)* completed a more recent pooled analysis of prospective cohort studies of dietary fiber intake and risk of colorectal cancer. From 13 prospective cohort studies included in the Pooling Project of Prospective Studies of Diet and Cancer, 725,628 subjects were followed for 6–20 years. Dietary fiber intake was inversely associated with risk of colorectal cancer in age-adjusted analyses. However, after accounting for other dietary risk factors, high-dietary fiber intake was not associated with a reduced risk of colorectal cancer.

Results of three intervention studies documented that dietary fiber did not protect against colon cancer *(40–42)*. These studies found no significant effect of high-fiber intakes on recurrence of colorectal adenomas. Possible explanations for these results include short-term fiber interventions and low fiber levels; the recurrence of adenoma may not be an appropriate measure of fiber's effectiveness in preventing colon cancer. In addition the fiber intake by the low-fiber control subjects exceeded that of the American population. Increasing dietary fiber consumption over a 3-year period did not alter the recurrence of adenomas. Despite the inconsistency of results from epidemiological studies, there appears to be sufficient scientific consensus dietary fiber may exert protective effects against colon cancer and that health professionals should be promoting increased consumption of dietary fiber *(43)*.

Recent follow-up analysis of the Polyp Prevention Trial (PPT) also found no effect of a low-fat, high-fiber, high-fruit and vegetable diet on adenoma recurrence 8 years after randomization *(44)*. Because the PPT study was conducted over a 4-year period, one possibility is that the beneficial effects of higher fiber intake could be detectable at later times. Although the experimental group continued to consume more fiber beyond year 4, there was no effect of fiber intervention on later polyp recurrence.

The European Prospective Investigation into Cancer and Nutrition (EPIC) is a prospective cohort study comparing dietary habits of more than a half-million people in 10 countries with colorectal cancer incidence *(45)*. This study found that populations whose total fiber intake averaged 33 g/day had a 25% lower incidence of colorectal cancer than those with average fiber intake of 12 g/day. Also, this study estimated that populations with low average fiber consumption could reduce by 40% colorectal cancer incidence by doubling their fiber intake. Dukas et al. *(46)* reported that in the Nurses' Health Study, women in the highest quintile of dietary fiber intake (median intake 20 g/day) were less likely to experience constipation than women in the lowest quintile (median intake 7 g/day).

Although prospective studies suggest dietary fiber intake may not protect against colorectal cancer, support exists for the protective properties of whole grain intake. Schatzkin et al. *(47)* investigated the relationship between whole grain intake and invasive colorectal cancer in the prospective National Institutes of Health-AARP Diet and Health Study. Total dietary fiber intake was not associated with colorectal cancer risk, whereas whole grain consumption was associated with a modest reduced risk. The association with whole grain intake was stronger for rectal than colon cancer.

The incidence of colorectal cancer is much higher in African Americans compared to native Africans. O'Keefe et al. *(48)* compared a randomly selected sample of African Americans ($n = 17$) to a group of native Africans ($n = 17$). Diet was evaluated by 3-day diet recall. Breath samples were collected and fecal samples were cultured for bacteria. Colonoscopic mucosal biopsies were taken to measure proliferation rates and colonic crypt cell proliferation rates were found higher in African Americans. Differences were also found in bacterial populations, although dietary fiber intakes were the same in both groups.

6.2. Breast Cancer

Limited epidemiological evidence is available concerning the effects of fiber intake and breast cancer risk. Since the fat and fiber contents of diet are generally inversely related, it is difficult to separate the independent effects of these nutrients, and most research has focused on the fat and breast cancer hypothesis. International comparisons show an inverse correlation between breast cancer death rates and consumption of fiber-rich foods *(49)*. An interesting exception to the high-fat diet hypothesis in breast cancer was observed in Finland, where intake of both fat and fiber is high and the breast cancer mortality rate is considerably lower than in the United States and other Western countries where the typical diet is high in fat *(50)*. The large amounts of fiber in the rural Finnish diet may modify the breast cancer risk associated with a high-fat diet. A pooled analysis of 12 case–control studies of dietary factors and risk of breast cancer found that high dietary fiber intake was associated with reduced risk of breast cancer *(51)*. Dietary fiber intake also has been linked to lower risk of benign proliferative epithelial disorders of the breast *(52)*. Not all studies found a relationship between dietary fiber intake and breast cancer incidence, including a US prospective cohort study *(53)*. A pooled analysis of eight prospective cohort studies of breast cancer found that fruit and vegetable consumption during adulthood was not significantly associated with reduced breast cancer risk *(54)*. However, a large case–control study reported protective effects with high intake of cereals and grains, vegetables, and beans *(55)*.

Jain et al. *(56)* found no association among total dietary fiber, fiber fractions, and risk of breast cancer. Still, nutrition differences, including dietary fiber intake, appeared to contribute to the higher rate of breast cancer experienced by younger African American women *(57)*. Additionally, a diet high in vegetables, fruits, and fiber did not reduce additional breast cancer events or mortality during 7.3 years of follow-up in the Women's Health Eating and Living (WHEL) randomized trial *(58)*. This study was conducted among survivors of early stage breast cancer. The intervention group was targeted with a telephone counseling program, cooking classes, and newsletters that promoted daily target intakes (five vegetable servings plus 16 oz of vegetable juice, three fruits, 30 g of fiber, and reduced fat intake). This intervention did not reduce additional breast cancer events or mortality during a 7.3 year follow-up period.

The effects of dietary fiber on breast cancer risk may be confounded by estrogen and progesterone receptor (ER/PR) status. Suzuki et al. *(59)* evaluated the association between dietary fiber and ER/PR-defined breast cancer risk stratified by postmenopausal hormone use, alcohol use, and family history of breast cancer in the population-based Swedish Mammography Screening Cohort, which included 51,823 postmenopausal women. Fiber intake was measured by food frequency questionnaire. These studies correlated significant risk reductions in breast cancer with intake of fruit and cereal fiber.

Overall, results of population studies appear to be mixed, with large US prospective studies finding little relationship between dietary fiber intake and breast cancer. Additionally, fruit and vegetable intake does not appear to be protective against breast cancer *(54)*. But, similar to colon cancer, typical intakes of dietary fiber in the US cohorts may be lower than levels found to be protective in European studies.

6.3. Other Cancers

Similar to colon and breast cancer, it is not clear whether fiber intake is protective against other types of cancer. In general, results of case–control studies are more positive than results with prospective trials. Cereal fiber intakes were found to reduce risk of gastric adenocarcinomas in the EPIC-EURGAST study *(60)*. Bandera et al. *(61)* conducted a meta-analysis of the association between dietary fiber and endometrial cancer. They found support for a protective effect from case–control studies, but no evidence was obtained for the single prospective study that had been conducted. Preliminary findings from the CPID study showed no association between fruit and vegetable consumption and risk of prostate and breast cancer *(62)*. Thus, although case–control studies show protection against cancer with dietary fiber intake, prospective, cohort studies do not demonstrate a preventive effect of fiber against cancer. A possible protective effect may be detectable by indirect methods including obesity protection.

7. OTHER COMPONENTS IN FIBER-CONTAINING FOODS

There is substantial scientific evidence suggesting vegetables, fruits, and whole grains reduce risk of chronic diseases including cancer *(63, 64)*. In epidemiological studies, it is often easier to count servings of whole foods than translate information on food frequency questionnaires to nutrient intakes. Additionally, recent studies suggest that analyses based on whole foods are better correlated with protection against chronic diseases than dietary fiber, antioxidants, or other biologically active components present in foods. Table 2 lists the many phytochemicals that have been shown to have cancer prevention actions. This suggests that the addition of purified dietary fiber to foodstuffs is less likely to be beneficial as opposed to changing American diets to include whole foods high in dietary fiber. The concept of synergy among components in whole foods is an important aspect of any dietary counseling.

Table 2
Phytochemicals, Beyond Fiber, with Cancer Protective Properties

Dietary fiber
Lignans
Isoflavones
Coumarins
Phytates
Dithiothiones
Carotenoids
Tocopherols
Ascorbate
Folate
Isothiocyantes
Indoles
Glucosinolate
Plant sterols
Protease inhibitors
Allium compounds
Flavonoids
Other phenolic compounds

A lot of what is known about the benefits of a higher fiber diet comes from epidemiological studies, and DRI recommendations for dietary fiber intake are based on epidemiological findings. However, discrepancies exist between epidemiological and metabolic studies. Foods in current databases may not be reflective of what was consumed more than a decade ago. This is particularly true for data on dietary fiber in foods that have been gathered largely in the past 15 years. Progress in standardization of methods used to determine total dietary fiber in US foods is necessary to improve fiber databases necessary for epidemiological studies. For example, the proportion of total fiber that is soluble varies by two to threefold across major methods of analysis. Thus, the use of databases to differentiate the effects of soluble vs. insoluble fiber with disease could produce statistically significant relationships, when in fact there are none.

Also, the use of specific fiber sources in metabolic studies may not be representative of normal diets that contain various sources of fiber.

8. CONCLUSIONS

The relationship between cancer and dietary fiber remains complex. Although not all data support the relationship, the difficulty in measuring dietary fiber and the poor databases for dietary fiber content of foods make it a difficult relationship to study. Stronger protective support has been found for whole foods high in dietary fiber, such as cereal fiber, fruits, and whole grains. Dietary fiber may be just part of the protective puzzle with other components including antioxidants, phenolic compounds, and associated substances also providing protection against colorectal cancer.

Other cancer sites are equally elusive as to their connection with dietary fiber intake. Since fiber intake is linked to lower body mass index, it will be protective against breast and prostate cancer. Also, breast cancer may be prevented by high fiber intakes, especially if the fibers consumed are high in phytoestrogens that alter sex hormone metabolism.

Despite many years of research and nutrition education, dietary fiber intakes are not increasing. We must continue to promote consumption of foods high in complex carbohydrates, including resistant starch, oligosaccharides, and dietary fiber. As many consumers depend on processed foods as the mainstay of their diets, efforts should be made to increase the fiber content of popular foods to assist consumers in obtaining recommended levels of unavailable carbohydrate. Differences in fiber composition must be considered since recent studies find that cereal fiber is most protective, while vegetable and fruit fiber are often not protective against cancer. But since dietary fiber intakes are so low, the ability to detect relationships between dietary fiber intake and cancer is limited.

REFERENCES

1. McCance, R.A., and Widdowson, E.M. (1955) Old thought and new work on breads white and brown. *Lancet* **2**, 205–10.
2. Burkitt, D.P. (1971) Epidemiology of cancer of the colon and rectum. *Cancer* **28**, 3–13.
3. Institute of Medicine of the National Academies. (2002) Dietary Reference Intakes: Energy, Carbohydrates, Fiber, Fat, Fatty Acids, Cholesterol, Protein and Amino Acids. Washington, DC: The National Academies Press.
4. Marlett, J.A., and Cheung, T.-F. (1997) Database and quick methods of assessing typical dietary fiber intakes using data for 228 commonly consumed foods. *J Am Diet Assoc* **97**, 1139–48.
5. Nutrient Concent of the US Food Supply, 2005 and Interactive Food Supply. USDA Center for Nutrition Policy and Promotion.
6. National Academy Press. (2001) Dietary Reference Intakes Proposed Definition of Dietary Fiber. Washington DC: National Academy Press, 1–64.
7. Asp, N.-G. (1994) Nutritional classification and analysis of food carbohydrates. *Am J Clin Nutr* **59**(Suppl 3), 679S–681S.
8. Marlett, J.A., and Longacre, M.J. (1996) Comparisons of in vitro and in vivo measures of resistant starch in selected grain products. *Cereal Chem* **73**, 63–68.
9. Murphy, M.M., Douglass, J.S., and Birkett, A. (2008) Resistant starch intakes in the United States. *J Am Diet Assoc* **108**, 67–78.

10. Fearton, E.F., and Jones, P.A. (1992) Progressing toward a molecular description of colorectal cancer development. *FASEB J* **6**, 2783–90.

11. Doll, R., and Peto, R. (1981) The causes of cancer: Quantitative estimates of avoidable risks of cancer in the United States today. *J Natl Cancer Inst* **66**, 1191–308.

12. Hill, M.J. (1998) Cereals, dietary fibre, and cancer. *Nutr Res* **18**, 653–59.

13. Topping, D.L., and Clifton, P.M. (2001) Short-chain fatty acids and human colonic function: Roles of resistant starch and nonstarch polysaccharides. *Physiol Rev* **81**, 1031–64.

14. Cummings, J.H., and Macfarlane, G.T. (1997) Colonic microflora: Nutrition and health. *Nutrition* **13**, 476–78.

15. Valazquez, O.C., Lederer, H.M., and Rombeau, J.L. (1996) Butyrate and the colonocyte – Implications for neoplasia. *Dig Dis Sci* **14**, 727–39.

16. Hague, A., Singh, B., and Paraskeva, C. (1997) Butyrate acts as a survival factor for colonic epithelial cells: Further fuel for the in vivo versus in vitro debate. *Gastroenterology* **112**, 1036–40.

17. Thornton, J.R. (1981) High colonic pH promotes colorectal cancer. *Lancet* **1**, 1083–87.

18. Hamer, H.M., Jonkers, D., Vanema, K., Vanhoutvin, S., Troost, F.J., and Brummer, R.J. (2008) Review article: The role of butyrate on colonic function. *Aliment Pharmacol Ther* **27**, 104–19.

19. Bordonaro, M., Lazarova, D.L., and Sartorelli, A.C. (2008) Butyrate and Wnt signaling: A possible solution to the puzzle of dietary fiber and colon cancer risk? *Cell Cycle* **7**, 1178–83.

20. Reddy, B., Engle, A., Katsifis, S., Simi, B., Bartram, H.P., Perrino, P., and Mahan, C. (1989) Biochemical epidemiology of colon cancer: Effect of types of dietary fiber on fecal mutagens, acid and neutral sterols in healthy subjects. *Cancer Res* **49**, 4629–35.

21. Jenab, M., and Thompson, L.U. (1998) The influence of phytic acid in wheat bran on early biomarkers of colon carcinogenesis. *Carcinogenesis* **19**, 1087–92.

22. Lu, F.J., Chu, L.H., and Gau, R.J. (1998) Free radical-scavenging properties of lignin. *Nutr Cancer* **30**, 31–38.

23. Haack, V.S., Chesters, J.G., Vollendorf, N.W., Story, J.A., and Marlett, J.A. (1998) Increasing amounts of dietary fiber provided by foods normalizes physiologic response of the large bowel without altering calcium balance or fecal steroid excretion. *Am J Clin Nutr* **68**, 615–22.

24. Cummings, J.H. (1993) The effect of dietary fiber on fecal weight and composition. In: Spiller G.A., ed. CRC Handbook of Dietary Fiber in Human Nutrition. 2nd ed., Boca Raton, FL: CRC Press, 263–349.

25. Spiller, G.A. (1993) Suggestions for a basis on which to determine a desirable intake of dietary fibre. In: G.A. Spillered. CRC Handbook of Dietary Fiber in Human Nutrition. Boca Raton, FL: CRC Press, 351–54.

26. Kurasawa, S., Haack, V.S., and Marlett, J.A. (2000) Plant residue and bacteria as bases for increased stool weight accompanying consumption of higher dietary fiber diets. *J Am Coll Nutr* **19**, 426–33.

27. Slavin, J.L., Nelson, N.L., McNamara, E.A., and Cashmere, K. (1985) Bowel function of healthy men consuming liquid diets with and without dietary fiber. *J Parenter Enteral Nutr* **9**, 317–21.

28. Oettle, G.J. (1991) Effect of moderate exercise on bowel habit. *Gut* **32**, 941–44.

29. Bingham, S.A., and Cummings, J.H. (1989) Effect of exercise and physical fitness on large intestinal function. *Gastroenterology* **97**, 1389–99.

30. Lampe, J.W., Fredstrom, S.B., Slavin, J.L., and Potter, J.D. (1993) Sex differences in colonic function: A randomized trial. *Gut* **34**, 531–36.

31. Tucker, D.M., Sandstead, H.H., Logan, G.M., Klevay, L.M., Mahalko, J., Johnson, L.K., Inman, L., and Inglett, G.E. (1981) Dietary fiber and personality factors as determinants of stool output. *Gastroenterology* **81**, 879–83.

32. Gibson, G.R., Macfarlane, G.T., and Cummings, J.H. (1993) Sulphate reducing bacteria ahnd hydrogen metabolism in the human intestine. *Gut* **34**, 437–39.

33. Christl, S.U., Gibson, G.R., and Cummings, J.H. (1992) Role of dietary sulphate in the regulation of methanogenesis in the human large intestine. *Gut* **33**, 1234–38.

34. Pitcher, M.C.L., Beatty, E.R., and Cummings, J.H. (2000) The contribution of sulphate reducing bacteria and 5-aminosalicylic acid to faecal sulphide in patients with ulcerative colitis. *Gut* **46**, 64–72.

35. Xie, J., and Itzkowitz, S.H. (2008) Cancer in inflammatory bowel disease. *World J Gastroenterol* **14**, 378–89.

36. Huycke, M., and Gaskins, H.R. (2004) Commensal bacteria, redox stress and colorectal cancer: Mechanisms and models. *Exp Biol Med* **299**, 586–97.

37. Cummings, J.H., Bingham, S.A., Heaton, K.W., and Eastwood, M.A. (1992) Fecal weight, colon cancer risk and dietary intake of nonstarch polysaccharides (dietary fiber). *Gastroenterology* **103**, 1783–89.

38. Howe, G.R., Benito, E., Castelleto, R., Cornee, J., Esteve, J., Gallagher, R.P., Iscovich, J.M., Deng-ao, J., Kaaks, R., and Kune, G.A. (1992) Dietary intake of fiber and decreased risk of cancers of the colon and rectum: Evidence from the combined analysis of 13 case-control studies. *J Natl Cancer Inst* **84**, 1887–96.

39. Park, Y., Hunter, D.J., Spiegelman, D., Bergkvist, L., Berrino, F., van den Brandt, P.A., Buring, J.E., Colditz, G.A., Freudenheim, J.L., Fuchs, C.S., Biovannucci, E., Goldbohm, R.A., Braham, S., Harnack, L., Hartman, A.M., Jacobs, D.R., Kato, I., Krogh, V., Leitzmann, M.F., McCullough, M.L., Miller, A.B., Pietinen, P., Rohan, T.E., Schatzkin, A., Willett, W.C., Wolk, A., Zeleniuch-Jacquotte, A., Zhang, S.M., and Smith-Warner, S.A. (2005) Dietary fiber intake and risk of colorectal cancer: A pooled analysis of prospective cohort studies. *J Am Med Assoc* **294**, 2849–57.

40. Schatzkin, A., Lanza, E., Corle, D., Lance, P., Iber, F., Cann, B., Shike, M., Weissfeld, J., Burt, R., Cooper, M.R., Kikendall, J.W., Cahill, J., and The Polyp Prevention Trial Study Group (2000) Lack of effect of a low-fat, high-fiber diet on the recurrence of colorectal adenomas. *New Eng J Med* **342**, 1149–55.

41. Alberts, D.S., Marinez, M.E., Kor, D.L., Guillen-Rodriguez, J.M., Marshall, J.R., Van Leeuwen, J.B., Reid, M.E., Ritenbaugh, C., Vargas, P.A., Bhattacharyya, A.B., Earnest, D.L., Sampliner, R.E., and The Phoenix Colon Cancer Prevention Physicians' Network (2000) Lack of effect of a high-fiber cereal supplement on the recurrence of colorectal adenomas. *New Eng J Med* **324**, 1156–62.

42. Bonithon-Kopp, C., Kronborg, O., Giacosa, A., Rath, U., Faivre, J., and For the European Cancer Prevention Organization Study Group (2000) Calcium and fibre supplementation in prevention of colorectal adenoma recurrence: A randomized intervention trial. *Lancet* **356**, 1300–06.

43. Kim, Y.I. (2000) AGA technical review: Impact of dietary fiber on colon cancer occurrence. *Gastroenterology* **118**, 1235–57.

44. Lanza, E., Yu, B., Murphy, G., Albert, P.S., Caan, B., Marshall, J.R., Lance, P., Paskett, E.D., Weissfeld, J., Slattery, M., Burt, R., Iber, F., Shike, M., Kikendall, J.W., Brewer, B.K., and Schatzkin, A. (2007) Polyp Prevention Trial Study Group. The polyp prevention trial continued follow-up study: No effect of a low-fat, high-fiber, high-fruit, and -vegetable diet on adenoma recurrence eight years after randomization. *Cancer Epidemiol Biomarkers Prev* **16**, 1745–52.

45. Bingham, S.A., Day, N.E., Luben, R., Ferrari, P., Slimani, N., Norat, T., Clavel-Chapelon, F., Kesse, E., Nieters, A., Boeing, H., Tjonneland, A., Overvad, K., Martinez, C., Dorronsoro, M., Gonzalez, C.A., Key, T.J., Trichopoulou, A., Naska, A., Vineis, P., Tumino, R., Krogh, V., Bueno-de-Masquita, H., Peeters, P.H.M., Berglund, G., Hallmans, G., Lund, E., Skele, G., Kaaks, R., and Riboll, E. (2003) Dietary fibre in food and protection against colorectal cancer in the European Prospective Investigation into Cancer and Nutrition (EPIC): An observational study. *Lancet* **361**, 1496–501.

46. Dukas, L., Willett, W.C., and Giovannucci, E.L. (2003) Association between physical activity, fiber intake, and other lifestyle variables and constipation in a study of women. *Am J Gastroenterol* **98**, 1790–96.

47. Schatzkin, A., Houw, T., Park, Y., Subar, A.F., Kipnis, V., Hollenbeck, A., Leitzmann, M.F., and Thompson, F.E. (2007) Dietary fiber and whole-grain consumption in relation to colorectal cancer in the NIH-AARP Diet and Health Study. *Am J Clin Nutr* **85**, 1353–60.

48. O'Keefe, S.J., Chung, D., Mahmoud, N., Sepulveda, A.R., Manafe, M., Arch, J., Adada, H., and van der Merwe, T. (2007) Why do African Americans get more colon cancer than Native Africans? *J Nutr* **137**, 175S–182S.

49. Prentice, R.L. (2000) Future possibilities in the prevention of breast cancer: Fat and fiber and breast cancer research. *Breast Cancer Res* **2**, 268–76.

50. Adlercreutz, H. (1998) Evolution, nutrition, intestinal microflora, and prevention of cancer. A hypothesis. *Proc Soc Exp Biol Med* **217**, 241–46.

51. Howe, G.R., Hirohata, T., Hislop, T.G., Iscovich, J.M., Katsouyanni, K., Lubin, F., Marubini, E., Modan, B., and Rohan, T. (1990) Dietary factors and risk of breast cancer: Combined analysis of 12 case-control studies. *J Natl Cancer Inst* **82**, 561–69.

52. Baghurst, P.A., and Rohan, T.E. (1995) Dietary fiber and risk of benign proliferative epithelial disorders of the breast. *Int J Cancer* **63**, 481–85.

53. Willett, W.C., Hunter, D.J., Stampfer, M.J., Coldiz, G., Manson, J.E., Spiegelman, D., Rosner, B., Hennekens, C.H., and Speizer, F.E. (1992) Dietary fat and fiber in relation to risk of breast cancer. An 8-year follow-up. *J Am Med Assoc* **268**, 2037–44.

54. Smith-Warner, S.A., Spiegelman, D., Yaun, S.S., Adami, H.O., Beeson, W.L., van den Brandt, P.A., Folson, A.R., Fraser, G.E., Freudenseim, J.L., Goldbohm, R.A., Graham, S., Miller, A.B., Potter, J.D., Rohan, T.E., Speizer, F.E., Toniolo, P., Willett, W.C., Wolk, A., Zeleniuch-Jacquotte, A., and Hunter, D.J. (2001) Intake of fruits and vegetables and risk of breast cancer: A pooled analysis of cohort studies. *J Am Med Assoc* **285**, 769–76.

55. Potischman, N., Swanson, C.A., Coates, R.J., Gammon, M.D., Brogan, D.R., Curtin, J., and Brinton, L.A. (1999) Intake of food groups and associated micronutrients in relation to risk of early-stage breast cancer. *Int J Cancer* **82**, 315–21.

56. Jain, T.P., Miller, A.B., Howe, G.R., and Rohan, T.E. (2002) No association among total dietary fiber, fiber fractions, and risk of breast cancer. *Cancer Epidemiol Biomarkers Prev* **11**, 507–508.

57. Forshee, R.A., Storey, M.L., and Ritenbaugh, C. (2003) Breast cancer risk and lifestyle differences among premenopausal and postmenopausal African-American women and white women. *Cancer* **97**(1 Suppl), 280–88.

58. Pierce, J.P., Natarajan, L., Caan, B.J., Parker, B.A., Greenberg, E.R., Flatt, S.W., Rock, C.L., Kealey, S., Al-Delaimy, W.K., Bardwell, W.A., Carlson, R.W., Emond, J.A., Faefber, S., Gould, E.B., Hajek, R.A., Hollenback, K., Jones, L.A., Karanja, N., Madlensky, L., Marshall, J., Newman, V.A., Ritenbaugh, C., Thomson, C.A., Wasserman, L., and Stefanick, M.L. (2007) Influence of a diet very high in vegetables, fruit, and fiber and low in fat on prognosis following treatment for breast cancer. The Women's Healthy Eating and Living (WHEL) Randomized Trial. *J Am Med Assoc* **298**, 289–98.

59. Suzuki, R., Rylander-Rudqvist, T., Ye, W., Saji, S., Adlercreutz, H., and Wolk, A. (2008) Dietary fiber intake and risk of postmenopausal breast cancer defined by estrogen and progesterone receptor status – a prospective cohort study among Swedish women. *Int J Cancer* **122**, 403–12.

60. Mendez, M.A., Pera, G., Agudo, A., Bueno-de-Mesquita, H., Palli, D., Boeing, H., Carneiro, F., Berrino, F., Sacerdote, C., Tumino, R., Panico, S., Berglund, G., Manjer, J., Johansson, I., Stenling, R., Martinez, C., Dorronsoro, M., Barricarte, A., Tormo, M.J., Quiros, J.R., Allen, N., Key, T.J., Bingham, S., Linseisen, J., Kaaks, R., Overvad, K., Jensen, J., Olsen, A., Tjonneland, A., Peeters, P.H.M., Numans, M.E., Ocke, M.C., Clavel-Chapelon, F., Boutron-Ruault, M., Trichopoulou, A., Lund, E., Slimani, N., Jenab, M., Perrair, P., Riboli, E., and Gonzalez, C.A. (2007) Cereal fiber intake may reduce risk of gastric adenocarcinomas: The EPIC-EURGAST Study. *Int J Cancer* **121**, 1618–23.

61. Bandera, E.B., Kushi, L.H., Moore, D.F., Gifkins, D.M., and McCullough, M.L. (2007) Association between dietary fiber and endometrial cancer: A dose-response meta-analysis. *Am J Clin Nutr* **86**, 1730–37.

62. Gonzales, C.A. (2006) The European Prospective Investigation into Cancer and Nutrition (EPIC). *Public Health Nutr* **9**(1A), 124–26.

63. Potter, J.D. (2000) Your mother was right: Eat your vegetables. *Asia Pac J Clin Nutr* **9**(Suppl S), S10–S12.

64. Slavin, J.L. (2004) Whole grains and human health. *Nutr Res Rev* **17**, 99–110.

9 Gut Microbiota, Probiotics, Prebiotics and Colorectal Cancer

Gemma E. Walton and Glenn R. Gibson

Key Points

1. Both probiotics and prebiotics are dietary ingredients that modulate the gut microbiota composition and activity. Probiotics are live microbial feed additions, whereas prebiotics are selectively metabolized by beneficial flora components.

2. One of the most common forms of cancer is colorectal. Because the human gut, particularly the colon, harbours an extremely profuse and metabolically active microbiota, there is interest in how the microbial fermentation affects colorectal cancer risk.

3. An important environmental factor that can play a large role in cancers of digestive tract is diet. The principal hypothesis is that fat and meat increase risk and cereals, fruit and vegetables (dietary fibre) decrease risk of cancer. With the current interest in the use of both probiotics and prebiotics to modulate this microbiota, it is feasible that such dietary intervention tools may find use in reducing risk.

4. Probiotics such as bifidobacteria and lactobacilli have many positive effects on the human digestive tract, including the inhibition of pathogens and having anti-cancer activities. However, enterococci, a Gram-positive cocci, and *Enterococcus faecalis* may have negative effects including the production of hydrogen peroxide and triggering inflammatory bowel disease.

5. *Clostridium butyricum*, a species belonging to the core *Clostridium* 1 cluster, has been found to produce butyrate-generating SCFA in the colon. When supplementation of *C. butyricum* and high-amylase maize starch were fed to rats, it was noted that the colonic pH was lower and became a more favourable condition against cancer.

6. Butyrate, a gut microbial metabolite, has been known to be associated with reduced risk colorectal cancer onset. Colonocytes metabolize butyrate through β-oxidation, enabling it to aid in cell maturation, differentiation and apoptosis. Butyrate is purported as an anti-tumoural agent. It has been shown to induce apoptosis of colon cancer cell lines and inhibit growth in vitro.

Key Words: Colorectal cancer; gut microbiota; lactic acid bacteria; microbial fermentation

1. INTRODUCTION

Cancer is essentially a disease resulting from the uncontrolled proliferation of cells at a particular site. The cells divide rapidly but are unable to undergo differentiation

From: *Nutrition and Health: Bioactive Compounds and Cancer*
Edited by: J.A. Milner, D.F. Romagnolo, DOI 10.1007/978-1-60761-627-6_9,
© Springer Science+Business Media, LLC 2010

and this leads towards the development of tumours. Normal cellular activity is lost and cancer cells invade surrounding tissues. They may also have the ability to spread from site to site where new tumours can develop through the process of metastasis.

One of the commonest forms of cancer is colorectal. Because the human gut, particularly the colon, harbours an extremely profuse and metabolically active microbiota, there is interest in how the microbial fermentation affects colorectal cancer risk. There are incidences where this can be both positive and negative. Epidemiological studies that suggest geographical variation in cancer incidence in various countries, communities and migrant groups, together with results from studies of social factors, have led to the observation that a large proportion of human cancers may have an environmental component *(1)*. An important environmental factor that can play a large role in cancers of digestive tract is diet. The principal hypothesis is that fat and meat increase risk and cereals, fruit and vegetables (dietary fibre) decrease risk of cancer. With the current interest in the use of both probiotics and prebiotics to modulate this microbiota, it is feasible that such dietary intervention tools may find use in reducing risk.

2. RATIONALE FOR AN INVOLVEMENT OF THE GUT MICROBIOTA IN COLORECTAL CANCER

There are population variances, with ethnic and racial differences, for the incidences of digestive cancers. Such differences could be considered to be the result of genetic variation. Nevertheless, migrant studies have largely implicated environmental factors. A study from Australia compared the cancer incidence of natives to that of migrants and found that individuals originally from low CRC risk countries, such as Yugoslavia and Poland, developed an increased risk of colorectal cancer *(2)*. A similar study in North America monitored cancer patients and controls of American origin, Chinese origin and native Chinese. The risk of colorectal cancer development increased proportionally to the duration of habitation within the USA. This was observed to correlate with altered diet, increased saturated fats and reduced exercise *(3, 4)*.

Epidemiological studies have also demonstrated that increased intakes of dietary fibre, fruit and vegetables are associated with a reduced risk of colorectal cancer *(5)*. Other factors such as consumption of supplements and lifestyle may influence outcome *(6, 7)*. The European prospective investigation into cancer and nutrition (EPIC) study has assessed the dietary intakes of over half a million individuals from 10 different European countries. These intakes have been observed alongside cancer status and a follow-up assessment over an average of almost 5 years. This work has led to a wealth of information regarding diet and colorectal cancer risk factors. The EPIC study provides a wide-scale study of people from different countries and has demonstrated an inverse correlation between dietary fibre intake and colorectal cancer risk *(8)*. Methods for protection by dietary fibre may include increased faecal bulking, dilution of colonic contents and reduced intestinal transit time *(9)*. An additional issue for protection could be increased carbohydrate availability and its fermentation in the colon. On the contrary, diets high in meat protein, particularly red and processed meats, have been associated with increased risk of colorectal cancer development *(10)*.

Diet impacts strongly with the colonic microflora and can mediate both changes in bacterial populations and their metabolic activities *(11)*. The ability of the microflora to alter the effects of carcinogens within the colon was observed by Reddy et al. *(12)*, whereby germ-free rats and conventional rats were exposed to carcinogens. Germ-free rats developed less dimethylhydrazine (DMH)-induced colonic tumours than conventional rats.

The ingestion of foods and excretion of bile can be converted by microbial metabolic pathways in the colon, leading to the production of carcinogenic and genotoxic compounds. Nevertheless, not all microorganisms are involved with such negative effects. Dietary intake can alter bacteria within the colon and their fermentation patterns. The metabolic activities of some bacteria can also lead to the production of various short-chain fatty acids (SCFAs) and anti-cancer compounds.

3. THE HUMAN GUT MICROBIOTA

Bacterial inhabitants of the colon have been estimated to comprise up to 1,000 different bacterial species *(13–15)*, belonging to at least 50 different genera *(16)*. The resident microflora of the colon makes this organ the most metabolically active in the human body *(17)*. Undoubtedly, this will have both negative and positive implications for chronic disorders like colorectal cancer. The colonic microbial ecosystem is able to exert many systemic effects in the human body through promotion and/or prevention of health and disease states.

At the birth of the probiotic concept, Metchnikoff *(18)* reported how putrefaction could be reduced through consumption of fermented milk products and proposed that such benefits resulted from antagonistic effects exerted by bacteria present in the yoghurt. He hypothesized that the colonic flora was, in the main, harmful to the host and responsible for much putrefaction. However, beneficial bacteria from the fermented milks were thought to repress more negative components. Today, it is widely understood that the colonic bacteria exert many effects on the human body, good and bad, hence there is a need to maintain an optimal community structure. The normal colonic microbiota provides a level of resistance via competition with potentially pathogenic organisms.

The genera bifidobacteria and lactobacilli are generally regarded as being helpful to host health. Their effects are exerted in many ways including inhibition of pathogens *(19)*, reduced cholesterol levels *(20)*, fortified immune response *(21)* and production of vitamins *(22)*. Through the fermentation of carbohydrates, bifidobacteria produce SCFAs, lowering the colonic pH and making the colonic environment less favourable to pathogens *(23)*. For example, *Bifidobacterium breve* isolated from healthy humans can inhibit harmful enzymes and ammonia production *(24)*. Different species of *Lactobacillus* have been involved in promoting a beneficial environment. These two genera have also been attributed to have anti-cancer activities possibly by binding to harmful amines within the colon, and thus preventing absorption *(25)*.

Enterococci are Gram-positive, facultative anaerobic cocci. Some species can produce hydrogen peroxide and superoxide, which are damaging to colonic epithelial cell DNA. Increased levels of genotoxicity have been observed in the faeces of rats with heightened levels of *E. faecalis (26)*. *Enterococcus faecalis* has also been associated with the triggering of inflammatory bowel disease, dysplasia and carcinoma in genetically susceptible mouse models *(27)*. Conversely, a non-pathogenic strain *E. faecalis* SF68 has been used as a probiotic for its ability to produce lactic acid in the colon and protect against diarrhoea *(28)*.

Bacteroides are Gram-negative, obligatory anaerobic rods. *Bacteroides fragilis* and *Bacteroides vulgatus* have been identified as the most common species in faecal samples of healthy individuals *(29)*. *Bacteroides fragilis* is associated with diarrhoeal disease due to toxin production *(30)*.

Clostridium spp. are Gram-positive, spore-forming, obligatory anaerobic rods. These microorganisms are often proteolytic. *Clostridium difficile* and *Clostridium perfringens* are known for producing a variety of harmful enzymes and toxins, thus making them potentially pathogenic *(31)*. Within the colon, *C. perfringens* participates in various putrefactive processes and has been implicated as a causative agent of gastroenteritis *(32)*. *Clostridium butyricum* is a species belonging to the core *Clostridium* 1 cluster. *Clostridium butyricum* produces butyrate-generating amounts of SCFA in the colon. Spores of *C. butyricum* were fed to rats and in combination with high-amylose maize starch. In rats receiving supplementation with high-amylase maize starch plus spores of *C. butyricum*, the colonic pH was lower than with high-amylase maize starch alone. Numbers of aberrant crypt foci (ACF), after injection with azoxymethane (AOM), were lower in this group as was β-glucuronidase activity. Butyrate production was also higher in the colons of rats receiving spores *(33)*. Hence, favourable colonic conditions against cancers were seen in rats receiving synbiotic treatment of *C. butyricum* and high-amylase maize starch. Although the genus *Clostridium* is normally considered as non-beneficial, the group consists of a range of species, some of which may even have a positive impact on the host.

There is a link between the colonic microflora and the health status. The gut microflora can thus be considered relevant to improved host health. Within the colon, a range of effects are exerted by the resident microbiota, some of which are considered beneficial, some benign and some harmful to the host. This has relevance for colorectal cancer but obviously there are several other determinants that may affect the outcome.

4. IN VITRO, ANIMAL AND HUMAN STUDIES: PREVENTION AND ONSET ASPECTS OF THE GUT MICROBIOTA IN COLORECTAL CANCER

Saccharolytic metabolism is the digestion of carbohydrates by bacteria for energy and a source of carbon. It is a major metabolic process for colonic bacteria. The end products of saccharolytic metabolism can be considered either benign or positive *(34)*, these are organic acids, principally acetate, propionate and butyrate. They are involved in supporting the growth of colonic epithelial cells and reducing absorption of toxic products. When carbohydrates are in short supply in the colon, the bacteria utilize energy from other compounds including proteins (see later).

Butyrate has received attention as a gut microbial metabolite associated with reduced risk colorectal cancer onset *(35–37)*. Colonocytes metabolize butyrate through β-oxidation, enabling it to aid in cell maturation, differentiation and apoptosis *(38)*. Butyrate is purported as an anti-tumoural agent. It has been shown to induce apoptosis of colon cancer cell lines and inhibit growth in vitro.

Perrin et al. *(39)* conducted experiments whereby rats were assigned to control diets or with added resistant starch or prebiotic fructooligosaccharides for 44 days. The rats were then injected with AOM and killed. Rats in the control diet had a larger number of ACF and reduced levels of butyrate in their colons. The authors stated that at least 2 weeks were needed for adaptation to the test diet.

Emenaker et al. *(40)* obtained freshly isolated primary invasive colonocytes from surgical specimens, which were treated with the SCFA acetate, propionate, or butyrate. All three SCFA significantly reduced cellular invasion, but butyrate was the most potent inhibitor. The SCFA exerted their effects by upregulating tumour inhibitor protein and tumour suppressor genes, whilst downregulating mutant p53 activity. Mutant p53 cells suppress apoptosis and hence can be involved in the process of uncontrolled proliferation *(41)*. Beyer-Selmeyer et al. *(42)* showed that fermentation of faecal bacteria with different dietary substrates yielded products with enhanced inhibitory effects on colon cancer cell lines. Again, butyrate exerted the most potent inhibitory effects on cell growth.

Avivi-Green et al. *(43)* studied the molecular events of butyrate-induced apoptosis in different cell lines including CaCo-2 cells (from a colonic carcinoma cell line) and RSB, a cell line obtained from a colonic tumour of an ulcerative colitis patient. Caspase-1 was cleaved in CaCo-2 cells, whereas in RSB cells butyrate dose-dependently induced caspase-3 cleavage. These results led to the conclusion that butyrate-induced apoptosis is activated via different pathways depending on the cell line and type of colon cancer. Kobayashi et al. *(44)* showed that sodium butyrate inhibited cell growth and stimulated the cell cycle control factor p21(waf1/cip1) independent of p53.

Butyrate is also thought to exert its actions by inhibiting histone deacetylase (HDAC), hence favouring histone acetylation. This histone modification allows DNA to become less tightly wound, thus enabling transcription factors to interact with target binding regions and stimulate transcription of genes coding for cell cycle checkpoints *(45)*. Thus, it appears that butyrate may exert its protective actions through regulation of genes involved in cell cycle control and through enzymatic inhibition of HDAC. Hence, these mechanisms may favour apoptosis in cells that are undergoing uncontrolled proliferation

Predominantly, colon cancer manifests itself in the distal regions of the bowel *(46)*. It is in these regions that dietary carbohydrate is less available and proteins become more important as fermentable energy sources. Bacteria ferment proteins and generate a number of by-products including ammonia, amines, phenols, and indoles, which are potentially toxic *(47)*. Ammonia, for example, has several cytopathic effects on colonic cells *(48)*. In particular, it stimulates cellular turnover and cell division, conditions that increase the vulnerability to DNA damage *(49)*.

Certain *Bacteroides* and *Clostridium* species can carry out proteolytic fermentation. Metabolic activities of bacteria are affected by diet; hence high-protein diets will lead to sustained proteolytic fermentation in the colon. Conversely, persistence of carbohydrates in the colon would reduce protein catabolism and favour saccharolytic fermentation.

5. INTERVENTION STUDIES: PROBIOTICS AND PREBIOTICS

Probiotics are live microbial feed supplements used to alter the colonic microflora and improve the microbial balance *(50)*. The bacteria used as probiotics are non-pathogenic and non-toxic to the host and must be able to adapt to the colonic environment. The most successful example of probiotics are the acid-tolerant strains of *Lactobacillus* and *Bifidobacterium,* which are found in a wide range of functional foods and dietary supplements including fermented milk drinks and dried powders *(51)*. Desired characteristics of a good probiotic are as follows: exerts a beneficial effect on the consumer non-pathogenic and non-toxic, contains a large number of viable cells, has the capacity to survive and metabolize in the gut, retain viability during storage and use and lastly, if incorporated into a food, has good sensory qualities *(52–55)*.

The word probiotic is translated from the Greek meaning "for life". An early definition was given by Parker *(56)*: "Organisms and substances which contribute to intestinal microbial balance". However, this definition was subsequently refined by Fuller *(19)* as follows: "A live microbial feed supplement which beneficially affects the host animal by improving its intestinal microbial balance." This definition removed the reference to particles and a probiotic would, therefore, incorporate into the diet living microorganisms beneficial for gut health. A further definition of probiotics was given as "a live microbial feed supplement that is beneficial to health" *(57)*. A WHO/FAO working party defined probiotics as "live microorganisms that, when administered in adequate amounts, confer a health benefit on the host" *(58, 59)*.

An alternative approach for microflora management is the use of dietary prebiotics, which are directed (at present) towards genus level changes in the gut microbiota composition. Here, the selective growth of indigenous gut bacteria is required. Prebiotics are "non-digestible food ingredients that beneficially affect the host by selectively stimulating the growth and/or activity of one or a limited number of bacteria already resident in the colon" *(60)*. Thus, the prebiotic approach advocates administration of non-viable entities and requires that many health promoting microorganisms, such as bifidobacteria and lactobacilli, are already present in the human colon. This definition was updated in 2004 and prebiotics are now defined as "selectively fermented ingredients that allow specific changes, both in the composition and/or activity in the gastrointestinal microflora, that confer benefits upon host well-being and health" *(61)*. The latter definition does not consider only the microflora changes of the human colonic ecosystem, but extends the definition to other areas of the gastrointestinal tract that may benefit from selective targeting of specific microorganisms. As mentioned earlier, the target genera have been lactobacilli and bifidobacteria. However, prebiotic success has predominantly been with the bifidobacteria because of their preference for oligosaccharides and their prevalence in the human colon compared to lactobacilli. Criteria required for a prebiotic effect are *(61)* resistance to gastric acidity, hydrolysis by mammalian enzymes and gastrointestinal absorption; fermentation by intestinal microflora; and selective stimulation of growth and/or activity of intestinal bacteria associated with health and well-being.

Any dietary material that enters the large intestine is a candidate prebiotic. This includes carbohydrates such as resistant starch and dietary fibre as well as proteins and lipids. However, current prebiotics are generally non-digestible oligosaccharides, many of which seem to confer the desired degree of selective fermentation. Oligosaccharides are sugars consisting of ~2–20 saccharide units, i.e. they are short-chain polysaccharides. Best success has been seen with fructooligosaccharides (e.g. inulin), galacto-oligosaccharides and lactulose *(61)*.

Synbiotics are a mixture of prebiotics and probiotics *(60)* used to enhance probiotic growth and survival of the colonic microflora. The colonic microbiota can be influenced through the diet and potentially modified through the consumption of prebiotics, probiotics or synbiotics. These dietary interventions may prove effective against colorectal cancer. Studies whereby the use of probiotics, prebiotics and synbiotics have been used to test anti-cancer activities are relevant (Table 1). Many of these experiments are based upon the AOM rat model for colorectal cancer *(62)*.

The prebiotic inulin was more effective as anti-cancer agent than oligofructose. This effect of inulin was attributed to a greater degree of polymerization, which allows for slower fermentation rate in a more distal part of the colon *(12, 63, 64)*.

To investigate the metabolism of inulin and galacto-oligosaccharides (GOS) with respect to bacterial growth, bifidobacterial stimulatory properties and anti-mutagenicity potential, McBain and Macfarlane *(65)* conducted a three-stage in vitro continuous culture of faecal microflora. Reductions in β-glucosidase and β-glucuronidase were observed in the presence of inulin, whereas GOS strongly suppressed these enzymes. In a separate study, the comet assay, was used to determine how heterocyclic amines affected faecal genotoxicity. It was observed that microflora had a strong impact on the genotoxic effects of IQ. Specifically, IQ had a genotoxic effect in liver and colon with germ-free rats showing less DNA damage compared to conventional rats *(66)*. Further work has shown that when *Lactobacillus bulgaricus* was administered, there was inhibition of DNA damage *(67)* documenting that intestinal microflora plays a crucial role in the genotoxicity of the cooked food mutagen 2-amino-3-methylimidazo [4,5-f]quinoline (IQ). Humblot et al. *(68)* showed that inulin could also be used to suppress DNA damage through reducing concentration of the enzyme β-glucuronidase. These studies indicated that bacteria may modulate the health risks caused by dietary carcinogens.

Studies have shown that incorporation of lactic acid bacteria into a diet is associated with reduced concentrations of harmful enzymes. In a human study *(69)*, healthy volunteers received probiotic *Lactobacillus acidophilus* daily. After 10 days of supplementation, there was a significant decline in the enzyme activities of β-glucuronidase, azoreductase and nitroreductase. Therefore, modulation of colonic bacteria can potentially reduce xenobiotic enzymes and proteolytic fermentation. This reduces the exposure of colonocytes to providing protection against development of colorectal cancer. Further benefits may also be achieved by increasing the production of SCFAs, particularly butyrate.

6. FUTURE RESEARCH DIRECTIONS

6.1. Improved Microbiota Characterization

Vargo et al. *(70)* used anaerobic culture techniques to compare the colonic microflora of healthy individuals with that of colorectal cancer patients. Results of these studies showed that in the colon cancer group, there was a larger number of aerobes in the

Table 1

Studies on Rats Establishing Potential for Dietary Factors and Pre, Pro and Synbiotics to Modulate Colorectal Cancer Risk Assessed Through ACF and Apoptosis (Apop)

Rats	Diet	Adaptation	Carcinogen	Promotion	Butyrate concentration	Change in cancer potential	Other effects	References
F344	Inulin FOS	2 weeks	AOM	7 weeks	N/A	↓↓ ACF ↓ ACF	N/A	Reddy et al. (12)
F344	Inulin	2 weeks	AOM	11 weeks	N/A	↓ ACF	Dose dependently	Verghese et al. (78)
Sprague Dawley	Inulin FOS	3 weeks	DMH	1 day	N/A	↑↑ apop ↑ apop	N/A	Hughes and Rowland (79)
Sprague Dawley	B. longum Inulin Synbiotic	1 week (AOM pre treatment)	AOM	12 weeks	N/A	↓ ACF ↓ ACF ↓↓ ACF	↓ β-glucuronidase ↓ Ammonia	Rowland et al. (62)
Sprague Dawley	Resistant starch + B. lactis	4 weeks	AOM	6 h	↑	sm.↑ apop ↑ apop	N/A	Le Leu et al. (80)

AOM = aoxymethane; DMH = dimethylhydrazine. Results are as compared to control rats not receiving the dietary treatment.

microflora and less anaerobic genera, such as *Eubacterium* and *Fusobacterium*, which are butyrate producers *(71)*. Legakis et al. *(72)* found that in a colon cancer group there were more *Bacteroides* spp., particularly *B. fragilis,* and more *Clostridium paraputrificum*. The later are bacteria associated with proteolytic activities. A study with Japanese polyp patients, cancer patients and healthy controls *(73)* showed there were elevated numbers of clostridia, but lower bifidobacteria levels, in subjects with polyps and colon cancer.

Attempts to characterize the gut microflora of patients with colorectal cancer have given rise to conflicting results. Such studies have largely relied upon traditional culturing techniques. Gut microbiology is usually carried out by plating faecal microorganisms onto selective agars designed to recover numerically predominant groups. However, the agars used are only semi-selective, do not recover non-culturable bacteria and allow operator subjectivity in terms of microbial characterization – which is usually based on limited phenotypic procedures. Data obtained using modern, more specific, molecular biological techniques are lacking. Molecular markers have been used to more effectively characterize the microflora involved in fermentation. This approach is accepted to have considerable advantages over conventional or phenotypic methodologies in that it avoids culturing the microflora and is less prone to error due to operator subjectivity. Studies are needed to more definitely identify the differences in gut microbiota composition between those suffering from, or prone to, colorectal cancer compared to controls. This knowledge would allow a more effective use of probiotics and prebiotics in prevention.

6.2. Prebiotics for Butyrate Production

Butyrate has received attention for its preventive attributes towards colorectal cancer. However, most probiotics are lactate- and acetate-producing bifidobacteria and lactobacilli. Therefore, probiotics and prebiotics are not generally used to generate butyrate. As molecular-based knowledge of the microbiota diversity improves, new probiotics with the ability to generate butyrate may become available.

Clostridium butyricum is one species that is able to produce butyrate in the colon *(74)*. Research has also led to knowledge of cross-feeding mechanisms *(75, 76)* by a few members of the *Clostridia* XIVa group (*Eubacterium hallii* and *Anaerostipes caccae*), whereby butyrate can be produced from the breakdown of lactate and acetate. This finding suggests that favouring the growth of organisms that produce lactate and acetate may be a viable strategy to increase the colonic production of butyrate.

6.3. Distally Targeted Effects

Bacteria that produce xenobiotic enzymes favourably colonize more distal areas of the large intestine (descending colon, sigmoid rectum), where colorectal cancer is most prevalent. Therefore, when investigating the effects of prebiotic, probiotic and synbiotic it is necessary to consider the site of fermentation. It is likely that most of these agents have their largest influence in proximal regions of the large intestine. The ability of prebiotics, probiotics and synbiotics to aid the development of a more saccharolytic environment in the distal regions of the large intestine would be more favourable for reducing colorectal cancer risk, perhaps through the use of mixtures of these agents.

7. CONCLUSIONS AND DIETARY RECOMMENDATIONS

Probiotics have been safely used in human nutrition for many generations. Prebiotics are also extremely safe, although their use is more recent. Research data supporting the use of probiotics and prebiotics in the prevention of colorectal cancer are limited. Therefore, there is a need for more human studies to confirm the preventive efficacy of these dietary strategies. It is conceivable that probiotics and prebiotics may reduce the risk of colon cancer rather than offering much therapeutic value. The recently completed EU-funded SYNCAN project documented the potential benefits deriving from the combined use of probiotics and prebiotics *(77)*. Taken together, we propose that a synbiotic approach should be exploited to develop preventative strategies against colon cancer.

REFERENCES

1. Higginson, J. (1993) Environmental carcinogenesis. *Cancer* **72**, 971–77.
2. Kune, S., Kune, G.A., and Watson, L. (1986) The Melbourne colorectal cancer study: Incidence findings by age, sex, site, migrants and religion. *Int J Epidemiol* **15**, 483–93.
3. Whittemore, A.S. (1989) Colorectal cancer incidence among Chinese in North America and the People's Republic of China: Variation with sex, age and anatomical site. *Int J Epidemiol* **18**, 563–68.
4. Whittemore, A.S., Wu-Williams, A.H., Lee, M., Zheng, S., Gallagher, R.P., Jiao, D.A., Zhou, L., Wang, X.H., Chen, K., and Jung, D. (1990) Diet, physical activity, and colorectal cancer among Chinese in North America and China. *J Nat Cancer Inst* **6**, 915–26.
5. Terry, P., Giovannucci, E., Michels, K.B., Bergkvist, L., Hansen, H., Holmberg, L., and Wolk, A. (2001) Fruit, vegetables, dietary fiber, and risk of colorectal cancer. *J Nat Cancer Inst* **93**, 525–33.
6. Flood, D.M., Weiss, N.S., Cook, L.S., Emerson, J.C., Schwartz, S.M., and Potter, J.D. (2000) Colorectal cancer incidence in Asian migrants to the United States and their descendants. *Cancer Causes Control* **11**, 403–11.
7. Dixon, L.B., Balder, H.F., Virtanen, M.J., Rashidkhani, B., Mannisto, S., Krogh, V., van Den Brandt, P.A., Hartman, A.M., Pietinen, P., Tan, F., Virtamo, J., Wolk, A., and Goldbohm, R.A. (2004) Dietary patterns associated with colon and rectal cancer: Results from the Dietary Patterns and Cancer (DIETSCAN) Project. *Am J Clin Nutr* **80**, 1003–11.
8. Bingham, S.A., Day, N.E., Luben, R., Ferrari, P., Slimani, N., Norat, T., Clavel-Chapelon, F., Kesse, E., Nieters, A., Boeing, H., Tjønneland, A., Overvad, K., Martinez, C., Dorronsoro, M., Gonzalez, C.A., Key, T.J., Trichopoulou, A., Naska, A., Vineis, P., Tumino, R., Krogh, V., Bueno-de-Mesquita, H.B., Peeters, P.H., Berglund, G., Hallmans, G., Lund, E., Skeie, G., Kaaks, R., and Riboli, E. (2003) Dietary fibre in food and protection against colorectal cancer in the European prospective investigation into cancer and nutrition (EPIC): An observational study. *Lancet* **361**, 1496–501.
9. Burkitt, D.P. (1969) Related disease – related cause? *Lancet* **2**, 1229–31.
10. English, D.R., MacInnis, R.J., Hodge, A.M., Hopper, J.L., Haydon, A.M., and Giles, G.G. (2005) Red meat, chicken, and fish consumption and risk of colorectal cancer. *Cancer Epidemiol Biomarker Prev* **13**, 1509–12.
11. Goldin, B.R. (1986) In situ bacterial metabolism and colon mutagens. *Ann Rev Microbiol* **40**, 367–93.
12. Reddy, B.S., Narisawa, T., Wright, P., Vukusich, D., Weisburger, J.H., and Wynder, E.L. (1975) Compound via MeSH, substance via MeSH, colon carcinogenesis with azoxymethane and dimethylhydrazine in germ-free rats. *Cancer Res* **35**, 287–90.
13. Hooper, L.V., and Gordon, J.I. (2001) Commensal host-bacterial relationships in the gut. *Science* **11**, 1115–18.

14. Eckburg, P.B., Bik, E.M., Bernstein, C.N., Purdom, E., Dethlefsen, L., Sargent, M., Gill, S.R., Nelson, K.E., and Relman, D.A. (2005) Diversity of the human intestinal microbial flora. *Science* **10**, 1635–38.

15. Egert, M., de Graaf, A.A., Smidt, H., de Vos, W.M., and Venema, K. (2006) Beyond diversity, functional microbiomics of the human colon. *Trend Microbiol* **14**, 86–91.

16. Collins, M.D., and Gibson, G.R. (1999) Probiotics, prebiotics and synbiotics, approaches for modulating the microbial ecology of the gut. *Am J Clin Nutr* **69**, 1052S–7S.

17. Mason, P. (2001) Prebiotics and probiotics. *Pharm J* **266**, 118–21.

18. Metchnikoff, E. (1907) The Prolongation of Life. London: William Heinemann.

19. Fuller, R. (1989) Probiotics in man and animals. *J Appl Bacteriol* **66**, 365–78.

20. Pereira, D.I., and Gibson, G.R. (2002) Cholesterol assimilation by lactic acid bacteria and bifidobacteria isolated from the human gut. *Appl Environ Microbiol* **68**, 4689–93.

21. Young, S.L., Simon, M.A., Baird, M.A., Tannock, G.W., Bibiloni, R., Spencely, K., Lane, J.M., Fitzharris, P., Crane, J., Town, I., Addo-Yobo, E., Murray, C.S., and Woodcock, A. (2004) Bifidobacterial species differentially affect expression of cell surface markers and cytokines of dendritic cells harvested from cord blood. *Clin Diagn Lab Immunol* **11**, 686–90.

22. Noda, H., Akasaka, N., and Ohsugi, M. (1994) Biotin production by bifidobacteria. *J Nutr Sci Vitaminol* **40**, 181–88.

23. Campbell, J.M., Fahey, G.C., Jr., and Wolf, B.W. (1997) Selected indigestible oligosaccharides affect large bowel mass, cecal and fecal short-chain fatty acids, pH and microflora in rats. *J Nutr* **127**, 130–36.

24. Park, H.Y., Bae, E.A., Han, M.J., Choi, E.C., and Kim, D.H. (1998) Inhibitory effects of *Bifidobacterium* spp. isolated from a healthy koream on harmful enzymes of human intestinal microflora. *Arch Pharm Res* **21**, 54–61.

25. Orrhage, K., Sillerstrom, E., Gustafsson, J.A., Nord, C.E., and Rafter, J. (1994) Binding of mutagenic heterocyclic amines by intestinal and lactic acid bacteria. *Mutat Res* **311**, 239–48.

26. Huycke, M.M., Abrams, V., and Moore, D.R. (2002) *Enterococcus faecalis* produces extracellular superoxide and hydrogen peroxide that damages colonic epithelial cell dna. *Carcinogen* **23**, 529–36.

27. Balish, E., and Warner, T. (2002) Enterococcus faecalis induces inflammatory bowel disease in interleukin-10 knockout mice. *Am J Pathol* **160**, 2253–57.

28. Wunderlich, P.F., Braun, L., Fumagalli, I., D'Apuzzo, V., Heim, F., Karly, M., Lodi, R., Politta, G., Vonbank, F., and Zeltner, L. (1989) Double-blind report on the efficacy of lactic acid-producing *Enterococcus* SF68 in the prevention of antibiotic-associated diarrhoea and in the treatment of acute diarrhoea. *J Int Med Res* **17**, 333–38.

29. Rigottier-Gois, L., Rochet, V., Garrec, N., Suau, A., and Doré, J. (2003) Enumeration of *Bacteroides* species in human faeces by fluorescent in situ hybridisation combined with flow cytometry using 16S rRNA probes. *Sys Appl Microbiol* **26**, 110–18.

30. Wu, S., Lim, K.C., Huang, J., Saidi, R.F., and Sears, C.L. (1998) *Bacteroides fragilis* enterotoxin cleaves the zonula adherens protein, E-cadherin. *Proc Nat Acad Sci* **95**, 14979–84.

31. Lyerly, D.M., Krivan, H.C., and Wilkins, T.D. (1988) *Clostridium difficile*, its disease and toxins. *Clin Microbiol Rev* **1**, 1–18.

32. Fernandez, M., Pistone Creydt, M.E., Uza, V., McClane, F.A., and Ibarra, B.A. (2005) *Clostridium perfringens* enterotoxin damages the human intestine in vitro. *Infec Imm* **73**, 8407–10.

33. Nakamura, J., Kubota, Y., Miyaoka, M., Saitoh, T., Mizuno, F., and Benno, Y. (2002) Comparison of four microbial enzymes in bacteroides isolated from human faeces. *Microbiol Immunol* **46**, 487–90.

34. Gibson, G.R. (1999) Dietary modulation of the human gut microflora using the prebiotics oligofructose and inulin. *J Nutr* **129**, 1438–41.

35. Roediger, W.E. (1980) Role of anaerobic bacteria in the metabolic welfare of the colonic mucosa in man. *Gut* **21**, 793–98.

36. Singh, B., Halestrap, A.P., and Paraskeva, C. (1997) Butyrate can act as a stimulator of growth or an inducer of apoptosis in human colonic epithelial cell lines depending on the presence of alternative energy sources. *Carcinogen* **18**, 1265–70.

37. Hill, M. (2003) Dietary fibre and colon cancer, Where do we go from here? *Proc Nutr Soc* **62**, 63–65.

38. Knudsen, K.E.B., Serena, A., Canibe, N., and Juntunen, K.S. (2003) New insight into butyrate metabolism. *Proc Nutr Soc* **62**, 81–86.

39. Perrin, P., Pierre, F., Patry, Y., Champ, M., Berreur, M., Pradal, G., Bornet, F., Meflah, K., and Menanteau, J. (2001) Only fibres promoting a stable butyrate producing colonic ecosystem decrease the rate of aberrant crypt foci in rats. *Gut* **48**, 53–61.
40. Emenaker, N.J., Calaf, G.M., Cox, D., Basson, M.D., and Qureshi, N. (2001) Short-chain fatty acids inhibit invasive human colon cancer by modulating uPA, TIMP-1, TIMP-2, mutant p53, Bcl-2, Bax, p21 and PCNA protein expression in an in vitro cell culture model. *J Nutr* **131**, 3041S–6S.
41. Pool-Zobel, B.L., Selvaraju, V., Sauer, J., Kautenburger, T., Kiefer, J., Richter, K.K., Soom, M., and Wolfl, S. (2005) Butyrate may enhance toxicological defence in primary, adenoma and tumor human colon cells by favourably modulating expression of glutathione S-transferases genes, an approach in nutrigenomics. *Carcinogen* **6**, 1064–76.
42. Beyer-Sehlmeyer, G., Glei, M., Hartman, E., Hughes, R., Persin, C., Böhm, V., Rowland, I., Schubert, R., Jahreis, G., and Pool-Zobel, B.L. (2003) Butyrate is only one of several growth inhibitors produced during gut flora-mediated fermentation of dietary fibre sources. *Br J Nutr* **90**, 1057–70.
43. Avivi-Green, A., Charcon, S.P., Mardar, Z., and Schwartz, B. (2002) Different molecular events account for butyrate-induced apoptosis in two human colon cancer cell lines. *J Nutr* **132**, 1812–18.
44. Kobayashi, H. (2003) Sodium butyrate inhibits cell growth and stimulates p21, WAF1, CIP1 proteins in human colonic adenocorcinoma cells independently of p53 status. *Nutr Canc* **46**, 202–11.
45. Hassig, C.A., Tong, J.K., and Schreiber, S.L. (1997) Fiber-derived butyrate and the prevention of colon cancer. *Chem Biol* **4**, 783–89.
46. Fuszek, P., Horvath, H.C., Speer, G., Papp, J., Haller, P., Fischer, S., Halasz, J., Jaray, B., Szekely, E., Schaff, Z., Papp, A., Bursics, A., Harsanyi, L., Lukovich, P., Kupcsulik, P., Hitre, E., and Lakatos, P.L. (2006) Location and age at onset of colorectal cancer in Hungarian patients between 1993 and 2004. The high number of advanced cases supports the need for a colorectal cancer screening program in Hungary. *Anticancer Res* **26**, 52–55.
47. Gibson, S.A.W., McFarlan, C., Hay, S., and MacFarlane, G.T. (1989) Significance of microflora in proteolysis in the colon. *Appl Environ Microbiol* **55**, 679–83.
48. Lin, H.C., and Visek, W.J. (1991) Colon mucosal cell damage by ammonia in rats. *J Nutr* **121**, 887–93.
49. Macfarlane, G.T., Gibson, G.R., and Cummings, J.H. (1992) Comparison of fermentation reactions in different regions of the human colon. *J Appl Bacteriol* **72**, 57–64.
50. Fuller, R., and Gibson, G.R. (1998) Probiotics and prebiotics, microflora management for improved gut health. *Clin Microbiol Infec* **4**, 477–80.
51. Tannock, G.W. (2001) Molecular assessment of intestinal microflora. *Am J Clin Nutr* **73**, 401–04.
52. Bezkorovainy, A. (2001) Probiotics, determinants of survival and growth in the gut. *Am J Clin Nutr* **73**, 399S–405S.
53. Dunne, C., O'Mahony, L., Murphy, L., Thornton, G., Morrissey, D., O'Halloran, S., Feeney, M., Flynn, S., Fitzgerald, G., Daly, C., Kiley, B., O'Sullivan, G.C., Shanahan, F., and Collins, K. (2001) In vitro selection criteria for probiotic bacteria of human origin, correlation with in vivo findings. *Am J Clin Nutr* **73**, 386S–92S.
54. Guarner, F., and Malagelada, J.R. (2003) Gut flora in health and disease. *Lancet* **361**, 512–19.
55. Goldin, B.R. (1998) Health benefits of probiotics. *Br J Nutr* **80**, S203–S07.
56. Parker, R.B. (1974) Probiotics, the other half of the antibiotic story. *Ann Nutr Health* **29**, 4–8.
57. Salminen, S., Bouley, C., Boutron-Ruault, M.C., Cummings, J.H., Franck, A., Gibson, G.R., Isolauri, I., Moreau, M.C., Roberfroid, M., and Rowland, I.R. (1998) Functional food science and gastrointestinal physiology and function. *Br J Nutr* **80**, S147–S71.
58. United Nations. Food and Agriculture Organization of the United Nations (UNFAO). (2001) Health and nutritional properties of probiotics in food including powder milk with live lactic acid bacteria, http//ftp.fao.org/es/esn/food/probio_report_en.pdf (4 Oct 2006).
59. United Nations. Food and Agriculture Organization of the United Nations (UNFAO). (2002) Guidelines for the evaluation of probiotics in Food. http,//ftp.fao.org/es/esn/food/wgreport2.pdf (4 Oct 2006).
60. Gibson, G.R., and Roberfroid, M.B. (1995) Dietary modulation of the human colonic microflora introducing the concept of probiotics. *J Nutr* **125**, 1401–12.
61. Gibson, G.R., Probert, H.M., van Loo, J.A.E., Rastall, R.A., and Roberfroid, M.B. (2004) Dietary modulation of the human colonic microbiota, Updating the concept of prebiotics. *Nutr Res Rev* **17**, 259–75.

62. Rowland, I.R., Rumney, C.J., Coutts, J.T., and Lievense, L.C. (1998) Effect of *Bifidobacterium longum* and inulin on gut bacterial metabolism and carcinogen-induced aberrant crypt foci in rats. *Carcinogen* **19**, 281–85.

63. Reddy, B.S., Hamis, R., and Rao, C.V. (1997) Effect of dietary oligofructose and inulin on colonic preneoplastic aberrant crypt foci inhibition. *Carcinogen* **18**, 1371–74.

64. Rafter, J. (2002) Lactic acid bacteria and cancer, mechanistic perspective. *Br J Nutr* **88**, S89–S94.

65. McBain, A.J., and Macfarlane, G.T. (2001) Modulation of genotoxic enzyme activities by non-digestible oligosaccharide metabolism in in-vitro human gut bacterial enzymes. *J Med Microbiol* **50**, 833–42.

66. Kassie, F., Rabot, S., Kundi, M., Chabicovsky, M., Qin, H.M., and Knasmuller, S. (2001) Intestinal microflora plays a crucial role in the genotoxicity of the cooked food mutagen 2-amino-3-methylimidazo [4,5-f]quinoline. *Carcinogen* **22**, 1721–25.

67. Zsivkovits, M., Fekadu, K., Sontag, G., Nabinger, U., Huber, W.W., Kundi, M., Chakarborty, A., Foissy, H., and Knasmuller, S. (2003) Prevention of heterocyclic damage in colon and liver of rats by different lactobacilli strains. *Carcinogen* **24**, 1913–18.

68. Humblot, C., Lhoste, E., Knasmuller, S., Gloux, K., Bruneau, A., Bensaada, M., Durao, J., Rabot, S., Andrieux, C., and Kassie, F. (2004) Protective effects of Brussels sprouts, oligosaccharides and fermented milk towards 2-amino-3-methylimidazo[4,5-f]quinoline (IQ)-induced genotoxicity in the human flora associated F344 rat, role of xenobiotic metabolising enzymes and intestinal microflora. *J Chromat* **25**, 231–37.

69. Goldin, B.R., and Gorbach, S.L. (1984) The effect of milk and lactobacillus feeding on human intestinal bacterial enzyme activity. *Am J Clin Nutr* **39**, 756–61.

70. Vargo, D., Moskovitz, M., and Floch, M.H. (1980) Faecal bacterial flora in cancer of the colon. *Gut* **21**, 701–05.

71. Barcenilla, A., Pryde, S.E., Martin, J.C., Duncan, S.H., Stewart, C.S., Henderson, C., and Flint, H.J. (2000) Phylogenic relationships of butyrate-producing bacteria from the human gut. *Appl Environ Microbiol* **66**, 1654–61.

72. Legakis, N.J., Ioannides, H., Tzannetis, S., Golematis, B., and Papavassiliou, J. (1981) Faecal bacterial flora in patients with colon cancer and control subjects. *Zentral Bakteriol Mikrobiol Hyg* **251**, 54–61.

73. Kubota, Y. (1990) Fecal intestinal flora in patients with colon adenoma and colon cancer. *Nipp Shok Gak Zas* **87**, 771–79.

74. Saint-Amans, S., Girbal, L., Andrade, J., Ahrens, K., and Soucaille, P. (2001) Regulation of cabon and electron flow in *Clostridium butyricum* VPI 3266 grown on glucose-glycerol mixtures. *J Bacteriol* **183**, 1748–54.

75. Belenguer, A., Duncan, S.H., Calder, A.G., Holtrop, G., Louis, P., Lobley, G.E., and Flint, H.J. (2006) Two routes of metabolic cross-feeding between *Bifidobacterium adolescentis* and butyrate-producing anaerobes from the human gut. *Appl Environ Microbiol* **72**, 3593–99.

76. Morrison, D.J., Mackay, W.G., Edwards, C.A., Preston, T., Dodson, B., and Weaver, L.T. (2006) Butyrate production from oligofructose fermentation by the human faecal flora, what is the contribution of extracellular acetate and lactate? *Br J Nutr* **96**, 570–77.

77. Rafter, J., Bennett, M., Caderni, G., Clune, Y., Hughes, R., Karlsson, P.C., Klinder, A., O'Riordan, M., O'Sullivan, G.C., Pool-Zobel, B., Rechkemmer, G., Roller, M., Rowland, I., Salvadori, M., Thijs, H., Van Loo, J., Watzl, B., and Collins, J.K. (2007) Dietary synbiotics reduce cancer risk factors in polypectomized and colon cancer patients. *Am J Clin Nutr* **85**, 488–96.

78. Verghese, M., Rao, D.R., Chawan, C.B., and Shackelford, L. (2002) Dietary inulin supresses azoxymethane-induced preneoplastic aberrant crypt foci in mature fisher 344 rats. *J Nutr* **132**, 2804–08.

79. Hughes, R., and Rowland, I.R. (2001) Stimulation of apoptosis by two prebiotic chicory fructans in the rat colon. *Carcinogen* **22**, 43–47.

80. Le Leu, R.K., Brown, I.L., Hu, Y., Bird, A.R., Jackson, M., Esterman, A., and Young, G.P. (2005) A synbiotic combination of resistant starch and *Bifidobacterium lactis* facilitates apoptotic deletion of carcinogen-damaged cells in rat colon. *J Nutr* **135**, 996–1001.

10 Meats, Protein and Cancer

Gunter G.C. Kuhnle and Sheila A. Bingham

Key Points

1. Several studies showed that dietary red meat, not white meat, was associated with a statistically significant increased risk for cancer of the esophagus, colon, lung and pancreas with an estimated risk increase of 29% per 100 g red meat and 21% per 50 g processed meat.
2. In randomised controlled diet intervention studies, it was shown that intake of red and processed meats, but not white meat, was associated with an increase in endogenously formed nitroso compounds, many of which are known carcinogens. This was concluded because the combined actions of heme, found in high concentrations in red meat, and free thiol groups can promote the endogenous formation of *N*-nitroso compounds.
3. Epidemiological studies have shown that changes in anaerobic fermentation related to dietary fiber can exert protective effects against meat-induced risk for colorectal cancer. A plausible explanation is that hydroxyl groups in fiber may scavenge nitrosating species and thus prevent the endogenous formation of nitroso compounds.
4. Polycyclic aromatic hydrocarbons (PAHs) are potentially carcinogenic chemical compounds that consist of fused aromatic rings and do not contain heteroatoms or carry substituents. They are products of incomplete combustion of organic matter and are present in most foods as a result of environmental contamination. PAH is found in relatively high concentrations in meat that is cooked over an open flame, due to the pyrolysis of the fat. The amount of PAHs produced is dependent upon the fat content in the meat and the temperature and proximity of the heat used to cook it. Lower cooking temperatures generally do not produce excessive amounts of PAHs.
5. The WCRF recommended that meat intake should be reduced to an average of 300 g/week with as little intake of processed meat as possible. Meat should be prepared carefully to avoid the formation of carcinogens such as HCA and PAH. The formation of these compounds can be avoided by using lower cooking temperatures and changing the concentration of carcinogenic precursors by marinating or reducing the amount of available water.

Key Words: Meats; protein; cancer; nitroso compounds; polycyclic aromatic hydrocarbons

1. INTRODUCTION

Globally, meat accounts for approximately 0.8 MJ/person/d with an almost 80-fold variation between different countries *(1)* and an average annual consumption of 38 kg/person/year. Consumption *per caput* appears to be closely related to wealth with

From: *Nutrition and Health: Bioactive Compounds and Cancer*
Edited by: J.A. Milner, D.F. Romagnolo, DOI 10.1007/978-1-60761-627-6_10,
© Springer Science+Business Media, LLC 2010

more than 90 kg/person/year in North America, Europe and Oceania whereas intake in Africa is on average less than 20 kg/person/year *(2)*. The large geographical variation of meat consumption coincides with high rates of several common cancers. Armstrong and Doll *(3)* conducted a detailed investigation into the effect of environmental factors on cancer incidence and mortality. They compared incidence rates with *per caput* commodity consumption and found a positive correlation between the intake of meat and protein and most types of cancer (Table 1), in particular for cancers of the colon and rectum. A comparison using more recent data also shows a significant ($p < 0.0001$) correlation between age-standardised cancer incidence rates and *per caput* meat consumption (Fig. 1).

Table 1
Correlation Coefficients Between Meat and Protein Consumption and Cancer Incidence and Mortality

	Meat		*Total protein*	
	Men	*Women*	*Men*	*Women*
Colon	0.85	0.89	0.54	0.62
Rectum	0.83	0.68	0.64	0.44
Breast	–	0.78	–	0.49
Corpus uteri	–	0.78	–	0.50
Ovary	–	0.40	–	0.32
Prostate	0.37	–	–0.11	–
Testis	0.50	–	0.34	–
Kidney	0.70	0.73	0.55	0.70
Liver	–0.40	–0.47	–0.46	–0.54
Nervous system	0.50	0.37	0.54	0.45

Adapted from Armstrong and Doll *(3)*.

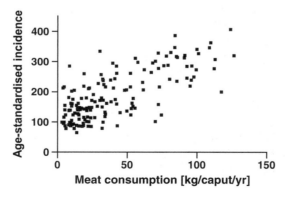

Fig. 1. Correlation between annual meat consumption and age-standardised cancer incidence rates (in males; incidence per 100,000 per year) for all cancers. The correlation is significant ($p < 0.0001$) with a Pearson's ρ of 0.739. Meat consumption data (2002) from FAO as cited by Speedy *(2)*; 2002 cancer incidence rates from WHO (Globocan).

In a recent prospective study in the NIH-AARP (American Association for Retired Persons) Diet and Health Study cohort,[1] significant associations between dietary meat and cancer of the colorectum, the liver, the pancreas (in males) and the lung were found (Fig. 2) *(4)*. Similarly, the WCRF's Second Expert Report *(5)* identified meat consumption as a risk factor for cancer, in particular of the colon and rectum, with an estimated relative risk of 1.29 (95% CI: 1.05–1.59) per 100 g (Fig. 3). Larson and Wolk *(6)* found

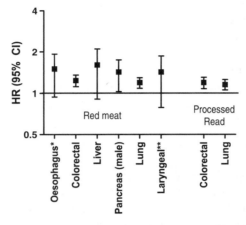

Fig. 2. Data from NIH-AARP prospective study. Hazard ratios (and 95% confidence intervals) for the first vs. fifth quintile of red and processed meat intake and cancer risk (*p*-trend < 0.05 except for *(*p* = 0.09) and **(*p* = 0.13)). Data from Cross et al. *(4)*.

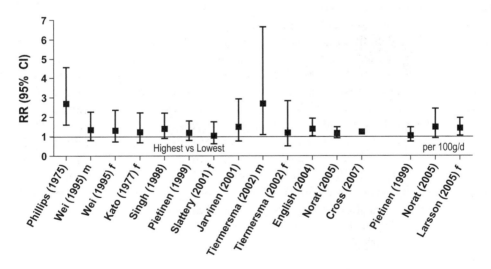

Fig. 3. Relative risk (95% CI) for colorectal cancer between highest and lowest exposure to dietary red meat and per 100 g/d consumption of red meat in cohort studies *(4, 13, 93–102)*. Data cited from the WCRF's Second Expert Report *(5)*. f/m indicates female/male cohort.

[1] Approximately 500,000 participants aged 50–71 years at baseline (1995–1996); 53,396 incident cancers were ascertained during 8.2 years of follow-up.

a relative risk of 1.28 (95% CI: 1.15–1.42) between the highest and lowest category of red meat consumption in a meta-analysis of prospective studies. There are fewer data available for other cancer sites, although several studies showed that dietary red meat was associated with a statistically significant increased risk for cancer of the esophagus (7–9), lung (4, 10) and pancreas (4, 11) and a statistically non-significant increased risk for endometrial cancer (12).

Several hypotheses have been proposed to explain the positive association between meat consumption and cancer. Main hypotheses focus on the heme content of meat, the endogenous formation of nitroso compounds and exposure to carcinogenic heterocylic amines (HCAs) and polycyclic aromatic hydrocarbons (PAHs). Each hypothesis will be discussed separately with special emphasis on gastric and bowel cancers, which have the strongest association with meat intake in epidemiological studies. Effects of dietary fat and iron are discussed, respectively, in Chapters 13 and 21.

2. HEME

In epidemiological studies investigating the association between meat and cancer, significant associations were only found for red and processed meats, but not for white meat. In the EPIC cohort with 478,000 participants, dietary red and processed meats were significantly associated with an increased risk for colorectal cancer (HR: 1.55; 95% CI: 1.19; 2.02; p-trend $= 0.001$; per 100 g/d increase) whereas no association was found with intake of white meat (13). A major difference between red and white meats is the heme content, mainly from myoglobin in muscle tissue. The heme content in red meat such as beef is more than 10 times higher than in white meat such as poultry (Table 2). Heme has shown to exert both cytotoxic and haemotoxic effects in in vitro cultures and in animal models. It can either act directly as cytolytic agent (14) or be converted into biliverdin by heme oxygenase (present in the intestinal epithelium) and further into bilirubin, which also has lytic properties (15, 16). Furthermore, it can act indirectly by catalysing the endogenous formation of radicals (17) and nitroso compounds (18) (see below). In rats fed a heme-rich diet, colonic epithelial proliferation increased significantly and the resulting faecal water[2] was highly cytotoxic when compared with faecal water of controls (14). In HT29 and primary tumour cells, haemoglobin and haemin were found to induce DNA damage and reduce metabolic activity and growth (19). However, most of these effects were observed with heme concentrations well above 100 μM (500–1000 μM for haemin), which are more than 1.5 times the concentrations found in stool samples after the ingestion of approximately 400 g of red meat and similar to the levels found after the ingestion of 10–20 ml of blood (20).

Several epidemiological studies have been conducted to investigate the effect of heme on the development of cancer, but the results so far are inconclusive. In the Iowa Women's Health Study, the risk for proximal colon cancer increased twofold between the highest and lowest quintile of heme intake (21) whereas in a Dutch cohort the risk

---

[2] The term "faecal water" refers either to the aqueous fraction of stool samples or an aqueous extract of stool samples.

Table 2
Heme Content in Foods as Haemoglobin Equivalent

	mg/g	nmol/g
Bacon	0.8	52.5
Beefsteak	7.5	466.4
Cheddarwurst	1.4	87.5
Chicken (dark)	0.5	28.1
Chicken (white)	0.3	16.9
Corned beef	2.6	162.5
Ham	0.8	46.9
Hamburger	4.6	287.5
Lamb	2.7	168.8
Pastrami	2.3	143.8
Pork chop	2.1	131.3
Pork sausage	1.9	118.8
Salami	2.6	162.5
Shrimp	0.0	1.3
Smoked pork	0.7	43.8
Sunfish	0.0	1.9
Tuna (brine)	0.1	5.0
Tuna (oil)	0.6	36.9
Turkey (dark)	1.2	74.4
Turkey (white)	0.3	21.3
Turnips	0.0	0.6
Venison	2.4	150
Wiener	2.1	131.3
Wild duck	2.1	131.3

Adapted from Schwartz et al. *(20)*.

increased but not to a statistically significant degree *(22)*. A Canadian study found no association between dietary iron and heme iron intake and colorectal cancer in women *(23)*. Similarly, no association has been found for dietary heme and breast *(24)* and endometrial cancers *(25)*. However, these studies estimated the heme intake as a fixed proportion of total iron from meat leading to inaccuracies in estimating exposure. To obtain more reliable information and identify associations between exposure to heme and cancer risk, more accurate data on the levels of heam in meat are necessary.

3. ENDOGENOUS NITROSATION

Red and processed meats, but not white meat, induce the endogenous formation of nitroso compounds in the gastrointestinal tract. This process is facilitated by heme *(18, 26)*. Of particular interest are endogenously formed *N*-nitroso compounds (NOC), many of which are known carcinogens *(27)*. Heme becomes easily nitrosylated under the anaerobic and reducing conditions of the gastrointestinal tract to form nitrosyl heme which is a NO donor *(28)* and can act as a nitrosating agent *(29)*. Nitroso-thiols are formed readily under acidic condition *(30)*, a process that is promoted by heme *(18)*. In turn, nitroso-thiols can act as NO donors and nitrosating species *(31)*. Thus, the combined actions of heme and free thiol groups can promote the endogenous formation of *N*-nitroso compounds. In a diet intervention study, it was shown that supplementation of heme, but not "inorganinc" iron, resulted in a significant increase in the formation of endogenously formed nitroso compounds *(26)*.

   N-nitroso compounds may be activated by cytochrome P450-dependent oxidorectuc-tases *(32)*, yielding alkyldiazonium ions which are considered to be the ultimate alkylating species. The alkylation of DNA is likely to be a major effect of these compounds *(33, 34)* and can induce GC → AT transitions in genes such as *ki-ras (35)* that are typically mutated in human cancers. In the absence of enzymatic activation, the nitrosation of amino acids such as glycine can yield intermediate bioactive metabolites such as di-azoacetate *(36)*. These compounds can induce the formation of DNA base adducts like O^6-carboxymethyl-2'-*deoxy*-guanosine (O^6CmeG; Fig. 4 for details). O^6CmeG is not repaired by O^6-alkylguanine transferase *(37)* and was shown to increase in colonic cells isolated from human volunteers on a high red meat diet *(38)*. The profile of mutations induced by diazoacetate in a plasmid containing human *p53* was very similar to the mutations detected in human gastrointestinal tract tumours *(39)*. In addition to their

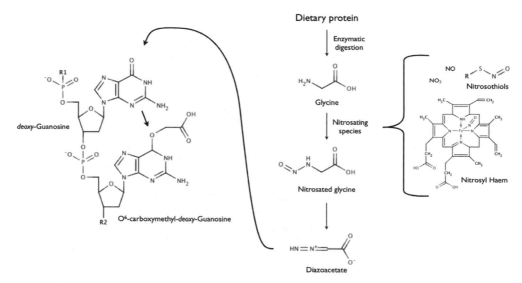

Fig. 4. Heme induced formation of DNA adducts. Enzymatic hydrolysis of dietary protein results in the formation of amino acids which subsequently can become nitrosated. The nitrosation process can be promoted by heme – which itself can become nitrosylated – and nitroso-thiols; these compounds can also act as nitrosating agents and NO donors. Nitrosated amino acids such as diazoacetate can then react with DNA bases and result in the formation of DNA adducts such as O^6-carboxymethyl-*deoxy*-guanosine (O^6CMeG).

alkylating properties, nitroso compounds, such as nitrosyl heme, can also cause an increase in nitric oxide (NO) concentrations in the gastrointestinal tract and trigger inflammatory responses. Under normal conditions, gastrointestinal NO plays an important role in mucosa defence by modulating immune response and blood flow, stimulation of mucus and bicarbonate secretion and reduction of the epithelial barrier *(40, 41)*. However, studies have shown that NO can lead to tissue injury *(41)* and its concentration is increased in inflammatory bowel disease (IBD) *(42, 43)*. In addition, reactive nitrogen species (RNS) derived from NO such as peroxynitrite, nitroxyl or nitrogen dioxide have a pathogenic potential by inducing oxidative and nitrative damages *(44)*.

Although NOC are known carcinogens *(27, 45)*, only little information from in vitro studies and animal experiments is available about the carcinogenic effect of endogenously formed NOC. However, in randomised controlled diet intervention studies with human volunteers, it was shown that intake of red and processed meats, but not white meat, was associated with an increase in endogenously formed nitroso compounds *(46–50)*. Presumably, heme, but not "inorganic" iron, promoted the formation of these compounds *(26)* via formation of nitrosyl heme *(18)*. The diet-dependent genotoxic effects of faecal waters have been investigated, and an increase in genotoxicity following a high meat diet has been shown in one study *(51)* but not in another *(52)*. However, in the preparation of faecal water, large quantities of NOC are lost so that genotoxic effects might be expected not to be detectable *(52)*. DNA adducts specific for endogenous nitroso compounds, such as nitrosated glycine, were found in cells exfoliated from volunteers who were on a high red meat diet *(38)*.

Because faeces are not routinely collected in epidemiological studies and the lack of suitable biomarkers of exposure, it is difficult to investigate the effect of endogenous nitrosation. Presently, it is only possible to estimate the endogenous formation of nitroso compounds using data from dietary studies with volunteers *(26, 47–49)*. Results from these studies were used to estimate an index of NOC exposure correlating the formation of nitroso compounds with dietary iron from meat (r = 0.95). In the European Prospective Investigation into Cancer and Nutrition (EPIC-EURGAST) study investigating the association between endogenous nitrosation and cancer, a statistically significant association between endogenous nitrosation and non-cardia gastric cancer was detected (HR: 1.42) for an increase of 40 μg/d of endogenously formed nitroso compounds. There was no association with exogenous NOC *(53)*.

4. HCA AND PAH

The activation of HCA and PAH by cytochrome P450-dependent oxidoreductases leads to the formation of reactive intermediates, which induce DNA mutations and tumours in animal models *(54–57)*. Well-studied HCA includes imidazoquinolines and quinoxalines (IQ compounds) and 2-amino-1-methyl-6-imidazo[4,5-*b*]bipyridine (PhIP). These compounds are formed during the preparation of food by *Maillard* reactions *(58)* between creatinine, free amino acids and monosaccharides. The biochemical processes leading to their formation depend on the presence of sufficient precursors, the cooking method (i.e. time, temperature) and the presence of water. The formation of HCA increases both with cooking time and temperature with more PhIP than MeIQ (2-amino-3,4-methylimidazo[4,5-*f*]quinoline) formed at high temperatures. Water transfers water-soluble precursors to the surface where HCA formation occurs and binding water decreases the amount of HCA formed *(59)*. MeIQ and PhIP mainly induce G:C → T:A transversions and G:C base pair deletions *(60)*. In cultured cells, HCA induced chromosomal aberrations *(61)* and sister chromatid exchanges *(62)*. In long-term animal experiments with the maximum tolerable dose (MTD), tumours were induced mainly in the liver but also in the intestine, skin, oral cavity, mammary gland, Zymbal gland and clitoral gland *(56)*. However, the concentrations used in these animal studies ranged from 100 to 800 ng/g, which are considerably higher than the concentrations found in prepared beef or chicken (0.2–40 ng/g) *(56)*. Carcinogenic HCA was found in urine of healthy volunteers eating normal diet, but not in urine of patients receiving parenteral diets *(63)*. Furthermore, DNA adducts have been found in human tissue from colon, rectum and kidney *(64, 65)*.

Lipophilic PAHs are products of incomplete combustion of organic matter and have therefore been present in the environment for thousands of years. These compounds were initially identified as the carcinogenic ingredients of tars and oils *(66)*. The compound benzo[*a*]pyrene (B[*a*]P) was among the first carcinogenic PAH compounds identified *(67)*. However, the carcinogenic risk of these compounds was suspected much earlier *(68)*, in particular in professions which came into close contact with combusted materials such as coke plant workers or chimney sweeps as described by Pott *(69)*. PAH is present in most foods as a result of environmental contamination, e.g. proximity to industrial plants or roads, and up to 94 ppb has been found in lettuce in Finland *(70)*. Depending on geographical location, levels for benzo[*a*]pyrene ranged from 3 to 25 ppb *(71)*, which are similar to levels detected in smoked meat (3–30 ppb) *(72)*. Conversely, meat cooked over an open flame may contain much higher amounts of PAHs. For example, in barbecued meat, total PAH concentrations of more than 160 ppb were detected *(73)*. PAH is formed by the pyrolysis of fat, either directly on the meat or through fat dripping into the flame, and then deposited onto the meat. The formation of PAH depends on the fat content and the proximity to the open heat source and can be reduced by cooking at a lower temperature *(55)*. Nevertheless, normal roasting or frying does not produce excessive amounts of PAH *(55)*. The average dietary intake, which is the main non-occupational source of PAH in non-smokers, has been estimated to be approximately 3 μg/d, with only small contributions from meat *(55)*.

The pro-mutagenic and carcinogenic effects of HCA and PAH have been investigated extensively using in vitro studies and animal models. The International Agency for Research on Cancer (IARC) published monographs on HCA *(74)* and PAH *(75)*; Table 3 gives an overview of some results and classifications. Many of these compounds require metabolic activation by P450-dependent oxidoreductases; therefore, even non-carcinogenic HCAs and PAHs can enhance carcinogenicity of these compounds by inducing metabolising enzymes *(68)*.

In vitro mutagenicity tests using *Salmonella typhimurium* (Ames test) showed that compounds like MeIQ (661,000 revertants/μg) and IQ (433,000 revertants/μg) exhibited a much higher mutagenicity than aflatoxin B_1 (28,000 revertants/μg), B[*a*]P (660

Table 3
Mutagenicity and Carcinogenicity Data for Some Heterocyclic Amines and Polycyclic Aromatic Hydrocarbons Found in or Associated with Dietary Meat from IARC Monographs (45, 74, 75). Apart from benzo[a]pyrene, most other PAHs were not classifiable

Compound	IARC evaluation and classification	Animal studies	Target organs	Other observations
Heterocyclic amines				
IQ	2A (probably carcinogenic to humans)	Mice, rats and monkeys	Liver, lungs, forestomach (mice), small and large intestines, Zymbal glands, mammary glands, squamous cell carcinoma (skin, clitoral gland)	IQ binds to DNA in most organs in monkeys and rodents; DNA damage, gene mutation and chromosomal abnormalities in rodents; induces DNA damage in human and animal cells in vitro; induces mutations in *Drosophila melanogaster* and bacteria
MeIQ	2B (possibly carcinogenic to humans)	Mice and rats	Liver, forestomach, Zymbal gland, oral cavity, colon, skin and mammary glands	MeIQ binds to DNA and induces DNA damage and sister chromatid exchange; induces DNA damage and gene mutation in animal cells in vitro and in bacteria

(*Continued*)

Table 3
(Continued)

MeIQx	2B (possibly carcinogenic to humans)	Mice, rats	Liver, lymphoma, leukaemia, lung, Zymbal gland, skin and clitoral gland	MeIQx binds to DNA in several tissues in rodents and induces chromosomal abnormalities; induced sister chromatid exchange in rodent cells in vitro; induced mutations in insects and in bacteria
PhIP	2B (possibly carcinogenic to humans)	Mice and rats	Lymphoma, small and large intestines, mammary glands and liver (intraperitoneal injection)	DNA adducts in vivo in rats and monkeys; DNA damage, gene mutation and chromosomal abnormalities in rodent cells in vitro; DNA damage and mutations in bacteria
Polyaromatic cyclic hydrocarbons				
Benzo[*a*]pyrene	1 (carcinogenic to humans)	Mice, rats, hamster and others	Skin, lung, forestomach, liver, lymphoreticular tissue, esophagus, tongue, upper respiratory tract, upper digestive tract and mammary glands	–

revertants/μg) or *N,N*-dimethylnitrosamine (0.23 revertants/μg), whereas the mutagenic activity of PhIP (1,800 revertants/μg) in this system was much lower *(54)*. In Big Blue® mice (BBM), the exposure to HCA (MeIQ, PhIP and AαC[3]) induced mainly mutations at G:C base pairs *(60)* with a significant sequence specificity: 5′-*GC*-3′ was the specific mutation site for MeIQ, 5′-*CGT*-3′ for AαC and G-runs for PhIP. The mouse model BBM carries approximately 40 copies of the *lacI* transgene *(76)*, which is widely used to assess spontaneous and induced mutations in *Escherichia coli* *(77)*. Following metabolic activation, HCA induces the formation of C-8 guanine base adducts, which induce genetic alterations *(54)*.

Activated PAH can readily react with DNA to form adducts, which ultimately induce mutations *(68)*. Notwithstanding the convincing evidence of the carcinogenic nature of HAC and PAH, this does not explain the marked difference between red, white and processed meats. In the EPIC-Heidelberg cohort, the median daily intake of HCA from fried chicken, turkey breast and turkey goulash (3.6 ng/d) was higher than from red meats such as beef steak or filet (1.1 ng/d), pork steak (0.8 ng/d), pork roast (0.2 ng/d) or processed meat such as Wieners *(78)*. Furthermore, rats fed a diet of cooked beef with high amounts of HCA did not show any mutations in the *p53* or *APC* genes nor any tumours *(79)*. The mutation profiles in human colorectal tumours were different from those expected following exposure to HCA or PAH *(80)*.

The exposure to HCA has been investigated using either biomarkers or dietary records. In a Swedish cohort, increased exposure to HCA was associated with lower age, overweight, sedentary lifestyle and smoking with a total average daily intake from all sources of 583 ng for women and 821 ng for men *(81)*. These levels of exposure are lower, but still comparable to the exposure observed in the United States with approximately 11–18 ng/kg/d *(82)*. In contrast, HCA intake from meat in the EPIC-Heidelberg cohort was much lower, with an average intake of 69 ng/d *(78)*.

The effect of HCA and PAH exposures on cancer has also been investigated. For example, the risk for post-menopausal breast cancer was found to be increased in women consuming the most grilled or barbecued meat (OR: 1.47; CI = 1.12–1.92 for highest vs. lowest tertile of intake), suggesting an effect of HCA and PAH *(83)*. Similarly, the intake of HCA and PAH from prepared meat was shown to be associated with an increased risk for pancreatic cancer (OR and 95% CI for each compound: PhIP, 1.8 (1.0–3.1); DiMeIQx, 2.0 (1.2–3.5); MeIQx, 1.5 (0.9–2.7) and B(*a*)P, 2.2 (1.2–4.0)) *(84)* and colorectal cancer and adenomas (OR and 95% CI for each compound: PhIP, 2.5 (1.1–5.5); DiMeIQx 2.2 (1.2–4.1) and MeIQx 2.1 (1.0–4.3)) *(85)*. In a sigmoidoscopy-based case–control study, an increased risk of large adenoma (6% per 10 ng of benzo[*a*]pyrene) was found, equivalent to 29% per 10 g of barbecued meat *(86)*. For lung cancer, a risk increase of 6% and 9% was found for each 10 g consumption of red and fried meats, respectively *(87)*. Whereas these studies relied on databases to estimate the exposure to HCA and PAH, detection of PhIP DNA adducts in pancreatic tissue was also associated with increased cancer risk (OR: 3.4; 95% CI: 1.5–7.5) *(88)*. However, other studies have

---

[3] 2-Amino-9*H*-pyrido[*2,3-b*]indole.

not reported significant associations between exposure to HCA and cancer risk *(89)* or explained differences in cancer risk between red and processed meats.

5. TOTALITY OF THE EVIDENCE

The evidence available from epidemiological studies, intervention studies and in vitro models clearly suggests that red and processed meats, but not white meat such as poultry, increase the risk for certain types of cancer, in particular colorectal and lung cancer, with an estimated risk increase of 29% per 100 g red meat and 21% per 50 g processed meat *(5)*. However, the mechanisms linking the consumption of meat to the development of cancer are still unclear; Fig. 5 shows a summary of the mechanisms that may explain how meat and protein consumptions influence cancer risk. Although environmental mutagens such as HCA and PAH are known to be potent carcinogens, the exposure to these agents alone does not explain the observed differences in cancer

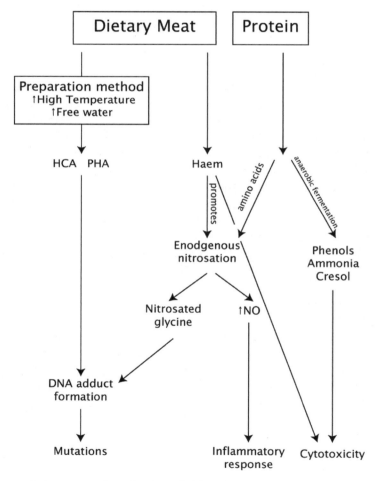

Fig. 5. Summary of the proposed mechanisms linking dietary meat and protein to cancer risk, in particular colorectal cancer.

risk between red and white meats. *N*-nitroso compounds are found in the colon and are formed endogenously because amines and amides are produced by bacterial decarboxylation of amino acids in the large gut *(46)*. The procarcinogenic and cytotoxic effects of heme have been shown in several in vitro and diet intervention studies, both as cytotoxic compound itself and in promoting endogenous nitrosation. Nevertheless, data from epidemiological studies are not sufficient to evaluate the effects of heme in larger populations because of lack of biomarkers of exposure. It is noteworthy that the intake of 60 g/d of red meat did not elevate endogenous NOC production above levels endogenously formed in the absence of any meat in the diet *(46)*.

6. FUTURE RESEARCH DIRECTIONS

Although the association between increased cancer risk and high consumption of red and processed meats has been documented *(3)*, the mechanisms responsible for this association remain elusive. Several plausible hypotheses have been proposed, but results have been inconclusive and in some instances contradicting. For example, it is unclear whether or not heterocyclic amines or heme can act as direct cytotoxic agents. To make recommendations that go beyond reducing meat intake, future research should focus on elucidating the mechanisms linking cancer incidence and meat consumption. If successful, these investigations may provide new strategies to attenuate the risk of cancer. Because studies have documented the DNA adduct-inducing effects of red meat *(38)*, future dietary intervention studies with large cohorts should investigate the meat-induced formation of DNA adducts. Furthermore, the development of a suitable urinary or serum biomarker for endogenous nitrosation may help explaining the effects of exposure to endogenously formed nitroso compounds. In general, the development of better biomarkers to assess exposure to potential carcinogens is crucial to advance the field of meat-related carcinogenicity *(90)*.

Information on dietary strategies that may attenuate meat-induced carcinogenesis is lacking. Epidemiological studies have shown that changes in anaerobic fermentation related to dietary fiber can exert protective effects against meat-induced risk for colorectal cancer *(13, 91)*. A plausible explanation is that hydroxyl groups in fiber may scavenge nitrosating species and thus prevent the endogenous formation of nitroso compounds. This protective effect of dietary fiber awaits further investigation. Another potentially protective class of compounds is flavonoids which may reduce meat-induced cancer risk by antagonizing endogenous nitrosation *(92)*; however, this effect has only been described in in vitro studies and should be investigated in clinical trials.

7. CONCLUSIONS AND RECOMMENDATIONS FOR INTAKE/DIETARY CHANGES

The data available allow an estimate of a risk increase for colorectal cancer of 29% per 100 g of red meat and 21% per 50 g of processed meat; however, similar data are not available for other cancer sites. Using available epidemiological evidence, the WCRF recommended that meat intake should be reduced to an average of 300 g per week with as little intake of processed meat as possible *(5)*. Meat should be prepared carefully to avoid the formation of carcinogens such as HCA and PAH. The formation of these compounds can be avoided by using lower cooking temperatures and changing the concentration of carcinogenic precursors by marinating or reducing the amount of available water. An effective way to reduce the production of carcinogens during cooking may be using starch to absorb water or coating of foods with breadcrumbs *(59)*. Although the cancer risks associated with high intake levels of red and processed meats are clearly established, experimental evidence suggests that meat consumption should be reduced substantially, rather than eliminated from the diet altogether. This change in dietary habit may have general applicability, but is of particular importance for those populations who are at higher risk of developing colorectal cancer.

REFERENCES

1. Food & Agriculture Organization of the United Nations (FAO) (2005) FAO Statistical Yearbook: Food & Agriculture Organization of the United Nations (FAO).
2. Speedy, A.W. (2003) Global production and consumption of animal source foods. *J Nut* **133**, 4048S–53S.
3. Armstrong, B., and Doll, R. (1975) Environmental factors and cancer incidence and mortality in different countries, with special reference to dietary practices. *Int J Cancer* **15**, 617–31.
4. Cross, A.J., Leitzmann, M.F., Gail, M.H., Hollenbeck, A.R., Schatzkin, A., and Sinha, R. (2007) A prospective study of red and processed meat intake in relation to cancer risk. *PLoS Med* **4**, 1973–84.
5. World Cancer Research Fund/American Institute for Cancer Research (2007) Food, Nutrition, Physical Activity, and the Prevention of Cancer: A Global Perspective. Washington, DC: AICR.
6. Larsson, S.C., and Wolk, A. (2006) Meat consumption and risk of colorectal cancer: A meta-analysis of prospective studies. *Int J Cancer* **119**, 2657–64.
7. Rolon, P.A., Castellsague, X., Benz, M., and Munoz, N. (1995) Hot and cold mate drinking and esophageal cancer in Paraguay. *Cancer Epidemiol Biomarkers Prev* **4**, 595–605.
8. De Stefani, E., Deneo-Pellegrini, H., Mendilaharsu, M., and Ronco, A. (1999) Diet and risk of cancer of the upper aerodigestive tract–I. Foods. *Oral Oncology* **35**, 17–21.
9. De Stefani, E., Deneo-Pellegrini, H., Ronco, A.L. et al. (2003) Food groups and risk of squamous cell carcinoma of the esophagus: A case-control study in Uruguay. *Br J Cancer* **89**, 1209–14.
10. Breslow, R.A., Graubard, B.I., Sinha, R., and Subar, A.F. (2000) Diet and lung cancer mortality: A 1987 National Health Interview Survey cohort study. *Cancer Causes Control* **11**, 419–31.
11. Khan, M.M., Goto, R., Kobayashi, K. et al. (2004) Dietary habits and cancer mortality among middle aged and older Japanese living in hokkaido, Japan by cancer site and sex. *Asian Pac J Cancer Prev* **5**, 58–65.
12. Zheng, W., Kushi, L.H., Potter, J.D. et al. (1995) Dietary intake of energy and animal foods and endometrial cancer incidence. The Iowa Women's Health Study. *Am J Epidemiol* **142**, 388–94.
13. Norat, T., Bingham, S., Ferrari, P. et al. (2005) Meat, fish, and colorectal cancer risk: The European prospective investigation into cancer and nutrition. *J Natl Cancer Inst* **97**, 906–16.
14. Sesink, A.L., Termont, D.S., Kleibeuker, J.H., and Van der Meer, R. (1999) Red meat and colon cancer: The cytotoxic and hyperproliferative effects of dietary heme. *Cancer Res* **59**, 5704–09.
15. Kirschnerzilber, I., Rabizadeh, E., and Shaklai, N. (1982) The interaction of hemin and bilirubin with the human red-cell membrane. *Biochim Biophys Acta* **690**, 20–30.
16. Rosenberg, D.W., and Kappas, A. (1989) Characterization of heme oxygenase in the small intestinal epithelium. *Arch Biochem Biophys* **274**, 471–80.
17. Everse, J., and Hsia, N. (1997) The toxicities of native and modified hemoglobins. *Free Radic Biol Med* **22**, 1075–99.
18. Kuhnle, G.G.C., Story, G.W., Reda, T. et al. (2007) Diet-induced endogenous formation of nitroso compounds. *Free Radic Biol Med* **43**, 1040–47.

19. Glei, M., Klenow, S., Sauer, J., Wegewitz, U., Richter, K., and Pool-Zobel, B.L. (2006) Hemoglobin and hemin induce DNA damage in human colon tumor cells HT29 clone 19A and in primary human colonocytes. *Mutat Res* **594**, 162–71.
20. Schwartz, S., and Ellefson, M. (1985) Quantitative fecal recovery of ingested hemoglobin-heme in blood: Comparisons by HemoQuant assay with ingested meat and fish. *Gastroenterology* **89**, 19–26.
21. Lee, D.-H., Anderson, K.E., Harnack, L.J., Folsom, A.R., and Jacobs, D.R., Jr. (2004) Heme iron, zinc, alcohol consumption, and colon cancer: Iowa women's health study. *J Natl Cancer Inst* **96**, 403–07.
22. Balder, H.F., Vogel, J., Jansen, M.C.J.F. et al. (2006) Heme and chlorophyll intake and risk of colorectal cancer in the Netherlands cohort study. *Cancer Epidemiol Biomarkers Prev* **15**, 717–25.
23. Kabat, G.C., Miller, A.B., Jain, M., and Rohan, T.E. (2007) A cohort study of dietary iron and heme iron intake and risk of colorectal cancer in women. *Br J Cancer* **97**, 118–22.
24. Kabat, G.C., Miller, A.B., Jain, M., and Rohan, T.E. (2007) Dietary iron and heme iron intake and risk of breast cancer: A prospective cohort study. *Cancer Epidemiol Biomarkers Prev* **16**, 1306–08.
25. Kabat, G.C., Miller, A.B., Jain, M., and Rohan, T.E. (2008) Dietary iron and haem iron intake and risk of endometrial cancer: A prospective cohort study. *Br J Cancer* **98**, 194–98.
26. Cross, A.J., Pollock, J.R.A., and Bingham, S.A. (2003) Haem, not protein or inorganic iron, is responsible for endogenous intestinal N-nitrosation arising from red meat. *Cancer Res* **63**, 2358–60.
27. Magee, P.N., and Barnes, J.M. (1956) The production of malignant primary hepatic tumours in the rat by feeding dimethylnitrosamine. *Br J Cancer* **10**, 114–22.
28. Sharma, V.S., Traylor, T.G., Gardiner, R., and Mizukami, H. (1987) Reaction of nitric oxide with heme proteins and model compounds of hemoglobin. *Biochemistry* **26**, 3837–43.
29. Bonnett, R., Charalambides, A.A., Martin, R.A., Sales, K.D., and Fitzsimmons, B.W. (1975) Reactions of nitrous acid and nitric oxide with porphyrins and haems. Nitrosylhaems as nitrosating agents. *J Chem Soc Chem Commun* 884–5.
30. Butler, A.R., and Rhodes, P. (1997) Chemistry, analysis, and biological roles of S-nitrosothiols. *Anal Biochem* **249**, 1–9.
31. Al-Kaabi, S.S., Williams, D.L.H., Bonnett, R., and Ooi, S.L. (1982) A kinetic investigation of the thionitrite from (±)-2-Acetylamino-2-carboxy-1,1-dimethylethanethiol as a possible nitrosating agent. *J Chem Soc, Perkin Trans* **2**, Physical Organic Chemistry: Physical Organic Chemistry, 227–30.
32. Yang, C.S., Smith, T., Ishizaki, H., and Hong, J.Y. (1991) Enzyme mechanisms in the metabolism of nitrosamines. *IARC Sci Publ* **105**, 265–74.
33. Saffhill, R., Margison, G.P., and O'Connor, P.J. (1985) Mechanisms of carcinogenesis induced by alkylating agents. *Biochim Biophys Acta* **823**, 111–45.
34. Harrison, K.L., Fairhurst, N., Challis, B.C., and Shuker, D.E. (1997) Synthesis, characterization, and immunochemical detection of O6-(carboxymethyl)-2'-deoxyguanosine: A DNA adduct formed by nitrosated glycine derivatives. *Chem ResToxicol* **10**, 652–9.
35. Bos, J.L. (1989) ras oncogenes in human cancer: A review. *Cancer Res* **49**, 4682–9.
36. Cupid, B.C., Zeng, Z., Singh, R., and Shuker, D.E.G. (2004) Detection of O6-carboxymethyl-2'-deoxyguanosine in DNA following reaction of nitric oxide with glycine and in human blood DNA using a quantitative immunoslot blot assay. *Chem Res Toxicol* **17**, 294–300.
37. Shuker, D.E., and Margison, G.P. (1997) Nitrosated glycine derivatives as a potential source of O6-methylguanine in DNA. *Cancer Res* **57**, 366–9.
38. Lewin, M.H., Bailey, N., Bandaletova, T. et al. (2006) Red meat enhances the colonic formation of the DNA adduct O6-carboxymethyl guanine: Implications for colorectal cancer risk. *Cancer Res* **66**, 1859–65.
39. Gottschalg, E., Scott, G.B., Burns, P.A., and Shuker, D.E. (2006) Potassium diazoacetate-induced p53 mutations in vitro in relation to formation of O6-carboxymethyl- and O6-methyl-2'-deoxyguanosine DNA adducts – relevance for gastrointestinal cancer. *Carcinogenesis* **28**(2): 356–362.
40. Wallace, J.L., and Miller, M.J.S. (2000) Nitric oxide in mucosal defense: A little goes a long way. *Gastroenterology* **119**, 512–20.
41. Martin, G.R., and Wallace, J.L. (2006) Gastrointestinal inflammation: A central component of mucosal defense and repair. *Exp Biol Med* **231**, 130–7.

42. Reinders, C.I., Jonkers, D., Jansson, E.Å., Stockbrügger, R.W., Stobberingh, E.E., and Hellström, P.M. (2007) Rectal nitric oxide and fecal calprotectin in inflammatory bowel disease. *Scand J Gastroenterol* **42**, 1151–7.

43. Bengmark, S. (2007) Bioecological control of inflammatory bowel disease. *Clin Nutr* **26**, 169–81.

44. Sawa, T., and Ohshima, H. (2006) Nitrative DNA damage in inflammation and its possible role in carcinogenesis. *Nitric Oxide* **14**, 91–100.

45. International Agency for Research on Cancer (IARC) (2007) Smokeless Tobacco and Some Tobacco-Specific N-nitrosamines. Lyon: World Health Organization, International Agency for Research on Cancer.

46. Bingham, S.A., Hughes, R., and Cross, A.J. (2002) Effect of white versus red meat on endogenous N-nitrosation in the human colon and further evidence of a dose response. *J Nutr Biochem* **132**, 3522S–5S.

47. Hughes, R., Cross, A.J., Pollock, J.R., and Bingham, S. (2001) Dose-dependent effect of dietary meat on endogenous colonic N-nitrosation. *Carcinogenesis* **22**, 199–202.

48. Silvester, K.R., Bingham, S.A., Pollock, J.R., Cummings, J.H., and O'Neill, I.K. (1997) Effect of meat and resistant starch on fecal excretion of apparent N-nitroso compounds and ammonia from the human large bowel. *Nutr Cancer* **29**, 13–23.

49. Bingham, S.A., Pignatelli, B., Pollock, J.R. et al. (1996) Does increased endogenous formation of N-nitroso compounds in the human colon explain the association between red meat and colon cancer? *Carcinogenesis* **17**, 515–23.

50. Lunn, J.C., Kuhnle, G.G.C., Frankenfeld, C. et al. (2007) The effect of haem in red and processed meat on the effect of N-nitroso compounds in the upper gastrointestinal tract. *Carcinogenesis* **28**, 685–90.

51. Rieger, M.A., Parlesak, A., Pool-Zobel, B.L., Rechkemmer, G., and Bode, C. (1999) A diet high in fat and meat but low in dietary fiber increases the genotoxic potential of 'faecal water'. *Carcinogenesis* **20**, 2311–6.

52. Cross, A.J., Greetham, H.L., Pollock, J.R., Rowland, I.R., and Bingham, S.A. (2006) Variability in fecal water genotoxicity, determined using the Comet assay, is independent of endogenous N-nitroso compound formation attributed to red meat consumption. *Environ Mol Mutagen* **47**, 179–84.

53. Jakszyn, P., Bingham, S., Pera, G. et al. (2006) Endogenous versus exogenous exposure to N-nitroso compounds and gastric cancer risk in the European Prospective Investigation into Cancer and Nutrition (EPIC-EURGAST) study. *Carcinogenesis* **27**, 1497–501.

54. Sugimura, T. (1997) Overview of carcinogenic heterocyclic amines. *Mutat Res* **376**, 211–9.

55. Phillips, D.H. (1999) Polycyclic aromatic hydrocarbons in the diet. *Mutat Res* **443**, 139–47.

56. Wakabayashi, K., and Sugimura, T. (1998) Heterocyclic amines formed in the diet: Carcinogenicity and its modulation by dietary factors. *J Nutr Biochem* **9**, 604–12.

57. Sinha, R., Rothman, N., Brown, E.D. et al. (1994) Pan-fried meat containing high levels of heterocyclic aromatic amines but low levels of polycyclic aromatic hydrocarbons induces cytochrome P4501A2 activity in humans. *Cancer Res* **54**, 6154–9.

58. Maillard, L.C. (1912) Action des acides aminés sur les sucres: Formation des mélanoïdines par voie méthodique. *C R Acad Sci* **154**, 66–8.

59. Skog, K.I., Johansson, M.A.E., and Jägerstad, M.I. (1998) Carcinogenic heterocyclic amines in model systems and cooked foods: A review on formation, occurrence and intake. *Food Chem Toxicol* **36**, 879–6.

60. Okonogi, H., Ushijima, T., Zhang, X.B. et al. (1997) Agreement of mutational characteristics of heterocyclic amines in lacI of the Big Blue mouse with those in tumor related genes in rodents. *Carcinogenesis* **18**, 745–8.

61. Ishidate, M, Jr., Sofuni, T., and Yoshikawa, K. (1981) Chromosomal aberration tests in vitro as a primary screening tool for environmental mutagens and/or carcinogens. *GANN Monogr Cancer Res* **27**, 95–108.

62. Tohda, H., Oikawa, A., Kawachi, T., and Sugimura, T. (1980) Induction of sister-chromatid exchanges by mutagens from amino acid and protein pyrolysates. *Mutat Res* **77**, 65–9.

63. Ushiyama, H., Wakabayashi, K., Hirose, M., Itoh, H., Sugimura, T., and Nagao, M. (1991) Presence of carcinogenic heterocyclic amines in urine of healthy-volunteers eating normal diet, but not of inpatients receiving parenteral-alimentation. *Carcinogenesis* **12**, 1417–22.

64. Friesen, M.D., Kaderlik, K., Lin, D.X. et al. (1994) Analysis of DNA-adducts of 2-Amino-1-methyl-6-phenylimidazo[4,5-B]pyridine in rat and human tissues by alkaline-hydrolysis and gas-chromatography electron-capture mass-spectrometry – validation by comparison with P-32 postlabeling. *Chem Res Toxicol* **7**, 733–9.

65. Totsuka, Y., Fukutome, K., Takahashi, M. et al. (1996) Presence of N-2-(deoxyguanosin-8-yl)-2-amino-3,8-demethylimidazo [4,5-f]quinoxaline (dG-C8-MeIQx) in human tissues. *Carcinogenesis* **17**, 1029–34.

66. Hieger, I.L.V.I.I.I. (1930) The spectra of cancer-producing tars and oils and of related substances. *Biochem J* **24**, 505–11.

67. Cook, J.W., Hewett, C., and Hieger, I. (1932) Coal tar constituents and cancer. *Nature* **130**, 926.

68. Jacob, J. (1996) The significance of polycyclic aromatic hydrocarbons as environmental carcinogens. *Pure Appl Chem* **68**, 301–8.

69. Pott, P. (1775) Chirurgical Observations Relative to the Cataract, the Polypus of the Nose, the Cancer of the Scrotum, the Different Kinds of Ruptures and the Mortifications of the Toes and Feet. London: Haves, Clarke and Collins.

70. Wickstrom, K., Pyysalo, H., Plaami-Heikkila, S., and Tuominen, J. (1986) Polycyclic aromatic compounds (PAC) in leaf lettuce. *Zeitschrift für Lebensmittel-Untersuchung und -Forschung* **183**, 182–5.

71. Grasso, P. (1984) Carcinogens in food. In: Searle, C.E., ed. Chemical Carcinogens. Washington, DC: American Chemical Society.

72. Gomaa, E.A., Gray, J.I., Rabie, S., Lopez-Bote, C., and Booren, A.M. (1993) Polycyclic aromatic hydrocarbons in smoked food products and commercial smoke flavourings. *Food Addit Contam* **10**, 503–21.

73. Panalaks, T. (1976) Determination and identification of polycyclic aromatic hydrocarbons in smoked and charcoal-broiled food products by high pressure liquid chromatography and gas chromatography. *J Environ Sci Health Part B* **11**, 299–315.

74. International Agency for Research on Cancer (IARC) (1993) Some naturally occurring substances: Food items and constituents, heterocyclic aromatic amines and mycotoxins. Lyon: World Health Organization, International Agency for Research on Cancer.

75. International Agency for Research on Cancer (IARC) (2008) Air Pollution, Part 1, Some Non-heterocyclic Polycyclic Aromatic Hydrocarbons and Some Related Industrial Exposures. Lyon: World Health Organization, International Agency for Research on Cancer.

76. Kohler, S.W., Provost, G.S., Fieck, A. et al. (1991) Spectra of spontaneous and mutagen-induced mutations in the laci Gene in transgenic mice. *Proc Natl Acad Sci U S A* **88**, 7958–62.

77. Horsfall, M.J., and Glickman, B.W. (1989) Mutational specificities of environmental carcinogens in the laci gene of escherichia-coli .1. The direct-acting analog N-nitroso-N-methyl-N-alpha-acetoxymethylamine. *Carcinogenesis* **10**, 817–22.

78. Rohrmann, S., Zoller, D., Hermann, S., and Linseisen, J. (2007) Intake of heterocyclic aromatic amines from meat in the European Prospective Investigation into Cancer and Nutrition (EPIC)-Heidelberg cohort. *Br J Nutr* **98**, 1112–5.

79. Shen, C.L., Purwal, M., San Francisco, S., and Pence, B.C. (1998) Absence of PhIP adducts, p53 and APC mutations, in rats fed a cooked beef diet containing a high level of heterocyclic amines. *Nutr Cancer* **30**, 227–31.

80. Kinzler, K.W., and Vogelstein, B. (1996) Lessons from hereditary colorectal cancer. *Cell* **87**, 159–70.

81. Ericson, U., Wirfalt, E., Mattisson, I., Gullberg, B., and Skog, K.I. (2007) Dietary intake of heterocyclic amines in relation to socio-economic, lifestyle and other dietary factors: Estimates in a Swedish population. *Publ Health Nutr* **10**, 616–27.

82. Keating, G.A., and Bogen, K.T. (2004) Estimates of heterocyclic amine intake in the US population. *J Chromatogr B: Biomed Appl* **802**, 127–33.

83. Steck, S.E., Gaudet, M.M., Eng, S.M. et al. (2007) Cooked meat and risk of breast cancer-lifetime versus recent dietary intake. *Epidemiology* **18**, 373–82.

84. Anderson, K.E., Kadlubar, F.F., Kulldorff, M. et al. (2005) Dietary Intake of Heterocyclic Amines and Benzo(a)Pyrene: Associations with Pancreatic Cancer. *Cancer Epidemiol Biomarkers Prev* **14**, 2261–5.

85. Sinha, R., Kulldorff, M., Chow, W.-H., Denobile, J., and Rothman, N. (2001) Dietary intake of heterocyclic amines, meat-derived mutagenic activity, and risk of colorectal adenomas. *Cancer Epidemiol Biomarkers Prev* **10**, 559–62.

86. Gunter, M.J., Probst-Hensch, N.M., Cortessis, V.K., Kulldorff, M., Haile, R.W., and Sinha, R. (2005) Meat intake, cooking-related mutagens and risk of colorectal adenoma in a sigmoidoscopy-based case-control study. *Carcinogenesis* **26**, 637–42.

87. Sinha, R., Kulldorff, M., Curtin, J., Brown, C.C., Alavanja, M.C.R., and Swanson, C.A. (1998) Fried, well-done red meat and risk of lung cancer in women (United States). *Cancer Causes Control* **9**, 621–30.

88. Zhu, J., Rashid, A., Cleary, K. et al. (2008) Detection of 2-amino-1-methyl-6-phenylimidazo [4,5-b]-pyridine (PhIP)-DNA adducts in human pancreatic tissues. *Biomarkers* **11**, 319–28.

89. Augustsson, K., Skog, K.I., Jagerstad, M., Dickman, P.W., and Steineck, G. (1999) Dietary heterocyclic amines and cancer of the colon, rectum, bladder, and kidney: A population based study. *Lancet* **353**, 604–12.

90. Cross, A.J., and Sinha, R. (2004) Meat-related mutagens/carcinogens in the etiology of colorectal cancer. *Environ Mol Mutagen* **44**, 44–55.

91. Le Leu, R., and Young, G.P. (2007) Fermentation of starch and protein in the colon. *Cancer Biol Ther* **6**, 259–60.

92. Lee, S.Y., Munerol, B., Pollard, S.E. et al. (2006) The reaction of flavanols with nitrous acid protects against N-nitrosamine formation and leads to the formation of nitroso derivatives which inhibit cancer cell growth. *Free Radic Biol Med* **40**, 323–34.

93. Phillips, R.L. (1975) Role of life-style and dietary habits in risk of cancer among seventh-day adventists. *Cancer Res* **35**, 3513–22.

94. Wei, H., Bowen, R., Cai, Q., Barnes, S., and Wang, Y. (1995) Antioxidant and antipromotional effects of the soybean isoflavone genistein. *Proc Soc Exp Biol Med* **208**, 124–30.

95. Kato, I., Akhmedkhanov, A., Koenig, K., Toniolo, P.G., Shore, R.E., and Riboli, E. (1997) Prospective study of diet and female colorectal cancer: The New York university women's health study. *Nutr Canc* **28**, 276–81.

96. Singh, P.N., and Fraser, G.E. (1998) Dietary risk factors for colon cancer in a low-risk population. *Am J Epidemiol* **148**, 761–74.

97. Pietinen, P., Malila, N., Virtanen, M. et al. (1999) Diet and risk of colorectal cancer in a cohort of Finnish men. *Cancer Causes Control* **10**, 387–96.

98. Järvinen, R., Knekt, P., Hakulinen, T., Rissanen, H., and Heliövaara, M. (2001) Dietary fat, cholesterol and colorectal cancer in a prospective study. *Br J Cancer* **85**, 357–61.

99. Tiemersma, E.W., Kampman, E., Bueno de Mesquita, H.B. et al. (2002) Meat consumption, cigarette smoking, and genetic susceptibility in the etiology of colorectal cancer: Results from a Dutch prospective study. *Cancer Causes Control* **13**, 383–93.

100. Slattery, M.L., Levin, T.R., Ma, K., Goldgar, D., Holubkov, R., and Edwards, S. (2003) Family history and colorectal cancer: Predictors of risk. *Cancer Causes Control* **14**, 879–87.

101. English, D.R., MacInnis, R.J., Hodge, A.M., Hopper, J.L., Haydon, A.M., and Giles, G.G. (2004) Red meat, chicken, and fish consumption and risk of colorectal cancer. *Cancer Epidemiol Biomarkers Prev* **13**, 1509–14.

102. Larsson, S.E., Rafter, J., Holmberg, L., Bergkvist, L., and Wolk, A. (2005) Red meat consumption and risk of cancers of the proximal colon, distal colon and rectum: The Swedish Mammography Cohort. *Int J Cancer* **113**, 829–34.

11 Saturated Fatty Acids and Cancer

Michele R. Forman and Somdat Mahabir

Key Points

1. Saturated fatty acids are a class of lipids that have a unique feature of no double bonds along the carbon chain due to the full saturation of the carbon atoms. Saturated fatty acids (SFAs) can have a chain length of 2–20 carbons and are referred to as short, medium, or long-chain SFAs. Short-chain SFAs contain 2–8 carbons in length, whereas long-chain SFAs contain 16–20 carbons in length.
2. Total SFA intake in the USA accounts for approximately 12% of energy intake. Several expert nutrition committees and USDA recommend that Americans consume less than 10% of calories from saturated fats.
3. Saturated fatty acids are found in the diet and can be synthesized de novo by the enzyme, fatty acid synthase (FAS). FAS is an important phenotype for many cancers and produces the SFA, palmitic acid, an energy source in tumor cells. However, in contrast with most SFAs, butyrate is a bioactive dietary component and product of colonic fermentation of dietary fibers that has chemopreventive potential for colon and other cancers.
4. Increased levels of FAS in tumor tissues relative to normal tissues have been reported in cancers of the lung, prostate, breast, ovary, endometrium, colon, and bladder. Development of FAS or Spot 14 inhibitors combined with dietary modulation of SFA intake may offer new opportunities in cancer prevention.
5. An important consideration regarding research on SFAs and cancer is the capacity of SFA to become desaturated. SFAs from lauric acid (C12:0) to stearic (C18:0) can be converted to its respective monounsaturated product through the action of $\Delta 9$-destaurase (stearoyl-CoA desaturase) with varying efficiency, which may have more down-stream effects. Thus, the inter-relationships between SFAs and other fatty acids are likely fundamental for understanding their role in carcinogenesis.

Key Words: Saturated fatty acids (SFAs); fatty acid synthase (FAS); palmitic acid; butyrate; epidemiology; cancer

1. SATURATED FATTY ACIDS AND CANCER

Fatty acids are a class of lipids consisting of three elements: carbon (C), hydrogen (H), and oxygen (O) arranged as a carboxyl group at one end. They are classified based on length of the carbon chain; whether or not there are any double bonds; the number of double bonds and their location relative to the carboxylic acid (COOH) end of the chain; and the geometric structure. In general, fatty acids have a carboxylic acid with

From: *Nutrition and Health: Bioactive Compounds and Cancer*
Edited by: J.A. Milner, D.F. Romagnolo, DOI 10.1007/978-1-60761-627-6_11,
© Springer Science+Business Media, LLC 2010

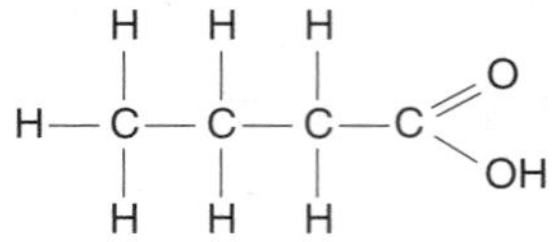

Fig. 1. Structural formula for butyric acid.

an unbranched carbon chain, classified either as *saturated fatty acids* (SFAs) or *unsaturated fatty acids*. The unique feature of SFAs is that they do not contain any double bonds along the single linkage carbon chain. This is because the carbon atoms that comprise the fatty acid chain are fully saturated with hydrogen atoms (Fig. 1). SFAs range from 2 to 20 or more carbons in length, and depending on the number of carbon atoms, they are referred to as short- or long-chain SFAs. In contrast, the unsaturated fatty acids are classified further as either monounsaturated (MUFA = one double bond) or polyunsaturated (PUFA = more than one double bond) (Table 1).

Table 1
Chemical Structure and Abbreviation for Saturated Fatty Acids

Saturated fatty acids	Chemical structure	Abbreviation
Butyric	$CH_3(CH_2)_2COOH$	C4:0
Caproic	$CH_3(CH_2)_4COOH$	C6:0
Caprylic	$CH_3(CH_2)_6COOH$	C8:0
Capric	$CH_3(CH_2)_8COOH$	C10:0
Lauric	$CH_3(CH_2)_{10}COOH$	C12:0
Myristic	$CH_3(CH_2)_{12}COOH$	C14:0
Palmitic	$CH_3(CH_2)_{14}COOH$	C16:0
Stearic	$CH_3(CH_2)_{16}COOH$	C18:0
Arachidic	$CH_3(CH_2)_{18}COOH$	C20:0

1.1. Sources of Dietary Saturated Fatty Acids

On average, SFAs account for 30–40% of fatty acids in animal tissues, with the main SFA being palmitic (15–25%), stearic (10–20%), myristic (0.5–1%), and lauric acid (<0.5%) *(1)*. Palmitic acid is the most common SFA in the human diet and the major one that is synthesized de novo *(2)*. Sources rich in stearic acid are animal fat and cocoa butter. Sources of myristic acid are milk fat and coconut. Coconut and palm kernel are excellent sources of lauric acid. Milk fat is a good source of several other SFAs *(2)*. Therefore, dietary fat composition affects availability, storage, and metabolism of SFA and partly influences fatty acid composition in cells, plasma, serum, and tissues.

1.2. De Novo Synthesis of Saturated Fatty Acids

While SFAs are part of the dietary supply in both plant- and animal-based foods, they are non-essential nutrients because they can be synthesized de novo. However, both dietary fatty acids and fatty acids synthesized de novo are necessary for normal physiological and cellular functions in humans. Fatty acid synthase (FAS) is an important enzyme that synthesizes fatty acids de novo *(3)*. In addition, Spot 14, originally identified as a protein induced by the action of thyroid hormones, is an important regulator of de novo synthesis of fatty acids *(4)*. Therefore, in addition to dietary sources, fatty acid composition in cells, body fluids, and tissues is influenced by the activity of FAS, Spot 14, and possibly other molecular factors.

1.3. Rationale

The total SFA intake in the USA accounts for approximately 12% of energy intake *(5, 6)*. Several expert nutrition committees and the USDA recommend that Americans consume less than 10% of calories from saturated fats *(7)*. In 1999–2000, only 41% of the USA population (≥ 2 years of age) met the recommendation for saturated fat *(5)*. In 2006, the American Heart Association amended its guidelines to reduce intake of saturated fat to less than 7% of energy intake *(8)*.

Epidemiological studies of SFA intake and cancer report inconsistent findings. The interpretation of these data is complicated by methodological issues. First, measurement errors related to the use of different questionnaires and incomplete values for total SFAs and specific fatty acids in food databases are an important problem. Second, discussion of the relative contribution of endogenous de novo synthesis of specific SFAs to cancer is lacking. Therefore, for cancer prevention, an important strategy might be modification of the type and amount of dietary fat consumed as well as approaches aimed at regulating the de novo synthesis of fatty acids. Development of FAS or Spot 14 inhibitors combined with dietary modulation of SFA intake may offer new opportunities in cancer prevention. New strategies should also consider the impact of genetic variants in regulation of fatty acid pathways *(3)*.

2. REVIEW OF THE EVIDENCE

2.1. SFA in Tumors

The enzyme FAS, which catalyzes the de novo synthesis of fatty acids, is strongly expressed in many cancers and has emerged as a phenotype common to most human cancers *(3, 9)*. Increased levels of FAS in tumor tissues relative to normal tissues have been reported in cancers of the lung *(10, 11)*, prostate *(12, 13)*, breast *(14, 15)*, ovary *(16)*, endometrium *(17)*, colon *(18)*, and bladder *(19)*. In human breast tumors, expression of Spot 14 is a marker of aggressive breast cancer *(20, 21)*. Thus, regulators of de novo fatty acid synthesis such as FAS and Spot 14 represent potential therapeutic targets in cancer prevention.

2.2. Cell Culture Studies

The major product of FAS in cancer cells is palmitic acid (C16:0), a SFA *(9)*; however, the fate of palmitic acid in tumor cells is unknown. Because inhibition of FAS kills cancer cells *(9)*, agents that inhibit FAS may be useful in cancer prevention. Cerulenin, a natural antifungal antibiotic, inhibits FAS and growth in human breast carcinoma cells *(22)*. In contrast, supraphysiologic levels of palmitic acid reverse the action of cerulenin, confirming that the antiproliferative effects of cerulenin are due to FAS inhibition *(22)*. Additionally, palmitic, stearic, and myristic acid inhibit adriamycin (a chemotherapeutic drug) – induced upregulation of p21, Bax, and p53 in response to DNA damage, while inhibition of FAS enhances these cellular events *(23)*. Myristic and palmitic acid are inducers of mammary cell differentiation *(24)*. In contrast, stearic and myristic acid induce apoptosis in HL-60 human leukemia cells, but the degree of induction of apoptosis is less than that seen for unsaturated fatty acids *(25)*.

Palmitic and lauric acid are potent inducers of COX-2 expression in murine macrophage-like cells *(26)*. The overexpression of COX-2 is observed in several tumor tissue and is associated with a proinflammatory response. Palmitic and lauric acids induce iNOS and IL-1α (both proinflammatory markers) in a dose-dependent manner *(26)*. Lauric acid activates NF$_K$B in a dose-dependent manner *(26)*.

An enzyme that is important in FA homeostasis is acetyl-CoA carboxylase (ACC), which catalyzes the carboxylation of acetyl-CoA to malonyl-CoA, a product that serves as a substrate for fatty acid synthesis. Inhibition of AAC activity reduced proliferation and survival of prostate cancer cells (LNCaP); however, the addition of palmitic acid to the culture medium completely abolishes the effect of ACC inhibition and prevents cell death *(27)*. An in vitro study with human breast (MCF-7, MDA-MB-231) and prostate (LNCaP) cancer cells reported that silencing of the ACC isoform α (ACCα) or FAS genes decreased the synthesis of palmitic acid. This was associated with the induction of apoptosis and ROS production, whereas the addition of palmitic acid or vitamin E to the culture medium completely prevented cell death *(28)*. These studies provided evidence that cancer cells are dependent on ACC activity, which is a rate-limiting enzyme for the synthesis of fatty acids necessary for proliferation and survival.

Besides palmitic acid, butyric acid has been studied extensively in cell culture studies of colonic carcinogenesis because it is both a bioactive dietary component and a product of microbial colonic fermentation of dietary fibers *(29)*. Colonic generation of butyrate is regarded as a mechanism by which dietary fiber protects against colon cancer. It has also been reported that butyrate treatment of colon cancer cells in vitro induces the Wnt signaling pathway which is associated with increased level of apoptosis *(29)*. Also, butyrate induces apoptosis in colorectal cancer cell lines *(30)*. In another study, butyrate enhanced toxicological defense in primary human colon tissue, premalignant LT97 adenoma, and human colon tumor cells by upregulating GSTs (GSTA2 and GSTT2) known to enhance the defense against oxidative stress *(31)*. These cell culture studies suggest butyrate may have protective effects against colon cancer, but contrast with the inconsistent epidemiologic findings related to the role of dietary fiber in the etiology of colon cancer. This discrepancy might be partly explained by different subtypes of colon cancer in which butyrate may differentially affect the induction of Wnt signaling pathway *(29)* or glutathione *S*-transferase genes *(31)*. Other factors that may modulate the effects of fiber include variations in the colonic bacteria that generate butyrate and levels of dietary butyrate.

Research on butyrate in other cancer cell lines and in vitro studies demonstrates that butyrate is not only a potent inhibitor of cellular proliferation, but is an inducer of differentiation and apoptosis. In vitro studies using rat intestinal smooth muscle cells have demonstrated that the effects of butyrate may be dose dependent. For example, low amounts of butyrate may stimulate cell proliferation while high amounts may inhibit it *(32)*. Also, butyrate had anti-inflammatory activities and downregulated HIF-1 transcriptional activity in cultured intestinal epithelial cells *(33)*. In an in vitro study of human lung carcinoma cell line (H460), butyrate inhibited proinflammatory cytokines signaling pathway and down-regulated 3 metastatic suppressors genes and 11 genes whose protein products promote metastasis *(34)*. In human MCF-7 breast cancer cells, treatment with sodium butyrate inhibited tumor growth by inducing apoptosis *(35)*. The induction of apoptosis by butyrate in the breast cancer cells was associated with down-regulation of expression of Bcl-2 mRNA and proteins. The Bcl-2 factors are involved in the regulation of apoptosis. In contrast, one study reported that butyric acid induced mammary cell differentiation *(24)*.

Butyrate has also been reported to inhibit proliferation and induce apoptosis of prostate cancer cells by altering the expression of cell cycle regulators and androgen receptor *(36)*. In bladder cancer cells, butyrate not only inhibited growth, but also enhanced the action of the anticancer drugs, cisplatin, mitomycin, and adriamycin *(37)*. Buytrate inhibited the growth of tongue cancer cells *(38)* and lymphoma cells *(39)* via the induction of cell cycle arrest and apoptosis.

One of the proposed mechanisms for the anticancer effects of butyrate is inhibition of histone deacetylase (HDAC) *(40)*. Histone deacetylation, a process that regulates chromatin remodeling, is an important epigenetic modification that controls gene expression. For example, treatment of prostate cancer cells with butyrate led to significant accumulation of acetylated histone H3 and H4 *(36)*.

3. ANIMAL STUDIES

3.1. Inhibition of FAS

Given that FAS is overexpressed in several tumors, studies have examined the effect of specific FAS inhibitors. The administration of C93, a pharmacologic inhibitor of FAS, blocked FAS activity in human lung cancer xenografts in nude mice and inhibited tumor growth without causing toxicity *(41)*. Similarly, administration of orlistat, an anti-obesity drug and pharmacologic inhibitor of FAS, antagonized the growth of prostate tumors in nude mice *(42)*. In a study of chemically induced lung cancer tumors in mice, pharmacologic inhibition of FAS was associated with reductions in both the number and size of tumors *(43)*.

3.2. Dietary Butyrate

In Sprague-Dawley rats weaned at 21 days of age and then injected with nitrosomethylurea (a mammary carcinogen) 3 days later, dietary butyrate was very effective in inhibiting mammary tumorigenesis *(44)*. The addition of 1 and 3% of butyrate to a high-fat diet containing 20% sunflower seed oil reduced tumor incidence by 20 and 52%, respectively, compared to the same diet without butyrate. In a separate study, sodium butyrate inhibited the enhancing effect of a high-margarine diet (20% margarine) on mammary tumorigenesis in rats *(45)*.

3.3. Dietary Myristic Acid

Feeding studies with *Cebus* monkeys suggested that myristic acid (14:0) was the SFA responsible for raising plasma cholesterol levels *(46)*. Similarly, dietary myristic acid was the principal SFA increasing serum cholesterol levels in humans *(47)*. Furthermore, myristic acid upregulated HMG-CoA reductase *(48)*, an enzyme important in endogenous cholesterol biosynthesis. Finally, myristic acid exerted antitumor effects against melanoma in a murine model *(49)*. These cumulative results provided excellent examples of how a nutrient consumed in trace amounts (myristic acid accounts for 0.5–1% of SFA intake) may affect phenotypic responses related to metabolism and cancer.

3.4. Coconut Fat

Coconut fat is rich in medium-chain SFA. In a study with female Wistar rats *(50)*, dams were supplemented daily with either coconut fat or fish oil (rich in *n*–3 PUFA) at a dose of 1 g/kg body weight as a single bolus orally prior to mating, and then throughout pregnancy and gestation. In the F2 generation at 90 days of age, 50% of the male offspring were inoculated with Walker 256 tumor cells and cancer cachexia was assessed. Fish oil, but not coconut fat supplementation, decreased cancer cachexia. A separate study investigated in rat mammary tumor model the effects of fatty acid supplementation on *N*-nitrosomethylurea-induced mammary tumor. Results documented that the incidence of mammary tumors in rats fed coconut oil, high lard, high-beef tallow, high corn oil, and low corn oil, after 28 weeks of treatment, was 43, 65, 50, 35, and 33%, respectively *(51)*. These data demonstrated that high dietary fat intake increased mammary carcinogenesis, but the type of fat modified the susceptibility to chemical carcinogenesis.

4. EPIDEMIOLOGIC STUDIES

In this section, we summarize the results of epidemiological studies that investigated how intake of SFA or specific SFA-containing food sources influences the risk of cancer. Results are difficult to interpret because of differences in collection of data for body mass, dietary fat and energy intakes, and energy expenditure across studies. These factors may confound the estimated risk for many cancers and make it difficult to separate the effects of SFAs from other dietary and lifestyle factors. We discuss the impact of "Western" diets, how dietary pattern analysis may assist in the detection of associations, use of dietary tools, and the impact of time interval for reporting food intake. Most dietary data discussed in this chapter were collected from either food frequency questionnaires (FFQ) or dietary history. However, interpretation of these data is difficult due to culture-specific food composition database, differences in distribution and availability of macro- and micro-nutrient intakes across geographical areas within and outside the USA. Nevertheless, diet–cancer meta-analyses may provide an opportunity to review the individual and aggregated estimates of risk taking into account heterogeneity, sample size, and confounding factors. Response rates may vary by study design, with different participation rates among control and case participants providing a source of bias. Taken together, care should be exercised to eliminate or reduce inaccurate dietary data collection methods which may bias the estimated risk of cancer *(52)*.

4.1. Endometrial Cancer (EC)

In a review *(53)* of research up to December 2006, case–control data suggested an increased risk of EC for SFA intake, but cohort data were insufficient to determine a significant association. Using random-effects models in a meta-analysis, the summary estimates for the odds ratio (OR) of EC in case–control studies was 1.28 (95% CI 1.12, 1.47) per 10 g/1,000 kcal of SFAs. A recent US population-based case–control study of 500 EC patients and 470 controls suggested a null association *(54)*. A Chinese population-based case–control study identified an elevated risk of EC for intakes of SFA and MUFA from animal protein intake but not for PUFA *(55)*. In an Italian hospital-based case–control study, diet–EC associations were explored for oleic, SAF, and PUFA *(56)*. Compared to those subjects in the lowest quintile of intake, participants in the highest quintile had a 2.1 higher odds of EC for cholesterol intake and a non-significant 30% higher odds for SFA *(56)*. Thus additional data, particularly from prospective studies, are needed before conclusions can be drawn regarding associations between intake of SFA and incidence of EC.

4.2. Ovarian Cancer (OC)

In a pooled analysis of 12 cohort studies that had 523,217 women including 2,132 OC patients, the summary risk estimate for SFA intake was 1.29 (95% CI 1.01, 1.66) for those women in the highest versus lowest deciles of intake *(57)*. No differences were found when the analysis was stratified by histological subtype of ovarian cancer. In a 2004 review of dietary foods high in fat and OC risk, the evidence for red meat was suggestive of increased risk based on 11 case–control studies and 3 of 4 cohort studies *(58)*. Yet it is noteworthy that the risk estimates in the cohort studies were not significant but above unity in all 11 case–control studies and moderate to strongly significant in 5 of these 11 studies. Of 7 studies that examined milk intake by fat content, 2 of 7 studies had significantly increased risk of OC for full-fat milk and 3 of these had an inverse association for low-fat or skim milk. Two of 3 studies of butter consumption were directly and significantly associated with risk and 1 Chinese study identified an increased risk for OC with animal fat intake (lard) *(58)*. Thus, future research on dietary intakes of SFA, meat, and dairy by fat content, and OC risk may help to shed light in this field.

4.3. Breast Cancer (BC)

In a meta-analysis of research through July, 2003 on SFA intake and BC risk, the summary estimator adjusted for total energy intake revealed a direct association with values of 1.19 (95% CI 1.06, 1.35) for all studies, 1.23 (95% CI 1.03, 1.46) for 23 case–control studies, and 1.15 (95% CI 1.02, 1.30) for 12 cohort studies *(59)*. Among the 37 studies (25 case–control, 12 cohort studies) that examined food sources rich in SFA and BC risk, the summary estimator was 1.21 (95% CI 0.98, 1.49).

In July 2003, Bingham et al. reported on the same women participants in the EPIC-Norfolk study, the hazard ratios (HR) for SFA and BC were 1.22 (95% CI 1.06, 1.40) based on 7-day food diaries and 1.10 (95% CI 0.94. 1.29) based on the FFQ (60). Both analyses were adjusted for non-fat energy, and the HR was significant across the third, fourth, and fifth quintiles of intake using food diary data. In other cohort studies, SFA was directly associated with HR of BC in the AARP Diet and Health Study cohort (61), but not associated with BC risk in the Swedish Women's Lifestyle and Health cohort study (62) and the Japan Collaborative Cohort (JACC) study (63). In an analysis of food sources and BC risk in the Malmo Diet and Cancer cohort, women consuming a high fiber–low fat diet had the lowest risk compared to those on a high fat–low fiber diet (64). Finally in a recent population-based case–control study, a positive association between oleic acid intake and BC risk was observed (65).

Higher levels of serum palmitic and stearic acids were associated with increased BC risk in nested case–control studies (66, 67). In a meta-analysis of biomarkers of dietary fatty acid intake and BC risk, levels of oleic and palmitic acid were significantly associated with risk, while total SFA was associated with risk in cohort studies of postmenopausal women only (68). In an analysis of data from the E3N-EPIC study, BC risk was associated with increasing levels of *trans*-monounsaturated fatty acids but not palmitoleic acid or other SFAs (69). Compared to estimated dietary intake, the use of biomarkers offers objective and qualitative measures in assessing the relationships between SFA and BC risk.

4.4. Prostate Cancer

The intake of SFAs is not associated with prostate cancer risk across multiple cohort studies (70–73). In Japanese men, prostate cancer rates are typically lower than the USA or Europe. Interestingly, in a Japanese cohort including 329 cancer patients, the intake of myristic and palmitic acid were associated with 1.62 (1.15, 2.29) and 1.53 (1.07, 2.20) higher risk of developing prostate cancer (74). Also in one cohort study (75) and one case–case comparison (76), SFA intake was associated with increased risk of advanced (stages C and D) cancer. In contrast, some case–control studies documented a direct association between intake of SFAs and prostate cancer risk (77, 78) while others did not (76, 79). Food sources of SFAs like meat and dairy products have not been consistently associated with prostate cancer risk (80–83). Among prostate cancer patients, the ratio of oleic to stearic acid *in the prostate* (84, 85) and SFA intake (86) predict biochemical failure (PSA $\geq$ 0.1 ng/ml) after prostatectomy or cancer recurrence, respectively. Two studies identified a 3.0-fold higher risk of dying from prostate cancer among men in the highest tertile of SFA intake compared to those men in the lowest (87, 88).

4.5. Pancreatic Cancer

The role of SFAs or food sources rich in SFAs in the etiology of pancreatic cancer and related mortality has been studied for more than 20 years. In an article on the epidemiology of pancreatic cancer (89), Ghadirian et al. reported positive associations for pancreatic cancer with dietary intake of oil and fat *(90–92)*, intake of meat and diary products *(93)*, and intake of fried foods *(94, 95)*. Several case–control studies identified energy balance as an important factor influencing risk of pancreatic cancer because both obesity and total energy intake, but not SFA intake, are directly related to the risk *(96)*. In studies conducted in Athens, Greece, the intake of PUFA was directly associated with risk of pancreatic cancer *(97)*. Interestingly, the use of proxy respondents due to the short survival of patients after diagnosis *(98, 99)* may be a source of bias when estimating associations between dietary history and risk of pancreatic cancer.

The Nurses' Health Study I, among whom 178 pancreatic cancer patients were diagnosed, reported no association between intake of meat or SFA and risk of pancreatic cancer, but the influence of cooking practices was highlighted as a potential area for further research *(100)*. In the Alpha-Tocopherol, Beta-Carotene (ATBC) Trial, among whom 163 of the male smokers developed pancreatic cancer, energy-adjusted SFA intakes were positively associated with pancreatic cancer (HR = 1.60, 95% CI 0.96, 2.64 (*P* for trend = 0.02)) *(101)*. A Japanese cohort study did not identify an association between meat intake and risk *(102)*, but the Swedish mammography cohort identified that red meat intake was directly related to risk (RR = 1.73, 95% CI 0.99, 2.98) *(103)*. Recent population-based case–control research identified an association with an OR of 1.9 (95% CI 1.4, 2.6) for SFA in the USA *(104)*. In a case–case comparison of diet and K-*ras* mutations, patients with the mutation who were daily consumers of milk and dairy products, but not meat, were at 5.0-fold higher risk than non-mutation carriers *(105)*. Finally, recent papers that examined dietary mutagen exposure from meat cookery and pancreatic cancer risk supported the hypothesis that meat intake, particularly meat cooked at high temperatures where heterocyclic amines (HCA) are produced, may play a role in pancreatic cancer development *(106, 107)*. Therefore, it may be difficult to separate the effects of SFA intake from those of HCA on risk of pancreatic cancer.

4.6. Colorectal Cancers (CRC)

Since the publication of the 1969 case–control study of Wynder and colleagues *(108)* suggesting that dietary fat was associated with CRC, numerous epidemiologic studies have examined the role of total fat intake in development of CRC. Nevertheless, only a few studies have examined the role of specific fatty acids. Japanese hospital-based *(109, 110)* and Scottish population-based *(111)* case–control studies reported a positive association between CRC and total SFAs intake; however, these findings were not observed in other case–control *(112)* or cohort studies *(113)*. Erythrocyte fatty acids, notably palmitic, total SFAs, and the ratio of SFA/PUFA were directly associated with CRC in the Japanese case–control study *(109)* but further research is required to test the association. A number of studies have examined the role of SFAs and gene variants of *APC, K-ras*, and *PPAR gamma*, with the magnitude of the interaction dependent on the frequency of gene variants and dietary SFA intake *(111, 114–116)*. Future research related to colon cancer should focus on interactions between molecular variants of the APC gene and diet *(115, 116)*; how the proportion of conjugated linoleic acid (CLA) versus SFAs in fatty and lean meats affect the risk *(117)*; and the role of heme proteins and nitrite from meat intake *(118)*.

4.7. Gastric and Esophageal Cancers

Population-based case–control studies on SFAs and risk of gastric and esophageal cancers reported dietary cholesterol, total fat, or SFAs may influence cancer risk. Dietary fat was associated with an OR of 2.18 (95% CI 1.27, 3.76) for esophageal cancer in one study (119). SFA intake was associated with OR of 1.0, 4.1, and 4.6 by tertile of intake for esophageal cancer and OR of 1.0, 1.2, 3.6 by tertile of intake for distal stomach cancer (120). When SFA was categorized in quartiles of intake, SFA intake in the highest quartile was associated with an OR of 4.37 (95% CI 1.89, 10.12) for distal gastric cancer in Mexico (121). In a Chinese-based case–control study, men, but not women, in the highest quartile of SFA intake had an OR of 3.24 (95% CI 1.11, 9.49) (122). Dietary fat intake was not associated with gastric cancer risk in a population-based case–control study in Spain (123) and in China (124). In hospital-based case–control studies, dietary fat intake was directly associated with increased risk of esophageal and gastric cardia cancers in the USA (125). Dietary SFA intake was directly associated with risk of gastric cancer in France (126), but null findings were obtained in Italy, Belgium, and Korea (127–129). In a 2006 meta-analysis of the association of processed meat consumption and stomach cancer risk, intake of processed meat (30 g/d (i.e., approximately ½ portion)) was associated with a RR of 1.15 (95% CI 1.04, 1.27) based on six cohort studies and with a RR of 1.38 (95% CI 1.19, 1.60) based on nine case–control studies (130). Too few studies have stratified analysis by anatomic site or histological subtype to examine the meat–gastric cancer associations by sub-group. Analysis of data from the EPIC cohort revealed an association between total meat and red meat (both calibrated as gram/day) with gastric noncardia cancer. In a nested case–control study, only participants with *H. pylori* infections experienced an increased risk from meat intake (131). In a Swedish population based case–control study, a high score on a "Western" diet was associated with increased risk of gastric cardia, not noncardia, cancer (OR = 1.8, 95% CI 1.1, 2.9) (132). A recent Canadian study reported that those who consumed a "Western" diet (soft drinks, processed meats, refined grains, and sugars) were at increased risk of gastric adenocarcinoma (OR = 1.86 ,95% CI 1.20, 2.89 in women; OR = 1. 44 (95% CI 1.03, 2.02 in men) (133). Further, evidence exists that socioeconomic status may be inversely associated with risk of gastric cardia cancer (134). Therefore, estimates of risk that are not adjusted for social position may not have detected a possible association.

4.8. Lung Cancer (LC)

In a 2002 pooled analysis of eight prospective cohort studies (N = 280,419 women and 149,862 men and 3,188 LC), no association was observed for LC and SFA (RR = 1.03, 95% CI 0.96, 1.11) before and after stratification by smoking status (135). In an earlier cohort study in New York State, SFA intake was directly associated with LC risk in a monotonic dose–response (P for trend = 0.01) for men, but not for women (136). In contrast, case–control data from a study in Uruguay revealed associations between SFA intake and adenocarcinoma of the lung (OR = 2.3, 95% CI 1.2, 4.4) (137). A monotonic dose–response between quintiles of SFA intake and LC risk was observed in lifetime nonsmokers and former female smokers in Missouri (OR = 5.3, 2.8, 1.9, 1.5; P, 0.001) (138).

Foods rich in SFAs have been examined in association with LC risk. Intake of red meat including pork was associated with elevated risk of squamous cell carcinoma *(139, 140)*, all LC incidence *(140–144)* and mortality *(145)*; whereas null associations appear in two studies *(146, 147)*. Red meat intake is neither significantly associated with histological type of LC nor by smoking status except in current smokers *(144)*. The associations between smoked and cured meat intake and LC incidence *(148, 149)* and mortality *(145)* were null in some studies, but elevated in others *(146)*. Total meat intake was associated with no *(146, 150, 151)* or elevated risk *(146)*. Dairy products were associated with reduced risk of adenocarcinoma *(140)*, all LC in women *(152, 153)*, and LC mortality *(145)*, but were not significant for all LC *(139)* and for squamous cell carcinoma *(140)*. In other studies, cheese intake was protective of LC incidence and mortality *(145, 146, 149, 150, 152)*; while whole milk was associated with elevated risk *(141, 152)*, protective of LC *(149, 154)*, or the association was null *(145, 146, 148)*. Low fat and skim milks were protective of LC mortality, but the estimates were not significant *(145)*. Yogurt was protective of LC risk *(149)* or elevated risk that did not reach significance *(155)*. Fatty foods were associated with LC risk in a case–control study in Uruguay *(156)* but not in Czechoslovakia *(140)*.

4.9. Head and Neck Cancers

The majority of studies that investigated the effects of dietary SFAs or food sources of SFAs on the incidence of head and neck cancers are designed as case–control studies with hospital-based controls. Foods rich in animal fat and SFAs such as pork meat and fried foods are associated with risk of oral cancer in Brazil *(157)*, Italy *(158, 159)*, Switzerland *(160)*, Spain *(161)*, and Uruguay *(162)*. Using the population data obtained from the Italian study *(159)*, dietary SFA intakes were directly associated with risk of oral and pharyngeal cancers in smokers *(163)* and in never smokers *(164)*. In another analysis of the same Italian study, SFA was positively associated with risk in contrast to monounsaturated fatty acids which were negatively associated with risk of oral and pharyngeal cancers *(165)*.

In one population-based case–control study, low intake of butter and preserved meats were associated with reduced risk of laryngeal cancers *(166)*. Diets associated with reduced risk included a high PUFA/SFA ratio *(166)*. Furthermore, a socioeconomic difference was revealed by cancer site where endolaryngeal cancers tended to occur more frequently among the higher SES, while the reverse was true for hypopharyngeal and epilaryngeal cancers *(167)*. Thus the absence of many population-based case–control and cohort studies of diet and head and neck cancers as well as the inability to disaggregate the effects of other components such as nitrosamines in the same food sources hamper progress in assessing the role of SFA in the etiology of head and neck cancers.

5. SUMMARY OF EVIDENCE

SFAs play a crucial role in the etiology and pathogenesis of several cancers. A major product of FAS is the SFA, palmitic acid. In cell culture studies, pharmacological inhibition of FAS activity induced death of cancer cells. Palmitic and lauric acid are potent inducers of pro-inflammatory responses associated with cancer development. In contrast, butyric acid may exert preventive effects against cancer.

Extensive cell culture data on butyrate and colon cancer consistently show that butyric acid may inhibit cell proliferation, increase apoptosis, and protect against oxidative stress. Similar results have been reported for breast, lung, bladder, and prostate cells. Nevertheless, epidemiological studies have not clearly demonstrated whether cancer dietary SFAs influence cancer risk. Also, it remains unclear whether the potential association between intake of processed, red, or total meat and incidence of gastric, esophageal, and colon cancers relates to fat intake or other components found in meats including salt used in the curative processing or presence of nitrosamines originated during the cooking process.

6. CONCLUSIONS AND RECOMMENDATIONS AND FUTURE RESEARCH DIRECTIONS

Sorting the effects of SFAs on cancer risk are complicated because the pool of SFAs available to cells comprises dietary fatty acids and those synthesized de novo. In addition, studies should take into account the role of genetic polymorphisms related to metabolism of SFAs. Epidemiological studies should assess the levels of SFAs in serum, plasma, and cell membranes in an effort to estimate the relative contribution of dietary and de novo SFAs. Epidemiological studies should integrate investigations with preclinical models. For example, there is a need for a comprehensive evaluation of different forms of SFAs to chemical-induced tumors in animals representing a spectrum of ages and both sexes.

There is emerging evidence that SFAs in the diet or synthesized de novo may alter/modulate molecular mechanisms relevant to carcinogenesis such as signaling pathways and gene expression. Elucidating the mechanisms by which SFAs regulate and/or are regulated by signaling pathways, gene expression, and inflammatory response will further our understanding of the etiology of SFAs in cancer, other chronic diseases, and inflammatory conditions. Another important consideration regarding research on SFAs and cancer is the capacity of SFAs to become desaturated. SFAs from lauric acid (C12:0) to stearic (C18:0) can be converted to its respective monounsaturated product through the action of $\Delta 9$-destaurase (stearoyl-CoA desaturase) with varying efficiency *(1)*, which may have more down-stream effects. Thus, the inter-relationships between SFAs and other fatty acids are likely fundamental for understanding their role in carcinogenesis.

In terms of cancer therapy, current evidence suggests that the fatty acid and lipogenic pathways may be targets for antineoplastic therapy due to the cross-talk of different types of FA and triglycerides. Future research should also address specific dietary recommendations for fatty acid intake among patients undergoing chemotherapeutic regimens.

REFERENCES

1. Rioux, V., and Legrand, P. (2007) Saturated fatty acids: Simple molecular structures with complex cellular functions. *Curr Opin Clin Nutr Metab Care* **10**, 752–58.
2. Dupont, J. (2006) Basic lipidology. In: Moffatt, R.J. and Stamford, B., eds. *Lipid Metabolism and Health*. Boca Raton, FL: Taylor & Francis.

3. Kridel, S., Lowther, W., and Pemble, C. (2007) Fatty acid synthase inhibitors: New directions for oncology. *Expert Opin Investig Drugs* **16**, 1817–29.

4. Young, C., and Anderson, S. (2008) Sugar and fat – that's where it's at: Metabolic changes in tumors. *Breast Cancer Res* **10**, (doi:10.1186/bcr1852).

5. Briefel, R., and Johnson, C. (2004) Secular trends in dietary intake in the United States. *Annu Rev Nutr* **24**, 401–31.

6. Allison, D., Egan, K., Barraj, L., Caughman, C., Infante, M., and Heimbach, J. (1999) Estimated intakes of trans fatty and other fatty acids in the US population. *J Am Diet Assoc* **99**, 166–74.

7. USDHSS. Dietary guidelines for Americans. (2005) US Department of Agriculture, US Government Printing office. Washington, DC.

8. Lichtenstein, A., Appel, L., Brands, M., Carnethon, M., Daniels, S., Franch, H., Franklin, B., Kris-Etherton, P., Harris, W., Howard, B., Karanja, N., Lefevre, M., Rudel, L., Sacks, F., Van Horn, L., Winston, M., and Wylie-Rosett, J. (2006) Diet and lifestyle recommendations revision 2006: A scientific statement from the American Heart Association Nutrition Committee. *Circulation* **114**, 82–96.

9. Kuhajda, F. (2007) Fatty acid synthase and cancer: New application of an old pathway. *Cancer Res* **66**, 5977–80.

10. Visca, P., Sebastiani, V., Botti, C., Diodoro, M., Lasagni, R., Romagnoli, F., Brenna, A., De Joannon, B., Donnorso, R., Lombardi, G., and Alo, P. (2004) Fatty acid synthase (FAS) is a marker of increased risk of recurrence in lung carcinoma. *Anticancer Res* **24**, 6.

11. Piyathilake, C., Frost, A., Manne, U., Bell, W., Weiss, H., Heimburger, D., and Grizzle, W. (2000) The expression of fatty acid synthase (FASE) is an early event in the development and progression of squamous cell carcinoma of the lung. *Hum Pathol* **31**, 1068–73.

12. Swinnen, J., Roskams, T., Joniau, S., Van Poppel, H., Oyen, R., Baert, L., Heyns, W., and Verhoeven, G. (2002) Overexpression of fatty acid synthase is an early and common event in the development of prostate cancer. *Int J Cancer* **98**, 19–22.

13. Rossi, S., Graner, E., Febbo, P., Weinstein, L., Bhattacharya, N., Onody, T., Bubley, G., Balk, S., and Loda, M. (2003) Fatty acid synthase expression defines distinct molecular signatures in prostate cancer. *Mol Cancer Res* **1**, 707–15.

14. Milgraum, L., Witters, L., Pasternack, G., and Kuhajda, F. (1997) Enzymes of the fatty acid synthesis pathway are highly expressed in in situ breast carcinoma. *Clin Cancer Res* **3**, 2115–20.

15. Nakamura, I., Kimijima, I., Zhang, G., Onogi, H., Endo, Y., Suzuki, S., Tuchiya, A., Takenoshita, S., Kusakabe, T., and Suzuki, T. (1999) Fatty acid synthase expression in Japanese breast carcinoma patients. *Int J Mol Med* **4**, 381–87.

16. Gansler, T., Hardman, W.R., Hunt, D., Schaffel, S., and Hennigar, R. (1997) Increased expression of fatty acid synthase (OA-519) in ovarian neoplasms predicts shorter survival. *Hum Pathol* **28**, 686–92.

17. Sebastiani, V., Visca, P., Botti, C., Santeusanio, G., Galati, G., Piccini, V., Capezzone de Joannon, B., Di Tondo, U., and Alo, P. (2004) Fatty acid synthase is a marker of increased risk of recurrence in endometrial carcinoma. *Gynecol Oncol* **92**, 101–05.

18. Notarnicola, M., Altomare, D., Calvani, M., Orlando, A., Bifulco, M., D'Attoma, B., and Caruso, M. (2006) Fatty acid synthase hyperactivation in human colorectal cancer: Relationship with tumor side and sex. *Oncology* **71**, 327–32.

19. Visca, P., Sebastiani, V., Pizer, E., Botti, C., De Carli, P., Filippi, S., Monaco, S., and Alo, P. (2003) Immunohistochemical expression and prognostic significance of FAS and GLUT1 in bladder carcinoma. *Anticancer Res* **23**, 335–39.

20. Wells, W., Schwartz, G., Morganelli, P., Cole, B., Gibson, J., and Kinlaw, W. (2006) Expression of "Spot 14" (THRSP) predicts disease free survival in invasive breast cancer: Immunohistochemical analysis of a new molecular marker. *Breast Cancer Res Treat* **98**, 231–40.

21. Kinlaw, W., Quinn, J., Wells, W., Roser-Jones, C., and Moncur, J. (2006) Spot 14: A marker of aggressive breast cancer and a potential therapeutic target. *Endocrinology* **147**, 4048.

22. Kuhajda, F., Jenner, K., Wood, F., Hennigar, R., Jacobs, L., Dick, J., and Pasternack, G. (1994) Fatty acid synthesis: A potential selective target for antineoplastic therapy. *Proc Natl Acad Sci U S A* **91**, 6379–83.

23. Zeng, L., Wu, G., Goh, K., Lee, Y., Ng, C., You, A., Wang, J., Jia, D., Hao, A., Yu, Q., and Li, B. (2008) Saturated fatty acids modulate cell response to DNA damage: Implication for their role in tumorigenesis. *PLoS ONE* **3**, e2329.

24. Dulbecco, R., Bologna, M., and Unger, M. (1980) Control of differentiation of a mammary cell line by lipids. *Proc Natl Acad Sci U S A* **77**, 1551–55.

25. Jung, K., Park, C., Hwang, Y., Rhee, H., Lee, J., Kim, H.-K., and Yang, C. (2006) Fatty acids, inhibitors for DNA binding of c-Myc/Max dimer, suppress proliferation and induce apoptosis of differentiated HL-60 human leukemia cell. *Leukemia* **20**, 122–27.

26. Lee, J., Sohn, K., Rhee, S., and Hwang, D. (2001) Saturated fatty acids, but not unsaturated fatty acids, induce the expression of cyclooxygenase-2 mediated through toll-like receptor 4. *J Biol Chem* **276**, 1663–89.

27. Beckers, A., Organe, S., Timmermans, L., Scheys, K., Peeters, A., Brusselmans, K., Verhoeven, G., and Swinnen, J. (2007) Chemical inhibition of acetyl-CoA carboxylase induces growth arrest and cytoxicity selectively in cancer cells. *Cancer Res* **67**, 8180–87.

28. Chajes, V., Cambot, M., Moreau, K., Lenoir, G., and Joulin, V. (2006) Acetyl-CoA carboxylase α is essential to breast cancer cell survival. *Cancer Res* **66**, 5287–94.

29. Bordonaro, M., Lazarova, D., and Sartorelli, A. (2008) Butyrate and wnt signalling. *Cell Cycle* **9**, 1178–83.

30. Hague, A., and Paraskeva, C. (1995) The short-chain fatty caid butyrate induces apoptosis in colorectal tumor cell lines. *Eur J Cancer Prev* **4**, 359–64.

31. Pool-Zobel, H., Selvaraju, V., Sauer, J., Kautenburger, T., Kiefer, J., Richter, K., Soom, M., and Wolfl, S. (2005) Butyrate may enhance toxicological defence in primary, adenoma and tumor human colon cells by favourably modulating expression of glutathione S-transferases genes, an approach in nutrigenomics. *Carcinogenesis* **26**, 1064–76.

32. Le Blay, G., Blottière, H., Ferrier, L., Le Foll, E., Bonnet, C., Galmiche, J., and Cherbut, C. (2000) Short-chain fatty acids induce cytoskeletal and extracellular protein modifications associated with modulation of proliferation on primary culture of rat intestinal smooth muscle cells. *Dig Dis Sci* **45**, 1623–30.

33. Miki, K., Unno, N., Nagata, T., Uchijima, M., Konno, H., Koide, Y., and Nakamura, S. (2004) Butyrate suppresses hypoxia-inducible factor-1 activity in intestinal epithelial cells under hypoxic conditions. *Shock* **22**, 446–52.

34. Joseph, J., Mudduluru, G., Antony, S., Vashistha, S., Ajitkumar, P., and Somasundaram, K. (2004) Expression profiling of sodium butyrate (NaB)-treated cells: Identification of regulation of genes related to cytokine signaling and cancer metastasis by NaB. *Oncogene* **23**, 6304.

35. Mandal, M., and Kumar, R. (1996) Bcl-2 expression regulates sodium butyrate-induced apoptosis in human MCF-7 breast cells. *Cell Growth Differ* **7**, 311–19.

36. Kim, J., Park, H., Im, J., Choi, W., and Kim, H.S. (2007) Sodium butyrate regulates androgen receptor expression and cell cycle arrest in human prostate cancer cells. *Anticancer Res* **27**, 3285–92.

37. Wang, D., Wang, Z., Tian, B., Li, X., Li, S., and Tian, Y. (2008) Two hour exposure to sodium butyrate sensitizes bladder cancer to anticancer drugs. *Int J Urol* **15**, 435–41.

38. Jeng, J.-H., Kuo, M.Y.-P., Lee, P.-H., Wang, Y.-J., Lee, M.-Y., Lee, J.-J., Lin, B.-R., Tai, T.-F., and Chang, M.-C. (2006) Toxic and metabolic effect of sodium butyrate on SAS tongue cancer cells: Role of cell cycle deregulation and redox changes. *Toxicol* **223**, 235–47.

39. Wang, Y.-F., Chen, N.-S., Chung, Y.-P., Chang, L.-H., Chiou, Y.-H., and Chen, C.-Y. (2006) Sodium buytrate induces apoptosis and cell cycle arrest in primary effusion lymphoma cells independently of oxidative stress and p21$^{CIP1/WAG1}$ induction. *Molec Cell Biochem* **285**, 51–59.

40. Dashwood, R., Myzak, M., and Ho, E. (2006) Dietary HDAC inhibitors: Time to rethink weak ligands in cancer chemoprevention. *Carcinogenesis* **27**, 344–49.

41. Orita, H., Coulter, J., Lemmon, C., Tully, E., Vadlamudi, A., Medghalchi, S., Kuhajda, F., and Gabrielson, E. (2007) Selective inhibition of fatty acid synthase for lung cancer treatment. *Clin Cancer Res* **13**, 7139–45.

42. Kridel, S., Axelrod, F., Rozenkrantz, N., and Smith, J. (2004) Orlistat is a novel inhibitor of fatty acid synthase with antitumor activity. *Cancer Res* **64**, 2070–75.

43. Orita, H., Coulter, J., Tully, E., Kuhajda, F., and Gabrielson, E. (2008) Inhibiting fatty acid synthase for chemoprevention of chemically induced lung tumors. *Clin Cancer Res* **14**, 2458–64.

44. Belobrajdic, D., and McIntosh, G. (2000) Dietary butyrate inhibits NMU-induced mammary cancer in rats. *Nutr Cancer* **36**, 217–23.

45. Yanagi, S., Yamashita, M., and Imai, H. (1993) Sodium butyrate inhibits the enhancing effect of high fat diet on mammary tumorigenesis. *Oncology* **50**, 201–04.

46. Hayes, K., and Khosla, P. (1992) Dietary fatty acid thresholds and cholesterolemia. *FASEB J* **6**, 2600–07.

47. Hegsted, D., McGandy, R., Myers, M., and Stare, F. (1965) Quantitative effects of dietary fat on serum cholesterol in man. *Am J Clin Nutr* **17**, 281–95.

48. Garcia-Pelayo, M., Garcia-Peregrin, E., and Martinez-Cayuela, M. (2004) Differential translational effects of myristic acid and eicosapentaenoic acid on 3-hydroxyl-3-methylglutaryl-CoA reducatase from Reuber H35 hepatoma cells. *Exp Biol Med* **228**, 781–86.

49. Galdiero, F., Carratelli, C., Nuzzo, I., Bentivoglio, C., De Martino, L., Gorga, F., Folgore, A., and Galdiero, M. (1994) Beneficial effects of myristic, stearic or oleic acid as part of liposomes on experimental infection and antitumor effect in a murine model. *Life Sci* **55**,

50. Folador, A., Hirabara, S., Bonatto, S., Aikawa, J., and Yamazaki, R. (2006) Effect of fish oil supplementation for 2 generations on changes in macrophage function induced by Walker 256 cancer cachexia in rats. *Int J Cancer* **120**, 344–50.

51. Chan, P.-C., Ferguson, K., and Dao, T. (1983) Effects of dietary fats on mammary carcinogenesis. *Cancer Res* **43**, 1079–83.

52. Kipnis, V., Midthune, D., Freedman, L., Bingham, S., Day, N.E., Riboli, E., Ferrari, P., and Carroll, R.J. (2002) Bias in dietary-report instruments and its implications for nutritional epidemiology. *Public Health Nutr* **5**, 915–23.

53. Bandera, E.V., Kushi, L.H., Moore, D.F., Gifkins, D.M., and McCullough, M.L. (2007) Dietary lipids and endometrial cancer: The current epidemiologic evidence. *Cancer Causes Control* **18**, 687–703.

54. Dalvi, T.B., Canchola, A.J., and Horn-Ross, P.L. (2007) Dietary patterns, Mediterranean diet, and endometrial cancer risk. *Cancer Causes Control* **18**, 957–66.

55. Xu, W.H., Dai, Q., Xiang, Y.B., Zhao, G.M., Ruan, Z.X., Cheng, J.R., Zheng, W., and Shu, X.O. (2007) Nutritional factors in relation to endometrial cancer: A report from a population-based case–control study in Shanghai, China. *Int J Cancer* **120**, 1776–81.

56. Lucenteforte, E., Talamini, R., Montella, M., Dal Maso, L., Tavani, A., Deandrea, S., Pelucchi, C., Greggi, S., Zucchetto, A., Barbone, F., Parpinel, M., Franceschi, S., La Vecchia, C., and Negri, E. (2008) Macronutrients, fatty acids and cholesterol intake and endometrial cancer. *Ann Oncol* **19**, 168–72.

57. Genkinger, J.M., Hunter, D.J., Spiegelman, D., Anderson, K.E., Beeson, W.L., Buring, J.E., Colditz, G.A., Fraser, G.E., Freudenheim, J.L., Goldbohm, R.A., Hankinson, S.E., Koenig, K.L., Larsson, S.C., Leitzmann, M., McCullough, M.L., Miller, A.B., Rodriguez, C., Rohan, T.E., Ross, J.A., Schatzkin, A., Schouten, L.J., Smit, E., Willett, W.C., Wolk, A., Zeleniuch-Jacquotte, A., Zhang, S.M., and Smith-Warner, S.A. (2006) A pooled analysis of 12 cohort studies of dietary fat, cholesterol and egg intake and ovarian cancer. *Cancer Causes Control* **17**, 273–85.

58. Schulz, M., Lahmann, P.H., Riboli, E., and Boeing, H. (2004) Dietary determinants of epithelial ovarian cancer: A review of the epidemiologic literature. *Nutr Cancer* **50**, 120–40.

59. Boyd, N.F., Stone, J., Vogt, K.N., Connelly, B.S., Martin, L.J., and Minkin, S. (2003) Dietary fat and breast cancer risk revisited: A meta-analysis of the published literature. *Br J Cancer* **89**, 1672–85.

60. Bingham, S., Luben, R., Welch, A., Wareham, N., Khaw, K., and Day, N. (2003) Are imprecise methods obscuring a relation between fat and breast cancer? *Lancet* **362**, 212–14.

61. Thiebaut, A.C., Kipnis, V., Chang, S.C., Subar, A.F., Thompson, F.E., Rosenberg, P.S., Hollenbeck, A.R., Leitzmann, M., and Schatzkin, A. (2007) Dietary fat and postmenopausal invasive breast cancer in the National Institutes of Health-AARP Diet and Health Study cohort. *J Natl Cancer Inst* **99**, 451–62.

62. Lof, M., Sandin, S., Lagiou, P., Hilakivi-Clarke, L., Trichopoulos, D., Adami, H.O., and Weiderpass, E. (2007) Dietary fat and breast cancer risk in the Swedish women's lifestyle and health cohort. *Br J Cancer* **97**, 1570–76.

63. Wakai, K., Tamakoshi, K., Date, C., Fukui, M., Suzuki, S., Lin, Y., Niwa, Y., Nishio, K., Yatsuya, H., Kondo, T., Tokudome, S., Yamamoto, A., Toyoshima, H., and Tamakoshi, A. (2005) Dietary intakes of fat and fatty acids and risk of breast cancer: A prospective study in Japan. *Cancer Sci* **96**, 590–99.

64. Mattisson, I., Wirfalt, E., Johansson, U., Gullberg, B., Olsson, H., and Berglund, G. (2004) Intakes of plant foods, fibre and fat and risk of breast cancer – a prospective study in the Malmo Diet and Cancer cohort. *Br J Cancer* **90**, 122–27.

65. Wang, J., John, E.M., Horn-Ross, P.L., and Ingles, S.A. (2008) Dietary fat, cooking fat, and breast cancer risk in a multiethnic population. *Nutr Cancer* **60**, 492–504.

66. Saadatian-Elahi, M., Toniolo, P., Ferrari, P., Goudable, J., Akhmedkhanov, A., Zeleniuch-Jacquotte, A., and Riboli, E. (2002) Serum fatty acids and risk of breast cancer in a nested case–control study of the New York University Women's Health Study. *Cancer Epidemiol Biomarkers Prev* **11**, 1353–60.

67. Chajès, V., Hultén, K., Van Kappel, A., Winkvist, A., Kaaks, R., Hallmans, G., Lenner, P., and Riboli, E. (1999) Fatty-acid composition in serum phospholipids and risk of breast cancer: An incident case–control study in Sweden. *Int J Cancer* **83**, 585–90.

68. Saadatian-Elahi, M., Norat, T., Goudable, J., and Riboli, E. (2004) Biomarkers of dietary fatty acid intake and the risk of breast cancer: A meta-analysis. *Int J Cancer* **111**, 584–91.

69. Chajes, V., Thiebaut, A.C., Rotival, M., Gauthier, E., Maillard, V., Boutron-Ruault, M.C., Joulin, V., Lenoir, G.M., and Clavel-Chapelon, F. (2008) Association between serum trans-monounsaturated fatty acids and breast cancer risk in the E3N-EPIC Study. *Am J Epidemiol* **167**, 1312–20.

70. Veierod, M.B., Laake, P., and Thelle, D.S. (1997) Dietary fat intake and risk of prostate cancer: A prospective study of 25,708 Norwegian men. *Int J Cancer* **73**, 634–38.

71. Crowe, F.L., Key, T.J., Appleby, P.N., Travis, R.C., Overvad, K., Jakobsen, M.U., Johnsen, N.F., Tjonneland, A., Linseisen, J., Rohrmann, S. et al. (2008) Dietary fat intake and risk of prostate cancer in the European Prospective Investigation into Cancer and Nutrition. *Am J Clin Nutr* **87**, 1405–13.

72. Park, S.Y., Murphy, S.P., Wilkens, L.R., Henderson, B.E., and Kolonel, L.N. (2007) Fat and meat intake and prostate cancer risk: The multiethnic cohort study. *Int J Cancer* **121**, 1339–45.

73. Schuurman, A.G., van den Brandt, P.A., Dorant, E., Brants, H.A., and Goldbohm, R.A. (1999) Association of energy and fat intake with prostate carcinoma risk: Results from The Netherlands Cohort Study. *Cancer* **86**, 1019–27.

74. Kurahashi, N., Inoue, M., Iwasaki, M., Sasazuki, S., and Tsugane, A.S. (2008) Dairy product, saturated fatty acid, and calcium intake and prostate cancer in a prospective cohort of Japanese men. *Cancer Epidemiol Biomarkers Prev* **17**, 930–37.

75. Giovannucci, E., Rimm, E.B., Colditz, G.A., Stampfer, M.J., Ascherio, A., Chute, C.C., and Willett, W.C. (1993) A prospective study of dietary fat and risk of prostate cancer. *J Natl Cancer Inst* **85**, 1571–79.

76. Bairati, I., Meyer, F., Fradet, Y., and Moore, L. (1998) Dietary fat and advanced prostate cancer. *J Urol* **159**, 1271–75.

77. De Stefani, E., Deneo-Pellegrini, H., Boffetta, P., Ronco, A., and Mendilaharsu, M. (2000) Alpha-linolenic acid and risk of prostate cancer: A case–control study in Uruguay. *Cancer Epidemiol Biomarkers Prev* **9**, 335–38.

78. Whittemore, A.S., Kolonel, L.N., Wu, A.H., John, E.M., Gallagher, R.P., Howe, G.R., Burch, J.D., Hankin, J., Dreon, D.M., West, D.W. et al. (1995) Prostate cancer in relation to diet, physical activity, and body size in blacks, whites, and Asians in the United States and Canada. *J Natl Cancer Inst* **87**, 652–61.

79. Andersson, S.O., Wolk, A., Bergstrom, R., Giovannucci, E., Lindgren, C., Baron, J., and Adami, H.O. (1996) Energy, nutrient intake and prostate cancer risk: A population-based case–control study in Sweden. *Int J Cancer* **68**, 716–22.

80. Rohrmann, S., Platz, E.A., Kavanaugh, C.J., Thuita, L., Hoffman, S.C., and Helzlsouer, K.J. (2007) Meat and dairy consumption and subsequent risk of prostate cancer in a US cohort study. *Cancer Causes Control* **18**, 41–50.

81. Allen, N.E., Key, T.J., Appleby, P.N., Travis, R.C., Roddam, A.W., Tjonneland, A., Johnsen, N.F., Overvad, K., Linseisen, J., Rohrmann, S., Boeing, H., Pischon, T., Bueno-de-Mesquita, H.B., Kiemeney, L., Tagliabue, G., Palli, D., Vineis, P., Tumino, R., Trichopoulou, A., Kassapa, C., Trichopoulos, D., Ardanaz, E., Larranaga, N., Tormo, M.J., Gonzalez, C.A., Quiros, J.R., Sanchez, M.J., Bingham, S., Khaw, K.T., Manjer, J., Berglund, G., Stattin, P., Hallmans, G., Slimani, N., Ferrari, P., Rinaldi, S., and Riboli, E. (2008) Animal foods, protein, calcium and prostate cancer risk: The European Prospective Investigation into Cancer and Nutrition. *Br J Cancer* **98**, 1574–81.

82. Michaud, D.S., Augustsson, K., Rimm, E.B., Stampfer, M.J., Willet, W.C., and Giovannucci, E. (2001) A prospective study on intake of animal products and risk of prostate cancer. *Cancer Causes Control* **12**, 557–67.

83. Rodriguez, C., McCullough, M.L., Mondul, A.M., Jacobs, E.J., Chao, A., Patel, A.V., Thun, M.J., and Calle, E.E. (2006) Meat consumption among Black and White men and risk of prostate cancer in the Cancer Prevention Study II Nutrition Cohort. *Cancer Epidemiol Biomarkers Prev* **15**, 211–16.

84. Kositsawat, J., Flanigan, R.C., Meydani, M., Choi, Y.K., and Freeman, V.L. (2007) The ratio of oleic-to-stearic acid in the prostate predicts biochemical failure after radical prostatectomy for localized prostate cancer. *J Urol* **178**, 2391–96, discussion 2396.

85. Freeman, V.L., Flanigan, R.C., and Meydani, M. (2007) Prostatic fatty acids and cancer recurrence after radical prostatectomy for early-stage prostate cancer. *Cancer Causes Control* **18**, 211–18.

86. Strom, S.S., Yamamura, Y., Forman, M.R., Pettaway, C.A., Barrera, S.L., and DiGiovanni, J. (2008) Saturated fat intake predicts biochemical failure after prostatectomy. *Int J Cancer* **122**, 2581–85.

87. Fradet, Y., Meyer, F., Bairati, I., Shadmani, R., and Moore, L. (1999) Dietary fat and prostate cancer progression and survival. *Eur Urol* **35**, 388–91.

88. Meyer, F., Bairati, I., Shadmani, R., Fradet, Y., and Moore, L. (1999) Dietary fat and prostate cancer survival. *Cancer Causes Control* **10**, 245–51.

89. Ghadirian, P., Lynch, H.T., and Krewski, D. (2003) Epidemiology of pancreatic cancer: An overview. *Cancer Detect Prev* **27**, 87–93.

90. Howe, G.R., Ghadirian, P., Bueno de Mesquita, H.B., Zatonski, W.A., Baghurst, P.A., Miller, A.B., Simard, A., Baillargeon, J., de Waard, F., Przewozniak, K. et al. (1992) A collaborative case–control study of nutrient intake and pancreatic cancer within the search programme. *Int J Cancer* **51**, 365–72.

91. Ghadirian, P., Simard, A., Baillargeon, J., Maisonneuve, P., and Boyle, P. (1991) Nutritional factors and pancreatic cancer in the francophone community in Montreal, Canada. *Int J Cancer* **47**, 1–6.

92. Ghadirian, P., Thouez, J.P., and PetitClerc, C. (1991) International comparisons of nutrition and mortality from pancreatic cancer. *Cancer Detect Prev* **15**, 357–62.

93. Falk, R.T., Pickle, L.W., Fontham, E.T., Correa, P., and Fraumeni, J.F., Jr. (1988) Life-style risk factors for pancreatic cancer in Louisiana: A case-control study. *Am J Epidemiol* **128**, 324–36.

94. Mack, T.M., Yu, M.C., Hanisch, R., and Henderson, B.E. (1986) Pancreas cancer and smoking, beverage consumption, and past medical history. *J Natl Cancer Inst* **76**, 49–60.

95. Ghadirian, P., Baillargeon, J., Simard, A., and Perret, C. (1995) Food habits and pancreatic cancer: A case-control study of the Francophone community in Montreal, Canada. *Cancer Epidemiol Biomarkers Prev* **4**, 895–99.

96. Silverman, D.T., Swanson, C.A., Gridley, G., Wacholder, S., Greenberg, R.S., Brown, L.M., Hayes, R.B., Swanson, G.M., Schoenberg, J.B., Pottern, L.M., Schwartz, A.G., Fraumeni, J.F., Jr., and Hoover, R.N. (1998) Dietary and nutritional factors and pancreatic cancer: A case-control study based on direct interviews. *J Natl Cancer Inst* **90**, 1710–19.

97. Kalapothaki, V., Tzonou, A., Hsieh, C.C., Karakatsani, A., Trichopoulou, A., Toupadaki, N., and Trichopoulos, D. (1993) Nutrient intake and cancer of the pancreas: A case-control study in Athens, Greece. *Cancer Causes Control* **4**, 383–89.

98. Lyon, J.L., Slattery, M.L., Mahoney, A.W., and Robison, L.M. (1993) Dietary intake as a risk factor for cancer of the exocrine pancreas. *Cancer Epidemiol Biomarkers Prev* **2**, 513–18.

99. Olsen, G.W., Mandel, J.S., Gibson, R.W., Wattenberg, L.W., and Schuman, L.M. (1991) Nutrients and pancreatic cancer: A population-based case-control study. *Cancer Causes Control* **2**, 291–97.

100. Michaud, D.S., Giovannucci, E., Willett, W.C., Colditz, G.A., and Fuchs, C.S. (2003) Dietary meat, dairy products, fat, and cholesterol and pancreatic cancer risk in a prospective study. *Am J Epidemiol* **157**, 1115–25.

101. Stolzenberg-Solomon, R.Z., Pietinen, P., Taylor, P.R., Virtamo, J., and Albanes, D. (2002) Prospective study of diet and pancreatic cancer in male smokers. *Am J Epidemiol* **155**, 783–92.

102. Lin, Y., Kikuchi, S., Tamakoshi, A., Yagyu, K., Obata, Y., Inaba, Y., Kurosawa, M., Kawamura, T., Motohashi, Y., and Ishibashi, T. (2006) Dietary habits and pancreatic cancer risk in a cohort of middle-aged and elderly Japanese. *Nutr Cancer* **56**, 40–49.

103. Larsson, S.C., Hakanson, N., Permert, J., and Wolk, A. (2006) Meat, fish, poultry and egg consumption in relation to risk of pancreatic cancer: A prospective study. *Int J Cancer* **118**, 2866–70.

104. Chan, J.M., Wang, F., and Holly, E.A. (2007) Pancreatic cancer, animal protein and dietary fat in a population-based study, San Francisco Bay Area, California. *Cancer Causes Control* **18**, 1153–67.

105. Morales, E., Porta, M., Vioque, J., Lopez, T., Mendez, M.A., Pumarega, J., Malats, N., Crous-Bou, M., Ngo, J., Rifa, J., Carrato, A., Guarner, L., Corominas, J.M., and Real, F.X. (2007) Food and nutrient intakes and K-ras mutations in exocrine pancreatic cancer. *J Epidemiol Community Health* **61**, 641–49.

106. Li, D., Day, R.S., Bondy, M.L., Sinha, R., Nguyen, N.T., Evans, D.B., Abbruzzese, J.L., and Hassan, M.M. (2007) Dietary mutagen exposure and risk of pancreatic cancer. *Cancer Epidemiol Biomarkers Prev* **16**, 655–61.

107. Stolzenberg-Solomon, R.Z., Cross, A.J., Silverman, D.T., Schairer, C., Thompson, F.E., Kipnis, V., Subar, A.F., Hollenbeck, A., Schatzkin, A., and Sinha, R. (2007) Meat and meat-mutagen intake and pancreatic cancer risk in the NIH-AARP cohort. *Cancer Epidemiol Biomarkers Prev* **16**, 2664–75.

108. Wynder, E.L., Kajitani, T., Ishikawa, S., Dodo, H., and Takano, A. (1969) Environmental factors of cancer of the colon and rectum. II. Japanese epidemiological data. *Cancer* **23**, 1210–20.

109. Kuriki, K., Wakai, K., Hirose, K., Matsuo, K., Ito, H., Suzuki, T., Saito, T., Kanemitsu, Y., Hirai, T., Kato, T., Tatematsu, M., and Tajima, K. (2006) Risk of colorectal cancer is linked to erythrocyte compositions of fatty acids as biomarkers for dietary intakes of fish, fat, and fatty acids. *Cancer Epidemiol Biomarkers Prev* **15**, 1791–98.

110. Kuriki, K., Hirose, K., Matsuo, K., Wakai, K., Ito, H., Kanemitsu, Y., Hirai, T., Kato, T., Hamajima, N., Takezaki, T., Suzuki, T., Saito, T., Tanaka, R., and Tajima, K. (2006) Meat, milk, saturated fatty acids, the Pro12Ala and C161T polymorphisms of the PPARgamma gene and colorectal cancer risk in Japanese. *Cancer Sci* **97**, 1226–35.

111. Theodoratou, E., Campbell, H., Tenesa, A., McNeill, G., Cetnarskyj, R., Barnetson, R.A., Porteous, M.E., Dunlop, M.G., and Farrington, S.M. (2008) Modification of the associations between lifestyle, dietary factors and colorectal cancer risk by APC variants. *Carcinogenesis*.

112. Nkondjock, A., Shatenstein, B., Maisonneuve, P., and Ghadirian, P. (2003) Can dietary fatty acids affect colon cancer risk? Reply to Leitzmann and Giovannucci. *Int J Epidemiol* **32**, 879–80.

113. Weijenberg, M.P., Luchtenborg, M., de Goeij, A.F., Brink, M., van Muijen, G.N., de Bruine, A.P., Goldbohm, R.A., and van den Brandt, P.A. (2007) Dietary fat and risk of colon and rectal cancer with aberrant MLH1 expression, APC or KRAS genes. *Cancer Causes Control* **18**, 865–79.

114. Tranah, G.J., Giovannucci, E., Ma, J., Fuchs, C., and Hunter, D.J. (2005) APC Asp1822Val and Gly2502Ser polymorphisms and risk of colorectal cancer and adenoma. *Cancer Epidemiol Biomarkers Prev* **14**, 863–70.

115. Slattery, M.L., Samowitz, W., Ballard, L., Schaffer, D., Leppert, M., and Potter, J.D. (2001) A molecular variant of the APC gene at codon 1822: Its association with diet, lifestyle, and risk of colon cancer. *Cancer Res* **61**, 1000–04.

116. Chen, S.P., Tsai, S.T., Jao, S.W., Huang, Y.L., Chao, Y.C., Chen, Y.L., Wu, C.C., Lin, S.Z., and Harn, H.J. (2006) Single nucleotide polymorphisms of the APC gene and colorectal cancer risk: A case-control study in Taiwan. *BMC Cancer* **6**, 83.

117. Eynard, A.R., and Lopez, C.B. (2003) Conjugated linoleic acid (CLA) versus saturated fats/cholesterol: Their proportion in fatty and lean meats may affect the risk of developing colon cancer. *Lipids Health Dis* **2**, 6.

118. Hogg, N. (2007) Red meat and colon cancer: Heme proteins and nitrite in the gut. A commentary on "diet-induced endogenous formation of nitroso compounds in the GI tract". *Free Radic Biol Med* **43**, 1037–39.

119. Mayne, S.T., Risch, H.A., Dubrow, R., Chow, W.H., Gammon, M.D., Vaughan, T.L., Farrow, D.C., Schoenberg, J.B., Stanford, J.L., Ahsan, H., West, A.B., Rotterdam, H., Blot, W.J., and Fraumeni, J.F., Jr. (2001) Nutrient intake and risk of subtypes of esophageal and gastric cancer. *Cancer Epidemiol Biomarkers Prev* **10**, 1055–62.

120. Chen, H., Tucker, K.L., Graubard, B.I., Heineman, E.F., Markin, R.S., Potischman, N.A., Russell, R.M., Weisenburger, D.D., and Ward, M.H. (2002) Nutrient intakes and adenocarcinoma of the esophagus and distal stomach. *Nutr Cancer* **42**, 33–40.

121. Lopez-Carrillo, L., Lopez-Cervantes, M., Ward, M.H., Bravo-Alvarado, J., and Ramirez-Espitia, A. (1999) Nutrient intake and gastric cancer in Mexico. *Int J Cancer* **83**, 601–05.

122. Qiu, J.L., Chen, K., Zheng, J.N., Wang, J.Y., Zhang, L.J., and Sui, L.M. (2005) Nutritional factors and gastric cancer in Zhoushan Islands, China. *World J Gastroenterol* **11**, 4311–16.

123. Gonzalez, C.A., Riboli, E., Badosa, J., Batiste, E., Cardona, T., Pita, S., Sanz, J.M., Torrent, M., and Agudo, A. (1994) Nutritional factors and gastric cancer in Spain. *Am J Epidemiol* **139**, 466–73.

124. Ji, B.T., Chow, W.H., Yang, G., McLaughlin, J.K., Zheng, W., Shu, X.O., Jin, F., Gao, R.N., Gao, Y.T., and Fraumeni, J.F., Jr. (1998) Dietary habits and stomach cancer in Shanghai, China. *Int J Cancer* **76**, 659–64.

125. Zhang, Z.F., Kurtz, R.C., Yu, G.P., Sun, M., Gargon, N., Karpeh, M., Jr., Fein, J.S., and Harlap, S. (1997) Adenocarcinomas of the esophagus and gastric cardia: The role of diet. *Nutr Cancer* **27**, 298–309.

126. Cornee, J., Pobel, D., Riboli, E., Guyader, M., and Hemon, B. (1995) A case-control study of gastric cancer and nutritional factors in Marseille, France. *Eur J Epidemiol* **11**, 55–65.

127. Franceschi, S., Bidoli, E., Negri, E., Zambon, P., Talamini, R., Ruol, A., Parpinel, M., Levi, F., Simonato, L., and La Vecchia, C. (2000) Role of macronutrients, vitamins and minerals in the aetiology of squamous-cell carcinoma of the oesophagus. *Int J Cancer* **86**, 626–31.

128. Kaaks, R., Tuyns, A.J., Haelterman, M., and Riboli, E. (1998) Nutrient intake patterns and gastric cancer risk: A case-control study in Belgium. *Int J Cancer* **78**, 415–20.

129. Kim, H.J., Kim, M.K., Chang, W.K., Choi, H.S., Choi, B.Y., and Lee, S.S. (2005) Effect of nutrient intake and Helicobacter pylori infection on gastric cancer in Korea: A case-control study. *Nutr Cancer* **52**, 138–46.

130. Larsson, S.C., Orsini, N., and Wolk, A. (2006) Processed meat consumption and stomach cancer risk: A meta-analysis. *J Natl Cancer Inst* **98**, 1078–87.

131. Gonzalez, C.A., Jakszyn, P., Pera, G., Agudo, A., Bingham, S., Palli, D., Ferrari, P., Boeing, H., del Giudice, G., Plebani, M. et al. (2006) Meat intake and risk of stomach and esophageal adenocarcinoma within the European Prospective Investigation Into Cancer and Nutrition (EPIC). *J Natl Cancer Inst* **98**, 345–54.

132. Bahmanyar, S., and Ye, W. (2006) Dietary patterns and risk of squamous-cell carcinoma and adenocarcinoma of the esophagus and adenocarcinoma of the gastric cardia: A population-based case-control study in Sweden. *Nutr Cancer* **54**, 171–78.

133. Campbell, P.T., Sloan, M., and Kreiger, N. (2008) Dietary patterns and risk of incident gastric adenocarcinoma. *Am J Epidemiol* **167**, 295–304.

134. Nagel, G., Linseisen, J., Boshuizen, H.C., Pera, G., Del Giudice, G., Westert, G.P., Bueno-de-Mesquita, H.B., Allen, N.E., Key, T.J., Numans, M.E. et al. (2007) Socioeconomic position and the risk of gastric and oesophageal cancer in the European Prospective Investigation into Cancer and Nutrition (EPIC-EURGAST). *Int J Epidemiol* **36**, 66–76.

135. Smith-Warner, S.A., Ritz, J., Hunter, D.J., Albanes, D., Beeson, W.L., van den Brandt, P.A., Colditz, G., Folsom, A.R., Fraser, G.E., Freudenheim, J.L. et al. (2002) Dietary fat and risk of lung cancer in a pooled analysis of prospective studies. *Cancer Epidemiol Biomarkers Prev* **11**, 987–92.

136. Bandera, E.V., Freudenheim, J.L., Marshall, J.R., Zielezny, M., Priore, R.L., Brasure, J., Baptiste, M., and Graham, S. (1997) Diet and alcohol consumption and lung cancer risk in the New York State Cohort (United States). *Cancer Causes Control* **8**, 828–40.

137. De Stefani, E., Deneo-Pellegrini, H., Mendilaharsu, M., Carzoglio, J.C., and Ronco, A. (1997) Dietary fat and lung cancer: A case-control study in Uruguay. *Cancer Causes Control* **8**, 913–21.

138. Alavanja, M.C., Brownson, R.C., and Benichou, J. (1996) Estimating the effect of dietary fat on the risk of lung cancer in nonsmoking women. *Lung Cancer* **14**(*Suppl 1*), S63–S74.

139. Kubik, A.K., Zatloukal, P., Tomasek, L., and Petruzelka, L. (2002) Lung cancer risk among Czech women: A case-control study. *Prev Med* **34**, 436–44.

140. Zatloukal, P., Kubik, A., Pauk, N., Tomasek, L., and Petruzelka, L. (2003) Adenocarcinoma of the lung among women: Risk associated with smoking, prior lung disease, diet and menstrual and pregnancy history. *Lung Cancer* **41**, 283–93.

141. Sankaranarayanan, R., Varghese, C., Duffy, S.W., Padmakumary, G., Day, N.E., and Nair, M.K. (1994) A case-control study of diet and lung cancer in Kerala, south India. *Int J Cancer* **58**, 644–49.

142. Alavanja, M.C., Field, R.W., Sinha, R., Brus, C.P., Shavers, V.L., Fisher, E.L., Curtain, J., and Lynch, C.F. (2001) Lung cancer risk and red meat consumption among Iowa women. *Lung Cancer* **34**, 37–46.

143. Kubik, A., Zatloukal, P., Tomasek, L., Pauk, N., Petruzelka, L., and Plesko, I. (2004) Lung cancer risk among nonsmoking women in relation to diet and physical activity. *Neoplasma* **51**, 136–43.

144. De Stefani, E., Brennan, P., Ronco, A., Fierro, L., Correa, P., Boffetta, P., Deneo-Pellegrini, H., and Barrios, E. (2002) Food groups and risk of lung cancer in Uruguay. *Lung Cancer* **38**, 1–7.

145. Breslow, R.A., Graubard, B.I., Sinha, R., and Subar, A.F. (2000) Diet and lung cancer mortality: A 1987 National Health Interview Survey cohort study. *Cancer Causes Control* **11**, 419–31.

146. Hu, J., Mao, Y., Dryer, D., and White, K. (2002) Risk factors for lung cancer among Canadian women who have never smoked. *Cancer Detect Prev* **26**, 129–38.

147. Kalandidi, A., Katsouyanni, K., Voropoulou, N., Bastas, G., Saracci, R., and Trichopoulos, D. (1990) Passive smoking and diet in the etiology of lung cancer among non-smokers. *Cancer Causes Control* **1**, 15–21.

148. Koo, L.C. (1988) Dietary habits and lung cancer risk among Chinese females in Hong Kong who never smoked. *Nutr Cancer* **11**, 155–72.

149. Kreuzer, M., Heinrich, J., Kreienbrock, L., Rosario, A.S., Gerken, M., and Wichmann, H.E. (2002) Risk factors for lung cancer among nonsmoking women. *Int J Cancer* **100**, 706–13.

150. Brennan, P., Fortes, C., Butler, J., Agudo, A., Benhamou, S., Darby, S., Gerken, M., Jokel, K.H., Kreuzer, M., Mallone, S., Nyberg, F., Pohlabeln, H., Ferro, G., and Boffetta, P. (2000) A multicenter case-control study of diet and lung cancer among non-smokers. *Cancer Causes Control* **11**, 49–58.

151. Takezaki, T., Hirose, K., Inoue, M., Hamajima, N., Yatabe, Y., Mitsudomi, T., Sugiura, T., Kuroishi, T., and Tajima, K. (2001) Dietary factors and lung cancer risk in Japanese: With special reference to fish consumption and adenocarcinomas. *Br J Cancer* **84**, 1199–206.

152. Mayne, S.T., Janerich, D.T., Greenwald, P., Chorost, S., Tucci, C., Zaman, M.B., Melamed, M.R., Kiely, M., and McKneally, M.F. (1994) Dietary beta carotene and lung cancer risk in US nonsmokers. *J Natl Cancer Inst* **86**, 33–38.

153. Kubik, A., Zatloukal, P., Tomasek, L., Pauk, N., Havel, L., Dolezal, J., and Plesko, I. (2007) Interactions between smoking and other exposures associated with lung cancer risk in women: Diet and physical activity. *Neoplasma* **54**, 83–88.

154. Kvale, G., Bjelke, E., and Gart, J.J. (1983) Dietary habits and lung cancer risk. *Int J Cancer* **31**, 397–405.

155. Nyberg, F., Agrenius, V., Svartengren, K., Svensson, C., and Pershagen, G. (1998) Dietary factors and risk of lung cancer in never-smokers. *Int J Cancer* **78**, 430–36.

156. De Stefani, E., Fontham, E.T., Chen, V., Correa, P., Deneo-Pellegrini, H., Ronco, A., and Mendilaharsu, M. (1997) Fatty foods and the risk of lung cancer: A case-control study from Uruguay. *Int J Cancer* **71**, 760–66.

157. Toporcov, T.N., Antunes, J.L., and Tavares, M.R. (2004) Fat food habitual intake and risk of oral cancer. *Oral Oncol* **40**, 925–31.

158. Bosetti, C., La Vecchia, C., Talamini, R., Negri, E., Levi, F., Fryzek, J., McLaughlin, J.K., Garavello, W., and Franceschi, S. (2003) Energy, macronutrients and laryngeal cancer risk. *Ann Oncol* **14**, 907–12.

159. Bosetti, C., Talamini, R., Levi, F., Negri, E., Franceschi, S., Airoldi, L., and La Vecchia, C. (2002) Fried foods: A risk factor for laryngeal cancer? *Br J Cancer* **87**, 1230–33.
160. Levi, F., Pasche, C., La Vecchia, C., Lucchini, F., Franceschi, S., and Monnier, P. (1998) Food groups and risk of oral and pharyngeal cancer. *Int J Cancer* **77**, 705–09.
161. Uzcudun, A.E., Retolaza, I.R., Fernandez, P.B., Sanchez Hernandez, J.J., Grande, A.G., Garcia, A.G., Olivar, L.M., De Diego Sastre, I., Baron, M.G., and Bouzas, J.G. (2002) Nutrition and pharyngeal cancer: Results from a case-control study in Spain. *Head Neck* **24**, 830–40.
162. Oreggia, F., De Stefani, E., Boffetta, P., Brennan, P., Deneo-Pellegrini, H., and Ronco, A.L. (2001) Meat, fat and risk of laryngeal cancer: A case-control study in Uruguay. *Oral Oncol* **37**, 141–45.
163. Franceschi, S., Favero, A., Conti, E., Talamini, R., Volpe, R., Negri, E., Barzan, L., and La Vecchia, C. (1999) Food groups, oils and butter, and cancer of the oral cavity and pharynx. *Br J Cancer* **80**, 614–20.
164. Fioretti, F., Bosetti, C., Tavani, A., Franceschi, S., and La Vecchia, C. (1999) Risk factors for oral and pharyngeal cancer in never smokers. *Oral Oncol* **35**, 375–78.
165. Franceschi, S., Levi, F., Conti, E., Talamini, R., Negri, E., Dal Maso, L., Boyle, P., Decarli, A., and La Vecchia, C. (1999) Energy intake and dietary pattern in cancer of the oral cavity and pharynx. *Cancer Causes Control* **10**, 439–44.
166. Esteve, J., Riboli, E., Pequignot, G., Terracini, B., Merletti, F., Crosignani, P., Ascunce, N., Zubiri, L., Blanchet, F., Raymond, L., Repetto, F., and Tuyns, A.J. (1996) Diet and cancers of the larynx and hypopharynx: The IARC multi-center study in southwestern Europe. *Cancer Causes Control* **7**, 240–52.
167. Lehmann, W., Raymond, L., Faggiano, F., Sancho-Garnier, H., Blanchet, F., Del Moral, A., Zubiri, L., Terracini, B., Berrino, F., Pequignot, G. et al. (1991) Cancer of the endolarynx, epilarynx and hypopharynx in south-western Europe: Assessment of tumoral origin and risk factors. *Adv Otorhinolaryngol* **46**, 145–56.

12 Conjugated Linoleic Acid and Cancer

Kent L. Erickson, Neil E. Hubbard,
Alexander D. Borowsky,
and Patrizia Damonte

Key Points

1. Conjugated linoleic acid (CLA) contains conjugated double bonds and is known as a family of isomers of linoleic acid that can be found in the meat and dairy products.
2. In vitro studies have shown that CLA can inhibit the growth of mammary, colon, colorectal, gastric, prostate, and malignant liver cell lines and has also been shown to induce the expression of apoptotic genes.
3. The incidence of mammary tumors induced by methylnitrosourea and forestomach tumors induced by benzo[a]pyrene was decreased by CLA in rodent models. CLA isomers may regulate tumorigenesis through different mechanisms by altering lipid metabolism, regulation of oncogene expression, regulation of cyclooxygenase-2 expression, and lipooxygenase metabolic pathways.
4. The specific effects of CLA appear to be dependent on which isomer is assessed. The effects of various isomers in vitro and in vivo have recently been reviewed. With respect to breast cancer, the $t10$, $c12$-CLA isomer was shown to enhance tumorigenesis in a transgenic mouse mammary tumor model when compared to the $c9$, $t11$-CLA isomer. In a parallel study, increased polyp diameter was associated with supplementation of the $t10$, $c12$-CLA diet compared to the $c9$, $t11$-CLA diet, which decreased colonic polyp number in the mouse MIN model of colon cancer.
5. Future studies should investigate the effects of CLA on developing cancer tissues, their progenitor cells, and stem cells. Moreover, animal studies should use models that better recapitulate human cancers in an effort to shorten the time for the development of clinical studies. Therefore, no recommendations for CLA consumption in the context of prevention or therapy can be made until such studies are undertaken.

Key Words: CLA; breast cancer; metastasis; mechanisms

1. INTRODUCTION

Conjugated linoleic acid (CLA) refers to a family of positional and geometric isomers of linoleic acid in which the double bonds are conjugated *(1)*. Most published studies focusing on CLA and health have used a mixture of isomers including the two major

From: *Nutrition and Health: Bioactive Compounds and Cancer*
Edited by: J.A. Milner, D.F. Romagnolo, DOI 10.1007/978-1-60761-627-6_12,
© Springer Science+Business Media, LLC 2010

forms of *cis*9, *trans*11-CLA (*c*9, *t*11-CLA) and *trans*10, *cis*12-CLA, (*t*10, *c*12-CLA). Some minor isomers include *t*7, *t*9-CLA, *c*9, *c*11-CLA, *t*9, *t*11-CLA, *c*10, *c*12-CLA, *t*10, *t*12-CLA, *t*11, *t*13-CLA, and *c*11, *c*13-CLA. Although CLA contains a *trans* double bond, some researchers claim that it is not as harmful as other *trans* fatty acids, but rather can be beneficial. Biological conversion of linoleic acid to CLA can occur in the rumen portion of the digestive system of ruminant animals. Thus, ruminant meat and dairy products are major dietary sources of *c*9, *t*11-CLA. Non-ruminants, such as humans, as well as ruminants are able to produce some isomers of CLA from vaccenic acid by Δ-9-desaturase *(2, 3)*. In addition, partially hydrogenated oils such as shortenings and margarines are major sources of *t*10, *c*12-CLA as well as other isomers. Using food duplicate methodologies, investigators have suggested that the average intake of CLA in the US population is <500 mg/day *(4)*. This level is probably significantly lower compared to that of centuries or even decades ago.

Since CLA was originally reported to be antimutagenic *(5)*, interest in the health benefits or side effects of CLA in humans has prompted continued research, especially with regard to cancer. Studies with several animal models have assessed effects of CLA on tumorigenesis at various sites. Several reviews have indicated that feeding CLA hindered the growth of numerous tumor types *(6–11)*. For example, CLA has been shown to have anti-carcinogenic effects in colon, prostate, and breast cancers as well as reduce the development, growth, and spread of breast tumors in several animal models *(12–14)*. Carcinogen-induced and transplantable models have been used extensively. Recently, transgenic mice have been used to assess the effects of dietary CLA *(15, 16)*. A number of in vitro studies with several cancer cell lines have incorporated additional dietary CLA isomers. Studies have shown that CLA can alter tumor cell growth by reducing cell proliferation and inducing apoptosis in human breast, colon, and gastric cancer cells *(17–19)*. Thus, the potential for altering dietary intake of CLA as a means for decreasing risk of mammary primary tumor growth and metastasis is a distinct possibility. Accordingly, the purpose of this chapter is to review selected mechanisms through which CLA could modulate tumorigenesis. Initially, we will review the effects on proliferation and metastasis. Although there are a number of potential mechanisms through which this could occur, we will focus on alteration of eicosanoid metabolism and extracellular matrix. In addition, we will explore the possibility that CLA could target the population of cells in the tumor now believed to give rise to the malignancy, the cancer stem cell population.

2. IN VITRO STUDIES

A number of studies have shown that CLA added directly to tumor cells in vitro can decrease proliferation and/or induce cell death. Most published reports on the effects of CLA in vitro were with tumor cell lines derived from mammary gland, prostate, and the digestive tract or their metastases. Many of these studies used *c*9, *t*11-CLA and *t*10, *c*12-CLA isomers; overall the *t*10, *c*12-CLA isomer was more potent at inhibiting tumor cell growth in vitro. In our studies, treatment with *t*10, *c*12-CLA but not *c*9, *t*11-CLA caused a significant change in cell morphology compared to controls of ethanol or linoleic acid (Fig. 1). A significant number of cells treated with *t*10, *c*12-CLA appeared to be

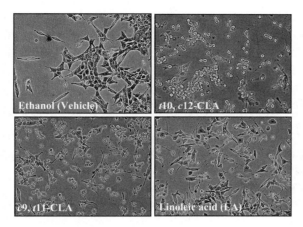

Fig. 1. Phase-contrast microscopy of mouse mammary tumor cell line 4526 grown in culture with the specific treatments indicated. Cells were photographed after 24 h of incubation. Magnification is ×100.

undergoing apoptosis while the control cells and cells treated with *c*9, *t*11-CLA maintained their typical morphology. When cell viability of these mouse mammary tumor cells was assessed after treatment with fatty acids, *t*10, *c*12-CLA showed the most toxic effect (Fig. 2; reproduced from *(20)*). Compared to vehicle control, 50 μM *t*10, *c*12-CLA reduced cell viability by 80% while the *c*9, *t*11-CLA isomer reduced viability by less than 20%. The *t*10, *c*12-CLA isomer also inhibited cell growth when tested with colon, colorectal, and gastric cancer cell lines. The *t*10, *c*12-CLA isomer was actually more growth inhibitory than *c*9, *t*11-CLA in most studies, but a few reported that *c*9, *t*11-CLA was more potent than *t*10, *c*12-CLA in inhibiting the growth of several colon cell lines (MIP-101, Caco-2, HT-29, DLD-1) *(21, 22)*. Culture conditions including the

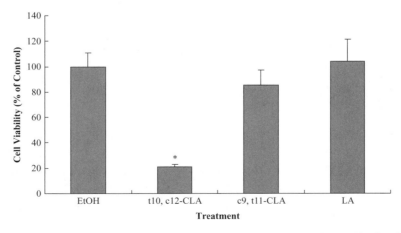

Fig. 2. Effect of fatty acids on cell viability. Cell viability was measured with MTT after fatty acid or ethanol treatment. *Significantly ($P < 0.05$) less than control or other fatty acid treatment; the mean ± SEM of six separate experiments. Reprinted from *(20)* with permission from Elsevier.

concentration of CLA, duration of treatment, and tumor type as well as the cell lines used seem to determine whether CLA isomers could inhibit cell growth. In most studies with prostate cell lines, both *t*10, *c*12-CLA and *c*9, *t*11-CLA inhibited cell growth *(22–25)*.

3. IN VIVO ANIMAL EXPERIMENTS

A number of dietary effects of mixed isomers of CLA have been shown in rodent models of tumorigenesis. As little as 0.1% dietary CLA reduced the appearance of mammary tumors induced by a chemical carcinogen *(26)*. The response to CLA was maximal at the relatively low dietary concentration of 1%, which may have important implications since this amount could theoretically be incorporated in human diet. Dietary CLA had a protective effect against mammary tumor initiation when fed to mice from time of weaning until carcinogen exposure *(26)*. This CLA treatment corresponds to the time of mammary gland maturation *(27)*. In contrast, feeding diets containing CLA to post-pubertal rats required a continuous intake of CLA in order to prevent carcinogen-induced mammary tumorigenesis *(28)*. For example, CLA-containing diets failed to prevent the development of mammary tumors when fed to 50-day-old rats after the injection of the carcinogen. Thus, a mixture of CLA isomers had a direct chemo-protective effect on the mammary gland during development as well as a suppressive influence on tumor progression.

Animals fed diets containing butter enriched in *c*9, *t*11-CLA, purified *c*9, *t*11-CLA, or a mixture of CLA isomers (0.8%) for 1 month had reduced mammary epithelial mass, size of the terminal end buds, and mammary tumor development *(29)*. These data demonstrated that purified *c*9, *t*11-CLA fed either as butter fat or as an isomer was as effective as a mixture of CLA isomers in reducing the number of MNU-induced mammary tumors. Feeding of 1% *c*9, *t*11-CLA or 2% vaccenic acid, which can be metabolized to *c*9, *t*11-CLA in animal tissues, reduced MNU-induced pre-malignant lesions by 50% when compared to the number of lesions found in the control group fed a diet containing regular butter *(2)*. Also, CLA concentrations in the tissues and the concentration of *c*9, *t*11-CLA in the mammary gland was fivefold greater in the vaccenic acid group than in the control group. These results showed that rats could metabolize vaccenic acid to *c*9, *t*11-CLA, which was effective in decreasing MNU-induced mammary tumorigenesis. The same investigators compared the efficacy of purified *c*9, *t*11-CLA and *t*10, *c*12-CLA in the prevention of mammary tumors in rats injected with MNU *(30)*. Both CLA isomers decreased the number of pre-malignant lesions by 35% at 6 weeks and decreased the number of mammary tumors by 40% at 24 weeks after MNU injections. The authors concluded that *c*9, *t*11- and *t*10, *c*12-CLA isomers were equally effective in reducing MNU-induced tumorigenesis. Rats fed diets with sunflower oil containing *c*9, *t*11-CLA or a mixture of isomers decreased tumor incidence by 45% *(31)*. Neither of the CLA-containing diets altered latency, the time between induction and detection of palpable tumors. Results from these studies showed that *c*9, *t*11- and *t*10, *c*12-CLA were as effective as the CLA mixture in reducing mammary tumors induced by MNU.

The incidence of chemically induced forestomach tumors in Kun Ming mice was significantly decreased with isomers of CLA *(32)*. Also, dietary mixed isomers of CLA

(1%) fed to rats for 30 weeks significantly decreased the incidence of colon cancer induced by 1,2-dimethylhydrazine *(33)*. However, CLA significantly increased hepatic metastasis from a chemically induced pancreatic tumor in male Syrian hamsters *(34)*. In this study, animals received the carcinogen weekly for 12 weeks and a diet with 3.3% CLA for 24 weeks.

In two studies, the *t*10, *c*12-CLA isomer was shown to contribute to an enhancement of tumorigenesis. In one study, the size of adenomas was significantly greater in the distal part of small intestine of Min mice fed *t*10, *c*12-CLA compared to those in the control group *(35)*. Min mice have a mutation of the APC gene leading to neoplasia at multiple sites of both the small and large intestine. The Min mouse, however, may not be a good model for human tumorigenesis where almost all tumors occur in the large intestine. In another study, FVB/J female mice with an alteration in erbB2 gene expression in mammary epithelium had accelerated mammary tumor development and decreased median tumor latency compared to FVB/J mice fed diets containing *t*10, *c*12-CLA *(15)*. While the *c*9, *t*11-CLA isomer seems to decrease tumorigenesis, studies with the *t*10, *c*12-CLA isomer demonstrate both enhancement and suppression of tumorigenesis depending on the site of the tumor, the type of tumor, and the means for induction.

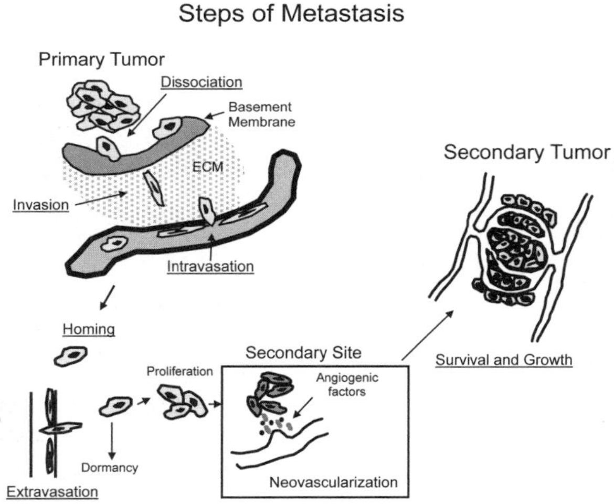

Fig. 3. Schematic representation of steps in tumor metastasis.

Since most deaths from breast cancer are due to metastasis, studies to determine the efficacy of CLA on any component of metastasis is crucial (Fig. 3). We demonstrated previously that CLA had a significant effect on the latency, metastasis, and pulmonary tumor burden of transplantable mammary tumors grown in mice fed 20% fat diets *(13)*. The latency of tumors for mice fed 0.5% or more CLA was increased to more than 19 days from 13 when compared with the control or mice fed a diet that contained 0.1% CLA (Fig. 4; reprinted from *(13)*). The volume of pulmonary tumor burden, as a result of spontaneous metastasis from the transplanted primary tumor, decreased proportionately with increasing concentrations of dietary CLA (Fig. 5; reprinted from *(13)*). With 0.5 and 1% CLA, pulmonary tumor burden was significantly decreased compared to mice

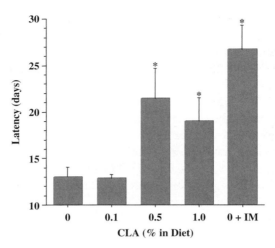

Fig. 4. Effect of dietary CLA on the latency of line 4526 mammary tumors. All diets contained 20% (w/w) total fat with the indicated concentration of CLA. IM represents a group of mice fed no CLA and treated with 20 μg/ml indomethacin in the drinking water. *Significantly (*P* <0.05) greater when compared with 0 and 0.1% CLA groups. **Significantly greater when compared with 0, 0.1, and 1% CLA groups. Reprinted from *(13)* with permission from Elsevier.

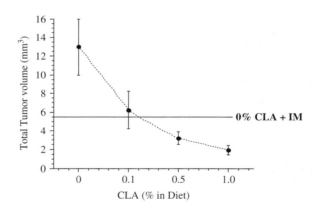

Fig. 5. Effect of increasing amounts of dietary CLA on the metastatic pulmonary tumor burden of mice with line 4,526 primary tumors. Decreased tumor burden was highly correlated with increasing dietary concentrations of CLA. Values are mean ± SEM. Reprinted from *(13)* with permission from Elsevier.

treated with the prostaglandin inhibitor, indomethacin (IM), and fed diets containing no CLA. We had previously shown that IM was a very potent reducer of mammary tumorigenesis in this prostaglandin producing transplantable tumor model *(36)*. Tumors of mice fed as little as 0.1% CLA and as much as 1% had significantly decreased numbers of pulmonary tumors when compared with mice fed diets containing no CLA. These data suggest that the protective effects of CLA on mammary tumorigenesis may extend to advanced stages, especially metastasis. Other studies with dietary CLA have shown that specific isomers may have differential effects on several biological processes. Thus, we sought to assess the effects of specific CLA isomers on mouse mammary tumor metastasis. For this purpose, we fed 20% (w/w) total fat diets which contained either no CLA, low or high levels of $c9$, $t11$-CLA, $t10$, $c12$-CLA, or a mixture of the two isomers *(37)*. Neither the separate isomers nor the mixture had an effect on the latency or growth of primary tumors when compared to the group fed diets without CLA. However, all CLA diets significantly decreased the total tumor burden in lungs of mice from both spontaneous metastasis and implantation and survival of the metastatic cells when compared with diets containing no CLA. Diets containing a greater concentration of either $c9$, $t11$ or $t10$, $c12$-CLA had a significantly greater effect compared to the lower concentrations of the same isomer when metastatic tumor size and total tumor load were assessed *(37)*. The diet containing a mixture of both isomers decreased metastasis similarly to the diets containing the lower concentration of single isomers. Thus, the $c9$, $t11$ and $t10$, $c12$-CLA exerted no additive effects and may decrease metastatic tumor burden through independent mechanisms (Fig. 3).

The concentration of CLA required to effectively alter mammary tumor metastasis may be dependent on other fats in the diet; alteration of the major types of fat can enhance or suppress tumor metastasis. When a fat blend that reflected the typical Western diet was used *(38)*, not only did 0.1% CLA added to the diet reduce the metastatic lung tumor burden, but when beef tallow was substituted for half of the vegetable fat blend (VFB) and 0.1% CLA added, the level of metastasis (BT) was even lower (Fig. 6;

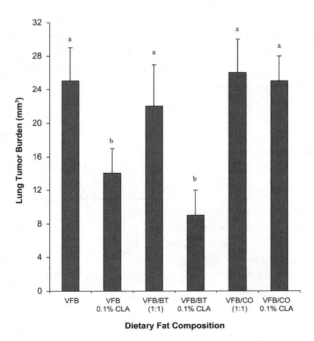

Fig. 6. Mice were fed diets for 3 weeks then injected i.v. in the tail vein with tumor cells. Metastasis was significantly decreased after treatment with 0.1% CLA in both the VFB and the VFB/BT groups. Reprinted from *(38)* with permission from the American Society for Nutrition.

reprinted from *(38))*. These results indicated that other fats in the diet such as beef tallow may increase the efficacy of dietary CLA in reducing mammary tumorigenesis.

4. STUDIES IN HUMANS

Only a few epidemiological human studies have investigated the relationship between CLA intake or tissue CLA concentrations and tumor incidence. One study showed a weak positive relationship between breast cancer incidence and the intake of CLA *(39)*. In this study, female subjects ranging from 55 to 69 years of age were followed for 6 years and answered self-administered questionnaires regarding dietary intake, smoking habits, family incidence of cancer, and other factors. During the course of the study, 941 of the 62,573 women reported breast cancer diagnoses. In two other studies, CLA levels in the serum and breast adipose tissue were used to analyze the relationship between breast cancer and exposure to CLA *(40, 41)*. In one study, the levels of serum and dietary CLA were significantly lower in postmenopausal breast cancer patients than in control subjects *(40)*. In another study, CLA levels in breast adipose tissue showed no direct correlation with breast cancer *(41)*.

5. MECHANISMS THROUGH WHICH CLA MAY ALTER BREAST TUMORIGENESIS

A number of studies have hypothesized several possible mechanisms through which CLA may alter breast tumorigenesis *(11)*. Mixtures of CLA isomers have been shown to alter most stages of mammary tumorigenesis through various molecular mechanisms including alteration of lipid peroxidation, tissue fatty acid composition, eicosanoid metabolism, gene expression, cell cycle regulation, cell proliferation, and apoptosis *(11)*. While CLA may exert many potent biological effects (Table 1), only a few will be discussed here.

Table 1
Potential Mechanisms Through Which CLA May Alter
Breast Tumorigenesis

Tumor cell proliferation/apoptosis
Cell cycle regulation
Immune function
Extracellular matrix degradation
Angiogenesis
Cell adhesion
Gene expression
Energy metabolism
Eicosanoid metabolism
Lipid peroxidation
Terminal end bud formation

6. ALTERATION OF LIPOXYGENASE PATHWAY

Because several studies have shown that alteration of cyclooxygenase or lipoxygenase metabolites by different fatty acids can change tumor cell growth by altering cell proliferation and apoptosis, we hypothesized that the effect of CLA on tumorigenesis may be due to alteration of these enzymes. Inhibition of the lipoxygenase, but not the cyclooxygenase pathway, decreased the viability of mouse mammary tumor cells 4526 *(20)*. Since *t*10, *c*12-CLA altered the growth of the mouse mammary tumor cell growth (Fig. 2), we assessed whether this effect was due to alteration of the lipoxygenase pathway. First, we determined whether *t*10, *c*12-CLA could alter the production of lipoxygenase metabolites, such as hydroxyeicosatetraenoic acids (HETE) or leukotrienes (LT). Even after stimulation with calcium ionophore, the tumor cells were unable to produce detectable HETE or LT other than 5-HETE *(20)*. Treatment of cells with *t*10, *c*12-CLA significantly decreased 5-HETE production while *c*9, *t*11-CLA or linoleic acid had no effect as compared to the control (Fig. 7; reprinted from *(20)*). Adding 5-HETE back to the media after *t*10, *c*12-CLA treatment reduced the *t*10, *c*12-CLA-stimulated decrease in tumor cell viability while 5-HETE alone had no effect. Adding 5-HETE to the media also significantly reduced *t*10, *c*12-CLA and *c*9, *t*11-CLA-induced effects on apoptosis and proliferation *(20)*. In a subsequent study designed to assess CLA alteration of the lipoxygenase pathway, the human mammary tumor cell line MDA-MB-231 was used *(42)*. As previously seen with mouse mammary cell lines, the treatment with *t*10, *c*12-CLA significantly decreased in a dose-dependent manner the viability of MDA-MB-231 cells. Also, the lipoxygenase inhibitor nordihydroguaiaretic acid reduced the viability of MDA-MB-231 cells in a dose-dependent manner and produced 5-, 12-, and 15-HETE

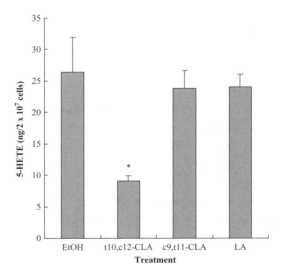

Fig. 7. Calcium ionophore-stimulated 5-HETE production after pre-incubation with 10 μM fatty acid. HETE production was measured with HPLC. 5-HETE was not detected without A23187 stimulation. Values represent the mean ± SEM for three separate experiments. *Significantly less (*P* <0.05) than other treatments. Reprinted from *(20)* with permission from Elsevier.

only after stimulation with calcium ionophore. Treatment with the $t10$, $c12$-CLA isomer reduced 5- and 15-HETE production by 70 and 50% *(42)*. Tumor cell viability was increased when 5-HETE was added with $t10$, $c12$-CLA compared to only $t10$, $c12$-CLA (Fig. 8; reprinted from *(42)*). It is possible that CLA isomers could reduce lipoxygenase metabolite production by competing with the substrate arachidonic acid (AA) *(42)*. Co-incubation of both $c9$, $t11$-CLA or $t10$, $c12$-CLA with AA significantly (P <0.05) reduced 5-HETE production in human breast tumor cells (Fig. 9; reprinted from *(42)*). Thus, one possible mechanism of CLA action on lipoxygenase could be competition with the substrate AA. CLA could also modulate the production of eicosanoid metabolites by altering the lipoxygenase enzyme system. To produce 5-HETE, fatty acid

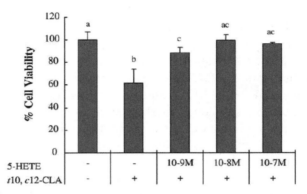

Fig. 8. Effect of 5-HETE on $t10$, $c12$-CLA altered tumor cell viability. MDA-MB-231 cells were pre-incubated with 100 μM $c9$, $t11$-CLA, $t10$, $c12$-CLA or LA for 30 min then 5-HETE added for an additional 48 h. Viability reported as percentage of control; means ± SEM for three separate experiments. Values not sharing the same superscript were significantly (P <0.05) different. Reprinted from *(42)* with permission from Elsevier.

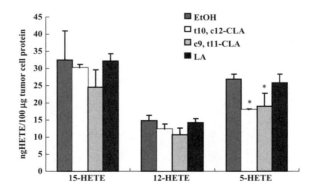

Fig. 9. Effect of select CLA isomers on conversion of arachidonic acid to 15-, 12-, and 5-HETE. 10 μM $c9$, $t11$-CLA, $t10$, $c12$-CLA, or LA and 2 μM arachidonic acid were co-incubated with 100 μg protein for 45 min, then HETE isolated and measured by RP-HPLC. *Significantly (P <0.05) less than control or other fatty acid treatment. Values are means ± SEM of three separate experiments. Reprinted from *(42)* with permission from Elsevier.

substrate has to first bind to 5-lipoxygenase activating protein (FLAP) making it available to 5-lipoxygenase to form 5-HETE *(43)*. Neither CLA isomer altered 5-lipoxygenase mRNA, but *t*10, *c*12-CLA did significantly reduce FLAP mRNA expression. In addition, FLAP over-expression in MDA-MB-231 cells reduced the ability of *t*10, *c*12-CLA to decrease cell viability (Fig. 10; reprinted from *(42)*). Based on this information, it may be concluded that at least the *t*10, *c*12 isomer alters mammary tumorigenesis through the lipoxygenase pathway by substrate competition and alteration of FLAP expression.

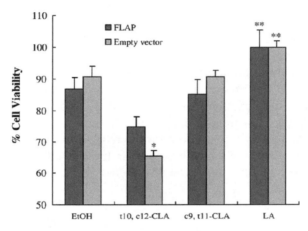

Fig. 10. Effect of FLAP over-expression on CLA reduction of MDA-MB-231 cell viability. Cells were transfected with FLAP or empty vector (twofold increase in FLAP expression) then treated with 100 μM of fatty acids for 48 h. Cell viability was measured by MTT. Values represent mean ± SEM for three separate experiments. *Significantly ($P < 0.05$) less than EtOH or **significantly ($P < 0.05$) greater than EtOH. Reprinted from *(42)* with permission from Elsevier.

7. EFFECTS OF CLA ON EXTRACELLULAR MATRIX

Most tumor cells have to degrade components of the extracellular matrix (ECM) to survive, migrate, and proliferate. A clue that CLA may alter tumor cell modification of ECM was the observation that the intake of mixed CLA isomers affected the latency, metastasis, and secondary tumor burden of a highly metastatic mammary tumor cell in mice *(13)*. The expression of one or several proteinases is necessary to aid in the destruction and remodeling of surrounding tissues and for migration to a secondary site (Fig. 3). In a recent study, we examined how dietary CLA could alter tumor cell metastasis by modulation of 2 ECM-modifying enzymes, MMP-2 and MMP-9 *(44)*. CLA decreased tumor cell invasion and migration when compared with tumor cells treated with linoleic acid. Most of the MMP-2 present in tumor cell lysates was in an inactive form. TIMP-2, the natural inhibitor of MMP-2, was enhanced by the addition of CLA to the diet *(44)*. Moreover, the amount of active MMP-9 decreased and mRNA levels of the MMP-9 inhibitor, TIMP-1, increased as dietary CLA levels rose. Protein levels of TIMP-1 were also increased by CLA. These results implied that CLA could affect the activation of the MMP-2 proenzyme, perhaps by altering the production of

MMP-2 activators or inhibitors, or both. Moreover, MMP-9 activity could be inhibited by TIMP-1. Therefore, the reduction of metastasis by CLA could be mediated by an alteration in metalloproteinases and their activities resulting in suppression of both invasion and migration of tumor cells *(13)*.

8. EFFECTS OF CLA ON BREAST CANCER STEM CELLS (CSC)

Current chemoprevention strategies focus on delivery of bioactive components in an attempt to slow down, stop, or block the tumorigenic process. Currently, available chemotherapeutic agents target growing and dividing tumor cells, but leave stem cells intact (Fig. 11). Stem cells are normally found in most tissues and generally divide very slowly. Stem cells in several organs, including the breast, can be likely candidates for accumulating the multiple mutations involved in the process of tumor progression because of their long life. Mutations accumulated in the cancer stem cell disrupt the tight control of stem cell functions, ultimately leading to deregulation of self-renewal, which drives the process of tumorigenesis and aberrant differentiation. The stem cell origin of breast tumors may also account for the reoccurrence of cancer after treatment as well as the heterogeneity of the cells present in the tumors. The role of stem cells in breast cancer has been recently reviewed elsewhere *(46)*.

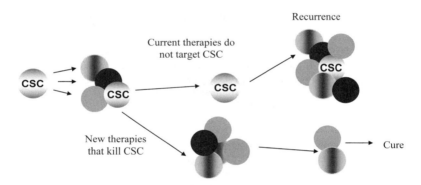

Fig. 11. Schematic diagram of possible therapy effects on tumors and tumor "stem cells."

A subset of cells with high-proliferative potential and the ability to differentiate is present in the mammary gland to sustain numerous possible pregnancies, a description that fits the definition of stem cells. Indirect evidence to support the hypothesis that CLA can alter breast stem cells was provided some years ago when it was shown that CLA targeted the terminal end buds (TEB) by reducing their number and proliferation *(27, 29)*. Because TEB are one major source of stem cells, we hypothesize that CLA may target this population of cells and reduce their number or proliferation. However, there has been no direct evidence that CLA can target either normal or cancer stem cells.

Until recently, it had not been feasible to study breast stem cells because their identification was difficult. However, considerable progress has been made in the field of stem cell biology in the past few years, and some of the approaches used in other systems such as hematopoietic have been applied recently to the mouse mammary gland.

We have used a combination of mammary transplantation with a derivative of genetically engineered mouse mammary gland to create a mouse model of ductal carcinoma in situ (DCIS) that precisely recapitulates human breast cancer. The model is referred to as mouse mammary intraepithelial neoplasia outgrowths (MINO). The MINO mouse can be a mammary pre-cancer "stem" model, harboring potential pre-cancer "stem" cells. Serial transplantation confirms that these mammary tissues meet the biologic definitions for "stemness," asynchronous division including self-renewal, as well as "pre-cancer," consistent progression to invasive carcinoma. The MINO tissue can be dissociated to single cells, grown in three-dimensional (non-adherent) culture, and can reconstitute the MINO pre-cancer phenotype when transplanted into the gland-free mammary fat pad (45). The dissociated MINO cells can be sorted by flow cytometry for stem markers. A resulting single cell suspension can be used to yield spheroid cell formations (mammospheres) plated in Matrigel. The ability to perform transplantation experiments using mammary epithelial cells transplanted into the cleared fat pad provides a powerful assay to identify and isolate functional stem cells (47–49).

We have begun to assess the effects of CLA on breast stem tissues. Some of these studies involved isolating stem tissues and whereas others utilized tissue transplantation and the MINO model described above. Transplantation of pre-neoplastic or putative neoplastic lesions (or selected cells) allowed evaluation of the effects of CLA on proliferative rates, malignant potential, metastatic potential, and response to therapy. In our pilot studies, tumor and MINO tissues were used to isolate single cells for in vitro culture and growth of spheroids called either tumorspheres or MINOspheres. A large proportion of spheroids have been shown to be a combination of stem cells and multipotent progenitor cells (50). To study the effects of CLA on tumorspheres, single cells were isolated from spontaneous polyoma virus middle T tumors and treated immediately with CLA to assess the effects on spheroid formation. Alternatively, spheroids were allowed to form first and then treated with CLA to assess cytotoxicity. CLA significantly reduced tumorsphere formation (Table 2). Linoleic acid actually enhanced tumorsphere formation, but not to a significant extent. When fatty acids were added only after tumorspheres had formed, the effects of both CLA and LA were not as pronounced (Table 2). Since the tumorspheres form from stem cells and progenitor cells, we can conclude that CLA may be toxic to tumor initiating cells present in the spheroids. Additional studies are needed to confirm these findings.

Table 2
Effect of Fatty Acids on Tumorsphere Formation and Cytotoxicity

Fatty acid	Tumorsphere formation	Cytotoxicity[a]
Control	100[b]	100
5 μM c9, t11-CLA	58 ± 8	80 ± 12
5 μM LA	108 ± 13	109 ± 10

[a]Cytotoxicity was assessed by adding fatty acids to cultures after tumorspheres had already formed in control media.
[b]Values represent relative percent of control.

To assess the effects of CLA on precancerous tissues, single cells were isolated and those cells positive for CD31 (endothelial cells), CD45 (hematopoietic in origin), and TER119 (erythroid) removed to enrich for an epithelial population. MINO cells were then suspended in Matrigel and spheroids grown in the presence of various fatty acids. Both c9, t11-CLA and t10, c12-CLA isomers inhibited the growth of MINOspheres in the Matrigel compared to control, LA, and AA treatments (Table 3). Therefore, CLA may be effective at not only reducing tumors but inducing toxicity in precancerous tissue.

Table 3
Effect of Fatty Acids on MINOsphere Formation in Matrigel

Fatty acid	MINOspheres formed
Control	100[a]
20 µM c9, t11-CLA	10 ± 4
20 µM t10, c12-CLA	11 ± 2
20 µM LA	102 ± 15
20 µM AA	104 ± 11

[a]Values represent relative percent of control.

9. CLA SPECIFICITY

CLA has been shown to have several health benefits altering the severity or slowing the progression of some diseases. In general, research data suggest that the effects of CLA may not be restricted to specific tissues and in the case of tumorigenesis, specific cancer sites. The best evidence that CLA does not appear to be specific in the carcinogenic process is the observation of reduced tumorigenesis at several sites in animal models. Notably, CLA can reduce tumorigenesis in the skin, breast, colon, stomach, and prostate. Although there are a couple of examples in which selected CLA isomers have increased tumorigenesis, most commonly CLA reduced tumorigenesis in all models tested to date. While there may be several mechanisms involved, CLA has specifically been shown to alter angiogenesis and apoptosis, two important processes involved in tumor progression (28). CLA was shown to alter angiogenesis in mammary tissue and more recently, it was shown to alter angiogenesis in normal brain tissue (51). Therefore, the effects of CLA on angiogenesis may not be specific to tumors. However, the effects of CLA may be more tissue specific during developmental stages. For example, CLA had a much greater effect at preventing mammary tumorigenesis when it was given to animals before mammary gland development rather at later stages (29).

The specific effects of CLA, however, do appear to be dependent on which isomer is assessed. We have recently reviewed the effects of various isomers in vitro and in vivo (11). With respect to breast cancer, the t10, c12-CLA isomer was shown to enhance tumorigenesis in a transgenic mouse mammary tumor model when compared to the c9, t11-CLA isomer (15). In a parallel study, increased polyp diameter was associated with supplementation of the t10, c12-CLA diet compared to the c9, t11-CLA diet, which decreased colonic polyp number in the mouse MIN model of colon cancer (52). There are numerous studies showing differences in isomer activities in vitro (*11*). More studies are needed to clarify the effects of supplementation with specific CLA isomers and possible positive and negative interactions among isomers present in mixtures.

10. CONCLUSIONS AND FUTURE RESEARCH DIRECTIONS

CLA isomers can be potent regulators of biological processes that affect human health including tumorigenesis. This conclusion is based on results of a number of animal studies. Nevertheless, future studies should investigate the effects of CLA on developing cancer tissues, their progenitor cells, and stem cells. Moreover, animal studies should use animal models that better recapitulate human cancers in an effort to shorten the time for the development of clinical studies. Therefore, no recommendations for CLA consumption in the context of prevention or therapy can be made until such studies are undertaken.

REFERENCES

1. Kelley, D.S., and Erickson, K.L. (2003) Modulation of body composition and immune cell functions by conjugated linoleic acid in humans and animal models: Benefits vs. risks. *Lipids* **38**(4), 377–86.
2. Banni, S., Angioni, E., Murru, E. et al. (2001) Vaccenic acid feeding increases tissue levels of conjugated linoleic acid and suppresses development of premalignant lesions in rat mammary gland. *Nutr Cancer* **41**(1–2), 91–97.
3. Kuhnt, K., Kraft, J., Moeckel, P., and Jahreis, G. (2006) Trans-11-18: 1 is effectively Delta9-desaturated compared with trans-12-18: 1 in humans. *Br J Nutr* **95**(4), 752–61.
4. Ritzenthaler, K.L., McGuire, M.K., Falen, R., Shultz, T.D., Dasgupta, N., and McGuire, M.A. (2001) Estimation of conjugated linoleic acid intake by written dietary assessment methodologies underestimates actual intake evaluated by food duplicate methodology. *J Nutr* **131**(5), 1548–54.
5. Ha, Y.L., Grimm, N.K., and Pariza, M.W. (1987) Anticarcinogens from fried ground beef: Heat-altered derivatives of linoleic acid. *Carcinogenesis* **8**(12), 1881–7.
6. Belury, M.A. (2002) Dietary conjugated linoleic acid in health: Physiological effects and mechanisms of action. *Annu Rev Nutr* **22**, 505–31.
7. Bhattacharya, A., Banu, J., Rahman, M., Causey, J., and Fernandes, G. (2006) Biological effects of conjugated linoleic acids in health and disease. *J Nutr Biochem* **17**(12), 789–810.
8. Ip, M.M., Masso-Welch, P.A., and Ip, C. (2003) Prevention of mammary cancer with conjugated linoleic acid: Role of the stroma and the epithelium. *J Mammary Gland Biol Neoplasia* **8**(1), 103–18.
9. Lee, K.W., Lee, H.J., Cho, H.Y., and Kim, Y.J. (2005) Role of the conjugated linoleic acid in the prevention of cancer. *Crit Rev Food Sci Nutr* **45**(2), 135–44.
10. Wahle, K.W., Heys, S.D., and Rotondo, D. (2004) Conjugated linoleic acids: Are they beneficial or detrimental to health? *Prog Lipid Res* **43**(6), 553–87.
11. Kelley, N.S., Hubbard, N.E., and Erickson, K.L. (2007) Conjugated linoleic acid isomers and cancer. *J Nutr* **137**(12), 2599–607.
12. Cunningham, D.C., Harrison, L.Y., and Shultz, T.D. (1997) Proliferative responses of normal human mammary and MCF-7 breast cancer cells to linoleic acid, conjugated linoleic acid and eicosanoid synthesis inhibitors in culture. *Anticancer Res* **17**(1A), 197–203.
13. Hubbard, N.E., Lim, D., Summers, L., and Erickson, K.L. (2000) Reduction of murine mammary tumor metastasis by conjugated linoleic acid. *Cancer Lett* **150**(1), 93–100.
14. Shultz, T.D., Chew, B.P., and Seaman, W.R. (1992) Differential stimulatory and inhibitory responses of human MCF-7 breast cancer cells to linoleic acid and conjugated linoleic acid in culture. *Anticancer Res* **12**(6B), 2143–5.

15. Ip, M.M., McGee, S.O., Masso-Welch, P.A. et al. (2007) The t10,c12 isomer of conjugated linoleic acid stimulates mammary tumorigenesis in transgenic mice overexpressing erbB2 in the mammary epithelium. *Carcinogenesis* **28**(6), 1269–76.

16. Meng, X., Shoemaker, S., McGee, S.O., and Ip, M.M. (2008) t10,c12-conjugated linoleic acid stimulates mammary tumor progression in her2/erbB2 mice through activation of both proliferative and survival pathways. *Carcinogenesis* **29**(5), 1013–21.

17. Cho, H.J., Kim, W.K., Kim, E.J. et al. (2003) Conjugated linoleic acid inhibits cell proliferation and ErbB3 signaling in HT-29 human colon cell line. *Am J Physiol* **284**(6), G996–G1005.

18. Liu, J.R., Chen, B.Q., Yang, Y.M. et al. (2002) Effect of apoptosis on gastric adenocarcinoma cell line SGC-7901 induced by cis-9, trans-11-conjugated linoleic acid. *World J Gastroenterol* **8**(6), 999–1004.

19. Majumder, B., Wahle, K.W., Moir, S. et al. (2002) Conjugated linoleic acids (CLAs) regulate the expression of key apoptotic genes in human breast cancer cells. *Faseb J* **16**(11), 1447–9.

20. Kim, J.H., Hubbard, N.E., Ziboh, V., and Erickson, K.L. (2005) Conjugated linoleic acid reduction of murine mammary tumor cell growth through 5-hydroxyeicosatetraenoic acid. *Biochim Biophys Acta* **1687**(1–3), 103–9.

21. Beppu, F., Hosokawa, M., Tanaka, L., Kohno, H., Tanaka, T., and Miyashita, K. (2006) Potent inhibitory effect of trans9, trans11 isomer of conjugated linoleic acid on the growth of human colon cancer cells. *J Nutr Biochem* **17**(12), 830–6.

22. Palombo, J.D., Ganguly, A., Bistrian, B.R., and Menard, M.P. (2002) The antiproliferative effects of biologically active isomers of conjugated linoleic acid on human colorectal and prostatic cancer cells. *Cancer letters* **177**(2), 163–72.

23. De la Torre, A., Debiton, E., Durand, D. et al. (2005) Conjugated linoleic acid isomers and their conjugated derivatives inhibit growth of human cancer cell lines. *Anticancer Res* **25**(6B), 3943–9.

24. Kim, E.J., Shin, H.K., Cho, J.S. et al. (2006) trans-10,cis-12 conjugated linoleic acid inhibits the G1-S cell cycle progression in DU145 human prostate carcinoma cells. *J Med Food* **9**(3), 293–9.

25. Ochoa, J.J., Farquharson, A.J., Grant, I., Moffat, L.E., Heys, S.D., and Wahle, K.W. (2004) Conjugated linoleic acids (CLAs) decrease prostate cancer cell proliferation: Different molecular mechanisms for cis-9, trans-11 and trans-10, cis-12 isomers. *Carcinogenesis* **25**(7), 1185–91.

26. Ip, C., Chin, S.F., Scimeca, J.A., and Pariza, M.W. (1991) Mammary cancer prevention by conjugated dienoic derivative of linoleic acid. *Cancer Res* **51**(22), 6118–24.

27. Ip, C., Scimeca, J.A., and Thompson, H. (1995) Effect of timing and duration of dietary conjugated linoleic acid on mammary cancer prevention. *Nutr Cancer* **24**(3), 241–7.

28. Ip, C., and Scimeca, J.A. (1997) Conjugated linoleic acid and linoleic acid are distinctive modulators of mammary carcinogenesis. *Nutr Cancer* **27**(2), 131–5.

29. Ip, C., Banni, S., Angioni, E. et al. (1999) Conjugated linoleic acid-enriched butter fat alters mammary gland morphogenesis and reduces cancer risk in rats. *J Nutr* **129**(12), 2135–42.

30. Ip, C., Dong, Y., Ip, M.M. et al. (2002) Conjugated linoleic acid isomers and mammary cancer prevention. *Nutr Cancer* **43**(1), 52–58.

31. Lavillonniere, F., Chajes, V., Martin, J.C., Sebedio, J.L., Lhuillery, C., and Bougnoux, P. (2003) Dietary purified cis-9,trans-11 conjugated linoleic acid isomer has anticarcinogenic properties in chemically induced mammary tumors in rats. *Nutr Cancer* **45**(2), 190–4.

32. Chen, B.Q., Xue, Y.B., Liu, J.R. et al. (2003) Inhibition of conjugated linoleic acid on mouse forestomach neoplasia induced by benzo (a) pyrene and chemopreventive mechanisms. *World J Gastroenterol* **9**(1), 44–49.

33. Park, H.S., Ryu, J.H., Ha, Y.L., and Park, J.H. (2001) Dietary conjugated linoleic acid (CLA) induces apoptosis of colonic mucosa in 1,2-dimethylhydrazine-treated rats: A possible mechanism of the anticarcinogenic effect by CLA. *Br J Nutr* **86**(5), 549–55.

34. Kilian, M., Mautsch, I., Gregor, J.I. et al. (2002) Influence of conjugated vs. conventional linoleic acid on liver metastasis and hepatic lipid peroxidation in BOP-induced pancreatic cancer in Syrian hamster. *Prostaglandins Leukot Essent Fatty Acids* **67**(4), 223–8.

35. Rajakangas, J., Basu, S., Salminen, I., and Mutanen, M. (2003) Adenoma growth stimulation by the trans-10, cis-12 isomer of conjugated linoleic acid (CLA) is associated with changes in mucosal NF-kappaB and cyclin D1 protein levels in the Min mouse. *J Nutr* **133**(6), 1943–8.

36. Hubbard, N.E., Chapkin, R.S., and Erickson, K.L. (1988) Inhibition of growth and linoleate-enhanced metastasis of a transplantable mouse mammary tumor by indomethacin. *Cancer Lett* **43**(1–2), 111–20.

37. Hubbard, N.E., Lim, D., and Erickson, K.L. (2003) Effect of separate conjugated linoleic acid isomers on murine mammary tumorigenesis. *Cancer Lett* **190**(1), 13–19.

38. Hubbard, N.E., Lim, D., and Erickson, K.L. (2006) Beef tallow increases the potency of conjugated linoleic acid in the reduction of mouse mammary tumor metastasis. *J Nutr* **136**(1), 88–93.

39. Voorrips, L.E., Brants, H.A., Kardinaal, A.F., Hiddink, G.J., van den Brandt, P.A., and Goldbohm, R.A. (2002) Intake of conjugated linoleic acid, fat, and other fatty acids in relation to postmenopausal breast cancer: The Netherlands Cohort Study on Diet and Cancer. *Am J Clin Nutr* **76**(4), 873–82.

40. Aro, A., Mannisto, S., Salminen, I., Ovaskainen, M.L., Kataja, V., and Uusitupa, M. (2000) Inverse association between dietary and serum conjugated linoleic acid and risk of breast cancer in postmenopausal women. *Nutr Cancer* **38**(2), 151–7.

41. Chajes, V., Lavillonniere, F., Ferrari, P. et al. (2002) Conjugated linoleic acid content in breast adipose tissue is not associated with the relative risk of breast cancer in a population of French patients. *Cancer Epidemiol Biomarkers Prev* **11**(7), 672–3.

42. Kim, J.H., Hubbard, N.E., Ziboh, V., and Erickson, K.L. (2005) Attenuation of breast tumor cell growth by conjugated linoleic acid via inhibition of 5-lipoxygenase activating protein. *Biochim Biophys Acta* **1736**(3), 244–50.

43. Dixon, R.A., Diehl, R.E., Opas, E. et al. (1990) Requirement of a 5-lipoxygenase-activating protein for leukotriene synthesis. *Nature* **343**(6255), 282–4.

44. Hubbard, N.E., Lim, D., and Erickson, K.L. (2007) Conjugated linoleic acid alters matrix metalloproteinases of metastatic mouse mammary tumor cells. *J Nutr* **137**(6), 1423–9.

45. Damonte, P., Hodgson, J.G., Chen, J.Q., Young, L.J., Cardiff, R.D., and Borowsky, A.D. (2008) Mammary carcinoma behavior is programmed in the precancer stem cell. *Breast Cancer Res* **10**(3), R50.

46. Farnie, G., and Clarke, R.B. (2006) Breast stem cells and cancer. *Ernst Schering Found Symp Proc* **5**, 141–53.

47. Borowsky, A. (2007) Special considerations in mouse models of breast cancer. *Breast Dis* **28**, 29–38.

48. Namba, R., Young, L.J., Abbey, C.K. et al. (2006) Rapamycin inhibits growth of premalignant and malignant mammary lesions in a mouse model of ductal carcinoma in situ. *Clin Cancer Res* **12**(8), 2613–21.

49. Namba, R., Young, L.J., Maglione, J.E. et al. (2005) Selective estrogen receptor modulators inhibit growth and progression of premalignant lesions in a mouse model of ductal carcinoma in situ. *Breast Cancer Res* **7**(6), R881–R89.

50. Liu, S., Ginestier, C., Charafe-Jauffret, E. et al. (2008) BRCA1 regulates human mammary stem/progenitor cell fate. *Proc Natl Acad Sci USA* **105**(5), 1680–5.

51. Sikorski, A.M., Hebert, N., and Swain, R.A. (2008 Jun 5) Conjugated Linoleic Acid (CLA) inhibits new vessel growth in the mammalian brain. *Brain Res* **1213**, 35–40. Epub 2008 Feb 16.

52. Mandir, N., and Goodlad, R.A. (2008 Apr) Conjugated linoleic acids differentially alter polyp number and diameter in the Apc(min/+) mouse model of intestinal cancer. *Cell Prolif* **41**(2), 279–91.

13 Cancer and *n*–3PUFAs: The Translation Initiation Connection

B.H. Aktas, M. Chorev, and J.A. Halperin

Key Points

1. A combination of epidemiological, case–control, and cohort studies in the second half of the past century underscored the possibility that high dietary intake of *n*–3 polyunsaturated fatty acids (*n*–3 PUFA) could have a protective effect against cancer.
2. Polyunsaturated fatty acids are classified as having at least 18 carbon chains that are linear and display sequential non-conjugated double bonds separated by single methylene units. The double bonds are solely in the *cis* configuration, with the two hydrogens and the two methylenes on opposite side of the double bond. The two polyunsaturated fatty acids of importance are linoleic (18:2 *n*–6) and linolenic (18:3 *n*–3).
3. Since *n*–3 PUFA incorporate into and are an integral part of membrane phospholipids they can exert profound effects on its physical properties, including permeability, lateral diffusion, lipid packing, and domain formation, and thereby affect function of membrane proteins intimately involved in intracellular signaling. Consistently, *n*–3 PUFA have been shown to influence G protein-coupled receptors and receptor tyrosine kinase signaling pathways, and ion channels, a diversity of cellular effects believed to contribute to their anti-cancer properties.
4. The long chain PUFA are highly susceptible to lipid peroxidation. Peroxidation products of the marine fatty acids have been proposed as mediators of their anti-cancer effects.
5. Evolutionary and cultural changes have shifted the human diet over time toward a lower *n*–3 to *n*–6 PUFA ratio to the point that the modern Western diet is overwhelmingly rich in *n*–6 PUFA. The observed increase in cancer rates in populations that until recently still relied on *n*–3 PUFA-rich diets may be a reflection of the potential impact of the dietary transition from *n*–3 to *n*–6 PUFA-rich diets.

Key Words: *n*–3 polyunsaturated fatty acids; *n*–6 polyunsaturated fatty acids; cellular effects; peroxidation; cancer

From: *Nutrition and Health: Bioactive Compounds and Cancer*
Edited by: J.A. Milner, D.F. Romagnolo, DOI 10.1007/978-1-60761-627-6_13,
© Springer Science+Business Media, LLC 2010

1. INTRODUCTION

1.1. Fatty Acid Biosynthesis

Metabolism of both dietary and de novo synthesized fatty acids generates the fatty acids required for normal physiology. Many physiologically relevant polyunsaturated fatty acids have long, linear, and even carbon-numbered chains of at least 18 carbons that display sequential non-conjugated double bonds separated by single methylene units. These double bonds are exclusively in the *cis* configuration, namely the two substituting hydrogens and the two substituting methylenes are on the opposite sides of the double bond.

The two fatty acids linoleic (18:2 *n*–6) and linolenic acid (18:3 *n*–3) are extremely important constituents of the membrane lipids and indispensable precursors in the biosynthesis of eicosanoid signaling molecules including prostaglandins, thromboxanes, leukotriens, and 5-hydroxyeicosatetraenoic acid *(1–4)*. Because they lack the enzymes required to introduce double bonds within the last seven carbons proximatel to the methyl end of the molecule, mammals can neither synthesize nor interconvert one to the other and must obtain them from the diet. As such they are termed essential fatty acids.

2. METABOLISM OF ESSENTIAL FATTY ACIDS

The 20-carbon or longer polyunsaturated *n*–6 or *n*–3 fatty acids are, respectively, derived from linoleic (18:2 *n*–6) or linolenic (18:3 *n*–3) acids. Linoleic acid is modified by a $\Delta 6$-desaturase that adds a double bond between carbons 6 and 7 from the carboxyl group generating γ-linolenic acid (18:3 *n*–6). This serves as a substrate for elongase generating the dihomo-γ-linolenic acid (20:3 *n*–6), which is longer by two carbons added next to the carboxyl group. A subsequent modification by $\Delta 5$-desaturase adds another double bond between carbons 5 and 6 from the carboxyl group yielding arachidonic acid (20:4 *n*–6). Arachidonic acid is a substrate for prostaglandin synthases, which produces the two double bonds containing prostanoids: prostaglandins, prostacyclins, and thromboxanes, and for lipoxygenases, which produces hydroxyeicosatetraenoic acids and the four double bonds containing leukotrienes. α-Linolenic acid (18:3 *n*–3) is similarly metabolized to eicosapentaenoic acid (20:5 *n*–3; EPA), the precursor of the three double bonds containing prostanoids *(5, 6)* and the five double bonds containing leukotrienes such as LTA_5, LTB_5, and LTC_5 *(7–9)*.

Although the metabolism of both *n*–6 and *n*–3 PUFA series utilizes the same elongase and desaturase enzymes, some observations suggest that the desaturase has higher affinity for *n*–3 than for *n*–6 PUFAs *(10)*. As a result, dietary *n*–3 PUFAs reduce the synthesis of arachidonic acid and the eicosanoids derived from it *(11–15)*. Animals cannot interconvert *n*–3 and *n*–6 PUFA, and lack the $\Delta 12$- and $\Delta 15$-desaturases necessary to convert oleic acid (18:1 *n*–9) to linoleic (18:2 *n*–6) and α-linolenic (18:3 *n*–3) acids, the two essential fatty acids. In contrast, algae have the full repertoire of enzymes to synthesize stearic (18:0 *n*–9) and oleic (18:1 *n*–9) acids, and to convert the latter to linoleic acid (18:2 *n*–6) by $\Delta 12$-desaturase and subsequently to α-linolenic acid (18:3 *n*–3) by $\Delta 15$-desaturase *(16)*. Fish obtain both *n*–6 and *n*–3 fatty acids from the algae they feed on, and the *n*–6/*n*–3 fatty acid distribution of fish oils is influenced by the availability of *n*–3 fatty acids producing plankton found in their habitat. Humans obtain their *n*–3 fatty acids by dietary intake of fish or fish oils. *n*–3 PUFAs are more abundant in cold water fatty fish than in warm water lean fish. It is also important to highlight that because the *n*–3 content of the fish fat is influenced by their food source, aquaculture fish fed with processed food may have a lower content of *n*–3 PUFAs.

3. EPIDEMIOLOGICAL, PROSPECTIVE, AND EXPERIMENTAL STUDIES

The incidence of some cancers in different populations around the world shows dramatic variation. For example, the incidence of prostate and breast cancer is much higher in the United States and Northern Europe than in Asia. This difference cannot be explained by ethnic or racial differences because 1–2 generations after Asian men or women migrate to the United States their age-adjusted risk of prostate and breast cancer rises to reach the risk of the white American population *(17, 18)*. Since diet and dietary habits represent some of the most conspicuous differences in the lifestyles of Western and Asian societies, the regional distribution of breast and prostate cancers together with other comparable observations fueled the speculation that dietary factors, especially the amount of fat consumed and its dietary origin, critically influence the genesis and/or progression of some cancers. A classical example frequently quoted in support of the fat–cancer risk association is that populations like Alaskan Eskimos and Greenland inhabitants, whose diets are based almost exclusively on cold water fish rich in *n*–3 PUFAs, reportedly have a low incidence of prostate and breast cancer *(19–22)*. Another example is that in countries historically considered to have low incidence of cancer, the increase in cancer rate coincides with the wider adoption of more Westernized diets including higher fat intake *(23–26)*. In Japan, for example, an increase in fat consumption between 1955 and 1987 from 9 to 25% of the total energy intake was paralleled by a progressive increase in the incidence of breast cancer *(27–29)*.

In recent years, increasing attention has been paid to an association between cancer risk and the intake of specific fatty acids rather than total fat intake, and notable among these have been fatty acids of marine origin. This is because most of the abovementioned populations with apparent low rates of cancer derive a very significant part of their diet from fish and marine animals, whose fat is rich in *n*–3 PUFA. In these populations, a progressive increase in cancer risk parallels a change in diet that results in a decline in *n*–3 PUFA concomitant with an increase in *n*–6 PUFA intake *(19, 20, 23, 30–33)*.

Although ecological studies of special populations seem to support a negative association between dietary *n*–3 PUFA intake and cancer risk, it is worth noting that the epidemiological evidence is purely inferential and correlative, which makes its interpretation difficult because of other confounding factors. For example, factors such as early age at menarche and at first pregnancy and prolonged lactation, known to reduce the risk of breast cancer, are also prevalent in the populations known to have low incidence of breast cancer and high consumption of *n*–3 PUFAs. These behavioral/cultural patterns may also be changing in response to Western influence. In summary, although nutritional epidemiology studies have intrinsic problems related to both methodology and the role of multifactorial confounding factors that are difficult to control, they were useful in bringing to the forefront the notion that dietary fat in general and the relative intake of n–3 PUFA of marine origin in particular could exert a protective effect against some cancers.

Case–control and cohort studies provide another approach to analyze possible correlations between diet and the risk of cancer. In case–control studies the diet and life style of the cancer patients are compared to those of control subjects whereas in cohort studies a group of healthy individuals is monitored for extended periods of time and the correlation between the incidence of cancer and the dietary habits is analyzed at the end of the study period.

In contrast with frequently quoted ecologic studies mentioned above, some case–control studies were unable to support a potential cancer protective effect of predominantly fish diets *(34, 35)*. In an extensive review of epidemiological, case–control, and cohort studies examining the association between consumption of fish and risk of breast, prostate, and other hormone-dependent cancers published by Terry et al. *(36)* the authors concluded that "... the development and progression of breast and prostate cancer appear to be affected by processes in which eicosapentaenoic acid (EPA) and docosahexaenoic acid (DHA) play important roles; yet whether the consumption of fish containing marine fatty acids can alter the risk of these or of other cancers is unclear". Importantly, these authors pointed out some critical factors that could have clouded the results of those studies. For example, the concentration of EPA and DHA contained in fish varies between species. Relative high concentrations are found in wild cold water fatty fish such as salmon, mackerel, sardines, and herring, whereas warm water lean fish usually have lower concentrations of n–3 PUFA and sometimes higher content of arachidonic acid (n–6 PUFA). Thus, case–control or cohort studies that only analyzed total fish consumption in relation to cancer risk regardless of the type of fish may generate conflicting results. Terry et al. *(36)* also pointed out that an analysis of published studies indicates that the duration of the follow-up period may also affect the results of a study since stronger inverse associations between cancer risk and consumption of n–3 PUFA of marine origin were found in studies with the longest follow-up periods. It seems, therefore, that a clearer picture of the potential association between fatty acids intake and cancer risk would emerge from studies with long follow-up periods that provide repeated diet assessment as well as detailed information on the stages of cancer growth and progression.

This was the case in a recent report from the Health Professionals Follow-up Study *(37)* that examined prospectively the consumption of fish and marine oils in relation to risk of prostate cancer in a cohort of 50,000 men followed up for 12 years. The participants responded to a semi-quantitative food frequency questionnaire mailed in four times during the 12-year period. The food questionnaire was validated measuring actual food intake for 1 week among a sample of 127 cohort members, and dietary intake of n–3 PUFA verified by analysis of the relative composition of fatty acids in a subcutaneous fat aspirate taken from a sample of men from this cohort. The results adjusted for other dietary and non-dietary risk factors showed that men consuming more than three servings of fish per week had almost half the risk of metastatic prostate cancer as compared with rare or non-consumers. Even more remarkable in that study was the finding that each additional daily intake of 0.5 g of marine oil further reduced the risk of metastatic prostate cancer by 24%. Interestingly, no association was found between fish intake and the overall risk (incidence) of prostate cancer among the cohort, an indication suggesting that the intake of fish or marine oils affects tumor progression and metastatic potential rather than the development of cancer. Comparable results suggesting that consumption of fatty fish may reduce the occurrence of renal cell carcinoma (RCC) in women were obtained in the population-based prospective Swedish Mammography Cohort Study in which 61,433 women aged 40–76 years were followed for an average of 15.3 years *(38)*. After adjustment for potential confounders, an inverse association of fatty but not lean fish consumption with the risk of RCC was found. Compared with no consumption, the multivariate rate ratio (RR) was 0.56 for women eating fatty fish once a week or more, and 0.26 for those women reporting consistent consumption of fatty fish in two food questionnaires at the beginning and end of the study.

Experimental studies have provided more consistent data showing that both EPA and DHA, the main *n*–3 PUFAs in fish oils, exert anti-cancer properties in cancer cell lines in vitro and in animal xenograft models of human cancer *(39–43)*. In our hands, daily oral administration of EPA doubled the life expectancy of p53$^{-/-}$ mice, which develop multiple cancers with 100% penetrance and die at $\approx$ 40 weeks of age (unpublished observation).

Taken together, human and experimental studies indicate that *n*–3 PUFAs may exert a protective anti-cancer effect that deserves further investigation. A critical unmet need for such future studies is to define the cellular and molecular mechanism(s) underlying the anti-cancer effect of *n*–3 PUFAs and to derive from this research much needed mechanism-specific biomarkers to conduct human studies.

4. PROPOSED MECHANISMS OF ANTI-CANCER ACTIVITY OF N–3 PUFAS

4.1. Effects on Membrane Structure and Function

Since *n*–3 PUFA incorporate into and are an integral part of membrane phospholipids they can exert profound effects on its physical properties, including permeability, lateral diffusion, lipid packing, and domain formation, and thereby affect function of membrane proteins intimately involved in intracellular signaling. Consistently, *n*–3 PUFAs have been shown to influence G protein-coupled receptors and receptor tyrosine kinase signaling pathways *(44, 45)*, and ion channels *(46)*, a diversity of cellular effects believed to contribute to their anti-cancer properties.

4.2. Effects on Angiogenesis

Neovascularization is essential for growth and metastasis of solid tumors and depends critically on the expression of angiogenic factors such as VEGF and their receptors. Some eicosanoids appear to promote angiogenesis and reduction in their levels may account for the anti-angiogenic activity of *n*–3 PUFAs *(47–49)*.

4.3. Inhibition of Eicosanoid Production from Arachidonic Acid

Eicosanoids including prostaglandins, leukotriens, and thromboxanes, which are derived from 20-carbon PUFAs, affect a wide variety of cellular processes including cell proliferation, differentiation, and apoptosis. Arachidonic acid, a 20-carbon fatty acid abundant in cell membrane phospholipids, is the major precursor of two double bond containing prostanoids. Cyclooxygenase (COX) catalyzes the first step in the conversion of arachidonic acid to prostaglandins and thromboxanes, and lipooxygenase catalyzes its conversion to four double bond containing leukotrienes.

Increased expression of COX and overproduction of some eicosanoids have been implicated in both the development of cancers and the promotion of angiogenesis. Prostaglandins derived from arachidonic acid by the COX-2 enzyme, notably prostaglandin E2 (PGE2), have been linked to carcinogenesis in studies on the proliferation of breast and prostate cancer cell lines in vitro, in experimental animal models leading to the development of mammary tumors, and in human studies on the effect of fish oil intake on the rate of epithelial cell proliferation *(50, 51)*.

Increasing the dietary intake of *n*–3 PUFA reduces the production of arachidonic acid *(52)* and thereby the generation of arachidonic acid-derived eicosanoids. In addition, both EPA and DHA can displace arachidonic acid in cell membrane phospholipids *(53)* and in diacylglycerols *(54)* and have been shown to inhibit COX-2 *(50)* and lipoxygenase. Thus, replacement and reduced formation of arachidonic acid, as well as inhibition of key enzymes in the eicosanoid synthesis pathways, are proposed mechanism underlying the anti-cancer effects of *n*–3 PUFA, a view supported in part by the apparent inhibitory effect on cancer cells growth of some non-steroidal anti-inflammatory drugs that inhibit COX activity.

4.4. Effect on Mevalonate Metabolism

3-Hydroxy-3-methylglutaryl coenzyme-A reductase catalyzes the synthesis of mevalonate and is the rate-limiting enzyme in the cholesterol biosynthesis. Products of this biosynthetic pathway play a critical role in the organization of signaling pathways that impinge on cell proliferation *(55)*. Expression of 3-hydroxy-3-methylglutaryl coenzyme A reductase and mevalonate production are suppressed *(56)* in the mammary glands of menhaden oil-fed female rats but the importance of this finding for the anti-breast cancer effects of *n*–3 PUFAs is not known.

4.5. Effect on Estrogen and Testosterone Metabolism

17β-Estradiol, the main mammalian endogenous estrogen, stimulates normal mammary development and promotes the neoplastic transformation of breast cells. Estradiol is metabolized along two major pathways, generating two different metabolites, 16-hydroxyestrone and 2-hydroxyestrone with the former considered to be more bioactive than the latter. 16-Hydroxyestrone produces aberrant hyper-proliferation in mammary explants and is considered a mediator of estrogen-induced transformation of breast epithelial cells *(57)*; also, clinical studies suggest that elevated C16-hydroxylation of estradiol may provide a biomarker for breast cancer risk *(58, 59)*. Osborne et al. *(60)* reported that feeding an *n*–3 PUFA-rich fish oil supplement to women reduced the extent of C16-hydroxylation, suggesting that a reduced production of 16-hydroxyestrone and perhaps increased generation of 2-hydroxyestrone may contribute to an anti-cancer effect of *n*–3 PUFAs in breast cancer.

Testosterone promotes proliferation and neoplastic transformation of prostate cells. Both *n*–3 and *n*–6 PUFAs interfere with testosterone metabolism by inhibiting the enzyme 5α-reductase and thereby the conversion of testosterone to dihydrotestosterone *(61)*. However, the anti-cancer properties of PUFAs in prostate cancer seem to be limited to the *n*–3 series.

4.6. Effect of Lipid Peroxidation

The long chain PUFAs are highly susceptible to lipid peroxidation. Peroxidation products of the marine fatty acids have been proposed as mediators of their anti-cancer effects *(62, 63)*. For example, in breast cancer cell lines, treatment with DHA increased lipid peroxides and enhanced the toxicity of anthracyclins (agents that generate oxidative stress); both effects were inhibited by the antioxidant vitamin E *(64)*. Similar results have been reported in animal models of experimental breast cancer *(65, 66)*. However, the mechanism(s) by which these oxidation products of *n*–3 PUFAs inhibit cancer cell growth is still debated *(67)*.

In summary, although effects on cell membrane, eicosanoid formation, estrogen and testosterone metabolism, and lipid peroxidation have been proposed as potential mediators of the anti-cancer effects of marine fish oils, these mechanisms are not embraced because of the lack of stringent and direct evidence for their causative role.

4.7. The Translation Initiation Connection

Recent work has identified translation initiation as a putative molecular target mediating the anti-cancer effects of *n*–3 PUFAs. Translation, the cellular process by which mRNAs are translated into proteins, is operationally divided in three phases: initiation, elongation, and termination. Translation initiation, a highly regulated process requiring the concerted participation of more than 20 proteins/cellular factors known as eukaryotic translation initiation factors (eIFs), plays a critical role in the control of growth, differentiation, and division in eukaryotic cells *(68–70)*. This is because structural features in the mRNAs coding for most proto-oncogenic, growth, and transcription factors and cell cycle regulatory proteins make their translation rather inefficient and critically dependent on the activity of translation initiation factors such as eIF2, eIF4E, eIF4A, and eIF4G. Long and complex 5′-untranslated regions (5′UTR) are associated with inefficient translation probably because the presence of stable secondary structures prevents ribosomes from scanning efficiently the entire 5′UTR to reach the AUG translation initiation codon *(71, 72)*. In contrast, mRNAs with short, simple, and less structured 5′-UTRs are translated more efficiently. Interestingly, the sequences of 5′UTRs of approximately 90% of vertebrate mRNAs are between 10 and 200 bases long, mostly without a complex secondary structure are therefore efficiently translated ("strong" mRNAs). On the other hand, most mRNAs encoding for cell growth regulatory proteins and proto-oncogenes contain atypical 5′UTRs which are more than 200 bases long, rich in Gs and Cs, and contain stable secondary structures that restrict their translational efficiency and render their translation highly dependent on the activity of translation initiation factors ("weak" mRNAs) *(73)*. Indeed, experimental evidence indicates that the rate of translation controls the expression of most cell growth regulatory proteins. For example, early mitogenic signals that turn on the transcription of cell growth regulatory genes simultaneously activate translation initiation factors such as eIF2 and eIF4E that are rate limiting for translation initiation. In this manner, extracellular signals that stimulate cell proliferation couple transcription with translation resulting in a dramatic increase in the expression of growth regulatory proteins at the G0–G1 transition and during the G1 phase of the cell cycle. Consistently, we and others have shown experimentally that reducing the rate of translation initiation preferentially inhibits the synthesis and expression of oncogenic proteins and cell growth regulatory proteins such as the G1-cyclins (cyclin D1, cyclin E, and cyclin A) while other "house keeping" proteins are minimally affected *(74)*.

5. TRANSLATION INITIATION AND CANCER

Cancer cells proliferate disregarding the checkpoints that restrain growth in normal cells. This ability is acquired through mutations that lead to inactivation of growth inhibitory genes such as Rb (retinoblastoma) or of tumor suppressor genes such as p53, and/or to activation of proto-oncogenes such as cyclin D1, c-myc, and Ras. Products of these genes regulate specific events in cell growth and division. Interestingly, over-expression of proteins that regulate translation initiation causes neoplastic transformation because the consequent increase in the rate of protein synthesis leads to a disproportionately higher translation of oncogenic proteins such as cyclin D1 and c-myc, which are over-expressed in a large number of human cancers *(75–77)*.

In human cancers, over-expression of the translation initiation factor eIF2α correlates with neoplastic transformation of mammary epithelial cells, and with the aggressiveness of non-Hodgkin's lymphomas *(78, 79)*. Over-expression of eIF4E reportedly is a prognostic tumor marker for breast cancers *(80)*, a predictor of recurrence in head and neck tumors *(81, 82)*, and is abundant in breast *(83)*, head and neck *(84)*, primary bladder *(85)*, colon carcinomas *(86)*, and in non-Hodgkin's lymphomas *(78)*. Also, in many human cancers, the translational efficiency of oncogenic proteins and growth factors such as c-myc, VEGF, and TGF-β is significantly enhanced through variations that simplify the structure of their mRNA thus enabling them to escape tight control of translation initiation *(87)*. For example, the mRNA for TGF-β has two alternative splicing forms, one with an 1100-nucleotide long and highly structured 5′-UTR and the other with a 230-nucleotide long and simpler 5′-UTR that has sevenfold higher translational efficiency. The shorter, translationally stronger TGF-β mRNA is almost exclusively seen in cancers, and is believed to contribute to the metastatic potential of some breast cancers *(88)*.

In contrast, inhibition of translation initiation interferes with both cell growth and malignant transformation *(89–91)*. For instance, over-expression of eIF4E-BP, a cellular inhibitor of translation initiation that blocks formation of the eIF4F complex, suppresses cancer cell proliferation and tumor growth *(89, 92–94)*. Similarly, pharmacological inhibitors of translation initiation such as clotrimazole, troglitazone, rapamycin, 4EGI-1 as well as anti-sense oligonucleotides targeting eIF4E reportedly inhibit cancer cell proliferation and/or tumor growth in animal models of human cancer *(95, 74, 96–100)*.

The previous paragraphs highlight the critical role played by translation initiation in the physiological control of cell growth as well as in both malignant transformation and maintenance of transformed phenotypes. The translation initiation machinery, therefore, represents an attractive target for cancer therapy *(101)*, and translation initiation inhibitors are now recognized as an emerging class of anti-cancer agents *(102)*.

5.1. Inhibition of Translation Initiation Mediates the Anti-cancer Effect of EPA

In the following sections, we will briefly describe the translation initiation process, and summarize the experimental evidence generated in our laboratories demonstrating that the anti-cancer effects of EPA are mediated by inhibition of translation initiation *(95, 103)*.

In the initiation phase of mRNA translation, the translation initiation factor eIF2 forms a ternary complex with GTP and the initiating methionyl-tRNA (Met-tRNA$_i$). The eIF2·GTP·Met-tRNA$_i$ recruits the 40S ribosomal subunit forming the 43S pre-initiation complex, which then binds to the mRNA cap through interaction with other translation initiation factors. The pre-initiation complex scans the 5′-UTR of mRNA for the initiator AUG codon, a process that requires the participation of several translation initiation factors including eIF4E, eIF4G, and the RNA helicase eIF4A. At the AUG codon, the 60S ribosomal subunit is recruited to join the 48S pre-initiation complex to form the catalytically competent 80S ribosome. Concomitantly, GTP that is associated with eIF2 is hydrolyzed to GDP. To initiate a new cycle of translation GDP needs to be exchanged for GTP. This GDP–GTP exchange, which is carried out while bound to eIF2, is catalyzed by the multi-subunit guanine nucleotide exchange factor eIF2B. Because phosphorylation of the alpha subunit of eIF2 (eIF2α) by eIF2α kinases increases its affinity for the GDP–GTP exchange factor eIF2B, phosphorylation of eIF2α inhibits translation initiation *(104)*. Since the stoichiometric ratio of eIF2B to eIF2 in the cytosol is quite low, even partial phosphorylation of eIF2α is sufficient to sequester the free eIF2B that is necessary for GDP–GTP exchange *(105, 106)*. Figure 1 summarizes the translation initiation process.

The eIF2α kinases phosphorylate eIF2α on its serine 51. At least two eIF2α kinases, interferon-inducible, double-stranded RNA-dependent protein kinase (PKR) and PKR-like ER-resident kinase (PERK), are activated by signals from a "stressed" endoplasmic reticulum (ER) triggering a cascade of events generally termed the ER-stress response *(107, 108)*. It is well established that partial depletion of ER Ca^{2+} stores rapidly activates eIF2α kinases that phosphorylate eIF2α thus limiting the availability of the ternary complex resulting in reduced rate of translation initiation and protein synthesis *(74, 105)*.

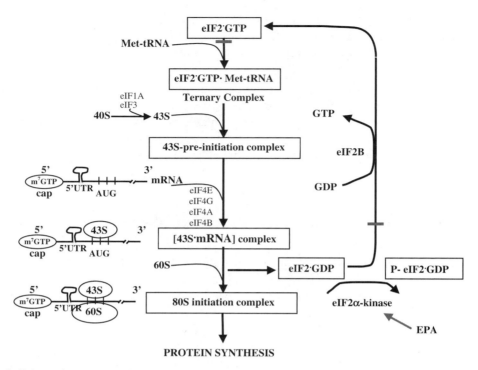

Fig. 1. Schematic representation of translation initiation highlighting the putative sites of action of the n–3 PUFAs.

5.2. EPA Depletes Intracellular Ca²⁺ Stores

Binding of many physiological agonists such as hormones, growth factors, and cytokines to their cognate cell membrane receptors induces a transient rise in cytosolic Ca^{2+} following its release from intracellular stores. When Ca^{2+} is released from intracellular stores, Ca^{2+} channels in the plasma membrane known as "store-operated calcium channels" (SOC) open to refill the intracellular stores by capacitative Ca^{2+} entry from the extracellular medium thus re-establishing intracellular Ca^{2+} homeostasis (109, 110).

The n–3 PUFA EPA has a dual effect on intracellular Ca^{2+} homeostasis. It induces Ca^{2+} release from the intracellular Ca^{2+} stores while inhibiting Ca^{2+} influx through SOC in the plasma membrane. These cellular effects require peroxidation of EPA because they are blocked by vitamin E (95). By simultaneously releasing Ca^{2+} from the ER stores and closing SOC, EPA partially depletes intracellular Ca^{2+} stores (Fig. 2a). Depletion of the intracellular Ca^{2+} stores by EPA was confirmed in our laboratory by transfecting cells with ER-targeted "chameleon" proteins that monitor the ER calcium content in real time. Figure 2b shows the ER-calcium depleting effect of EPA, as determined with ER-targeted "chameleon" proteins.

As mentioned above, partial depletion of intracellular Ca^{2+} stores activates eIF2α kinases and inhibits translation initiation. Inhibition of translation initiation by EPA was demonstrated by polysome-profiling cell lysates through sucrose density gradient

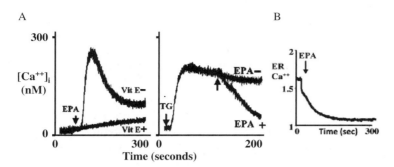

Fig. 2. EPA releases Ca^{2+} from ER stores and closes SOC. Fura-2 loaded cells were treated with EPA in the presence or absence of vitamin E (**a**) in Ca^{2+}-free media or with TG in Ca^{2+}-containing media to open SOC and then treated with or without EPA (**b**). ER-targeted chameleon expressing cells were treated with EPA excited at 440 nM and FRET was measured by determining the emission ratio at 530 nM (YFP) vs. 480 nM (CFP) (**c**). **a** and **b** from *(95)*.

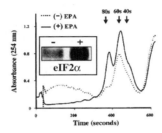

Fig. 3. EPA shifts the cell polysome profile from heavy to lighter polysomes. Lysates of exponentially growing cell were processed by sucrose density gradient centrifugation and then read from the bottom at 214 nm. The *inset* shows phosphorylation of eIF2α by EPA.

centrifugation. Treatment of cells with EPA shifts the polysome profile from heavy polyribosomal fractions toward light polysomes and free ribosomal subunits *(95)* (Fig. 3). This shift of the cellular polysome profile toward lighter fractions indicates reduction in the loading of the mRNAs with ribosomes and is recognized as the hallmark of inhibition of translation initiation.

5.3. EPA-Mediated Phosphorylation of eIF2α Results in Inhibition of Translation Initiation

Inhibition of translation initiation by EPA is mediated by eIF2α kinase-dependent phosphorylation of eIF2α. This conclusion is based on the experimental findings in cancer cell lines treated with EPA, which (a) causes phosphorylation of eIF2α (inset to Fig. 3), (b) inhibits translation initiation in wild-type cells but not in cells expressing a dominant negative mutant of the eIF2α kinase PKR, and (c) does not affect translation initiation, protein synthesis or cell growth in cells transfected with a constitutively active but phosphorylation resistant mutant of eIF2α (eIF2α-S51A) *(95)*.

Inhibitory phosphorylation of eIF2α on its serine 51 residue is catalyzed by four eIF2α kinases: PKR, PERK, HRI, and GCN2. Each of these enzymes is activated in response to different perturbations in the cellular environment with the common end result of shutting off mRNA translation via phosphorylation of eIF2α. It has been proposed that phosphorylation of eIF2α in response to a decrease in the calcium content of the ER is mediated by PERK. This conclusion was based on experiments with thapsigargin (TG), a specific inhibitor of the SERCA-ATPase. By inhibiting active calcium influx into the ER, TG breaks the steady-state cellular calcium homeostasis and induces a net Ca^{2+} leakage from the ER into the cytosol leading to a reduction of the ER-calcium content. This effect is associated with restorative calcium influx from the extracellular medium that occurs through SOC that open up to refill the calcium content of the ER. The operation of these channels is revealed by a sustained increase in cytosolic calcium that follows the addition of TG to cell incubated in a calcium containing but not in a calcium-free medium. In contrast, EPA-mediated release of Ca^{2+} from the ER is not mediated by inhibition of the SERCA-ATPase (Halperin et al. unpublished observation) and is associated with closing rather than opening of the SOC. Indeed, sequential addition of TG followed by EPA revealed that EPA inhibits calcium influx via the SOC, as we have shown in previous studies (95) (Fig. 2). These differences are functionally important because by releasing Ca^{2+} from the ER while closing SOC, EPA induces a sustained partial depletion of ER-calcium while the effect of TG is only transient (74). Given the peculiar nature of the EPA effect on intracellular Ca^{2+} homeostasis, we investigated whether PERK was necessary for EPA-induced phosphorylation of eIF2α. To this end, we compared the effects of EPA and TG on phosphorylation of eIF2α in PERK$^{+/+}$ and PERK$^{-/-}$ cells (kindly provided by David Ron). The results showed that in sharp contrast with TG, EPA-induced phosphorylation of eIF2α was PERK independent (Fig. 4). This difference between EPA and TG seems to be directly related to the differential effect of EPA and TG on intracellular Ca^{2+} homeostasis because simultaneous treatment of cells with TG and sulindac sulfide, a specific inhibitor of SOC channels, caused phosphorylation of eIF2α in a PERK independent manner, identical to the effect of EPA (Fig. 5, bottom left panel). These data confirm that EPA inhibits translation initiation because it releases Ca^{2+} from ER and inhibits Ca^{2+} influx through SOC channels thus causing partial and sustained depletion of ER-Ca^{2+} stores (Fig. 5).

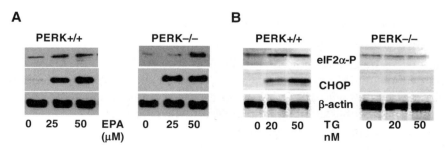

Fig. 4. EPA-induced eIF2a phosphorylation is PERK independent. PERK$^{+/+}$ and PERK $^{-/-}$ cells were treated with EPA (**a**) or TG (**b**) lysed and blotted with antibodies to pS51-eIF2α, CHOP, and β-actin.

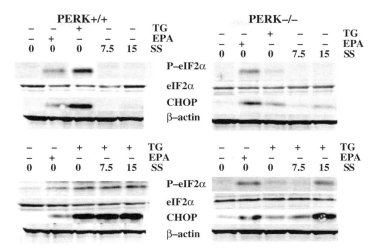

Fig. 5. Simultaneous release of Ca^{2+} from ER and closing of SOC channels renders eIF2α phosphorylation independent of PERK. PERK$^{+/+}$ and PERK$^{-/-}$ mouse embryonic fibroblasts were treated with vehicle, EPA (50 mM), TG (0.2 mM), sulindac sulfide (SS, 7.5 and 15 mM) or combination of SS and TG for 1 h to determine phosphorylation of eIF2α or 8 h to determine induction of CHOP expression. Cell lysates were blotted with the indicated antibodies.

5.4. EPA Downregulates Expression of Oncogenic Proteins and Upregulates Expression of Pro-apoptotic and Tumor Suppressor Proteins

Phosphorylation of eIF2α is a rate-limiting step controlling the overall rate of translation. However, unique structural features in the 5′UTR of mRNAs provide an additional mechanism for regulation of gene-specific expression. In previous sections, we described how mRNAs with complex 5′UTRs that predominantly encode for oncogenic proteins are translationally weak and therefore preferentially downregulated when eIF2α is phosphorylated.

Interestingly, a limited subset of mRNAs with well-defined structural features in their mRNA are paradoxically upregulated when eIF2α is phosphorylated. A characteristic example of this paradoxical translational upregulation is represented by the activating transcription factor-4 (ATF-4). The 5′UTR of ATF-4 mRNA contains multiple upstream open reading (uORF) frames that behave as ribosomal traps rendering its translation inefficient when the eIF2·GTP·Met-tRNA$_i$ ternary complex is abundant. In contrast, the translation efficiency of ATF-4 is increased when the availability of the ternary complex is limited, as it occurs when eIF2α is phosphorylated. This in turn results in the transcriptional upregulation of pro-apoptotic CHOP and the ER-chaperon BiP, which are under the transcriptional control of ATF-4.

More recently, we have identified a comparable mechanism responsible for translational upregulation of the tumor suppressor gene, BRCA1. Specifically, breast cancer cells express a BRCA1 mRNA isoform (mRNAb) in which the BRCA1 uORF is preceded by a 5′-UTR remarkably similar to the 5′UTR of ATF-4. Conversely, non-transformed breast epithelial cells express a BRCA1 transcript with a simple 5′UTR

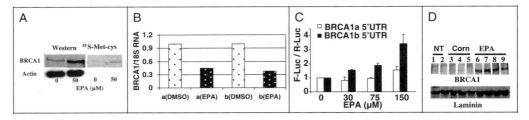

Fig. 6. EPA upregulates expression of BRCA1 in MCF-7 human breast cancer cells. (**a**) EPA increases BRCA1 expression and de novo synthesis. (**b**) Real-time PCR for BRCA1 mRNAa and mRNAb in the EPA-treated cells from **a**. (**c**) The 5′-UTR of BRCA1 mRNAb but not of BRCA1 mRNAa confers to reporter gene translational upregulation by EPA. (**d**) Orthotopic breast tumors were formed in nude mice by inoculating MCF-7 breast cancer cells. Tumor-bearing mice were fed with menhaden (fish) or corn oil diet and expression of BRCA1 in the tumor was determined by Western blot.

(mRNAa) *(111)*. Importantly, in the transition from in situ to progressive breast cancer, expression switches from mRNAa to mRNAb that reduces the translational efficiency and thereby the expression of BRCA1, a tumor suppressor protein. We have shown experimentally that (1) EPA induces upregulation of BRCA1 expression in MCF-7 breast cancer cells (Fig. 6a), (2) the EPA-induced expression of BRCA1 is translational because synthesis of BRCA1 protein is increased without a concomitant increase in the levels of its mRNA (Fig. 6), and (3) fusion to a reporter gene of the 5′UTR of BRCA1 mRNAb, which contains multiple uORF, renders the reporter sensitive to translational upregulation by EPA (Fig. 6). This translational upregulation was not observed when the reporter gene was fused to the 5′UTR of BRCA1 mRNAa, which does not contain multiple uORF. Suppression of BRCA1 expression in aggressive breast cancers *(112, 113)* is unique in that somatic mutations, loss of heterozygosity (LOH) *(114)*, or promoter methylation cannot explain its lack of expression in vast majority of spontaneous breast cancers *(112, 115–123)*. Importantly, restoration of BRCA1 expression reverts malignant phenotype in breast cancer cells *(124)*. These findings have led us to propose that the anti-breast cancer effect of n–3 PUFAs is mediated, at least in part, by upregulation of BRCA1 expression secondary to phosphorylation of eIF2α.

In summary, we have identified the molecular mechanism of the anti-cancer activity of n–3 PUFAs such as EPA in vitro and most likely in vivo. By partially depleting ER Ca^{2+} stores, these natural nutrients inhibit translation initiation, preferentially downregulate the synthesis and expression of oncogenic proteins and thereby block progression of the cell cycle into the G1 phase. These activities are associated with increased apoptosis mediated, at least in part, by upregulation of pro-apoptotic and tumor suppressor genes via specific transcription factors and tumor suppressing genes encoded by mRNAs with multiple uORF in the 5′UTR. Figure 7 summarizes the proposed mechanism of the anti-cancer effect of n–3 PUFAs such as EPA.

6. CONCLUSIONS

n–3 PUFAs were readily available nutrients in the primitive food chain. The recently identified effect of n–3 PUFAs on the translational regulation of genes that control cell

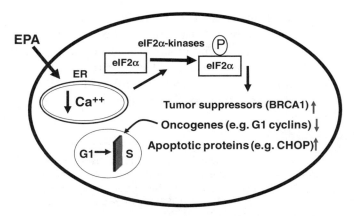

Fig. 7. Proposed mechanisms of the anti-cancer effect of *n*–3 PUFAs such as EPA. Through partial depletion of ER Ca^{2+} stores, EPA inhibits translation initiation, preferentially downregulates the synthesis and expression of oncogenic proteins and thereby blocks progression of the cell cycle into the G1 phase. These activities are associated with increased apoptosis mediated, at least in part, by upregulation of pro-apoptotic (CHOP) and tumor suppressor genes via specific transcription factors and tumor-suppressing genes encoded by mRNAs with multiple uORF in the 5′-UTR.

proliferation and survival can be conceived as an environmental clue to maintain a correct restrain on physiological cell growth at periods of excessive food abundance. Evolutionary and cultural changes have shifted the human diet over time toward a lower *n*–3 to *n*–6 PUFA ratio to the point that the modern Western diet is overwhelmingly rich in *n*–6 PUFAs. The observed increase in cancer rates in populations that until recently still relied on *n*–3 PUFA-rich diets may be a reflection of the potential impact of the dietary transition from *n*–3 to *n*–6 PUFA-rich diets.

Efforts to restore an adequate balance of *n*–3 to *n*–6 PUFAs in the modern diet might be hampered by the precipitous decline of wild marine fish stocks. Indeed, it seems that current wild marine sources would not be capable to sustain a progressive increase in dietary *n*–3 PUFAs in the growing world population. Fish produced in aquaculture farms may not represent a viable alternative to increase the *n*–3 PUFA content of the modern diet because their feeding with industrial food rich in *n*–6 PUFAs may reduce very long chain *n*–3 PUFA content of aquaculture fish. There may be hope, however, since genes that can convert *n*–6 to *n*–3 fatty acids such as *fat-1* can be transgenically introduced into both plants and animals, as recently reported in mice *(125)*.

Thus, given the magnitude of the potential public health benefits that could derive from increasing the *n*–3 PUFAs of the human diet, and the multi-factorial economic, cultural, and practical difficulties implicated in achieving that goal, extensive intervention studies are needed to determine conclusively whether *n*–3 PUFA-rich diets reduce cancer risk in a manner that justifies the effort. The conduction and success of such human trials critically depends on the availability of biomarkers that will provide clear-cut and efficient end points thus limiting their duration and facilitating the interpretation of their results. The generation of such biomarkers is an important contribution of the research summarized in this chapter. Indeed, preliminary results in human cancer patients indicate that administration of EPA-rich fish oils induces phosphorylation of eIF2α in vivo. Thus, the theoretical and practical tools are now available for the conduction of prospective trials to validate the molecular target of the putative anti-cancer effects of n–3 PUFAs in human cancers and, if confirmed, conduct adequate trials to assess the preventive and perhaps therapeutic effects of these nutrients.

REFERENCES

1. Hansen, A.E., Haggard, M.E., Boelsche, A.N., Adam, D.J., and Wiese, H.F. (1958) Essential fatty acids in infant nutrition. III. Clinical manifestations of linoleic acid deficiency. *J Nutr* **66**, 565–76.
2. Collins, F.D. et al. (1971) Plasma lipids in human linoleic acid deficiency. *Nutr Metab* **13**, 150–67.
3. Holman, R.T., Johnson, S.B., and Hatch, T.F. (1982) A case of human linolenic acid deficiency involving neurological abnormalities. *Am J Clin Nutr* **35**, 617–23.
4. Paulsrud, J.R., Pensler, L., Whitten, C.F., Stewart, S., and Holman, R.T. (1972) Essential fatty acid deficiency in infants induced by fat-free intravenous feeding. *Am J Clin Nutr* **25**, 897–904.
5. Needleman, P., Raz, A., Minkes, M.S., Ferrendelli, J.A., and Sprecher, H. (1979) Triene prostaglandins: Prostacyclin and thromboxane biosynthesis and unique biological properties. *Proc Natl Acad Sci U S A* **76**, 944–48.
6. Fischer, S., and Weber, P.C. (1984) Prostaglandin I3 is formed in vivo in man after dietary eicosapentaenoic acid. *Nature* **307**, 165–68.
7. Prescott, S.M. (1984) The effect of eicosapentaenoic acid on leukotriene B production by human neutrophils. *J Biol Chem* **259**, 7615–21.
8. Lee, T.H. et al. (1984) Characterization and biologic properties of 5,12-dihydroxy derivatives of eicosapentaenoic acid, including leukotriene B5 and the double lipoxygenase product. *J Biol Chem* **259**, 2383–89.
9. Strasser, T., Fischer, S., and Weber, P.C. (1985) Leukotriene B5 is formed in human neutrophils after dietary supplementation with icosapentaenoic acid. *Proc Natl Acad Sci U S A* **82**, 1540–43.
10. Brenner, R.R. (1974) The oxidative desaturation of unsaturated fatty acids in animals. *Mol Cell Biochem* **3**, 41–52.
11. Chen, Q., and Nilsson, A. (1993) Desaturation and chain elongation of n-3 and n-6 polyunsaturated fatty acids in the human CaCo-2 cell line. *Biochim Biophys Acta* **1166**, 193–201.
12. Emken, E.A. (1994) Metabolism of dietary stearic acid relative to other fatty acids in human subjects. *Am J Clin Nutr* **60**, 1023S–1028S.
13. Emken, E.A., Adlof, R.O., Duval, S.M., and Nelson, G.J. (1998) Effect of dietary arachidonic acid on metabolism of deuterated linoleic acid by adult male subjects. *Lipids* **33**, 471–80.
14. Emken, E.A., Adlof, R.O., Duval, S.M., and Nelson, G.J. (1999) Effect of dietary docosahexaenoic acid on desaturation and uptake in vivo of isotope-labeled oleic, linoleic, and linolenic acids by male subjects. *Lipids* **34**, 785–91.
15. Sauerwald, T.U. et al. (1996) Effect of dietary alpha-linolenic acid intake on incorporation of docosahexaenoic and arachidonic acids into plasma phospholipids of term infants. *Lipids* **31**(Suppl), S131–S35.
16. Sayanova, O.V., and Napier, J.A. (2004) Eicosapentaenoic acid: Biosynthetic routes and the potential for synthesis in transgenic plants. *Phytochemistry* **65**, 147–58.
17. Ziegler, R.G. et al. (1993) Migration patterns and breast cancer risk in Asian–American women. *J Nat Cancer Inst* **85**, 1819–27.
18. Deapen, D., Liu, L., Perkins, C., Bernstein, L., and Ross, R.K. (2002) Rapidly rising breast cancer incidence rates among Asian–American women. *Int J Cancer* **99**, 747–50.
19. Bjarnason, O., Day, N., Snaedal, G., and Tulinius, H. (1974) The effect of year of birth on the breast cancer age-incidence curve in Iceland. *Int J Cancer* **13**, 689–96.
20. Nielson, N.H., and Hansen, J.P. (1980) Breast cancer in greenland – selected epidemiological, clinical, and histological features. *Clin Oncol* **1980**, 287–99.

21. Lanier, A.P., Bulkow, L.R., and Ireland, B. (1989) Cancer in Alaskan Indians, Eskimos, and Aleuts, 1969–1983: Implications for etiology and control. *Public Health Rep* **104**, 658–64.

22. Lanier, A.P., Bender, T.R., Blot, W.J., Fraumeni, J.F., Jr., and Hurlburt, W.B. (1976) Cancer incidence in Alaska natives. *Int J Cancer* **18**, 409–12.

23. Lanier, A.P. et al. (1996) Alaska Native cancer update: Incidence rates 1989–1993. *Cancer Epidemiol Biomarkers Prev* **5**, 749–51.

24. Tsuji, K., Harashima, E., Nakagawa, Y., Urata, G., and Shirataka, M. (1996) Time-lag effect of dietary fiber and fat intake ratio on Japanese colon cancer mortality. *Biomed Environ Sci* **9**, 223–28.

25. You, W.C. et al. (2002) Rapid increase in colorectal cancer rates in urban Shanghai, 1972–1997, in relation to dietary changes. *J Cancer Epidemiol Prev* **7**, 143–46.

26. Bruce, W.R., Giacca, A., and Medline, A. (2000) Possible mechanisms relating diet and risk of colon cancer. *Cancer Epidemiol Biomarkers Prev* **9**, 1271–79.

27. Wynder, E.L., Fujita, Y., Harris, R.E., Hirayama, T., and Hiyama, T. (1991) Comparative epidemiology of cancer between the United States and Japan. A second look. *Cancer* **67**, 746–63.

28. Hirayama, T. (1978) Epidemiology of breast cancer with special reference to the role of diet. *Prev Med* **7**, 173–95.

29. Karmali, R.A. et al. (1987) The effects of dietary w-3 fatty acids on the DU-145 transplantable human prostatic tumor. *Anticancer Res* **7**, 1173–80.

30. Kaizer, L., Boyd, N.F., Kriukov, V., and Tritchler, D. (1989) Fish consumption and breast cancer risk: An ecological study. *Nutr Cancer* **12**, 61–68.

31. Armstrong, B., and Doll, R. (1975) Environmental factors and cancer incidence and mortality in different countries, with special reference to dietary practices. *Int J Cancer* **15**, 617–31.

32. Sasaki, S., Horacsek, M., and Kesteloot, H. (1993) An ecological study of the relationship between dietary fat intake and breast cancer mortality. *Prev Med* **22**, 187–202.

33. Jansson, B., Seibert, B., and Speer, J.F. (1975) Gastrointestinal cancer. Its geographic distribution and correlation to breast cancer. *Cancer* **36**, 2373–84.

34. Willett, W.C. (1997) Specific fatty acids and risks of breast and prostate cancer: Dietary intake. *Am J Clin Nutr* **66**, 1557S–1563S.

35. MacLean, C.H. et al. (2006) Effects of omega-3 fatty acids on cancer risk: A systematic review. *JAMA* **295**, 403–15, DOI: %R 10.1001/jama.295.4.403.

36. Terry, P.D., Rohan, T.E., and Wolk, A. (2003) Intakes of fish and marine fatty acids and the risks of cancers of the breast and prostate and of other hormone-related cancers: A review of the epidemiologic evidence. *Am J Clin Nutr* **77**, 532–43.

37. Augustsson, K. et al. (2003) A prospective study of intake of fish and marine fatty acids and prostate cancer. *Cancer Epidemiol Biomarkers Prev* **12**, 64–67.

38. Wolk, A., Larsson, S.C., Johansson, J.E., and Ekman, P. (2006) Long-term fatty fish consumption and renal cell carcinoma incidence in women. *JAMA* **296**, 1371–76.

39. Grammatikos, S.I., Subbaiah, P.V., Victor, T.A., and Miller, W.M. (1994) n-3 and n-6 fatty acid processing and growth effects in neoplastic and non-cancerous human mammary epithelial cell lines. *Br J Cancer* **70**, 219–27.

40. Falconer, J.S. et al. (1994) Effect of eicosapentaenoic acid and other fatty acids on the growth in vitro of human pancreatic cancer cell lines. *Br J Cancer* **69**, 826–32.

41. Whelan, J., Petrik, M.B., McEntee, M.F., and Obukowicz, M.G. (2002) Dietary EPA reduces tumor load in ApcMin/+ mice by altering arachidonic acid metabolism, but conjugated linoleic acid, gamma – and alpha-linolenic acids have no effect. *Adv Exp Med Biol* **507**, 579–84.

42. Calviello, G. et al. (1998) Dietary supplementation with eicosapentaenoic and docosahexaenoic acid inhibits growth of Morris hepatocarcinoma 3924A in rats: Effects on proliferation and apoptosis. *Int J Cancer* **75**, 699–705.

43. Rose, D.P., Connolly, J.M., and Coleman, M. (1996) Effect of omega-3 fatty acids on the progression of metastases after the surgical excision of human breast cancer cell solid tumors growing in nude mice. *Clinical Cancer Res* **2**, 1751–56.

44. Mitchell, D., Niu, S., and Litman, B. (2003) DHA-rich phospholipids optimize G-Protein-coupled signaling. *J Pediatr* **143**, S80–S86.

45. Zhang, Y.W., Morita, I., Yao, X.S., and Murota, S. (1999) Pretreatment with eicosapentaenoic acid prevented hypoxia/reoxygenation-induced abnormality in endothelial gap junctional intercellular communication through inhibiting the tyrosine kinase activity. *Prostaglandins Leukot Essent Fatty Acids* **61**, 33–40.

46. Xiao, Y.-F. et al. (2001) Single point mutations affect fatty acid block of human myocardial sodium channel alpha subunit Na+ channels. *PNAS* **98**, 3606–11.

47. Form, D.M., and Auerbach, R. (1983) PGE2 and angiogenesis. *Proc Soc Exp Biol Med* **172**, 214–18.

48. Connolly, J.M., Coleman, M., and Rose, D.P. (1997) Effects of dietary fatty acids on DU145 human prostate cancer cell growth in athymic nude mice. *Nutr Cancer* **29**, 114–19.

49. Tang, G., Blanco, M.C., Fox, J.G., and Russell, R.M. (1995) Supplementing ferrets with canthaxan-thin affects the tissue distributions of canthaxanthin, other carotenoids, vitamin A and vitamin E. *J Nutr* **125**, 1945–51.

50. Rose, D.P., and Connolly, J.M. (1999) Omega-3 fatty acids as cancer chemopreventive agents. *Pharmacol Ther* **83**, 217–44.

51. Benoit, V. et al. (2004) Regulation of HER-2 oncogene expression by cyclooxygenase-2 and prostaglandin E2. *Oncogene* **23**, 1631–35.

52. Christiansen, E.N., Lund, J.S., Rortveit, T., and Rustan, A.C. (1991) Effect of dietary n-3 and n-6 fatty acids on fatty acid desaturation in rat liver. *Biochim Biophys Acta* **1082**, 57–62.

53. Rose, D.P., Rayburn, J., Hatala, M.A., and Connolly, J.M. (1994) Effects of dietary fish oil on fatty acids and eicosanoids in metastasizing human breast cancer cells. *Nutr Cancer* **22**, 131–41.

54. Madani, S., Hichami, A., Charkaoui-Malki, M., and Khan, N.A. (2004) Diacylglycerols containing omega 3 and omega 6 fatty acids bind to RasGRP and modulate MAP kinase activation. *J Biol Chem* **279**, 1176–83.

55. Elson, C.E. (1995) Suppression of mevalonate pathway activities by dietary isoprenoids: Protective roles in cancer and cardiovascular disease. *J Nutr* **125**, 1666S–1672S.

56. El-Sohemy, A., and Archer, M.C. (1997) Regulation of mevalonate synthesis in rat mammary glands by dietary n-3 and n-6 polyunsaturated fatty acids. *Cancer Res* **57**, 3685–87.

57. Fishman, J., Osborne, M.P., and Telang, N.T. (1995) The role of estrogen in mammary carcinogenesis. *Ann N Y Acad Sci* **768**, 91–100.

58. Telang, N.T., Inoue, S., Bradlow, H.L., and Osborne, M.P. (1997) Negative growth regulation of oncogene-transformed mammary epithelial cells by tumor inhibitors. *Adv Exp Med Biol* **400A**, 409–18.

59. Telang, N.T., Katdare, M., Bradlow, H.L., and Osborne, M.P. (1997) Estradiol metabolism: An endocrine biomarker for modulation of human mammary carcinogenesis. *Environ Health Perspect* **105**, 559–64.

60. Osborne, C.K. (1988) Effects of estrogens and antiestrogens on cell proliferation: Implications for the treatment of breast cancer. *Cancer Treat Res* **39**, 111–29.

61. Liang, T., and Liao, S. (1992) Inhibition of steroid 5 alpha-reductase by specific aliphatic unsaturated fatty acids. *Biochem J* **285**, 557–62.

62. Welsch, C. (1997) The role of lipid peroxidation in growth suppression of human breast carcinoma by dietary fish oil. *Adv Exp Med Biol* **400B**, 849–60.

63. Gonzalez, M.J. (1995) Fish oil, lipid peroxidation and mammary tumor growth. *J Am Coll Nutr* **14**, 325–35.

64. Gonzalez, M.J., Schemmel, R.A., Dugan, L., Jr., Gray, J.I., and Welsch, C.W. (1993) Dietary fish oil inhibits human breast carcinoma growth: A function of increased lipid peroxidation. *Lipids* **28**, 827–32.

65. Hardman, W.E., Munoz, J., Jr., and Cameron, I.L. (2002) Role of lipid peroxidation and antioxidant enzymes in omega 3 fatty acids induced suppression of breast cancer xenograft growth in mice. *Cancer Cell Int* **2**, 10.

66. Colas, S. et al. (2005) Alpha-tocopherol suppresses mammary tumor sensitivity to anthracyclines in fish oil-fed rats. *Nutr Cancer* **51**, 178–83.

67. Welsch, C.W. (1995) Review of the effects of dietary fat on experimental mammary gland tumorige-nesis: Role of lipid peroxidation. *Free Radic Biol Med* **18**, 757–73.

68. Mamane, Y. et al. (2004) eIF4E – from translation to transformation. *Oncogene* **23**, 3172–79.

69. Li, S. et al. (2002) Translational control of cell fate: Availability of phosphorylation sites on translational repressor 4E-BP1 governs its proapoptotic potency. *Mol Cell Biol* **22**, 2853–61.

70. Gingras, A.C., Raught, B., and Sonenberg, N. (1999) eIF4 initiation factors: Effectors of mRNA recruitment to ribosomes and regulators of translation. *Annu Rev Biochem* **68**, 913–63.

71. Koromilas, A.E., Lazaris-Karatzas, A., and Sonenberg, N. (1992) mRNAs containing extensive secondary structure in their 5′ non-coding region translate efficiently in cells overexpressing initiation factor eIF-4E. *EMBO J* **11**, 4153–58.

72. Rousseau, D., Kaspar, R., Rosenwald, I., Gehrke, L., and Sonenberg, N. (1996) Translation initiation of ornithine decarboxylase and nucleocytoplasmic transport of cyclin D1 mRNA are increased in cells overexpressing eukaryotic initiation factor 4E. *Proc Natl Acad Sci U S A* **93**, 1065–70.

73. Kozak, M. (1991) An analysis of vertebrate mRNA sequences: Intimations of translational control. *J Cell Biol* **115**, 887–903.

74. Aktas, H. et al. (1998) Depletion of intracellular Ca^{2+} stores, phosphorylation of eIF2alpha, and sustained inhibition of translation initiation mediate the anticancer effects of clotrimazole. *Proc Natl Acad Sci U S A* **95**, 8280–85.

75. Duan, D.R. et al. (1995) Inhibition of transcription elongation by the VHL tumor suppressor protein. *Science* **269**, 1402–06.

76. Shilatifard, A., Lane, W.S., Jackson, K.W., Conaway, R.C., and Conaway, J.W. (1996) An RNA polymerase II elongation factor encoded by the human ELL gene. *Science* **271**, 1873–76.

77. Lazaris-Karatzas, A., Montine, K.S., and Sonenberg, N. (1990) Malignant transformation by a eukaryotic initiation factor subunit that binds to mRNA 5′ cap. *Nature* **345**, 544–47.

78. Wang, S. et al. (1999) Expression of the eukaryotic translation initiation factors 4E and 2alpha in non-Hodgkin's lymphomas. *Am J Pathol* **155**, 247–55.

79. Raught, B. et al. (1996) Expression of a translationally regulated, dominant-negative CCAAT/enhancer-binding protein b isoform and up-regulation of the eukaryotic translation initiation factor 2a are correlated with neoplastic transformation of Mammary epithelial cells. *Cancer Res* **56**, 4382–86.

80. Li, B.D. et al. (2002) Prospective study of eukaryotic initiation factor 4E protein elevation and breast cancer outcome. *Ann Surg* **235**, 732–38, discussion 738–739.

81. Nathan, C.A. et al. (1997) Elevated expression of eIF4E and FGF-2 isoforms during vascularization of breast carcinomas. *Oncogene* **15**, 1087–94.

82. Rosenwald, I.B., Hutzler, M.J., Wang, S., Savas, L., and Fraire, A.E. (2001) Expression of eukaryotic translation initiation factors 4E and 2alpha is increased frequently in bronchioloalveolar but not in squamous cell carcinomas of the lung. *Cancer* **92**, 2164–71.

83. Li, B.D., McDonald, J.C., Nasssar, R., and DeBenedetti, A. (1998) Clinical outcome in stage I to III breast carcinoma and eIF4E overexpression. *Ann Surg* **227**, 756–63.

84. Nathan, C.A. et al. (2002) Molecular analysis of surgical margins in head and neck squamous cell carcinoma patients. *Laryngoscope* **112**, 2129–40.

85. Crew, J.P. et al. (2000) Eukaryotic initiation factor-4E in superficial and muscle invasive bladder cancer and its correlation with vascular endothelial growth factor expression and tumour progression. *Br J Cancer* **82**, 161–66.

86. Berkel, H.J., Turbat-Herrera, E.A., Shi, R., and de Benedetti, A. (2001) Expression of the translation initiation factor eIF4E in the polyp-cancer sequence in the colon. *Cancer Epidemiol Biomarkers Prev* **10**, 663–66.

87. Scott, P.A. et al. (1998) Differential expression of vascular endothelial growth factor mRNA vs protein isoform expression in human breast cancer and relationship to eIF-4E. *Br J Cancer* **77**, 2120–28.

88. Arrick, B.A., Grendell, R.L., and Griffin, L.A. (1994) Enhanced translational efficiency of a novel transforming growth factor beta 3 mRNA in human breast cancer cells. *Mol Cell Biol* **14**, 619–28.

89. Rousseau, D., Gingras, A.C., Pause, A., and Sonenberg, N. (1996) The eIF4E-binding proteins 1 and 2 are negative regulators of cell growth. *Oncogene* **13**, 2415–20.

90. Graff, J.R. et al. (1995) Reduction of translation initiation factor 4E decreases the malignancy of ras-transformed cloned rat embryo fibroblasts. *Int J Cancer* **60**, 255–63.

91. Sonenberg, N. (1994) mRNA translation: Influence of the 5′ and 3′ untranslated regions. *Curr Opin Genet Dev* **4**, 310–15.

92. Avdulov, S. et al. (2004) Activation of translation complex eIF4F is essential for the genesis and maintenance of the malignant phenotype in human mammary epithelial cells. *Cancer Cell* **5**, 553–63.

93. Rastinejad, F., Conboy, M.J., Rando, T.A., and Blau, H.M. (1993) Tumor suppression by RNA from the 3′ untranslated region of a-tropomyosin. *Cell* **75**, 1107–17.

94. Davis, S., and Watson, J.C. (1996) In vitro activation of the interferon-induced, double-stranded RNA-dependent protein kinase PKR by RNA from the 3′ untranslated regions of human alpha-tropomyosin. *Proc Natl Acad Sci U S A* **93**, 508–13.

95. Palakurthi, S.S. et al. (2000) Inhibition of translation initiation mediates the anticancer effect of the n-3 polyunsaturated fatty acid eicosapentaenoic acid. *Cancer Res* **60**, 2919–25.

96. Barnhart, B.C., and Simon, M.C. (2007) Taking aim at translation for tumor therapy. *J Clin Invest* **117**, 2385–88.

97. Graff, J.R. et al. (2007) Therapeutic suppression of translation initiation factor eIF4E expression reduces tumor growth without toxicity. *J Clin Invest* **117**, 2638–48.

98. Mathis, J.M. et al. (2006) Cancer-specific targeting of an adenovirus-delivered herpes simplex virus thymidine kinase suicide gene using translational control. *J Gene Med* **8**, 1105–20.

99. Palakurthi, S.S., Aktas, H., Grubissich, L.M., Mortensen, R.M., and Halperin, J.A. (2001) Anticancer effects of thiazolidinediones are independent of peroxisome proliferator-activated receptor gamma and mediated by inhibition of translation initiation. *Cancer Res* **61**, 6213–18.

100. Aissat, N. et al. (2008) Antiproliferative effects of rapamycin as a single agent and in combination with carboplatin and paclitaxel in head and neck cancer cell lines. *Cancer Chemother Pharmacol* **62**, 305–13.

101. Clemens, M.J., and Bommer, U.A. (1999) Translational control: The cancer connection. *Int J Biochem Cell Biol* **31**, 1–23.

102. Dua, K., Williams, T.M., and Beretta, L. (2001) Translational control of the proteome: Relevance to cancer. *Proteomics* **1**, 1191–99.

103. Aktas, H., and Halperin, J.A. (2004) Translational regulation of gene expression by omega-3 fatty acids. *J Nutr* **134**, 2487S–2491S.

104. Pain, V.M. (1996) Initiation of protein synthesis in eukaryotic cells. *Eur J Biochem* **236**, 747–71.

105. Brostrom, C.O., Chin, K.V., Wong, W.L., Cade, C., and Brostrom, M.A. (1989) Inhibition of translational initiation in eukaryotic cells by calcium ionophore. *J Biol Chem* **264**, 1644–49.

106. Srivastava, S.P., Davies, M.V., and Kaufman, R.J. (1995) Calcium depletion from the endoplasmic reticulum activates the double-stranded RNA-dependent protein kinase (PKR) to inhibit protein synthesis. *J Biol Chem* **270**, 16619–24.

107. Harding, H.P., Zhang, Y., Bertolotti, A., Zeng, H., and Ron, D. (2000) Perk is essential for translational regulation and cell survival during the unfolded protein response. *Mol Cell* **5**, 897–904.

108. Kaufman, R.J. (1999) Stress signaling from the lumen of the endoplasmic reticulum: Coordination of gene transcriptional and translational controls. *Genes Dev* **13**, 1211–33.

109. Berridge, M.J. (1995) Capacitative calcium entry. *Biochem J* **312**, 1–11.

110. Putney, J.W., Jr. (1997) Type 3 inositol 1,4,5-trisphosphate receptor and capacitative calcium entry. *Cell Calcium* **21**, 257–61.

111. Sobczak, K., and Krzyzosiak, W.J. (2002) Structural determinants of BRCA1 translational regulation. *J Biol Chem* **277**, 17349–58.

112. Esteller, M. et al. (2000) Promoter hypermethylation and BRCA1 inactivation in sporadic breast and ovarian tumors. *J Natl Cancer Inst* **92**, 564–69.

113. Zheng, W. et al. (2000) Reduction of BRCA1 expression in sporadic ovarian cancer. *Gynecol Oncol* **76**, 294–300.

114. Futreal, P.A. et al. (1994) BRCA1 mutations in primary breast and ovarian carcinomas. *Science* **266**, 120–22.

115. Miyamoto, K. et al. (2002) Promoter hypermethylation and post-transcriptional mechanisms for reduced BRCA1 immunoreactivity in sporadic human breast cancers. *Jpn J Clin Oncol* **32**, 79–84.

116. Magdinier, F., Ribieras, S., Lenoir, G.M., Frappart, L., and Dante, R. (1998) Down-regulation of BRCA1 in human sporadic breast cancer; analysis of DNA methylation patterns of the putative promoter region. *Oncogene* **17**, 3169–76.

117. Dobrovic, A., and Simpfendorfer, D. (1997) Methylation of the BRCA1 gene in sporadic breast cancer. *Cancer Res* **57**, 3347–50.

118. Dumitrescu, R.G., and Cotarla, I. (2005) Understanding breast cancer risk – where do we stand in 2005? *J Cell Mol Med* **9**, 208–21.

119. Wilson, C.A. et al. (1999) Localization of human BRCA1 and its loss in high-grade, non-inherited breast carcinomas. *Nat Genet* **21**, 236–40.

120. Lambie, H. et al. (2003) Prognostic significance of BRCA1 expression in sporadic breast carcinomas. *J Pathol* **200**, 207–13.

121. Yang, Q. et al. (2002) BRCA1 in non-inherited breast carcinomas (Review). *Oncol Rep* **9**, 1329–33.

122. Taylor, J. et al. (1998) An important role for BRCA1 in breast cancer progression is indicated by its loss in a large proportion of non-familial breast cancers. *Int J Cancer* **79**, 334–42.

123. Thompson, M.E., Jensen, R.A., Obermiller, P.S., Page, D.L., and Holt, J.T. (1995) Decreased expression of BRCA1 accelerates growth and is often present during sporadic breast cancer progression. *Nat Genet* **9**, 444–50.

124. Holt, J.T. et al. (1996) Growth retardation and tumour inhibition by BRCA1. *Nat Genet* **12**, 298–302.

125. Kang, J.X., Wang, J., Wu, L., and Kang, Z.B. (2004) Transgenic mice: Fat-1 mice convert n-6 to n-3 fatty acids. *Nature* **427**, 504.

14 n-6 Polyunsaturated Fatty Acids and Cancer

Marie Lof, Susan Olivo-Marston, and Leena Hilakivi-Clarke

Key Points

1. It is important to consume a balanced diet containing about 25–35% energy from fat. In order to reduce the risk of disease related to high fat intake, a restricted total calorie intake would be beneficial, while consuming approximately 30% total calories from fat.
2. A high fat intake is generally associated with cardiovascular diseases, cancer, and other chronic diseases. However, a diet low in fat and high in carbohydrates may also be associated with the diseases because it may reduce HDL cholesterol and increase serum triacylglycerol concentrations.
3. The recommended ratio of n-6 polyunsaturated (PUFA) fats to n-3 polyunsaturated fat is 1–2:1. Populations that consume low levels of n-6 PUFA and high levels of n-3 PUFA appear to have reduced incidence of heart disease, diabetes, arthritis, and cancer.
4. High n-6 PUFA intake is associated with cancer because it promotes preexisting tumor growth and accelerates cancer metastasis. The eicosanoids in n-6 PUFA have also been found to increase cell proliferation and be inflammatory.
5. A high intake of n-6 PUFA has been directly related to breast cancer; however, this is seen in animal studies, whereas no effect has been found in human studies. It is certain that dietary fat intake may directly affect breast cancer risk, but the effect may depend on the type of fat and age when the fats were consumed.

Key Words: Dietary n-3 PUFA; n-6 PUFA; inflammation; cancer; cardiovascular diseases

1. INTRODUCTION

People living in the Western world consume on average 30–35% energy from various types of fats including saturated fatty acids (SFAs), monosaturated fatty acids (MUFAs), and polyunsaturated fatty acids (PUFAs). The main biochemical difference that distinguishes these fats is the length of the fatty acid chain and absence (SFA) or presence of one (MUFA) or more (PUFA) double bonds. Cells of the human body can synthesize SFA and MUFA, but lack the enzymes necessary to synthesize n-6 and n-3 PUFA. Consequently, these essential fatty acids (EFA) have to be obtained from the diet.

From: *Nutrition and Health: Bioactive Compounds and Cancer*
Edited by: J.A. Milner, D.F. Romagnolo, DOI 10.1007/978-1-60761-627-6_14,
© Springer Science+Business Media, LLC 2010

Although fat is one of the three required macronutrients in the human diet, the other two being protein and carbohydrate, current recommendations for typical western diets suggest intake of fat should be restricted. For example, high fat intake is generally associated with increased risk of cardiovascular diseases, cancer, and other chronic diseases *(1)*. Nevertheless, replacing fat with high carbohydrate diet is not advisable since high intake of carbohydrates may reduce high density lipoprotein (HDL)-associated cholesterol and increase serum triacylglycerol concentrations leading to higher levels of glucose and insulin. These changes increase the risk of coronary heart disease, diabetes *(2)*, and cancer *(3, 4)*. Therefore, maintaining a balanced diet that contains ~25–35% energy from fat (fat requirement changes during the life span, being highest at a younger age and during pregnancy) is probably ideal for overall health. The best way to reduce fat consumption and avoid development of diseases linked to high fat intake is to restrict total daily energy intake, while keeping dietary fat content at ~30% of the total energy intake. Moderate calorie restriction is suggested to be linked to multiple health benefits, including longer life span *(5)*.

2. POLYUNSATURATED FATTY ACIDS

The mean dietary intake of PUFA is 10–15% of total fat intake, most of it in the form of *n*-6 PUFA. The focus of this chapter is on *n*-6 PUFA, which can be found in plant seed oils, such as safflower, sunflower, corn, and soybean oil. Nuts and grains also are high in *n*-6 PUFA. Fish and other seafood contain high levels of *n*-3 PUFA. Linseed/flaxseed, rapeseed/canola, and soybean oils contain notable levels of *n*-3 PUFA in addition to containing sufficient amounts of *n*-6 PUFA. To maintain optimal health, it has been proposed that the intake of *n*-6 and *n*-3 PUFA should be at the ratio of 1–2 *n*-6 PUFA to 1 *n*-3 PUFA; however, in Western diets the ratio is currently 15–20:1 *(6)*. *n*-6/*n*-3 PUFA ratio in the hunter gatherers living 40,000 years ago was 1:1 and it is still 4:1 in Japan *(7)*. There are several reasons for proposing to increase *n*-3 PUFA and reduce *n*-6 PUFA intake in the West. First, populations consuming very high levels of *n*-3 PUFA appear healthier; they have reduced incidence of heart disease, diabetes, arthritis, cancer, and other diseases than those populations whose diet is composed of high levels of *n*-6 PUFA and low levels of *n*-3 PUFA *(7)*. Second, as described in more detail below, *n*-6 PUFA-derived eicosanoids are known to increase cell proliferation and be inflammatory, while *n*-3 PUFA eicosanoids are anti-inflammatory and induce apoptosis *(8)*. Because Western diets are clearly higher in *n*-6 PUFA than *n*-3 PUFA, more arachidonic acid (AA)-derived eicosanoids are formed than those derived from *n*-3 PUFA. Consequently, individual on western diets may have higher levels of inflammatory eicosanoids exerting harmful effects on various target tissues.

The primary metabolite of linoleic acid (LA, 18:2) is AA, which is generated from LA by the action of $\Delta 6$ and $\Delta 5$ desaturase and elongase enzymes (Fig. 1). The metabolism of PUFA takes place mainly in the liver. AA is a key component of cell membrane structural lipids. However, upon activity of phospholipase A2, AA is mobilized from the cell membrane and metabolized to eicosanoids, such as thromboxane A_2, prostacyclin, and leukotriene B_4 (Fig. 1). Levels of *n*-6 PUFA intake alone do not determine how much AA-derived eicosanoids are produced since the 18- and 20-carbon long fatty acids of *n*-3 PUFA and MUFA compete for a common $\Delta 6$ and $\Delta 5$ desaturase enzymes, which have

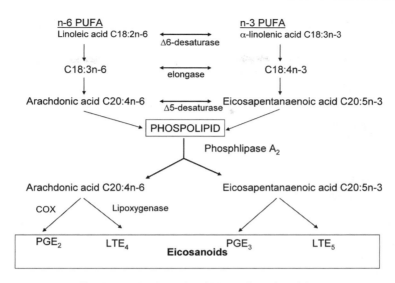

Fig. 1. Metabolism of *n*-6 PUFA linoleic acid.

different affinity for various fatty acids in the order of *n*-3 PUFA>*n*-6 PUFA>MUFA *(9, 10)*. High intakes of LA can inhibit eicosanoid production by competing for available desaturases *(11)*.

Although *n*-6 PUFA-derived eicosanoids are generally related to adverse health effects, low intake or impaired absorption of these fatty acids results in growth retardation *(12)*. Clinical signs of *n*-6 PUFA deficiency include scale skin rash and increased transepidermal water loss *(13)* and defects in the normal function of the kidneys, muscle, and other organs *(14, 15)*. These observations emphasize the fact that these fatty acids play critical roles in normal epithelial cell functions. *n*-6 PUFA deficiency also has been associated with impaired immune responses *(16)*. Defects related to low intake of *n*-3 PUFA are described in Chapter 11.

3. *n*-6 PUFA AND CANCER

High fat intake is thought to increase cancer risk, promote the growth of existing tumors, and accelerate cancer metastasis. However, data that do not to support a role of high fat intake in cancer causation also exist. There is also evidence that high intakes of *n*-6 PUFA and high *n*-6/*n*-3 PUFA ratios increase the risk of prostate *(17)*, colon *(18)*, and breast cancer *(19)*. Other cancers might also be influenced by *n*-6 PUFA intake, such as skin cancer, which is linked to high levels of AA *(20)*, or pancreatic cancer *(21)*. The growth of four different human pancreatic cancer cell lines in a xenograft mouse model was increased by a diet high in *n*-6 PUFA *(21)*. Although these findings seem to indicate a strong positive correlation between intake of *n*-6 PUFA and pancreatic cancer risk, human studies have not confirmed this association *(22)*.

It is not clear whether endometrial and ovarian cancers are linked to high intakes of PUFA *(23–25)*, although some evidence suggests that high levels of cyclooxygenase-2 (COX-2) – which is up-regulated by *n*-6 PUFA and converts AA to prostaglandins

(PG) – are associated with increased risk of both cancers *(26, 27)*. Both *n*-6 PUFA and *n*-3 PUFA decrease human lung tumor cell growth in vitro in a concentration-dependent manner while inducing cell death at concentrations of 100 μM or higher *(28)*. These contrasting findings highlight the lack of consensus concerning the effects of *n*-6 PUFA intake on cancer risk.

We shall review the experimental data generated using in vitro and in animal models of colon, prostate, and breast cancers, which according to epidemiological studies may be influenced by high intakes of *n*-6 PUFA intake. This will be followed by discussion of epidemiological studies that have investigated whether intake of PUFA is associated with breast cancer risk.

Animal studies have shown that diets containing high levels of *n*-6 PUFA increase colon carcinogenesis *(29, 30)*. However, findings obtained in vitro with human colon cancer cells have failed to detect an increase in cell proliferation following treatment with LA or AA *(18)*. Since the in vitro data strongly implicate AA-derived eicosanoids, particularly prostaglandin E2 (PGE2) in the growth of colon cancer cells *(31, 32)*, the association between high *n*-6 PUFA intake and increased colon cancer risk in human populations is biologically feasible.

Findings generated with cell lines do not clearly link *n*-6 PUFA to increased prostate cancer risk. In one study, LA stimulated the growth of PC-3 human prostate cancer cells, but had no effect on proliferation of DU 145 cells *(33)*. Another study reported that growth of PC-3, LNCaP, and TSU prostate cell lines and rat metastatic Mat-Ly-Lu and rat non-metastatic epithelial cell lines EPYP1, EPYP2, and EPYP3 was stimulated following exposure to physiological doses (1–100 ng/ml) of LA *(34)*. Nude mice injected with LAPC-4 prostate cancer cells exhibited increased tumor growth when fed a diet high in *n*-6 PUFA, compared to mice fed *n*-3 PUFA *(35)*. However, according to a review by Astorg *(36)*, the evidence linking high intake of LA or AA to prostate cancer is scarce.

Exposure to LA or AA induces proliferation of rat and mouse breast cancer cells, but among human breast cancer cells, only those negative for the estrogen receptor (ER), such as MDA-MB-231 and MDA-MB-465 cells, are stimulated *(37, 38)*. In contrast, the growth of ER-positive MCF-7 or ZR-75-1 human breast cancer cells is either inhibited or not affected at all *(37, 39)*. Although this could be interpreted to indicate that *n*-6 PUFAs stimulate only the growth of ER-negative breast cancer cells, findings in humans indicate that *n*-6 PUFA intake does not correlate with ER status of breast tumors *(40)*. Furthermore, diets high in *n*-6 PUFA promoted the growth of carcinogen-induced, ER-positive mammary tumors in rat models *(41, 42)*. The intake of *n*-6 PUFA has been linked to changes in estrogen levels, which are expected to promote activation of ER in the mammary gland and tumors inducing cell proliferation. High intake of *n*-6 PUFA also increases the risk of developing metastasis *(43–45)*.

4. DIETARY *n*-6 PUFA INTAKE AND BREAST CANCER RISK IN WOMEN

Since the early 1980s, numerous epidemiological studies have investigated the possible association between total dietary fat intakes during adulthood, mostly shortly before breast cancer diagnosis, and breast cancer risk. Epidemiological and some case–control studies suggest that a high consumption of total dietary fat increases breast cancer risk *(19)*, but the results from prospective cohort studies are inconsistent *(19, 46)*.

In 2001 and 2003, a pooled analysis from eight studies and a meta-analysis from 45 cohort studies examined the relationships between dietary *n*-6 PUFA and breast cancer risk. Results of the pooled analysis did not show any association between total fat and breast cancer, whereas the meta-analysis showed a summary relative risk of 1.13 (95% CI: 1.04–1.23) for total fat. Results of the eight prospective cohorts are summarized in Table 1. Only one study showed a positive association between breast cancer and total fat *(47)*, while most of them found a null association *(40, 48–52)*.

The role of the subtypes of fat for development of breast cancer has also attracted a lot of interest over the years, and these associations were evaluated in the recent pooled analysis and meta-analysis *(19, 46)*. Prospective cohort studies on total fat and intake of PUFAs within this area published thereafter are presented in Table 1. To summarize, several case–control studies have reported a statistically significant reduced risk for breast cancer with higher PUFA intakes *(19)*, but only two of a total of eight prospective cohorts have confirmed this. We found that among postmenopausal women, high PUFA intake was protective *(40)*. However, these studies did not necessarily separate *n*-6 PUFA intake from that of *n*-3 PUFA intake – the two EFAs often have opposite effects on breast cancer risk.

A few studies have investigated the effect of *n*-3 PUFA and *n*-6 PUFA separately on breast cancer risk, and the most recent epidemiological studies in this area are summarized in Table 2. Although not consistent, there is some evidence indicating that *n*-3 PUFA may protect against breast cancer, while *n*-6 PUFA appears to have an opposite effect. Three of the studies reported a protective effect of *n*-3 PUFA and especially marine *n*-3 PUFA *(50, 51, 53)*. One Swedish nested case–control study reported a threefold increased breast cancer risk on the consumption of *n*-6 PUFAs *(54)*. Two analyses within American cohorts found no association between long-chain *n*-3 PUFA and breast cancer risk *(49, 55)*. There are also two studies which investigated whether the ratio between *n*-6 and *n*-3 PUFAs impacts the risk of developing breast cancer. Data generated in the Singaporean study suggested that high consumption of *n*-6 PUFA was associated with an increased risk of breast cancer among women consuming low levels of marine *n*-3 PUFA *(56)*. A study done in Sweden reported a non-significantly reduced risk of developing postmenopausal breast cancer among women who consumed high levels of PUFA and lower levels of *n*-6 PUFA *(54)*.

There are several possible reasons for the inconsistent results for the numerous epidemiological studies regarding total dietary fat, subtypes of dietary fat, and breast cancer risk. For instance, they could be due to methodological difficulties in classification of total fat intake. Epidemiological studies often use food frequency questionnaires to assess dietary fat intake, although food diaries are superior to food frequency questionnaires in detecting positive associations between dietary fat intake and breast cancer *(57, 58)*. Another possible explanation may be the differences in the age of women when their dietary intakes were assessed. Most studies so far have investigated the association between dietary fat intakes during postmenopausal years,

Table 1
Prospective Cohort Studies on Intakes of Total Fat, MUFA, PUFA, and SFA and Breast Cancer Risk Conducted During 2002–2007

Authors, year	Population, cases/cohort	Exposure difference	RR (95% CI)	Adjustments
Voorips et al. (51).	Netherlands, postmenopausal 941/62573	5th vs. 1st quintile		Age, history of benign breast disease, maternal breast cancer, breast cancer in one or more sisters, age at menarche, age at menopause, oral contraceptives, parity, age at first birth, Quetelet index, education, alcohol use, smoking, and total energy intake
Total fat			1.16 (0.87–1.56)	
PUFA			0.88 (0.65–1.21)	
Byrne et al. (48).	US, postmenopausal 1071/44,697	5th vs. 1st quintile		Age, height, age at menarche, age at menopause, use of postmenopausal hormones, parity, age at first birth, BMI at age 18, weight change since age 18, total energy intake, alcohol intake, vitamin A, and family history of breast cancer
Total fat			0.94 (0.77–1.15)	
MUFA+PUFA			1.16 (0.92–1.46)	
Wirfält et al. (54).	Sweden, postmenopausal, 237 cases and 673 controls within a prospective cohort of 12,803 postmenopausal women	5th vs. 1st quintile		Past food habit change, energy intake, BMI, height, waist circumference, age at birth of first child, current hormone therapy, alcohol habits, and educational habits
Total fat			1.51 (0.92–2.49)	
PUFA			3.02 (1.75–5.21)	
Gago-Dominguez et al. (56).	Singapore, pre-and postmenopausal, 314/35298	4th vs. 1st quartile		Age, year of recruitment, dialect group, education, primary school, daily alcohol drinker, family history of breast cancer, age at menarche, and number of live births
Total fat			0.94 (0.68–1.31)	
PUFA			1.27 (0.92–1.74)	

Study	Population, cases/cohort	Comparison	RR (95% CI)	Adjustment
Wakai et al. (50).	Japan, pre-and postmenopausal, 129/26291	4th vs. 1st quartile		Age, study area, educational level, family history of breast cancer, age at menarche, age at menopause, age at first birth, parity, use of exogenous female hormones, alcohol consumption, smoking, consumption of green leafy vegetables, daily walking, height, BMI, and energy intake
Total fat			0.80 (0.46–1.38)	
PUFA			1.10 (0.63–1.90)	
Kim et al. (49).	US, postmenopausal, 3537/80375	Per 5 energy percent continuous increment		Energy intake, age, alcohol intake, time period, height, parity, age at first birth, weight change since age 18, BMI at age 18, age at menopause, use of hormone replacement therapy, family history of breast cancer, benign breast disease, and age at menarche
Total fat			0.98 (0.95–1.00)	
PUFA			0.94 (0.82–1.02)	
Thiebaut et al. (47).	US, postmenopausal, 3501/188736	5th vs. 1st quintile		Age, alcohol and non-alcohol energy intakes, smoking history, age at first birth and number of children, age at menopause, menopausal hormone use, and BMI
Total fat			1.11 (1.00–1.24)	
PUFA			1.12 (1.01–1.25)	
Lof et al. (40).	Sweden, pre-and postmenopausal, 974/44569	5th vs. 1st quintile		Education, parity, age at menarche, use of oral contraceptives, age at first birth by parity, first degree relative with breast cancer, non-alcohol total energy intake, total fat intake, BMI, and alcohol intake. Attained age was utilized as time scale
Total fat	<50 years of attained age		1.46 (0.87–2.47)	
PUFA			1.06 (0.64–1.75)	
Total fat	≥50 years of attained age		0.76 (0.47–1.22)	
PUFA			0.54 (0.35–0.85)	

MUFA, monounsaturated fat; PUFA, polyunsaturated fat; SFA, saturated fat; RR, rate ratio; CI, confidence interval; BMI, body mass index.

Table 2
Epidemiological studies on dietary intake of *n*-3 and *n*-6 fatty acids and breast cancer risk between 1999 and 2007

Authors, year	Population, cases/entire cohort or controls	Exposure difference	RR (95% CI)	Adjustments
Holmes et al. (*200*).	US, pre-and postmenopausal, 2097/77519			Energy intake, age, vitamin A, alcohol intake, time period, height, parity, age at first birth, weight change since age 18, BMI, age at menopause, menopausal status, use of hormonal replacement therapy, family history, benign breast disease, and age at menarche
n-3 Fish fatty acids		0.1 energy percent (continuous)	1.08 (1.03–1.13)	
EPA		0.03 energy% (continuous)	1.06 (1.02–1.10)	
DHA		0.03 energy% (continuous)	1.04 (1.01–1.06)	
Mannisto et al. (*201*).	Finland, premenopausal, 119 cases/178 controls	5th vs. 1st quintile		Age, area, age at menarche, age at first full-term pregnancy, use of oral contraceptives, use of estrogen replacement therapy, family history of breast cancer, history of benign breast disease, education, alcohol intake, smoking, leisure activity, and waist/hip ratio
n-3			0.7 (0.3–1.7)	
n-6			0.7 (0.3–1.6)	
Voorrips et al. (*51*).	Netherlands, postmenopausal, 941/62573	5th vs. 1st quintile		Age, history of benign breast disease, maternal breast cancer, breast cancer in one or more sisters, age at menarche, age at menopause, oral contraceptives, parity, age at first birth, Quetelet index, education, alcohol use, smoking, and total energy intake
Linolenic			0.70 (0.51–0.97)	
EPA			0.98 (0.72–1.35)	
DHA			1.00 (0.72–1.37)	

Study	Population	Comparison	OR (95% CI)	Adjusted for
Wirfalt et al. (54).	Sweden, postmenopausal, 237 cases and 673 controls within a prospective cohort of 12,803 postmenopausal women	5th vs. 1st quintile		Past food habit change, energy intake, BMI, height, waist circumference, age at birth of first child, current hormone therapy, alcohol habits, and educational habits
n-3			1.81 (1.09–2.99)	
n-6			3.02 (1.78–5.13)	
n-3/n-6			0.66 (0.41–1.08)	
Cho et al. (55).	US, premenopausal, 714/90655	5th vs. 1st quintile		Age, height, parity, age at first birth, BMI, age at menarche, family history of breast cancer, history of benign breast disease, oral contraceptive use, menopausal status, alcohol, and protein and energy intake
Long-chain n-3			1.01 (0.78–1.31)	
Gago-Dominguez et al. (56).	Singapore, pre-and postmenopausal, 314/35298	4th vs. 1st quartile		Age, year of recruitment, dialect group, education, primary school, daily alcohol drinker, family history of breast cancer, age at menarche, and number of live births
n-3 total			0.87 (0.64–1.18)	
n-3, marine			0.72 (0.53–0.98)	
n-3, other foods			1.00 (0.73–1.36)	
n-6			1.22 (0.89–1.67)	

Table 2
(Continued)

Authors, year	Population, cases/entire cohort or controls	Exposure difference	RR (95% CI)	Adjustments
Wakai et al. (50).	Japan, pre-and postmenopausal, 129/26291	4th vs. 1st quartile		Age, study area, educational level, family history of breast cancer, age at menarche, age at menopause, age at first birth, parity, use of exogenous female hormones, alcohol consumption, smoking, consumption of green leafy vegetables, daily walking, height, BMI, and energy intake
n-3			0.69 (0.40–1.18)	
n-6			1.02 (0.59–1.74)	
n-6/n-3			1.31 (0.78–2.19)	
Long-chain n-3			0.50(0.30–0.85)	
Kim et al. (49). Long-chain n-3	US, postmenopausal, 3537/80375	Per 0.1 energy percent continuous increment	1.00 (1.00–1.01)	Energy intake, age, alcohol intake, time period, height, parity, age at first birth, weight change since age 18, BMI at age 18, age at menopause, use of hormone replacement therapy, family history of breast cancer, benign breast disease, and age at menarche

DHA, docosahexaenoic acid; EPA, eicosapentaenoic acid.

but those that have investigated intakes during premenopausal years have generated opposing data.

4.1. Premenopausal vs. Postmenopausal Fat Intake/Obesity and Breast Cancer Risk

The relationship between obesity and breast cancer risk is strongly dependent on the menopausal status at the time of diagnosis. Among premenopausal women, obesity is inversely associated with breast cancer risk, while overweight postmenopausal women are at increased risk of developing this disease *(59)*. Since high fat intake is linked to obesity, it is reasonable to assume that there could be a differential effect of dietary fat intake on pre- and postmenopausal breast cancer risk, perhaps similar to the one established for obesity. However, the majority of the studies have investigated fat intake among postmenopausal women only, limiting the knowledge regarding the role for dietary fat intake for development of premenopausal breast cancers.

Cho et al. have conducted the largest study investigating the effects of fat intake on breast cancer risk among 90,655 premenopausal women *(55)*. No association was found for total fat intake, but women consuming the highest quintile of animal fat had an increased risk for breast cancer (RR: 1.33; 95% CI 1.02–1.73). We have investigated, in a cohort study, whether intakes of total dietary fat and fat subtypes during premenopausal years affect subsequent breast cancer risk in a cohort of 44,569 Swedish women *(40)*. Of these women, 432 developed breast cancer before age 50 and 542 after that age. We found no association between total fat, MUFA, PUFA, or SFA and breast cancer risk for the entire cohort. However, among women diagnosed with breast cancer at 50 years of age or above, higher MUFA and PUFA intakes were associated with a statistically significant 50% reduction in risk *(40)* (Table 2). We also found a statistically significant interaction between age at diagnosis (<50 vs. ≥50) and intakes of PUFA ($P = 0.049$) as well as of unsaturated fat (combining MUFA and PUFA) ($P = 0.040$). Our results indicate that intake of dietary fat (MUFA and PUFA) in premenopausal years may have differential effects on breast cancer risk diagnosed before or after menopause.

4.2. PUFA and Breast Cancer Recurrence

Attempts to link dietary fat intake to prognosis have generally provided null findings. For example, adoption of a diet that was very high in vegetables, fruits, and fibers and low in fats, among survivors of early stage breast cancer, did not reduce breast cancer recurrence or mortality during a 7.3-year follow-up period *(60)*. We were unable to identify any studies which would have investigated the effect of PUFA intake on survival from breast cancer. Indirect evidence indicates that there might be a link, because among women treated for breast cancer, those who had the highest levels of AA in their circulation exhibited highest levels of 8-OhdG, which is a biomarker of oxidative damage *(61)*. Obesity is the only dietary factor which has been consistently shown to impair breast cancer prognosis *(62, 63)*.

5. TIMING OF DIETARY PUFA EXPOSURES AND BREAST CANCER RISK

In general, when the effects of dietary exposures on cancer are investigated in humans, the studies have explored whether the diet consumed at the time of diagnosis is associated with the risk of having developed cancer. In animal studies, diets are provided after cancer is initiated by a carcinogen exposure or due to a genetic modification in transgenic mice. Recent studies indicate that dietary exposures during periods limited to in utero development, prepuberty, or pregnancy, to a variety of bioactive food components, differentially affect later breast cancer risk *(64)*. These dietary exposures include *n*-6 PUFAs, *n*-3 PUFAs, monounsaturated fatty acids, and obesity-inducing high-fat diet (OID) containing high levels of saturated fats.

5.1. In Utero Exposure

Maternal exposure to a high *n*-6 PUFA fat diet during pregnancy increases female offspring's mammary tumorigenesis in many different model systems, which include carcinogen exposure in rats *(65, 66)*, spontaneous tumor development in mice *(67)*, and mammary tumors in genetically modified mice caused by an activation of an oncogene *(68)*. In contrast, an exposure to *n*-3 PUFA during fetal development *(69)* or olive oil *(66)*, which is high in monounsaturated fatty acids, reduces later mammary tumorigenesis. Human studies indicate that high birth weight, which might result from high maternal fat intake during pregnancy, is associated with increased breast cancer risk *(70–79)*.

5.2. Prepubertal Dietary Fat Exposure

There is some limited evidence that a prepubertal dietary exposure to *n*-3 PUFAs reduces mammary cancer in rats *(80)*. However, the protective effect is seen only if *n*-3 PUFAs are fed in the low fat context, and increased risk is seen if rats are fed *n*-3 PUFAs in the high fat background *(80)*. The *n*-6 to *n*-3 PUFA ratio in both diets was of 2:1, indicating that it is the total amount of *n*-3 PUFAs rather than the ratio which is critical in determining the effect on breast cancer risk following exposures before puberty. Since prepubertal exposure to a high-fat corn oil diet, containing mostly *n*-6 PUFAs, has no effect on later risk *(80)*, the adverse impact of high-fat *n*-3 PUFA diet reflects the intake of the particular type of fat. In humans, high body mass index during childhood is inversely linked to breast cancer risk *(81, 82)*.

5.3. Pregnancy n-6 PUFA Exposures

In animal studies, dietary fat intake during pregnancy has been shown to affect dams' mammary tumorigenesis. Rats fed a diet high in *n*-6 PUFAs during pregnancy had a fourfold higher tumor incidence compared to the control group *(83)*. The increase in mammary tumorigenesis in high-fat PUFA-fed dams is accompanied by a twofold increase in E2 levels *(83)*. Another study showed that rat dams who gain an excessive amount of weight during pregnancy exhibit a significantly increased DMBA-induced mammary tumorigenesis *(84)*. The exposure that results in an excessive pregnancy weight gain – an obesity-inducing diet – increased circulating leptin levels *(84)*. These findings are consistent with studies done in pregnant women showing that those who gained more weight than recommended by the obstetricians are at over 60% increased risk of developing breast cancer *(85)*.

6. MECHANISMS MEDIATING THE EFFECTS OF *n-6* PUFAS ON CANCER RISK

At present time, it is not known why high intake of *n-6* PUFAs increases the risk of some cancers. We will review the potential role of *n-6* PUFA-derived eicosanoids, cyclooxygenase 2 (COX-2, i.e., the enzyme responsible of converting AAs to eicosanoids), genes activated or down-regulated by *n-6* PUFAs, alterations in hormone levels, and obesity as possible mechanisms of action in increasing cancer risk. Other pathways might also be involved, such as *n-6* PUFA-induced increase in inflammatory events, as indicated by elevated levels of interleukins IL-1β and IL-6 and tumor necrosis factor α (TNF-α) by *n-6* PUFA *(86)*. Further, high *n-6* PUFA intake elevates lipid peroxidation *(87)*, which causes DNA adduct formation and oxidative damage.

6.1. n-6 PUFA-Derived Eicosanoids

Free AA is metabolized to eicosanoids by COX or lipoxygenase (LOX) enzymes (Fig. 1). Metabolism by COX enzymes results AA to be converted to the 2-series of prostaglandins (PGE$_2$) and thromboxane (TX), while 5-, 12-, and 15-LOX enzymes generate four series of leukotrienes (LT), 12-HETE, and lipoxin A$_4$, respectively. These eicosanoids can cause a thrombotic and atherogenic state by affecting platelet aggregation, hemodynamics, and coronary vascular tone *(88)*. They also may affect cancer risk and promote the growth of tumor and induce metastasis *(89)*.

Prostaglandins are a diverse group of hormones and have received most attention as potential mediators of increased cancer risk by *n-6* PUFA intake, but also as regulators of normal physiological functions. For example, in the gastrointestinal tract prostaglandins not only protect the gastric mucosa and regulate motility but they may also play a role in inflammatory bowel disease (IBD) *(90)* and colorectal cancers *(91)*. After their synthesis, prostaglandins are released outside the cell where they either bind to cell surface prostanoid receptors or are transported across the cell membrane into the cytoplasmic compartment by PG transporters and "eliminated" by different types of enzymes. PGE$_2$ receptors belong to the family of Rhodopsin-type receptors which are coupled to G-proteins *(92)*. There are four main prostanoid receptors, designated EP$_1$, EP$_2$, EP$_3$, and EP$_4$, which differ from each other by their pharmacological properties and secondary messenger pathways (Fig. 2). However, the mechanisms by which PGs and their receptors exert their biological functions remain poorly understood.

The actions of PGE$_2$ through different receptors are described by Dey et al. *(93)* and some of them might explain how *n-6* PUFA affects the processes involved in neoplasia. Overall, activation of EP$_1$ or EP$_{2/4}$ receptors by PGE$_2$ induces intracellular Ca^{2+} or cAMP, while EP$_3$ receptors reduce intracellular cAMP.

EP$_1$: EP$_1$ activates protein kinase Cα (PKCα), PKB/Akt, and c-Src pathways and can also transactivate HER-2/Neu tyrosine kinase receptor and epidermal growth factor

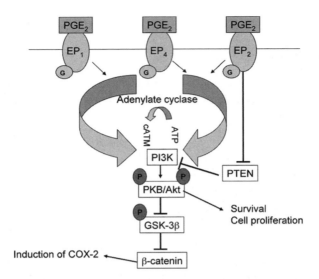

Fig. 2. Prostaglandin E_2 binds to prostanoid receptors EP_1, EP_2, and EP_4 which activate PI3K/Akt pathway, leading to increased cell survival and proliferation and induction of COX-2.

receptor (EGFR) via c-Src *(94, 95)*. These target genes are involved in cancer. For example, PKC family members phosphorylate various protein targets in diverse cellular signaling pathways, leading to cell transformation and de-regulation of cell cycle checkpoint. C-Src is a proto-oncogene which is linked to several cancers. Perhaps most important of the EP1 targets is the PI3K/AKT pathway which regulates the signaling of multiple biological processes such as apoptosis, metabolism, cell proliferation, and cell growth. Reflecting activation of these genes, EP_1 has been linked to colon carcinogenesis *(96)*, breast cancer *(97)*, cholangiocarcinoma *(98)*, and ovarian cancer *(99)*. It has been reported that EP_1 is up-regulated during early tumorigenesis and it might participate in promoting cellular proliferation and the antiapoptotic effects observed in cancer cells, suggesting that these receptors play a role in cancer *(100)*.

EP 2: PGE_2 has been shown to promote the growth of esophageal squamous cell carcinoma via EP_2 *(101)*. Further, PGE_2-induced VEGF secretion in prostate cancer cells is mediated through EP_2-, and possibly EP_4-, dependent cAMP signaling pathways *(102)*. A recent study has linked EP_2 receptor activation to cellular proliferation: upon activation the $G_{\alpha s}$ subunit of EP_2 receptors can directly associate with the regulator of G-protein signaling domain of Axin, which inactivates and releases GSK-3β from the Axin complex causing β-catenin activation and nuclear translocation *(103)*. Further, similar to EP_1, PGE_2 signaling through EP_2 receptors can activate both PI3K and Akt by using the free βγsubunit of G-protein *(103)*. An observation that signaling through EP_2 receptors decreases the inhibitory tyrosine phosphorylation of PTEN might explain increased activation of PI3K via EP_2. *PTEN* acts as an antagonist to PI3K signaling by dephosphorylating lipid messenger PIP3 (phosphatidylinositol 3,4,5-trisphosphate) *(104)*.

EP₄: Antagonists of the PGE receptor subtype 4, EP_4, inhibit experimental metastasis in a murine model of hormone-resistant, metastatic breast cancer *(105)*. PGE_2-EP_4

receptor coupling induces TNFα, cyclin D, and angiogenesis mediated by MAP kinases *(93)*. In addition, EP4 activates PI3K/Akt pathway *(106)*.

EP$_3$: Selective activation of each of the three variants of the EP3 receptor suppresses tumor cell function by activating a G *(12)*-RhoA pathway *(107)*. Early onset of the growth of malignant melanoma was significantly promoted in EP$_3$ knockouts *(108)*. In contrast to the view that activation of EP3 reduces tumorigenesis, EP$_3$ receptors have also been shown to activate the Ras signaling pathway which is closely linked to cancer *(109)*.

Findings in gastrointestinal cancers relating to expression of EP receptors summarize well their expression in cancers in general. A differential expression of EP receptors has been observed in gastrointestinal cancers which are caused, for example, by a carcinogen exposure in rats or due to genetic modifications in ApcΔ716 mouse *(110, 111)*. EP$_1$ and EP$_2$ are generally increased, EP$_4$ is not altered, and EP$_3$ is reduced in the colon during early stages of tumorigenesis in rodents and humans *(93, 112)*. These studies implicate EP$_1$, EP$_2$, and EP$_4$ receptors in tumorigenesis, although they do not provide any evidence for a causative association. Further, it is not known what role dietary intake of *n*-6 PUFAs plays in affecting gastrointestinal carcinogenesis via the EP receptors.

6.2. Cyclooxygenases (COXs)

COX enzymes, which convert AA to prostaglandins, have been suggested to be involved in increasing cancer risk. COX exists in three isoforms: COX-1, COX-2, and COX-3. COX-1 is a constitutively expressed enzyme which performs various house-keeping functions to regulate vascular homeostasis, water re-absorption, gastric acid secretion, platelet aggregation, and renal blood flow. COX-3 is a splice variant of COX-1 and is mostly expressed in the brain and the heart *(113)*. COX-2 in turn is an inducible enzyme by, for example, mitogens, cytokines, and growth factors. PGE$_2$ can also induce COX-2, i.e., a positive feedback loop operates to generate prostaglandins when free AA is available. These enzymes exist as integral membrane glycoprotein homodimers and are present on the luminal surfaces of the endoplasmic reticulum and nuclear envelop within cells *(114)*.

Of the three COX enzymes, COX-2 is the one suggested to be linked to cancer *(115)*, by increasing PGE$_2$ synthesis in response to various factors which themselves are associated with increased cancer risk, i.e., mitogens, etc. Findings showing that non-steroidal anti-inflammatory drugs (NSAIDs) which inhibit COX-2 activity also inhibit tumorigenesis *(116)* are supportive of this view. Conversely, COX-2 over-expression in mice is sufficient to induce, for example, mammary tumors *(117)*. In addition, elevated expression of COX-2 has been linked to development of colon cancer *(29, 118)*, prostate cancer *(119)*, UV-related non-melanoma skin cancers *(120)*, ovarian cancer *(99)*, and several other cancers.

Some data cast doubt as to whether *n*-6 PUFA-induced up-regulation of COX-2 is a causative factor in cancer. Rats fed *n*-3 PUFAs exhibit increased incorporation of *n*-3 PUFAs into the membrane phospholipids and a subsequent inhibition of COX-2 expression *(29, 121)*. In agreement, we have found that prepubertal exposure to either the low or high-fat *n*-3 PUFA diet decreases the expression of COX-2 *(80)*. Since the high-fat *n*-3

PUFA diet increased, while the low-fat *n*-3 PUFA diet decreased mammary tumorigenesis *(80)*, COX-2 expression is unlikely to be correlated with increased tumorigenesis in the high-fat *n*-3 PUFA-fed rats. The fact that COX-2 is up-regulated in multiple cancers, in the absence of solid evidence to link these cancers to increased dietary intake of *n*-6 PUFAs, can also be interpreted to be against the role of COX-2 in mediating the effects of *n*-6 PUFA on cancer. We conclude that high levels of COX-2 expression in tumors occur independently from dietary intake of *n*-6 PUFAs, and changes in COX-2 expression by *n*-6 PUFA intake may not be sufficient to further modify cancer growth.

6.3. Gene Expression

Besides the genes directly linked to eicosanoids, such as COX-2 or the prostanoid receptors and their target genes (Fig. 2), several other genes influenced by PUFA intake have been identified. One of them is peroxisome proliferator-activated receptor γ (PPARγ). 15d-PGJ *(2)*, a metabolite of *n*-6 PUFA pathway, is a natural ligand for PPARγ *(122)*. This nuclear receptor which heterodimerizes with retinoid receptors to induce downstream signaling cascade, leading to increased cellular differentiation, is linked to reduced cancer risk *(123)*. PPARγ induces differentiation of pre-adipocytes *(124, 125)* and inhibits proliferation of epithelial cells, including mammary cells *(126)*. Due to its action in adipocytes *(124, 125, 127)* PPARγ reduces insulin resistance *(128–130)*. It has been reported that 15d-PGJ *(2)*, by acting through PPARγ, significantly inhibited estrogen-mediated proliferation of MCF-7 cells and caused accumulation of p21 and p27 proteins *(131)*. This single observation is in concert with other reports showing that PPARγ agonists reduce mammary tumor risk *(132)*; however, once breast tumors arise, PPARγ activation promotes tumor growth *(133)*. PPARγ coactivators, PGC-1α and 1β, play an important role in regulating glucose and lipid homeostasis and mitochondrial oxidation of fatty acids *(134)*. It also has been proposed that PPARγ is mainly expressed in well-differentiated and ER-positive breast carcinomas and modulates estrogenic actions *(131, 135)*.

Microarray studies have compared differences in gene expression in normal or carcinogen-exposed rat colon *(136)*, normal mammary glands *(137)*, and in mammary cancer cells exposed to either *n*-6 or *n*-3 PUFA *(138)*. In the colon, dietary exposure to *n*-3 PUFA fish oil up-regulated genes involved in apoptosis and differentiation *(136)*, when compared to colon of rats fed *n*-6 PUFA corn oil diet. The effects of *n*-6 PUFAs LA and AA and *n*-3 PUFAs EPA and DHA have been studied in human breast cancer cell lines MDA-MB-231, MDA-MB-435s, MCF-7, and HCC2218; the analysis identified differences in genes covering a broad spectrum of biological functions, such as cellular nutrition, cell division, cell proliferation, metastasis, and transcription factors *(138)*. We have determined differences in gene expression in mammary glands of adult rats fed low or high *n*-3 PUFA diets or low or high *n*-6 PUFA diets during prepubertal period *(80)*. Findings from these studies are discussed below (see Section 7.2). In summary, the differences induced in colon or mammary cells exposed to *n*-6 or *n*-3 PUFAs indicate that these fatty acids alter multiple different signaling pathways, any of which could be causally linked to differences in tumorigenesis between animals fed *n*-6 or *n*-3 PUFAs.

6.4. Estrogen Levels and PUFA

High fat intake and obesity have been associated with elevated circulating estrogen levels *(139)*. More than one biological pathway exists to link consumption of a diet high in *n*-6 PUFAs to increases in estrogen levels. High dietary intake of *n*-6 PUFAs promotes COX-2 activity, while *n*-3 PUFAs have an opposite effect *(140, 141)*. High levels of COX-2 expression result in higher levels of PGE_2, which in turn increases CYP19 aromatase expression through increases in intracellular cyclic AMP levels and activation of promoter II *(142, 143)*. This may occur via EP2 and EP4 which activate the cAMP→PKA→CREB pathway leading to enhanced CYP19 transcription and increased aromatase activity *(142)*. Thus, PGE_2 produced via COX may act locally in paracrine and autocrine fashion to increase the biosynthesis of estrogen by aromatase to promote hormone-dependent breast cancer development. Another potential pathway PUFA intake can affect circulating hormone levels is through modifying the expression of tumor suppressor gene BRCA1. *n*-3 PUFAs induce up-regulation of BRCA1 in cell culture model *(144)*, and BRCA1 in turn can selectively inhibit aromatase expression *(142, 145)*, leading to reduced estrogen levels.

High total fat intake and the resulting increase in fat depots may increase estrogenic signaling due to high aromatase activity in the adipocytes, leading to conversion of testosterone to estrogens. Estrogens, in turn, promote the growth of ER-positive malignant mammary cells, increasing breast cancer risk *(146)*. However, the data are controversial regarding total fat intake and high circulating estrogen levels, particularly in premenopausal women *(139)*.

6.5. Fat Intake and Obesity

One possible mechanism of action of dietary fats on breast cancer risk is through obesity. Obesity increases the risk of developing postmenopausal breast cancer in women *(147)* and animal models *(148)*. Obesity is a complex state which may have many different causes, but it always reflects a positive energy balance resulting from an energy intake being higher than energy consumption. Dietary fat is the most energy-rich nutrient – fat contains 9 kcal/g, while protein and carbohydrates each contain 4 kcal/g – making it easier to "overeat" than other macronutrients.

Different fats have different effects on the location where in the body fat depots are stored. Fat accumulates in the abdominal area as subcutaneous and visceral fat, also called central fat, or in the buttocks, legs, and arms as peripheral fat. Abdominal fat storage is typical for men and postmenopausal women *(149, 150)*, and it is linked to increased risk of developing metabolic syndrome, insulin resistance, and type 2 diabetes *(151, 152)*. These changes, in turn, are associated with increased breast cancer risk, even more so than obesity itself *(151, 153)*. Saturated fatty acids are stored as visceral fat, while monounsaturated fatty acids are stored as peripheral subcutaneous fat *(154)*. Dietary intake of *n*-6 PUFA also is associated with abdominal obesity *(155)*, while the peripheral fat depots contain higher levels of *n*-3 PUFA *(156)*. Further, dietary intake of PUFAs is linked to the size of adipocytes, while saturated fat intake increases both the size and the number of fat cells *(156)*. These findings suggest that SFA and *n*-6 PUFA may increase breast cancer risk through inducing central obesity. However, impaired insulin sensitivity is linked to reduced levels of PUFA in the skeletal muscle phospholipids, and increased AA levels in turn are related to increased insulin sensitivity *(157, 158)*. Thus, it is not apparent whether *n*-6 PUFA intake might affect breast cancer risk through changes in insulin signaling, since the results generated in different studies do not present a cohesive picture. It also is important to note that prostanoid receptors EP1, EP2, and EP4 all affect PI3K/Akt signaling cascade, which is linked to the development of insulin resistance.

7. MECHANISMS MEDIATING THE EFFECTS OF TIMING OF DIETARY PUFA EXPOSURES ON BREAST CANCER RISK

7.1. In Utero Exposures

It is not known how modifications in maternal diet during pregnancy can alter offspring's later susceptibility to develop breast cancer, but they may involve epigenetic changes *(159)* and changes in stem cell behavior *(160)*. However, the causality between the epigenetic changes in different tissues in adult animals induced by in utero hormonal manipulations and increased cancer risk, or between changes in stem cell behavior and breast cancer risk, remains to be established.

Many of the dietary compounds fed to pregnant dams which alter mammary cancer risk among their offspring modify pregnancy hormone levels. These hormonal changes may be central in explaining how in utero environment can alter later breast cancer risk, because this environment participates in programming the normal mammary gland development *(160)*. In humans, high birth weight correlates with increased pregnancy levels of estrogens *(161)*, leptin *(162, 163)*, and insulin-like growth factors (IGFs) *(164, 165)*, and other changes are likely. In our animal model, high-saturated fat diet which led to high birth weight significantly increased pregnancy leptin levels, but did not modify estrogen levels and non-significantly increased IGF-1 levels *(166)*. An exposure to *n*-6 PUFA high-fat diet during pregnancy elevated dam's E2 levels *(65, 83)*, but so did a high-fat *n*-3 PUFA diet *(167)* which reduced female offspring's risk to develop carcinogen-induced mammary tumors. The effects of maternal consumption of a diet high in monounsaturated fatty acids on pregnancy hormonal environment have not been studied. In summary, an increase in fetal estrogenic environment is unlikely to be the common link among different maternal dietary exposures and their effects on offspring's mammary cancer risk. It is possible that an alteration in some other hormone or growth factor is common to all the dietary exposures which modify susceptibility to cancer development. Alternatively, many hormonal factors in the fetal environment can influence later breast cancer risk.

Maternal diet during pregnancy, through affecting fetal environment in yet unspecified way, might cause alterations in the morphology of the mammary gland. We have shown that in utero exposures to excess estradiol *(65)* or obesity-inducing high-fat diet which increases birth weight *(166)* as well as high-fat *n*-6 PUFA diet *(65)* increases the number of targets in the mammary epithelial tree for malignant transformation, while high-fat *n*-3 PUFA diet reduces them *(69)*. These targets are terminal end buds (TEBs) which contain high numbers of proliferating cells and lead the invasion of mammary epithelial tree through the mammary fat pad *(168)*. Changes in TEBs may result from changes in mammary stem cell behavior, which in turn is regulated by few key signaling pathways, including Notch, Wnt, and Hedgehog *(169–171)*. In addition, Musashi-1 might be important in regulating these pathways and stem cell behavior *(172)*. A recent study indicates that the number of stem cells is causally linked to increased breast cancer risk *(173)*, but it is not known whether in utero dietary exposures alter mammary stem cell number and/or behavior.

7.2. Prepubertal Dietary Fat Exposures

Similar to the in utero dietary fat exposures, prepubertal exposures may affect later mammary cancer risk by altering circulating hormone levels. However, in contrast to in utero period when elevated E2 levels increase later susceptibility to develop breast cancer, elevated estrogen levels around puberty reduce breast cancer risk *(174, 175)*. This is suggested to be due to elimination of targets for malignant transformation, i.e., TEBs, and increased lobulo-alveolar differentiation, which prepubertal exposure to E2 induces *(175)*. However, prepubertal dietary exposures to low- and high-fat *n*-3 PUFA diets both reduce the number of TEBs and increase lobular differentiation, although they have opposite effect on mammary tumorigenesis *(80)*. These observations suggest that TEBs alone do not determine later susceptibility to mammary cancer. Alterations in stem cell behavior within the TEBs may also be involved.

To determine which signaling pathways are differentially expressed in the mammary glands of rats fed prepubertally diets containing *n*-6 or *n*-3 PUFAs, we have performed gene microarray analysis *(137)*. This comparison identified seven genes which were different between low-fat *n*-3 PUFA and both low- and high-fat *n*-6 PUFA groups, and also between high-fat *n*-3 PUFA and both *n*-6 PUFA groups (see Table 3). Among the genes was serine/threonine glycogen synthase kinase 3b (*Gsk3b*) which is the key component of the canonical WNT and PI3K-AKT signaling pathways. The role of Gsk3b in breast cancer is not well characterized, but it is the gene which has been involved in the signaling through prostanoid receptors EP1, EP2, and EP4 (see Fig. 2). Many changes also have been observed between pubertally low-fat and high-fat *n*-3 PUFA-fed rats *(137)*. Specifically, mammary glands of low-fat *n*-3 PUFA rats exhibited increased expression of antioxidant genes and genes linked to increased cellular differentiation, and reduced expression of genes which induce survival or promote cell proliferation, when compared to high-fat *n*-3 PUFA-fed rats. These changes may be causally linked to low mammary cancer risk in the low-fat *n*-3 PUFA-fed rats.

7.3. Pregnancy

Age at first pregnancy affects later breast cancer risk: completed pregnancy before age 20 protects a woman from developing breast cancer, while women giving birth first time after age 35 exhibit a lifelong increase in risk *(176)*. The levels of estrogens during pregnancy further modify breast cancer risk: a higher risk has been reported among women whose pregnancy estrogen levels were elevated. Higher pregnancy estrogenicity and increased breast cancer incidence are seen in women who suffered from severe nausea or vomiting during pregnancy *(177)*, gave birth to heavy infants *(178)*, were exposed

Table 3
Differences in gene expression in the mammary glands of 50-day-old rats fed *n*-3 or *n*-6 PUFA-containing diets prepubertally

Gene		High-fat n-3/n-6 PUFA	Low-fat n-3/n-6 PUFA	Gene function
Nucleoporin 62	Nup62	3.63[a]	2.22	Nuclear pore transport
Vacuolar protein sorting 13A	Vps13a	4.77	5.01	Regulation of protein cycling through the trans-Golgi network
Nuclear protein E3-3	RGD708545	2.15	4.41	Unknown
Developmentally regulated protein TPO1	Tpo1	3.42	3.03	Myelin biogenesis
Glycogen synthase kinase 3 beta	Gsk3b	6.28	4.51	Wnt signaling and energy metabolism
Heme oxygenase (decyling) 2	Hmox2	3.08	3.75	Oxidative stress
Mitochondrial ribosomal protein L53	Mrpl53	2.19	4.32	Mitochondrial protein synthesis

[a]Fold difference, $p < 0.05$.

to the synthetic estrogen DES during pregnancy *(179)* or exhibited excessive pregnancy weight gain *(85)*. In addition, results obtained in a nested case–control study indicate that women with higher estrone levels during the third trimester of pregnancy had two times higher incidence of breast cancer than those with more modest levels *(180)*. Conversely, lower levels of estrogens during pregnancy seem to decrease breast cancer risk. Maternal levels of circulating alpha-fetoprotein, a glycoprotein that binds to estrogens and suppresses its activity *(181, 182)* during pregnancy, are inversely associated with breast cancer risk *(183, 184)*.

Pregnancy induces a marked differentiation of the mammary epithelial tree, and this is thought to partly explain its protective effects *(185)*. Alternatively, changes in the gene signaling patterns in the mammary gland induced by pregnancy provide protection against breast cancer. For example, the expression of nuclear receptors ER-α, progesterone receptor (PR), and epidermal growth factor receptor (EGFR) is lower in the mammary glands of parous than nulliparous animals *(186, 187)*. Microarray analysis which compared gene expression in the mammary glands of multiple strains of pregnant and nulliparous mice and rats identified a panel of genes that were differentially expressed by pregnancy. These genes fell into three categories: those regulating cell proliferation, differentiation, or immune responses *(188)*.

Animals which undergo mimicked pregnancy through having been exposed to similar levels of estradiol and progesterone as detected during a normal pregnancy, develop fewer mammary tumors than vehicle-exposed controls *(189)*, and exhibit higher protein levels of p53, p21, and mdm2 than the vehicle-exposed controls *(190)*.

If the changes in gene/protein expression noted in parous rats and mice are causally related to their reduced mammary cancer risk, when compared to nulliparous animals, an exposure to excessive hormone levels during pregnancy, which increase mammary carcinogenesis, might be expected to reverse the protective gene/protein expression changes. We found this to be the case in a study in which rat dams were treated with estradiol or leptin during pregnancy, both of which increased their mammary tumorigenesis (de Assis et al., unpublished data). In addition, some genes which have earlier been reported to be down-regulated following pregnancy, for example, pleiotrophin, by twofold *(188)* were up-regulated by twofold in the mammary glands of estradiol and leptin-treated parous rats, while α-lactalbumin which was up-regulated by 13-fold in the mammary glands of parous rats and mice *(188)* was down-regulated twofold in our study involving estradiol and leptin-treated parous rats. As discussed above, leptin is closely linked to body weight and weight gain during pregnancy, and it is an estrogen-regulated gene. Specifically, leptin induces transcriptional activation of the aromatase gene in MCF-7 cells *(191)*, activates the ERα signaling pathway through the MAPK pathway *(192)*, and can interfere with the action of antiestrogens by decreasing ERα ubiquitination and increasing ERα half-life *(193)*. Thus, elevated pregnancy hormone levels linked to maternal obesity and excessive pregnancy weight gain *(83, 84, 161–163)* may counteract molecular changes linked to pregnancy's ability to reduce breast cancer risk.

Even if pregnancy-induced differentiation of the mammary epithelial tree – i.e., increased presence of lobulo-alveolar structures – does not explain the changes in breast cancer risk, it is possible that differentiation of mammary stem cells does. It has been proposed that pregnancy hormones induce a molecular switch in mammary stem cells which inhibits cell proliferation in response to subsequent exposure to hormones or carcinogens *(194)*. Some of these pregnancy-induced mammary epithelial stem cells fail to undergo apoptosis during post-lactational remodeling, and if transformed to malignancy prior to pregnancy, might give rise to breast cancers *(195)*.

In conclusion, intake of a high-fat *n*-6 PUFA or saturated fatty acid diet during pregnancy increases dams later mammary cancer risk *(83, 84)*. It remains to be determined whether these findings are caused by elevated pregnancy E2 and/or leptin levels. Further, the signaling pathways mediating the effects of pregnancy dietary fat exposures on later breast cancer risk also need to be identified.

8. CONCLUSIONS

Findings obtained in animal studies provide strong evidence to suggest that high dietary intake of *n*-6 PUFAs during pregnancy increases mammary tumorigenesis among dams *(83)* and their female offspring *(65)*. Thus, a short-term exposure during critical developmental periods to this fatty acid can have a lifelong negative impact on breast cancer risk. In addition, an exposure during pregnancy to an obesity-inducing diet in which the fat source is a mix of SFA, MUFA, and PUFA, and which causes excessive pregnancy weight gain and high birth weight, increases mammary cancer risk both in dams *(84)* and in offspring *(85)*. These findings are consistent with human studies showing that excessive pregnancy weight gain increases mothers' breast cancer risk *(85)*, and that high birth weight is associated with increased breast cancer risk *(70–79)*. It is not known whether *n*-6 PUFA intake during pregnancy affects breast cancer in humans. The mechanisms mediating the effects of pregnancy *n*-6 PUFA exposures on mammary cancer risk in animal models remain mostly unknown, but probably are linked to increased mammary epithelial cell proliferation and inhibition of functional differentiation.

The picture is very different regarding pubertal fat exposures and breast cancer. High-fat *n*-6 PUFA diet before puberty onset has no effect on mammary tumorigenesis in rats, when compared to low-fat *n*-6 PUFA diet *(196)*. In humans, childhood obesity provides a lifelong protection against breast cancer *(81, 82)*. These findings suggest that for a reason that needs to be identified, fat exposures around puberty reduce susceptibility to breast cancer risk. To complicate things further, this does not apply to prepubertal dietary exposure to high-fat *n*-3 PUFA which increases later mammary tumorigenesis in rats *(80)*. A low-fat *n*-3 PUFA diet during prepuberty has an opposite effect *(80)*, i.e., it reduces the risk, similarly than exposures to this fatty acid during adult life in animal models *(44, 197)* and humans have been reported to do (see Table 3). We propose that the protective effects of childhood obesity reflect changes in circulating hormone levels which regulate mammary epithelial cell proliferation and differentiation, although what these changes are, remain to be discovered. The effects of *n*-3 PUFAs, in turn, might be caused by changes in antioxidant genes and genes regulating cell survival and apoptosis *(137)*.

There is a discrepancy regarding *n*-6 PUFA intake during adult life and effects on mammary cancer in animal studies and human populations. In animals, *n*-6 PUFA consistently promotes the growth of existing mammary tumor cells *(43–45)*. However, in women PUFA intake is mostly without effect. One possibility is that humans obtain *n*-6 PUFAs from dietary sources which contain several other compounds that could reverse the harmful effects of this fatty acid. For example, milk fat is composed of 65% of saturated fats, 4% polyunsaturated fats, and 28% monounsaturated fats. Although lard is high in saturated fats (39%), it also contains a high proportion of monounsaturated (50%) and polyunsaturated fats (11%). Other explanation is that in humans *n*-6 PUFA intake is often assessed using food frequency questionnaires which are poor instruments to obtain accurate information on specific dietary intakes *(198, 199)*. There are multiple mechanisms potentially mediating the breast cancer promoting effects of *n*-6 PUFAs and at present time is not clear if one particular pathway is more significant that another.

To summarize, dietary fat intake may affect breast cancer risk, but the direction of the effect depends on the type of fat and the age when different fats are consumed.

REFERENCES

1. Kuller, L.H. (2006) Nutrition, lipids, and cardiovascular disease. *Nutr Rev* **64**, S15–S26.
2. Livesey, G., Taylor, R., Hulshof, T., and Howlett, J. (2008) Glycemic response and health—a systematic review and meta-analysis: Relations between dietary glycemic properties and health outcomes. *Am J Clin Nutr* **87**, 258S-68S.

3. Mulholland, H.G., Murray, L.J., Cardwell, C.R., and Cantwell, M.M. (2008) Dietary glycaemic index, glycaemic load and endometrial and ovarian cancer risk: A systematic review and meta-analysis. *Br J Cancer* **99**, 434–41.

4. Pisani, P. (2008) Hyper-insulinaemia and cancer, meta-analyses of epidemiological studies. *Arch Physiol Biochem* **114**, 63–70.

5. Ingram, D.K., Young, J., and Mattison, J.A. (2007) Calorie restriction in nonhuman primates: Assessing effects on brain and behavioral aging. *Neuroscience* **145**, 1359–64.

6. Kang, J.X. (2005) From fat to fat-1: A tale of omega-3 fatty acids. *J Membr Biol* **206**, 165–72.

7. Simopoulos, A.P. (2008) The importance of the omega-6/omega-3 fatty acid ratio in cardiovascular disease and other chronic diseases. *Exp Biol Med (Maywood)* **233**, 674–88.

8. Calder, P.C. (2005) Polyunsaturated fatty acids and inflammation. *Biochem Soc Trans* **33**, 423–27.

9. Brenner, R.R. (1974) The oxidative desaturation of unsaturated fatty acids in animals. *Mol Cell Biochem* **3**, 41–52.

10. Castuma, J.C., Brenner, R.R., and Kunau, W. (1977) Specificity of delta 6 desaturase – effect of chain length and number of double bonds. *Adv Exp Med Biol* **83**, 127–34.

11. Ou, J., Tu, H., Shan, B., Luk, A., DeBose-Boyd, R.A., Bashmakov, Y., Goldstein, J.L., and Brown, M.S. (2001) Unsaturated fatty acids inhibit transcription of the sterol regulatory element-binding protein-1c (SREBP-1c) gene by antagonizing ligand-dependent activation of the LXR. *Proc Natl Acad Sci U S A* **98**, 6027–32.

12. Wainwright, P.E., Jalali, E., Mutsaers, L.M., Bell, R., and Cvitkovic, S. (1999) An imbalance of dietary essential fatty acids retards behavioral development in mice. *Physiol Behav* **66**, 833–39.

13. Ziboh, V.A. (1996) The significance of polyunsaturated fatty acids in cutaneous biology. *Lipids* **31**(Suppl), S249-S53.

14. Soares, A.F., Santiago, R.C., Alessio, M.L., Descomps, B., and Castro-Chaves, C. (2005) Biochemical, functional, and histochemical effects of essential fatty acid deficiency in rat kidney. *Lipids* **40**, 1125–33.

15. Ayre, K.J., and Hulbert, A.J. (1996) Effects of changes in dietary fatty acids on isolated skeletal muscle functions in rats. *J Appl Physiol* **80**, 464–71.

16. Boissonneault, G.A., and Johnston, P.V. (1983) Essential fatty acid deficiency, prostaglandin synthesis and humoral immunity in Lewis rats. *J Nutr* **113**, 1187–94.

17. Kobayashi, N., Barnard, R.J., Henning, S.M., Elashoff, D., Reddy, S.T., Cohen, P., Leung, P., Hong-Gonzalez, J., Freedland, S.J., Said, J., Gui, D., Seeram, N.P., Popoviciu, L.M., Bagga, D., Heber, D., Glaspy, J.A., and Aronson, W.J. (2006) Effect of altering dietary omega-6/omega-3 fatty acid ratios on prostate cancer membrane composition, cyclooxygenase-2, and prostaglandin E2. *Clin Cancer Res* **12**, 4662–70.

18. Dommels, Y.E., Haring, M.M., Keestra, N.G., Alink, G.M., van Bladeren, P.J., and van Ommen, B. (2003) The role of cyclooxygenase in n-6 and n-3 polyunsaturated fatty acid mediated effects on cell proliferation, PGE(2) synthesis and cytotoxicity in human colorectal carcinoma cell lines. *Carcinogenesis* **24**, 385–92.

19. Boyd, N.F., Stone, J., Vogt, K.N., Connelly, B.S., Martin, L.J., and Minkin, S. (2003) Dietary fat and breast cancer risk revisited: A meta-analysis of the published literature. *Br J Cancer* **89**, 1672–85.

20. Harris, R.B., Foote, J.A., Hakim, I.A., Bronson, D.L., and Alberts, D.S. (2005) Fatty acid composition of red blood cell membranes and risk of squamous cell carcinoma of the skin. *Cancer Epidemiol Biomarkers Prev* **14**, 906–12.

21. Funahashi, H., Satake, M., Hasan, S., Sawai, H., Newman, R.A., Reber, H.A., Hines, O.J., and Eibl, G. (2008) Opposing effects of n-6 and n-3 polyunsaturated fatty acids on pancreatic cancer growth. *Pancreas* **36**, 353–62.

22. Chan, J.M., Wang, F., and Holly, E.A. (2007) Pancreatic cancer, animal protein and dietary fat in a population-based study, San Francisco Bay Area, California. *Cancer Causes Control* **18**, 1153–67.

23. Xu, W.H., Dai, Q., Xiang, Y.B., Zhao, G.M., Ruan, Z.X., Cheng, J.R., Zheng, W., and Shu, X.O. (2007) Nutritional factors in relation to endometrial cancer: A report from a population-based case-control study in Shanghai, China. *Int J Cancer* **120**, 1776–81.

24. Bertone, E.R., Rosner, B.A., Hunter, D.J., Stampfer, M.J., Speizer, F.E., Colditz, G.A., Willett, W.C., and Hankinson, S.E. (2002) Dietary fat intake and ovarian cancer in a cohort of US women. *Am J Epidemiol* **156**, 22–31.

25. Pan, S.Y., Ugnat, A.M., Mao, Y., Wen, S.W., and Johnson, K.C. (2004) A case-control study of diet and the risk of ovarian cancer. *Cancer Epidemiol Biomarkers Prev* **13**, 1521–27.

26. Ferrandina, G., Legge, F., Ranelletti, F.O., Zannoni, G.F., Maggiano, N., Evangelisti, A., Mancuso, S., Scambia, G., and Lauriola, L. (2002) Cyclooxygenase-2 expression in endometrial carcinoma: Correlation with clinicopathologic parameters and clinical outcome. *Cancer* **95**, 801–07.

27. Seo, S.S., Song, Y.S., Kang, D.H., Park, I.A., Bang, Y.J., Kang, S.B., and Lee, H.P. (2004) Expression of cyclooxygenase-2 in association with clinicopathological prognostic factors and molecular markers in epithelial ovarian cancer. *Gynecol Oncol* **92**, 927–35.

28. Trombetta, A., Maggiora, M., Martinasso, G., Cotogni, P., Canuto, R.A., and Muzio, G. (2007) Arachidonic and docosahexaenoic acids reduce the growth of A549 human lung-tumor cells increasing lipid peroxidation and PPARs. *Chem Biol Interact* **165**, 239–50.

29. Singh, J., Hamid, R., and Reddy, B.S. (1997) Dietary fat and colon cancer: Modulation of cyclooxygenase-2 by types and amount of dietary fat during the postinitiation stage of colon carcinogenesis. *Cancer Res* **57**, 3465–70.

30. Dommels, Y.E., Alink, G.M., van Bladeren, P.J., and van, O.B. (2002) Dietary n-6 and n-3 polyunsaturated fatty acids and colorectal carcinogenesis: Results from cultured colon cells, animal models and human studies. *Environ Toxicol Pharmacol* **12**, 233–44.

31. Chell, S.D., Witherden, I.R., Dobson, R.R., Moorghen, M., Herman, A.A., Qualtrough, D., Williams, A.C., and Paraskeva, C. (2006) Increased EP4 receptor expression in colorectal cancer progression promotes cell growth and anchorage independence. *Cancer Res* **66**, 3106–13.

32. Qualtrough, D., Kaidi, A., Chell, S., Jabbour, H.N., Williams, A.C., and Paraskeva, C. (2007) Prostaglandin F(2alpha) stimulates motility and invasion in colorectal tumor cells. *Int J Cancer* **121**, 734–40.

33. Rose, D.P., and Connolly, J.M. (1991) Effects of fatty acids and eicosanoid synthesis inhibitors on the growth of two human prostate cancer cell lines. *Prostate* **18**, 243–54.

34. Pandalai, P.K., Pilat, M.J., Yamazaki, K., Naik, H., and Pienta, K.J. (1996) The effects of omega-3 and omega-6 fatty acids on in vitro prostate cancer growth. *Anticancer Res* **16**, 815–20.

35. Kelavkar, U.P., Hutzley, J., Dhir, R., Kim, P., Allen, K.G., and McHugh, K. (2006) Prostate tumor growth and recurrence can be modulated by the omega-6:omega-3 ratio in diet: Athymic mouse xenograft model simulating radical prostatectomy. *Neoplasia* **8**, 112–24.

36. Astorg, P., and Dietary, N.- (2004) 6 and N-3 polyunsaturated fatty acids and prostate cancer risk: A review of epidemiological and experimental evidence. *Cancer Causes Control* **15**, 367–86.

37. Rose, D.P. (1997) Effects of dietary fatty acids on breast and prostate cancers: Evidence from in vitro experiments and animal studies. *Am J Clin Nutr* **66**, 1513S-1522S.

38. Wicha, M.S., Liotta, L.A., and Kidwell, W.R. (1979) Effects of free fatty acids on the growth of normal and neoplastic rat mammary epithelial cells. *Cancer Res* **39**, 426–35.

39. Chamras, H., Ardashian, A., Heber, D., and Glaspy, J.A. (2002) Fatty acid modulation of MCF-7 human breast cancer cell proliferation, apoptosis and differentiation. *J Nutr Biochem* **13**, 711–16.

40. Lof, M., Sandin, S., Lagiou, P., Hilakivi-Clarke, L., Trichopoulos, D., Adami, H.O., and Weiderpass, E. (2007) Dietary fat and breast cancer risk in the Swedish women's lifestyle and health cohort. *Br J Cancer* **97**, 1570–76.

41. Hopkins, G.J., and Carroll, K.K. (1979) Relationship between amount and type of dietary fat in promotion of mammary carcinogenesis induced by 7,12-dimethylmenz(a)anthracene. *J Natl Cancer Inst* **62**, 1009–12.

42. Cohen, L.A., Chen-Backlund, J.Y., Sepkovic, D.W., and Sugie, S. (1993) Effect of varying proportions of dietary menhaden and corn oil on experimental rat mammary tumor promotion. *Lipids* **28**, 449–56.

43. Welsch, C.W. (1992) Relationship between dietary fat and experimental mammary tumorigenesis: A review and critique. *Cancer Res* **52**, 2040–48.

44. Freedman, L.S., Clifford, C.K., and Messina, M. (1990) Analysis of dietary fat, calories, body weight, and the development of mammary tumors in rats and mice: A review. *Cancer Res* **50**, 5710–19.

45. Fay, M.P., and Freedman, L.S. (1997) Meta-analyses of dietary fats and mammary neoplasms in rodent experiments. *Breast Cancer Res Treat* **46**, 215–23.

46. Smith-Warner, S.A., Spiegelman, D., Adami, H.-O., Beeson, W.L., van den Brandt, P.A., Folsom, A.R., Fraser, G.E., Freudenheim, J.L., Goldbohm, R.A., Graham, S., Kushi, L.H., Miller, A.B., Rohan, T.E., Speizer, F.E., Toniolo, P., Willett, W.C., Wolk, A., Zeleniuh-Jacquette, A., and Hunter, D.J. (2001) Types of dietary fat and breast cancer: A pooled analysis of cohort studies. *Int J Cancer* **92**, 767–74.

47. Thiebaut, A.C., Kipnis, V., Chang, S.C., Subar, A.F., Thompson, F.E., Rosenberg, P.S., Hollenbeck, A.R., Leitzmann, M., and Schatzkin, A. (2007) Dietary fat and postmenopausal invasive breast cancer in the National Institutes of Health-AARP Diet and Health Study cohort. *J Natl Cancer Inst* **99**, 451–62.

48. Byrne, C., Rockett, H., and Holmes, M.D. (2002) Dietary fat, fat subtypes, and breast cancer risk: Lack of an association among postmenopausal women with no history of benign breast disease. *Cancer Epidemiol Biomarkers Prev* **11**, 261–65.

49. Kim, E.H., Willett, W.C., Colditz, G.A., Hankinson, S.E., Stampfer, M.J., Hunter, D.J., Rosner, B., and Holmes, M.D. (2006) Dietary fat and risk of postmenopausal breast cancer in a 20-year follow-up. *Am J Epidemiol* **164**, 990–97.

50. Wakai, K., Tamakoshi, K., Date, C., Fukui, M., Suzuki, S., Lin, Y., Niwa, Y., Nishio, K., Yatsuya, H., Kondo, T., Tokudome, S., Yamamoto, A., Toyoshima, H., and Tamakoshi, A. (2005) Dietary intakes of fat and fatty acids and risk of breast cancer: A prospective study in Japan. *Cancer Sci* **96**, 590–99.

51. Voorrips, L.E., Brants, H.A., Kardinaal, A.F., Hiddink, G.J., van den Brandt, P.A., and Goldbohm, R.A. (2002) Intake of conjugated linoleic acid, fat, and other fatty acids in relation to postmenopausal breast cancer: The Netherlands Cohort Study on Diet and Cancer. *Am J Clin Nutr* **76**, 873–82.

52. Zhang, S.M., Lee, I.M., Manson, J.E., Cook, N.R., Willett, W.C., and Buring, J.E. (2007) Alcohol consumption and breast cancer risk in the Women's Health Study. *Am J Epidemiol* **165**, 667–76.

53. Terry, P.D., Rohan, T.E., and Wolk, A. (2003) Intakes of fish and marine fatty acids and the risks of cancers of the breast and prostate and of other hormone-related cancers: A review of the epidemiologic evidence. *Am J Clin Nutr* **77**, 532–43.

54. Wirfalt, E., Mattisson, I., Gullberg, B., Johansson, U., Olsson, H., and Berglund, G. (2002) Postmenopausal breast cancer is associated with high intakes of omega6 fatty acids (Sweden. *Cancer Causes Control* **13**, 883–93.

55. Cho, E., Spiegelman, D., Hunter, D.J., Chen, W.Y., Stampfer, M.J., Colditz, G.A., and Willett, W.C. (2003) Premenopausal fat intake and risk of breast cancer. *J Natl Cancer Inst* **95**, 1079–85.

56. Gago-Dominguez, M., Yuan, J.M., Sun, C.L., Lee, H.P., and Yu, M.C. (2003) Opposing effects of dietary n-3 and n-6 fatty acids on mammary carcinogenesis: The Singapore Chinese Health Study. *Br J Cancer* **89**, 1686–92.

57. Bingham, S.A., Luben, R., Welch, A., Wareham, N., Khaw, K.T., and Day, N. (2003) Are imprecise methods obscuring a relation between fat and breast cancer?. *Lancet* **362**, 212–14.

58. Freedman, L.S., Potischman, N., Kipnis, V., Midthune, D., Schatzkin, A., Thompson, F.E., Troiano, R.P., Prentice, R., Patterson, R., Carroll, R., and Subar, A.F. (2006) A comparison of two dietary instruments for evaluating the fat-breast cancer relationship. *Int J Epidemiol* **35**, 1011–21.

59. Carmichael, A.R. (2006) Obesity as a risk factor for development and poor prognosis of breast cancer. *BJOG* **113**, 1160–66.

60. Pierce, J.P., Natarajan, L., Caan, B.J., Parker, B.A., Greenberg, E.R., Flatt, S.W., Rock, C.L., Kealey, S., Al Delaimy, W.K., Bardwell, W.A., Carlson, R.W., Emond, J.A., Faerber, S., Gold, E.B., Hajek, R.A., Hollenbach, K., Jones, L.A., Karanja, N., Madlensky, L., Marshall, J., Newman, V.A., Ritenbaugh, C., Thomson, C.A., Wasserman, L., and Stefanick, M.L. (2007) Influence of a diet very high in vegetables, fruit, and fiber and low in fat on prognosis following treatment for breast cancer: The Women's Healthy Eating and Living (WHEL) randomized trial. *JAMA* **298**, 289–98.

61. Thomson, C.A., Giuliano, A.R., Shaw, J.W., Rock, C.L., Ritenbaugh, C.K., Hakim, I.A., Hollenbach, K.A., Alberts, D.S., and Pierce, J.P. (2005) Diet and biomarkers of oxidative damage in women previously treated for breast cancer. *Nutr Cancer* **51**, 146–54.

62. Majed, B., Moreau, T., Senouci, K., Salmon, R.J., Fourquet, A., and Asselain, B. (2008) Is obesity an independent prognosis factor in woman breast cancer?. *Breast Cancer Res Treat* **111**, 329–42.

63. Obermair, A., Kurz, C., Hanzal, E., Bancher-Todesca, D., Thoma, M., Bodisch, A., Kubista, E., Kyral, E., Kaider, A., Sevelda, P. et al. (1995) The influence of obesity on the disease-free survival in primary breast cancer. *Anticancer Res* **15**, 2265–69.

64. de, A.S., and Hilakivi-Clarke, L. (2006) Timing of dietary estrogenic exposures and breast cancer risk. *Ann N Y Acad Sci* **1089**, 14–35.

65. Hilakivi-Clarke, L., Clarke, R., Onojafe, I., Raygada, M., Cho, E., and Lippman, M.E. (1997) A maternal diet high in n-6 polyunsaturated fats alters mammary gland development, puberty onset, and breast cancer risk among female rat offspring. *Proc Natl Acad Sci U S A* **94**, 9372–77.

66. Stark, A.H., Kossoy, G., Zusman, I., Yarden, G., and Madar, Z. (2003) Olive oil consumption during pregnancy and lactation in rats influences mammary cancer development in female offspring. *Nutr Cancer* **46**, 59–65.

67. Walker, B.E. (1990) Tumors in female offspring of control and diethylstilbestrol-exposed mice fed high-fat diets. *J Nat Cancer Inst* **82**, 50–54.

68. Luijten, M., Thomsen, A.R., van den Berg, J.A., Wester, P.W., Verhoef, A., Nagelkerke, N.J., Adlercreutz, H., van Kranen, H.J., Piersma, A.H., Sorensen, I.K., Rao, G.N., and van Kreijl, C.F. (2004) Effects of soy-derived isoflavones and a high-fat diet on spontaneous mammary tumor development in Tg.NK (MMTV/c-neu) mice. *Nutr Cancer* **50**, 46–54.

69. Hilakivi-Clarke, L., Cho, E., Cabanes, A., DeAssis, S., Olivo, S., Helferich, W., Lippman, M.E., and Clarke, R. (2002) Dietary modulation of pregnancy estrogen levels and breast cancer risk among female rat offspring. *Clin Cancer Res* **8**, 3601–10.

70. Michels, K.B., Trichopoulos, D., Robins, J.M., Rosner, B.A., Manson, J.E., Hunter, D., Colditz, G.A., Hankinson, S.E., Speizer, F.E., and Willett, W.C. (1996) Birthweight as a risk factor for breast cancer. *Lancet* **348**, 1542–46.

71. Sanderson, M., Williams, M., Malone, K.E., Stanford, J.L., Emanuel, I., White, E., and Daling, J.R. (1996) Perinatal factors and risk of breast cancer. *Epidemiology* **7**, 34–37.

72. Ahlgren, M., Sorensen, T., Wohlfahrt, J., Haflidadottir, A., Holst, C., and Melbye, M. (2003) Birth weight and risk of breast cancer in a cohort of 106,504 women. *Int J Cancer* **107**, 997–1000.

73. McCormack, V.A., dos Santos Silva, I., De Stavola, B.L., Mohsen, R., Leon, D.A., and Lithell, H.O. (2003) Fetal growth and subsequent risk of breast cancer: Results from long term follow up of Swedish cohort. *BMJ* **326**, 248.

74. Stavola, B.L., Hardy, R., Kuh, D., Silva, I.S., Wadsworth, M., and Swerdlow, A.J. (2000) Birthweight, childhood growth and risk of breast cancer in a British cohort. *Br J Cancer* **83**, 964–68.

75. Hilakivi-Clarke, L., Forsen, T., Eriksson, J.G., Luoto, R., Tuomilehto, J., Osmond, C., and Barker, D.J. (2001) Tallness and overweight during childhood have opposing effects on breast cancer risk. *Br J Cancer* **85**, 1680–84.

76. Ahlgren, M., Melbye, M., Wohlfahrt, J., and Sorensen, T.I. (2004) Growth patterns and the risk of breast cancer in women. *N Engl J Med* **351**, 1619–26.

77. McCormack, V.A., dos Santos Silva, I., Koupil, I., Leon, D.A., and Lithell, H.O. (2005) Birth characteristics and adult cancer incidence: Swedish cohort of over 11,000 men and women. *Int J Cancer* **115**, 611–17.

78. Vatten, L.J., Nilsen, T.I., Tretli, S., Trichopoulos, D., and Romundstad, P.R. (2005) Size at birth and risk of breast cancer: Prospective population-based study. *Int J Cancer* **114**, 461–64.

79. Michels, K.B., Xue, F., Terry, K.L., and Willett, W.C. (2006) Longitudinal study of birthweight and the incidence of breast cancer in adulthood. *Carcinogenesis* **27**, 2464–68.

80. Olivo, S.E., and Hilakivi-Clarke, L. (2005) Opposing effects of prepubertal low and high fat n-3 polyunsaturated fatty acid diets on rat mammary tumorigenesis. *Carcinogenesis* **26**, 1563–72.

81. Wu, A.H., Wan, P., Hankin, J., Tseng, C.C., Yu, M.C., and Pike, M.C. (2002) Adolescent and adult soy intake and risk of breast cancer in Asian-Americans. *Carcinogenesis* **23**, 1491–96.

82. Shu, X.O., Jin, F., Dai, Q., Wen, W., Potter, J.D., Kushi, L.H., Ruan, Z., Gao, Y.T., and Zheng, W. (2001) Soyfood intake during adolescence and subsequent risk of breast cancer among Chinese women. *Cancer Epidemiol Biomarkers Prev* **10**, 483–88.

83. Hilakivi-Clarke, L., Onojafe, I., Raygada, M., Cho, E., Clarke, R., and Lippman, M. (1996) Breast cancer risk in rats fed a diet high in n-6 polyunsaturated fatty acids during pregnancy. *J Natl Cancer Inst* **88**, 1821–27.

84. de Assis, S., Wang, M., Goel, S., Foxworth, A., Helferich, W.G., and Hilakivi-Clarke, L. (2005) Excessive weight gain during pregnancy increases carcinogen-induced mammary tumorigenesis in Sprague-Dawley and lean and obese Zucker rats. *J Nutr* **136**, 998–1004.

85. Kinnunen, T.I., Luoto, R., Gissler, M., Hemminki, E., and Hilakivi-Clarke, L. (2004) Pregnancy weight gain and breast cancer risk. *BMC Womens Health* **4**, 7–17.

86. Zhao, G., Etherton, T.D., Martin, K.R., Gillies, P.J., West, S.G., and Kris-Etherton, P.M. (2007) Dietary alpha-linolenic acid inhibits proinflammatory cytokine production by peripheral blood mononuclear cells in hypercholesterolemic subjects. *Am J Clin Nutr* **85**, 385–91.

87. Eritsland, J. (2000) Safety considerations of polyunsaturated fatty acids. *Am J Clin Nutr* **71**, 197S-201S.

88. Benatti, P., Peluso, G., Nicolai, R., and Calvani, M. (2004) Polyunsaturated fatty acids: Biochemical, nutritional and epigenetic properties. *J Am Coll Nutr* **23**, 281–302.

89. Rose, D.P. (1997) Dietary fatty acids and cancer. *Am J Clin Nutr* **66**, 998S–1003S.

90. Ahrenstedt, O., Hallgren, R., and Knutson, L. (1994) Jejunal release of prostaglandin E2 in Crohn's disease: Relation to disease activity and first-degree relatives. *J Gastroenterol Hepatol* **9**, 539–43.

91. Eberhart, C.E., Coffey, R.J., Radhika, A., Giardiello, F.M., Ferrenbach, S., and Dubois, R.N. (1994) Up-regulation of cyclooxygenase 2 gene expression in human colorectal adenomas and adenocarcinomas. *Gastroenterology* **107**, 1183–88.

92. Breyer, R.M., Bagdassarian, C.K., Myers, S.A., and Breyer, M.D. (2001) Prostanoid receptors: Subtypes and signaling. *Annu Rev Pharmacol Toxicol* **41**, 661–90.

93. Dey, I., Lejeune, M., and Chadee, K. (2006) Prostaglandin E2 receptor distribution and function in the gastrointestinal tract. *Br J Pharmacol* **149**, 611–23.

94. Su, J.L., Shih, J.Y., Yen, M.L., Jeng, Y.M., Chang, C.C., Hsieh, C.Y., Wei, L.H., Yang, P.C., and Kuo, M.L. (2004) Cyclooxygenase-2 induces EP1- and HER-2/Neu-dependent vascular endothelial growth factor-C up-regulation: A novel mechanism of lymphangiogenesis in lung adenocarcinoma. *Cancer Res* **64**, 554–64.

95. Han, C., and Wu, T. (2005) Cyclooxygenase-2-derived prostaglandin E2 promotes human cholangiocarcinoma cell growth and invasion through EP1 receptor-mediated activation of the epidermal growth factor receptor and Akt. *J Biol Chem* **280**, 24053–63.

96. Watanabe, K., Kawamori, T., Nakatsugi, S., Ohta, T., Ohuchida, S., Yamamoto, H., Maruyama, T., Kondo, K., Ushikubi, F., Narumiya, S., Sugimura, T., and Wakabayashi, K. (1999) Role of the prostaglandin E receptor subtype EP1 in colon carcinogenesis. *Cancer Res* **59**, 5093–96.

97. Thorat, M.A., Morimiya, A., Mehrotra, S., Konger, R., and Badve, S.S. (2008) Prostanoid receptor EP1 expression in breast cancer. *Mod Pathol* **21**, 15–21.

98. Zhang, L., Jiang, L., Sun, Q., Peng, T., Lou, K., Liu, N., and Leng, J. (2007) Prostaglandin E2 enhances mitogen-activated protein kinase/Erk pathway in human cholangiocarcinoma cells: Involvement of EP1 receptor, calcium and EGF receptors signaling. *Mol Cell Biochem* **305**, 19–26.

99. Rask, K., Zhu, Y., Wang, W., Hedin, L., and Sundfeldt, K. (2006) Ovarian epithelial cancer: A role for PGE2-synthesis and signalling in malignant transformation and progression. *Mol Cancer* **5**, 62.

100. Kawamori, T., Kitamura, T., Watanabe, K., Uchiya, N., Maruyama, T., Narumiya, S., Sugimura, T., and Wakabayashi, K. (2005) Prostaglandin E receptor subtype EP(1) deficiency inhibits colon cancer development. *Carcinogenesis* **26**, 353–57.

101. Yu, L., Wu, W.K., Li, Z.J., Wong, H.P., Tai, E.K., Wu, Y.C., Li, H.T., and Cho, C.H. (2008) EP2 receptor-mediated activation of extracellular signal-regulated kinase/activator protein-1 signaling is required for the mitogenic action of prostaglandin E2 in esophageal squamous-cell carcinoma. *J Pharmacol Exp Ther* **327**, 258–67.

102. Wang, X., and Klein, R.D. (2007) Prostaglandin E2 induces vascular endothelial growth factor secretion in prostate cancer cells through EP2 receptor-mediated cAMP pathway. *Mol Carcinog* **46**, 912–23.

103. Castellone, M.D., Teramoto, H., Williams, B.O., Druey, K.M., and Gutkind, J.S. (2005) Prostaglandin E2 promotes colon cancer cell growth through a Gs-axin-beta-catenin signaling axis. *Science* **310**, 1504–10.

104. White, E.S., Atrasz, R.G., Dickie, E.G., Aronoff, D.M., Stambolic, V., Mak, T.W., Moore, B.B., and Peters-Golden, M. (2005) Prostaglandin E(2) inhibits fibroblast migration by E-prostanoid 2 receptor-mediated increase in PTEN activity. *Am J Respir Cell Mol Biol* **32**, 135–41.

105. Fulton, A.M., Ma, X., and Kundu, N. (2006) Targeting prostaglandin E EP receptors to inhibit metastasis. *Cancer Res* **66**, 9794–97.

106. Regan, J.W. (2003) EP2 and EP4 prostanoid receptor signaling. *Life Sci* **74**, 143–53.

107. Macias-Perez, I.M., Zent, R., Carmosino, M., Breyer, M.D., Breyer, R.M., and Pozzi, A. (2008) Mouse EP3 alpha, beta, and gamma receptor variants reduce tumor cell proliferation and tumorigenesis in vivo. *J Biol Chem* **283**, 12538–45.

108. Axelsson, H., Lonnroth, C., Wang, W., Svanberg, E., and Lundholm, K. (2005) Cyclooxygenase inhibition in early onset of tumor growth and related angiogenesis evaluated in EP1 and EP3 knockout tumor-bearing mice. *Angiogenesis* **8**, 339–48.

109. Yano, T., Zissel, G., Muller-Qernheim, J., Jae, S.S., Satoh, H., and Ichikawa, T. (2002) Prostaglandin E2 reinforces the activation of Ras signal pathway in lung adenocarcinoma cells via EP3. *FEBS Lett* **518**, 154–58.

110. Sonoshita, M., Takaku, K., Sasaki, N., Sugimoto, Y., Ushikubi, F., Narumiya, S., Oshima, M., and Taketo, M.M. (2001) Acceleration of intestinal polyposis through prostaglandin receptor EP2 in Apc(Delta 716) knockout mice. *Nat Med* **7**, 1048–51.

111. Kawamori, T., Uchiya, N., Sugimura, T., and Wakabayashi, K. (2003) Enhancement of colon carcinogenesis by prostaglandin E2 administration. *Carcinogenesis* **24**, 985–90.

112. Shoji, Y., Takahashi, M., Kitamura, T., Watanabe, K., Kawamori, T., Maruyama, T., Sugimoto, Y., Negishi, M., Narumiya, S., Sugimura, T., and Wakabayashi, K. (2004) Downregulation of prostaglandin E receptor subtype EP3 during colon cancer development. *Gut* **53**, 1151–58.

113. Chandrasekharan, N.V., Dai, H., Roos, K.L., Evanson, N.K., Tomsik, J., Elton, T.S., and Simmons, D.L. (2002) COX-3, a cyclooxygenase-1 variant inhibited by acetaminophen and other analgesic/antipyretic drugs: Cloning, structure, and expression. *Proc Natl Acad Sci U S A* **99**, 13926–31.

114. Otto, J.C., and Smith, W.L. (1995) Prostaglandin endoperoxide synthases-1 and -2. *J Lipid Mediat Cell Signal* **12**, 139–56.

115. Muller-Decker, K., and Furstenberger, G. (2007) The cyclooxygenase-2-mediated prostaglandin signaling is causally related to epithelial carcinogenesis. *Mol Carcinog* **46**, 705–10.

116. Harris, R.E., Alshafie, G.A., bou-Issa, H., and Seibert, K. (2000) Chemoprevention of breast cancer in rats by celecoxib, a cyclooxygenase 2 inhibitor. *Cancer Res* **60**, 2101–03.

117. Liu, C.H., Chang, S.H., Narko, K., Trifan, O.C., Wu, M.-T., Smith, E., Haudenschild, C., Lane, T.F., and Hla, T. (2001) Overexpression of cyclooxygenase-2 is sufficient to induce tumorigenesis in transgenic mice. *J Biol Chem* **276**, 18563–69.

118. Reddy, B.S., and Rao, C.V. (2002) Novel approaches for colon cancer prevention by cyclooxygenase-2 inhibitors. *J Environ Pathol Toxicol Oncol* **21**, 155–64.

119. Hussain, T., Gupta, S., and Mukhtar, H. (2003) Cyclooxygenase-2 and prostate carcinogenesis. *Cancer Lett* **191**, 125–35.

120. Rundhaug, J.E., and Fischer, S.M. (2008) Cyclo-oxygenase-2 plays a critical role in UV-induced skin carcinogenesis. *Photochem Photobiol* **84**, 322–29.

121. Badawi, A.F., El-Sohemy, A., Stephen, L.L., Ghoshal, A.K., and Archer, M.C. (1998) The effect of dietary n-3 and n-6 polyunsaturated fatty acids on the expression of cyclooxygenase 1 and 2 and levels of p21 in rat mammary glands. *Carcinogenesis* **19**, 903–10.

122. Willson, T.M., Lambert, M.H., and Kliewer, S.A. (2001) Peroxisome proliferator-activated receptor gamma and metabolic disease. *Annu Rev Biochem* **70**, 341–67.

123. Wang, T., Xu, J., Yu, X., Yang, R., and Han, Z.C. (2006) Peroxisome proliferator-activated receptor gamma in malignant diseases. *Crit Rev Oncol Hematol* **58**, 1–14.

124. Hosono, T., Mizuguchi, H., Katayama, K., Koizumi, N., Kawabata, K., Yamaguchi, T., Nakagawa, S., Watanabe, Y., Mayumi, T., and Hayakawa, T. (2005) RNA interference of PPARgamma using

fiber-modified adenovirus vector efficiently suppresses preadipocyte-to-adipocyte differentiation in 3T3-L1 cells. _Gene_ **348**, 157–65.

125. Fu, M., Rao, M., Bouras, T., Wang, C., Wu, K., Zhang, X., Li, Z., Yao, T.P., and Pestell, R.G. (2005) Cyclin D1 inhibits peroxisome proliferator-activated receptor gamma-mediated adipogenesis through histone deacetylase recruitment. _J Biol Chem_ **280**, 16934–41.

126. Jarrar, M.H., and Baranova, A. (2007) PPARgamma activation by thiazolidinediones (TZDs) may modulate breast carcinoma outcome: The importance of interplay with TGFbeta signalling. _J Cell Mol Med_ **11**, 71–87.

127. Imai, T., Takakuwa, R., Marchand, S., Dentz, E., Bornert, J.M., Messaddeq, N., Wendling, O., Mark, M., Desvergne, B., Wahli, W., Chambon, P., and Metzger, D. (2004) Peroxisome proliferator-activated receptor gamma is required in mature white and brown adipocytes for their survival in the mouse. _Proc Natl Acad Sci U S A_ **101**, 4543–47.

128. Kubota, N., Terauchi, Y., Miki, H., Tamemoto, H., Yamauchi, T., Komeda, K., Satoh, S., Nakano, R., Ishii, C., Sugiyama, T., Eto, K., Tsubamoto, Y., Okuno, A., Murakami, K., Sekihara, H., Hasegawa, G., Naito, M., Toyoshima, Y., Tanaka, S., Shiota, K., Kitamura, T., Fujita, T., Ezaki, O., Aizawa, S., Kadowaki, T. et al. (1999) PPAR gamma mediates high-fat diet-induced adipocyte hypertrophy and insulin resistance. _Mol Cell_ **4**, 597–609.

129. Yamauchi, T., Kamon, J., Waki, H., Terauchi, Y., Kubota, N., Hara, K., Mori, Y., Ide, T., Murakami, K., Tsuboyama-Kasaoka, N., Ezaki, O., Akanuma, Y., Gavrilova, O., Vinson, C., Reitman, M.L., Kagechika, H., Shudo, K., Yoda, M., Nakano, Y., Tobe, K., Nagai, R., Kimura, S., Tomita, M., Froguel, P., and Kadowaki, T. (2001) The fat-derived hormone adiponectin reverses insulin resistance associated with both lipoatrophy and obesity. _Nat Med_ **7**, 941–46.

130. Jones, J.R., Barrick, C., Kim, K.A., Lindner, J., Blondeau, B., Fujimoto, Y., Shiota, M., Kesterson, R.A., Kahn, B.B., and Magnuson, M.A. (2005) Deletion of PPARgamma in adipose tissues of mice protects against high fat diet-induced obesity and insulin resistance. _Proc Natl Acad Sci U S A_ **102**, 6207–12.

131. Suzuki, T., Hayashi, S., Miki, Y., Nakamura, Y., Moriya, T., Sugawara, A., Ishida, T., Ohuchi, N., and Sasano, H. (2006) Peroxisome proliferator-activated receptor gamma in human breast carcinoma: A modulator of estrogenic actions. _Endocr Relat Cancer_ **13**, 233–50.

132. Yin, Y., Russell, R.G., Dettin, L.E., Bai, R., Wei, Z.L., Kozikowski, A.P., Kopelovich, L., and Glazer, R.I. (2005) Peroxisome proliferator-activated receptor delta and gamma agonists differentially alter tumor differentiation and progression during mammary carcinogenesis. _Cancer Res_ **65**, 3950–57.

133. Saez, E., Rosenfeld, J., Livolsi, A., Olson, P., Lombardo, E., Nelson, M., Banayo, E., Cardiff, R.D., Izpisua-Belmonte, J.C., and Evans, R.M. (2004) PPAR gamma signaling exacerbates mammary gland tumor development. _Genes Dev_ **18**, 528–40.

134. Puigserver, P., and Spiegelman, B.M. (2003) Peroxisome proliferator-activated receptor-gamma coactivator 1 alpha (PGC-1 alpha): Transcriptional coactivator and metabolic regulator. _Endocr Rev_ **24**, 78–90.

135. Kim, H.J., Kim, J.Y., Meng, Z., Wang, L.H., Liu, F., Conrads, T.P., Burke, T.R., Veenstra, T.D., and Farrar, W.L. (2007) 15-deoxy-Delta12,14-prostaglandin J2 inhibits transcriptional activity of estrogen receptor-alpha via covalent modification of DNA-binding domain. _Cancer Res_ **67**, 2595–602.

136. Davidson, L.A., Nguyen, D.V., Hokanson, R.M., Callaway, E.S., Isett, R.B., Turner, N.D., Dougherty, E.R., Wang, N., Lupton, J.R., Carroll, R.J., and Chapkin, R.S. (2004) Chemopreventive n-3 polyunsaturated fatty acids reprogram genetic signatures during colon cancer initiation and progression in the rat. _Cancer Res_ **64**, 6797–804.

137. Olivo, S., Zhou, Y., Lee, R., Cabanes, A., Khan, G., Zwart, A., Wang, Y., Clarke, R., and Hilakivi-Clarke, L. (2008) Gene signaling pathways mediating the opposite effects of prepubertal low and high fat n-3 polyunsaturated fatty acid diets on mammary cancer risk. _Cancer Prev Res_ **1**, 532–45.

138. Hammamieh, R., Chakraborty, N., Miller, S.A., Waddy, E., Barmada, M., Das, R., Peel, S.A., Day, A.A., and Jett, M. (2007) Differential effects of omega-3 and omega-6 Fatty acids on gene expression in breast cancer cells. _Breast Cancer Res Treat_ **101**, 7–16.

139. Wu, A.H., Pike, M.C., and Stram, D.O. (1999) Meta-analysis: Dietary fat intake, serum estrogen levels, and the risk of breast cancer. _J Natl Cancer Inst_ **91**, 529–34.

140. Salhab, M., Singh-Ranger, G., Mokbel, R., Jouhra, F., Jiang, W.G., and Mokbel, K. (2007) Cyclooxygenase-2 mRNA expression correlates with aromatase expression in human breast cancer. *J Surg Oncol* **96**, 424–28.

141. Brueggemeier, R.W., Su, B., Sugimoto, Y., Diaz-Cruz, E.S., and Davis, D.D. (2007) Aromatase and COX in breast cancer: Enzyme inhibitors and beyond. *J Steroid Biochem Mol Biol* **106**, 16–23.

142. Subbaramaiah, K., Hudis, C., Chang, S.H., Hla, T., and Dannenberg, A.J. (2008) EP2 and EP4 receptors regulate aromatase expression in human adipocytes and breast cancer cells. Evidence of a BRCA1 and p300 exchange. *J Biol Chem* **283**, 3433–44.

143. Diaz-Cruz, E.S., and Brueggemeier, R.W. (2006) Interrelationships between cyclooxygenases and aromatase: Unraveling the relevance of cyclooxygenase inhibitors in breast cancer. *Anticancer Agents Med Chem* **6**, 221–32.

144. Bernard-Gallon, D.J., Vissac-Sabatier, C., Antoine-Vincent, D., Rio, P.G., Maurizis, J.C., Fustier, P., and Bignon, Y.J. (2002) Differential effects of n-3 and n-6 polyunsaturated fatty acids on BRCA1 and BRCA2 gene expression in breast cell lines. *Br J Nutr* **87**, 281–89.

145. Lu, M., Chen, D., Lin, Z., Reierstad, S., Trauernicht, A.M., Boyer, T.G., and Bulun, S.E. (2006) BRCA1 negatively regulates the cancer-associated aromatase promoters I.3 and II in breast adipose fibroblasts and malignant epithelial cells. *J Clin Endocrinol Metab* **91**, 4514–19.

146. Dickson, R.B., and Lippman, M.E. (1987) Estrogenic regulation of growth and polypeptide growth factor secretion in human breast carcinoma. *Endo Rev* **8**, 29–39.

147. van den Brandt, P.A., Spiegelman, D., Yaun, S.S., Adami, H.O., Beeson, L., Folsom, A.R., Fraser, G., Goldbohm, R.A., Graham, S., Kushi, L., Marshall, J.R., Miller, A.B., Rohan, T., Smith-Warner, S.A., Speizer, F.E., Willett, W.C., Wolk, A., and Hunter, D.J. (2000) Pooled analysis of prospective cohort studies on height, weight, and breast cancer risk. *Am J Epidemiol* **152**, 514–27.

148. Bachman, A.N., Curtin, G.M., Doolittle, D.J., and Goodman, J.I. (2006) Altered methylation in gene-specific and GC-rich regions of DNA is progressive and nonrandom during promotion of skin tumorigenesis. *Toxicol Sci* **91**, 406–18.

149. Poehlman, E.T., Toth, M.J., and Gardner, A.W. (1995) Changes in energy balance and body composition at menopause: A controlled longitudinal study. *Ann Intern Med* **123**, 673–75.

150. Wake, D.J., Strand, M., Rask, E., Westerbacka, J., Livingstone, D.E., Soderberg, S., Andrew, R., Yki-Jarvinen, H., Olsson, T., and Walker, B.R. (2007) Intra-adipose sex steroid metabolism and body fat distribution in idiopathic human obesity. *Clin Endocrinol (Oxf)* **66**, 440–46.

151. Vona-Davis, L., Howard-McNatt, M., and Rose, D.P. (2007) Adiposity, type 2 diabetes and the metabolic syndrome in breast cancer. *Obes Rev* **8**, 395–408.

152. Weiss, R. (2007) Fat distribution and storage: How much, where, and how?. *Eur J Endocrinol* **157**(Suppl 1), S39–S45.

153. Garmendia, M.L., Pereira, A., Alvarado, M.E., and Atalah, E. (2007) Relation between insulin resistance and breast cancer among Chilean women. *Ann Epidemiol* **17**, 403–09.

154. Sabin, M.A., Crowne, E.C., Stewart, C.E., Hunt, L.P., Turner, S.J., Welsh, G.I., Grohmann, M.J., Holly, J.M., and Shield, J.P. (2007) Depot-specific effects of fatty acids on lipid accumulation in children's adipocytes. *Biochem Biophys Res Commun* **361**, 356–61.

155. Garaulet, M., Perez-Llamas, F., Perez-Ayala, M., Martinez, P., de Medina, F.S., Tebar, F.J., and Zamora, S. (2001) Site-specific differences in the fatty acid composition of abdominal adipose tissue in an obese population from a Mediterranean area: Relation with dietary fatty acids, plasma lipid profile, serum insulin, and central obesity. *Am J Clin Nutr* **74**, 585–91.

156. Garaulet, M., Hernandez-Morante, J.J., Lujan, J., Tebar, F.J., and Zamora, S. (2006) Relationship between fat cell size and number and fatty acid composition in adipose tissue from different fat depots in overweight/obese humans. *Int J Obes (Lond)* **30**, 899–905.

157. Clore, J.N., Harris, P.A., Li, J., Azzam, A., Gill, R., Zuelzer, W., Rizzo, W.B., and Blackard, W.G. (2000) Changes in phosphatidylcholine fatty acid composition are associated with altered skeletal muscle insulin responsiveness in normal man. *Metabolism* **49**, 232–38.

158. Borkman, M., Storlien, L.H., Pan, D.A., Jenkins, A.B., Chisholm, D.J., and Campbell, L.V. (1993) The relation between insulin sensitivity and the fatty-acid composition of skeletal-muscle phospholipids. *N Engl J Med* **328**, 238–44.

159. Tang, W.Y., and Ho, S.M. (2007) Epigenetic reprogramming and imprinting in origins of disease. *Rev Endocr Metab Disord* **8**, 173–82.

160. Hilakivi-Clarke, L. (2007) Nutritional modulation of terminal end buds: Its relevance to breast cancer prevention. *Curr Cancer Drug Targets* **7**, 465–74.

161. Gerhard, I., Vollmar, B., Runnebaum, B., Klinga, K., Haller, U., and Kubli, F. (1987) Weight percentile at birth: II prediction by endocrinological and sonographic measurements. *Eur J Obstet Gynecol Reprod Biol* **26**, 313–28.

162. Catalano, P.M., and Kirwan, J.P. (2001) Maternal factors that determine neonatal size and body fat. *Curr Diab Rep* **1**, 71–77.

163. Domali, E., and Messinis, I.E. (2002) Leptin in pregnancy. *J Matern Fetal Neonatal Med* **12**, 222–30.

164. Delvaux, T., Buekens, P., Thoumsin, H., Dramaix, M., and Collette, J. (2003) Cord C-peptide and insulin-like growth factor-I, birth weight, and placenta weight among North African and Belgian neonates. *Am J Obstet Gynecol* **189**, 1779–84.

165. Vatten, L.J., Nilsen, S.T., Odegard, R.A., Romundstad, P.R., and Austgulen, R. (2002) Insulin-like growth factor I and leptin in umbilical cord plasma and infant birth size at term. *Pediatrics* **109**, 1131–35.

166. de Assis, S., Galam, K., and Hilakivi-Clarke, L. (2006) High birth weight increases mammary tumorigenesis in rats. *Int J Cancer* **119**, 1537–46.

167. Kerdelhue, B., and Jolette, J. (2002) The influence of the route of administration of 17beta-estradiol, intravenous (pulsed) versus oral, upon DMBA-induced mammary tumour development in ovariectomised rats. *Breast Cancer Res Treat* **73**, 13–22.

168. Russo, J., and Russo, I.H. (1987) Biological and molecular bases of mammary carcinogenesis. *Lab Invest* **57**, 112–37.

169. Liu, B.Y., McDermott, S.P., Khwaja, S.S., and Alexander, C.M. (2004) The transforming activity of Wnt effectors correlates with their ability to induce the accumulation of mammary progenitor cells. *Proc Natl Acad Sci U S A* **101**, 4158–63.

170. Dontu, G., Jackson, K.W., McNicholas, E., Kawamura, M.J., Abdallah, W.M., and Wicha, M.S. (2004) Role of Notch signaling in cell-fate determination of human mammary stem/progenitor cells. *Breast Cancer Res* **6**, R605–R15.

171. Farnie, G., and Clarke, R.B. (2007) Mammary stem cells and breast cancer—role of Notch signalling. *Stem Cell Rev* **3**, 169–75.

172. Wang, X.Y., Yin, Y., Yuan, H., Sakamaki, T., Okano, H., and Glazer, R.I. (2008) Musashi1 modulates mammary progenitor cell expansion through proliferin-mediated activation of the Wnt and Notch pathways. *Mol Cell Biol* **28**, 3589–99.

173. Liu, S., Ginestier, C., Charafe-Jauffret, E., Foco, H., Kleer, C.G., Merajver, S.D., Dontu, G., and Wicha, M.S. (2008) BRCA1 regulates human mammary stem/progenitor cell fate. *Proc Natl Acad Sci U S A* **105**, 1680–85.

174. Grubbs, C.J., Farneli, D.R., Hill, D.L., and McDonough, K.C. (1985) Chemoprevention of n-nitro-n-methylurea-induced mammary cancers by pretreatment with 17beta-estradiol and progesterone. *J Natl Cancer Inst* **74**, 927–31.

175. Cabanes, A., Wang, M., Olivo, S., de Assis, S., Gustafsson, J.A., Khan, G., and Hilakivi-Clarke, L. (2004) Prepubertal estradiol and genistein exposures up-regulate BRCA1 mRNA and reduce mammary tumorigenesis. *Carcinogenesis* **25**, 741–48.

176. MacMahon, B., Cole, P., Lin, T.M., Lowe, C.R., Mirra, A.P., Ravnihar, B., Salber, E.J., Valaoras, V.G., and Yuasa, S. (1970) Age at first birth and breast cancer. *Bull World Health Organ* **43**, 209–21.

177. Enger, S.M., Ross, R.K., Henderson, B., and Bernstein, L. (1997) Breastfeeding history, pregnancy experience and risk of breast cancer. *Br J Cancer* **76**, 118–23.

178. Wohlfahrt, J., and Melbye, M. (1999) Maternal risk of breast cancer and birth characteristics of offspring by time since birth. *Edidemiology* **10**, 441–44.

179. Colton, T., Greenberg, R., Noller, K., Resseguie, L., Bennekom, C.V., Heeren, T., and Zhang, Y. (1993) Breast cancer in mothers prescribed diethylstilbestrol in pregnancy. *JAMA* **269**, 2096–100.

180. Peck, J.D., Hulka, B.S., Poole, C., Savitz, D.A., Baird, D., and Richardson, B.E. (2002) Steroid hormone levels during pregnancy and incidence of maternal breast cancer. *Cancer Epidemiol Biomarkers Prev* **11**, 361–68.

181. Allen, S.H., Bennett, J.A., Mizejewski, G.J., Andersen, T.T., Ferraris, S., and Jacobson, H.I. (1993) Purification of alpha-fetoprotein from human corad serum with demonstration of its antiestrogenic activity. *Biochim Biophys Acta* **1202**, 135–42.

182. Vakharia, D., and Mizejewski, G.J. (2000) Human alpha-fetoprotein peptides bind estrogen receptor and estradiol, and suppress breast cancer. *Breast Cancer Res Treat* **63**, 41–52.

183. Melbye, M., Wohlfahrt, J., Lei, U., Norgaard-Pedersen, B., Mouridsen, H.T., Lambe, M., and Michels, K.B. (2000) Alpha-fetoprotein levels in maternal serum during pregnancy and maternal breast cancer incidence. *J Natl Cancer Inst* **92**, 1001–05.

184. Richardson, B.E., Hulka, B.S., Peck, J.L., Hughes, C.L., van den Berg, B.L., Christianson, R.E., and Calvin, J.A. (1998) Levels of maternal serum alpha-fetoprotein (AFP) in pregnant women and subsequent breast cancer risk. *Am J Epidemiol* **148**, 719–27.

185. Russo, J., Balogh, G.A., Heulings, R., Mailo, D.A., Moral, R., Russo, P.A., Sheriff, F., Vanegas, J., and Russo, I.H. (2006) Molecular basis of pregnancy-induced breast cancer protection. *Eur J Cancer Prev* **15**, 306–42.

186. Thordarson, G., Jin, E., Guzman, R.C., Swanson, S.M., Nandi, S., and Talamantes, F. (1995) Refractoriness to mammary tumorigenesis in parous rats: Is it caused by persistent changes in the hormonal environment or permanent biochemical alterations in the mammary epithelia?. *Carcinogenesis* **16**, 2847–53.

187. Yang, J., Yoshizawa, K., Nandi, S., and Tsubura, A. (1999) Protective effects of pregnancy and lactation against N-methyl-N-nitrosourea-induced mammary carcinomas in female Lewis rats. *Carcinogenesis* **20**, 623–28.

188. D'Cruz, C.M., Moody, S.E., Master, S.R., Hartman, J.L., Keiper, E.A., Imielinski, M.B., Cox, J.D., Wang, J.Y., Ha, S.I., Keister, B.A., and Chodosh, L.A. (2002) Persistent parity-induced changes in growth factors, TGF-beta3, and differentiation in the rodent mammary gland. *Mol Endocrinol* **16**, 2034–51.

189. Rajkumar, L., Guzman, R.C., Yang, J., Thordarson, G., Talamantes, F., and Nandi, S. (2001) Short-term exposure to pregnancy levels of estrogen prevents mammary carcinogenesis. *Proc Natl Acad Sci USA* **98**, 11755–59.

190. Li, Z., and Li, L. (2006) Understanding hematopoietic stem-cell microenvironments. *Trends Biochem Sci* **31**, 589–95.

191. Catalano, S., Marsico, S., Giordano, C., Mauro, L., Rizza, P., Panno, M.L., and Ando, S. (2003) Leptin enhances, via AP-1, expression of aromatase in the MCF-7 cell line. *J Biol Chem* **278**, 28668–76.

192. Catalano, S., Mauro, L., Marsico, S., Giordano, C., Rizza, P., Rago, V., Montanaro, D., Maggiolini, M., Panno, M.L., and Ando, S. (2004) Leptin induces, via ERK1/ERK2 signal, functional activation of estrogen receptor alpha in MCF-7 cells. *J Biol Chem* **279**, 19908–15.

193. Garofalo, C., Sisci, D., and Surmacz, E. (2004) Leptin interferes with the effects of the antiestrogen ICI 182,780 in MCF-7 breast cancer cells. *Clin Cancer Res* **10**, 6466–75.

194. Sivaraman, L., Stephens, L.C., Markaverich, B.M., Clark, J.A., Krnacik, S., Conneely, O.M., O'Malley, B.W., and Medina, D. (1998) Hormone-induced refractoriness to mammary carcinogenesis in Wistar-Furth rats. *Carcinogenesis* **19**, 1573–81.

195. Wagner, K.U., and Smith, G.H. (2005) Pregnancy and stem cell behavior. *J Mammary Gland Biol Neoplasia* **10**, 25–36.

196. Coffey, R.J., Derynck, R., Wilcox, J.N., Bringman, T.S., Goustin, A.S., Moses, H.L., and Pittelkow, M.R. (1987) Production and autoinduction of transforming growth factor α in human keratinocytes. *Nature* **328**, 817–20.

197. Rose, D.P., and Connolly, J.M. (1993) Effects of dietary omega-3 fatty acids on human breast cancer growth and metastases in nude mice. *J Natl Cancer Inst* **85**, 1743–47.

198. Brunner, E., Stallone, D., Juneja, M., Bingham, S., and Marmot, M. (2001) Dietary assessment in Whitehall II: Comparison of 7 d diet diary and food-frequency questionnaire and validity against biomarkers. *Br J Nutr* **86**, 405–14.

199. Day, N.E., Wong, M.Y., Bingham, S., Khaw, K.T., Luben, R., Michels, K.B., Welch, A., and Wareham, N.J. (2004) Correlated measurement error—implications for nutritional epidemiology. *Int J Epidemiol* **33**, 1373–81.
200. Holmes, M.D., Hunter, D.J., Colditz, G.A., Stampfer, M.J., Hankinson, S.E., Speizer, F.E., Rosner, B., and Willett, W.C. (1999) Association of dietary intake of fat and fatty acids with risk of breast cancer. *JAMA* **281**, 914–20.
201. Mannisto, S., Pietinen, P., Virtanen, M., Kataja, V., and Uusitupa, M. (1999) Diet and the risk of breast cancer in a case-control study: Does the threat of disease have an influence on recall bias?. *J Clin Epidemiol* **52**, 429–39.

III ROLE OF DIETARY BIOACTIVE COMPONENTS IN CANCER PREVENTION AND/OR TREATMENT: CAROTENOIDS, VITAMINS AND MINERALS

15 Carotenoids

Brian L. Lindshield and John W. Erdman

Key Points

1. Carotenoids are 40 carbon pigmented compounds, of which approximately 600 have been identified throughout nature. The six main carotenoids found in diet, blood, and tissue are lycopene, β-carotene, α-carotene, β-cryptoxanthin, lutein, and zeaxanthin.
2. The production of retinoids, which promote cell differentiation and inhibit cell proliferation, could be one mechanism for the anticancer activity of carotenoids. However, carotenoids' multiple conjugated double bonds also make them excellent scavengers of free radicals and thus antioxidants.
3. Epidemiological studies consistently support an inverse relationship between fruit and vegetable consumption and cancer risk. Blood β-carotene concentration has been used as a biomarker of fruit and vegetable intake because β-carotene is plentiful in most fruits and vegetables.
4. Epidemiological studies examine the relationship between tomato/lycopene consumption, serum lycopene levels, and prostate cancer. The prostate is an androgen-responsive tissue, thus the androgens, testosterone, and dihydrotestosterone stimulate proliferation and development of most prostate tumors. Androgens appear to alter lycopene metabolism and, in turn, lycopene may alter androgen metabolism by decreasing the expression of androgen-producing enzymes.
5. To reduce the risk of prostate cancer, it is recommended that men consume at least two servings of tomatoes a week. For β-carotene, it is important to eat the recommended daily servings of fruits and vegetables, especially those high in β-carotene.

Key Words: Carotenoids; cancer prevention; antioxidants; prostate cancer; fruits and vegetables

1. INTRODUCTION

1.1. Rationale for the Use of Carotenoids in Cancer Prevention and/or Treatment

Carotenoids are 40 carbon pigmented compounds, of which approximately 600 have been identified throughout nature. The six main carotenoids found in diet, blood, and tissue are lycopene, β-carotene, α-carotene, β-cryptoxanthin, lutein, and zeaxanthin (see Table 1 and Fig. 1) *(1)*. β-carotene, α-carotene, and β-cryptoxanthin are provitamin A carotenoids, meaning that they can be cleaved to form vitamin A. The production of retinoids, which promote cell differentiation and inhibit cell proliferation, could be one

From: *Nutrition and Health: Bioactive Compounds and Cancer*
Edited by: J.A. Milner, D.F. Romagnolo, DOI 10.1007/978-1-60761-627-6_15,
© Springer Science+Business Media, LLC 2010

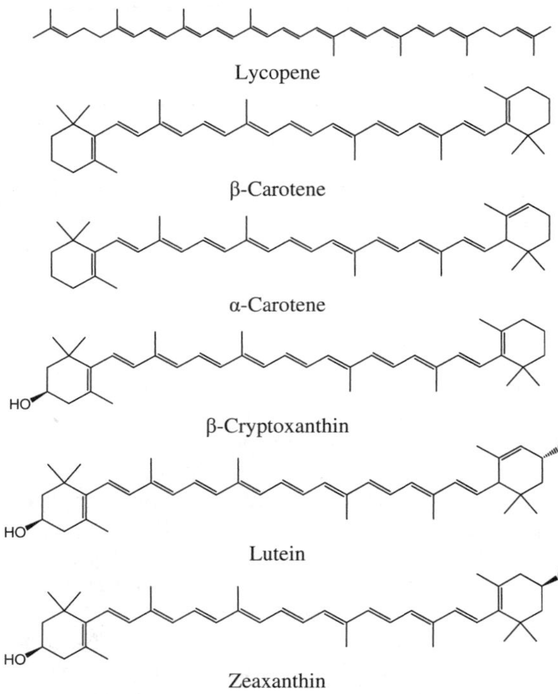

Fig. 1. Structures of the six main cartenoids.

Table 1
The Six Primary Carotenoids, Their Color, and Good Dietary Sources

Carotenoid	Color	Good food sources
Lycopene	Red	Tomatoes, watermelon, guava, pink grapefruit
β-Carotene	Yellow-orange	Carrots, sweet potatoes, pumpkin, spinach, apricots
α-Carotene	Light yellow	Carrots, pumpkin
β-Cryptoxanthin	Orange	Sweet red peppers, tangerines, papaya, persimmons
Lutein	Yellow	Kale, spinach, corn, collard greens, broccoli, eggs
Zeaxanthin	Yellow	

mechanism for the anticancer activity of carotenoids. However, carotenoids' multiple conjugated double bonds also make them excellent scavengers of free radicals and thus antioxidants. Most research on carotenoids and cancer has been focused on lycopene and prostate cancer and β-carotene and lung cancer. Because of space limitation and wealth of data available on carotenoids, in this chapter we will focus on the review of data documenting the potential benefits of lycopene and β-carotene against these forms of cancer.

An epidemiological review by Peto et al. first raised the possibility that β-carotene supplementation could markedly decrease cancer incidence (2). In 1995, a landmark epidemiological study was published related to lycopene and tomatoes. In the Health

Professional Follow-up Study, a prospective cohort study in the USA, lycopene intake as well as the consumption of raw tomatoes, tomato sauce, and pizza were all significantly associated with a decreased risk of prostate cancer (3). Thus, epidemiological evidence spurred further research on lycopene and β-carotene and these sites of cancer. There was an enthusiastic and rapid transition from epidemiological studies investigating β-carotene and lung cancer to intervention studies. However, the research approach investigating the potential of lycopene/tomatoes to decrease prostate cancer has progressed at a more cautious and safer pace based on lessons learned from prior research on β-carotene and lung cancer.

2. IN VITRO STUDIES AND ANIMAL EXPERIMENTS

2.1. β-Carotene

To the best of our knowledge, results of the first lung cancer animal model (4–6) and in vitro (7) studies were published in 1991–1992. These investigations suggest that as the intake of β-carotene shifts from dietary to high pharmacological levels, the effect on lung cancer development also shifts from beneficial to detrimental in combination with smoke or carcinogen exposure (8–15).

2.2. Lycopene/Tomato Extracts

A number of investigators examined the effects of lycopene or tomato extract treatment on prostate cancer cells in vitro (Table 2). In general, the results suggest that lycopene is taken up by prostate cells in culture and decreases their proliferation. It is important to note that many studies use supraphysiological lycopene concentrations. It is difficult to exceed 2 μM lycopene concentrations in human serum even when supplementing the diet with tomato products (16). Therefore, in vitro results obtained using lycopene treatment concentrations exceeding ~2 μM need to be interpreted with caution. In addition, another factor that should be considered is that lycopene rapidly degrades in vitro. For example, 4 h after lycopene treatment in tetrahydrofuran (THF) vehicle, only approximately 20% of the original lycopene concentration remained in media with very little cell absorption (17, 18). The rapid degradation of lycopene observed in cell culture is a problem because most cell culture studies are 2–3 days in duration. Some evidence suggests that lycopene's metabolites/oxidation products may be bioactive (19); thus, it is difficult to discern using cell culture models whether the decrease in proliferation is due to lycopene itself or its metabolic products.

In addition to in vitro studies, there have been a number of investigations that examined the potential for lycopene to prevent the development of chemically induced prostate cancer (20, 21) or decrease the growth of prostate tumors in animal models (22–25) (Table 3). Overall, lycopene alone has produced modest beneficial effects in animal prostate cancer models. One critical issue to note is that rats and mice are poor carotenoid absorbers and metabolize carotenoids quite differently than humans. Therefore, pharmacological carotenoid levels are provided to achieve similar tissue concentrations to those found in humans (26).

Table 2
Lycopene/Tomato Extracts and In Vitro Prostate Cell Outcomes

Cell line (references)	Treatment	Vehicle	Outcomes
PC-3 and PC-3MM2 (108)	Lyc	Chloroform	1 µM ↓ proliferation in PC-3, but not PC-3MM2
LNCaP (109)	Lyc	THF	(0.3–3.0 µM) NE on proliferation or necrosis, altered mitochondrial function, and induced apoptosis
LNCaP (110)	Lyc Beadlets	DMSO	(0.1, 1, and 5 µM) ↓ proliferation; 5 µM ↓cell cycle progression and induced apoptosis
LNCaP (111)	Lyc Beadlets	DMSO	(0.1–50 µM) ↓ proliferation; NE – DNA damage marker (8-OHdG) at ≤1 µM; ↑ 8-OHdG at ≥5 µM; ↓ antioxidant marker (MDA) at ≤1 µM; ↑ MDA ≥5 µM
LNCaP (112)	Tomato paste extracts	DMSO	5 µM ↓ proliferation and cell cycle progression; ↑ apoptosis
LNCaP (113)	LycoRed[a]	Proprietary vehicle	1 and 10 µM ↓ proliferation; significant dose response (1–100 nM)
PC-3, DU 145, LNCaP (114)	Lyc	THF	5, 10, 20 µM all significantly ↓ proliferation in PC-3 and DU-145, but not LNCaP
Normal human prostate epithelial cells (115)	Lyc	THF	0.1, 0.5 µM NE; 1, 2, and 5 µM significantly ↓ proliferation; 5 µM altered cell cycle; 5, but not 0.5 µM, ↓ cell cycle protein (cyclin D1)
PC-3, DU 145, LNCaP (25)	Lyc	THF	10–50 µM; 20–50 µM ↓ cell proliferation in PC-3 and DU 145; NE on LNCaP; 32 µM altered cell cycle
LNCaP (17)	Lyc	Micelles	Lyc stabile in micelles
DU 145 (116)	Lyc	Acetone	NE on proliferation up to 10 µM of Lyc
Dunning AT3 and DTE (117)	Lyc	α-Cyclodextrin water-soluble carrier	0.2, 2.0, and 10 µM ↓ AT3 proliferation, NE on DTE cells

	LycopenTMa LycoTrueTMb		
PC-3 and LNCaP (118)	LycopenTMa LycoTrueTMb	FBS THF	1 and 10 µM LycopenTM ↓ LNCaP proliferation; LycoTrueTM (nM) alters cell cycle, ↓ proliferation (BrdU incorporation) in both cell lines, ↑apoptosis in LNCaP only
PC-3 (119)	Lyc	THF	20, 40, 60 µM significantly ↓ proliferation, alter IGF-1 axis
LNCaP, primary prostate epithelial cell cultures (97)	Lyc	THF	1–20 µM dose-dependent ↓ in proliferation (BrdU incorporation) and apoptosis (FITC-stained nuclei to PI-stained nuclei) in both cell lines
LNCaP (120)	Lyc	THF	0.075, 0.75, 7.45 µM ↓ proliferation in both cell lines, less effect on C4-2 cells, NE on PSA mRNA or protein levels
PC-3, DU 145, LNCaP (121)	Lyc Beadlets	Media	Lycopene-accumulated LNCaP>PC-3 >DU-145; Lyc did not bind to AR
PC3AR (122)	Lyc	Rat serum	Unknown concentration; NE on cell numbers, gap junction communication protein (Cx43) RNA or protein levels
PC-3 and DU 145 (18)	Lyc	FBS, THF, micelles	FBS was a better delivery route than THF or micelles
DU-145 and PC-3 (123)	Lyc	THF	1 µM when combined with 50 µM α-tocopherol synergistically ↓ proliferation
LNCaP (124)	Lyc	Unknown	1 and 10 µM; only 10 µM significantly ↓ cell numbers

Abbreviations: 8-OHdG, 8-hydroxydeoxyguanosine; AR, androgen receptor; BrdU, bromodeoxyuridine; Cx43, connexin 43; DMSO, dimethylsulfoxide; FBS, fetal bovine serum; FITC, fluorescein isothiocyanate; Lyc, lycopene; MDA, malondialdehyde; NE, no effect; PI, propidium iodide; PSA, prostate-specific antigen; THF, tetrahydrofuran.

[a]LycoRed and LycopenTM are produced by LycoRed Ltd. (Beer Sheva, Israel).

[b]LycoTrueTM is produced by Waters Solutions (Caldwell, ID).

Table 3
Lycopene in Prostate Cancer Animal Models

Model	Amount (mg/kg)	Admin	Groups	Duration	Outcomes
DMBA-induced (20)	15(LycoRed[a])	Diet	During DMBA administration / After DMBA administration	20 wk / 40 wk	After ↓ PIN incidence; both during and after ↓ PCNA levels
DMBA-induced (20)	5, 15, 45 (LycoRed[a])	Diet	After DMBA administration	40 wk	NE – PCa stage, BrdU labeling
PhIP-induced (20)	45	Diet	After PhIP administration	50 wk	NE – PCa stage
NMU-induced (21)	250 10% ToP	Diet	Given when NMU started	60 wk	Lyc NS ↓, ToP ↓ PCa death
Dunning R3327-H (23)	25 or 250	Diet	25, 250 Lyc, 10% ToP, preferred 4 wk before implant	17–18 wk after implant	Both Lyc doses and ToP ↓ tumor areas; ToP ↓, Lyc NS ↓ tumor wts
Dunning MatLyLu (24)	200	Diet	Lyc / Lyc + Vit. E / Preferred 4 wk before implant	46 d after implant	Lyc NS ↑ tumor necrosis, NE on tumor wts / Lyc + Vit. E ↑ necrosis, NE tumor wts
Du145 xenograph (25)	10, 100, 300 BW	Gavage	0, 10, 100, 300	8 wk	100, 300 ↓ tumor volume and wts
PC-346C orthotopic (22)	5, 50 BW	Gavage	5, 50 Lyc alone and 5 Lyc + low Vit. E	95 d	Both Lyc doses NE on tumor volume, PSA, or survival; Lyc + Vit. E ↓ tumor volume, PSA, and ↑ survival

Abbreviations: Admin, Administration method; BrdU, bromodeoxyuridine; BW, body weight; d, days; DMBA, 7,12-dimethylbenz[a]anthracene; implant, implantation; NE, no effect; NS, not significant; NMU, N-methyl-N-nitrosourea; NS, nonsignificant; PCa, prostate cancer; PCNA, proliferating cell nuclear antigen; PhIP, 2-amino-1-methyl-6-phenylimidazol[4,5-b]pyridine; ToP, tomato powder; Vit. E, vitamin E; wk, weeks; wts, weights.
[a]LycoRed is produced by LycoRed Ltd. (Beer Sheva, Israel).

3. EPIDEMIOLOGICAL STUDIES

3.1. β-Carotene

Epidemiological studies consistently support an inverse relationship between fruit and vegetable consumption (many are rich sources of β-carotene) and cancer risk *(27)*. Blood β-carotene concentration has been used as a biomarker of fruit and vegetable intake, because β-carotene is plentiful in most fruits and vegetables. Zeigler et al. argued that blood β-carotene concentration was the best available biomarker of fruit and vegetable intake. However, β-carotene itself may not be responsible for decreased lung cancer risk with increased fruit and vegetable intake *(28)*. A meta-analysis found that high vs. low dietary β-carotene intake (relative risk (RR) = 0.92 (0.83–1.02)) and serum β-carotene concentrations (RR = 0.84 (0.66–1.07)) were not associated with significant decreases in lung cancer risk *(29)*.

3.2. Tomatoes/Lycopene

Epidemiological studies examining the relationship between tomato/lycopene consumption, serum lycopene levels, and prostate cancer were identified using PubMed and references in prior reviews *(30, 31)*, publications *(32, 33)*, and a meta-analysis *(34)*. We identified 19 case–control studies that examined the relationship between lycopene/tomato intake and prostate cancer risk (Table 4). One study found a nonsignificant decrease *(35)*, seven studies *(36–42)* were neutral, five studies *(43–47)* found a nonsignificant increase, and seven studies *(48–56)* reported a significant decrease in prostate cancer risk with increased lycopene/tomato intake. We also identified six cohort studies that examined the relationship between lycopene/tomato intake and prostate cancer *(3, 57–61)*, with one study also producing a follow-up publication *(62)* (Table 5). Out of the six studies, two were neutral *(57, 60)*, four studies *(3, 58, 59, 61)* and the follow-up publication *(62)* reported a significant decrease in prostate cancer risk with increased lycopene/tomato intake. We identified 14 studies that examined the relationship between serum lycopene concentrations and prostate cancer risk (Table 6). One study found a nonsignificant increase *(32)*, three studies were neutral *(33, 63, 64)*, seven studies reported a nonsignificant decrease *(65–71)*, and three studies found a significant decrease *(72–74)*. When viewed as a whole, the majority of the studies suggest a moderate decrease in prostate cancer risk with increased dietary tomato/lycopene consumption and/or serum levels.

4. INTERVENTION STUDIES

4.1. β-Carotene

In the mid-1980s two large, randomized, placebo-controlled trials began recruiting subjects to determine whether β-carotene supplementation would decrease lung cancer incidence in high-risk populations. In the Alpha-Tocopherol Beta-Carotene Cancer Prevention Trial (ATBC), Finnish male smokers received daily supplements of placebo, 50 mg of *dl*-α-tocopheryl acetate, 20 mg of β-carotene, or both antioxidants *(75)*. In the

Table 4
Lycopene/Tomato Consumption Case–Control Studies

Location (references)	Cases	Relative risk	Exposure servings/wk or mg/day (Lyc)	Adjusted factors
Canada (35)	215	L – 1.73 (0.92–3.26) P(trend) = 0.21	4th vs. 1st quartile	Age, education, family history, group, and calories
Hawaii (37)	452	T – 0.9 <70 yrs P(trend) = 0.35 T – 1.1 ≥70 yrs P(trend) = 0.57	4th vs. 1st quartile	Age, ethnicity
Great Britain (38)	328	RT – 1.06 (0.55–1.62) P(trend) = 0.88 CT – 0.92 (0.59–1.42) P(trend) = 0.64 L – 0.99 (0.68–1.45) P(trend) = 0.88	≥5 vs. ≤1 ≥2 vs. <1 ≥0.7 vs. <0.4	Age, calories, social class
Canada (39)	1,623	T – 1.0 (0.7–1.3) P(trend) = 0.29	≥7 vs. <1	Age, location, race, smoking, BMI, diet, income, family history
Uruguay (40)	175	L – 1.2 (0.7–2.2) P(trend) = 0.90	>3.3 vs. ≤1.3	Age, residence, urban/rural status, education, family history, BMI
Washington (36)	628	RT – 1.22 (0.83–1.80) P(trend) = 0.26 CT – 0.90 (0.57–1.42) P(trend) = 0.68 L – 0.89 (0.60–1.31) P(trend) = 0.96	≥3 vs. ≤1 ≥3 vs. <1 ≥9.9 vs. <4.9	Age, race, dietary fat, energy, family history, BMI, PSA, education
Italy (41)	1,294	L – 0.94 (0.72–1.23)	7.5 Median	Age, study site, education, physical activity, BMI, family history, calories
US and Canada (42)	1,619	T – 1.08 (0.75–1.56) P(trend) = 0.85	>5 vs. <1[a]	Age, education, ethnicity, geographic area, calories
Minnesota (43)	223	T – 0.71 NS	≥3.5 vs. <0.8	Age
USA (44)	932	RT – 0.8 P(trend) = 0.16 CT – 1.3 P(trend) = 0.71 L (combined sources) = 0.9 P(trend) = 0.07	≥5 vs. 0 ≥5 vs. 0 ≥5 vs. 0	Age, study site, calories, race

Location	N	Result (OR/RR, 95% CI, P)	Comparison	Adjusted for
New Zealand (45)	317	RT – 1.01 (0.66–1.53) P(trend) = 0.93	≥1.7 vs. ≤0.6[a]	Age, height, NSAIDs, socioeconomic status
		T – 0.82 (0.53–1.26) P(trend) = 0.30	≥3 vs. <1[a]	
		L – 0.76 (0.5–1.17) P(trend) = 0.30	>2.0 vs. <0.7	
Japan (46)	140	T – 0.86 (0.37–2.01) P(trend) = 0.87	≥4.7 vs. ≤ 1.3[a]	Age, smoking, calories
South Carolina (47)	416	L – 0.71 (0.46–1.08) P(trend) = 0.32	≥8.1 vs. ≤2.6[b]	Age, geographic region, family history
Canada (48)	617	T – 0.64 (0.45–0.91) P = 0.04	≥5 vs. ≤1[a]	Age, calories, vasectomy, smoking, marital status, study location, BMI, education, multivitamin use, grains, fruit, vegetables, plants, carotenoids, folic acid, fiber, conjugated linoleic acid, vitamin E, vitamin C, total fat, linoleic acid
		L – 1.01 (0.76–1.35)	>12.7 vs. <2.1	
Greece (49, 50)	320	RT – 0.65 P(trend) = 0.14	>7.5 vs. <5	Age, height, BMI, education, calories
		CT – 0.52 P(trend) = 0.005	≥7 vs. <3.3	
Australia (51)	858	T – 0.8 (0.6–1.0) P(trend) = 0.03	≥6.5 vs. <3.5	State, age group, year, country of birth, socioeconomic status, family history, calories
		L – 0.8 (0.6–1.2) P(trend) = 0.30	≥11.1 vs. <4.1	
China (52, 53)	130	T – 0.16 (0.07–0.38) P(trend) = 0.002	≥1.7 vs. ≤0.3	Age, location, education, family income, marital status, # of children, family history, BMI, tea consumption, calories, fat intake
		L – 0.18 (0.08–0.41) P(trend) = 0.009	>4.9 vs. <1.6	
New York (54)	433	L – 0.62 (0.42–0.92) P(trend) = 0.08	>8.9 vs. ≤3.9	Age, education, BMI, smoking, calories
North Carolina (55)	77	L – 0.49 (0.24–0.99) P(trend) = 0.05	>1.5 vs. <0.7	Age, calories
Iran (56)	130	T – 0.45 (0.09–2.12) P = 0.3	>4.7 vs. ≤0.5[a]	Occupation, ethnicity, marital status, family history, smoking, alcohol

Abbreviations: BMI, body mass index; L, lycopene; CT, cooked tomatoes; NS, not significant; RT, raw tomatoes; T, tomatoes.

[a]Intake data was converted to servings based on National Labeling Education Act tomato size of 148 g.

[b]Serving of lycopene per week.

Table 5
Lycopene/Tomato Consumption and Prostate Cancer Cohort Studies

Location	Cases	Relative risk	Exposure servings/wk or mg/d (Lyc)	Adjusted factors
California (58)	180	0.60 (0.37–0.97) P = 0.02	≥5 vs. <1	Age, education, meat, poultry, fish, legumes, fruit
USA (3)	773	T – 0.65 (0.44–0.95) P(trend) = 0.01 TS – 0.66 (0.49–0.90) P(trend) = 0.03 L – 0.79 (0.64–0.99) P(trend) = 0.04	>10 vs. <1.5 2–4 vs. 0 10.0 vs. 1.5	Age, calories, family history, vasectomy status, animal fat, retinol
Iowa (59)	101	L – 0.5 (0.3–0.9) P(trend) = 0.03	NG	Age, energy
USA (62)	2,481	TS – 0.77 (0.66–0.9) P(trend) <0.001 L – 0.84 (0.73–0.96) P(trend) = 0.003	≥ 2 vs. <0.25 18.8 vs. 3.4	Age, time period, family history, BMI at 21, calories, calcium, phosphorous, fructose, vitamin D, vitamin E, total fat, α-linolenic acid
The Netherlands (60)	642	L – 0.98 (0.71–1.34) P(trend) = 0.58	2.0 vs. 0.1	Age, family history, socioeconomic status, and alcohol from white or fortified wine
USA (57)	1,338	T – 0.99 (0.81–1.21) P(trend) = 0.36 L – 0.95 (0.79–1.13) P(trend) = 0.33	10.3 vs. 2.3 17.6 vs. 5.1	Age, energy, race, study center, family history, BMI, smoking, physical activity, vitamin E supplements, total fat intake, red meat intake, diabetes history, aspirin use, previous number of screening exams
Europe (61)	562	L – 0.65 (0.51–0.84) P(trend) = 0.001	4.0 vs. 0.6	Age, sex, calories, education, BMI, physical activity, smoking, alcohol consumption

Abbreviations: BMI, body mass index; L, lycopene; T, tomatoes; TS, tomato sauce.

Table 6
Serum Lycopene and Prostate Cancer Epidemiologic Studies

Location	Cases	Relative risk	Control median Lyc (μg/dl)	Cases median Lyc (μg/dl)	Adjusted factors
Maryland (66, 67)	103	0.5 (0.2–1.29) P(trend) = 0.26	32	30	Age, nationality, religion, marital status, alcohol status, blood pressure, serum cholesterol, BMI
Hawaii (63)	142	1.1 (0.5–2.2) P(trend) = 0.86	13.4	13.4	Age, education, smoking, time since last meal
USA (68)	578	0.75 (0.54–1.06) P(trend) = 0.12	38.8	36.9	Age, smoking, exercise, BMI, follow-up time, plasma cholesterol, alcohol, multivitamin use
Canada (72)	12	P = 0.004	23.3	13.1	Age, smoking, fruit, vegetables, beans
USA (69)	418	0.65 P(trend) = 0.09	Blacks 15.4 Whites 18.7	Blacks 14.5 Whites 16.9	Age, study center, month of blood draw
Arizona (73)	65	0.17 (0.04–0.78) P(trend) = 0.005	16.4[a]	12.0[a]	Age, race, education, alcohol, smoking, family history, calories
USA (70)	182	0.83 (0.46–1.48) P(trend) = 0.72	35.7	34.2	Age, race, date of blood donation, total lipid levels, hours since last meal, education, smoking

Maryland (70)	142	0.79 (0.41–1.54) P(trend) = 0.49	42.1	38.4	Age, race, date of blood donation, total lipid levels, hours since last meal, education, smoking, BMI
USA (71)	450	0.66 (0.38–1.13) P(trend) = 0.33	39.0	37.5	Age, cholesterol, selenium and vitamin E supplements, family history, BMI, height, vigorous exercise, vasectomy, smoking
USA (65)	205	1.04 (0.61–1.77) P(trend) = 0.83	30.9[b]	30.7[b]	Exposure population, randomization center, age, sex, smoking, year of randomization
Texas (32)	118	1.3 (0.63–2.71)	25.2	27.4	Age, smoking, height, BMI, family history
USA (64)	692	1.14 (0.82–1.58) P(trend) = 0.28	62.2	64.4	Age, time since initial screening, blood draw year, study center
Europe (33)	966	0.97 (0.70–1.34) P(trend) = 0.41	27.0[b]	27.1[b]	BMI, smoking, alcohol, exercise, marital status, education
Arkansas (74)	193	0.45 (0.24–0.85) P(trend) = 0.042	31.1	27.4	Age, race, BMI, education, smoking

Abbreviations: BMI, body mass index; Lyc, lycopene.
[a]Mean.
[b]Geometric mean.

Beta-Carotene and Retinol Efficacy Trial (CARET), American male and female smokers or asbestos-exposed workers received 30 mg of β-carotene and 25,000 IU of retinyl palmitate or placebo daily *(76)*. The research community was shocked when ATBC and CARET were terminated early in the mid-1990s because of significant increases in lung cancer incidence among those receiving β-carotene supplements *(75, 76)*.

It is important to note that 6 years after ATBC and CARET were terminated, follow-up found that β-carotene supplementation was no longer associated with a significant increase in lung cancer risk *(77, 78)*. In addition, no other β-carotene supplementation clinical trials (Physician's Health Study *(79)*, Women's Health Study *(80)*, Australian asbestos workers *(81)*, and Linxian China Study *(82)*) found a significant increase in lung cancer risk with β-carotene supplementation. A recent pooled-effects random meta-analysis of all of these β-carotene supplementation clinical trials found that β-carotene supplementation was associated with a nonsignificant increase in lung cancer risk (RR = 1.10 (0.89–1.36)) *(29)*. However, another meta-analysis that only considered ATBC, CARET, Physician's Health Study, and Women's Health Study found that in current smokers β-carotene supplementation was associated with a significant increase in lung cancer risk (RR = 1.24 (1.10–1.39)) *(83)*. The primary difference between these two meta-analyses is that the influence of the ATBC and CARET results is greater in the second meta-analysis that does not include as many studies.

4.2. Tomatoes/Lycopene

We identified 13 small clinical trials/intervention studies investigating the potential of lycopene or tomato consumption to decrease prostate cancer risk/progression (Table 7). These studies have mostly targeted men with prostate cancer scheduled for a prostatectomy, with benign prostatic hyperplasia, or at high risk of developing prostate cancer. Almost all of these men have reported an improved or stabilized PSA response (decreased concentration, reduced velocity, stabilization) as an outcome related to disease progression or prostate health. Prostate-specific antigen (PSA) is a protease that is believed to be important in aiding in sperm motility by thinning ejaculate *(84)* and has been used as a prostate cancer screening marker since 1987 *(85)*. Overall, 10 trials have reported improved or stabilized PSA response *(86–97)* with lycopene or tomato consumption, whereas a few studies found no benefit *(98–100)*. It is important that these trials be viewed in the context of their small size and general lack of an appropriate control group.

5. TISSUE SPECIFICITY AND TOTALITY OF THE EVIDENCE

5.1. β-Carotene

β-carotene consumption has not been reported to reduce the risk of a specific cancer site, thus no tissue specificity can be advocated for this bioactive compound. In 2007, the American Institute for Cancer Research (AICR) released its second expert report and judgments based on systemic reviews of the world's research literature *(101)*. The panel ranked the evidence (limited-suggestive, probable, convincing) that

Table 7
Lycopene Clinical Trials

Product (references)	Subjects (references)	Groups	Duration	Outcome(s)
Tomato sauce intervention (86, 87)	Men with localized PCa prior to prostatectomy	n = 32 30 mg/day Lyc	3 wk	↓ leukocyte and prostate 8-OHdG, ↓ PSA concentrations, ↑ prostate apoptotic index; NE – prostate Bcl-2, ↓ prostate bax vs. baseline
Lyc-O-Mato[a] (15 mg Lyc) 2X daily (88, 89)	Men with localized PCa prior to prostatectomy	Sup (n = 15) No Sup (n = 11)	3 wk	↑ tumors confined to prostate; NE – PSA, IGF-1, IGFBP-3, tumor connexin 43, bcl-2, bax, leukocyte 5-OHmdU levels vs. no Sup
Lyc (2 mg/day) 2× daily (90)	Men with metastatic PCa	Castration (n = 27) Lyc + Castration (n = 27)	2 yr	↓ PSA, improved PSA and bone scan response, urinary flow rate, survival vs. castration alone
LycoRed[a] (10 mg)/day (91)	Men with metastatic hormone-refractory PCa	Lycopene (n = 20)	3 mo	Some improvements in PSA and disease symptoms
Lyc-O-Mato[a] (4 mg Lyc)/day (92)	Men with HG-PIN	Control (n = 20) Lyc (n = 20)	1 yr	Improved PSA and disease progression vs. control
Lyc-O-Mato[a] (98)	Men with biochemically relapsed PCa	15, 30, 45, 60, 90, 120 mg Lyc/day	1 yr	NE – PSA response vs. baseline
Tomato paste (50 g)/day (93)	Men with BPH	n = 43	10 wk	↓ PSA vs. baseline

Product (references)	Subjects (references)	Groups	Duration	Outcome(s)
Lyc-O-Mato[a] (15 mg Lyc) 2× daily (99)	Men at high risk of PCa (HG-PIN or atypical foci) or more than 1 non-cancerous biopsy	Multivitamin (n = 40) Multivitamin + Lyc (n = 30)	4 mo	NE – PSA
Tomato paste or juice (100)	Men with androgen-independent PCa	n = 46 (15 mg Lyc) 2×/day	4 mo	NE – PSA or outcomes
Lyc-O-Mato[a] (94)	Men with PCa and rising PSA	n = 38 (15 mg Lyc) 2×/day	6 mo	NE – PSA response, but PSA stabilization did occur
Tomato products (95)	Men with recurrent, asymptomatic PCa	n = 40 (25 mg Lyc/day)	4 wk	Some evidence of ↓ PSA and serum VEGF; NE – serum IGF-I
Lyc (15 mg/day) (96)	Men with BPH	Placebo (n = 18) Lyc (n =19)	6 mo	↓ PSA, improved symptoms on International Prostate Symptom Score Questionnaire, prevented prostate enlargement that occurred in placebo; NE – IGF-I, IGFBP-3 vs. baseline
LycoPlus (10 mg/day) (97)	Men with PCa	n = 37	Ave. 10.4 mo	↓ PSA velocity; NE PSA doubling time

Abbreviations: 5-OHmdU, 5-hydroxymethyl-deoxyuridine; 8-OHdG, 8-hydroxydeoxyguanosine; BPH, benign prostatic hyperplasia; HG-PIN, high-grade prostatic intraepithelial neoplasia; IGF-I, insulin-like growth factor 1; IGFBP-3, insulin-like growth factor binding protein 3; Lyc, lycopene; mo, month; NE, no effect; PCa, prostate cancer; PSA, prostate-specific antigen; Sup, supplementation; VEGF, vascular epithelial growth factor; wk, week; yr, year.
[a]LycoRed and Lyc-O-Mato are produced by LycoRed Ltd. (Beer Sheva, Israel).

foods/micronutrients were associated with increased or decreased risk at multiple cancer sites. The panel labeled the evidence convincing "that β-carotene supplements cause lung cancer in current smokers *(101)*." β-carotene supplements were not identified as being detrimental to other sites of cancer. In addition, dietary β-carotene was not ranked as altering the risk of any cancer site *(101)*.

5.2. Lycopene/Tomatoes

The prostate is an androgen-responsive tissue, thus the androgens, testosterone, and dihydrotestosterone stimulate proliferation and development of most prostate tumors. Androgens appear to alter lycopene metabolism and, in turn, lycopene may alter androgen metabolism by decreasing the expression of androgen-producing enzymes *(24, 102)*. Castration of male rats leads to a two-fold increase in hepatic lycopene concentrations, an effect that is normalized by testosterone replacement *(103, 104)*. Furthermore, lycopene in vitro is secreted as exosomes from prostate cancer cells *(105)* and assimilated into prostasomes *(106)*. For these reasons, research has primarily focused on the prostate as lycopene/tomato consumption site of action.

A 2004 meta-analysis of published epidemiological studies found that the highest lycopene/tomato consumption levels or serum lycopene concentrations were associated with an 11–29% decrease in prostate cancer risk *(34)*. A more recent publication estimates that higher serum lycopene concentrations are associated with a nonsignificant 16% decrease in prostate cancer risk *(33)*. Based on much of the research reviewed in this chapter, a 2004 petition was submitted to the FDA for a health claim for tomatoes, lycopene, and cancer. After reviewing the evidence, FDA issued the following qualified health claim: "very limited and preliminary scientific research suggest that eating one-half to one cup of tomatoes and/or tomato sauce a week may reduce the risk of prostate cancer *(107)*." The FDA rejected all requests for lycopene health claims and concluded "that there was no credible evidence to support lycopene consumption, either as a food ingredient, a component of food, or as a dietary supplement, and any of the cancers evaluated in the studies *(107)*." The American Institute for Cancer Research panel concluded that "foods containing lycopene (particularly tomato products) probably protect against prostate cancer," while not assigning an evidence ranking to consumption of lycopene alone, due to a lack of evidence to support its effectiveness *(101)*. The prostate is the only site assigned an evidence ranking by the committee.

6. FUTURE RESEARCH DIRECTIONS

The appropriate efficacious lycopene dosage has not been addressed in the literature. The majority of animal studies and human intervention trials have not performed dose–response studies, instead choosing a single dose based on past research. The optimal lycopene dose needs to be established in appropriate prostate cancer models to determine whether lycopene supplementation is efficacious. These findings along with evidence from small clinical trials will determine whether lycopene alone is worth further pursuing. Carotenoid metabolism and its resulting health implications should also be examined, and research on other carotenoids may be warranted.

7. CONCLUSIONS AND RECOMMENDATIONS FOR INTAKE/DIETARY CHANGES

We do not recommend lycopene supplementation because it has not been proven to be efficacious for prostate cancer treatment or prevention. However, we suggest that men "Try for 5, Push for 2" tomato product servings/week. We base the "Try for 5" recommendation on the inverse relationship often seen in epidemiological studies of tomato consumption and prostate cancer when comparing men who consume 5 servings/week to those who consume ≤1 serving/week *(3, 43, 48, 56, 58)*. The second part of the recommendation is to "Push for 2," or consumption of at least 2 servings/week as a minimum consumption level will move men out of the reference group, where low tomato intake has been associated with increased prostate cancer risk.

For β-carotene, we encourage people to consume sources of dietary β-carotene such as fruits and vegetables, which are commonly associated with decreased chronic disease risk. In support of our recommendation, the AICR panel claimed "that foods containing carotenoids probably protect against lung cancer *(101)*." We do not recommend and especially discourage smokers from taking high-dose β-carotene supplements because clinical trials suggest enhanced lung cancer incidence, with no indication of chronic disease prevention. However, consumers should not be apprehensive of β-carotene in multivitamins or of taking β-carotene to provide vitamin A. β-carotene is commonly used as a vitamin A source because β-carotene supplementation does not lead to vitamin A toxicity. Normally, β-carotene levels in these supplements are far lower than concentrations that led to the adverse outcomes observed in the ATBC and CARET studies.

As alluded to in the introduction, the research approach used to investigate the effects of lycopene/tomatoes on prostate cancer has been more cautious than that used in the β-carotene and lung cancer studies. Typically, results of preclinical and phase I and II clinical trials need to demonstrate safety and efficacy before a large clinical trial may be undertaken. These steps will hopefully prevent potential negative outcomes like those observed in the ATBC and CARET trials from occurring again in future investigations.

REFERENCES

1. Lindshield, B.L., and Erdman, J.W. (2006) Carotenoids. In: Bowman B.A., and Russell R.M., eds. Present Knowledge in Nutrition. 9th ed., 184–97, Washington, DC: International Life Sciences Institute.
2. Peto, R., Doll, R., Buckley, J.D., and Sporn, M.B. (1981) Can dietary beta-carotene materially reduce human cancer rates? *Nature* **290**, 201–08.
3. Giovannucci, E., Ascherio, A., Rimm, E.B., Stampfer, M.J., Colditz, G.A., and Willett, W.C. (1995) Intake of carotenoids and retinol in relation to risk of prostate cancer. *J Natl Cancer Inst* **87**, 1767–76.
4. Castonguay, A., Pepin, P., and Stoner, G.D. (1991) Lung tumorigenicity of NNK given orally to A/J mice: Its application to chemopreventive efficacy studies. *Exp Lung Res* **17**, 485–99.
5. Moon, R.C., Rao, K.V., Detrisac, C.J., and Kelloff, G.J. (1992) Animal models for chemoprevention of respiratory cancer. *J Natl Cancer Inst Monogr* **52**, 45–49.
6. Murakoshi, M., Nishino, H., Satomi, Y. et al. (1992) Potent preventive action of alpha-carotene against carcinogenesis: Spontaneous liver carcinogenesis and promoting stage of lung and skin carcinogenesis in mice are suppressed more effectively by alpha-carotene than by beta-carotene. *Cancer Res* **52**, 6583–87.
7. Schwartz, J., and Shklar, G. (1992) The selective cytotoxic effect of carotenoids and alpha-tocopherol on human cancer cell lines in vitro. *J Oral Maxillofac Surg* **50**, 367–73, discussion 73–4.

8. Wang, X.D., Liu, C., Bronson, R.T., Smith, D.E., Krinsky, N.I., and Russell, M. (1999) Retinoid signaling and activator protein-1 expression in ferrets given beta-carotene supplements and exposed to tobacco smoke. *J Natl Cancer Inst* **91**, 60–66.

9. Russell, R.M. (2004) The enigma of beta-carotene in carcinogenesis: What can be learned from animal studies. *J Nutr* **134**, 262S–8S.

10. Palozza, P., Simone, R., and Mele, M.C. (2008) Interplay of carotenoids with cigarette smoking: Implications in lung cancer. *Curr Med Chem* **15**, 844–54.

11. Liu, C., Russell, R.M., and Wang, X.D. (2004) Low dose beta-carotene supplementation of ferrets attenuates smoke-induced lung phosphorylation of JNK, p38 MAPK, and p53 proteins. *J Nutr* **134**, 2705–10.

12. Goralczyk, R., Bachmann, H., Wertz, K. et al. (2006) beta-carotene-induced changes in RARbeta isoform mRNA expression patterns do not influence lung adenoma multiplicity in the NNK-initiated A/J mouse model. *Nutr Cancer* **54**, 252–62.

13. Kuntz, E., Borlak, J., Riss, G. et al. (2007) Transcriptomics does not show adverse effects of beta-carotene in A/J mice exposed to smoke for 2 weeks. *Arch Biochem Biophys* **465**, 336–46.

14. Fuster, A., Pico, C., Sanchez, J. et al. (2008) Effects of 6-month daily supplementation with oral beta-carotene in combination or not with benzo[a]pyrene on cell-cycle markers in the lung of ferrets. *J Nutr Biochem* **19**, 295–304.

15. Goralczyk, R., Wertz, K., Lenz, B. et al. (2005) Beta-carotene interaction with NNK in the AJ-mouse model: Effects on cell proliferation, tumor formation and retinoic acid responsive genes. *Biochim Biophys Acta* **1740**, 179–88.

16. Allen, C.M., Schwartz, S.J., Craft, N.E., Giovannucci, E.L., De Groff, V.L., and Clinton, S.K. (2003) Changes in plasma and oral mucosal lycopene isomer concentrations in healthy adults consuming standard servings of processed tomato products. *Nutr Cancer* **47**, 48–56.

17. Xu, X., Wang, Y., Constantinou, A.I., Stacewicz-Sapuntzakis, M., Bowen, P.E., and van Breemen, R.B. (1999) Solubilization and stabilization of carotenoids using micelles: Delivery of lycopene to cells in culture. *Lipids* **34**, 1031–36.

18. Lin, C.Y., Huang, C.S., and Hu, M.L. (2007) The use of fetal bovine serum as delivery vehicle to improve the uptake and stability of lycopene in cell culture studies. *Br J Nutr* **98**, 226–32.

19. Lindshield, B.L., Canene-Adams, K., and Erdman, J.W., Jr. (2007) Lycopenoids: Are lycopene metabolites bioactive? *Arch Biochem Biophys* **458**(2), 136–40.

20. Imaida, K., Tamano, S., Kato, K. et al. (2001) Lack of chemopreventive effects of lycopene and curcumin on experimental rat prostate carcinogenesis. *Carcinogenesis* **22**, 467–72.

21. Boileau, T.W., Liao, Z., Kim, S., Lemeshow, S., Erdman, J.W., Jr., and Clinton, S.K. (2003) Prostate carcinogenesis in N-methyl-N-nitrosourea (NMU)-testosterone-treated rats fed tomato powder, lycopene, or energy-restricted diets. *J Natl Cancer Inst* **95**, 1578–86.

22. Limpens, J., Schroder, F.H., de Ridder, C.M. et al. (2006) Combined lycopene and vitamin E treatment suppresses the growth of PC-346C human prostate cancer cells in nude mice. *J Nutr* **136**, 1287–93.

23. Canene-Adams, K., Lindshield, B.L., Wang, S., Jeffery, E.H., Clinton, S.K., and Erdman, J.W., Jr. (2007) Combinations of tomato and broccoli enhance antitumor activity in dunning R3327-H prostate adenocarcinomas. *Cancer Res* **67**, 836–43.

24. Siler, U., Barella, L., Spitzer, V. et al. (2004) Lycopene and vitamin E interfere with autocrine/paracrine loops in the Dunning prostate cancer model. *Faseb J* **18**, 1019–21.

25. Tang, L., Jin, T., Zeng, X., and Wang, J.S. (2005) Lycopene inhibits the growth of human androgen-independent prostate cancer cells in vitro and in BALB/c nude mice. *J Nutr* **135**, 287–90.

26. Lee, C.M., Boileau, A.C., Boileau, T.W. et al. (1999) Review of animal models in carotenoid research. *J Nutr* **129**, 2271–77.

27. Block, G., Patterson, B., and Subar, A. (1992) Fruit, vegetables, and cancer prevention: A review of the epidemiological evidence. *Nutr Cancer* **18**, 1–29.

28. Ziegler, R.G., Mayne, S.T., and Swanson, C.A. (1996) Nutrition and lung cancer. *Cancer Causes Control* **7**, 157–77.

29. Gallicchio, L., Boyd, K., Matanoski, G. et al. (2008) Carotenoids and the risk of developing lung cancer: A systematic review. *Am J Clin Nutr* **88**, 372–83.

30. Giovannucci, E. (1999) Tomatoes, tomato-based products, lycopene, and cancer: Review of the epidemiologic literature. *J Natl Cancer Inst* **91**, 317–31.
31. Giovannucci, E. (2002) A review of epidemiologic studies of tomatoes, lycopene, and prostate cancer. *Exp Biol Med (Maywood)* **227**, 852–59.
32. Chang, S., Erdman, J.W., Jr., Clinton, S.K. et al. (2005) Relationship between plasma carotenoids and prostate cancer. *Nutr Cancer* **53**, 127–34.
33. Key, T.J., Appleby, P.N., Allen, N.E. et al. (2007) Plasma carotenoids, retinol, and tocopherols and the risk of prostate cancer in the European Prospective Investigation into Cancer and Nutrition study. *Am J Clin Nutr* **86**, 672–81.
34. Etminan, M., Takkouche, B., and Caamano-Isorna, F. (2004) The role of tomato products and lycopene in the prevention of prostate cancer: A meta-analysis of observational studies. *Cancer Epidemiol Biomarkers Prev* **13**, 340–45.
35. Meyer, F., Bairati, I., Fradet, Y., and Moore, L. (1997) Dietary energy and nutrients in relation to preclinical prostate cancer. *Nutr Cancer* **29**, 120–26.
36. Cohen, J.H., Kristal, A.R., and Stanford, J.L. (2000) Fruit and vegetable intakes and prostate cancer risk. *J Natl Cancer Inst* **92**, 61–68.
37. Le Marchand, L., Hankin, J.H., Kolonel, L.N., and Wilkens, L.R. (1991) Vegetable and fruit consumption in relation to prostate cancer risk in Hawaii: A reevaluation of the effect of dietary beta-carotene. *Am J Epidemiol* **133**, 215–19.
38. Key, T.J., Silcocks, P.B., Davey, G.K., Appleby, P.N., and Bishop, D.T. (1997) A case-control study of diet and prostate cancer. *Br J Cancer* **76**, 678–87.
39. Villeneuve, P.J., Johnson, K.C., Kreiger, N., and Mao, Y. (1999) Risk factors for prostate cancer: Results from the Canadian National Enhanced Cancer Surveillance System. The Canadian Cancer Registries Epidemiology Research Group. *Cancer Causes Control* **10**, 355–67.
40. Deneo-Pellegrini, H., De Stefani, E., Ronco, A., and Mendilaharsu, M. (1999) Foods, nutrients and prostate cancer: A case-control study in Uruguay. *Br J Cancer* **80**, 591–97.
41. Bosetti, C., Talamini, R., Montella, M. et al. (2004) Retinol, carotenoids and the risk of prostate cancer: A case-control study from Italy. *Int J Cancer* **112**, 689–92.
42. Kolonel, L.N., Hankin, J.H., Whittemore, A.S. et al. (2000) Vegetables, fruits, legumes and prostate cancer: A multiethnic case-control study. *Cancer Epidemiol Biomarkers Prev* **9**, 795–804.
43. Schuman, L.M., Mandel, J.S., Radke, A., Seal, U., and Halberg, F. (1982) Some selected features of the epidemiology of prostatic cancer: Minneapolis-St. Paul, Minnesota case-control study, 1976–1979. In: Magnas K., ed. Trends in Cancer Incidence: Causes and Practical Implications. 345–54, Washington, DC: Hemisphere Publishing Corp..
44. Hayes, R.B., Ziegler, R.G., Gridley, G. et al. (1999) Dietary factors and risks for prostate cancer among blacks and whites in the United States. *Cancer Epidemiol Biomarkers Prev* **8**, 25–34.
45. Norrish, A.E., Jackson, R.T., Sharpe, S.J., and Skeaff, C.M. (2000) Prostate cancer and dietary carotenoids. *Am J Epidemiol* **151**, 119–23.
46. Sonoda, T., Nagata, Y., Mori, M. et al. (2004) A case-control study of diet and prostate cancer in Japan: Possible protective effect of traditional Japanese diet. *Cancer Sci* **95**, 238–42.
47. Sanderson, M., Coker, A.L., Logan, P., Zheng, W., and Fadden, M.K. (2004) Lifestyle and prostate cancer among older African–American and Caucasian men in South Carolina. *Cancer Causes Control* **15**, 647–55.
48. Jain, M.G., Hislop, G.T., Howe, G.R., and Ghadirian, P. (1999) Plant foods, antioxidants, and prostate cancer risk: Findings from case-control studies in Canada. *Nutr Cancer* **34**, 173–84.
49. Tzonou, A., Signorello, L.B., Lagiou, P., Wuu, J., Trichopoulos, D., and Trichopoulou, A. (1999) Diet and cancer of the prostate: A case-control study in Greece. *Int J Cancer* **80**, 704–08.
50. Bosetti, C., Tzonou, A., Lagiou, P., Negri, E., Trichopoulos, D., and Hsieh, C.C. (2000) Fraction of prostate cancer incidence attributed to diet in Athens, Greece. *Eur J Cancer Prev* **9**, 119–23.
51. Hodge, A.M., English, D.R., McCredie, M.R. et al. (2004) Foods, nutrients and prostate cancer. *Cancer Causes Control* **15**, 11–20.
52. Jian, L., Du, C.J., Lee, A.H., and Binns, C.W. (2005) Do dietary lycopene and other carotenoids protect against prostate cancer? *Int J Cancer* **113**, 1010–14.

53. Jian, L., Lee, A.H., and Binns, C.W. (2007) Tea and lycopene protect against prostate cancer. *Asia Pac J Clin Nutr* **16**(Suppl 1), 453–57.

54. McCann, S.E., Ambrosone, C.B., Moysich, K.B. et al. (2005) Intakes of selected nutrients, foods, and phytochemicals and prostate cancer risk in western New York. *Nutr Cancer* **53**, 33–41.

55. Goodman, M., Bostick, R.M., Ward, K.C. et al. (2006) Lycopene intake and prostate cancer risk: Effect modification by plasma antioxidants and the XRCC1 genotype. *Nutr Cancer* **55**, 13–20.

56. Pourmand, G., Salem, S., Mehrsai, A. et al. (2007) The risk factors of prostate cancer: A multicentric case-control study in Iran. *Asian Pac J Cancer Prev* **8**, 422–28.

57. Kirsh, V.A., Mayne, S.T., Peters, U. et al. (2006) A prospective study of lycopene and tomato product intake and risk of prostate cancer. *Cancer Epidemiol Biomarkers Prev* **15**, 92–98.

58. Mills, P.K., Beeson, W.L., Phillips, R.L., and Fraser, G.E. (1989) Cohort study of diet, lifestyle, and prostate cancer in Adventist men. *Cancer* **64**, 598–604.

59. Cerhan, J., Chiu, B., Putnam, S. et al. (1998) A cohort study of diet and prostate cancer risk. *Cancer Epidemiol Biomarkers Prev* **7**, 175.

60. Schuurman, A.G., Goldbohm, R.A., Brants, H.A., and van den Brandt, P.A. (2002) A prospective cohort study on intake of retinol, vitamins C and E, and carotenoids and prostate cancer risk (Netherlands). *Cancer Causes Control* **13**, 573–82.

61. Agudo, A., Cabrera, L., Amiano, P. et al. (2007) Fruit and vegetable intakes, dietary antioxidant nutrients, and total mortality in Spanish adults: Findings from the Spanish cohort of the European Prospective Investigation into Cancer and Nutrition (EPIC-Spain). *Am J Clin Nutr* **85**, 1634–42.

62. Giovannucci, E., Rimm, E.B., Liu, Y., Stampfer, M.J., and Willett, W.C. (2002) A prospective study of tomato products, lycopene, and prostate cancer risk. *J Natl Cancer Inst* **94**, 391–98.

63. Nomura, A.M., Stemmermann, G.N., Lee, J., and Craft, N.E. (1997) Serum micronutrients and prostate cancer in Japanese Americans in Hawaii. *Cancer Epidemiol Biomarkers Prev* **6**, 487–91.

64. Peters, U., Leitzmann, M.F., Chatterjee, N. et al. (2007) Serum lycopene, other carotenoids, and prostate cancer risk: A nested case-control study in the prostate, lung, colorectal, and ovarian cancer screening trial. *Cancer Epidemiol Biomarkers Prev* **16**, 962–68.

65. Goodman, G.E., Schaffer, S., Omenn, G.S., Chen, C., and King, I. (2003) The association between lung and prostate cancer risk, and serum micronutrients: Results and lessons learned from beta-carotene and retinol efficacy trial. *Cancer Epidemiol Biomarkers Prev* **12**, 518–26.

66. Comstock, G.W., Helzlsouer, K.J., and Bush, T.L. (1991) Prediagnostic serum levels of carotenoids and vitamin E as related to subsequent cancer in Washington County, Maryland. *Am J Clin Nutr* **53**, 260S–4S.

67. Hsing, A.W., Comstock, G.W., Abbey, H., and Polk, B.F. (1990) Serologic precursors of cancer. Retinol, carotenoids, and tocopherol and risk of prostate cancer. *J Natl Cancer Inst* **82**, 941–46.

68. Gann, P.H., Ma, J., Giovannucci, E. et al. (1999) Lower prostate cancer risk in men with elevated plasma lycopene levels: Results of a prospective analysis. *Cancer Res* **59**, 1225–30.

69. Vogt, T.M., Mayne, S.T., Graubard, B.I. et al. (2002) Serum lycopene, other serum carotenoids, and risk of prostate cancer in US Blacks and Whites. *Am J Epidemiol* **155**, 1023–32.

70. Huang, H.Y., Alberg, A.J., Norkus, E.P., Hoffman, S.C., Comstock, G.W., and Helzlsouer, K.J. (2003) Prospective study of antioxidant micronutrients in the blood and the risk of developing prostate cancer. *Am J Epidemiol* **157**, 335–44.

71. Wu, K., Erdman, J.W., Jr., Schwartz, S.J. et al. (2004) Plasma and dietary carotenoids, and the risk of prostate cancer: A nested case-control study. *Cancer Epidemiol Biomarkers Prev* **13**, 260–69.

72. Rao, A.V., Fleshner, N., and Agarwal, S. (1999) Serum and tissue lycopene and biomarkers of oxidation in prostate cancer patients: A case-control study. *Nutr Cancer* **33**, 159–64.

73. Lu, Q.Y., Hung, J.C., Heber, D. et al. (2001) Inverse associations between plasma lycopene and other carotenoids and prostate cancer. *Cancer Epidemiol Biomarkers Prev* **10**, 749–56.

74. Zhang, J., Dhakal, I., Stone, A. et al. (2007) Plasma carotenoids and prostate cancer: A population-based case-control study in Arkansas. *Nutr Cancer* **59**, 46–53.

75. Heinonen, O.P., Huttunen, J.K., Albanes, D. et al. (1994) The effect of vitamin E and beta carotene on the incidence of lung cancer and other cancers in male smokers. The Alpha-Tocopherol, Beta Carotene Cancer Prevention Study Group. *N Engl J Med* **330**, 1029–35.

76. Omenn, G.S., Goodman, G.E., Thornquist, M.D. et al. (1996) Effects of a combination of beta carotene and vitamin A on lung cancer and cardiovascular disease. *N Engl J Med* **334**, 1150–55.

77. Virtamo, J., Pietinen, P., Huttunen, J.K. et al. (2003) Incidence of cancer and mortality following alpha-tocopherol and beta-carotene supplementation: A postintervention follow-up. *JAMA* **290**, 476–85.

78. Goodman, G.E., Thornquist, M.D., Balmes, J. et al. (2004) The Beta-Carotene and Retinol Efficacy Trial: Incidence of lung cancer and cardiovascular disease mortality during 6-year follow-up after stopping beta-carotene and retinol supplements. *J Natl Cancer Inst* **96**, 1743–50.

79. Goodman, D.S., and Huang, H.S. (1965) Biosynthesis of vitamin A with rat intestinal enzymes. *Science* **149**, 879–80.

80. Lee, I.M., Cook, N.R., Manson, J.E., Buring, J.E., and Hennekens, C.H. (1999) Beta-carotene supplementation and incidence of cancer and cardiovascular disease: The Women's Health Study. *J Natl Cancer Inst* **91**, 2102–06.

81. de Klerk, N.H., Musk, A.W., Ambrosini, G.L. et al. (1998) Vitamin A and cancer prevention II: Comparison of the effects of retinol and beta-carotene. *Int J Cancer* **75**, 362–67.

82. Kamangar, F., Qiao, Y.L., Yu, B. et al. (2006) Lung cancer chemoprevention: A randomized, double-blind trial in Linxian, China. *Cancer Epidemiol Biomarkers Prev* **15**, 1562–64.

83. Tanvetyanon, T., and Bepler, G. (2008) Beta-carotene in multivitamins and the possible risk of lung cancer among smokers versus former smokers: A meta-analysis and evaluation of national brands. *Cancer* **113**, 150–57.

84. De Angelis, G., Rittenhouse, H.G., Mikolajczyk, S.D., Blair Shamel, L., and Semjonow, A. (2007) Twenty years of PSA: From prostate antigen to tumor marker. *Rev Urol* **9**, 113–23.

85. Barry, M.J. (2001) Clinical practice. Prostate-specific-antigen testing for early diagnosis of prostate cancer. *N Engl J Med* **344**, 1373–77.

86. Chen, L., Stacewicz-Sapuntzakis, M., Duncan, C. et al. (2001) Oxidative DNA damage in prostate cancer patients consuming tomato sauce-based entrees as a whole-food intervention. *J Natl Cancer Inst* **93**, 1872–79.

87. Kim, H.S., Bowen, P., Chen, L. et al. (2003) Effects of tomato sauce consumption on apoptotic cell death in prostate benign hyperplasia and carcinoma. *Nutr Cancer* **47**, 40–47.

88. Kucuk, O., Sarkar, F.H., Sakr, W. et al. (2001) Phase II randomized clinical trial of lycopene supplementation before radical prostatectomy. *Cancer Epidemiol Biomarkers Prev* **10**, 861–68.

89. Kucuk, O., Sarkar, F.H., Djuric, Z. et al. (2002) Effects of lycopene supplementation in patients with localized prostate cancer. *Exp Biol Med (Maywood)* **227**, 881–85.

90. Ansari, M.S., and Gupta, N.P. (2003) A comparison of lycopene and orchidectomy vs orchidectomy alone in the management of advanced prostate cancer. *BJU Int* **92**, 375–78, discussion 8.

91. Ansari, M.S., and Gupta, N.P. (2004) Lycopene: A novel drug therapy in hormone refractory metastatic prostate cancer. *Urol Oncol* **22**, 415–20.

92. Mohanty, N.K., Saxena, S., Singh, U.P., Goyal, N.K., and Arora, R.P. (2005) Lycopene as a chemopreventive agent in the treatment of high-grade prostate intraepithelial neoplasia. *Urol Oncol* **23**, 383–85.

93. Edinger, M.S., and Koff, W.J. (2006) Effect of the consumption of tomato paste on plasma prostate-specific antigen levels in patients with benign prostate hyperplasia. *Braz J Med Biol Res* **39**, 1115–19.

94. Vaishampayan, U., Hussain, M., Banerjee, M. et al. (2007) Lycopene and soy isoflavones in the treatment of prostate cancer. *Nutr Cancer* **59**, 1–7.

95. Grainger, E.M., Schwartz, S.J., Wang, S. et al. (2008) A combination of tomato and soy products for men with recurring prostate cancer and rising prostate specific antigen. *Nutr Cancer* **60**, 145–54.

96. Schwarz, S., Obermuller-Jevic, U.C., Hellmis, E., Koch, W., Jacobi, G., and Biesalski, H.K. (2008) Lycopene inhibits disease progression in patients with benign prostate hyperplasia. *J Nutr* **138**, 49–53.

97. Barber, N.J., Zhang, X., Zhu, G. et al. (2006) Lycopene inhibits DNA synthesis in primary prostate epithelial cells in vitro and its administration is associated with a reduced prostate-specific antigen velocity in a phase II clinical study. *Prostate Cancer Prostatic Dis* **9**, 407–13.

 98. Clark, P.E., Hall, M.C., Borden, L.S., Jr. et al. (2006) Phase I–II prospective dose-escalating trial of lycopene in patients with biochemical relapse of prostate cancer after definitive local therapy. *Urology* **67**, 1257–61.

 99. Bunker, C.H., McDonald, A.C., Evans, R.W., de la Rosa, N., Boumosleh, J.M., and Patrick, A.L. (2007) A randomized trial of lycopene supplementation in Tobago men with high prostate cancer risk. *Nutr Cancer* **57**, 130–37.

100. Jatoi, A., Burch, P., Hillman, D. et al. (2007) A tomato-based, lycopene-containing intervention for androgen-independent prostate cancer: Results of a Phase II study from the North Central Cancer Treatment Group. *Urology* **69**, 289–94.

101. Anonymous (2007) Food, Nutrition, Physical Activity, and the Prevention of Cancer: A Global Perspective. Washington, DC: World Cancer Research Fund/American Institute for Cancer Research.

102. Herzog, A., Siler, U., Spitzer, V. et al. (2005) Lycopene reduced gene expression of steroid targets and inflammatory markers in normal rat prostate. *Faseb J* **19**, 272–74.

103. Boileau, T.W., Clinton, S.K., and Erdman, J.W., Jr. (2000) Tissue lycopene concentrations and isomer patterns are affected by androgen status and dietary lycopene concentration in male F344 rats. *J Nutr* **130**, 1613–18.

104. Boileau, T.W., Clinton, S.K., Zaripheh, S., Monaco, M.H., Donovan, S.M., and Erdman, J.W., Jr. (2001) Testosterone and food restriction modulate hepatic lycopene isomer concentrations in male F344 rats. *J Nutr* **131**, 1746–52.

105. Goyal, A., Delves, G.H., Chopra, M., Lwaleed, B.A., and Cooper, A.J. (2006) Prostate cells exposed to lycopene in vitro liberate lycopene-enriched exosomes. *BJU Int* **98**, 907–11.

106. Goyal, A., Delves, G.H., Chopra, M., Lwaleed, B.A., and Cooper, A.J. (2006) Can lycopene be delivered into semen via prostasomes? In vitro incorporation and retention studies. *Int J Androl* **29**, 528–33.

107. Kavanaugh, C.J., Trumbo, P.R., and Ellwood, K.C. (2007) The US Food and Drug Administration's evidence-based review for qualified health claims: Tomatoes, lycopene, and cancer. *J Natl Cancer Inst* **99**, 1074–85.

108. Forbes, K., Gillette, K., and Sehgal, I. (2003) Lycopene increases urokinase receptor and fails to inhibit growth or connexin expression in a metastatically passaged prostate cancer cell line: A brief communication. *Exp Biol Med (Maywood)* **228**, 967–71.

109. Hantz, H.L., Young, L.F., and Martin, K.R. (2005) Physiologically attainable concentrations of lycopene induce mitochondrial apoptosis in LNCaP human prostate cancer cells. *Exp Biol Med (Maywood)* **230**, 171–79.

110. Hwang, E.S., and Bowen, P.E. (2004) Cell cycle arrest and induction of apoptosis by lycopene in LNCaP human prostate cancer cells. *J Med Food* **7**, 284–89.

111. Hwang, E.S., and Bowen, P.E. (2005) Effects of lycopene and tomato paste extracts on DNA and lipid oxidation in LNCaP human prostate cancer cells. *Biofactors* **23**, 97–105.

112. Hwang, E.S., and Bowen, P.E. (2005) Effects of tomato paste extracts on cell proliferation, cell-cycle arrest and apoptosis in LNCaP human prostate cancer cells. *Biofactors* **23**, 75–84.

113. Kim, L., Rao, A.V., and Rao, L.G. (2002) Effect of lycopene on prostate LNCaP cancer cells in culture. *J Med Food* **5**, 181–87.

114. Kotake-Nara, E., Kushiro, M., Zhang, H., Sugawara, T., Miyashita, K., and Nagao, A. (2001) Carotenoids affect proliferation of human prostate cancer cells. *J Nutr* **131**, 3303–06.

115. Obermuller-Jevic, U.C., Olano-Martin, E., Corbacho, A.M. et al. (2003) Lycopene inhibits the growth of normal human prostate epithelial cells in vitro. *J Nutr* **133**, 3356–60.

116. Burgess, L.C., Rice, E., Fischer, T. et al. (2008) Lycopene has limited effect on cell proliferation in only two of seven human cell lines (both cancerous and noncancerous) in an in vitro system with doses across the physiological range. *Toxicol In Vitro* **22**, 1297–300.

117. Gunasekera, R.S., Sewgobind, K., Desai, S. et al. (2007) Lycopene and lutein inhibit proliferation in rat prostate carcinoma cells. *Nutr Cancer* **58**, 171–77.

118. Ivanov, N.I., Cowell, S.P., Brown, P., Rennie, P.S., Guns, E.S., and Cox, M.E. (2007) Lycopene differentially induces quiescence and apoptosis in androgen-responsive and – independent prostate cancer cell lines. *Clin Nutr* **26**, 252–63.

119. Kanagaraj, P., Vijayababu, M.R., Ravisankar, B., Anbalagan, J., Aruldhas, M.M., and Arunakaran, J. (2007) Effect of lycopene on insulin-like growth factor-I, IGF binding protein-3 and IGF type-I receptor in prostate cancer cells. *J Cancer Res Clin Oncol* **133**, 351–59.

120. Peternac, D., Klima, I., Cecchini, M.G., Schwaninger, R., Studer, U.E., and Thalmann, G.N. (2008) Agents used for chemoprevention of prostate cancer may influence PSA secretion independently of cell growth in the LNCaP model of human prostate cancer progression. *Prostate* **68**, 1307–18.

121. Liu, A., Pajkovic, N., Pang, Y. et al. (2006) Absorption and subcellular localization of lycopene in human prostate cancer cells. *Mol Cancer Ther* **5**, 2879–85.

122. Gitenay, D., Lyan, B., Talvas, J. et al. (2007) Serum from rats fed red or yellow tomatoes induces Connexin43 expression independently from lycopene in a prostate cancer cell line. *Biochem Biophys Res Commun* **364**, 578–82.

123. Pastori, M., Pfander, H., Boscoboinik, D., and Azzi, A. (1998) Lycopene in association with alpha-tocopherol inhibits at physiological concentrations proliferation of prostate carcinoma cells. *Biochem Biophys Res Commun* **250**, 582–85.

124. Richards, L.R., Benghuzzi, H., Tucci, M., and Hughes, J. (2003) The synergistic effect of conventional and sustained delivery of antioxidants on LNCaP prostate cancer cell line. *Biomed Sci Instrum* **39**, 402–07.

16 Vitamin A

A. Catharine Ross

Key Points

1. Retinoids are one of the most effective classes of agents for promoting cell differentiation, and therefore are of strong interest for cancer prevention and cancer therapy. Nevertheless, despite a great deal of testing, their use in cancer chemoprevention has been limited by the side effects associated with most compounds.
2. Vitamin A, also known as retinol, and retinoic acid (RA) are widely recognized as important factors in the maintenance of healthy cells and tissues. RA possesses a fundamental ability to regulate cell growth, generally by slowing the rate of the cell cycle, and to induce immature and transformed cells to differentiate toward a more mature phenotype.
3. Retinol is an essential nutrient that serves as the substrate for the production, within various cells, of retinal required for rhodopsin biosynthesis, and for the production of RA, which functions as a critical regulator of cellular functions in essentially all tissues. RA is now recognized as a potent regulator of gene expression.
4. Metabolism is central to the biological basis of vitamin A's actions in cancer prevention. Retinoid metabolism is closely regulated through a variety of homeostatic mechanisms including transport proteins, intracellular chaperone proteins, nuclear receptors, and enzymes. The apparent "goal" of the body's homeostatic mechanisms is to maintain steady levels of plasma retinol and RA, which in turn assure a well-regulated exposure of extrahepatic tissues to these molecules.
5. There is no compelling evidence that changing current recommendations for dietary vitamin A would be helpful in reducing cancer risk. A recent report on the topic of "Multivitamin/Mineral Supplements and Chronic Disease Prevention" concluded that while supplement use has grown and now more than half of the adult population of the USA uses multivitamin/mineral supplements, most of the studies that were reviewed do not provide strong evidence for health-related effects.

Key Words: Vitamin A; retinol; retinoic acid; retinoid; gene expression; cell differentiation; epidemiology; nutrition; dietary recommendations

1. INTRODUCTION

Vitamin A (retinol) and its active metabolite, retinoic acid (RA), are widely recognized as important factors in the maintenance of healthy cells and tissues. RA possesses a fundamental ability to regulate cell growth, generally by slowing the rate of the cell cycle, and to induce immature and transformed cells to differentiate toward a

From: *Nutrition and Health: Bioactive Compounds and Cancer*
Edited by: J.A. Milner, D.F. Romagnolo, DOI 10.1007/978-1-60761-627-6_16,
© Springer Science+Business Media, LLC 2010

more mature phenotype. These intrinsic biological properties appear to be nearly ideal for the chemoprevention of cancer, possibly even for the treatment of established cancers. However, when vitamin A is consumed at elevated levels, it accumulates over time within tissues and can be damaging to the integrity of cellular membranes, culminating in symptoms of hypervitaminosis A. Thus, natural vitamin A is not well suited for long-term systemic therapy. The idea of producing "retinoids" *(1)* – i.e., synthetic analogues structurally related to retinol and RA, that would potentially be beneficial in the fight against cancer while also less toxic, has motivated the field of vitamin A and retinoid research for three decades. Numerous retinoids are significantly growth inhibitory to rapidly proliferating and transformed cells. These results have served as a strong impetus for studies in preclinical models and for clinical trials. As discussed in this chapter, results have been promising in the treatment of some premalignant diseases, such as leukoplakia, but for established cancers, results have generally been disappointing. However, an outstanding success has been achieved with the discovery that all-*trans*-RA (at-RA) is effective in the treatment of acute promyelocytic leukemia (APL) *(2)*. In a high proportion of APL patients, at-RA induces a complete remission. Retinoids have also become widely used in the treatment of diseases of the skin, such as cystic acne, which have proved refractory to other therapies.

Clinical studies have also revealed some unintended consequences of retinoids used for therapy on the metabolism of natural vitamin A. In a trial of fenretinide (4-HPR) for prevention of breast cancer recurrence, 4-HPR-treated women reported problems with dark adaptation (night blindness) *(3)*, a well-known sign of vitamin A deficiency *(4)*. Plasma analysis revealed low levels of retinol, despite no evidence of low-dietary vitamin A, and subsequent studies revealed that 4-HPR disrupted the plasma protein complex that transports retinol *(5)*, which is likely to increase its turnover rate. Such findings serve to underline that the metabolism of dietary vitamin A and synthetic retinoids used for therapy are highly intertwined. Some retinoids used for treatment, such as at-RA, are chemically indistinguishable from their naturally formed biological counterparts, but due to high dosage they still can perturb the normal metabolism of vitamin A. Indeed, at-RA at pharmacological dosage also rapidly reduces the concentration of plasma retinol *(6)*. Thus, to avoid unintended consequences, greater attention must be paid to understanding the interactions of diet-derived vitamin A and retinoids used or proposed for use as therapeutic drugs.

The purpose of this chapter is to review the biological basis for a role of vitamin A in cancer prevention and treatment, the types of evidence and the totality of evidence that this nutrient can reduce cancer risk, and the status of nutritional recommendations for vitamin A intakes that are optimal in terms of reducing the risk of cancer.

2. RATIONALE FOR WHY VITAMIN A CAN AFFECT CANCER PREVENTION AND/OR TREATMENT

Retinol is an essential nutrient that serves as the substrate for the production, within various cells, of retinal required for rhodopsin biosynthesis, and for the production of RA, which functions as a critical regulator of cellular functions in essentially all tissues. RA is now recognized as a potent regulator of gene expression. While the effects of

RA on gene expression are cell-type specific, three general outcomes on cell physiology have been reported for a wide variety of cells: a reduced rate of cell proliferation, enhanced cell differentiation, and in some cells with some retinoids, induction of apoptosis.

Today's understanding of retinoids and their potential role in cancer prevention is based on decades of prior research. The idea that vitamin A may be important for cancer prevention can be traced back to the 1920s, when Wolbach and Howe reported on histopathological changes in the epithelial tissues of rats fed a vitamin A-deficient diet (7). The mucosal linings of various epithelial tissues were squamous, dry, and keratinized in the vitamin A-deficient state. In other studies, vitamin A-deficient animals were more likely to develop metaplasia and spontaneous tumors (8). The field of vitamin A research then advanced to studies of specific metabolites, with the identification of retinal as the form essential for vision and of RA as an important, but quantitatively small, active metabolite of retinol. In 1960, Dowling and Wald (9) reported that at-RA can replace retinol for nearly all of the essential functions of vitamin A, except in vision where retinal is required. These studies helped lead to the current understanding of retinol as a precursor molecule from which all of the active forms of vitamin A are produced by metabolism. By the 1970–1980s when cell culture models became increasingly important in biomedical research, seminal studies were reported on the ability of RA to inhibit cell growth and induce cell differentiation. In relatively undifferentiated F9 embryonal carcinoma cells, RA induced formation of parietal endoderm (10), while in HL-60 myeloid leukemia cells, RA induced a myeloid, granulocytic phenotype (11). In 1987, the discovery of two families of nuclear retinoid receptors, RAR and RXR, provided a conceptual understanding of how retinoids may work as transcription factors in the regulation of gene expression (12, 13). In rapid succession, three RAR and three RXR genes were cloned and characterized, and their expression patterns were determined to elucidate where and under what conditions retinoid-activated nuclear receptors might function. These discoveries opened the way to a molecular understanding of retinoid actions. X-ray crystallographic studies of the RAR and RXR ligand-binding domains, with and without bound ligand, provided important information on how retinoid receptors interact with their ligand molecule, and suggested that significant conformational changes are induced by the binding of the retinoid to the ligand-binding domain of the receptor protein (14). This information then facilitated the production of new agonistic and antagonistic ligands, some with significant receptor specificity, such as the "rexinoids" specific for binding to RXRs.

Overall, many studies have led to the current understanding that RA is naturally involved in a great number of biological processes. The "fingerprint" of RA can be found in nearly every metabolic pathway (15).

Retinoid molecules of natural and synthetic origin. Major nutritional and pharmacologic retinoids are listed in Table 1. While the term retinoid once was used to distinguish structurally related synthetic analogues of vitamin A compounds, it now applies to all molecules of this structural group, whether produced in vivo from vitamin A or produced by chemical synthesis. In this chapter, the term vitamin A is used when the nutritional form is specifically meant, including retinyl esters and retinol and their natural metabolites. Vitamin A compounds exist in multiple oxidation states, in different

Table 1
Major Nutritional and Synthetically Derived Retinoids

Nutritional forms and physiologically produced metabolites	Structurally identical physiological and synthetic forms	Synthetic retinoids used in animal and human studies
Retinol (plasma; precursor to other forms)		
3,4-didehydroretinol (skin)		
Retinyl esters (storage)		Retinyl acetate; retinyl palmitate (RP)
Retinal (vision)		
All-*trans*-retinoic acid (ligand for RAR receptors; regulator of cell growth, cell differentiation, and apoptosis)	Yes	All-*trans*-RA (at-RA)
13-*cis*-RA (metabolite in plasma)	Yes	13-*cis*-RA
9-*cis*-RA (putative metabolite and ligand for RXR receptors)	?	9-*cis*-RA
Retinoyl glucuronides (water soluble; excreted metabolites)	Yes	Retinoyl glucuronides
		Axerophthene, anhydroretinol (hydrocarbons)
		Retinyl ethers
		Polyprenoic acid (acyclic retinoid)
		Arotinoids
		Retinobenzoic acids
		Rexinoids
		Hydroxyphenyl retinamide

isomeric forms, and in unconjugated or conjugated states. The principal oxidation states are alcohol, aldehyde, and carboxylic acid. Natural forms exist in the all-*trans* configuration, while the 11-*cis*-isomer of retinal, formed from retinol in retinal pigment epithelial cells, is an essential component of the visual pigment rhodopsin.

The mode of formation of *cis* isomers of RA in vivo, and even their physiological significance, is unclear. 13-*cis*-RA is a normal metabolite present in plasma *(16)*. Although 13-*cis*-RA as a drug has shown activity in chemoprevention studies, and is often used in treating diseases of the skin, 13-*cis*-RA does not transactivate nuclear receptors as all-*trans*-RA does. Exogenous 13-*cis*-RA might act as a pro-drug that is slowly converted to at-RA *(17)*. Although exogenous 9-*cis*-RA clearly binds to and transactivates nuclear retinoid receptors (see below), mainly of the RXR family, it is not certain that 9-*cis*-RA is an endogenous metabolite of vitamin A. Doubts have been raised based on finding very low or undetectable levels of this molecule in tissues where it would be expected and the possibility that it is formed artifactually during isolation. To date, no isomerase has been reported that catalyzes the formation of 9-*cis*-RA. This isomer could be generated nonenzymatically from all-*trans*-RA or 13-*cis*-RA, as to some extent all isomers of RA exist in equilibrium mixtures. The binding of at-RA to cellular retinoic acid-binding proteins stabilizes the all-*trans* isomer, but 9-*cis*-RA is not bound by these proteins. Therefore, even if 9-*cis*-RA is formed in vivo it may be quickly degraded. Other possible ligands for the RXR receptors have been suggested, including long-chain polyunsaturated fatty acids and phytanic acid.

The family of synthetic retinoids covers a great variety of forms. Detailed discussions of their synthesis and properties can be found in references *(18, 19)*. These retinoids exist in various oxidation states, as *cis* and all-*trans* isomers, in locked conformations, and with various substitutions and linkages (Table 1, Fig. 1). Some of the synthetic retinoids are chemically identical to natural metabolites of vitamin A, with at-RA as a prime example.

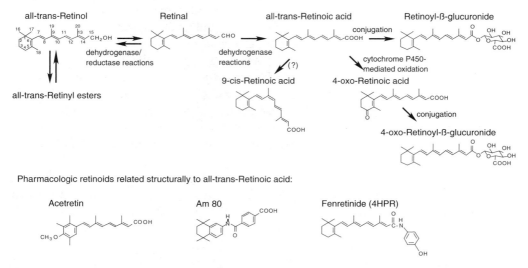

Fig. 1. Examples of naturally occurring and synthetic retinoids. The conversion of retinol to retinal and at-RA constitutes the major pathway of bioactivation for dietary vitamin A. Cytochrome P-450-mediated oxidation and subsequent conjugation contributes to catabolism of RA, whether generated from diet or administered for treatment. Retinol is also eliminated by this route (not shown). The *lower* panel shows three examples of synthetic retinoids, illustrating the substitution of an aromatic ring for the natural β-ionone ring of retinoic acid (acetretin); introduction of a heteroatom and creation of a locked conformation (Am80); and an amide analogue, 4-HPR, which has been tested extensively in cell, animal, and human clinical studies.

Metabolism as a major factor in retinoid homeostasis. Metabolism is central to the biological basis of vitamin A's actions in cancer prevention. Retinoid metabolism is closely regulated through a variety of homeostatic mechanisms, discussed below, which include transport proteins, intracellular chaperone proteins, nuclear receptors, and enzymes. The apparent "goal" of the body's homeostatic mechanisms is to maintain steady levels of plasma retinol and RA, which in turn assure a well-regulated exposure of extrahepatic tissues to these molecules. At the molecular level, at-RA itself regulates several genes/enzymes that are central to controlling the levels of retinol and RA, thus acting in an autoregulatory manner (20, 21). Although the retinoid homeostatic system is remarkably efficient over a wide range of dietary vitamin A intakes, it clearly cannot compensate for an inadequate vitamin A intake, and it can be overwhelmed by an excess of vitamin A and by exogenous retinoids. In unbound "free" form, retinoids disrupt cellular membranes (22), while an excess of RA induces gene responses that are inappropriate to the normal functioning of cells. The signs and clinical symptoms of hypervitaminosis A and retinoid toxicity are very similar (23). The maintenance of physiological levels of retinol and RA is essential for normal embryonic development, as both vitamin A deficiency and excess (of either retinol or RA) are teratogenic, causing developmental abnormalities of the head, limbs, heart, and other visceral organs (24). In the postnatal period, a well-regulated supply of vitamin A is necessary for lung maturation, development of immunity to natural pathogens and vaccines, and growth (25). In adults, an adequate intake of vitamin A is essential for maintaining the integrity of the skin, ciliated epithelia, and reproductive organs. These changes are sufficiently reproducible that the ability of retinoids to reverse epithelial metaplasia has been used as a bioassay for retinoid activity. Overall, a diet with an adequate but not excessive level of vitamin A is required across the lifespan for the well-regulated production of its active metabolites. An understanding of vitamin A metabolism is essential both for formulating optimal nutritional recommendations and for predicting how pharmacological retinoids, which at doses currently used significantly alter plasma retinol, are likely to affect the metabolism of natural vitamin A. Moreover, aberrant retinoid signaling appears to be a condition of many transformed cells and tumor tissues (see later). Figure 1 outlines the major pathways of vitamin A metabolism. Specific players in retinoid metabolism and homeostasis are described next.

RBP. Retinol-binding protein is the principal transport protein for plasma retinol. Retinol is released from liver bound to RBP, circulates in plasma within a narrow concentration range of approximately 1–3 μmol/l, and is taken up by target organs (26). In situations of a nutrition deficiency of vitamin A, during inflammation, and as a result of retinoid treatment, plasma retinol is markedly reduced. A recently identified plasma membrane transporter, Stra6, binds RBP and transports the retinol molecule into cells (27). This mechanism appears especially important in the retina. The RBP gene (RBP4) is also expressed in extrahepatic tissues. Kinetic studies have shown that retinol normally circulates several times between liver and extrahepatic tissues before undergoing irreversible oxidation, and thus the synthesis of RBP in extrahepatic tissues is likely to be important for reverse retinol transport back to the liver. RBP has also been shown to have adipokine-like properties and to be a factor in the regulation of glucose metabolism (28), suggesting novel interactions between vitamin A and energy homeostasis.

Cellular retinoid-binding proteins. The cellular retinol-binding proteins known as CRBP-I and CRBP-II are structurally and functionally similar, while CRBP-III is homologous but less well understood. As chaperone proteins, CRBP-I and CRBP-II guide retinol to the esterifying enzyme lecithin:retinol acyltransferase (LRAT) in the liver and intestine, respectively *(29)*, while also playing a role in retinol oxidation–reduction *(30)*. When CRBP-I knock-out mice were stressed by a low-vitamin A diet, they quickly lost retinol from the liver and retina, showing that CRBP is an important "efficiency factor" for the conservation of vitamin A *(31)*.

Intracellular RA is chaperoned by two cellular retinoic acid-binding proteins, CRABP-I and CRABP-II, which are differentially expressed in various tissues. These proteins bind at-RA selectively. They appear to regulate the availability and delivery of at-RA to nuclear receptor proteins. Additionally, in some cell types, CRABP-II appears to function as a transcriptional regulator associated with RAR-alpha-mediated gene expression *(32)*.

Absorption, storage, enzymatic activation, and elimination of retinoids. In the intestine, dietary vitamin A in foods and supplements is digested and absorbed, converted in enterocytes into esterified retinol, and packaged into chylomicrons, which are secreted into the lymphatics and then enter the circulation. Chylomicron remnants deliver most of their vitamin A to the liver, but a small proportion is released to extrahepatic tissues during chylomicron metabolism. The majority of whole-body vitamin A exists in esterified form, stored in the liver, mainly in stellate cells. This form of vitamin A is inactive but readily mobilized, and thus constitutes an important storage form that, when hydrolyzed, provides retinol for delivery throughout the body. Many extrahepatic tissues esterify and store retinyl esters in smaller pools, which may be crucial for the local generation of bioactive retinoids.

In contrast to retinol, retinoids possessing a carboxylic acid moiety are absorbed by the portal route bound to albumin. While diet contains little RA, the majority of retinoids used for cancer prevention and therapy are carboxylic acids (Fig. 1), and thus most clinically important retinoids are absorbed by the portal route. The plasma concentration of physiologically formed RA is normally in the low nanomolar range, but following vitamin A or retinoid treatment concentrations are significantly higher *(33, 34)*.

Retinol is esterified in the intestine, liver, eye, lung, testis, and other tissues by LRAT. In the liver, LRAT is sensitively regulated according to individual's vitamin A status, and RA is likely to mediate changes in LRAT gene expression. LRAT mRNA and enzyme activity are very low in vitamin A-deficient animals, while LRAT expression is rapidly induced after retinol or RA is administered *(29)*. The feedback regulation of LRAT by RA thus serves to divert retinol into storage, increasing the retinyl ester pool and decreasing the quantity of retinol available for oxidative metabolism (Fig. 2a).

Retinol oxidation is essential for activating the vitamin A molecule into its active forms, retinal and RA *(21, 30)*. A variety of enzymes with retinol dehydrogenase (RDH) and retinal dehydrogenase (RALDH) activities have been described as capable of forming retinal and at-RA. Multiple enzymes in each of these families exist, with different expression patterns, suggesting that RA formation is regulated in complex manner and by pathways that may differ among tissues. While retinol and retinal can be interconverted, the oxidation of retinal to at-RA is irreversible.

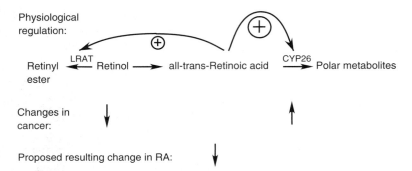

Fig. 2. Regulation of retinol esterification and oxidation by at-RA and proposed changes in cancer. Based on nutritional studies *(29)*, LRAT is kept in a tonic active state when RA is adequate, thus diverting retinol into storage, while CYP26 expression is rapidly and transiently up-regulated when the concentration of RA becomes elevated. In cancer, aberrant expression or the absence of LRAT leads to a lack of retinyl esters, from which bioactive retinoids are formed, and may induce overexpression of CYP26, leading to excessive degradation of RA *(56)*.

RA is catabolized in a sequential phase 1–phase 2 manner, with hydroxylation at C-4 or C-18 preceding conjugation, yielding metabolites such as RA-β-glucuronide *(21)*. A significant advance in understanding the oxidation of at-RA was made when the CYP26 gene family of RA-4-hydroxylases was cloned. at-RA was already known to induce its own metabolism. The CYP26A1 gene promoter has been shown to respond directly to all-*trans*-RA (see gene transactivation, see below). The isoform known as CYP26A1 is expressed in the liver and is highly inducible by RA *(35)*. It is also expressed at lower levels in extrahepatic tissues of the adult *(35)* and in the embryo where its expression pattern is consistent with a role in limiting signaling by all-*trans*-RA *(36)*. CYP26B1 is expressed in a pattern that overlaps with but still differs from CYP26A1. Other members of the cytochrome P-450 gene family have been suggested to play roles in the catabolism of RA, but less is known of their physiological significance. Once RA has been oxidized, it is conjugated to form water-soluble metabolites, which are readily excreted *(37)*. The expression of CYP26A1 and the efficiency of RA oxidation and formation of water-soluble metabolites in the liver was found to be significantly increased when rats were fed a vitamin A-supplemented diet *(37)* (Fig. 2b).

It has been suggested that at least some of the reactions of RA production and catabolism occur in a "cassette" manner, in which metabolic products formed by one enzyme are immediately channeled to become the substrates of other enzymes, resulting in further processing *(30)*. This may contribute to the overall efficiency of metabolism, and may explain why certain metabolites, such as all-*trans*-retinal, do not accumulate in most tissues, although the rate of flux through the pathway may be significant.

Retinoid receptors. Retinoic acid and its analogues are high-affinity ligands for nuclear hormone receptors of the retinoid receptor family. This family is comprised of two subfamilies, RAR (α, β, and γ) and RXR (α, β, and γ), which serve as transcription factors in the regulation of a large number of genes (see *(15, 38, 39)* for reviews). All-*trans*-RA is the principal natural ligand for the RAR. While exogenous 9-*cis*-RA, as mentioned earlier, binds effectively to the RXR its physiological role is not certain.

In some studies, the RAR–RXR complex with an RAR ligand is required for transactivation, but apparently a ligand for the RXR is not required. RXR proteins also form heterodimeric partners with several other nuclear receptors of the steroid hormone superfamily, including the vitamin D receptor, thyroid hormone receptor, receptors involved in the metabolism and regulatory functions of fatty acids, sterols and bile acids, and certain xenobiotics, and orphan receptors. One possible mode of regulation among different nuclear hormone receptors that interact with RXR may be the competition for a limited pool of RXR protein.

The RAR and RXR proteins are modular in structure, comprised of six defined regions, named A–F, and intermediate hinge regions, present in all of the receptors *(40)*. While the proteins in each receptor subfamily are well conserved overall, each subtype (α, β, and γ) of RAR and RXR differs somewhat, and isoforms, generated by the use of alternative promoters and/or differential RNA splicing, result in a further diversification of the receptors in different cells. For example, the RARβ receptor is expressed in four isoforms, where the mRNA for RARβ1 and RARβ3 is transcribed from an upstream 5' promoter, P1, while RARβ2 and RARβ4 mRNA are transcribed from another promoter, P2, located 20 mb downstream. Isoforms 1 vs. 3, and 2 vs. 4, are then formed by alternative splicing, resulting in proteins with different A regions but identical B–F regions in the 4 RARβ isoforms *(41)*. Other RAR protein and the RXR proteins also exist in isoforms. These differences are well conserved suggesting that the individual subtypes could have important but differential roles in gene regulation.

Mode of action of retinoids as regulators of gene transcription. Retinoids similar to at-RA, having a carboxylic acid functional group and an extended conformation, are potent ligands for the RAR family of nuclear retinoid receptors and often regulate gene expression when added to cells at concentrations in the low nanomolar range. Biochemical and structural studies have shown that a single retinoid molecule binds with high affinity to the ligand-binding domain (LBD) of the RAR, with the ligand's negatively charged carboxyl group coordinated with specific amino acids within the LBD pocket, so that the retinoid is positioned in a precise manner. X-ray crystallographic studies of the apo (with RA ligand) and holo (empty) forms of the LBD have shown that particular regions, especially alpha helix 12, are mobile. Helix 12 assumes an "open flap" position in the apo protein, but the flap is closed when RA is bound, forming an interior pocket *(40)*. Each RAR protein interacts with an RXR protein to form a heterodimeric complex of RAR–RXR, and the complex binds to specific DNA sequences through zinc fingers in the DNA-binding domain of each RAR and RXR. The ligand induced change in the position of RAR helix-12 results in an overall change in protein conformation that is critical for altering the surface interactions of the RAR–RXR complex with other proteins of the transcription regulatory complex, including coactivator/corepressor proteins or "mediators," that in turn regulate the basal transcriptional machinery including DNA-dependent RNA polymerase II (Pol-II) *(40)*. In the current general model, the RAR–RXR complex in the nonliganded state is already bound to DNA response elements (below) in a repressive state, associated with corepressors (e.g., N-CoR and SMRT) which recruit histone deacetylases, and thus result in a more compact and transcriptionally inactive form of chromatin. Ligand-dependent factors such as the receptor interacting protein RIP-140 may also be involved in keeping genes in a repressed state *(42)*. The binding of ligand(s) to the RAR–RXR complex is then thought to alter the conformation of the RAR–RXR complex in such a way that coactivator proteins are recruited. With the binding of coactivators (N-CoA, p300, or CBP) histone acetyl transferase activity is recruited to the complex resulting in the modification of histones, changes in chromatin structure, and recruitment of basal transcriptional factors, including Pol-II, which form the preinitiation complex required for the start of gene transcription *(40)*.

The canonical retinoic acid response element (RARE) motif is composed of two direct repeats of the hexameric nucleotide sequences, a/gggtca, separated by a spacer (n) of 2 or 5 nucleotides: a/gggtca(n)$_{2,5}$-a/ggtca *(40)*. Some RARE are located in the 5′ regulatory region of target genes near to the transcription start site, but others have also been found within introns or in regions quite distal from the basal promoter. However, while this general model is now well established, it is very likely that regulation in vivo is much more complex. Many more genes have been described to respond physiologically to RA than have been shown to contain an RARE and respond directly through ligand binding to RAR–RXR *(15)*. Moreover, there are undoubtedly additional layers of regulation that affect receptor function, including receptor protein phosphorylation, degradation, and shuttling of receptor proteins between the nuclear and cytoplasmic compartments *(39)*. Furthermore, RAR proteins sometime interact with other families of transcription factors. The antiproliferative activity demonstrated for RA may involve competition of the liganded RAR/RXR complex with the Jun-Fos (AP-1) transcription factor complex for binding to specific DNA sequences. Protein–protein interactions with a number of transcription factors of other gene families have also been noted *(39)*.

3. IN VITRO STUDIES IN CELLS AND ANIMALS – PREVENTION AND TREATMENT

Retinoids exert many of their effects on three major cellular processes: cell proliferation and growth regulation; cell differentiation, characterized by programs of cell-type specific gene expression; and, in some cells and with some retinoids, the induction of apoptosis. Most experiments have been conducted with cycling cells, often either transformed or malignant cells, and have been designed to test whether cell growth is inhibited and/or cell differentiation is promoted by retinoids. A wide variety of cell models have been studied. A few examples are given in Table 2, as the literature is too extensive to review comprehensively, and the principal findings of growth arrest and improved differentiation have been quite consistent regardless of the cell model studied.

In dividing cells, retinoids almost always reduce the rate of cell proliferation. The decision of cells to proliferate or differentiate is typically made in G1/G0 of the cell cycle. Mechanistic studies have shown reduced expression of genes and proteins encoding cyclins and cyclin-dependent kinases, increased expression of cyclin-dependent kinase inhibitory proteins, and increased expression of the retinoblastoma tumor suppressor protein (pRb), accompanied by a reduction in its phosphorylation status. In different cell models, the specific cyclin most affected has differed, for example, cyclins of the D family in some cells, cyclin E in others, etc., and, similarly, different cyclin inhibitory proteins have been the predominant ones increased, e.g., p27, p57, p21, p16, or p19. In nearly all cell models in which the cell cycle is inhibited, pRb expression

Table 2
Representative Cell Culture Studies Demonstrating Mechanisms Through Which Retinoids
May Inhibit Human Cancer Cells

Cell type	Major finding in RA-treated cells	References
HL-60 myeloblastic leukemia cells	Activation of extracellular signal-regulated kinase (ERK)-2 mitogen-activated protein kinase (MAPK) as an early event, required for growth arrest and induction of differentiation	Yen et al. (43)
THP-1 leukemia cell line	Increased Rb mRNA and protein levels while reducing Rb phosphorylation state; cyclin E reduced; p27 increased; functional differentiation of cells into macrophage-like phenotype	Chen and Ross (44)
CA-OV3 RA-sensitive ovarian carcinoma cells	Increased the levels of p27 and S10 phospho-p27, needed for RA-induced growth inhibition	Radu et al. (45)
Nt2/D1 embryonal carcinoma, germ cell cancer cells	Reduced cyclin D1/D2 transcription rates and protein levels, reduced Ki-67 staining and cell number	Freemantle et al. (46)
BEAS-2B human bronchial epithelial cells, and cells transformed by tobacco carcinogen	Inhibited transformation of carcinogen-treated cells and induced proteosome-mediated degradation of members of cyclin D family	Boyle et al. (47, 48)
CHP126 neuroblastoma cells	Cell cycle arrest and induced neurite outgrowth induced by 9-cis-RA, concomitant with reduction in cyclin-dependent kinase-activating kinase (CAK) phosphorylation of pRb and RXRα proteins	Zhang et al. (49)
NB4 APL leukemia cells	Inhibited the action of cyclin-dependent kinase-activating kinase (CAK) on PML–RARα protein and induced degradation of the CAK complex protein MAT1	Wang et al. (50)

has been increased, and/or its phosphorylation reduced (hypophosphorylation). Reduced phosphorylation enhances the ability of this "pocket" protein to sequester factors such as E2F required for progression of the cell cycle from the G1/G0 phase through the restriction point and into the S phase of the cell cycle (Fig. 3). These changes result in a prolongation of the G1 phase of the cell cycle and a reduced rate of entry into the S phase of the cycle. The results of many studies are consistent in showing a reduction in cell cycle progression and in cell counts in retinoid-treated cells as compared to untreated cells.

Retinoic acid has also been shown to regulate the cyclin-dependent kinase-activating kinase (CAK), which regulates exit from the G1 phase of the cell cycle (Table 2). The CAK complex can interact with and phosphorylate pRb and at least certain retinoid receptors. When neuroblastoma cells were treated with 1–5 μM 9-*cis*-RA, CAK activity was reduced, as shown by decreased CAK activity, hypophosphorylation of Rb and RXRα, reduced proliferation and morphological evidence of neuronal cell differentiation *(49)*. In NB4 cells, a model of APL leukemia, at-RA reduced CAK abundance and activity, the level of the aberrant receptor PML–RARα, which these cells express, and these changes were associated with a reduction in cell proliferation and induction of myeloid cell-type differentiation *(50)*. An RA-induced induction of proteolysis was observed in these studies and in others reviewed by Dragnev et al. *(51)*.

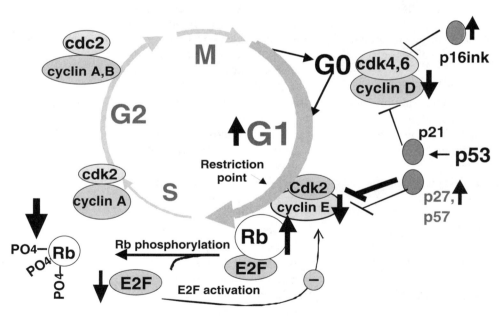

Fig. 3. Prominent effects of RA on the cell division cycle. A schematic of the cell cycle, with frequently observed effects in cells treated with RA shown as *up and down arrows*. Cdk, cyclin-dependent kinase; Rb, retinoblastoma protein; E2FE, transcription factor involved in G1 to M (mitosis)-transition. Generally consistent effects of RA include reduction in expression of G0 and G1 cyclins; increase in cyclin-dependent kinase inhibitors (p16, p21, p27, p57); increased Rb and decreased hyperphosphorylated form of Rb; increased fraction of G1 and decreased fraction of S (synthesis) and M phase cells.

Retinoids almost always either induce cell differentiation or they drive cells into apoptosis. Cell differentiation may be the consequence of the increased time in the G1 phase of the cell cycle when cell cycling is slowed, allowing some cells to "escape" the cell cycle and enter a program of differentiation. The features of cell differentiation observed depend, unsurprisingly, on the cell model studied, but they nearly always include alteration in gene expression as well as phenotypic changes consistent with a more mature cell type. The induction of apoptosis is a more varied finding and may depend on the retinoid used, type of cell, stage of differentiation, or presence of other regulatory factors. CD437, a retinoid with selectivity for RAR-γ, and fenretinide (4-HPR), a retinoid that appears to function independently of receptor binding, have been shown to induce apoptosis in several cancer cell models (52, 53). Recently, new rexinoids were tested. In B lymphoma cells, certain features of the RXR domain structure and RXR signaling were found to be essential for the induction of caspase activation and apoptosis (54).

The interpretation of results from cell culture studies needs to be made cautiously, and especially so if the retinoid concentrations employed have exceeded those normally found in vivo. Additionally, due to the lipophilic nature of most retinoids, an organic solvent such as ethanol or dimethylsulfoxide is required to dissolve the retinoids prior to their dispersion into tissue culture medium. Whereas the concentration of RA in human plasma is on the order of 10–50 nM, many experiments with culture cells have utilized RA concentrations of 1 μM or higher, with a serum concentration of 5–10%. Nevertheless, cell studies have been important for identifying alterations in retinoid signaling in tumor cells, some of which have been confirmed in cancer tissue specimens.

Aberrant retinoid signaling in cancer cells and tissues. A number of cancer cell lines, compared to nontransformed cells, have exhibited aberrant retinoid signaling (55–57). One of the most often affected genes is RAR-β, especially the isoform RARβ2. Loss of expression of RAR-β2 during cancer development is often associated with tumorigenesis and with retinoid resistance, while conversely, induction of its expression can suppress carcinogenesis (57). Expression of another isoform, RAR-β4, which includes only a short four amino acid section of the N-terminal A-domain that is important for protein–protein interactions and phosphorylation (39, 41), is increased in various types of cancer (56). RAR-β4 transgenic mice developed hyperplasia and neoplasia in various tissues, and induction of RAR-β4 expression increased the growth of tumor cells that do not express RAR-β2. In patients during breast cancer progression, RAR-β2 is reduced or lost (58) and hypermethylation of the 5′-region is thought to be responsible for the silencing of the RARβ gene. Silencing of RAR-β2 by gene methylation was reported to be an early event in head and neck carcinogenesis (59) and in other cancers (56).

Other receptors, enzymes, and retinoid-binding proteins have been reported to be aberrantly expressed or silenced in cancer cells and cancer tissue specimens (56). Besides RAR-β, other retinoid-related factors that are often reduced include LRAT, CRBP-I, RALDH2, and ALDH genes, required for retinoid storage and activation. Conversely, the catabolism of RA may be increased by overexpression of CYP26, as has been observed in colorectal cancer cells (56).

The totality of evidence thus suggests that the abnormal biology of cancer cells is often associated with abnormalities in vitamin A-related metabolism. However, whether these changes are consequence of transformation or whether impaired retinoid storage is part of cancer induction must still be determined.

Animal studies. A number of animal models of carcinogenesis have been used to determine if vitamin A or retinoids can reduce the onset or severity of tumors. Numerous models were employed in the 1970–1980s as previously reviewed *(60)*, and several results were promising enough to serve as an impetus for human clinical trials. Most animal studies used chemical carcinogens, either direct acting or requiring activation to induce tumors, while retinoids were supplied at levels of 1–2 mmol retinoid per kg of diet, sometimes starting before carcinogen exposure. Retinoid treatment did not abrogate tumor formation but several retinoids reproducibly reduced the number, multiplicity, or size of tumors. A few of the early studies investigated dietary vitamin A (retinol, retinyl palmitate (RP), or retinyl acetate) for chemoprevention, but at the doses tested the growth of the animals was significantly impaired or signs of vitamin A toxicity were observed, and so few later studies investigated these forms. Studies then turned to diets supplemented with at-RA, 13-*cis*-RA, or 9-*cis*-RA, or novel retinoids such as fenretinide/4-HPR. Several of these compounds were reported to inhibit the growth of bladder, mammary gland, and other tumors *(60)*. 4-HPR proved to be much better tolerated.

A recent study represents a different approach. McDaniel et al. *(61)* developed a human food-based rodent diet, composed with fruits and vegetables that give rise to vitamin A during digestion, to investigate the effects of vitamin A on adolescent rat mammary gland development and the subsequent risk for mammary carcinogenesis, induced by treatment with methylnitrosourea (MNU). A diet enriched in RP was used for comparison. The adolescent growth period was studied, as it is characterized by rapid body growth, sexual maturation, and mammary gland development, correlating with puberty in humans. Compared with adolescent rats that consumed an adequate diet, rats that consumed the natural foods diet and the RP diet had a reduced multiplicity of mammary cancers, associated with a reduction in alveolar gland development. The food-based diet also suppressed the onset of sexual maturation and inhibited markers of mammary alveoli formation more than the RP diet. Six months after treatment with MNU, latency and incidence of mammary tumors did not differ among dietary groups, but tumor multiplicity was reduced in rats fed either natural food-based or RP diets during adolescence. The results of this study suggest that the amount and source of vitamin A consumed in the adolescent period can influence the onset of puberty, mammary gland alveolar development, and risk of breast cancer. Since it has been suggested that a diet rich in fruits and vegetables may reduce breast cancer risk, these experimental results appear congruent. It is possible that components of the diet besides vitamin A contributed to the observed effects, although the results with the RP-enriched diet were similar to those for the whole foods-based diet.

Another recent approach has been to focus on RXR-selective agonists (rexinoids). Liby et al. *(62)* reported that in the A/J mouse model of lung cancer, a rexinoid known as NRX194204 significantly reduced the number and size of lung surface tumors and total tumor volume by 64–81%. This compound also delayed tumorigenesis in mouse mammary tumor virus-*neu* mice. The latter finding is encouraging, as in a study of *neu* mice treated long term with an implanted RA pellet, tumor growth was reported to be increased *(32)*.

Overall, animal studies of retinoids are continuing, with focus on newer diets approaches and new retinoids that seem promising at lower doses. The majority of evidence from animal studies supports a reduction in tumorigenesis with retinoid treatment, with a minority of studies showing no effect or an increase.

4. EPIDEMIOLOGICAL AND INTERVENTIONAL STUDIES

Hong and Itri *(63)* have thoroughly reviewed epidemiological, therapeutic, and prevention trials of human cancers involving vitamin A and a number of synthetic retinoids through the mid-1990s. Ross *(64)* has reviewed the epidemiology literature on dietary vitamin A and cancer risk. While epidemiological studies have long pointed to an inverse association between vitamin A and cancer risk, many of these studies concerned carotenoids. The preponderance of data supported reduced cancer risk from the consumption of a diet rich in fruits and vegetables, and therefore carotene, but there was little evidence for a relationship with dietary retinol. Both reviews noted strengths and weaknesses of epidemiological studies with vitamin A. Survey studies of vitamin A intake are inherently complicated due to vitamin A being consumed in part as carotenoids, often grouped with other antioxidant vitamins, and in part as preformed retinol in foods of animal origin and supplements. Food frequency questionnaires are imperfect tools for capturing vitamin A intake. Most are only qualitative or semi-quantitative, and thus the inferred data on vitamin A consumption is likely to be weak. Associations of cancer risk with serum retinol were also weak *(63, 64)*. In fact, a weak relationship could be anticipated because serum retinol concentrations are maintained at a relatively constant level over a wide range of vitamin A status *(21)*. Moreover, if a lower retinol level is measured after disease has developed it could be a consequence of cancer rather than a predictor. More recent reports from epidemiological studies on the prevention of prostate *(65)* and breast cancers *(66)* concluded that higher dietary intakes of fruits and vegetables and vitamin A were not associated with prevention of these cancers. Thus, overall the epidemiological evidence for reducing cancer risk by consuming foods containing provitamin A carotenoids or preformed vitamin A is quite weak.

Interventional studies of retinoids for cancer chemoprevention or therapy have been conducted for over three decades. For established cancers, most clinical trials have been disappointing. A review of phase III clinical trials of lung cancer prevention concluded that β-carotene, retinol, and 13-*cis*-RA (as well as other agents tested) did not demonstrate beneficial, reproducible results *(67)*. Retinol combined with zinc did not reduce liver cancer mortality in a randomized double-blind study of hepatocellular cancer in Linxian, China *(68)*. A Cochrane review of trials in which at-RA and 4-HPR were tested for prevention of progression of cervical neoplasia concluded the retinoids were not effective *(69)*.

For premalignancies, vitamin A and retinoids may have a benefit. A Cochrane review of various interventions for treating oral leukoplakia concluded that treatment with β-carotene, lycopene, and vitamin A or retinoids, was associated with significant rates of clinical resolution, compared with placebo or no treatment, although there was no evidence that any of the treatments prevented malignant transformation of leukoplakia *(70)*. For premalignant actinic keratoses, topical retinoids have provided some benefit *(71)*.

However, in a chemoprevention study using biomarkers to assess proliferative changes in the bronchial epithelium of former smokers, 13-*cis*-RA and α-tocopherol, but not 9-*cis*-RA, reduced the intermediate marker of cell proliferation, Ki-67 *(72)*. In another study of current and former smokers, 50,000 IU/d of retinol for 6 months did not up-regulate RAR-β, which as noted above is frequently silenced in cancer, or improve surrogate biomarkers of bronchial dysplasia *(73)*.

One type of cancer stands out for being a remarkable success. The demonstration that APL patients treated with at-RA can result in a high rate of response and complete remission was first demonstrated in a clinical study in Shanghai, China *(2)*, and has since been replicated in several trials in the USA, Europe, and Asia *(74)*. This unanticipated result has led to the use of at-RA for "differentiation therapy," as an important clinical treatment for this disease. APL is a unique form of cancer because a high proportion of patients have a specific chromosomal translocation that results in a break in the RARα gene, located on chromosome 17, and its fusion with another gene, often the PML gene on chromosome 15. In most cases, two abnormal fusion products, RARα–PML and PML–RARα, are formed from this t(15:17) translocation. PML is also a transcription factor. The PML–RARα protein binds to DNA but functions as a dominant negative receptor, interfering with normal RARα signaling *(75)*. Treatment with at-RA is thought to induce the differentiation of precursor cells that have retained a normal copy of the RAR gene, facilitating their progressive differentiation to more mature granulocytic cells, while leukemic cells containing the mutation are induced to undergo apoptosis. Despite the success of at-RA in inducing of cell differentiation, prolonged treatment with at-RA is not well tolerated. About 15% of patients treated with at-RA developed a severe and sometimes fatal thromboembolytic condition, referred to as retinoic acid syndrome *(76)*. Other patients have relapsed after treatment and become refractory to at-RA *(77)*. Clinical protocols have been revised to shorten the length of treatment with at-RA while combining it with other forms of chemotherapy, such as with arsenic trioxide or cisplatin.

Tissue specificity. Essentially all nucleated cells express RAR and RXR proteins. It is usual for one or more of these receptor forms to be predominant within a cell type; however, two or more forms may be co-expressed. For example, RARγ is more highly expressed in skin, while RARα has a broader tissue distribution. Although there are hints that the individual receptor types may differ somewhat in their functions, no single receptor has been shown to be indispensable, and the general mechanism of RA action does not appear to be tissue specific. Rather, the differences in tissue response to RA are likely to depend on factors such as ligand availability and the state of chromatin accessibility. Ligand availability is closely related to nutritional status, as an adequate supply of retinol substrate is a prerequisite for the endogenous production of RA. Substrate uptake could depend on the state of vascularization of the tissue or tumor and on the expression of enzymes required for RA production. Thus, *metabolic factors* leading to retinoid availability, as well as *cell-intrinsic properties* like nuclear receptor subtypes and relative amounts, coactivator/corepressor expression levels, and chromatin availability, are likely to interact in ways that determine tissue-specific patterns of retinoid-regulated gene expression.

Totality of the evidence. The totality of evidence suggests that production of RA from its natural nutritional precursor, retinol, is under sensitive control by retinoid-binding proteins, LRAT, CYP26, and other enzymes. Together, the actions of these proteins serve to maintain a consistent level and tissue distribution of at-RA that, presumably, is appropriate for the cell type and the organism as a whole.

Good nutrition plays a key role in providing adequate, but not excessive, amounts of substrate (retinol stored as retinyl ester) for bioactivation, thus regulating the production of retinal and RA. From these overall features of retinoid metabolism it can be inferred that maintaining a one's dietary intake of vitamin A in a healthful range is a key component for maintaining tissues in an optimally differentiated state.

As noted above, exogenous RA or other retinoids may be helpful in the chemoprevention of premalignancies, but agents like at-RA are not acceptable for long-term treatment. In the case of fenretinide/4-HPR, which is relatively well tolerated, another problem has surfaced, namely low plasma retinol due to impairment of the RBP–retinol transport system (3, 78). This illustrates that retinoids have the potential to alter the metabolism of diet-derived vitamin A in ways that were not anticipated. It is quite possible that the "best" retinoids are those formed in situ, in a well-regulated process from diet-derived substrates. Thus maintaining an adequate but not excessive dietary intake, and thus an adequate but not excessive pool of retinol substrate in tissues, should be a first principle of good nutrition.

5. FUTURE RESEARCH DIRECTIONS

The differentiation promoting activity of at-RA and other retinoids is still very attractive for cancer treatment. It can be confidently concluded that retinoids do "work" in isolated cells, so how can they be made more effective in vivo? A major challenge is to harness and direct the power of these agents into effective dietary and/or clinical interventions. Several novel ideas for targeting retinoids to tissues are under investigation in preclinical models. Patches, biofilms, the delivery of retinoid on nanoparticles, aerosolized retinoids, etc., all are based on the concept of maintaining a local exposure, in a targeted manner, while minimizing the diffuse spread and total-body exposure to retinoids that occurs when they are administered systemically. New combinations of retinoids with other therapies, similar to the combined use of conventional chemotherapeutic drugs or arsenic trioxide with at-RA in the treatment of APL, also could be promising. Recently, retinoids have gained new interest from the perspective of stem cell biology and regenerative medicine, due to their strong differentiation-promoting actions on immature progenitor cells. For example, retinol promoted differentiation in progenitor cells of mouse pancreas, increasing β-cell differentiation and insulin production (79). The generally positive effects of retinoids that have been observed in cell culture models suggest that they could be used effectively to promote the differentiation of stem, precursor, or progenitor cells ex vivo, prior to the transfer of cells to the patient.

6. CONCLUSIONS AND RECOMMENDATIONS FOR INTAKE/DIETARY CHANGES

The current nutritional recommendations for dietary vitamin A (retinol) are well supported by biological evidence that consumption of retinol at the recommended levels is both safe and adequate for supporting vision and maintaining the other systemic functions of vitamin A. The Recommended Dietary Allowance (RDA) for vitamin A is based on a factorial model that includes intake of enough vitamin A to build up adequate, but not excessive, tissue vitamin A reserves *(80)*. The Tolerable Upper Intake Level (UL) was established by the Institute of Medicine in 2002 *(80)* as a way to inform the public that excessive intakes of certain nutrients (above ~ 3,000 μg/day of preformed retinol) could lead over time to adverse effects. For vitamin A, the UL for adults was set at 3,000 μg/day of preformed retinol because higher amounts may cause liver damage, increase the risk of birth defects in women of child-bearing age, and possibly increase the risk of osteoporosis. To eliminate these risks, a person could chose to consume more of his or her vitamin A intake in the form of β-carotene, instead of preformed retinol, since consumption of β-carotene at nutritional levels poses no risk of toxicity. Based on the cancer literature reviewed in this chapter, there is no compelling evidence to suggest that increasing the intake of dietary vitamin A above currently recommended levels (i.e., RDA levels) will reduce the risk of developing cancer. Many epidemiological studies have, however, shown that cancer risk is reduced in individuals who consume a diet high in fruits and vegetables, which contains vitamin A as β-carotene, is relatively low in fats, and also contains a mixture of phytonutrients, some of which may have anticancer properties of their own. This type of diet provides most if not all of the vitamin A therein in the form of carotenoids. The 2002 IOM report on vitamin A included sample calculations to show that an RDA level of vitamin A can be obtained from a well-selected vegetarian or vegan diet, as well as from a mixed-type omnivorous diet. The published examples provide evidence that consumption of retinol per se is not required to meet the RDA for vitamin A.

Conversely, high intakes of retinol are potentially deleterious. Case reports and experimental studies have thoroughly documented adverse effects of hypervitaminosis A, while new and accumulating data from epidemiological studies suggest that intakes of retinol from diet and supplements at levels even moderately above the RDA may increase bone loss *(81)*. Based on research in animals, high dietary vitamin A and treatment with RA are expected to affect retinoid homeostasis by inducing genes in the cytochrome P-450 family that result in increased retinoid catabolism.

Overall, there is no compelling evidence that changing current recommendations for dietary vitamin A would be helpful in reducing cancer risk. A report of an NIH State-of-the-Science Conference on the topic of "Multivitamin/Mineral Supplements and Chronic Disease Prevention" (which was not specific to vitamin A or to cancer prevention) concluded that while supplement use has grown and now more than half of the adult population of the USA uses multivitamin/mineral supplements, most of the studies that were reviewed do not provide strong evidence for health-related effects. The report also noted weaknesses in the methodologies for assessing nutrient intake from supplements and from fortified foods *(82)*. At present there is no scientific rationale to suggest that personalized nutritional recommendations for vitamin A would be beneficial. Thus it seems prudent to follow the Dietary Guidelines, which stress obtaining nutrients from whole foods in a mixed diet, at levels near the RDA. The "5-a-Day" recommendation for including five servings of fruits and vegetables, provided these servings include green leafy and yellow vegetables, should supply all the dietary vitamin A now known to be required to meet the body's requirement for this micronutrient.

ACKNOWLEDGMENTS

Research support from NIH NCI grant R01-90214 is gratefully acknowledged. Acknowledgment is extended to the authors of many publications of importance in this area whose work is not cited. It was necessary to select examples, and thus many excellent contributions are not mentioned.

REFERENCES

1. Sporn, M.B., and Roberts, A.B. (1985) Introduction: What is a retinoid? In: Retinoids, Differentiation, and Disease. London: Pitman.
2. Huang, M., Ye, Y., Chen, S. et al. (1988) Use of all-trans retinoic acid in the treatment of acute promyelocytic leukemia. *Blood* **72**, 567–72.
3. Formelli, F., Carsana, R., Costa, A. et al. (1989) Plasma retinol level reduction by the synthetic retinoid fenretinide: A one year follow-up study of breast cancer patients. *Cancer Res* **49**, 6149–52.
4. Ross, A.C., and Harrison, E.H. (2007) Vitamin A: Nutritional aspects of retinoids and carotenoids. In: Zempleni, J., Rucker, R.B., McCormick, D.B., and Suttie, J.W., eds. Handbook of Vitamins. 4th ed., 1–40, Boca Raton: Taylor & Francis Group.
5. Berni, R., Clerici, M., Malpeli, G., Cleris, L., and Formelli, F. (1993) Retinoids: In vitro interaction with retinol-binding protein and influence on plasma retinol. *FASEB J* **7**, 1179–84.
6. Ritter, S.J., and Smith, J.E. (1996) Multiple retinoids alter liver bile salt-independent retinyl ester hydrolase activity, serum vitamin A and serum retinol-binding protein of rats. *Biochim Biophys Acta* **1291**, 228–36.
7. Wolbach, S.B., and Howe, P.R. (1925) Tissue changes following deprivation of fat-soluble A vitamin. *J Exp Med* **42**, 753–77.
8. Wong, Y.-C., and Buck, R.C. (1971) An electron microscopic study of metaplasia of the rat trachea epithelium in vitamin A deficiency. *Lab Invest* **24**, 55–66.
9. Dowling, J.E., and Wald, G. (1960) The biological function of vitamin A acid. *Proc Natl Acad Sci U S A* **46**, 587–608.
10. Strickland, S., and Mahdavi, V. (1978) The induction of differentiation in teratocarcinoma stem cells by retinoic acid. *Cell* **15**, 393–403.
11. Breitman, T.R., Collins, S.J., and Keene, B.R. (1981) Terminal differentiation of human promyelocytic leukemic cells in primary culture in response to retinoic acid. *Blood* **57**, 1000–04.
12. Giguère, V., Ong, E.S., Segui, P., and Evans, R.M. (1987) Identification of a receptor for the morphogen retinoic acid. *Nature* **330**, 624–29.
13. Petkovich, M., Brand, N.J., Krust, A., and Chambon, P. (1987) A human retinoic acid receptor which belongs to the family of nuclear receptors. *Nature* **330**, 444–50.
14. Blondel, A., Renaud, J.P., Fischer, S., Moras, D., and Karplus, M. (1999) Retinoic acid receptor: A simulation analysis of retinoic acid binding and the resulting conformational changes. *J Mol Biol* **291**, 101–15.
15. Balmer, J.E., and Blomhoff, R. (2002) Gene expression regulation by retinoic acid. *J Lipid Res* **43**, 1773–808.
16. Eckhoff, C., and Nau, H. (1990) Identification and quantitation of all-*trans*- and 13-*cis*-retinoic acid and 13-*cis*-4-oxoretinoic acid in human plasma. *J Lipid Res* **31**, 1445–54.
17. Blaner, W.S. (2001) Cellular metabolism and actions of 13-cis-retinoic acid. *J Am Acad Dermatol* **45**, S129–S35.
18. Dawson, M.I., and Zhang, X. (2002) Discovery and design of retinoic acid receptor and retinoid X receptor class- and subtype-selective synthetic analogs of all-trans-retinoic acid and 9-cis-retinoic acid. *Curr Med Chem* **9**, 6232–637.
19. Benbrook, D.M. (2002) Refining retinoids with heteroatoms. *Mini Rev Med Chem* **2**, 277–83.
20. Kurlandsky, S.B., Duell, E.A., Kang, S., Voorhees, J.J., and Fisher, G.J. (1996) Auto-regulation of retinoic acid biosynthesis through regulation of retinol esterification in human keratinocytes. *J Biol Chem* **271**, 15346–52.

21. Ross, A.C., Zolfaghari, R., and Weisz, J. (2001) Vitamin A: Recent advances in the biotransformation, transport, and metabolism of retinoids. *Curr Opin Gastroent* **17**, 184–92.
22. Goodall, A.H., Fisher, D., and Lucy, J.A. (1980) Cell fusion, haemolysis and mitochondrial swelling induced by retinol and derivatives. *Biochim Biophys Acta* **595**, 9–14.
23. Russell, R.M. (2000) The vitamin A spectrum: From deficiency to toxicity. *Am J Clin Nutr* **71**, 878–84.
24. Soprano, D.R., and Soprano, K.J. (1995) Retinoids as teratogens. *Annu Rev Nutr* **15**, 111–32.
25. Ross, A.C. (2005) Introduction to vitamin A: A nutritional and life cycle perspective. In: Carotenoids and Retinoids: Molecular Aspects and Health Issues. 23–41, Champaign, IL: AOCS Press.
26. Soprano, D.R., and Blaner, W.S. (1994) Plasma retinol-binding protein. In: Sporn, M.B., Roberts, A.B., and Goodman, D.S., eds. The Retinoids: Biology, Chemistry and Medicine. 257–81, New York: Raven Press.
27. Kawaguchi, R., Yu, J., Honda, J. et al. (2007) A membrane receptor for retinol binding protein mediates cellular uptake of vitamin A. *Science* **315**, 820–25.
28. Craig, R.L., Chu, W.S., and Elbein, S.C. (2007) Retinol binding protein 4 as a candidate gene for type 2 diabetes and prediabetic intermediate traits. *Mol Genet Metab* **90**, 338–44.
29. Ross, A.C., and Zolfaghari, R. (2004) Regulation of hepatic retinol metabolism: Perspectives from studies on vitamin A status. *J Nutr* **134**, 269S–75S.
30. Napoli, J.L. (2000) Enzymology and biogenesis of retinoic acid. In: Livrea, M.A., ed. Vitamin A and Retinoids: An Update of Biological Aspects and Clinical Applications. 17–27, Basel: Birkhèuser Verlag.
31. Ghyselinck, N.B., Båvik, C., Sapin, V. et al. (1999) Cellular retinol-binding protein I is essential for vitamin A homeostasis. *EMBO J* **18**, 4903–14.
32. Budhu, A.S., and Noy, N. (2002) Direct channeling of retinoic acid between cellular retinoic acid-binding protein II and retinoic acid receptor sensitizes mammary carcinoma cells to retinoic acid-induced growth arrest. *Mol Cell Biol* **22**, 2632–41.
33. Eckhoff, C., Collins, M.D., and Nau, H. (1991) Human plasma all-*trans*-, 13-*cis*- and 13-*cis*-4-oxoretinoic acid profiles during subchronic vitamin A supplementation: Comparison to retinol and retinyl ester plasma levels. *J Nutr* **121**, 1016–25.
34. Teerlink, T., Copper, M.P., Klaassen, I., and Braakhuis, B.J.M. (1997) Simultaneous analysis of retinol, all-*trans*- and 13-*cis*-retinoic acid and 13-cis-4-oxoretinoic acid in plasma by liquid chromatography using on-column concentration after single-phase fluid extraction. *J Chromatogr B Biomed Sci Appl* **694**, 83–92.
35. Wang, Y., Zolfaghari, R., and Ross, A.C. (2002) Cloning of rat cytochrome P450RAI (CYP26) cDNA and regulation of its gene expression by all-*trans*-retinoic acid in vivo. *Arch Biochem Biophys* **401**, 235–43.
36. Ribes, V., Fraulob, V., Petkovich, M., and Dolle, P. (2007) The oxidizing enzyme CYP26a1 tightly regulates the availability of retinoic acid in the gastrulating mouse embryo to ensure proper head development and vasculogenesis. *Dev Dyn* **236**, 644–53.
37. Cifelli, C.J., and Ross, A.C. (2007) Chronic vitamin A status and acute repletion with retinyl palmitate are determinants of the distribution and catabolism of all-trans-retinoic acid in rats. *J Nutr* **137**, 63–70.
38. Altucci, L., and Gronemeyer, H. (2001) Nuclear receptors in cell life and death. *Trends Endocr Metab* **12**, 460–68.
39. Rochette-Egly, C. (2003) Nuclear receptors: Integration of multiple signalling pathways through phosphorylation. *Cell Signal* **15**, 355–66.
40. Bastien, J., and Rochette-Egly, C. (2004) Nuclear retinoid receptors and the transcription of retinoid-target genes. *Gene* **328**, 1–16.
41. Zelent, A., Mendelsohn, C., Kastner, P. et al. (1991) Differentially expressed isoforms of the mouse retinoic acid receptor β are generated by usage of two promoters and alternative splicing. *EMBO J* **10**, 71–81.
42. Wei, L.N. (2004) Retinoids and receptor interacting protein 140 (RIP140) in gene regulation. *Curr Med Chem* **11**, 1241–53.

43. Yen, A., Robertson, M.S., Varvayanis, S., and Lee, A.T. (1998) Retinoic acid induced mitogen-activated protein (MAP)/extracellular regulated kinase (ERK)-dependent MAP kinase activation needed to elicit HL-60 cell differentiation and growth arrest. *Cancer Res* **58**, 3163–72.

44. Chen, Q.Y., and Ross, A.C. (2004) Retinoic acid regulates cell cycle progression and cell differentiation in human monocytic THP-1 cells. *Exp Cell Res* **297**, 68–81.

45. Radu, M., Soprano, D.R., and Soprano, K.J. (2008) S10 phosphorylation of p27 mediates atRA induced growth arrest in ovarian carcinoma cell lines. *J Cell Physiol* **217**, 558–68.

46. Freemantle, S.J., Veseva, A.V., Ewings, K.E. et al. (2007) Repression of cyclin D1 as a target for germ cell tumors. *Int J Oncol* **30**, 333–40.

47. Boyle, J.O., Langenfeld, J., Lonardo, F. et al. (1996) Cyclin D1 proteolysis: A retinoid chemoprevention signal in normal, immortalized, and transformed human bronchial epithelial cells. *J Natl Cancer Inst* **91**, 373–79.

48. Ma, Y., Feng, Q., Sekula, D., Diehl, J.A., Freemantle, S.J., and Dmitrovsky, E. (2005) Retinoid targeting of different D-type cyclins through distinct chemoprevention mechanisms. *Cancer Res* **65**, 6476–83.

49. Zhang, S., He, Q., Peng, H., Tedeschi-Blok, N., Triche, T.J., and Wu, L. (2004) MAT1-modulated cyclin-dependent kinase-activating kinase activity cross-regulates neuroblastoma cell G1 arrest and neurite outgrowth. *Cancer Res* **64**, 2977–83.

50. Wang, J., Barsky, L.W., Cavicioni, E. et al. (2006) Retinoic acid induces leukemia cell G1 arrest and transition into differentiation by inhibiting cyclin-dependent kinase-activating kinase binding and phosphorylation of PML/RARα. *FASEB J* **20**, E1495–E505.

51. Dragnev, K.H., Petty, W.J., and Dmitrovsky, E. (2003) Retinoid targets in cancer therapy and chemoprevention. *Cancer Biol Ther* **2**(Supp 1), S150–S56.

52. Sun, S.Y., Yue, P., Chandraratna, R.A.S., Tesfaigzi, Y., Hong, W.K., and Lotan, R. (2000) Dual mechanisms of action of the retinoid CD437: Nuclear retinoic acid receptor-mediated suppression of squamous differentiation and receptor-independent induction of apoptosis in UMSCC22B human head and neck squamous cell carcinoma cells. *Mol Pharm* **58**, 508–14.

53. Golubkov, V., Garcia, A., and Markland, F.S. (2005) Action of fenretinide (4-HPR) on ovarian cancer and endothelial cells. *Anticancer Res* **25**, 249–53.

54. Qin, S., Okawa, Y., Atangan, L.I., Brown, G., Chandraratna, R.A., and Zhao, Y. (2008) Integrities of A/B and C domains of RXR are required for rexinoid-induced caspase activations and apoptosis. *J Steroid Biochem Mol Biol* Aug 9. [Epub ahead of print].

55. Soprano, D.R., Qin, P., and Soprano, K.J. (2004) Retinoic acid receptors and cancers. *Annu Rev Nutr* **24**, 201–21.

56. Mongan, N.P., and Gudas, L. (2007) Diverse actions of retinoid receptors in cancer prevention and treatment. *Differentiation* **75**, 853–70.

57. Xu, X.C. (2007) Tumor-suppressive activity of retinoic acid receptor-beta in cancer. *Cancer Lett* **253**, 14–24.

58. Widschwendter, M., Berger, J., Müller, H.M., Zeimet, A.G., and Marth, C. (2001) Epigenetic down-regulation of the retinoic acid receptor-beta2 gene in breast cancer. *J Mammary Gland Biol Neoplasia* **6**, 193–201.

59. Youssef, E.M., Lotan, D., Issa, J.P. et al. (2004) Hypermethylation of the retinoic acid receptor-beta(2) gene in head and neck carcinogenesis. *Clin Cancer Res* **10**, 1733–42.

60. Moon, R.C., Mehta, R.G., and Rao, K.V.N. (1994) Retinoids and cancer in experimental animals. In: Sporn, M.B., Roberts, A.B., and Goodman, D.S., eds. The Retinoids: Biology, Chemistry and Medicine. 573–96, New York: Raven Press.

61. McDaniel, S.M., O'Neill, C., Metz, R.P. et al. (2007) Whole-food sources of vitamin A more effectively inhibit female rat sexual maturation, mammary gland development, and mammary carcinogenesis than retinyl palmitate. *J Nutr* **137**, 1415–22.

62. Liby, K., Royce, D.B., Risingsong, R. et al. (2007) A new rexinoid, NRX194204, prevents carcinogenesis in both the lung and mammary gland. *Clin Cancer Res* **13**, 6237–43.

63. Hong, W.K., and Itri, L.M. (1994) Retinoids and human cancer. In: Sporn, M.B., Roberts, A.B., and Goodman, D.S., eds. The Retinoids: Biology, Chemistry and Medicine. 597–630, New York: Raven Press.

64. Ross, A.C. (1994) Vitamin A and cancer. In: Carroll, K.K., and Kritchevsky, D., eds. Nutrition and Disease Update Cancer. 27–109, Champaign, IL: AOCS Press.

65. Ambrosini, G.L., de Klerk, N.H., Fritschi, L., Mackerras, D., and Musk, B. (2008) Fruit, vegetable, vitamin A intakes, and prostate cancer risk. *Prostate Cancer Prostatic Dis* **11**, 61–66.

66. Michels, K.B., Mohllajee, A.P., Roset-Bahmanyar, E., Beehler, G.P., and Moysich, K.B. (2007) Diet and breast cancer: A review of the prospective observational studies. *Cancer* **109**(Suppl 12), 2712–49.

67. Gray, J., Mao, J.T., Szabo, E. et al. (2007) Lung cancer chemoprevention: ACCP evidence-based clinical practice guidelines (2nd Edition). *Chest* **132**(Suppl 3), 56S–68S.

68. Qu, C.X., Kamangar, F., Fan, J.H. et al. (2007) Chemoprevention of primary liver cancer: A randomized, double-blind trial in Linxian, China. *J Natl Cancer Inst* **99**, 1240–47.

69. Helm, C.W., Lorenz, D.J., Meyer, N.J., Rising, W.R., and Wulff, J.L. (2007) Retinoids for preventing the progression of cervical intra-epithelial neoplasia. *Cochrane Database Syst Rev* Oct 17; CD003296.

70. Lodi, G., Sardella, A., Bez, C., Demarosi, F., and Carrassi, A. (2006) Interventions for treating oral leukoplakia. *Cochrane Database Syst Rev* (4) Oct 18; CD001829.

71. Weinberg, J.M. (2006) Topical therapy for actinic keratoses: Current and evolving therapies. *Rev Recent Clin Trials* **1**, 53–60.

72. Hittelman, W.N., Lui, D.D., Kurie, J.M. et al. (2007) Proliferative changes in the bronchial epithelium of former smokers treated with retinoids. *J Natl Cancer Inst* **99**, 1603–12.

73. Lam, S., Xu, X., Parker-Klein, H. et al. (2003) Surrogate end-point biomarker analysis in a retinol chemoprevention trial in current and former smokers with bronchial dysplasia. *Int J Oncol* **23**, 1607–13.

74. Soignet, S., Fleischauer, A., Polyak, T., Heller, G., and Warrell, R.P., Jr. (1997) All-*trans* retinoic acid significantly increases 5-year survival in patients with acute promyelocytic leukemia: Long-term follow-up of the New York study. *Cancer Chemother Pharm* **40**(Suppl), S25–S29.

75. Collins, S.J. (2008) Retinoic acid receptors, hematopoiesis and leukemogenesis. *Curr Opin Hematol* **15**, 346–51.

76. Patatanian, E., and Thompson, D.F. (2008) Retinoic acid syndrome: A review. *J Clin Pharm Ther* **33**, 331–38.

77. Gallagher, R.E. (2002) Retinoic acid resistance in acute promyelocytic leukemia. *Leukemia* **16**, 1940–58.

78. Baglietto, L., Torrisi, R., Arena, G. et al. (2000) Ocular effects of fenretinide, a vitamin A analog, in a chemoprevention trial of bladder cancer. *Cancer Detect Prev* **24**, 369–75.

79. Öström, M., Kloffler, K.A., Edfalk, S. et al. (2008) Retinoic acid promotes the generation of pancreatic endocrine progenitor cells and their further differentiation into β-cells. *PLoS One* **3**, e4821.

80. Institute of Medicine (2002) Dietary Reference Intakes for Vitamin A, Vitamin K, Arsenic, Boron, Chromium, Copper, Iodine, Iron, Manganese, Molybdenum, Nickel, Silicon, Vanadium, and Zinc. Washington: National Academy Press.

81. Promislow, J.H.E., Goodman-Gruen, D., Slymen, D.J., and Barrett-Connor, E. (2002) Retinol intake and bone mineral density in the elderly: The Rancho Bernardo Study. *J Bone Miner Res* **17**, 1349–58.

82. No authors listed (2006) NIH state-of-the-science conference statement on multivitamin/mineral supplements and chronic disease prevention. *NIH Consens State Sci Statements* **23**, 1–30.

17 Vitamin D and Cancer Chemoprevention

James C. Fleet

Key Points

1. Although vitamin D is a nutrient whose functions are most closely linked to the control of calcium and bone metabolism, it is also proposed to have a variety of other biological roles, including anti-cancer effects.
2. There is considerable controversy as to what constitutes optimal vitamin D status. While most accept that serum 25OHD levels < 25 nmol/l are deficient and lead to rickets in growing children, some argue that serum 25OHD levels > 80 nmol/l are necessary to optimize bone health and prevent other chronic diseases like cancer.
3. Epidemiological studies have shown that high UVB exposure is associated with lower risk of a wide variety of cancers. From these observations, researchers have hypothesized a link between UVB exposure–vitamin D status and cancer risk.
4. One way that cancer can influence the effects of $1,25(OH)_2$ D is by influencing its metabolism. Several groups have shown that CYP27b1 activity, and the ability to produce $1,25(OH)_2$ D locally, is lost as cancer develops.
5. Very few intervention studies have been conducted in the area of vitamin D and cancer. In addition, the development of effective vitamin D interventions for cancer prevention or treatment may be limited by the changes in vitamin D metabolism and signaling that have been documented to occur during carcinogenesis.

Key Words: Vitamin D; UVB; CYP27b1; 1,25(OH)2D; cancer prevention

1. INTRODUCTION

Although vitamin D is a nutrient whose functions are most closely linked to the control of calcium and bone metabolism *(1)*, it is also proposed to have a variety of other biological roles, including anti-cancer effects. The idea that high vitamin D status is protective against cancer was proposed nearly 30 years ago when Garland and Garland hypothesized that the North–South geographic gradient in colon cancer rates first observed by Apperly *(2)* (high in North, low in South) was due to differences in the ultraviolet B (UVB) light-induced production of vitamin D in the skin *(3)*. This hypothesis

From: *Nutrition and Health: Bioactive Compounds and Cancer*
Edited by: J.A. Milner, D.F. Romagnolo, DOI 10.1007/978-1-60761-627-6_17,
© Springer Science+Business Media, LLC 2010

was later extended to the protection of prostate cancer by Schwartz and Hulka who hypothesized that vitamin D deficiency is an underlying factor for increased prostate cancer risk due to advancing age, Black race, and northern latitudes *(4)*. These are all factors associated with decreased synthesis of vitamin D in the skin *(5)*. Low UVB radiation exposure has now been associated with greater risk of cancers of the prostate *(6)*, breast *(7)*, lung *(8)*, and at a variety of other sites *(9)*. In addition, in Norwegian men fatality for breast, colon, or prostate cancers was 30% lower in subjects when the cancer was diagnosed in the summer/fall *(10)* when skin production and vitamin D status are highest *(11)*. These types of studies suggest that higher vitamin D status is a potentially important and modifiable protective factor for a number of different cancers.

2. UNDERSTANDING VITAMIN D AND CANCER REQUIRES AN OVERVIEW OF VITAMIN D BIOLOGY

To fully appreciate the UV–Vitamin D–cancer connection, it is important to review our current understanding of vitamin metabolism and action.

2.1. Vitamin D Metabolism

In addition to vitamin D from the diet, vitamin D can be obtained by a nonenzymatic process in the skin from 7-dehydrocholesterol when skin is exposed to UV light in the range of 290–315 nm (UVB) (Fig. 1). Regardless of whether vitamin D comes from the skin or the diet, vitamin D is transported in the circulation by the vitamin D-binding protein (DBP) *(12)*. Vitamin D is rapidly converted to the more stable metabolite 25 hydroxyvitamin D (25OHD) in the liver by the enzyme, vitamin D-25-hydroxylase *(13)*. Serum 25OHD concentration is the best short-term indicator (1–2 month window) for vitamin D adequacy as its production reflects both absorption from the diet and cutaneous synthesis *(14)*. In the presence of adequate sunlight exposure there is no dietary requirement for vitamin D. However, a dietary requirement for vitamin D exists for people with highly pigmented skin, in those who cover their skin for religious or health reasons, in institutionalized people, in homebound elderly, and in areas where wintertime UVB irradiation is inadequate (e.g., the Northern part of the United States) *(14, 15)*.

There is considerable controversy as to what constitutes optimal vitamin D status. While most accept that serum 25OHD levels < 25 nmol/l are deficient and lead to rickets in growing children, some argue that serum 25OHD levels > 80 nmol/l are necessary to optimize bone health and prevent other chronic diseases like cancer *(16)*. Thus, although serum 25OHD levels of 50–60 nmol/l are average values seen in the United States, some researchers believe that they are inadequate for optimal health.

25OHD is thought to have minimal biological activity; instead it must be further metabolized. Studies on the hormonal response to changes in dietary calcium intake reveal that the vitamin D metabolite, 1,25 dihydroxyvitamin D ($1,25(OH)_2$ D), is the active form of vitamin D (Fig. 2, right side); it is well established that this metabolite regulates calcium homeostasis *(17)*. In this scenario low calcium intake reduces

Skin

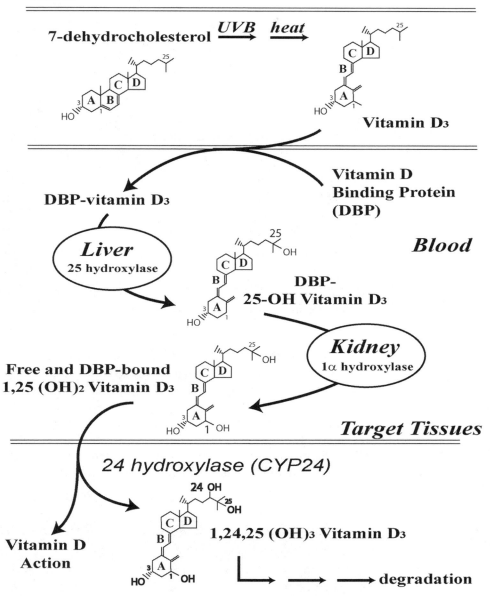

Fig. 1. Classical view of vitamin D metabolism.

serum calcium, which then stimulates production and release of parathyroid hormone (PTH) into the circulation. PTH can stimulate the renal enzyme, 25 hydroxyvitamin D-1α hydroxylase (CYP27B1), that catalyzes the conversion of 25OHD to $1,25(OH)_2$ D *(18, 19)*. The $1,25(OH)_2$ D produced by the kidney and released into the serum acts on intestine, bone, and kidney to regulate calcium homeostasis through a mechanism

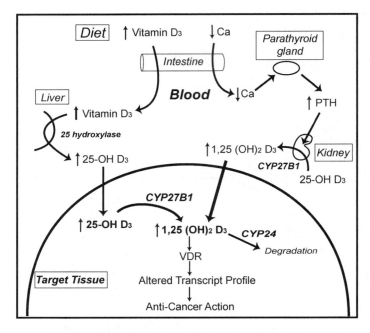

Fig. 2. Endocrine and autocrine vitamin D signaling.

that requires the nuclear vitamin D receptor (VDR) *(20–23)*. The vitamin D signaling system is "fine tuned" within each target tissue through the 1,25(OH)$_2$ D-mediated transcription of the gene encoding another important enzyme, the 25 hydroxyvitamin D-24 hydroxylase (CYP24) *(24)*. This enzyme catalyzes the first step in the metabolic inactivation of 1,25(OH)$_2$ D. Like low calcium intake, low vitamin D status (serum 25OHD < 25 nmol/l) influences serum 1,25(OH)$_2$ D level. In this case, the lack of substrate (25OHD) limits 1,25(OH)$_2$ D production *(25, 26)*. However, when serum 25OHD is within the normal range (40–90 nmol/l) it has no impact on serum 1,25(OH)$_2$ D level *(25, 26)*.

2.2. Regulation of Gene Expression Through the Vitamin D Receptor (VDR)

It is well established that the primary molecular action of 1,25(OH)$_2$ D is to initiate gene transcription by binding to the vitamin D receptor (VDR), a member of the steroid hormone receptor superfamily of ligand-activated transcription factors *(20, 27)*. The VDR has >500-fold higher affinity for 1,25(OH)$_2$ D compared to 25OHD *(28)*. Figure 3 summarizes the molecular processes leading to 1,25(OH)$_2$ D-mediated gene transcription through the VDR.

The VDR is found in both the cytoplasm and the nucleus of vitamin D target cells. Binding of 1,25(OH)$_2$ D to the VDR in the cytoplasm promotes dimerization with the retinoid X receptor (RXR) and subsequent migration of the RXR–VDR–ligand complex to the nucleus *(29–32)*. Once in the nucleus, the 1,25(OH)$_2$ D–VDR–RXR complex

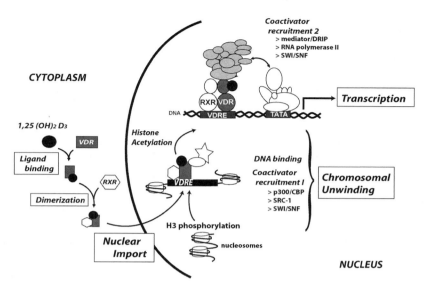

Fig. 3. Summary of vitamin D-mediated gene transcription through the vitamin D receptor (VDR).

regulates gene transcription by interacting with specific DNA-binding sites (vitamin D response elements, VDRE) in the promoters of vitamin D-responsive genes *(20, 27)*. To overcome the constraints imposed on transcription by higher order chromatin structure, the VDR–RXR dimer recruits protein complexes with histone acetyl transferase (HAT) activity [e.g., CBP/p300, SRC1 *(33, 34)*] as well as ATP-dependent remodeling activity [e.g., the BAF57 subunit of SWI/SNF directly interacts with SRC1 and steroid hormone receptors *(35)*]. The VDR–RXR dimer also recruits the mediator complex to the promoter and utilizes it to recruit and activate the basal transcription unit containing RNA polymerase II *(36)*. Deletion of VDR from mice causes reductions in the expression of vitamin D-responsive genes in traditional target tissues, such as the intestine, and severe disruption of calcium and bone metabolism *(21, 22)*.

2.3. VDR Gene Polymorphisms May Affect Vitamin D Action

Three major regions of polymorphism exist within the VDR gene that may account for individual differences in vitamin D responsiveness *(37, 38)*. First, there are three restriction fragment length polymorphisms (RFLP) (*Bsm*I, *Apa*I RFLPs in the intron between exons 8 and 9; *Taq*I RFLP in exon 9) and one nucleotide repeat polymorphism (a poly adenylate repeat in the 3′ UTR) in the 3′ end of the gene that are in linkage disequilibrium (i.e., they are inherited as a block and are thought to provide the same genetic information). These polymorphisms do not alter the coding of the VDR protein, but the BAtS haplotype reflects nucleotide changes in that regions that may make the VDR mRNA more stable *(39)* and lead to production of more VDR protein. Presumably this would lead to more robust responses to $1,25(OH)_2$ D. In addition, two polymorphisms have been identified in the VDR gene promoter that can disrupt the binding of the transcription factors Cdx2 or GATA to the promoter. Like the 3′ polymorphisms, the Cdx2 and GATA polymorphisms are in linkage disequilibrium so it is difficult to separate their biological effects in human association studies. Theoretically, the disruption of either the Cdx2 or the GATA-binding sites would also reduce the production of VDR protein and reduce cellular responsiveness to 1,25(OH)$_2$ D. However, it bears noting that Cdx2 is an intestine-specific transcription factor (40) so the impact of polymorphisms in this site may be limited to the biology of the enterocyte or the colonocyte. Finally, the only known polymorphism that affects the sequence of the VDR protein is a start site RFLP that can be determined with the enzyme FokI. This polymorphism disrupts the translation start site of VDR (the F allele) and leads to the production of a VDR that is shorter due to deletion of three amino acids from the N-terminus of the protein. The shorter VDR is more transcriptionally active, perhaps due to increased interactions of the VDR with TFIIB, an essential component of the basal transcription unit that includes RNA polymerase II (41). Consistent with this, Colin et al. (42) showed that peripheral blood mononuclear cells from subjects who were homozygous for the gene polymorphism coding the shorter VDR (FF) were growth arrested by treatment with 1,25(OH)$_2$ D to a greater extent than cells from subjects who carried the allele coding the long VDR(ff).

2.4. 1,25(OH)$_2$ D Rapidly Activates Signal Transduction Pathways Independent of Its Role in Transcription

There is now compelling evidence that 1,25(OH)$_2$ D induces signal transduction pathways within various cell types and that this action is distinct from the VDR-mediated gene transcription processes described above. I have previously reviewed the history of this field and interested readers are encouraged to read this review (43). However, a brief summary of this work shows that 1,25(OH)$_2$ D rapidly (within seconds and minutes) stimulates events normally associated with the activation of membrane receptors for growth factors and peptide hormones including: (1) phospholipase C (PLC) and phospholipase D activity; (2) phosphoinositide turnover leading to the generation of the second messengers inositol 1,3,4-triphosphate (IP3) and 1,2-diacylglycerol (DAG); (3) intracellular calcium by increasing calcium uptake and the release of intracellular calcium stores; (4) adenylate cyclase activity to increase cAMP levels and stimulate protein kinase A (PKA) activity; (5) calcium-dependent protein kinase C (PKC) isoform activity (α, β, δ) and cellular redistribution; and (6) Jun-activated kinase and extracellular response-activated kinase (ERK) mitogen-activated protein kinase (MAPK) family activation (44–46). While early reports suggested that these rapid actions depended upon the interaction of 1,25(OH)$_2$ D with a unique membrane-associated rapid response steroid-binding receptor (MARRS) (47), other data suggest that the traditional VDR may also be mediating these rapid actions through associations that occur at the plasma membrane (48). Collectively, these lines of evidence suggest that viewing vitamin D biology through the prism of the traditional, nuclear receptor-mediated transcriptional responses may be limited. However, since there are few studies that directly link rapid, nongenomic actions of vitamin D to cancer, we will not explore this question in detail for this review.

3. EPIDEMIOLOGICAL STUDIES EXAMINING THE RELATIONSHIP BETWEEN VITAMIN D AND CANCER

As noted in the introduction, epidemiological studies have shown that high UVB exposure is associated with lower risk of a wide variety of cancers. From these observations, researchers have hypothesized a link between UVB exposure–vitamin D status and cancer risk (3, 4). However, the relationship between vitamin D and cancer would be more compelling if it could be made more directly, e.g., between dietary intake or serum vitamin D metabolites and cancer-related outcomes.

While this goal is logical, there are some challenges to making direct links between cancer and vitamin D in human populations that deserve mention before discussing the research in this area. First, dietary intakes of vitamin D from food are generally low, and in the United States, most of the vitamin D within the body originates from skin production (49). As a result, it is not clear that a dietary evaluation will be informative unless it includes supplemental vitamin D use, and even then, a considerable contribution to vitamin D status from UVB exposure will be missing from the epidemiological association. Related to this, a number of other confounding factors have been identified that should be included as covariates in association studies due to their ability to influence skin vitamin D production and status (e.g. age, skin tone, season) (50). Second, the assessment of vitamin D metabolites in serum in population-based studies is difficult (51). Some of these discrepancies result from analytical sources; until recently there was considerable variability in the quality of assays to measure 25OHD (52) and this may have confounded the interpretation of earlier association studies. Third, since the biological half lives of vitamin D metabolites are relatively short, single measurements of 25OHD (half-life = several weeks) or $1,25(OH)_2$ D (half-life = several hours) may not be representative of either lifelong exposure or of exposure during critical periods of cancer development. For example, some hypothesize that environmental exposures during the periods of rapid prostate growth during fetal development or adolescence will influence adult prostate cancer risk. Assessment of vitamin D status in the adult will not capture the impact of vitamin D during these growth periods. Fourth, the relationship between vitamin D and cancer may be modified by polymorphisms in genes whose protein products control vitamin D action or metabolism. Thus, the appearance of an association may be population dependent. Finally, it is important to recognize that cancer is not a uniform disease within a given tissue, much less across tissues. For example, the molecular signature of distal colon cancer is characterized by a sequential accumulation of mutations in the genes APC, K-Ras, SMAD4, and p53 [i.e., the Vogelstein model (53)) while the molecular signature of proximal colon cancer is characterized by mutations in DNA mismatch repair genes (54). As a result, the nature of the disease may influence our ability to see a relationship between vitamin D and cancer. Very few studies make such fine distinctions based on the tumor characteristics.

The following paragraphs summarize the population-based studies relating vitamin D intake or status to the three best-studied cancers (breast, colon, prostate). One study that examined the effects of vitamin D status on the incidence and mortality from a number of cancers bears noting at the beginning of this discussion. Using data from a subset of 1,095 men from the Health Professionals Follow-Up Study (HPFS), Giovannucci et al.

(50) identified the factors contributing to plasma 25OHD levels and used six parameters from this analysis to make a vitamin D status prediction index that was then independently validated. They subsequently related this plasma 25OHD prediction index to the incidence of 4,286 incident cancers and 2,025 deaths from cancer occurring in the HPFS cohort between 1986 and 2000 (only organ-confined prostate cancer and nonmelanoma skin cancer were excluded). They found an inverse association between an increment of 25 nmol/l in predicted plasma 25OHD and both cancer incidence and mortality that was strongest for several major digestive cancers: colorectal (RR = 0.63), pancreatic (RR = 0.49), esophageal (RR = 0.37), and oral/pharyngeal (RR = 0.31) cancers. Suggestive inverse relationships were seen for leukemia (RR = 0.44) and stomach cancer (RR = 0.58), while nonstatistically significant inverse relationships were seen for lung, renal, non-Hodgkin lymphoma, and advanced prostate cancer incidence. While this study used an indirect measure of vitamin D status, it overcomes the difficulty and cost of measuring plasma 25OHD directly in large population trials and may have the advantage of being less susceptible to the variability inherent in single sample measurements that result from recent exposures.

3.1. Prostate Cancer

Two studies examining vitamin D intake and prostate cancer risk failed to find an association *(55, 56)*. However, several studies show that high dietary calcium intake increases the risk of advanced prostate cancer *(57–59)*; this increased risk would presumably result from the well-documented suppression of serum $1,25(OH)_2$ D levels caused by high dietary calcium intake. Ahonen et al. *(60)* reported a 70% increase in prostate cancer risk in Finnish men with 25OHD levels below the median, especially in younger men (<52 years) who entered the study with low serum 25OHD (adjusted odds ratio = 3.5). In contrast, others studied have not detected a relationship between prediagnostic serum vitamin D metabolites and prostate cancer risk *(61, 62)*. More recently, Ahn et al. *(63)* found no effect of vitamin D status on overall prostate cancer risk, but saw a positive relationship between vitamin D status and aggressive prostate cancer in a population of men with prevalent disease. However, 58% of the cases in this study were diagnosed within the second year of follow-up suggesting the disease was prevalent before the start of the study. Other factors related to vitamin D signaling may better reflect the complexity of mechanisms for vitamin D-mediated prostate cancer prevention. Corder et al. *(64)* found that prostate cancer risk was decreased in men with higher serum $1,25(OH)_2D$ levels, especially if serum 25OHD levels were low. Similarly, Li et al. *(65)* found that combined low serum 25OHD and $1,25(OH)_2$ D increased the risk of aggressive prostate cancer, while low serum 25OHD in men with the ff genotype of the *Fok*I polymorphism in the VDR gene increased the risk of total and aggressive prostate cancer.

3.2. Colon Cancer

The earliest study to evaluate the relationship between vitamin D intake and colorectal cancer risk study showed that total vitamin D intake was significantly inversely related to colon cancer risk (OR = 0.54, <106 vs. >917 IU/day, 203 male cases) *(66)*. More recent studies have shown similar protection against colorectal cancer in women (OR = 0.88 for total vitamin D, <92 vs. >477 IU/day) and subjects in the Veterans Administration health care system (per 100 IU intake, OR = 0.94) as well as for distal colon adenoma in women (OR = 0.67, <137 vs. >601 IU/day) *(67)*. Consistent with this, serum 25OHD has been shown to be protective against colon cancer in older women (threefold lower risk when serum 25OHD > 50 nmol/l) *(68)*, rectal cancer in Finish men (OR = 0.37, 146 cases, ≤24 vs. > 48 nmol/l) *(69)*, cancer of the distal colon and rectum in women older than 60-year-old (OR = 0.53, 193 cases, <37 vs. > 88 nmol/l) *(70)*, and colon cancer independent of location (OR = 0.54, <35 vs. >92 nmol/l) *(71)*, although there is some suggestion that the benefit in terms of adenoma risk is limited to women *(72)*. The benefit afforded by high vitamin D status also appears to extend to a reduction in overall mortality (HR = 0.52, 304 cases) and colorectal cancer-specific mortality (HR = 0.61) in subjects with colorectal cancer *(73)*.

3.3. Breast Cancer

Mammographic breast density, a marker of breast cancer risk, in pre- and post-menopausal women (OR = 0.24, <5 vs. >200 IU/day) *(74)* and in women with a strong family history of breast cancer (OR = 0.5, <164 vs. >737 IU/day, *n* = 157 cases) *(75)* was lower when vitamin D intake was high. Similarly, breast density showed a modest seasonal variation *(76)* and density was lowest in women with the highest vitamin D status *(77)*. Protection from breast cancer has also been observed with high vitamin D intake in premenopausal women (OR = 0.5–0.72) *(78–80)* and postmenopausal women with estrogen receptor positive tumors (OR = 0.74) *(81)*. Although one large case–control study found that serum 25OHD has been inversely related to breast cancer risk (OR = 0.31, <30 vs. >75 nmol/l), the effect has been weaker (OR = 0.74) *(82)*, limited to whites *(83)*, or not present *(84)* in other reports. There is no firm consensus regarding the impact of VDR polymorphisms on breast cancer risk. Some show that the "b" allele of the *Bsm*I RFLP *(85–87)* or 3′ UTR, long poly A repeat polymorphism *(88)*, increases breast cancer risk. In one study, women with low 25OHD coupled to the bb genotype were 6.8 times more likely to have breast cancer than subjects with >50 nmol 25OHD/l in plasma and carrying the "B" allele.

3.4. Summary of Population-Based Studies

Although there is some inconsistency in the literature, the majority of the population-based data support a hypothesis that high vitamin D status or intake over a lifetime is protective against prostate, colon, and breast cancers. The data supporting this link are strongest for the colon, moderate for the breast, and weakest for the prostate. The impact of VDR polymorphisms on cancer risk in these tissues is not uniform and results from these studies are often inconsistent. However, there is some suggestion that vitamin D status and VDR polymorphisms interact to influence breast and prostate cancer risk.

3.5. *The Paradox of Protection from Cancer by Higher Vitamin D Status*

While $1,25(OH)_2$ D is the most biologically active metabolite of vitamin D and binds to the VDR 1,000 times more avidly than 25OHD, it is the serum 25OHD level that usually associates with cancer risk in epidemiologic trials *(50)*. This observation suggests that there is a benefit to high vitamin D status that is independent of its renal conversion to $1,25(OH)_2$D and the appearance of $1,25(OH)_2$D in the serum.

The hypothesis to explain the paradox of cancer protection by high serum 25OHD levels is that there is local production of $1,25(OH)_2$ D mediated by extra-renal expression of the enzyme CYP27B1 in nonclassical vitamin D target tissues like the prostate, breast, and colon (Fig. 2, left side). In addition to the high CYP27B1 level seen in kidney, low CYP27B1 protein and message levels have been reported in other tissues *(89)* including mammary epithelial cells *(90)*, prostate epithelial cells *(91–93)*, mouse prostate *(94)*, and colonocytes *(95, 96)*. This "local production" hypothesis is consistent with studies showing that the CYP27B1 is substrate starved (the enzyme operates well below its K_m and thus is sensitive to increased substrate availability *(97)*) and with studies showing that CYP27B1 expression and activity correlate well with the ability of prostate cell lines (primary and cancer) to arrest growth in response to 25OHD treatment *(91–93)*. While these observations support the plausibility of the "local production" hypothesis, definitive proof identifying increased local conversion in vivo and the value of local CYP27B1 expression in animal models is currently lacking.

4. ANTI-CANCER ACTIONS OF VITAMIN D: CELL AND MOLECULAR STUDIES

Cancer is a complex and heterogeneous disease that is characterized by the accumulation of mutations in genes that control cellular processes such as cell proliferation, differentiation, apoptosis, cell migration, and DNA repair. This model of sequential acquired mutation is best characterized for the cancer of the distal colon where mutations in four specific genes accumulate as the colon cancer moves through the stages of initiation, promotion, and progression, i.e., APC loss of function, k-ras activation, SMAD loss of function, and p53 loss of function *(53)*. However, such a well-described course of events does not define cancers of the proximal colon where mutations in genes encoding mismatch repair enzymes are more common *(54)*. In other types of cancer, the molecular etiology is even less clear. As a result, researchers interested in cancer preventions should appreciate that what one learns in one form of cancer may not apply to another. In addition, since the cancer cell changes dramatically from the initiation steps through to the development of tumor or the metastasis of tumor cells to other tissues, the impact of an agent on cancer cells may also be stage-specific dependent (see below).

With this in mind, the traditional thinking has been that the target cells for the anti-cancer action of vitamin D are tumor cells and the normal cell types within tissues that transform into tumor cells. The best-studied noncalcium regulatory effects of $1,25(OH)_2$ D is the growth arrest of proliferating epithelial cells from the skin, breast, colon, and prostate. This phenomenon was first reported by Colston et al., who showed a dose-dependent decrease in growth rate of melanoma cells treated with $1,25(OH)_2$

D *(98)*. Growth inhibitory properties of 1,25(OH)$_2$ D were subsequently reported for tumor-derived cells from the colon *(99)*, breast *(100)*, and prostate *(101)*. Others have reported that 1,25(OH)$_2$ D influences apoptosis; however, this effect is not uniformly observed. For example, while MCF-7 breast cancer cells *(102)* and a variety of colon cancer cell lines *(103)* become apoptotic after 1,25(OH)$_2$ D treatment], the prostate cancer cell line LNCaP does not *(104)* even though 1,25(OH)$_2$ D treatment causes LNCaP cell growth arrest.

Most cell-based vitamin D research has focused on the impact of 1,25(OH)$_2$ D on normal or cancer-derived prostate epithelial cells, but there is evidence that other cells within the tissue or tumor microenvironment may also be vitamin D targets. For example, communication between the epithelial cells and the stromal cells surrounding them is emerging as critical for the progression of prostate cancer *(105)*. Lou et al. *(106)* have reported that 1,25(OH)$_2$ D can suppress the growth of prostate stromal cell lines in vitro but is not clear if this is relevant in vivo or if it alters stromal–epithelial cell communication. Similarly, the recent observations that inflammation is a critical part of carcinogenesis in many organs, including the prostate *(107, 108)*, suggest that the immune system is an important target for inhibiting prostate carcinogenesis. Using data from a variety of disease states, 1,25(OH)$_2$D modulates the number or activity of many types of immune cells *(109)*. In general, 1,25(OH)$_2$D promotes immunotolerence and immunosuppression by altering dendritic cell differentiation and the function of tolerogenic dendritic cells *(110)*, suppressing NFkβ signaling necessary for T helper cell activation *(111)*, and increasing the activity of regulatory T cells necessary for immunosuppression *(112)*. These actions would be expected to protect tissues from pro-inflammatory stresses that promote carcinogenesis. However, the interaction between vitamin D, inflammation, and cancer has not been critically tested.

4.1. Potential Gene Targets Mediating the Anti-cancer Effects of Vitamin D

The VDR-regulated genes that may impede carcinogenesis are not known with certainty, yet some clues exist. Consistent with the strong antiproliferative effects that 1,25(OH)$_2$ D has on cells, 1,25(OH)$_2$ D directly regulates the gene encoding the cyclin-dependent kinase inhibitor p21 in U937 monocytic cells *(113)* and 1,25(OH)$_2$ D-induced prostate epithelial cell growth is blocked by antisense RNA or siRNA against p21 *(114, 115)*. However, Zhuang et al. *(104)* found increased p21 protein but not mRNA in 1,25(OH)$_2$ D-treated LNCaP cells, suggesting the effect on p21 is not mediated directly at the promoter level. Consistent with these data, 1,25(OH)$_2$ D treatment increased IGF-binding protein 3 (IGFBP-3) gene expression, which then increased prostatic p21 level indirectly by suppressing IGF-1 signaling *(116)* [IGF1 signaling has been proposed to play a significant stimulatory role in prostate carcinogenesis *(117)*]. Several other groups have shown that 1,25(OH)$_2$ D and vitamin D analogs induce production of IGFBP3 in prostate cancer cells and primary prostate epithelial cells *(118, 119)* through a direct effect mediated by VDR binding to VDREs in the IGFBP3 gene promoter *(120)*.

Recently, an alternate hypothesis has emerged to account for vitamin D-mediated growth arrest, i.e., disruption of β-catenin transcriptional activity that is the downstream mediator of the pro-proliferative effects of Wnt signaling. Under normal conditions, β-catenin is held in the cytoplasm of cells by the protein APC. The release of β-catenin from APC permits its translocation to the nucleus where it then partners with TCF4 to stimulate the transcription of genes whose protein products control cell cycle [e.g., c-myc, cyclin D1, PPARδ *(121)*]. Palmer et al. *(122)* found that $1,25(OH)_2$ D treatment induced the translocation of β-catenin away from the nucleus to the membrane resulting in reduced expression of c-myc and other genes regulated by the β-catenin/TCF transcriptional complex in SW480 colon cancer cells. Shah et al. later showed that the AF-2 domain of the VDR can interact directly with the C-terminal end of β-catenin and that this interaction is unrelated to the traditional transcriptional effects of VDR *(123)*. The VDR–β-catenin interaction also may account for the inhibitory effects that $1,25(OH)_2$ D treatment exerts on the expression of dickkopf-4, a Wnt regulator that enhances cell migration and whose expression is increased in human colon cancer *(124)*. In addition, $1,25(OH)_2$ D treatment can also enhance expression of the Wnt antagonist dickkopf-1, although this effect is thought to be indirect and mediated through the $1,25(OH)_2$ D-mediated induction of E-cadherin *(125)*. Although it has not been definitively proven, the ability of $1,25(OH)_2$ D to interfere with β-catenin action through a VDR-mediated mechanism suggests that vitamin D may be an effective countermeasure to the loss of APC function that occurs in the early stage of distal colon cancer.

DNA microarrays have been used in 14 studies to identify the transcript-level changes relevant to vitamin D and cancer using normal or transformed cells of the prostate *(126–129)*, breast *(130–133)*, colon *(134)*, and ovary *(135)*. However, the most complete genomic profiling of vitamin D action has been reported in squamous cell carcinoma (SCC) cell lines *(136–139)*. These studies show that $1,25(OH)_2$ D treatment influences more cellular processes than cell cycle arrest including the up-regulation of DNA repair systems (gadd45α, p53 target genes), modulation of signal transduction pathways (e.g., amphiregulin, AP-4, STAT3, and fra-1), cell adhesion proteins (e.g., integrin α7B, E-cadherin), and protection from pro-oxidative stress (e.g., thioredoxin reductase, VDUP1). Although only a small number of differentially expressed transcripts have been reported for $1,25(OH)_2$ D-treated prostate cells using microarrays, these include genes encoding proteins that modulate prostaglandin synthesis (COX-2), metabolism (15-prostaglandin dehydrogenase), and action (the prostaglandin receptors EP2 and FP) and suggest that vitamin D suppresses the pro-inflammatory prostaglandin signaling pathway *(126, 140)*. In addition, other research has shown that $1,25(OH)_2$ D is antiangiogenic and that this may be caused by disruption of HIF-1-mediated transcription that activates angiogenesis through VEGF *(141)*. Collectively, these data reveal that the biological impact of $1,25(OH)_2$ D extends beyond the simple modulation of cell cycle (see Fig. 4 for summary).

4.2. $1,25(OH)_2$ D Action May Not Be Uniform Across All Stages of Cancer (from Normal Tissue to Metastatic Tumors)

Although we generally focus on the impact that vitamin D has on the development of cancer, in terms of prevention it is just as important to understand the impact that cancer has on vitamin D action. For example, Matusiak et al. *(142)* found that VDR protein level declines as a function of colon tumor dedifferentiation. This suggests

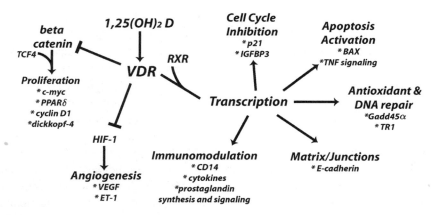

Fig. 4. Summary of putative molecular targets mediating vitamin D action in cancer prevention.

that the development of colon cancer may lead to lower responses to $1,25(OH)_2$ D. This is consistent with evidence that activated Ras, a common mutation in many cancers including colon cancer, can impair vitamin D transcriptional activity. For example, H-Ras transformation has also been shown to reduce VDR levels in HC-11 mammary cells *(143)*. In addition, H-Ras-transformed kerotinocytes *(144)* have reduced VDR transcriptional activity due to phosphorylation of the VDR heterodimeric partner RXRα at serine 260 and disruption of co-activator recruitment to the VDR–RXR heterodimer *(145)*.

Another way that cancer can influence the effects of $1,25(OH)_2$ D is by influencing its metabolism. Several groups have shown that CYP27b1 activity, and the ability to produce $1,25(OH)_2$ D locally, is lost as cancer develops. Hsu *(91)* found that CYP27b1 was present in normal prostate epithelial cells but that its activity was reduced in cells isolated from subjects with benign prostatic hypertrophy and nearly absent in cells from subjects with prostate cancer. As a result, while normal prostate epithelial cells could respond to treatment with 25OH D by growth arresting, prostate cancer cells with low CYP27b1 expression could not. This observation was confirmed by Chen et al. *(92)* who also showed that transgenic expression of CYP27b1 restored the growth inhibitory response to 25OH D in LNCaP prostate cancer cells that normally have low CYP27b1 activity. CYP27B1 expression is also absent in metastases from colon tumors in humans *(96)*. However, cancer-associated reductions in CYP27b1 levels are not uniformly observed for all cancers. Friedrich et al. *(146)* found that CYP27b1 was present in normal breast tissue, but its levels were actually higher in malignant breast tissue.

Some have also hypothesized that the enzyme responsible for the degradation of vitamin D metabolites, the 25 hydroxyvitamin D-24 hydroxylase (CYP24), is influenced by cancer. CYP24 was identified as a putative oncogene because the CYP24 gene was amplified in breast tumors *(147)*. Consistent with this observation, Anderson et al. *(148)* reported that CYP24 mRNA expression was increased in colorectal cancer as compared to adjacent normal tissue. Matusiak and Benya *(149)* subsequently found that CYP24 protein was present in the nuclei of normal tissue, increased in aberrant crypt foci and polyps, and finally shifted to the cytoplasm in tumors and metastatic colon cancer. This suggests that increased $1,25(OH)_2$ D metabolism may be a feature of advanced cancer.

The overall impact of these changes to vitamin D metabolism and signaling would affect cancer prevention in two ways. First, the protection provided by high vitamin D status will depend upon the level of CYP27b1 in the developing tumor; if CYP27b1 activity is lost, so will the protection due to high vitamin D status. Second, when CYP24 activity is elevated and/or VDR level or signaling is reduced, higher cellular levels of $1,25(OH)_2$ D will be needed to influence the biology of the cancer cell. It is unclear whether this is possible through local production of the hormone and increases in serum $1,25(OH)_2$ D levels are likely to have a negative impact on calcium metabolism. Hypercalcemia associated with $1,25(OH)_2$ D treatment has been a major motivation to produce vitamin D analogs that separate the calcemic and noncalcemic effects of $1,25(OH)_2$ D. However, vitamin D analog effectiveness may be limited if a cancer leads to reduced VDR expression. Figure 5 summarizes the putative effects of cancer on vitamin D signaling.

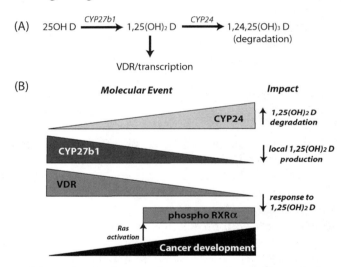

Fig. 5. A summary of the molecular impact of cancer on vitamin D metabolism. (**a**) $1,5(OH)2$ D transcriptional activity is dependent upon the balance between production and degradation. (**b**) Impact of cancer development on the expression and activity of proteins that mediate vitamin D metabolism (CYP27B1, CYP24) and signaling (VDR, RXRα).

5. ANTI-CANCER EFFECTS OF VITAMIN D: ANIMAL STUDIES

There are several types of questions that can be asked related to vitamin D and cancer in animal models. First, one can examine the impact of vitamin D status or vitamin D signaling in normal tissues. The information from these studies is relevant to the question of whether the normal biology of a healthy tissue is dependent upon vitamin D or its metabolites. Second, one can use an animal model for a tissue-specific cancer to evaluate the impact of vitamin D status on the progression or promotion of tumor development. These models can also be used to assess the therapeutic potential of vitamin D analogs as drugs. The challenge with both of these scenarios is to accurately assess how well the animal model reflects human biology and carcinogenesis. Readers interested in the relative merits of various models should look elsewhere for a detailed discussion of this topic. However, several points bear noting (1) the molecular basis for most chemically induced cancer models is unknown and so it is not clear how when they mimic the molecular etiology of human cancer; (2) the cancer phenotypes observed in genetically modified mouse models vary dramatically, and consequently, some models may only be useful as late-stage or aggressive cancer models (e.g., TRAMP model for prostate cancer), while others with a mild phenotype may only be useful as early-stage models (e.g., PTEN$^{+/-}$ model for prostate cancer); (3) genetically modified mice have very specific cancer phenotypes, and therefore, they may only model a subset of the cancers found in a specific tissue (e.g., APC min mouse is a model for distal but not proximal colon cancer); and (4) many cancer models develop cancer in multiple tissues and thus results may not be representative (e.g., APC min mice develop most of their tumors in the small intestine but they are often used as a model of colon cancer even though the phenotype there is very mild). However, new models are being created each year and these often overcome the limitations of earlier models.

A number of studies exist that suggest vitamin D has a role in the normal physiology of the colon, breast, and prostate. This concept was originally developed in a study by Xue et al. *(150)* and the studies by this group were recently reviewed *(151)*. This group showed that feeding a "Western diet" containing high fat (20% by weight vs. 5%), low calcium (0.05% vs. 0.5%), and low vitamin D (110 IU/kg vs. 1,000 IU/kg) for 9 weeks to C57BL/6 mice from weaning increased the epithelial cell-labeling index (by BrdU labeling) in the pancreas, dorsal lobe of the prostate, terminal ducts of the mammary gland, and the colon. Longer (18 months) feeding studies also revealed colon tumors may develop without the need for carcinogen exposure in the "Western diet"-fed mice. While these phenotypes can be reversed by increasing both the calcium (0.7%) and the vitamin D (2,400 IU/kg) levels of the diet, these studies do not speak specifically to the independent role that vitamin D may play in carcinogenesis.

Other studies supporting a role for vitamin D in normal tissue biology come from the VDR knockout mouse. There are more proliferating cells in the descending colon of VDR knockout mice and many of these proliferating cells are outside the normal proliferating cell zone in the bottom of the colonic crypt *(152)*. The descending colon of the VDR knockout mouse also has higher levels of 8-hydroxy-2′deoxyguanosine, a marker of oxidative stress that suggests the DNA in colonocytes from VDR null mice may be more susceptible to mutation. VDR knockout mice have hyperproliferation in the ductal epithelial cells of the mammary gland leading to accelerated mammary gland development during pregnancy and they also exhibit delayed postlactation involution suggesting defects in apoptosis in the absence of VDR-mediated signaling *(153)*. While no evidence yet exists on the impact of VDR deletion on cancer development in the colon or prostate, MMTV-neu mice with only one active VDR allele have a shorter latency and increased incidence of mammary tumor formation *(153)*.

Few studies have been conducted to evaluate the impact of nutritional vitamin D or vitamin D status on cancer in animal models. Our recent report on the impact of dietary vitamin D intake on serum 25OHD levels in rats and mice shows that "optimal" serum levels of 25OHD are achieved at dietary vitamin D levels of 200–400 IU/kg diet, and dietary levels of 50 IU/kg or less cause early signs of vitamin D deficiency *(25)*. Several groups have demonstrated that complete vitamin D deficiency has a negative impact on tumor growth or burden in colon cancer models *(154–156)*, but severe vitamin D deficiency is not common in humans. Using higher dietary vitamin D_3 levels between 250 and 10,000 IU/kg diet, Comer et al. *(157)* found that dietary vitamin D had no impact on dimethylhydrazine (DMH)-induced colon tumor incidence or colonocyte proliferation in Fisher 344 mice. However, Beaty et al. *(158)* found that a diet with 4,000 IU vitamin D/kg reduced the crypt cell proliferation index (compared to a 1,000 IU/kg diet) and the combination of 1.5% dietary calcium and 4,000 IU vitamin D/kg diet reduced tumor number and incidence by 45% in the rat DMH-induced colon cancer model. Given the documented benefits of high dietary calcium on colon cancer, it is not clear from this study that dietary vitamin D exerts an independent effect on colon cancer. Finally, UVB exposure (6 week, 10 min $3\times$ per week) was able to increase serum 25OHD levels in mice by 80% and this reduced tumor size and tumor cell growth in mice with mammary tumor cell xenographs *(159)*. The UVB exposure was also associated with increased skin cell proliferation and epidermal thickening, but it is not yet clear if using diet to raise serum 25OHD to a similar extent would reduce tumor endpoints.

In contrast to the limited number of animal experiments examining the impact of vitamin D intake or status on cancer, many studies are available where animals have been treated with the active vitamin D hormone ($1,25(OH)_2$ D) or with vitamin D analogs. Many of the studies that treat animals with $1,25(OH)_2$ D are confounded by the effect that the hormone has on serum calcium. For example, daily treatment with $1,25(OH)_2$ D (2 μg/d, 3 week) can significantly reduce prostate weight in mice. However, this effect is accompanied by severe hypercalcemia (16.4 vs. 9.7 mg/dl) and weight loss making it difficult to attribute the prostate effects to the vitamin D hormone. Similar confounded results have been reported for rats implanted with the Dunning prostate tumor *(160)*, LNCaP prostate cancer cell xenographs *(161)*, and in the APC min mouse model of colon cancer *(162)*. However, by using vitamin D analogs designed to eliminate the side effect of hypercalcemia, one can get a clearer picture of the therapeutic potential of vitamin D against cancer. The use of the analog 1 alpha hydroxy-24-ethylcholesterol D_5 can reduce both the incidence (by 50–80% depending upon dose) and number of N-methyl-N-nitrosourea (NMU)-induced mammary tumors in rats. In a dimethylbenz(a)anthracene (DMBA)-induced model of breast cancer this analog influences the promotion but not the initiation phase of cancer *(163)*. Other analogs have inhibited LNCaP xenograph tumor growth in mice *(164)*, reduced normal cell proliferation while enhancing programmed cell death in the rat prostate *(165)*, reduced the formation of DMH-induced formation of aberrant crypt foci in colon, and reduced the number of large and small colon tumors in rats *(166)*. Vitamin D analogs have also been shown to limit the early precancerous lesions and suppress pro-inflammatory events associated with azoxymethane and dextran sulfate sodium treatment *(167)* as well as the recruitment of immune cells in a mouse model of autoimmune prostatitis *(168)*. Taken together, these data demonstrate that vitamin D analogs can activate vitamin D signaling pathways that reduce both early and late events associated with carcinogenesis in animal models.

6. HUMAN INTERVENTION STUDIES

Very few intervention studies have been conducted in the area of vitamin D and cancer. In addition, the development of effective vitamin D interventions for cancer prevention or treatment may be limited by the changes in vitamin D metabolism and signaling that have been documented to occur during carcinogenesis (see section above).

To date most intervention studies have used the active hormonal form of vitamin D, $1,25(OH)_2$ D, or analogs based on this structure, as treatments for established cancer. The major barrier to this intervention is that $1,25(OH)_2$ D strongly stimulates the calcium regulatory machinery and leads to hypercalcemia that may cause muscle, cardiac, and neural dysfunction *(169)*. To overcome these side effects, researchers have developed unique dosing strategies for $1,25(OH)_2$ D or created vitamin D analogs that have growth inhibitory properties but which do not influence calcium metabolism (i.e., noncalcemic analogs). Alternate dosing strategies (e.g., treatment holidays rather than daily doses) lead to periods where the patient has normal serum calcium levels. Phase 1 and 2 clinical trials suggested this approach could help men with androgen-independent prostate cancer in combination with docetaxel chemotherapy *(170, 171)*. Unfortunately the phase I clinical trial with this treatment regime was terminated early due to an increase in unexplained deaths in the treatment group (ASCENT-2 trial data not yet published). Vitamin D analog therapy has not yet reached the clinic either, largely due to the inability to completely separate the calcemic and anti-cancer actions of $1,25(OH)_2$ D. This is likely due to the fact that both calcium metabolism and cancer are regulated by the same VDR. Isolating these effects may be difficult since we know very little of the details by which vitamin D is delivered to, and influences, the cancer cell. Readers interested in vitamin D analogs should refer to one of the many reviews on this subject *(172–174)*.

In terms of nutritional vitamin D, the largest study to date was the Women's Health Initiative *(175)*. Over 36,000 women were randomized to a combined vitamin D (400 IU/day) and calcium (1,000 mg/day) treatment or placebo group and followed for an average of 7 years. The incidence of pathologically confirmed colorectal cancer was a secondary outcome for this study. Although the baseline levels of serum 25OHD in a subset of these subjects ($n = 623$) showed a significant effect of prediagnostic vitamin D status on colorectal cancer risk (2.53-fold increase in risk when serum 25OHD was <31 nmol/l vs. a reference group with serum 25OHD > 58.4 nmol/l), the combined treatment had no impact on the development of colorectal cancer in the intervention arm of the study. This study has been criticized for several reasons including the short duration of follow-up, the low dose of vitamin D used (leading to only a 28% increase in serum 25OH D levels in the intervention group), the low compliance rate for subjects (only 59% took 80% or more of their treatment), and a high rate of nonstudy supplied supplement use (69% of all subjects took a personal calcium supplement). However, a recent reanalysis of the WHI data revealed that in women randomized to concurrent estrogen therapy, the calcium plus vitamin D intervention was protective only in women who did not receive the estrogen intervention (OR = 0.71, *p*-value for estrogen $\times$ calcium/vitamin D supplement = 0.018) *(176)*.

Another recent calcium and vitamin D intervention study also looked at cancer incidence as a secondary endpoint *(177)*. One thousand one hundred and seventy nine women (>55 years) received one of three treatments, calcium (1,400–1,500 mg/d, $n = 416$), calcium plus vitamin D_3 (1,100 IU vitamin D_3, $n = 403$), or placebo ($n = 266$) for 4 years and the incidence of all cancers between years 2 and 4 was recorded. While the number of cancers was small (41 cases), the relative risk for cancer in the vitamin D plus calcium group (but not the calcium only group) was significantly reduced (RR = 0.23). The average serum 25OH D level was high in this study group (72 ± 20 nmol/l), but the vitamin D intervention increased serum 25OHD by 35%.

Finally, Woo et al. *(178)* recently examined the impact of a 2,000 IU supplementation with vitamin D_3 on the rise in prostate-specific antigen (PSA) in 15 men whose treatment for prostate cancer had failed and who had rising PSA levels in the absence of symptoms. Fourteen of the 15 men had a prolonged doubling time for the rise in PSA and the mean doubling time for the study group rose from 14.3 to 25 mo. In nine subjects, the rise in PSA stopped or regressed. This suggests that optimizing vitamin D status may slow the progression of established prostate cancer.

7. TOTALITY OF THE EVIDENCE

At this point there is strong evidence from cell-based studies in support of the hypothesis that vitamin D metabolites have anti-cancer actions. At the population level, the strongest evidence is indirect – the incidence of many cancers is lower when UVB exposure indices are high. Direct relationships between high vitamin D status and low cancer risk are strongest for the colon and weaker for the breast and prostate. Nevertheless, these data are generally supportive of an inverse relationship between vitamin D status and cancer risk. Animal models generally support these observations, but most of the work in animals has been done using vitamin D analogs and models that are best for testing chemotherapeutic rather than chemopreventative agents. A critical missing link in all of these studies is that they do not allow us to state whether the relationship between vitamin D and cancer is resulting from a condition of deficiency (i.e., serum 25OHD levels <40 nmol/l) or due to raising vitamin D status to the proposed "optimal" levels (>80 nmol 25OHD/l). It is my opinion that totality of the evidence is supportive of a relationship, but that this evidence has not yet reached the level of certainty necessary to define public health messages regarding either a target vitamin D status level or a vitamin D supplementation level.

8. FUTURE RESEARCH DIRECTIONS

We have made remarkable progress in understanding the relationship between vitamin D status and cancer risk but many more questions remain. While it is impossible to identify all of the research questions relevant to the future of vitamin D and cancer research, I will attempt to identify a few interesting issues in the following passage.

From the mechanistic perspective, we need to determine the molecular targets of vitamin D action as well as translate these findings to preclinical models and patient populations. This includes a careful evaluation of the cellular targets of vitamin D action (e.g., is vitamin D-mediated immunosuppression important for cancer prevention?) as well as the gene targets regulated by vitamin D through the VDR. Regarding the gene targets, we currently have insight into what these targets may be from cell culture studies. However, we do not know if the targets that seem relevant for one cancer type (e.g., disruption of β-catenin signaling in colonocytes) are relevant to other cancers nor do we know whether the gene targets identified in cultured cells with high levels of $1,25(OH)_2$ D treatment are relevant in vivo. Similarly, we have insight from cell culture studies suggesting certain oncogenic gene mutations may limit vitamin D action and the utility of both nutritional vitamin D and vitamin D analogs as therapeutic agents. As we gain more insight into the molecular etiologies of various cancers, we need to incorporate this information into our cell, animal, and population-based work on the vitamin D–cancer connection. For example, while early case–control studies lumped cancers of the proximal colon, distal colon, and rectum together, we now understand that the molecular nature of these cancers make them distinct diseases that may be influenced differently by vitamin D (e.g., only distal colon cancer may be limited by Ras-activating mutations that blunt VDR-dependent gene transcription). Future population-based association studies need to use larger populations and incorporate clinical and molecular diagnostic information into their analysis.

Unlike the early days of vitamin D research, when the symptoms of deficiency would develop quickly and the benefits of intervention could be rapidly observed, cancer is a slow developing disease. For this reason, many of the questions related to early prevention and later therapeutic benefits will be impossible to address in human populations (e.g., a lifelong intervention project would be prohibitively expensive). For this reason, the use of mouse models that have been genetically manipulated to mimic various types and stages of human cancer will be necessary to adequately test the value of altering vitamin D status for cancer prevention and treatment. This will also be necessary to link the mechanistic cell-based studies to the complex, multicellular environment of whole tissues and tumors.

9. CONCLUSIONS AND RECOMMENDATIONS FOR INTAKE/DIETARY CHANGES

There are strong links between the molecular actions of vitamin D and cancer biology, as well as between indicators of vitamin D status and cancer risk. Unfortunately, careful studies directly defining the levels of vitamin D intake for cancer prevention and treatment are limited. As a result, it is premature to define uniform recommendations that will ensure prevention of all cancers in all individuals and will also have benefits at all stages of carcinogenesis. However, it is clear that many people have vitamin D status that is low by traditional standards (e.g., 10–15% of Caucasians and 30–40% of African-Americans have serum 25OHD levels less than 37.5 nmol/l) *(179, 180)* and these individuals would benefit from increased vitamin D intake. In addition, there is growing data to suggest that increasing vitamin D status beyond the US national average (i.e., to serum 25OHD >80 nmol/l) has a benefit to traditional *(16)* and cancer *(50)* endpoints. Few natural food sources are high in vitamin D (e.g., fatty fish and vitamin D-supplemented dairy products) and the current consensus is that individuals cannot easily meet their vitamin D needs by diet alone, especially when they need to raise their vitamin D status dramatically when they have documented low vitamin D status or if one is trying to reach the proposed optimal serum 25OH D levels (>80 nmol/l). Thus, supplementation has been recommended as the most efficient means to raise or maintain high vitamin D status. Nevertheless, the response of serum 25OHD level to supplemental vitamin D intake is influenced by a subject's baseline vitamin D status (i.e., larger serum response to supplemental vitamin D in subjects with low vitamin D status). Based on current evidence on the impact of supplemental vitamin D_3 on serum 25OHD levels, the average American would benefit from a supplement of 800–1,000 IU vitamin D_3 per day. Individuals with low initial vitamin D status may need substantially more vitamin D (>2,000 IU vitamin D_3 per day), but would be advised to do this under the supervision of a physician. There is some controversy regarding whether the supplements should be vitamin D_3 or vitamin D_2 *(13, 181)*; vitamin D_2 is traditionally used in US supplements and can increase serum 25OHD levels, but some believe that the form naturally produced in humans, vitamin D_3, should be used. Many multivitamin and mineral supplements are now including 800 IU vitamin D_2 in their formulations. For those wishing to supplement with more vitamin D, a dedicated vitamin D supplement should be used. For normal, healthy individuals, high vitamin D intake (up to 10,000 IU/day for 3 months) is safe *(182)*. However, the safety of vitamin D supplements in patients with cancer or groups with challenges to calcium homeostasis (i.e., people with renal insufficiency) has not been assessed. These groups should be cautious supplementing at levels greater than 1,000 IU per day until further evidence becomes available.

REFERENCES

1. Fleet, J.C. (2006) Molecular regulation of calcium metabolism. In: Weaver, C.M., and Heaney, R.P., eds. Calcium in Human Health. 163–90, Totowa, NJ: Humana Press.
2. Apperly, F.L. (1941) The relation of solar radiation to cancer mortality in North American. *Cancer Res* **1**, 191–95.
3. Garland, C.F., and Garland, F.C. (1980) Do sunlight and vitamin D reduce the likelihood of colon cancer? *Int J Epidemiol* **9**(3), 227–31.
4. Schwartz, G.G., and Hulka, B.S. (1990) Is vitamin D deficiency a risk factor for prostate cancer? (Hypothesis). *Anticancer Res* **10**(5A), 1307–11.
5. Holick, M. (1997) Photobiology of vitamin D. In: Feldman, D., Glorieux, F., and Pike, J., eds. Vitamin D. 33–39, San Diego, CA: Academic Press.
6. Hanchette, C.L., and Schwartz, G.G. (1992) Geographic patterns of prostate cancer mortality. Evidence for a protective effect of ultraviolet radiation. *Cancer* **70**(12), 2861–69.
7. Mohr, S.B., Garland, C.F., Gorham, E.D., Grant, W.B., and Garland, F.C. (2008) Relationship between low ultraviolet B irradiance and higher breast cancer risk in 107 countries. *Breast J* **14**(3), 255–60.
8. Porojnicu, A.C., Dahlback, A., and Moan, J. (2008) Sun exposure and cancer survival in Norway: Changes in the risk of death with season of diagnosis and latitude. *Adv Exp Med Biol* **624**, 43–54.
9. Boscoe, F.P., and Schymura, M.J. (2006) Solar ultraviolet-B exposure and cancer incidence and mortality in the United States, 1993–2002. *BMC Cancer* **6**, 264.
10. Robsahm, T.E., Tretli, S., Dahlback, A., and Moan, J. (2004) Vitamin D3 from sunlight may improve the prognosis of breast-, colon- and prostate cancer (Norway). *Cancer Causes Control* **15**(2), 149–58.
11. Webb, A.R., Kline, L., and Holick, M.F. (1988) Influence of season and latitude on the cutaneous synthesis of vitamin D3: Exposure to winter sunlight in Boston and Edmonton will not promote vitamin D3 synthesis in human skin. *J Clin Endocrinol Metab* **67**(2), 373–78.

12. White, P., and Cooke, N. (2000) The multifunctional properties and characteristics of vitamin D-binding protein. *Trends Endocrinol Metab* **11**(8), 320–27.

13. Trang, H.M., Cole, D.E., Rubin, L.A., Pierratos, A., Siu, S., and Vieth, R. (1998) Evidence that vitamin D3 increases serum 25-hydroxyvitamin D more efficiently than does vitamin D2. *Am J Clin Nutr* **68**(4), 854–58.

14. Holick, M.F. (2003) Vitamin D: A millenium perspective. *J Cell Biochem* **88**(2), 296–307.

15. Glerup, H., Mikkelsen, K., Poulsen, L., Hass, E., Overbeck, S., Thomsen, J. et al. (2000) Commonly recommended daily intake of vitamin D is not sufficient if sunlight exposure is limited. *J Intern Med* **247**(2), 260–68.

16. Vieth, R., Bischoff-Ferrari, H., Boucher, B.J., Dawson-Hughes, B., Garland, C.F., Heaney, R.P. et al. (2007) The urgent need to recommend an intake of vitamin D that is effective. *Am J Clin Nutr* **85**(3), 649–650.

17. Song, Y., Peng, X., Porta, A., Takanaga, H., Peng, J.B., Hediger, M.A. et al. (2003) Calcium transporter 1 and epithelial calcium channel messenger ribonucleic acid are differentially regulated by 1,25 dihydroxyvitamin D3 in the intestine and kidney of mice. *Endocrinology* **144**(9), 3885–94.

18. Zierold, C., Mings, J.A., and DeLuca, H.F. (2003) Regulation of 25-hydroxyvitamin D3-24-hydroxylase mRNA by 1,25-dihydroxyvitamin D3 and parathyroid hormone. *J Cell Biochem* **88**(2), 234–37.

19. Armbrecht, H.J., Boltz, M.A., and Hodam, T.L. (2003) PTH increases renal 25(OH)D3-1alpha-hydroxylase (CYP1alpha) mRNA but not renal 1,25(OH)2D3 production in adult rats. *Am J Physiol Renal Physiol* **284**(5), F1032–F36.

20. Haussler, M.R., Whitfield, G.K., Haussler, C.A., Hsieh, J.C., Thompson, P.D., Selznick, S.H. et al. (1998) The nuclear vitamin D receptor: Biological and molecular regulatory properties revealed. *J Bone Miner Res* **13**(3), 325–49.

21. Song, Y., Kato, S., and Fleet, J.C. (2003) Vitamin D receptor (VDR) knockout mice reveal VDR-independent regulation of intestinal calcium absorption and ECaC2 and calbindin D9k mRNA. *J Nutr* **133**(2), 374–80.

22. Van Cromphaut, S.J., Dewerchin, M., Hoenderop, J.G., Stockmans, I., Van Herck, E., Kato, S. et al. (2001) Duodenal calcium absorption in vitamin D receptor-knockout mice: Functional and molecular aspects. *Proc Natl Acad Sci U S A* **98**(23), 13324–29.

23. Song, Y., and Fleet, J.C. (2007) Intestinal resistance to 1,25 dihydroxyvitamin D in mice heterozygous for the vitamin D receptor knockout allele. *Endocrinology* **148**, 1396–402.

24. Omdahl, J.L., Morris, H.A., and May, B.K. (2002) Hydroxylase enzymes of the vitamin D pathway: Expression, function, and regulation. *Annu Rev Nutr* **22**, 139–66.

25. Fleet, J.C., Gliniak, C., Zhang, Z., Xue, Y., Smith, K.B., McCreedy, R. et al. (2008) Serum metabolite profiles and target tissue gene expression define the effect of cholecalciferol intake on calcium metabolism in rats and mice. *J Nutr* **138**(6), 1114–20.

26. Need, A.G., O'Loughlin, P.D., Morris, H.A., Coates, P.S., Horowitz, M., and Nordin, B.E. (2008) Vitamin D metabolites and calcium absorption in severe vitamin D deficiency. *J Bone Miner Res.*

27. Pike, J.W., Zella, L.A., Meyer, M.B., Fretz, J.A., and Kim, S. (2007) Molecular actions of 1,25-dihydroxyvitamin D3 on genes involved in calcium homeostasis. *J Bone Miner Res* **22**(Suppl 2), V16–V19.

28. Bouillon, R., Okamura, W.H., and Norman, A.W. (1995) Structure-function relationships in the vitamin D endocrine system. *Endocrine Rev* **16**(2), 200–57.

29. Barsony, J., Pike, J.W., DeLuca, H.F., and Marx, S.J. (1990) Immunocytology with microwave-fixed fibroblasts shows 1 alpha,25-dihydroxyvitamin D3-dependent rapid and estrogen-dependent slow reorganization of vitamin D receptors. *J Cell Biol* **111**(6 Pt 1), 2385–95.

30. Prufer, K., and Barsony, J. (2002) Retinoid X receptor dominates the nuclear import and export of the unliganded vitamin D receptor. *Mol Endocrinol* **16**(8), 1738–51.

31. Barsony, J., Renyi, I., and McKoy, W. (1997) Subcellular distribution of normal and mutant vitamin D receptors in living cells. *J Biol Chem* **272**, 5774–82.

32. Prufer, K., Racz, A., Lin, G.C., and Barsony, J. (2000) Dimerization with retinoid X receptors promotes nuclear localization and subnuclear targeting of vitamin D receptors. *J Biol Chem* **275**(52), 41114–23.

33. Freedman, L.P. (1999) Increasing the complexity of coactivation in nuclear receptor signaling. *Cell* **97**, 5–8.

34. Chen, H., Lin, R.J., Xie, W., Wilpitz, D., and Evans, R.M. (1999) Regulation of hormone-induced histone hyperacetylation and gene activation via acetylation of an acetylase. *Cell* **98**(5), 675–86.

35. Belandia, B., Orford, R.L., Hurst, H.C., and Parker, M.G. (2002) Targeting of SWI/SNF chromatin remodelling complexes to estrogen-responsive genes. *EMBO J* **21**(15), 4094–103.

36. Rachez, C., Lemon, B.D., Suldan, Z., Bromleigh, V., Gamble, M., Naar, A.M. et al. (1999) Ligand-dependent transcription activation by nuclear receptors requires the DRIP complex. *Nature* **398**, 824–28.

37. Uitterlinden, A.G., Fang, Y., van Meurs, J.B., Pols, H.A., and van Leeuwen, J.P. (2004) Genetics and biology of vitamin D receptor polymorphisms. *Gene* **338**(2), 143–56.

38. Rukin, N.J., and Strange, R.C. (2007) What are the frequency, distribution, and functional effects of vitamin D receptor polymorphisms as related to cancer risk? *Nutr Rev* **65**(8 Pt 2), S96–S101.

39. Morrison, N.A., Qi, J.C., Tokita, A., Kelly, P.J., Crofts, L., Nguyen, T.V. et al. (1994) Prediction of bone density from vitamin D receptor alleles. *Nature* **367**(6460), 284–87.

40. Fleet, J.C. (2007) Using genomics to understand intestinal biology. *J Physiol Biochem* **63**(1), 83–96.

41. Jurutka, P., Remus, L., Whitfield, K., Thompson, P., Hsieh, J., Zitzer, H. et al. (2000) The polymorphic N terminus in human vitamin D receptor isoforms influences transcriptional activity by modulating interaction with transcription factor IIB. *Mol Endocrinol* **14**, 401–20.

42. Colin, E.M., Weel, A.E., Uitterlinden, A.G., Buurman, C.J., Birkenhager, J.C., Pols, H.A. et al. (2000) Consequences of vitamin D receptor gene polymorphisms for growth inhibition of cultured human peripheral blood mononuclear cells by 1, 25-dihydroxyvitamin D3. *Clin Endocrinol (Oxf)* **52**(2), 211–16.

43. Fleet, J.C. (2004) Rapid, membrane-initiated actions of 1,25 dihydroxyvitamin d: What are they and what do they mean? *J Nutr* **134**(12), 3215–18.

44. Farach-Carson, M.C., and Nemere, I. (2003) Membrane receptors for vitamin D steroid hormones: Potential new drug targets. *Curr Drug Targets* **4**(1), 67–76.

45. Sitrin, M.D., Bissonnette, M., Bolt, M.J., Wali, R., Khare, S., Scaglione-Sewell, B. et al. (1999) Rapid effects of 1,25(OH)2 vitamin D3 on signal transduction systems in colonic cells. *Steroids* **64**(1–2), 137–42.

46. Chen, A.P., Davis, B.H., Bissonnette, M., Scaglione-Sewell, B., and Brasitus, T.A. (1999) 1,25-dihydroxyvitamin D-3 stimulates activator protein-1-dependent CaCo-2 cell differentiation. *J Biol Chem* **274**(50), 35505–13.

47. Khanal, R.C., and Nemere, I. (2008) Regulation of intestinal calcium transport. *Annu Rev Nutr* **28**, 179–96.

48. Huhtakangas, J.A., Olivera, C.J., Bishop, J.E., Zanello, L.P., and Norman, A.W. (2004) The vitamin D receptor is present in caveolae-enriched plasma membranes and binds 1{alpha},25(OH)2-vitamin D3 in vivo and in vitro. *Mol Endocrinol* **18**, 2660–71.

49. Holick, M.F. (2005) The influence of vitamin D on bone health across the life cycle. *J Nutr* **135**(11), 2726S–2727S.

50. Giovannucci, E., Liu, Y., Rimm, E.B., Hollis, B.W., Fuchs, C.S., Stampfer, M.J. et al. (2006) Prospective study of predictors of vitamin D status and cancer incidence and mortality in men. *J Natl Cancer Inst* **98**(7), 451–59.

51. Millen, A.E., and Bodnar, L.M. (2008) Vitamin D assessment in population-based studies: A review of the issues. *Am J Clin Nutr* **87**(4), 1102S–1105S.

52. Lips, P., Chapuy, M.C., Dawson-Hughes, B., Pols, H.A., and Holick, M.F. (1999) An international comparison of serum 25-hydroxyvitamin D measurements. *Osteoporos Int* **9**(5), 394–97.

53. Fearon, E.R., and Vogelstein, B. (1990) A genetic model for colorectal tumorigenesis. *Cell* **61**(5), 759–67.

54. Gervaz, P., Bucher, P., and Morel, P. (2004) Two colons-two cancers: Paradigm shift and clinical implications. *J Surg Oncol* **88**(4), 261–66.
55. Huncharek, M., Muscat, J., and Kupelnick, B. (2008) Dairy products, dietary calcium and vitamin D intake as risk factors for prostate cancer: A meta-analysis of 26,769 cases from 45 observational studies. *Nutr Cancer* **60**(4), 421–41.
56. Park, S.Y., Murphy, S.P., Wilkens, L.R., Stram, D.O., Henderson, B.E., and Kolonel, L.N. (2007) Calcium, vitamin D, and dairy product intake and prostate cancer risk: The Multiethnic Cohort Study. *Am J Epidemiol* **166**(11), 1259–69.
57. Chan, J.M., Stampfer, M.J., Ma, J., Gann, P.H., Gaziano, J.M., and Giovannucci, E.L. (2001) Dairy products, calcium, and prostate cancer risk in the Physicians' Health Study. *Am J Clin Nutr* **74**(4), 549–54.
58. Chan, J.M., Giovannucci, E., Andersson, S.O., Yuen, J., Adami, H.O., and Wolk, A. (1998) Dairy products, calcium, phosphorous, vitamin D, and risk of prostate cancer (Sweden). *Cancer Causes Control* **9**(6), 559–66.
59. Allen, N.E., Key, T.J., Appleby, P.N., Travis, R.C., Roddam, A.W., Tjonneland, A. et al. (2008) Animal foods, protein, calcium and prostate cancer risk: The European Prospective Investigation into Cancer and Nutrition. *Br J Cancer* **98**(9), 1574–81.
60. Ahonen, M.H., Tenkanen, L., Teppo, L., Hakama, M., and Tuohimaa, P. (2000) Prostate cancer risk and prediagnostic serum 25-hydroxyvitamin D levels (Finland). *Cancer Causes Control* **11**(9), 847–52.
61. Braun, M.M., Helzlsouer, K.J., Hollis, B.W., and Comstock, G.W. (1995) Prostate cancer and prediagnostic levels of serum vitamin D metabolites (Maryland, United States). *Cancer Causes Control* **6**(3), 235–39.
62. Nomura, A.M., Stemmermann, G.N., Lee, J., Kolonel, L.N., Chen, T.C., Turner, A. et al. (1998) Serum vitamin D metabolite levels and the subsequent development of prostate cancer (Hawaii, United States). *Cancer Causes Control* **9**(4), 425–32.
63. Ahn, J., Peters, U., Albanes, D., Purdue, M.P., Abnet, C.C., Chatterjee, N. et al. (2008) Serum vitamin D concentration and prostate cancer risk: A nested case-control study. *J Natl Cancer Inst* **100**(11), 796–804.
64. Corder, E.H., Guess, H.A., Hulka, B.S., Friedman, G.D., Sadler, M., Vollmer, R.T. et al. (1993) Vitamin D and prostate cancer: A prediagnostic study with stored sera. *Cancer Epidemiol Biomarkers Prev* **2**(5), 467–72.
65. Li, H., Stampfer, M.J., Hollis, J.B., Mucci, L.A., Gaziano, J.M., Hunter, D. et al. (2007) A prospective study of plasma vitamin D metabolites, vitamin D receptor polymorphisms, and prostate cancer. *PLoS Med* **4**(3), e103.
66. Kearney, J., Giovannucci, E., Rimm, E.B., Ascherio, A., Stampfer, M.J., Colditz, G.A. et al. (1996) Calcium, vitamin D, and dairy foods and the occurrence of colon cancer in men. *Am J Epidemiol* **143**(9), 907–17.
67. Oh, K., Willett, W.C., Wu, K., Fuchs, C.S., and Giovannucci, E.L. (2007) Calcium and vitamin D intakes in relation to risk of distal colorectal adenoma in women. *Am J Epidemiol* **165**(10), 1178–86.
68. Garland, C.F., Comstock, G.W., Garland, F.C., Helsing, K.J., Shaw, E.K., and Gorham, E.D. (1989) Serum 25-hydroxyvitamin D and colon cancer: Eight-year prospective study. *Lancet* **2**(8673), 1176–78.
69. Tangrea, J., Helzlsouer, K., Pietinen, P., Taylor, P., Hollis, B., Virtamo, J. et al. (1997) Serum levels of vitamin D metabolites and the subsequent risk of colon and rectal cancer in Finnish men. *Cancer Causes Control* **8**(4), 615–25.
70. Feskanich, D., Ma, J., Fuchs, C.S., Kirkner, G.J., Hankinson, S.E., Hollis, B.W. et al. (2004) Plasma vitamin D metabolites and risk of colorectal cancer in women. *Cancer Epidemiol Biomarkers Prev* **13**(9), 1502–08.
71. Wu, K., Feskanich, D., Fuchs, C.S., Willett, W.C., Hollis, B.W., and Giovannucci, E.L. (2007) A nested case control study of plasma 25-hydroxyvitamin D concentrations and risk of colorectal cancer. *J Natl Cancer Inst* **99**(14), 1120–29.

72. Peters, U., Hayes, R.B., Chatterjee, N., Shao, W., Schoen, R.E., Pinsky, P. et al. (2004) Circulating vitamin D metabolites, polymorphism in vitamin D receptor, and colorectal adenoma risk. *Cancer Epidemiol Biomarkers Prev* **13**(4), 546–52.

73. Ng, K., Meyerhardt, J.A., Wu, K., Feskanich, D., Hollis, B.W., Giovannucci, E.L. et al. (2008) Circulating 25-hydroxyvitamin d levels and survival in patients with colorectal cancer. *J Clin Oncol* **26**(18), 2984–91.

74. Berube, S., Diorio, C., Verhoek-Oftedahl, W., and Brisson, J. (2004) Vitamin D, calcium, and mammographic breast densities. *Cancer Epidemiol Biomarkers Prev* **13**(9), 1466–72.

75. Tseng, M., Byrne, C., Evers, K.A., and Daly, M.B. (2007) Dietary intake and breast density in high-risk women: A cross-sectional study. *Breast Cancer Res* **9**(5), R72.

76. Brisson, J., Berube, S., Diorio, C., Sinotte, M., Pollak, M., and Masse, B. (2007) Synchronized seasonal variations of mammographic breast density and plasma 25-hydroxyvitamin d. *Cancer Epidemiol Biomarkers Prev* **16**(5), 929–33.

77. Knight, J.A., Vachon, C.M., Vierkant, R.A., Vieth, R., Cerhan, J.R., and Sellers, T.A. (2006) No association between 25-hydroxyvitamin D and mammographic density. *Cancer Epidemiol Biomarkers Prev* **15**(10), 1988–92.

78. Shin, M.H., Holmes, M.D., Hankinson, S.E., Wu, K., Colditz, G.A., and Willett, W.C. (2002) Intake of dairy products, calcium, and vitamin d and risk of breast cancer. *J Natl Cancer Inst* **94**(17), 1301–11.

79. Lin, J., Manson, J.E., Lee, I.M., Cook, N.R., Buring, J.E., and Zhang, S.M. (2007) Intakes of calcium and vitamin D and breast cancer risk in women. *Arch Intern Med* **167**(10), 1050–59.

80. Abbas, S., Linseisen, J., and Chang-Claude, J. (2007) Dietary vitamin D and calcium intake and premenopausal breast cancer risk in a German case-control study. *Nutr Cancer* **59**(1), 54–61.

81. McCullough, M.L., Rodriguez, C., Diver, W.R., Feigelson, H.S., Stevens, V.L., Thun, M.J. et al. (2005) Dairy, calcium, and vitamin D intake and postmenopausal breast cancer risk in the Cancer Prevention Study II Nutrition Cohort. *Cancer Epidemiol Biomarkers Prev* **14**(12), 2898–904.

82. Bertone-Johnson, E.R., Chen, W.Y., Holick, M.F., Hollis, B.W., Colditz, G.A., Willett, W.C. et al. (2005) Plasma 25-hydroxyvitamin D and 1,25-dihydroxyvitamin D and risk of breast cancer. *Cancer Epidemiol Biomarkers Prev* **14**(8), 1991–97.

83. Janowsky, E.C., Lester, G.E., Weinberg, C.R., Millikan, R.C., Schildkraut, J.M., Garrett, P.A. et al. (1999) Association between low levels of 1,25-dihydroxyvitamin D and breast cancer risk. *Public Health Nutr* **2**(3), 283–91.

84. Freedman, D.M., Chang, S.C., Falk, R.T., Purdue, M.P., Huang, W.Y., McCarty, C.A. et al. (2008) Serum levels of vitamin D metabolites and breast cancer risk in the prostate, lung, colorectal, and ovarian cancer screening trial. *Cancer Epidemiol Biomarkers Prev* **17**(4), 889–94.

85. Trabert, B., Malone, K.E., Daling, J.R., Doody, D.R., Bernstein, L., Ursin, G. et al. (2007) Vitamin D receptor polymorphisms and breast cancer risk in a large population-based case-control study of Caucasian and African-American women. *Breast Cancer Res* **9**(6), R84.

86. Lowe, L.C., Guy, M., Mansi, J.L., Peckitt, C., Bliss, J., Wilson, R.G. et al. (2005) Plasma 25-hydroxy vitamin D concentrations, vitamin D receptor genotype and breast cancer risk in a UK Caucasian population. *Eur J Cancer* **41**(8), 1164–69.

87. Guy, M., Lowe, L.C., Bretherton-Watt, D., Mansi, J.L., Peckitt, C., Bliss, J. et al. (2004) Vitamin D receptor gene polymorphisms and breast cancer risk. *Clin Cancer Res* **10**(16), 5472–81.

88. Wedren, S., Magnusson, C., Humphreys, K., Melhus, H., Kindmark, A., Stiger, F. et al. (2007) Associations between androgen and Vitamin D receptor microsatellites and postmenopausal breast cancer. *Cancer Epidemiol Biomarkers Prev* **16**(9), 1775–83.

89. Zehnder, D., Bland, R., Williams, M.C., McNinch, R.W., Howie, A.J., Stewart, P.M. et al. (2001) Extrarenal expression of 25-hydroxyvitamin d(3)-1 alpha-hydroxylase. *J Clin Endocrinol Metab* **86**(2), 888–94.

90. Kemmis, C.M., Salvador, S.M., Smith, K.M., and Welsh, J. (2006) Human mammary epithelial cells express CYP27B1 and are growth inhibited by 25-hydroxyvitamin D-3, the major circulating form of vitamin D-3. *J Nutr* **136**(4), 887–92.

91. Hsu, J.Y., Feldman, D., McNeal, J.E., and Peehl, D.M. (2001) Reduced 1alpha-hydroxylase activity in human prostate cancer cells correlates with decreased susceptibility to 25-hydroxyvitamin D3-induced growth inhibition. *Cancer Res* **61**(7), 2852–56.

92. Chen, T.C., Wang, L., Whitlatch, L.W., Flanagan, J.N., and Holick, M.F. (2003) Prostatic 25-hydroxyvitamin D-1alpha-hydroxylase and its implication in prostate cancer. *J Cell Biochem* **88**(2), 315–22.

93. Whitlatch, L.W., Young, M.V., Schwartz, G.G., Flanagan, J.N., Burnstein, K.L., Lokeshwar, B.L. et al. (2002) 25-Hydroxyvitamin D-1alpha-hydroxylase activity is diminished in human prostate cancer cells and is enhanced by gene transfer. *J Steroid Biochem Mol Biol* **81**(2), 135–40.

94. Anderson, P.H., Hendrix, I., Sawyer, R.K., Zarrinkalam, R., Manavis, J., Sarvestani, G.T. et al. (2008) Co-expression of CYP27B1 enzyme with the 1.5 kb CYP27B1 promoter-luciferase transgene in the mouse. *Mol Cell Endocrinol* **285**(1–2), 1–9.

95. Bareis, P., Kallay, E., Bischof, M.G., Bises, G., Hofer, H., Potzi, C. et al. (2002) Clonal Differences in Expression of 25-Hydroxyvitamin D(3)-1alpha- hydroxylase, of 25-Hydroxyvitamin D(3)-24-hydroxylase, and of the Vitamin D Receptor in Human Colon Carcinoma Cells: Effects of Epidermal Growth Factor and 1alpha,25-Dihydroxyvitamin D(3). *Exp Cell Res* **276**(2), 320–27.

96. Matusiak, D., Murillo, G., Carroll, R.E., Mehta, R.G., and Benya, R.V. (2005) Expression of vitamin D receptor and 25-hydroxyvitamin D3-1{alpha}-hydroxylase in normal and malignant human colon. *Cancer Epidemiol Biomarkers Prev* **14**(10), 2370–76.

97. Vieth, R., McCarten, K., and Norwich, K.H. (1990) Role of 25-hydroxyvitamin D3 dose in determining rat 1,25-dihydroxyvitamin D3 production. *Am J Physiol* **258**(5 Pt 1), E780–E89.

98. Colston, K., Colston, M.J., and Feldman, D. (1981) 1,25-dihydroxyvitamin D3 and malignant melanoma: The presence of receptors and inhibition of cell growth in culture. *Endocrinology* **108**(3), 1083–86.

99. Lointier, P., Wargovich, M.J., Saez, S., Levin, B., Wildrick, D.M., and Boman, B.M. (1987) The role of vitamin D3 in the proliferation of a human colon cancer cell line in vitro. *Anticancer Res* **7**(4B), 817–21.

100. Gross, M., Kost, S.B., Ennis, B., Stumpf, W., and Kumar, R. (1986) Effect of 1,25-dihydroxyvitamin D3 on mouse mammary tumor (GR) cells: Evidence for receptors, cellular uptake, inhibition of growth and alteration in morphology at physiologic concentrations of hormone. *J Bone Miner Res* **1**(5), 457–67.

101. Skowronski, R.J., Peehl, D.M., and Feldman, D. (1993) Vitamin D and prostate cancer: 1,25 dihydroxyvitamin D3 receptors and actions in human prostate cancer cell lines. *Endocrinology* **132**(5), 1952–60.

102. Simboli-Campbell, M., Gagnon, A.M., Franks, D.J., and Welsh, J.E. (1994) 1,25-Dihydroxyvitamin D3 Translocates Protein Kinase Cß to Nucleus and Enhances Plasma Membrane Association of Protein Kinase C-alpha in Renal Epithelial Cells. *J Biol Chem* **269**, 3257–64.

103. Diaz, G.D., Paraskeva, C., Thomas, M.G., Binderup, L., and Hague, A. (2000) Apoptosis is induced by the active metabolite of vitamin D3 and its analogue EB1089 in colorectal adenoma and carcinoma cells: Possible implications for prevention and therapy. *Cancer Res* **60**(8), 2304–12.

104. Zhuang, S.H., and Burnstein, K.L. (1998) Antiproliferative effect of 1alpha,25-dihydroxyvitamin D3 in human prostate cancer cell line LNCaP involves reduction of cyclin-dependent kinase 2 activity and persistent G1 accumulation. *Endocrinology* **139**(3), 1197–207.

105. Hill, R., Song, Y., Cardiff, R.D., and Van Dyke, T. (2005) Selective evolution of stromal mesenchyme with p53 loss in response to epithelial tumorigenesis. *Cell* **123**(6), 1001–11.

106. Lou, Y.R., Laaksi, I., Syvala, H., Blauer, M., Tammela, T.L., Ylikomi , T.et al. (2004) 25-hydroxyvitamin D3 is an active hormone in human primary prostatic stromal cells. *FASEB J* **18**(2), 332–34.

107. Coussens, L.M., and Werb, Z. (2002) Inflammation and cancer. *Nature* **420**(6917), 860–67.

108. Haverkamp, J., Charbonneau, B., and Ratliff, T.L. (2007) Prostate inflammation and its potential impact on prostate cancer: A current review. *J Cell Biochem*.

109. Cantorna, M.T., Zhu, Y., Froicu, M., and Wittke, A. (2004) Vitamin D status, 1,25-dihydroxyvitamin D3, and the immune system. *Am J Clin Nutr* **80**(6 Suppl), 1717S–1720S.

110. Adams, J.S., Liu, P.T., Chun, R., Modlin, R.L., and Hewison, M. (2007) Vitamin D in defense of the human immune response. *Ann N Y Acad Sci* **1117**, 94–105.

111. Griffin, M.D., Dong, X., and Kumar, R. (2007) Vitamin D receptor-mediated suppression of RelB in antigen presenting cells: A paradigm for ligand-augmented negative transcriptional regulation. *Arch Biochem Biophys* **460**(2), 218–26.

112. Cantorna, M.T., and Mahon, B.D. (2004) Mounting evidence for vitamin D as an environmental factor affecting autoimmune disease prevalence. *Exp Biol Med (Maywood)* **229**(11), 1136–42.

113. Liu, M., Lee, M.H., Cohen, M., Bommakanti, M., and Freedman, L.P. (1996) Transcriptional activation of the Cdk inhibitor p21 by vitamin D leads to the induced differentiation of the myelomonocytic cell line U937. *Genes Dev* **10**, 142–53.

114. Moffatt, K.A., Johannes, W.U., Hedlund, T.E., and Miller, G.J. (2001) Growth inhibitory effects of 1alpha, 25-dihydroxyvitamin D(3) are mediated by increased levels of p21 in the prostatic carcinoma cell line ALVA-31. *Cancer Res* **61**(19), 7122–29.

115. Rao, A., Coan, A., Welsh, J.E., Barclay, W.W., Koumenis, C., and Cramer, S.D. (2004) Vitamin D receptor and p21/WAF1 are targets of genistein and 1,25-dihydroxyvitamin D3 in human prostate cancer cells. *Cancer Res* **64**(6), 2143–47.

116. Boyle, B.J., Zhao, X.Y., Cohen, P., and Feldman, D. (2001) Insulin-like growth factor binding protein-3 mediates 1 alpha,25- dihydroxyvitamin d(3) growth inhibition in the LNCaP prostate cancer cell line through p21/WAF1. *J Urol* **165**(4), 1319–24.

117. Monti, S., Proietti-Pannunzi, L., Sciarra, A., Lolli, F., Falasca, P., Poggi, M. et al. (2007) The IGF axis in prostate cancer. *Curr Pharm Des* **13**(7), 719–27.

118. Huynh, H., Pollak, M., and Zhang, J.C. (1998) Regulation of insulin-like growth factor (IGF) II and IGF binding protein 3 autocrine loop in human PC-3 prostate cancer cells by vitamin D metabolite 1,25(OH)2D3 and its analog EB1089. *Int J Oncol* **13**(1), 137–43.

119. Sprenger, C.C., Peterson, A., Lance, R., Ware, J.L., Drivdahl, R.H., and Plymate, S.R. (2001) Regulation of proliferation of prostate epithelial cells by 1,25- dihydroxyvitamin D3 is accompanied by an increase in insulin-like growth factor binding protein-3. *J Endocrinol* **170**(3), 609–18.

120. Peng, L.H., Malloy, P.J., and Feldman, D. (2004) Identification of a functional vitamin D response element in the human insulin-like growth factor binding protein-3 promoter. *Mol Endocrinol* **18**(5), 1109–19.

121. Macleod, K. (2000) Tumor suppressor genes. *Curr Opin Genet Dev* **10**(1), 81–93.

122. Palmer, H.G., Gonzalez-Sancho, J.M., Espada, J., Berciano, M.T., Puig, I., Baulida, J. et al. (2001) Vitamin D(3) promotes the differentiation of colon carcinoma cells by the induction of E-cadherin and the inhibition of beta-catenin signaling. *J Cell Biol* **154**(2), 369–87.

123. Shah, S., Islam, M.N., Dakshanamurthy, S., Rizvi, I., Rao, M., Herrell, R. et al. (2006) The molecular basis of vitamin D receptor and beta-catenin crossregulation. *Mol Cell* **21**(6), 799–809.

124. Pendas-Franco, N., Garcia, J.M., Pena, C., Valle, N., Palmer, H.G., Heinaniemi, M. et al. (2008) DICKKOPF-4 is induced by TCF/beta-catenin and upregulated in human colon cancer, promotes tumour cell invasion and angiogenesis and is repressed by 1alpha,25-dihydroxyvitamin D(3). *Oncogene.*

125. Aguilera, O., Pena, C., Garcia, J.M., Larriba, M.J., Ordonez-Moran, P., Navarro, D. et al. (2007) The Wnt antagonist DICKKOPF-1 gene is induced by 1alpha,25-dihydroxyvitamin D3 associated to the differentiation of human colon cancer cells. *Carcinogenesis* **28**(9), 1877–84.

126. Krishnan, A.V., Shinghal, R., Raghavachari, N., Brooks, J.D., Peehl, D.M., and Feldman, D. (2004) Analysis of vitamin D-regulated gene expression in LNCaP human prostate cancer cells using cDNA microarrays. *Prostate* **59**(3), 243–51.

127. Qiao, S., and Tuohimaa, P. (2004) The role of long-chain fatty-acid-CoA ligase 3 in vitamin D3 and androgen control of prostate cancer LNCaP cell growth. *Biochem Biophys Res Commun* **319**(2), 358–68.

128. Peehl, D.M., Shinghal, R., Nonn, L., Seto, E., Krishnan, A.V., Brooks, J.D. et al. (2004) Molecular activity of 1,25-dihydroxyvitamin D3 in primary cultures of human prostatic epithelial cells revealed by cDNA microarray analysis. *J Steroid Biochem Mol Biol* **92**(3), 131–41.

129. Guzey, M., Luo, J., and Getzenberg, R.H. (2004) Vitamin D3 modulated gene expression patterns in human primary normal and cancer prostate cells. *J Cell Biochem* **93**(2), 271–85.

130. Towsend, K., Trevino, V., Falciani, F., Stewart, P.M., Hewison, M., and Campbell, M.J. (2006) Identification of VDR-responsive gene signatures in breast cancer cells. *Oncology* **71**(1–2), 111–23.

131. Lee, H.J., Liu, H., Goodman, C., Ji, Y., Maehr, H., Uskokovic, M. et al. (2006) Gene expression profiling changes induced by a novel Gemini Vitamin D derivative during the progression of breast cancer. *Biochem Pharmacol* **72**(3), 332–43.

132. Lyakhovich, A., Aksenov, N., Pennanen, P., Miettinen, S., Ahonen, M.H., Syvala, H. et al. (2000) Vitamin D induced up-regulation of keratinocyte growth factor (FGF-7/KGF) in MCF-7 human breast cancer cells. *Biochem Biophys Res Commun* **273**(2), 675–80.

133. Swami, S., Raghavachari, N., Muller, U.R., Bao, Y.P., and Feldman, D. (2003) Vitamin D growth inhibition of breast cancer cells: Gene expression patterns assessed by cDNA microarray. *Breast Cancer Res Treat* **80**(1), 49–62.

134. Palmer, H.G., Sanchez-Carbayo, M., Ordonez-Moran, P., Larriba, M.J., Cordon-Cardo, C., and Munoz, A. (2003) Genetic signatures of differentiation induced by 1alpha,25-dihydroxyvitamin D3 in human colon cancer cells. *Cancer Res* **63**(22), 7799–806.

135. Zhang, X.T., Krutchinsky, A., Fukuda, A., Chen, W., and Yamamura, S. (2005) Chalt BT et al. MED1/TRAP220 exists predominantly in a TRAP/mediator subpopulation enriched in RNA polymerase II and is required for ER-mediated transcription. *Mol Cell* **19**(1), 89–100.

136. Akutsu, N., Lin, R., Bastien, Y., Bestawros, A., Enepekides, D.J., Black, M.J. et al. (2001) Regulation of gene Expression by 1alpha,25-dihydroxyvitamin D3 and Its analog EB1089 under growth-inhibitory conditions in squamous carcinoma Cells. *Mol Endocrinol* **15**(7), 1127–39.

137. Lin, R., Nagai, Y., Sladek, R., Bastien, Y., Ho, J., Petrecca, K. et al. (2002) Expression profiling in squamous carcinoma cells reveals pleiotropic effects of vitamin D(3) analog EB1089 signaling on cell proliferation, differentiation, and immune system regulation. *Mol Endocrinol* **16**(6), 1243–56.

138. Wang, T.T., Tavera-Mendoza, L.E., Laperriere, D., Libby, E., MacLeod, N.B., Nagai, Y. et al. (2005) Large-scale in silico and microarray-based identification of direct 1,25-dihydroxyvitamin D3 target genes. *Mol Endocrinol* **19**(11), 2685–95.

139. Tashiro, K., Abe, T., Oue, N., Yasui, W., and Ryoji, M. (2004) Characterization of vitamin D-mediated induction of the CYP 24 transcription. *Mol Cell Endocrinol* **226**(1–2), 27–32.

140. Moreno, J., Krishnan, A.V., and Feldman, D. (2005) Molecular mechanisms mediating the antiproliferative effects of Vitamin D in prostate cancer. *J Steroid Biochem Mol Biol* **97**(1–2), 31–36.

141. Ben Shoshan, M., Amir, S., Dang, D.T., Dang, L.H., Weisman, Y., and Mabjeesh, N.J. (2007) 1alpha,25-dihydroxyvitamin D3 (Calcitriol) inhibits hypoxia-inducible factor-1/vascular endothelial growth factor pathway in human cancer cells. *Mol Cancer Ther* **6**(4), 1433–39.

142. Matusiak, D., Murillo, G., Carroll, R.E., Mehta, R.G., and Benya, R.V. (2005) Expression of vitamin D receptor and 25-hydroxyvitamin D3-1{alpha}-hydroxylase in normal and malignant human colon. *Cancer Epidemiol Biomarkers Prev* **14**(10), 2370–76.

143. Escaleira, M.T., and Brentani, M.M. (1999) Vitamin D3 receptor (VDR) expression in HC-11 mammary cells: Regulation by growth-modulatory agents, differentiation, and Ha-ras transformation. *Breast Cancer Res Treat* **54**(2), 123–33.

144. Solomon, C., White, J.H., and Kremer, R. (1999) Mitogen-activated protein kinase inhibits 1,25-dihydroxyvitamin D3- dependent signal transduction by phosphorylating human retinoid X receptor alpha. *J Clin Invest* **103**(12), 1729–35.

145. Macoritto, M., Nguyen-Yamamoto, L., Huang, D.C., Samuel, S., Yang, X.F., Wang, T.T. et al. (2008) Phosphorylation of the human retinoid X receptor alpha at serine 260 impairs coactivator(s) recruitment and induces hormone resistance to multiple ligands. *J Biol Chem* **283**(8), 4943–56.

146. Friedrich, M., Diesing, D., Cordes, T., Fischer, D., Becker, S., Chen, T.C. et al. (2006) Analysis of 25-hydroxyvitamin D3-1alpha-hydroxylase in normal and malignant breast tissue. *Anticancer Res* **26**(4A), 2615–20.

147. Albertson, D.G., Ylstra, B., Segraves, R., Collins, C., Dairkee, S.H., Kowbel, D. et al. (2000) Quantitative mapping of amplicon structure by array CGH identifies CYP24 as a candidate oncogene. *Nat Genet* **25**(2), 144–46.

148. Anderson, M.G., Nakane, M., Ruan, X., Kroeger, P.E., and Wu-Wong, J.R. (2006) Expression of VDR and CYP24A1 mRNA in human tumors. *Cancer Chemother Pharmacol* **57**(2), 234–40.

149. Matusiak, D., and Benya, R.V. (2007) CYP27A1 and CYP24 expression as a function of malignant transformation in the colon. *J Histochem Cytochem* **55**(12), 1257–64.

150. Xue, L., Lipkin, M., Newmark, H., and Wang, J. (1999) Influence of dietary calcium and vitamin D on diet-induced epithelial cell hyperproliferation in mice. *J Natl Cancer Inst* **91**(2), 176–81.

151. Lamprecht, S.A., and Lipkin, M. (2003) Chemoprevention of colon cancer by calcium, vitamin D and folate: Molecular mechanisms. *Nat Rev Cancer* **3**(8), 601–14.

152. Kallay, E., Pietschmann, P., Toyokuni, S., Bajna, E., Hahn, P., Mazzucco, K. et al. (2001) Characterization of a vitamin D receptor knockout mouse as a model of colorectal hyperproliferation and DNA damage. *Carcinogenesis* **22**(9), 1429–35.

153. Rowling, M.J., Gliniak, C., Welsh, J., and Fleet, J.C. (2007) High dietary vitamin D prevents hypocalcemia and osteomalacia in CYP27B1 knockout mice. *J Nutr* **137**(12), 2608–15.

154. Sitrin, M.D., Halline, A.G., Abrahams, C., and Brasitus, T.A. (1991) Dietary calcium and vitamin D modulate 1,2-dimethylhydrazine-induced colonic carcinogenesis in the rat. *Cancer Res* **51**(20), 5608–13.

155. Llor, X., Jacoby, R.F., Teng, B.B., Davidson, N.O., Sitrin, M.D., and Brasitus, T.A. (1991) K-ras mutations in 1,2-dimethylhydrazine-induced colonic tumors: Effects of supplemental dietary calcium and vitamin D deficiency. *Cancer Res* **51**(16), 4305–09.

156. Tangpricha, V., Spina, C., Yao, M., Chen, T.C., Wolfe, M.M., and Holick, M.F. (2005) Vitamin D deficiency enhances the growth of MC-26 colon cancer xenografts in Balb/c mice. *J Nutr* **135**(10), 2350–54.

157. Comer, P.F., Clark, T.D., and Glauert, H.P. (1993) Effect of dietary vitamin D3 (cholecalciferol) on colon carcinogenesis induced by 1,2-dimethylhydrazine in male Fischer 344 rats. *Nutr Cancer* **19**(2), 113–24.

158. Beaty, M.M., Lee, E.Y., and Glauert, H.P. (1993) Influence of dietary calcium and vitamin D on colon epithelial cell proliferation and 1,2-dimethylhydrazine-induced colon carcinogenesis in rats fed high fat diets. *J Nutr* **123**(1), 144–52.

159. Valrance, M.E., Brunet, A.H., and Welsh, J. (2007) Vitamin D receptor-dependent inhibition of mammary tumor growth by EB1089 and ultraviolet radiation in vivo. *Endocrinology* **148**(10), 4887–94.

160. Chen, T.C., Holick, M.F., Lokeshwar, B.L., Burnstein, K.L., and Schwartz, G.G. (2003) Evaluation of vitamin D analogs as therapeutic agents for prostate cancer. *Recent Results Cancer Res* **164**, 273–88.

161. Oades, G.M., Senaratne, S.G., Clarke, I.A., Kirby, R.S., and Colston, K.W. (2003) Nitrogen containing bisphosphonates induce apoptosis and inhibit the mevalonate pathway, impairing Ras membrane localization in prostate cancer cells. *J Urol* **170**(1), 246–52.

162. Huerta, S., Irwin, R.W., Heber, D., Go, V.L., Koeffler, H.P. Uskokovic, M.R. et al. (2002) 1alpha,25-(OH)(2)-D(3) and its synthetic analogue decrease tumor load in the Apc(min) Mouse. *Cancer Res* **62**(3), 741–46.

163. Mehta, R.G. (2004) Stage-specific inhibition of mammary carcinogenesis by 1alpha-hydroxyvitamin D5. *Eur J Cancer* **40**(15), 2331–37.

164. Vegesna, V., O'Kelly, J., Said, J., Uskokovic, M., Binderup, L., and Koeffle, H.P. (2003) Ability of potent vitamin D3 analogs to inhibit growth of prostate cancer cells in vivo. *Anticancer Res* **23**(1A), 283–89.

165. Crescioli, C., Ferruzzi, P., Caporali, A., Scaltriti, M., Bettuzzi, S., Mancina, R. et al. (2004) Inhibition of prostate cell growth by BXL-628, a calcitriol analogue selected for a phase II clinical trial in patients with benign prostate hyperplasia. *Eur J Endocrinol* **150**(4), 591–603.

166. Otoshi, T., Iwata, H., Kitano, M., Nishizawa, Y., Morii, H., Yano, Y. et al. (1995) Inhibition of intestinal tumor development in rat multi-organ carcinogenesis and aberrant crypt foci in rat colon carcinogenesis by 22-oxa-calcitriol, a synthetic analogue of 1 alpha, 25-dihydroxyvitamin D3. *Carcinogenesis* **16**(9), 2091–97.

167. Fichera, A., Little, N., Dougherty, U., Mustafi, R., Cerda, S., Li, Y.C. et al. (2007) A vitamin D analogue inhibits colonic carcinogenesis in the AOM/DSS model. *J Surg Res* **142**(2), 239–45.

168. Penna, G., Amuchastegui, S., Cossetti, C., Aquilano, F., Mariani, R., Sanvito, F. et al. (2006) Treatment of experimental autoimmune prostatitis in nonobese diabetic mice by the vitamin D receptor agonist elocalcitol. *J Immunol* **177**(12), 8504–11.
169. Schwartz, G.G. (2008) Vitamin D and Intervention Trials in Prostate Cancer: From Theory to Therapy. *Ann Epidemiol.*
170. Beer, T.M., Munar, M., and Henner, W.D. (2001) A Phase I trial of pulse calcitriol in patients with refractory malignancies: Pulse dosing permits substantial dose escalation. *Cancer* **91**(12), 2431–39.
171. Beer, T.M., Ryan, C.W., Venner, P.M., Petrylak, D.P., Chatta, G.S., Ruether, J.D. et al. (2007) Double-blinded randomized study of high-dose calcitriol plus docetaxel compared with placebo plus docetaxel in androgen-independent prostate cancer: A report from the ASCENT Investigators. *J Clin Oncol* **25**(6), 669–74.
172. Brown, A.J. (2000) Mechanisms for the selective actions of vitamin D analogues. *Curr Pharm Des* **6**(7), 701–16.
173. Norman, A.W., Mizwicki, M.T., and Okamura, W.H. (2003) Ligand structure-function relationships in the vitamin D endocrine system from the perspective of drug development (including cancer treatment). *Recent Results Cancer Res* **164**, 55–82.
174. Vijayakumar, S., Mehta, R.R., Boerner, P.S., Packianathan, S., and Mehta, R.G. (2005) Clinical trials involving vitamin D analogs in prostate cancer. *Cancer J* **11**(5), 362–73.
175. Wactawski-Wende, J., Kotchen, J.M., Anderson, G.L., Assaf, A.R., Brunner, R.L., O'Sullivan, M.J. et al. (2006) Calcium plus vitamin D supplementation and the risk of colorectal cancer. *N Engl J Med* **354**(7), 684–96.
176. Ding, E.L., Mehta, S., Fawzi, W.W., and Giovannucci, E.L. (2008) Interaction of estrogen therapy with calcium and vitamin D supplementation on colorectal cancer risk: Reanalysis of Women's Health Initiative randomized trial. *Int J Cancer* **122**(8), 1690–94.
177. Lappe, J.M., Travers-Gustafson, D., Davies, K.M., Recker, R.R., and Heaney, R.P. (2007) Vitamin D and calcium supplementation reduces cancer risk: Results of a randomized trial. *Am J Clin Nutr* **85**(6), 1586–91.
178. Woo, T.C., Choo, R., Jamieson, M., Chander, S., and Vieth, R. (2005) Pilot study: Potential role of vitamin D (Cholecalciferol) in patients with PSA relapse after definitive therapy. *Nutr Cancer* **51**(1), 32–36.
179. Nesby-O'Dell, S., Scanlon, K.S., Cogswell, M.E., Gillespie, C., Hollis, B.W., Looker, A.C. et al. (2002) Hypovitaminosis D prevalence and determinants among African American and white women of reproductive age: Third National Health and Nutrition Examination Survey, 1988–1994. *Am J Clin Nutr* **76**(1), 187–92.
180. Looker, A.C., Dawson-Hughes, B., Calvo, M.S., Gunter, E.W., and Sahyoun, N.R. (2002) Serum 25-hydroxyvitamin D status of adolescents and adults in two seasonal subpopulations from NHANES III. *Bone* **30**(5), 771–77.
181. Holick, M.F., Biancuzzo, R.M., Chen, T.C., Klein, E.K., Young, A., Bibuld, D. et al. (2008) Vitamin D2 is as effective as vitamin D3 in maintaining circulating concentrations of 25-hydroxyvitamin D. *J Clin Endocrinol Metab* **93**(3), 677–81.
182. Hathcock, J.N., Shao, A., Vieth, R., and Heaney, R. (2007) Risk assessment for vitamin D. *Am J Clin Nutr* **85**(1), 6–18.

18 Folate

Cornelia M. Ulrich, Xinran Xu, Amy Liu, and Jia Chen

Key Points

1. Folate is a generic descriptor for a water-soluble B-complex vitamin that functions in one-carbon transfer reactions and exists in multiple chemical forms. Most naturally occurring folates are polyglutamated forms, which enable their retention in the cell. However, folic acid is the most oxidized and stable form of folate, rarely found in food, yet used commonly in vitamin supplements and fortified foods.
2. The nutrient folate is a B vitamin that provides methyl groups for one-carbon transfer reactions, including those supporting the synthesis of nucleotides and methylation reactions. A higher folate status has been consistently associated with decreased cancers risks of the colorectum, esophagus, and possibly pancreas. A decreased breast cancer risk with higher folate intakes among alcohol consumers has also been suggested.
3. Folate is also important for the synthesis of *S*-adenosylmethionine (SAM), the universal donor of methyl groups necessary for DNA methylation. Together with changes in the histone code, DNA methylation is an important epigenetic mode of gene silencing.
4. Recently, two trials involving the prevention of recurring colorectal polyps have proven that folic acid and aspirin administration did not prevent the recurrence of colorectal adenomas. Conversely, animal studies have proven an inverse relationship between folate deficiency and increased colorectal cancer. The unexpected results of the human prevention trials were interpreted in light of the accumulating evidence from the animal studies.
5. Results from a simulation investigating a dual role of folate in carcinogens conducted by Luebeck et al. indicate that the effects of folate on colon carcinogenesis are age- and dose-dependent, with predominantly increased risk if the amount of folate given were to increase cellular replication rates by 20%. However, a lack of quantitative estimates of the response of tissues or cancer precursors to folate or folic acid supplementation limits this modeling.

Key Words: Folate; methylation diets; DNA methylation; cancer risk

From: *Nutrition and Health: Bioactive Compounds and Cancer*
Edited by: J.A. Milner, D.F. Romagnolo, DOI 10.1007/978-1-60761-627-6_18,
© Springer Science+Business Media, LLC 2010

1. INTRODUCTION

1.1. What Is Folate?

Folate is a generic descriptor for a water-soluble B-complex vitamin that functions in one-carbon transfer reactions and exists in multiple chemical forms. Most naturally occurring folates are polyglutamated, which enables their retention in the cell. Folic acid is the most oxidized and stable form of folate, rarely found in food, yet used commonly in vitamin supplements and fortified foods *(1)*. Folic acid has about 1.7-fold greater bioavailability than naturally occurring folates, which has led to the designation of "dietary folate equivalents" (or DFE) for combined analyses *(2)*. Folate is essential for transferring single-carbon units in critical biochemical reactions such as the biosynthesis of methionine, thymidylate, purines, and glycine, and in the metabolism of serine, formate, and histidine. Figure 1 illustrates the principal reactions of folate-mediated

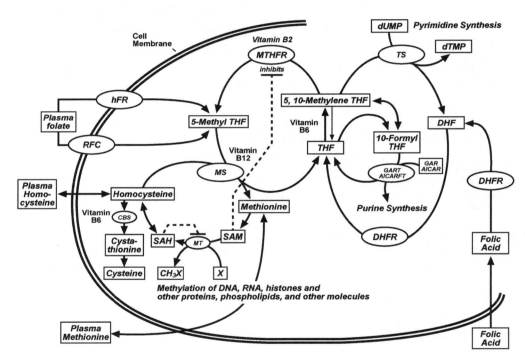

Fig. 1. Overview of folate-mediated one-carbon metabolism (simplified), links to methylation reactions, and nucleotide synthesis. Modified with permission from Ulrich, Robien and McLeod *(3)*. THF = tetrahydrofolate; DHF = dihydrofolate; RFC = reduced folate carrier; hFR = human folate receptor; MTHFR = 5,10-methylenetetrahydrofolate reductase; DHFR = dihydrofolate reductase; GART = glycinamide ribonucleotide transformylase; AICARFT = 5-amino-imidazole-4-carboxamide ribonucleotide transformylase; AICAR = 5-aminoimidazole-4-carboxamide ribonucleotide; GAR = glycinamide ribonucleotide; SAM (AdoMet) = S-adenosylmethionine; SAH (Ado-Hcy) = S-adenosylhomocysteine; dUMP = deoxyuridine monophosphate; dTMP = deoxythymidine monophosphate; MS = methionine synthase; TS = thymidylate synthase; MT = methyltransferases; X = a variety of substrates for methylation.

one-carbon metabolism (FOCM) in the cytosol, as well as major transport mechanisms. However, additional components of FOCM can be found in the mitochondria as well as possibly the nucleus *(4, 5)*.

2. BIOLOGIC MECHANISMS LINKING FOLATE TO CANCER RISK

Cancers arise as consequences of both genetic and epigenetic alterations, and importantly folate can influence both processes. Folate probably plays a role in carcinogenesis as part of its function in nucleotide synthesis: both thymidylate synthesis and purine synthesis depend on folate-mediated one-carbon transfers. Many experimental studies unequivocally link folate deficiency to decreased synthesis of both thymidylate and purines *(6)*. A consequence of decreased thymidylate synthesis is the misincorporation of uracil into DNA. During the repair process in the subsequent DNA replication cycles, chromosomal damage and genomic instability can occur. These effects have been well studied in relation to the efficacy of chemotherapeutic drugs that target folate metabolism, including methotrexate and 5-fluorouracil *(7, 8)*.

Folate is also important for the synthesis of *S*-adenosylmethionine (SAM), the universal donor of methyl groups necessary for DNA methylation. Together with changes in the histone code, DNA methylation is an important epigenetic mode of gene silencing *(9–11)*. However, the link between DNA methylation and cancer risk is not straightforward: DNA methylation can occur in gene promoter regions as well as in non-coding, predominantly repetitive, genomic sequences. To date, the mechanisms that initiate and regulate DNA methylation at these different genomic locations are poorly understood, although *BRAF* mutations may play a role *(9)*. Cancer tissues are characterized both by global DNA hypomethylation at repetitive sequences and by promoter-specific hypermethylation with consequent gene silencing. Global DNA hypomethylation may result in chromosomal instability, loss of imprinting, reactivation of transposons, or proto-oncogenes *(9)*. Yet, reduced methylation may also protect against C to T mutations *(12, 13)*. The influence of folate deficiency in reducing global genomic methylation is generally well supported by both experimental and human data *(14–18)*. However, current data are sparse and inconsistent on whether folate status impacts the methylation of specific gene promoters *(19–24)*. Similarly, the role of folate status in affecting a subset of cancers characterized by widespread gene promoter methylation (the CpG island methylator phenotype [CIMP]) is poorly understood and of potential importance to the folate–cancer connection *(25–27)*.

3. FOLATE STATUS AND CANCER RISK: EPIDEMIOLOGIC EVIDENCE

3.1. *Studies of Dietary Intake and Folate Biomarkers*

The relationship between folate intake or biomarkers thereof and risk of cancer has been studied extensively with respect to numerous types of cancer. Both case–control studies and prospective cohort studies have been conducted and, for several cancer sites, meta-analyses or pooled analyses have been published. While meta-analyses rely on combining the published risk estimates, such as relative risk (RR) or odds ratio (OR), pooled analyses combine individual-level data and thus permit a more comprehensive examination of the risk estimates, confounding factors, and potential effect modification. However, one needs to consider that these pooled or meta-analyses are performed retrospectively and can be subject to study heterogeneity and publication bias. Especially in the case of studying folate status and cancer risk, the nutritional status of the study population (i.e., with respect to folic acid fortification status, supplement use, and alcohol consumption) may result in differing results that are not easily combined. If the dose–response relationship between folate and cancer risk is non-linear, associations may be lost, and there is evidence from Martinez and colleagues that, indeed, the folate–cancer relationship differs depending on whether individuals use supplements or not *(28)*. Nevertheless, these analyses offer increased statistical power for detecting associations and provide more robust risk estimates.

Epidemiological studies have generally assessed folate status as an exposure of interest either with measures of self-reported dietary intakes, such as food-frequency questionnaires (FFQ), diet records, or 24-h recalls, or by measurement of circulating biomarkers (i.e., plasma folate or erythrocyte folate level). As discussed above, there are key differences between natural folates as found in unfortified foods vs. folic acid as it is added to supplements or, as of January 1998, to grain products in the United States and many countries *(29–31)*. This poses a challenge for the calculation of "total dietary intakes." Most studies to date have not used DFE to account for the differences in bioavailability between folic acid and natural folates. This may contribute to errors in estimating total folate intake and should not be neglected. Also, in many prospective studies the assessment of supplement use is very limited, again offering a potential source of error in evaluating total dietary folate, particularly as supplement use in many Western populations is high *(32–34)*.

Biomarkers of folate status that have been examined in epidemiological studies include red blood cell (RBC) folate and serum/plasma folate concentrations. RBC folate is generally considered a better measure of longer-term folate intakes *(2)*. In addition to the direct measurement of folate in plasma or cells, homocysteine (Hcy) concentrations have been used as a surrogate marker of folate availability. A limitation of this approach is that Hcy concentrations can depend on other factors, including vitamin B_{12} status and genetic factors.

Here we present a brief summary of the epidemiological evidence available to date, organized by cancer sites and strength of evidence. First, we discuss cancer sites that have been most extensively studied and for which results from pooled and meta-analyses are available. We also briefly summarize what is known for cancer sites for which no such summary analyses have been performed.

4. EVIDENCE FROM POOLED OR META-ANALYSES

4.1. Colorectal Cancer

Table 1 illustrates results from six meta-analyses and one pooled analysis that have been conducted up to mid 2008 and evaluate the risk of cancers of the colorectum,

Table 1
Meta- and Pooled Analyses of Folate Status and Cancer Risk

Cancer site	Author (references)	Folate measurement	No. of studies included	No. of cases	No. of controls[a]	Summary RR or OR	Comparison
Colorectal	Sanjoaquin et al. (35)	Dietary intake	5 cohorts	2,394	177,689	0.75 (0.64–0.89)	Highest vs. lowest quintile
		Total intake	3 cohorts	2,689	175,059	0.95 (0.81–1.11)	Highest vs. lowest quintile
		Dietary intake	7 case–controls	6,166	9,676	0.76 (0.60–0.96)	Highest vs. lowest quartile
		Total intake	3 case–controls	958	1,499	0.81 (0.62–1.05)	Highest vs. lowest quartile
Breast	Larsson et al. (36)	Dietary intake	8 cohorts	8,367	302,959	0.97 (0.88–1.07)	200 μg/day increments
		Total intake	6 cohorts	8,165	306,209	1.01 (0.97–1.05)	200 μg/day increments
		Dietary intake	13 case–controls	8,558	10,812	0.80 (0.72–0.89)	200 μg/day increments
		Total intake	3 case–controls	2,184	3,233	0.93 (0.81–1.07)	200 μg/day increments
		Plasma or serum levels	3 cohorts	970	1,979	0.81 (0.59–1.10)	Highest vs. lowest category
		Plasma or serum levels	2 case–controls	269	366	0.41 (0.15–1.10)	Highest vs. lowest category
	Lewis et al. (37)	Dietary intake	9 cohorts	11,227	331,462	0.99 (0.98–1.01)	100 μg/day increments
		Dietary intake	13 case–controls	8,566	10,834	0.91 (0.87–0.96)	100 μg/day increments

(Continued)

Table 1
(Continued)

Cancer site	Author (references)	Folate measurement	No. of studies included	No. of cases	No. of controls[a]	Summary RR or OR	Comparison
Gastric	Larsson et al. (38)	Dietary intake	2 cohorts	438	64,556	1.01 (0.72–1.42)	Highest vs. lowest category
		Dietary intake	9 case–controls	3,205	5,574	0.88 (0.67–1.14)	Highest vs. lowest category
Lung[b]	Cho et al. (39)	Dietary intake	8 cohorts	3,155	430,281	0.88 (0.74–1.04)	Highest vs. lowest quintile
		Total intake	5 cohorts	1,734	430,281	1.02 (0.83–1.26)	Highest vs. lowest quintile
Esophageal	Larsson et al. (38)	Dietary intake	7 case–controls	1,496	3,747	0.62 (0.53–0.72)	Highest vs. lowest category
Pancreatic	Larsson et al. (38)	Dietary intake	4 cohorts and 1 case–control	722	236,788	0.49 (0.35–0.67)	Highest vs. lowest category
		Dietary intake	4 cohorts	618	236,535	0.52 (0.36–0.75)	Highest vs. lowest category

[a]For cohort study, the numbers are total participant in the study.
[b]This is a pooled analyses.

breast, stomach, lung, esophagus, and pancreas. Colorectal cancer has been studied most extensively in relation to folate exposures. The meta-analysis by Sanjoaquin et al. suggests that in both cohort and case–control studies a significant inverse association exists for dietary folate (=folate from foods alone). Nevertheless, this association is much attenuated when total folate consumption (=folate from foods and supplements) is investigated *(35)*. Risk estimates for dietary folate (highest vs. lowest quintile) were 0.75 (95% CI: 0.64–0.89) in cohort studies and 0.76 (95% CI: 0.60–0.96) for case–control studies. For total intakes, risk estimates were 0.96 (0.81–1.11) in cohort and 0.81 (0.62–1.05) in case–control studies. In the case–control studies, significant heterogeneity ($p < 0.01$) was noted. A concern is that these studies calculated "total folate" intake by summing dietary folate with folate derived from supplement use (synthetic folic acid). As discussed previously, using this crude approach rather than using DFE to account for the greater bioavailability of folic acid can result in miscalculations and bias risk estimates toward null effects.

Subsequent to the publication of this meta-analysis, additional evidence has become available from prospective cohort studies. The Swedish Mammography Cohort reported an inverse association for colon, but not for rectal cancer *(40)*. A similar inverse association was reported for dietary, but not total folate intake, from subjects enrolled in a cancer prevention trial with aspirin and vitamin E *(41)*. Moreover, several studies have investigated biomarkers of folate status, including serum, plasma, and RBC levels. The Physicians' Health Study reported a marginal increased risk with deficient plasma folate concentrations (<3 ng/ml) *(42)*. However, a recent Swedish prospective study suggested a bell-shaped association between plasma folate concentrations and risk of colorectal cancer *(43)*.

4.2. Breast Cancer

The association between folate status and breast cancer risk is less consistent. A meta-analysis summarizing studies published until 2006 *(36)* suggests that higher folate intake (both dietary and total) in increments of 200 μg/d is not associated with breast cancer risk in prospective studies ($n = 8$), whereas an inverse association with dietary folate is suggested from case–control studies ($n = 13$, summary OR: 0.80; 95% CI: 0.72–0.89). A second meta-analysis *(37)* with partly overlapping studies included in the first meta-analysis showed similar results. For a 100 μg/d increase in folate intake, summary odds ratios for dietary folate were 0.91 (95% CI: 0.87–0.96) for the case–control studies and 0.99 (95% CI: 0.98–1.01) for the cohort studies. In these studies, total folate intakes generally did not use DFE. Subsequent cohort studies from France and Sweden suggested an inverse association with risk reductions between 22 and 40% *(44, 45)*, no association (Nurses' Health Study) *(46)*, or even an increase in risk with high intakes of supplemental folic acid (Prostate, Lung, Colorectal, and Ovarian Cancer Screening Trial) *(47)* were also observed.

Three issues need to be considered when interpreting the association between folate intake and breast cancer risk. First, some inconsistencies may be due to an interaction with alcohol intake, a known folate antagonist. Several cohort studies indicate that higher folate intake attenuates the elevated risk associated with moderate alcohol consumption and that low-folate intake in combination with high alcohol intake increases risk *(36, 48–50)*. It is possible that a more severe reduction of one-carbon status may be needed to detect an association with breast cancer. Second, the relationship between folate status and breast cancer may be complex in that a non-linear, inverted U-shaped relationship could exist *(51)*. While folate- or one-carbon deficiency is thought to increase risk, there is also evidence that very high intake, most likely from supplements, may result in elevated risk *(47)*. Finally, as discussed in more detail below, concerns have been raised over differential effects of folate, depending on the timing of its administration during carcinogenesis *(52)*. Our unpublished data from the Vital Study suggest that higher, long-term intakes of folate are protective, whereas more recent high intakes may not be advantageous *(53)*.

4.3. Other Cancers with Meta-analyses

For gastric cancer, a meta-analysis of nine case–control and two cohort studies (3,205 cases of gastric cancer) *(38)* revealed no significant association between folate intakes and cancer risk. However, geographical heterogeneity may have contributed to this lack of association, since the summary risk estimates for the highest vs. lowest categories of folate were 0.68 (95% CI: 0.58–0.80) for studies done in the United States ($n = 4$), 1.15 (95% CI: 0.91–1.45) in European studies ($n = 4$), and 0.89 (95% CI: 0.40–1.96) for those undertaken elsewhere ($n = 3$). Biomarkers of folate status were not associated with overall gastric cancer risk overall, or by anatomical subset/histological type in the European Prospective Investigation into Cancer and Nutrition (EPIC) cohort (>500,000 participants) *(54)*.

Similarly, epidemiological studies of lung cancer currently do not unequivocally support a protective role of folate intake in cancer risk. A pooled analysis of eight prospective cohort studies *(39)* reported an ~30–40% significantly reduced risk for dietary and total folate in analyses adjusted for age only; however, upon multivariate adjustment, dietary folate was associated with a non-significant 12% risk reduction and total folate with no risk reduction at all. No effect modification by sex, smoking habits, and cancer type was noted. More recently, the VITAL cohort reported no association between use of supplementary folic acid and risk of lung cancer *(55)*.

On the other hand, a strong inverse association between increasing folate intakes and esophageal cancer appears well supported. A meta-analysis conducted in 2006 *(38)* reported a risk reduction for the highest relative to the lowest category of dietary folate intake with summary odds ratios of 0.66 for esophageal squamous cell carcinoma (95% CI: 0.53–0.83), 0.50 for esophageal adenocarcinoma (95% CI: 0.39–0.65), and 0.62 for esophageal cancer (95% CI: 0.53–0.72).

Pancreatic cancer is characterized by very high mortality (median survival 3 months) and to date, few risk factors are established. A meta-analysis of five studies *(36)* reported a significantly reduced risk between high- and low-dietary folate for this severe type of cancer (OR 0.49; 95% CI: 0.35–0.67). However, studies on folate biomarkers and pancreatic cancer risk are less consistent, perhaps because of small sample sizes *(56, 57)*.

5. EVIDENCE FOR CANCERS WITH SUPPORTING DATA FROM PROSPECTIVE STUDIES

This section briefly summarizes the evidence of folate–cancer relationships for cancer types for which prospective studies as well as case–control studies, but no pooled- or meta-analyses, have been undertaken.

For ovarian cancer, three prospective cohort studies have reported results that range in risk estimates from 0.67 to 1.73; none of these investigations reached statistical significance *(58–61)*. However, these studies suggested a reduced risk at relatively high levels of folate intake, specifically among women consuming at least moderate amounts of alcohol. For example, the Swedish Mammography Cohort (266 cases among 61,084 women) *(61)* reported that dietary folate intake was inversely associated with total epithelial ovarian cancer risk with borderline significance (RR 0.67, 95% CI: 0.43–1.04; p trend = 0.08), which was increased among women who consumed more than 20 g of alcohol per week (RR 0.26, 95% CI: 0.11–0.60; p trend = 0.001).

For liver cancer, a cohort study among Chinese individuals at high risk due to hepatitis B antigen positivity *(62)* demonstrated that higher RBC folate concentrations were associated with a strongly reduced risk of hepatocarcinoma (RR 0.33; 95% CI: 0.13–0.86). The association with serum folate did not reach statistical significance. This may be partially explained by the fact that RBC folate is considered a more reliable biomarker of long-term folate status while serum folate concentration may be subject to transient influences.

Some, although not all, case–control studies support an inverse association between dietary folate and non-Hodgkin's lymphoma (NHL) *(63–65)*. However, two cohort studies failed to observe significant associations *(66, 67)*.

6. ADDITIONAL CANCER TYPES, LARGELY WITH EVIDENCE BASED ON CASE–CONTROL STUDIES

For cervical cancer, case–control studies have not provided consistent evidence supporting a role of folate intake on risk of preinvasive cervical lesions or cervical cancer, although many studies were small in size and partly hospital based *(68–76)*. Biomarker studies have been suggestive, but inconsistent, results. For example, low RBC folate concentrations have been associated with an elevated risk of cervical cancer in a population tested thoroughly for high-risk human papillomaviruses (HPV) and cervical intraepithelial neoplasia *(77)* and may also enhance the carcinogenic progression from HPV infections *(78)*. Nevertheless, other studies reported no association between biomarkers of folate status and risk of cervical cancer *(79–82)*. Several small randomized trials have not provided clear evidence for a protective role of folate against cervical carcinogenesis *(83–86)*.

Few studies have investigated associations between folate and leukemia, possibly because of the challenges associated with measuring relevant folate intakes in children and the low incidence of adult leukemia. A small case–control study from Western Australia reported a protective association of maternal folic acid supplementation during pregnancy with respect to childhood acute lymphoblastic leukemia *(87)*; a second study did not replicate these findings, confidence limits were wide *(88)*. A role of folate in the development of leukemia has been proposed largely because of studies on genetic polymorphisms, as discussed later on.

More recently, case–control studies of head and neck cancer suggest an inverse association between dietary folate or folate biomarkers and cancer risk *(89–91)*. However, the biomarkers were measured after diagnosis and well-designed studies are needed. Promising data on an inverse association between folate status and endometrial cancer are also available from several case–control studies of significant sample size *(92–94)*, although not all studies observed such effects *(95)*.

In summary, the role of folate on cancer risk has been most extensively studied for colorectal and breast cancer. The evidence for colorectal cancer is consistent and strong, whereas for breast cancer an interaction of folate with alcohol intake may be critical. For several other types of cancer, inverse associations between folate status and cancer risk have been suggested. This may be clinically relevant for pancreatic and esophageal cancers, which are malignancies with few modifiable risk factors and high mortality. In general, for many cancer sites, suggestive inverse associations with folate require follow-up studies with larger and better-designed protocols.

Limitations of the observational evidence summarized here are the general lack of a meaningful estimation of dietary folate and supplemental folic acid intakes by use of the DFE, and the potential for confounding effects due to folate present in many foods. Primary food sources of folate have been "healthy foods" including fruits and vegetables, which are sources of many bioactive components. However, with the advent of folic-acid fortification, this concern is less important. Further, studies on genetic variants in folate metabolism can strengthen the inference of causality for folate in carcinogenesis.

7. STUDIES OF GENETIC POLYMORPHISMS IN FOLATE-MEDIATED ONE-CARBON METABOLISM AND CANCER RISK

The role of folate genetics and nutrigenetics has already been discussed in several recent publications *(96–98)*. Folate metabolism is likely a key example for the necessity to take into account interactions between environmental factors and genetic background.

As shown in Fig. 1, folate-mediated one-carbon metabolism involves several micronutrients, including vitamins B_{12}, B_6, and B_2, as cofactors of various enzymes, and several overlapping biochemical pathways. Clearly, this complex biologic system with its many feedback mechanisms and regulatory processes has evolved to ensure robustness and tight regulation of chemical reactions that are critical for cellular functioning, including nucleotides and methylation reactions *(1, 99)*. It is thus conceivable that multiple disturbances within these pathways or "stress" on the system may be needed to effectively alter phenotypic outcomes. For example, "stress" may be exerted by low intakes of folate or other nutrients; by the administration of chemotherapeutic drugs that inhibit enzymes involved in folate metabolism; or by the presence of genetic polymorphisms that alter enzyme function. These changes may occur in combination and lead to additive effects that are larger than those measured following isolated changes. For example, genetic polymorphisms in the 5,10-methylenetetrahydrofolate reductase *(MTHFR)* are most strongly associated with certain biomarkers (e.g., homocysteine), when folate status is low. This provides a rationale for investigating gene–gene and gene–nutrient interactions within folate-mediated one-carbon metabolism.

7.1. Polymorphisms in One-Carbon Metabolism and Their Functional Impact

A large number of genetic polymorphisms in FOCM have been identified. Few of these have been associated with confirmed phenotypic changes such as effects on activity or transcription of the protein (=functional polymorphisms). To date, most published studies have utilized functional polymorphisms, rather than tag SNPs that cover the genetic variability of a gene with greater comprehensiveness. Table 2 summarizes the most common FOCM polymorphisms, which alter the amino-acid sequence or transcription/translation of key enzymes. Our recent work suggests that, because of robustness in the pathway or biologic system, the biological effects of these polymorphisms will be small or moderate at best *(100)*. Nevertheless, small lifelong effects on biologic mechanisms, such as thymidylate synthesis or DNA methylation, may affect cancer risk. Also, the high prevalence of these polymorphisms in the general population may result in significant attributable risks.

Here, we will briefly summarize the associations for MTHFR, which is a central enzyme in folate and homocysteine metabolism, by catalyzing the irreversible reduction of 5,10-methylene THF to 5-methylene THF. 5,10-Methylene THF is involved both in the synthesis of purines and in the conversion of deoxyuridylate monophosphate to deoxythymidylate monophosphate (dTMP, needed for DNA synthesis). As discussed previously, low-folate status (and thus low 5,10-methylene THF) can result in misincorporation of uracil into DNA, resulting in increased mutations, as well as chromosome breakage *(101)*. With reduced MTHFR activity, one would expect a greater provision of 5,10-methylene THF for nucleotide synthesis, which is supported by biochemical data as well as predictions from a mathematical simulation model of folate metabolism *(100, 102)*. On the other hand, reduced MTHFR activity can lower the ratio of SAM/SAH, with likely impact on DNA methylation *(12, 103, 104)*.

Two polymorphisms in the *MTHFR* gene, 677C>T (rs1801133) and 1298A>C (rs1801131), have been widely investigated in relation to risk of various cancer types. Individuals with homozygote *677TT* variant genotypes have ~70% lower enzyme activity compared to wild-type individuals *(677CC)*, with heterozygotes retaining about 65% enzyme activity *(105)*. The functional relevance of the 1298A>C

Table 2
Key Polymorphisms Involved in Folate-Mediated One-Carbon Metabolism (Amino-Acid Changes or Other Functional Evidences)

Genes	Enzyme	Chromosome	Polymorphism	rs number	AA change
MTHFR	5,10-Methylenetetrahydro-folate reductase	1p36.3	677C>T 1298A>C	rs1801133 rs1801131	Ala222Val Glu429Ala
TS	Thymidylate synthase	18p11.32	5′-UTR 28 bp tandem repeat; G>C SNP at 12th nucleotide in the 2nd repeat of the 3R allele (3RG > 3RC); 3′-UTR 6 bp deletion (1464del6)		
DHFR	Dihydrofolate reductase	5q11.2-q13.2	intron1-19 bp deletion		
MTR(MS)	Methionine synthase	1q43	2756A>G	rs1805087	Asp919Gly
MTRR	Methionine synthase reductase	5p15.3-p15.2	66A>G	rs1801394	Ile22Met
cSHMT	Serine hydroxymethyltransferase	17p11.2	1420C>T	rs1979277	Leu474Phe
RFC1	Reduced folate carrier	21q22.3	80G>A	rs1051266	Arg27His
BHMT	Betaine-homocysteine methyltransferase	5q13.1-q15	742G>A	rs3733890	Arg239Gln
CBS	Cystathionine β-synthase	21q22.3	31 bp VNTR		
MTHFD1	Methylenetetrahydrofolate dehydrogenase	14q24	401G>A 1958G>A	rs1950902 rs2236225	Arg134Lys Arg653Gln
TCN2	Transcobalamin II	22q12.2	776C>G	rs1950902	Pro259Arg

polymorphism is less clearly described, with about 60% activity for *1298CC* compared to wild-type *1298AA* reported in some studies *(106)*. Despite the lesser impact of 1298A>C and the high linkage disequilibrium between the two SNPs, they appear to contribute independently to changes in folate and homocysteine concentrations *(107, 108)*.

Meta-analyses on *MTHFR* polymorphisms and cancer risk are summarized in Table 3. Whereas the *677TT* genotype is associated with reduced colorectal cancer risk, an elevated risk of gastric cancer has been observed. These differences may suggest different etiologic mechanisms of these diseases associated with one-carbon metabolism, perhaps because of an interaction with *Helicobacter pylori* infections in the case of gastric cancer. Pooled and meta-analyses for breast and lung cancer show no significant associations.

The value of meta-analyses for *MTHFR* polymorphism–cancer relationships is, however, questionable. Their major limitation to date is that they have not been able to take folate status into account, nor one-carbon-status in general, which includes other nutrients as well as alcohol intake. Gene–diet interactions have been repeatedly and consistently reported for *MTHFR C677T* and a plausible biologic mechanism exists *(97, 98)*. Thus, the solitary evaluation of the *MTHFR* gene is not particularly meaningful. In fact, the combination of results from study populations with divergent nutritional status may mask any true biological effects.

In terms of other genetic variabilities, perhaps the most interesting enzyme in FOCM is thymidylate synthase (TS). A polymorphic 28-bp tandem repeat located in the 5′-UTR of the *TS* gene acts as a transcriptional enhancer element *(117)*. The *3R* allele has been associated with approximately 2–4 times increased gene expression compared to the *2R* allele *(118, 119)* and the *2R/2R* genotype may reduce risk of colorectal cancer *(120, 121)* as well as adult ALL *(122)*. An embedded SNP within the 3R allele may also have functional significance, yet few studies have investigated this polymorphism, perhaps because of the complexities in genotyping *(123)*. Finally, a 6 bp deletion (1494del6) polymorphism located in the 3′-UTR of the *TS* gene has been associated with reduced mRNA stability *(124, 125)* and perhaps interacts with one-carbon nutrients in relation to colorectal neoplasia *(126)*. Polymorphisms in *TS* have generally not been studied with sufficient sample sizes to account for possible genotypic combinations. However, a rigorous investigation of genetic variability in TS seems warranted, given its role in thymidylate synthesis as well as a target for a major chemotherapeutic drug, 5-fluorouracil.

Many other studies on genetic variants in FOCM and their relation to cancer risk have been undertaken (for reviews, see *(127, 128, 97)*). Overall, this substantial body of literature supports the notion that genetic variability in FOCM plays a critical role in cancer etiology, particularly for cancers of the gastrointestinal tract. However, larger and more systematic investigations are needed to reach sufficient statistical power for investigating rare variants and gene–gene as well as gene–diet interactions. There are also efforts underway to incorporate the comprehensive biologic knowledge of this biologic pathway into the statistical analysis by use of a mathematical simulation model of folate metabolism *(129, 130)*. Initial results from this model are consistent with experimental data, thus allowing for predictions on the impact of polymorphisms on biomarkers of

Table 3
Summary of Meta-Analysis Results of *MTHFR* Polymorphisms and Cancer Risk by Site

Cancer site	Author (references)	SNP	No. of studies included	Case–control	Summary OR	P for hetero-geneity
Colorectal	Huang et al. (109)	C677T	23	10,131/15,362	0.93 (0.89–0.98) T vs. C allele	0.22
					0.82 (0.75–0.89) TT vs. CC	
		A1298C	14	4,764/6,592	0.93 (0.85–1.01) C vs. A allele	0.09
					0.80 (0.65–0.98) CC vs. AA	
Breast	Hubner et al. (110)	C677T	25	12,243/17,688	0.83 (0.75–0.93) TT vs. CC	0.12
	Lewis et al. (37)	C677T	17	6,373/8,434	1.04 (0.94–1.16) TT vs. CC	
	Zintzaras et al. (111)	C677T	18	5,476/7,336	1.02 (0.95–1.10) T vs. C allele	0.08
		A1298C	10	3,768/5,276	0.97 (0.90–1.04) C vs. A allele	0.21
Lung	Mao et al. (112)	C677T	8	5,111/6,415	1.12 (0.97–1.28) T vs. C allele	0.0001
		A1298C	7	5,087/6,232	1.00 (0.92–1.08) C vs. A allele	0.24
ALL[a]	Pereira et al. (113)	C677T	12	2,191/3,437	Childhood: 0.85 (0.70–1.04) TT vs. CC	0.12
					Adult: 0.41 (0.24–0.72) TT vs. CC	0.24
		A1298C	10	2,067/3,193	Childhood: 0.83 (0.55–1.25) CC vs. AA	0.01
					Adult: 0.46 (0.03–7.46) CC vs. AA	
	Zintzaras et al. (114)	C677T	9	1,576/1,958	All: 0.88 (0.76–1.02) T vs. C allele	0.09
					Childhood: 0.74 (0.57–0.96) T vs. C allele	0.07
		A1298C	8	561/892	0.88 (0.72–1.07) C vs. A allele	0.01
Gastric	Boccia et al. (115)	C677T	16 for meta / 9 for pooled	2,727/4,640 / 1,540/2,577	1.52 (1.31–1.77) TT vs. CC	0.37
					1.49 (1.14–1.95) TT vs. CC	0.06
		A1298C	7 for meta / 5 for pooled	1,223/2,015 / 1,146/1,549	0.94 (0.65–1.35)	
					0.90 (0.69–1.34) CC vs. AA allele	0.50
	Zintzaras et al. (116)	C677T	8	1,584/2,785	1.27 (1.13–1.44) T vs. C allele	0.12
		A1298C	4	760/1,624	1.00 (0.84–1.20) C vs. A allele	0.47

[a] Acute lymphoblastic leukemia.

cancer risk *(100, 129–132)*. Hopefully, linking the two approaches will provide a more powerful tool for the statistical analyses.

8. FOLATE IN CANCER PREVENTION

8.1. Evidence from Animal Models

As discussed above, there is strong epidemiologic evidence supporting an inverse relationship between dietary folate intake and risk of colorectal cancer. In general, animal studies support a causal relationship between folate deficiency and increased colorectal cancer risk. Furthermore they demonstrate the importance of dosage and timing in examining the effects of folate on carcinogenesis *(133, 134)*. For example, studies in the *APC/Min* mouse (an established model of intestinal carcinogenesis) show that increasing dietary folate concentrations significantly reduced the number of ileal polyps and colonic aberrant crypt foci in a dose-dependent manner after 3 months of folic-acid administration *(135)*. However, the association was reversed at the 6-month time point, suggesting that folic acid may have enhanced the growth of intestinal precursor lesions. These intriguing findings suggest that folic-acid supplementation may enhance the development and progression of already existing, undiagnosed, premalignant lesions. This complex role of folate in carcinogenesis may also be mimicked in breast cancer development. Three animal studies, all using a well-established rat model of MNU-induced mammary tumor *(136–138)*, indicate that mild folate deficiency significantly inhibits mammary tumorigenesis, while folic-acid supplementation does not alter the development or progression of the disease.

8.2. Human Prevention Trials

Recently, results of two large trials investigating the efficacy of folic acid in the prevention of recurring (or, more accurately, metachronous) colorectal polyps have been published. The Aspirin/Folate Polyp Prevention Trial continued to add complexity to the picture of folate and cancer *(139)*. In this randomized controlled trial of folic acid for chemoprevention of colorectal polyps, about 1,000 participants with a history of colorectal adenomas were randomly assigned to 1 mg folic acid/day ± aspirin. Follow-up colonoscopies were scheduled approximately 3 years after the initial endoscopy and supplementation continued until a second surveillance exam, about 6–8 years post-randomization. Folic acid administration did not prevent the recurrence of colorectal adenomas, with rate ratios of 1.04 at the first and 1.13 (95% CI: 0.93–1.37) at the second follow-up. In contrast, at the second follow-up, the folic acid group showed a significantly increased risk of advanced adenomas (RR 1.67, 95% CI: 1.00–2.80), together with a more than 2-fold elevated risk for having at least 3 adenomas (RR 2.32, 95% CI: 1.23–4.35). These unexpected results have been interpreted in light of the accumulating evidence from animal studies, suggesting growth-promoting effects of folate on premalignant lesions *(134)*: It has been hypothesized that the increased risk of advanced and multiple adenomas in the intervention group may have occurred, because early precursor lesions were present in the mucosa of these patients, not detected during endoscopy, and their growth was supported by folic acid *(52)*.

Consistent with this hypothesis is that patients with adenoma are at increased risk of a second adenoma, probably because of the presence of precursor lesions such as aberrant crypt foci or microadenoma. Thus, for correct interpretation, the Aspirin/Folate Polyp Prevention Trial was designed to investigate the secondary prevention on colorectal adenoma, rather than the primary prevention. Of particular concern was that, in this trial, the risk of cancers other than those of the colorectum was significantly elevated. Although the numbers were small, this increase (largely due to prostate cancer) requires further follow-up.

Recently, results from the ukCAP trial, which parallels the Aspirin/Folate Polyp Prevention Trial, have also been published *(140)*. In this trial, 853 Europeans with a prior history of adenoma were randomized to 500 µg folic acid with follow-up colonoscopies targeted at 3 years, yet sometimes completed earlier. The trial reported relative risks of 1.07 (0.85–1.34) for the incidence of any adenoma in the folic-acid intervention arm and 0.98 (0.68–1.40) for advanced adenoma and, similar to the Aspirin/Folate Polyp Prevention Trial, no evidence for cardiovascular protection. The relative risks from ukCAP are nearly identical to those of the Aspirin/Folate Polyp Prevention Trial at its first, 3-year follow-up (e.g., 1.07 vs. 1.04 for any adenoma). A longer follow-up will be necessary to obtain information on whether elevated risks will emerge, matching those observed at 6–8 years in the Aspirin/Folate Polyp Prevention trial. This time frame may be necessary for the development of a larger colorectal polyp. Tumor multiplicity was not assessed in ukCAP, but hopefully a longer follow-up will be considered for evaluation of this critical end point. Finally, it is important to consider that the ukCAP trial took place in a population that has not (yet) been subjected to folic-acid fortification of grain products (estimated at 150–200 µg/day in the US population) and, thus, findings may not parallel those obtained in the United States if there is a dose-dependent effect.

Findings from these failed cancer prevention trials raise an important question. If there is both a mutation-suppressing and a growth-promoting effect of folate on carcinogenesis, what are the net effects of folate supplementation on colon cancer rates in the population? Mason et al. have researched national cancer data and reported a potential increase since folate fortification was implemented in both the United States and Canada *(141)*. Complementing this ecologic study, Luebeck et al. have used an established model of colon cancer development *(142)* to investigate a dual role of folate in carcinogenesis *(143)*. Results from this simulation indicate that the effects of folate on colon carcinogenesis are age- and dose-dependent, with predominantly increased risk if the amount of folate given were to increase cellular replication rates by 20% *(143)*. However, a lack of quantitative estimates of the response of tissues or cancer precursors to folate or folic-acid supplementation limits this modeling.

9. RECOMMENDATIONS

Can folate be considered an agent that can prevent cancer? For a number of tumor sites, the epidemiologic data are quite compelling. In addition, the molecular and epidemiological studies on polymorphisms in folate metabolism support a causal role for this nutrient in carcinogenesis. Convincing biological mechanisms have been proposed and substantiated by experimental studies. However, the prevention trials to date have been unsuccessful and raise concerns about potential harmful effects of folic-acid administration among individuals with a prior history of cancer lesions. Perhaps the most likely explanations for the discrepancies in findings are dual roles of folate on the cancer process may depend on timing of exposure and dose. For example, folate may be effective in the primary prevention of colorectal, and perhaps, pancreatic and esophageal cancers. However, after establishment of precursor lesions, supplementation with folate may have procarcinogenic effects. This information needs to be evaluated carefully when developing public health recommendations, including those on whether or not to initiate national folic acid fortification programs.

REFERENCES

1. Wagner, C. (1995) Biochemical Role of Folate in Cellular metabolism. Folate in Health and Disease. New York: Marcel Dekker.
2. Institute of Medicine (1998) Dietary Reference Intakes: Thiamin, Riboflavin, Niacin, Vitamin B6, Folate, Vitamin B12, Pantothenic Acid, Biotin, and Choline. Washington, DC: National Academy Press.
3. Ulrich, C.M., Robien, K., and McLeod, H.L. (2003) Cancer pharmacogenetics: Polymorphisms, pathways and beyond. *Nat Rev Cancer* **3**, 912–20.
4. Stover, P.J. (2004) Physiology of folate and vitamin B12 in health and disease. *Nutr Rev* **62**, S3–S12, discussion S13.
5. Woeller, C.F., Anderson, D.D., Szebenyi, D.M., and Stover, P.J. (2007) Evidence for small ubiquitin-like modifier-dependent nuclear import of the thymidylate biosynthesis pathway. *J Biol Chem* **282**, 17623–31.
6. Choi, S.W., and Mason, J.B. (2002) Folate status: Effects on pathways of colorectal carcinogenesis. *J Nutr* **132**, 2413S–2418S.
7. Chu, E., and Allegra, C. (1996) Antifolates. In: Chabner, B., and Longo, D., eds. Cancer Chemotherapy and Biotherapy. 109–48, Philadelphia: Lippincott-Raven Publishers.
8. Danenberg, P.V., Malli, H., and Swenson, S. (1999) Thymidylate synthase inhibitors. *Semin Oncol* **26**, 621–31.
9. Laird, P.W. (2005) Cancer epigenetics. *Hum Mol Genet* **14**(Spec No 1), R65–R76.
10. Jones, P.A., and Baylin, S.B. (2002) The fundamental role of epigenetic events in cancer. *Nat Rev Gene* **3**, 415–28.
11. Toyota, M., and Issa, J.P. (2005) Epigenetic changes in solid and hematopoietic tumors. *Semin Oncol* **32**, 521–31.
12. Ulrich, C.M., Curtin, K., Samowitz, W., Bigler, J., Potter, J.D., Caan, B., and Slattery, M.L. (2005) MTHFR variants reduce the risk of G:C->A:T transition mutations within the p53 tumor suppressor gene in colon tumors. *J Nutr* **135**, 2462–67.
13. Jones, P.A., and Gonzalgo, M.L. (1997) Altered DNA methylation and genome instability: A new pathway to cancer? *Proc Natl Acad Sci USA* **94**, 2103–05.
14. Rampersaud, G.C., Kauwell, G.P., Hutson, A.D., Cerda, J.J., and Bailey, L.B. (2000) Genomic DNA methylation decreases in response to moderate folate depletion in elderly women. *Am J Clin Nutr* **72**, 998–1003.
15. Kim, Y.I. (2004) Folate and DNA methylation: A mechanistic link between folate deficiency and colorectal cancer? *Cancer Epidemiol Biomarkers Prev* **13**, 511–19.
16. Davis, S., Stacpoole, P.W., Bailey, L.B., and Gregory, J.F., 3rd. (2002) C677T MTHFR genotype & homocysteine remethylation; effects of folate depletion. *Exp Biol.*
17. Shelnutt, K.P., Kauwell, G.P., Gregory, J.F., 3rd., Maneval, D.R., Quinlivan, E.P., Theriaque, D.W., Henderson, G.N., and Bailey, L.B. (2004) Methylenetetrahydrofolate reductase 677C–>T

polymorphism affects DNA methylation in response to controlled folate intake in young women. *J Nutr Biochem* **15**, 554–60.

18. Pufulete, M., Al-Ghnaniem, R., Khushal, A., Appleby, P., Harris, N., Gout, S., Emery, P.W., and Sanders, T.A. (2005) Effect of folic acid supplementation on genomic DNA methylation in patients with colorectal adenoma. *Gut* **54**, 648–53.

19. van den Donk, M., van Engeland, M., Pellis, L., Witteman, B.J., Kok, F.J., Keijer, J., and Kampman, E. (2007) Dietary folate intake in combination with MTHFR C677T genotype and promoter methylation of tumor suppressor and DNA repair genes in sporadic colorectal adenomas. *Cancer Epidemiol Biomarkers Prev* **16**, 327–33.

20. Waterland, R.A., and Jirtle, R.L. (2003) Transposable elements: Targets for early nutritional effects on epigenetic gene regulation. *Mol Cell Biol* **23**, 5293–300.

21. Dolinoy, D.C., Huang, D., and Jirtle, R.L. (2007) Maternal nutrient supplementation counteracts bisphenol A-induced DNA hypomethylation in early development. *Proc Natl Acad Sci USA* **104**, 13056–61.

22. Paz, M.F., Avila, S., Fraga, M.F., Pollan, M., Capella, G., Peinado, M.A., Sanchez-Cespedes, M., Herman, J.G., and Esteller, M. (2002) Germ-line variants in methyl-group metabolism genes and susceptibility to DNA methylation in normal tissues and human primary tumors. *Cancer Res* **62**, 4519–24.

23. Oyama, K., Kawakami, K., Maeda, K., Ishiguro, K., and Watanabe, G. (2004) The association between methylenetetrahydrofolate reductase polymorphism and promoter methylation in proximal colon cancer. *Anticancer Res* **24**, 649–54.

24. van Engeland, M., Weijenberg, M.P., Roemen, G.M., Brink, M., de Bruine, A.P., Goldbohm, R.A., van den Brandt, P.A., Baylin, S.B., de Goeij, A.F., and Herman, J.G. (2003) Effects of dietary folate and alcohol intake on promoter methylation in sporadic colorectal cancer: The Netherlands cohort study on diet and cancer. *Cancer Res* **63**, 3133–37.

25. Curtin, K., Slattery, M.L., Ulrich, C.M., Bigler, J., Levin, T.R., Wolff, R.K., Albertsen, H., Potter, J.D., and Samowitz, W.S. (2007) Genetic polymorphisms in one-carbon metabolism: Associations with CpG island methylator phenotype (CIMP) in colon cancer and the modifying effects of diet. *Carcinogenesis* **28**, 1672–79.

26. Slattery, M.L., Curtin, K., Sweeney, C., Levin, T.R., Potter, J., Wolff, R.K., Albertsen, H., and Samowitz, W.S. (2007) Diet and lifestyle factor associations with CpG island methylator phenotype and BRAF mutations in colon cancer. *Int J Cancer* **120**, 656–63.

27. Kawakami, K., Ooyama, A., Ruszkiewicz, A., Jin, M., Watanabe, G., Moore, J., Oka, T., Iacopetta, B., and Minamoto, T. (2008) Low expression of gamma-glutamyl hydrolase mRNA in primary colorectal cancer with the CpG island methylator phenotype. *Br J Cancer* **98**, 1555–61.

28. Martinez, M.E., Giovannucci, E., Jiang, R., Henning, S.M., Jacobs, E.T., Thompson, P., Smith-Warner, S.A., and Alberts, D.S. (2006) Folate fortification, plasma folate, homocysteine and colorectal adenoma recurrence. *Int J Cancer* **119**, 1440–46.

29. Honein, M.A., Paulozzi, L.J., Mathews, T.J., Erickson, J.D., and Wong, L.Y. (2001) Impact of folic acid fortification of the US food supply on the occurrence of neural tube defects. *JAMA* **285**, 2981–86.

30. Quinlivan, E.P., and Gregory, J.F., 3rd. (2003) Effect of food fortification on folic acid intake in the United States. *Am J Clin Nutr* **77**, 221–25.

31. Jacques, P.F., Selhub, J., Bostom, A.G., Wilson, P.W., and Rosenberg, I.H. (1999) The effect of folic acid fortification on plasma folate and total homocysteine concentrations. *N Engl J Med* **340**, 1449–54.

32. Brownie, S., and Myers, S. (2004) Wading through the quagmire: Making sense of dietary supplement utilization. *Nutr Rev* **62**, 276–82.

33. Harrison, R.A., Holt, D., Pattison, D.J., and Elton, P.J. (2004) Are those in need taking dietary supplements? A survey of 21 923 adults. *Br J Nutr* **91**, 617–23.

34. Huang, H.-Y., Caballero, B., Chang, S., Alberg, A.J., Semba, R.D., Schneyer, C.R., Wilson, R.F., Cheng, T.-Y., Vassy, J., Prokopowicz, G., Barnes, G.J., 2nd., and Bass, E.B. (2006) The efficacy and safety of multivitamin and mineral supplement use to prevent cancer and chronic disease in adults: A systematic review for a National Institutes of Health state-of-the-science conference. *Ann Intern Med* **145**, 372–85.

35. Sanjoaquin, M.A., Allen, N., Couto, E., Roddam, A.W., and Key, T.J. (2005) Folate intake and colorectal cancer risk: A meta-analytical approach. *Int J Cancer* **113**, 825–28.
36. Larsson, S.C., Giovannucci, E., and Wolk, A. (2007) Folate and risk of breast cancer: A meta-analysis. *J Natl Cancer Inst* **99**, 64–76.
37. Lewis, S.J., Harbord, R.M., Harris, R., and Smith, G.D. (2006) Meta-analyses of observational and genetic association studies of folate intakes or levels and breast cancer risk. *J Natl Cancer Inst* **98**, 1607–22.
38. Larsson, S.C., Giovannucci, E., and Wolk, A. (2006) Folate intake, MTHFR polymorphisms, and risk of esophageal, gastric, and pancreatic cancer: A meta-analysis. *Gastroenterology* **131**, 1271–83.
39. Cho, E., Hunter, D.J., Spiegelman, D., Albanes, D., Beeson, W.L., van den Brandt, P.A., Colditz, G.A., Feskanich, D., Folsom, A.R., Fraser, G.E., Freudenheim, J.L., Giovannucci, E., Goldbohm, R.A., Graham, S., Miller, A.B., Rohan, T.E., Sellers, T.A., Virtamo, J., Willett, W.C., and Smith-Warner, S.A. (2006) Intakes of vitamins A, C and E and folate and multivitamins and lung cancer: A pooled analysis of 8 prospective studies. *Int J Cancer* **118**, 970–78.
40. Larsson, S.C., Giovannucci, E., and Wolk, A. (2005) A prospective study of dietary folate intake and risk of colorectal cancer: Modification by caffeine intake and cigarette smoking. *Cancer Epidemiol Biomarkers Prev* **14**, 740–43.
41. Zhang, S.M., Moore, S.C., Lin, J., Cook, N.R., Manson, J.E., Lee, I.M., and Buring, J.E. (2006) Folate, vitamin B6, multivitamin supplements, and colorectal cancer risk in women. *Am J Epidemiol* **163**, 108–15.
42. Ma, J., Stampfer, M.J., Giovannucci, E., Artigas, C., Hunter, D.J., Fuchs, C., Willett, W.C., Selhub, J., Hennekens, C.H., and Rozen, R. (1997) Methylenetetrahydrofolate reductase polymorphism, dietary interactions, and risk of colorectal cancer. *Cancer Res* **57**, 1098–102.
43. Van Guelpen, B., Hultdin, J., Johansson, I., Hallmans, G., Stenling, R., Riboli, E., Winkvist, A., and Palmqvist, R. (2006) Low folate levels may protect against colorectal cancer. *Gut* **55**, 1461–66.
44. Lajous, M., Lazcano-Ponce, E., Hernandez-Avila, M., Willett, W., and Romieu, I. (2006) Folate, vitamin B6, and vitamin B12 intake and the risk of breast cancer among Mexican women. *Cancer Epidemiol Biomarkers Prev* **15**, 443–48.
45. Ericson, U., Sonestedt, E., Gullberg, B., Olsson, H., and Wirfalt, E. (2007) High folate intake is associated with lower breast cancer incidence in postmenopausal women in the Malmo Diet and Cancer cohort. *Am J Clin Nutr* **86**, 434–43.
46. Cho, E., Holmes, M., Hankinson, S.E., and Willett, W.C. (2007) Nutrients involved in one-carbon metabolism and risk of breast cancer among premenopausal women. *Cancer Epidemiol Biomarkers Prev* **16**, 2787–90.
47. Stolzenberg-Solomon, R.Z., Chang, S.C., Leitzmann, M.F., Johnson, K.A., Johnson, C., Buys, S.S., Hoover, R.N., and Ziegler, R.G. (2006) Folate intake, alcohol use, and postmenopausal breast cancer risk in the Prostate, Lung, Colorectal, and Ovarian Cancer Screening Trial. *Am J Clin Nutr* **83**, 895–904.
48. Zhang, S., Hunter, D.J., Hankinson, S.E., Giovannucci, E.L., Rosner, B.A., Colditz, G.A., Speizer, F.E., and Willett, W.C. (1999) A prospective study of folate intake and the risk of breast cancer. *JAMA* **281**, 1632–37.
49. Sellers, T.A., Kushi, L.H., Cerhan, J.R., Vierkant, R.A., Gapstur, S.M., Vachon, C.M., Olson, J.E., Therneau, T.M., and Folsom, A.R. (2001) Dietary folate intake, alcohol, and risk of breast cancer in a prospective study of postmenopausal women. *Epidemiology* **12**, 420–28.
50. Rohan, T.E., Jain, M.G., Howe, G.R., and Miller, A.B. (2000) Dietary folate consumption and breast cancer risk. *J Natl Cancer Inst* **92**, 266–69.
51. Ulrich, C.M. (2007) Folate and cancer prevention: A closer look at a complex picture. *Am J Clin Nutr* **86**, 271–73.
52. Ulrich, C.M., and Potter, J.D. (2007) Folate and cancer—timing is everything. *JAMA* **297**, 2408–9.
53. Maruti, S.S., Ulrich, C.M., and White, E. (2009) Folate and one-carbon metabolism nutrients from supplements and diet in relation to breast cancer risk. *Am J Clin Nutr* **89**, 624–33.

54. Vollset, S.E., Igland, J., Jenab, M., Fredriksen, A., Meyer, K., Eussen, S., Gjessing, H.K., Ueland, P.M., Pera, G., Sala, N., Agudo, A., Capella, G., Del Giudice, G., Palli, D., Boeing, H. (2007) The association of gastric cancer risk with plasma folate, cobalamin, and methylenetetrahydrofolate reductase polymorphisms in the European Prospective Investigation into Cancer and Nutrition. *Cancer Epidemiol Biomarkers Prev* **16**, 2416–24.

55. Slatore, C.G., Littman, A.J., Au, D.H., Satia, J.A., and White, E. (2008) Long-term use of supplemental multivitamins, vitamin C, vitamin E, and folate does not reduce the risk of lung cancer. *Am J Respir Crit Care Med* **177**, 524–30.

56. Stolzenberg-Solomon, R.Z., Albanes, D., Nieto, F.J., Hartman, T.J., Tangrea, J.A., Rautalahti, M., Selhub, J., Virtamo, J., and Taylor, P.R. (1999) Pancreatic cancer risk and nutrition-related methylgroup availability indicators in male smokers. *J Natl Cancer Inst* **91**, 535–41.

57. Schernhammer, E., Wolpin, B., Rifai, N., Cochrane, B., Manson, J.A., Ma, J., Giovannucci, E., Thomson, C., Stampfer, M.J., and Fuchs, C. (2007) Plasma folate, vitamin B6, vitamin B12, and homocysteine and pancreatic cancer risk in four large cohorts. *Cancer Res* **67**, 5553–60.

58. Navarro Silvera, S.A., Jain, M., Howe, G.R., Miller, A.B., and Rohan, T.E. (2006) Dietary folate consumption and risk of ovarian cancer: A prospective cohort study. *Eur J Cancer Prev* **15**, 511–15.

59. Tworoger, S.S., Hecht, J.L., Giovannucci, E., and Hankinson, S.E. (2006) Intake of folate and related nutrients in relation to risk of epithelial ovarian cancer. *Am J Epidemiol* **163**, 1101–11.

60. Kelemen, L.E., Sellers, T.A., Vierkant, R.A., Harnack, L., and Cerhan, J.R. (2004) Association of folate and alcohol with risk of ovarian cancer in a prospective study of postmenopausal women. *Cancer Causes Control* **15**, 1085–93.

61. Larsson, S.C., Giovannucci, E., and Wolk, A. (2004) Dietary folate intake and incidence of ovarian cancer: The Swedish Mammography Cohort. *J Natl Cancer Inst* **96**, 396–402.

62. Welzel, T.M., Katki, H.A., Sakoda, L.C., Evans, A.A., London, W.T., Chen, G., O'Broin, S., Shen, F.M., Lin, W.Y., and McGlynn, K.A. (2007) Blood folate levels and risk of liver damage and hepatocellular carcinoma in a prospective high-risk cohort. *Cancer Epidemiol Biomarkers Prev* **16**, 1279–82.

63. Koutros, S., Zhang, Y., Zhu, Y., Mayne, S.T., Zahm, S.H., Holford, T.R., Leaderer, B.P., Boyle, P., and Zheng, T. (2008) Nutrients contributing to one-carbon metabolism and risk of non-Hodgkin lymphoma subtypes. *Am J Epidemiol* **167**, 287–94.

64. Lim, U., Schenk, M., Kelemen, L.E., Davis, S., Cozen, W., Hartge, P., Ward, M.H., and Stolzenberg-Solomon, R. (2005) Dietary determinants of one-carbon metabolism and the risk of non-Hodgkin's lymphoma: NCI-SEER case-control study, 1998–2000. *Am J Epidemiol* **162**, 953–64.

65. Polesel, J., Dal Maso, L., La Vecchia, C., Montella, M., Spina, M., Crispo, A., Talamini, R., and Franceschi, S. (2007) Dietary folate, alcohol consumption, and risk of non-Hodgkin lymphoma. *Nutr Cancer* **57**, 146–50.

66. Lim, U., Weinstein, S., Albanes, D., Pietinen, P., Teerenhovi, L., Taylor, P.R., Virtamo, J., and Stolzenberg-Solomon, R. (2006) Dietary factors of one-carbon metabolism in relation to non-Hodgkin lymphoma and multiple myeloma in a cohort of male smokers. *Cancer Epidemiol Biomarkers Prev* **15**, 1109–14.

67. Zhang, S.M., Hunter, D.J., Rosner, B.A., Giovannucci, E.L., Colditz, G.A., Speizer, F.E., and Willett, W.C. (2000) Intakes of fruits, vegetables, and related nutrients and the risk of non-Hodgkin's lymphoma among women. *Cancer Epidemiol Biomarkers Prev* **9**, 477–85.

68. Wang, J.T., Ma, X.C., Cheng, Y.Y., Ding, L., and Zhou, Q. (2006) A case-control study on the association between folate and cervical cancer. *Zhonghua Liu Xing Bing Xue Za Zhi* **27**, 424–27.

69. VanEenwyk, J., Davis, F.G., and Bowen, P.E. (1991) Dietary and serum carotenoids and cervical intraepithelial neoplasia. *Int J Cancer* **48**, 34–38.

70. Ziegler, R.G., Jones, C.J., Brinton, L.A., Norman, S.A., Mallin, K., Levine, R.S., Lehman, H.F., Hamman, R.F., Trumble, A.C., Rosenthal, J.F. et al. (1991) Diet and the risk of in situ cervical cancer among white women in the United States. *Cancer Causes Control* **2**, 17–29.

71. Liu, T., Soong, S.J., Wilson, N.P., Craig, C.B., Cole, P., Macaluso, M., and Butterworth, C.E., Jr. (1993) A case control study of nutritional factors and cervical dysplasia. *Cancer Epidemiol Biomarkers Prev* **2**, 525–30.

72. Kwasniewska, A., Charzewska, J., Tukendorf, A., and Semczuk, M. (1998) Dietary factors in women with dysplasia colli uteri associated with human papillomavirus infection. *Nutr Cancer* **30**, 39–45.

73. Brock, K.E., Berry, G., Mock, P.A., MacLennan, R., Truswell, A.S., and Brinton, L.A. (1988) Nutrients in diet and plasma and risk of in situ cervical cancer. *J Natl Cancer Inst* **80**, 580–85.

74. Hernandez, B.Y., McDuffie, K., Wilkens, L.R., Kamemoto, L., and Goodman, M.T. (2003) Diet and premalignant lesions of the cervix: Evidence of a protective role for folate, riboflavin, thiamin, and vitamin B12. *Cancer Causes Control* **14**, 859–70.

75. Kjellberg, L., Hallmans, G., Ahren, A.M., Johansson, R., Bergman, F., Wadell, G., Angstrom, T., and Dillner, J. (2000) Smoking, diet, pregnancy and oral contraceptive use as risk factors for cervical intra-epithelial neoplasia in relation to human papillomavirus infection. *Br J Cancer* **82**, 1332–38.

76. Thomson, S.W., Heimburger, D.C., Cornwell, P.E., Turner, M.E., Sauberlich, H.E., Fox, L.M., and Butterworth, C.E. (2000) Correlates of total plasma homocysteine: Folic acid, copper, and cervical dysplasia. *Nutrition* **16**, 411–16.

77. Piyathilake, C.J., Macaluso, M., Brill, I., Heimburger, D.C., and Partridge, E.E. (2007) Lower red blood cell folate enhances the HPV-16-associated risk of cervical intraepithelial neoplasia. *Nutrition* **23**, 203–10.

78. Butterworth, C.E., Jr., Hatch, K.D., Macaluso, M., Cole, P., Sauberlich, H.E., Soong, S.J., Borst, M., and Baker, V.V. (1992) Folate deficiency and cervical dysplasia. *JAMA* **267**, 528–33.

79. Potischman, N., Brinton, L.A., Laiming, V.A., Reeves, W.C., Brenes, M.M., Herrero, R., Tenorio, F., de Britton, R.C., and Gaitan, E. (1991) A case-control study of serum folate levels and invasive cervical cancer. *Cancer Res* **51**, 4785–89.

80. Yeo, A.S., Schiff, M.A., Montoya, G., Masuk, M., van Asselt-King, L., and Becker, T.M. (2000) Serum micronutrients and cervical dysplasia in Southwestern American Indian women. *Nutr Cancer* **38**, 141–50.

81. Weinstein, S.J., Ziegler, R.G., Frongillo, E.A., Jr., Colman, N., Sauberlich, H.E., Brinton, L.A., Hamman, R.F., Levine, R.S., Mallin, K., Stolley, P.D., and Bisogni, C.A. (2001) Low serum and red blood cell folate are moderately, but nonsignificantly associated with increased risk of invasive cervical cancer in US women. *J Nutr* **131**, 2040–48.

82. Ziegler, R.G., Weinstein, S.J., and Fears, T.R. (2002) Nutritional and genetic inefficiencies in one-carbon metabolism and cervical cancer risk. *J Nutr* **132**, 2345S–2349S.

83. Butterworth, C.E., Jr., Hatch, K.D., Gore, H., Mueller, H., and Krumdieck, C.L. (1982) Improvement in cervical dysplasia associated with folic acid therapy in users of oral contraceptives. *Am J Clin Nutr* **35**, 73–82.

84. Butterworth, C.E., Jr., Hatch, K.D., Soong, S.J., Cole, P., Tamura, T., Sauberlich, H.E., Borst, M., Macaluso, M., and Baker, V. (1992) Oral folic acid supplementation for cervical dysplasia: A clinical intervention trial. *Am J Obstet Gynecol* **166**, 803–09.

85. Childers, J.M., Chu, J., Voigt, L.F., Feigl, P., Tamimi, H.K., Franklin, E.W., Alberts, D.S., and Meyskens, F.L., Jr. (1995) Chemoprevention of cervical cancer with folic acid: A phase III Southwest Oncology Group Intergroup study. *Cancer Epidemiol Biomarkers Prev* **4**, 155–59.

86. Zarcone, R., Bellini, P., Carfora, E., Vicinanza, G., and Raucci, F. (1996) Folic acid and cervix dysplasia. *Minerva Ginecol* **48**, 397–400.

87. Thompson, J.R., Gerald, P.F., Willoughby, M.L., and Armstrong, B.K. (2001) Maternal folate supplementation in pregnancy and protection against acute lymphoblastic leukaemia in childhood: A case-control study. *Lancet* **358**, 1935–40.

88. Dockerty, J.D., Herbison, P., Skegg, D.C., and Elwood, M. (2007) Vitamin and mineral supplements in pregnancy and the risk of childhood acute lymphoblastic leukaemia: A case-control study. *BMC Public Health* **7**, 136.

89. Almadori, G., Bussu, F., Galli, J., Cadoni, G., Zappacosta, B., Persichilli, S., Minucci, A., Giardina, B., and Maurizi, M. (2005) Serum levels of folate, homocysteine, and vitamin B12 in head and neck squamous cell carcinoma and in laryngeal leukoplakia. *Cancer* **103**, 284–92.

90. Eleftheriadou, A., Chalastras, T., Ferekidou, E., Yiotakis, I., Kyriou, L., Tzagarakis, M., Ferekidis, E., and Kandiloros, D. (2006) Association between squamous cell carcinoma of the head and neck and serum folate and homocysteine. *Anticancer Res* **26**, 2345–48.

91. Suzuki, T., Matsuo, K., Hirose, K., Hiraki, A., Kawase, T., Watanabe, M., Yamashita, T., Iwata, H., and Tajima, K. (2008) One-carbon metabolism-related gene polymorphisms and risk of breast cancer. *Carcinogenesis* **29**, 356–62.

92. Xu, W.H., Shrubsole, M.J., Xiang, Y.B., Cai, Q., Zhao, G.M., Ruan, Z.X., Cheng, J.R., Zheng, W., and Shu, X.O. (2007) Dietary folate intake, MTHFR genetic polymorphisms, and the risk of endometrial cancer among Chinese women. *Cancer Epidemiol Biomarkers Prev* **16**, 281–87.

93. McCann, S.E., Freudenheim, J.L., Marshall, J.R., Brasure, J.R., Swanson, M.K., and Graham, S. (2000) Diet in the epidemiology of endometrial cancer in western New York (United States). *Cancer Causes Control* **11**, 965–74.

94. Negri, E., La Vecchia, C., Franceschi, S., Levi, F., and Parazzini, F. (1996) Intake of selected micronutrients and the risk of endometrial carcinoma. *Cancer* **77**, 917–23.

95. Potischman, N., Swanson, C.A., Brinton, L.A., McAdams, M., Barrett, R.J., Berman, M.L., Mortel, R., Twiggs, L.B., Wilbanks, G.D., and Hoover, R.N. (1993) Dietary associations in a case-control study of endometrial cancer. *Cancer Causes Control* **4**, 239–50.

96. Little, J., Sharp, L., Duthie, S., and Narayanan, S. (2003) Colon cancer and genetic variation in folate metabolism: The clinical bottom line. *J Nutr* **133**, 3758S–3766S.

97. Ulrich, C. (2006) Genetic variability in folate-mediated one-carbon metabolism and cancer risk. In: Choi, S.W. and Friso, S., eds. Nutrient-Gene Interactions in Cancer. 75–91, Boca Raton, FL: Taylor & Francis Group.

98. Ulrich, C.M. (2005) Nutrigenetics in cancer research–folate metabolism and colorectal cancer. *J Nutr* **135**, 2698–702.

99. Nijhout, H.F., Reed, M.C., Budu, P., and Ulrich, C.M. (2004) A mathematical model of the folate cycle: New insights into folate homeostasis. *J Biol Chem* **279**, 55008–16.

100. Ulrich, C.M., Neuhouser, M.L., Liu, A.Y., Boynton, A., Gregory, G.F., 3rd., Shane, B.S., James, S.J., Reed, M.C., and Nijhout, H.F. (2008) Mathematical modeling of folate metabolism: Predicted effects of genetic polymorphisms on mechanisms and biomarkers relevant to carcinogenesis. *Cancer Epidemiol Biomarkers Prev* **17**, 1822–31.

101. Blount, B.C., Mack, M.M., Wehr, C.M., MacGregor, J.T., Hiatt, R.A., Wang, G., Wickramasinghe, S.N., Everson, R.B., and Ames, B.N. (1997) Folate deficiency causes uracil misincorporation into human DNA and chromosome breakage: Implications for cancer and neuronal damage. *Proc Natl Acad Sci USA* **94**, 3290–95.

102. Quinlivan, E.P., Davis, S.R., Shelnutt, K.P., Henderson, G.N., Ghandour, H., Shane, B., Selhub, J., Bailey, L.B., Stacpoole, P.W., and Gregory, J.F., 3rd. (2005) Methylenetetrahydrofolate reductase 677C–>T polymorphism and folate status affect one-carbon incorporation into human DNA deoxynucleosides. *J Nutr* **135**, 389–96.

103. Stern, L.L., Mason, J.B., Selhub, J., and Choi, S.W. (2000) Genomic DNA hypomethylation, a characteristic of most cancers, is present in peripheral leukocytes of individuals who are homozygous for the C677T polymorphism in the methylenetetrahydrofolate reductase gene. *Cancer Epidemiol Biomarkers Prev* **9**, 849–53.

104. Davis, C.D., and Uthus, E.O. (2004) DNA methylation, cancer susceptibility, and nutrient interactions. *Exp Biol Med* **229**, 988–95.

105. Frosst, P., Blom, H.J., Milos, R., Goyette, P., Sheppard, C.A., Matthews, R.G., Boers, G.J., den Heijer, M., Kluijtmans, L.A., van den Heuvel, L.P., and Rozen, R. (1995) A candidate genetic risk factor for vascular disease: A common mutation in methylenetetrahydrofolate reductase [letter]. *Nat Genet* **10**, 111–13.

106. Weisberg, I.S., Jacques, P.F., Selhub, J., Bostom, A.G., Chen, Z., Curtis Ellison, R., Eckfeldt, J.H., and Rozen, R. (2001) The 1298A–>C polymorphism in methylenetetrahydrofolate reductase (MTHFR): In vitro expression and association with homocysteine. *Atherosclerosis* **156**, 409–15.

107. Bailey, L.B., and Gregory, J.F., 3rd. (1999) Polymorphisms of methylenetetrahydrofolate reductase and other enzymes: Metabolic significance, risks and impact on folate requirement. *J Nutr* **129**, 919–22.

108. Ulvik, A., Ueland, P.M., Fredriksen, A., Meyer, K., Vollset, S.E., Hoff, G., and Schneede, J. (2007) Functional inference of the methylenetetrahydrofolate reductase 677 C > T and 1298A > C polymorphisms from a large-scale epidemiological study. *Hum Genet* **121**, 57–64.

109. Huang, Y., Han, S., Li, Y., Mao, Y., and Xie, Y. (2007) Different roles of MTHFR C677T and A1298C polymorphisms in colorectal adenoma and colorectal cancer: A meta-analysis. *J Hum Genet* **52**, 73–85.

110. Hubner, R.A., and Houlston, R.S.M.T.H.F.R. (2007) C677T and colorectal cancer risk: A meta-analysis of 25 populations. *Int J Cancer* **120**, 1027–35.

111. Zintzaras, E. (2006) Methylenetetrahydrofolate reductase gene and susceptibility to breast cancer: A meta-analysis. *Clin Genet* **69**, 327–36.

112. Mao, R., Fan, Y., Jin, Y., Bai, J., and Fu, S. (2008) Methylenetetrahydrofolate reductase gene polymorphisms and lung cancer: A meta-analysis. *J Hum Genet* **53**, 340–48.

113. Pereira, T.V., Rudnicki, M., Pereira, A.C., Pombo-de-Oliveira, M.S., and Franco, R.F. (2006) 5,10-Methylenetetrahydrofolate reductase polymorphisms and acute lymphoblastic leukemia risk: A meta-analysis. *Cancer Epidemiol Biomarkers Prev* **15**, 1956–63.

114. Zintzaras, E., Koufakis, T., Ziakas, P.D., Rodopoulou, P., Giannouli, S., and Voulgarelis, M. (2006) A meta-analysis of genotypes and haplotypes of methylenetetrahydrofolate reductase gene polymorphisms in acute lymphoblastic leukemia. *Eur J Epidemiol* **21**, 501–10.

115. Boccia, S., Hung, R., Ricciardi, G., Gianfagna, F., Ebert, M.P., Fang, J.Y., Gao, C.M., Gotze, T., Graziano, F., Lacasana-Navarro, M., Lin, D., Lopez-Carrillo, L., Qiao, Y.L., Shen, H., Stolzenberg-Solomon, R., Takezaki, T., Weng, Y.R., Zhang, F.F., van Duijn, C.M., Boffetta, P., and Taioli, E. (2008) Meta- and pooled analyses of the methylenetetrahydrofolate reductase C677T and A1298C polymorphisms and gastric cancer risk: A huge-GSEC review. *Am J Epidemiol* **167**, 505–16.

116. Zintzaras, E. (2006) Association of methylenetetrahydrofolate reductase (MTHFR) polymorphisms with genetic susceptibility to gastric cancer: A meta-analysis. *J Hum Genet* **51**, 618–24.

117. Kaneda, S., Takeishi, K., Ayusawa, D., Shimizu, K., Seno, T., and Altman, S. (1987) Role in translation of a triple tandemly repeated sequence in the 5′-untranslated region of human thymidylate synthase mRNA. *Nucleic Acids Res* **15**, 1259–70.

118. Horie, N., Aiba, H., Oguro, K., Hojo, H., and Takeishi, K. (1995) Functional analysis and DNA polymorphism of the tandemly repeated sequences in the 5′-terminal regulatory region of the human gene for thymidylate synthase. *Cell Struct Funct* **20**, 191–97.

119. Pullarkat, S.T., Stoehlmacher, J., Ghaderi, V., Xiong, Y.-P., Ingles, S.A., Sherrod, A., Warren, R., Tsao-Wei, D., Groshen, S., and Lenz, H.-J. (2001) Thymidylate synthase gene polymorphism determines response and toxicity of 5-FU chemotherapy. *Pharmacogenomics J* **1**, 65–70.

120. Chen, J., Hunter, D.J., Stampfer, M.J., Kyte, C., Chan, W., Wetmur, J.G., Mosig, R., Selhub, J., and Ma, J. (2003) Polymorphism in the thymidylate synthase promoter enhancer region modifies the risk and survival of colorectal cancer. *Cancer Epidemiol Biomarkers Prev* **12**, 958–62.

121. Ulrich, C.M., Curtin, K., Potter, J.D., Bigler, J., Caan, B., and Slattery, M.L. (2005) Polymorphisms in the reduced folate carrier, thymidylate synthase, or methionine synthase and risk of colon cancer. *Cancer Epidemiol Biomarkers Prev* **14**, 2509–16.

122. Skibola, C.F., Smith, M.T., Hubbard, A., Shane, B., Roberts, A.C., Law, G.R., Rollinson, S., Roman, E., Cartwright, R.A., and Morgan, G.J. (2002) Polymorphisms in the thymidylate synthase and serine hydroxymethyltransferase genes and risk of adult acute lymphocytic leukemia. *Blood* **99**, 3786–91.

123. Mandola, M.V., Stoehlmacher, J., Muller-Weeks, S., Cesarone, G., Yu, M.C., Lenz, H.J., and Ladner, R.D. (2003) A novel single nucleotide polymorphism within the 5′ tandem repeat polymorphism of the thymidylate synthase gene abolishes USF-1 binding and alters transcriptional activity. *Cancer Res* **63**, 2898–904.

124. Ulrich, C.M., Bigler, J., Velicer, C., Greene, E., Farin, F., and Potter, J.D. (2000) Searching expressed sequence tag databases: Discovery and confirmation of a common polymorphism in the thymidylate synthase gene. *Cancer Epidemiol Biomarkers Prev* **9**, 1381–85.

125. Mandola, M.V., Stoehlmacher, J., Zhang, W., Groshen, S., Yu, M.C., Iqbal, S., Lenz, H.J., and Ladner, R.D.A. (2004) 6 bp polymorphism in the thymidylate synthase gene causes message instability and is associated with decreased intratumoral TS mRNA levels. *Pharmacogenetics* **14**, 319–27.

126. Ulrich, C.M., Bigler, J., Bostick, R., Fosdick, L., and Potter, J.D. (2002) *Thymidylate synthase* promoter polymorphism, interaction with folate intake, and risk of colorectal adenomas. *Cancer Res* **62**, 3361–64.

127. Xu, X., Liu, A.Y., and Ulrich, C.M. (2009) Folate and cancer: Epidemiological perspective. In: Bailey, L., ed. Folate in Health and Disease, 2nd Edition.

128. Liu, A.Y., and Ulrich, C.M. (2009) Genetic Variability in folate-mediated one-carbon metabolism and risk of colorectal neoplasia. In: Lindor, L., and Potter, J.D., eds. Genetic Susceptibility to Colorectal Cancer. Springer, New York, 223–42.

129. Ulrich, C.M., Nijhout, H.F., and Reed, M.C. (2006) Mathematical modeling: Epidemiology meets systems biology. *Cancer Epidemiol Biomarkers Prev* **15**, 827–29.

130. Reed, M.C., Nijhout, H.F., Neuhouser, M.L., Gregory, J.F., 3rd., Shane, B., James, S.J., Boynton, A., and Ulrich, C.M. (2006) A mathematical model gives insights into nutritional and genetic aspects of folate-mediated one-carbon metabolism. *J Nutr* **136**, 2653–61.

131. Nijhout, H.F., Reed, M., Anderson, D., Mattingly, J., James, S.J., and Ulrich, C.M. (2006) Long-range allosteric interactions between the folate and methionine cycles stabilize DNA methylation rate. *Epigenetics* **1**, 81–87.

132. Nijhout, H.F., Reed, M.C., Lam, S.L., Shane, B., Gregory, J.F., 3rd., and Ulrich, C.M. (2006) In silico experimentation with a model of hepatic mitochondrial folate metabolism. *Theor Biol Med Model* **3**, 40.

133. Kim, Y.I. (2006) Folate: A magic bullet or a double edged sword for colorectal cancer prevention? *Gut* **55**, 1387–89.

134. Kim, Y.I. (2004) Folate, colorectal carcinogenesis, and DNA methylation: Lessons from animal studies. *Environ Mol Mutagen* **44**, 10–25.

135. Song, J., Medline, A., Mason, J.B., Gallinger, S., and Kim, Y.I. (2000) Effects of dietary folate on intestinal tumorigenesis in the apcMin mouse. *Cancer Res* **60**, 5434–40.

136. Baggott, J.E., Vaughn, W.H., Juliana, M.M., Eto, I., Krumdieck, C.L., and Grubbs, C.J. (1992) Effects of folate deficiency and supplementation on methylnitrosourea-induced rat mammary tumors. *J Natl Cancer Inst* **84**, 1740–44.

137. Kotsopoulos, J., Sohn, K.J., Martin, R., Choi, M., Renlund, R., McKerlie, C., Hwang, S.W., Medline, A., and Kim, Y.I. (2003) Dietary folate deficiency suppresses N-methyl-N-nitrosourea-induced mammary tumorigenesis in rats. *Carcinogenesis* **24**, 937–44.

138. Kotsopoulos, J., Medline, A., Renlund, R., Sohn, K.J., Martin, R., Hwang, S.W., Lu, S., Archer, M.C., and Kim, Y.I. (2005) Effects of dietary folate on the development and progression of mammary tumors in rats. *Carcinogenesis* **26**, 1603–12.

139. Cole, B.F., Baron, J.A., Sandler, R.S., Haile, R.W., Ahnen, D.J., Bresalier, R.S., McKeown-Eyssen, G., Summers, R.W., Rothstein, R.I., Burke, C.A., Snover, D.C., Church, T.R., Allen, J.I., Robertson, D.J., Beck, G.J., Bond, J.H., Byers, T., Mandel, J.S., Mott, L.A., Pearson, L.H., Barry, E.L., Rees, J.R., Marcon, N., Saibil, F., Ueland, P.M., and Greenberg, E.R. (2007) Folic acid for the prevention of colorectal adenomas: A randomized clinical trial. *JAMA* **297**, 2351–59.

140. Logan, R.F., Grainge, M.J., Shepherd, V.C., Armitage, N.C., and Muir, K.R. (2007) Aspirin and folic acid for the prevention of recurrent colorectal adenomas. *Gastroenterology*. **134**, 29–38.

141. Mason, J.B., Dickstein, A., Jacques, P.F., Haggarty, P., Selhub, J., Dallal, G., and Rosenberg, I.H. (2007) A temporal association between folic acid fortification and an increase in colorectal cancer rates may be illuminating important biological principles: A hypothesis. *Cancer Epidemiol Biomarkers Prev* **16**, 1325–29.

142. Luebeck, E.G., and Moolgavkar, S.H. (2002) Multistage carcinogenesis and the incidence of colorectal cancer. *Proc Natl Acad Sci USA* **99**, 15095–100.

143. Luebeck, E.G., Moolgavkar, S.H., Liu, A.Y., Boynton, A., and Ulrich, C.M. (2008) Does folic-acid supplementation prevent or promote colorectal cancer? Results from model-based predictions. *Cancer Epidemiol Biomarkers Prev* **17**, 1360–67.

19 Selenium

Margaret P. Rayman

Key Points

1. Evidence is accruing that the level of intake of selenium (Se) affects the risk of cancer and may even inhibit its spread from a primary tumour. Se exists in a number of dietary forms all of which are capable of being converted to hydrogen selenide (H_2Se), a crucial molecule in Se metabolism. The nutritional functions of Se are carried out by the selenoproteins which contain Se in the form of selenocysteine (Sec).

2. A number of parallel and/or consecutive mechanisms are likely to be involved in the anti-cancer effects of Se. Evidence exists for involvement of the selenoproteins, of methylated precursors that can generate methyl selenol and of redox-cycling superoxide and hydrogen peroxide generated by oxidation of hydrogen selenide, all of which have been associated with anti-cancer effects. Thus Se compounds can modify critical sulfhydryl groups to inhibit or promote tumor cell metabolism and cell transformation.

3. Selenoenzymes are involved in antioxidant protection and anti-inflammatory effects, and may enhance the cell-mediated immune response. Se compounds can cause cell cycle arrest and apoptosis, enhance DNA repair and reduce cancer cell migration. Importantly in relation to prostate cancer, Se can down-regulate the androgen receptor.

4. While there has been fairly general acceptance that a Se metabolite, methyl selenol, is a proximal anti-carcinogen at supra-nutritional doses, data linking cancer risk with the presence of seleno-protein polymorphisms and hypermethylation of promotor regions of selenoprotein genes has also implicated selenoproteins in anti-cancer effects. Numerous cohort and nested case–control studies have shown that higher Se status is associated with a lower risk of malignancies or death from cancer. However, such evidence is subject to some uncertainty owing to the effect of inflammation on plasma or serum Se concentration which can long precede the appearance of clinical symptoms.

5. Randomized clinical trials are not subject to such effects. Data from the Nutritional Prevention of Cancer randomized trial have shown a significant protective effect of supplementation with 200 μg Se/d, as high-Se yeast, on cancer incidence and mortality with the most notable effect being on prostate cancer, with lesser effects on colorectal and lung cancers. Significant effects were confined to males, were most pronounced in former smokers and in those with plasma Se < 105 μg Se/L at baseline, a level common in European populations. By contrast, the Selenium and Vitamin E Cancer Prevention Trial (SELECT) that gave 200 μg Se/d, as selenome-thionine, to men of replete Se status [serum Se 136 (range 123–150) μg /L] showed no benefit of Se supplementation over placebo. The need for further randomised trials in populations of low baseline Se status, in women, and with a lower Se dose, e.g. 100 μg Se/d, is argued. Trials with the methyl selenol precursor, Se-methylselenocysteine, also appear warranted as do trials in

From: *Nutrition and Health: Bioactive Compounds and Cancer*
Edited by: J.A. Milner, D.F. Romagnolo, DOI 10.1007/978-1-60761-627-6_19,
© Springer Science+Business Media, LLC 2010

subjects of known selenoprotein SNP genotype, as we can no longer assume that each person's Se requirement to reduce cancer risk is the same.

6. In the meantime, there is no justification for increasing Se intake in persons with plasma Se above around 125 μg Se/L, though a case can certainly be made that an increased intake may benefit those whose plasma Se falls below 105 μg Se/L. However, definitive guidelines on optimal intake await further research and, for individuals rather than populations, these must ultimately be genotype related.

Key Words: Selenium; cancer; mechanism; selenomethyl-selenocysteine; single-nucleotide polymorphisms; epidemiology; hypermethylation; acute phase response

1. INTRODUCTION

Evidence is accruing that the level of intake of selenium (Se) affects the risk of cancer and may even inhibit its spread from a primary tumour. The nature of the Se species involved in anti-cancer processes and the extent to which the selenoproteins are relevant is still a matter of speculation and much ongoing experimental work.

Se is an unusual trace element in having its own codon in mRNA that specifies its insertion into selenoproteins as selenocysteine (Sec), by means of a mechanism requiring a large Sec-insertion complex. Unlike the other 20 amino acids, Sec is biosynthesised on its own tRNA, Sec tRNA[Ser]Sec, from selenophosphate as the Se source. The insertion of Sec is specified by the UGA codon in mRNA. However, as UGA is also a stop codon, the presence of a stem-loop structure in mRNA – a SECIS (Sec Insertion Sequence) element – downstream from UGA in the 3′-mRNA-untranslated region, is also required for UGA to be read as selenocysteine. SECIS elements function by recruiting additional factors including the SECIS-binding protein, the Sec-specific elongation factor and Sec tRNA[Ser]Sec to form the large Sec-insertion complex required for the synthesis of selenoproteins and known as the selenosome *(1–3)*. This complex insertion machinery for selenoprotein production has implications for our Se requirements for cancer prevention. The human selenoproteome consists of 25 selenoproteins *(4)*.

Se exists in a number of dietary forms all of which are capable of being converted to hydrogen selenide (H_2Se), a central molecule in Se metabolism that can be further metabolised to selenoproteins, methylated or converted to selenosugars in the excretory pathway or oxidised to generate superoxide and hydrogen peroxide (Fig. 1) *(5)*. Selenomethionine (SeMet) is the main dietary form, particularly from grain or cereal sources. It can be metabolised to hydrogen selenide for conversion into selenoproteins but can also be incorporated indiscriminately into any body protein in place of methionine where it can remain until released by catabolism when it can undergo further metabolism. Selenocysteine is ingested in selenoproteins from animal sources and again must be metabolised to hydrogen selenide before further utilisation. Other food sources, notably plants from the *Allium* and *Brassica* families, contain *Se*-methyl-selenocysteine and γ-glutamyl-*Se*-methyl-selenocysteine which are readily converted to the potent anti-carcinogen, methylselenol (CH_3SeH), without the need for conversion to hydrogen selenide *(5)*. With regard to inorganic sources, a little selenate is present in vegetables *(5)* but selenite, though a component of some Se supplements and the form chosen for many human, animal and in vitro studies is basically absent from

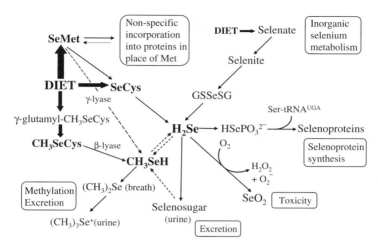

Fig. 1. Metabolic pathway of dietary Se in humans [Rayman et al. *(111)*] Abbreviations: SeMet, selenomethionine; SeCys, selenocysteine; γ-glutamyl-CH$_3$SeCys, γ-glutamyl-*Se*-methyl-selenocysteine; CH$_3$SeCys, *Se*-methyl-selenocysteine; H$_2$Se, hydrogen selenide; CH$_3$SeH, methyl selenol; (CH$_3$)$_2$Se, dimethyl selenol; (CH$_3$)$_3$Se$^+$, trimethyl selenonium ion; GSSeSG, selenodiglutathione; HSePO$_3$ $^{2-}$, selenophosphate; SeO$_2$, selenium dioxide.

the food chain. Synthetic Se compounds such as methyl seleninic acid that readily yield methylselenol in vitro have been developed for use in model systems.

2. RATIONALE FOR AN EFFECT OF SELENIUM ON CANCER PREVENTION AND TREATMENT

A number of parallel and/or consecutive mechanisms are likely to be involved in the anti-cancer effects of Se. Evidence exists for involvement of the selenoproteins, of methylated precursors that can generate methyl selenol and of redox-cycling superoxide and hydrogen peroxide generated by oxidation of hydrogen selenide, all of which have anti-cancer effects. The anti-carcinogenic mechanisms by which Se acts have previously been reviewed *(6–10)*. Anti-cancer mechanisms are summarised in Fig. 2 and further discussed below.

2.1. Modification of Critical Sulfhydryl Groups

Se can act very generally through its redox-active compounds (e.g. methylated Se metabolites) which can affect cellular proteins by modification of critical cysteine residues, particularly when clustered *(6, 11)*. This may in turn have downstream effects on signal transduction and gene transcription *(12)*. Se adducts of the selenotrisulfide (S–Se–S) or selenenylsulfide (S–Se) type may form while disulfide bonds may be made or broken. Ganther has proposed that Se catalysis of reversible cysteine/disulfide trans-formations that occur in a number of redox-regulated proteins, [e.g. p53 *(13)*, protein kinase C (PKC) *(14)*] including transcription factors, may be a chemopreventive mech-anism *(11)*. For instance, PKC regulates tumor promotion and cell growth by inducing

- Modification of critical sulfhydryl groups to inhibit (e.g. protein kinase C, NF-κB, AP-1) or promote (p53) redox-sensitive factors that impair tumor cell metabolism and cell transformation

- Antioxidant protection (selenoenzymes/selenoproteins)

- Anti-inflammatory effect (partly *via* selenoenzymes/selenoproteins e.g. SEPS1)

- Enhancement of cell-mediated immune response

- Maintenance of genome stability – prevention of DNA damage/enhancement of DNA repair

- Cell cycle arrest – decreases cell proliferation

    S/G2 cell cycle arrest (H_2Se)

    G1 cell cycle arrest (methyl selenol)

- Apoptosis (necrosis)

    caspase-mediated (methyl selenol)

    genotoxic-mediated (H_2Se)

    ER-stress-mediated

- Reduced tumor cell invasion/migration capacity (both selenite and methyl selenol)

- Inhibition of angiogenesis: effect on gene expression of MMPs and TIMPs (methyl selenol and H_2Se)

- Activation of p53 tumor-suppressive activity

- Inactivation of protein kinase C

- Upregulation of phase II carcinogen-detoxifying enzymes

- Androgen receptor down-regulation (relevant to prostate cancer)

Fig. 2. Anti-carcinogenic mechanisms of Se (see text for details and references).

activation of transcription factors and by increasing the expression of key enzymes, such as ornithine decarboxylase, inducible nitric oxide synthase and cyclooxygenase-2 *(14)*. Thus inactivation of PKC by redox-active selenometabolites can inhibit tumor promotion, cell growth, invasion and metastasis and promote the induction of apoptosis *(14)*.

A further example of the effect of redox modification of thiol/disulfide bonds is that it results in protein misfolding or unfolding *(15)*. Newly synthesized proteins are particularly vulnerable before they are properly folded in the endoplasmic reticulum (ER). Thus, it is highly plausible that Se metabolites can produce ER stress, which if too severe, exceeding the capacity for repair, will trigger the signal for apoptosis *(15)*. It appears that low doses of Se (e.g. as methylseleninic acid, a methyl selenol precursor) preferentially activate the rescue arm of the ER stress response [likely involving selenoprotein S, SEPS1 *(16)*, whereas high doses lead to the assembly of the apoptotic machinery. Se may have a dichotomous effect such that it favours survival response in normal cells but facilitates the apoptotic response in cancer cells *(15)*.

2.2. Antioxidant Protection (Selenoenzymes/Selenoproteins)

Se, as selenoenzymes reduces oxidative stress. Selenoenzymes can reduce hydrogen peroxide and lipid hydroperoxide intermediates in the cyclooxygenase and lipoxygenase pathways preventing further conversion to reactive oxygen species (ROS) that can cause oxidative stress, damaging DNA and other macromolecules and promoting cancer *(17)*.

That the ability of Se in selenoproteins to reduce oxidative stress is relevant to its anti-cancer effects is suggested by the modification of these effects by other antioxidant nutrients. Thus the strongest effect of Se on cancer risk has been shown among those with the lowest levels of dietary antioxidant vitamins and carotenoids *(18–24)* and particularly at low α-tocopherol concentrations *(25, 26)*. Smoking modifies the effect of Se on cancer risk, demonstrating the operation of an antioxidant mechanism *(27, 28)*.

A further indication of a link between the antioxidant capacity of Se and cancer risk is seen in the modification of that Se-dependent risk by a polymorphism in manganese superoxide dismutase (SOD2), the primary antioxidant enzyme in mitochondria. SOD2 has a polymorphism (Val16Ala, rs4880) that has been shown to alter the secondary structure of the mitochondrial import sequence of the superoxide dismutase protein such that the Ala16 variant is imported more efficiently into the mitochondrial matrix, resulting in higher enzyme activity *(29)*. Men carrying the Ala allele are therefore likely to produce more hydrogen peroxide which promotes prostate cancer cell proliferation and migration and induces matrix metalloproteinases required for tumour invasion *(30–32)*. There is an interaction between Se status and this polymorphism owing to the requirement for a selenoenzyme, GPx, to remove the hydrogen peroxide (there being no catalase in mitochondria). Thus men in the bottom quartile of Se status who were SOD2 Ala homozygotes had a significantly higher risk of aggressive prostate cancer than Val/Ala or Val/Val men (1.89; 95% CI 1.01, 3.56) but if they were in the top quartile, their risk was significantly lower, presumably because they could both efficiently remove superoxide *and* make enough GPx to deal with the extra hydrogen peroxide formed *(33)*. The interdependence of SOD2, Se status and prostate cancer risk implies a role for the antioxidant selenoenzymes.

2.3. Anti-inflammatory Effect (Partly via Selenoenzymes/Selenoproteins)

Inflammation is known to promote tumour growth *(34)*. Macrophage activation is a crucial step in the inflammatory process that forms the underlying basis of cancer progression *(35)*.

Se reduces inflammation by a number of mechanisms in at least some of which selenoproteins are known to be involved (Fig. 3). Se aids in the shunting of arachidonic acid towards endogenous anti-inflammatory mediators as an adaptive response to protect cells against pro-inflammatory gene expression induced by oxidative stress. Thus Se supplementation in macrophages increases the production of 15d-PGJ$_2$ (by the COX-1 pathway), an endogenous inhibitor of a key kinase of the NF-κB cascade, IκB-kinase

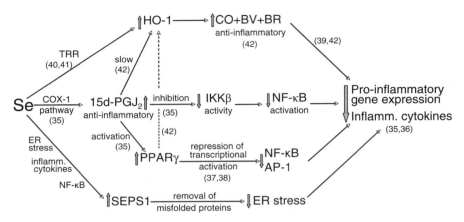

Fig. 3. Some mechanisms by which Se reduces inflammation resulting from oxidative stress *(39–42)*. Abbreviations: ER, endoplasmic reticulum; SEPS1, selenoprotein S; 15d-PGJ2, 15-deoxy-Δ12, 14-prostaglandin J2; IKKβ, IκB-kinase β; TRR, thioredoxin reductase; BV, billiverdin; BR, billirubin.

β (IKKβ) *(36)*. This effect results in decreased activation of NF-κB and down-regulates expression of inflammatory genes such as COX-2, TNF-α, IL-6 and VCAM-1 *(36, 37)*. In a second Se-dependent anti-inflammatory mechanism acting through 15d-PGJ$_2$, Se-supplemented macrophages activate the peroxisome proliferator-activated nuclear receptor-γ (PPAR-γ) *(36)*, repressing inflammatory gene expression *(38, 39)*.

HO-1 is an inducible enzyme that is upregulated in oxidative stress with cytoprotective and anti-inflammatory functions linked to its removal of the pro-oxidant, heme, and its production of the antioxidant bilirubin and the vasodilatory, anti-inflammatory carbon monoxide (CO) *(40)*. Se has been shown to upregulate HO-1 by a number of pathways resulting in reduced expression of pro-inflammatory genes *(41, 42)* (see Fig. 3) *(43, 44)*.

Selenoprotein S (SEPS1) is an endoplasmic reticulum (ER) membrane protein involved in the control of inflammation and genetic variation in selenoprotein S has been shown to influence the inflammatory response *(45, 46)*. By regulating cellular redox balance, SEPS1 protects the ER against the deleterious effects of oxidative stress. It has a role in the removal of stressor-induced misfolded proteins from the ER, preventing the accumulation of these proteins and the subsequent stress response that leads to activation of NF-κB, pro-inflammatory cytokine gene transcription and the inflammation cascade. Impairment of SEPS1 is directly associated with increased cellular cytokine production and release. There appears to be a regulatory loop whereby cytokines stimulate the expression of SEPS1 which in turn suppresses cytokine production *(45)*.

2.4. Enhancement of Cell-Mediated Immune Response

Cytotoxic lymphocytes and natural killer cells are able to destroy tumour cells. We know that Se is important to immune regulation but there is little understanding of how it acts at the molecular level. A recent study has shed some light on this process. Mice with selenoproteinless T cells were generated by cell type-specific ablation of the Sec tRNA([Ser]Sec) gene (*Trsp*) *(47)*. The resultant selenoprotein deficiency caused defects in the development of functionally mature T cells and their T-cell-receptor-dependent activation. Furthermore, selenoprotein deficiency led to oxidant hyperproduction in T cells, suppressing T cell proliferation in response to T-cell-receptor stimulation. Seleno-protein expression in T cells appears to be crucial for their ability to proliferate in response to T-cell receptor stimulation.

Se supplementation (as sodium selenite) enhanced the immune response of healthy volunteers and cancer patients *(48, 49)*. Thus supplementation of healthy volunteers with a "selenium replete" status with 200 µg/d Se for 8 wk increased the ability of human peripheral blood lymphocytes to respond to stimulation with alloantigen *(48)*. The supplementation regimen resulted in 118% increase in cytotoxic lymphocyte-mediated tumor cytotoxicity and 82.3% increase in natural killer cell activity as compared to baseline values. The effect appeared to be related to the ability of Se to enhance the expression of receptors for the growth regulatory lymphokine interleukin-2, and consequently, the rate of cell proliferation and differentiation into cytotoxic cells. Patients supplemented with 200 µg/d Se during therapy for squamous cell carcinoma of the head and neck, e.g. surgery, radiation or surgery and radiation, had a significantly enhanced cell-mediated immune response in contrast to patients in the placebo arm of the study who showed a decline in immune responsiveness during therapy *(50)*.

2.5. Maintenance of Genome Stability – Prevention of DNA Damage/Induction of DNA Repair

Se (presumably as selenoenzymes) can prevent damage to DNA that causes single- and double-strand breaks. Thus Se (as sodium selenite) and overexpression of GPx1 protected mammalian cells against UV-induced DNA damage *(51)*. Protection appeared to be dependent on functional activity of BRCA1, a protein involved in maintaining the integrity of the human genome which helps to repair DNA double-strand breaks. In a further set of studies, Se, as SeMet, protected normal fibroblasts from subsequent DNA damage by selective induction of the DNA repair branch of the p53 pathway involving interaction with BRCA1 and Redox-factor 1 (Ref1) *(52)*.

Given the requirement for functional BRCA1 activity found in the studies described above, it is perhaps surprising that Se appears to protect women born with a mutation in *BRCA1* that presumably leads to an abnormal BRCA1 protein. These women carry a lifetime risk of breast cancer of 80% and a lifetime risk of ovarian cancer of 40% *(53)*. When blood lymphocytes from *BRCA1* carriers are exposed to bleomycin, a known mutagen that induces double-strand breaks, an increased frequency of chromosome breaks per cell occurs, i.e. 0.58 in *BRCA1* carriers *vs.* 0.39 in non-carriers *(53)*. In 32 female *BRCA1* carriers supplemented with Se (276 µg/d as sodium selenite) for 1–3 months, the frequency of chromosome breaks per cell was significantly reduced from 0.63 before supplementation with Se to 0.40 after supplementation with Se, bringing it to the level in non-carrier controls. Thus Se may have the potential to reduce breast cancer risk in these women.

The effect of Se status on protection from DNA damage was investigated in New Zealand men, aged 50–75 year, judged to be at risk of prostate cancer (PSA >

4). The comet assay, carried out in blood leukocytes from those with serum Se below the mean, showed a significant inverse relationship with overall accumulated DNA damage ($p = 0.02$) *(54)*. As mean serum Se was measured as 98 ± 17 μg/L, this suggests that serum levels above 98 μg/L are required for the prevention of DNA damage in New Zealand men.

2.6. Cell Cycle Arrest – Decreases Cell Proliferation

Se compounds have been shown to cause a block in progression of the cell cycle. The resulting inhibition of growth may allow DNA repair to take place. In the case of selenite, the mechanism probably involves interaction with glutathione resulting in conversion to selenide and then oxidative metabolism to superoxide and hydrogen peroxide which can cause DNA strand breaks, triggering S-phase/G2 cycle arrest *(55–58)*. By contrast, methyl selenol precursors can induce G1 cell cycle arrest without single-strand breaks and with or without caspase induction and p53 involvement *(8, 56–58)*.

2.7. Apoptosis (Necrosis)

One of the most significant mechanisms by which Se reduces cancer risk is by the induction of apoptosis in cancer cells. In the case of selenite, in vitro experiments reveal a genotoxic mechanism involving superoxide and hydrogen peroxide which cause DNA single-strand breaks culminating apparently in necrosis or apoptosis, depending on the study *(57, 59)*. The caspases are not involved *(6)*. By contrast, methylated forms of Se (*Se*-methylselenocysteine, methylseleninic acid or methylselenocyanate) may not cause DNA strand breaks and induce apoptosis apparently by activating key enzymes in the caspase pathway *(8, 55, 57, 59, 60)*.

A further mechanism by which methylated Se can induce apoptosis is by the creation of endoplasmic reticulum (ER) stress. While low doses of Se preferentially activate the rescue arm of the ER stress response, high doses lead to the assembly of the apoptotic machinery. Se appears to have a dichotomous effect: it favours survival response in normal cells and facilitates apoptotic response in cancer cells *(15)*.

2.8. Reduced Tumor Cell Migration and Invasion

Cancer cell invasion requires coordinated processes, such as changes in cell–cell and cell–matrix adhesion, degradation of the extracellular matrix and cell migration *(61)*. Se, in a number of forms, inhibits the invasion of tumor cells, reducing the risk of metastasis:

– Dietary supplementation of selenomethionine reduced experimental metastasis of melanoma cells in mice and inhibited the growth of metastatic tumours that formed in the lungs *(62)*.
– Dietary supplementation of selenite, at 2- and 4-ppm, reduced pulmonary metastasis of B16BL6 melanoma cells in C57BL/6 mice and inhibited the growth of the metastatic tumours in the lungs *(63)*.
– Selenite inhibited invasion of HT1080 human fibrosarcoma cells and adhesion of the cells to the collagen matrix *(61)*.

– In HT1080 human fibrosarcoma cells, exposure to sub-micromolar concentrations of methylselenol (from seleno-L-methionine and methioninase) inhibited the migration and invasion rate of the tumor cells by up to 53 and 76%, respectively, when compared with the control tumor cells *(64)*.

2.9. Inhibition of Angiogenesis

Blood vessel formation, or angiogenesis, is required for the growth and metastasis of tumours. Two proteins critical for angiogenesis are matrix metalloproteinase-2 (MMP-2) produced by vascular endothelial cells, which degrades the extracellular matrix, and vascular endothelial growth factor (VEGF) produced by cancer epithelial cells *(65, 66)*.

Thus, in the rat mammary carcinoma model system, increased Se intake (as Se-enriched garlic, sodium selenite or *Se*-methylselenocysteine) significantly reduced intratumoral microvessel density and inhibited the expression of vascular endothelial growth factor (VEGF) *(66)*. By contrast, treatment caused no change in microvessel density of the uninvolved mammary glands.

In vitro data also show that both selenite and monomethyl Se inhibit the invasion of tumor cells by their effect on endothelial matrix metalloproteinase (MMP) and/or VEGF expression:

– Selenite inhibited the invasion of HT1080 human fibrosarcoma cells, adhesion of cells to the collagen matrix and reduced the expression of MMP-2 and -9 and urokinase-type plasminogen activator, which are involved in matrix degradation, while increasing the expression of a tissue inhibitor of metalloproteinase-1 (TIMP-1) *(61)*.
– Short-term exposure of human umbilical vein endothelial cells (HUVECs) to the methylselenol precursors, methylseleninic acid (MSeA) and methylselenocyanate (MSeCN) decreased the MMP-2 gelatinolytic activity in a concentration-dependent manner largely through a decrease of the MMP-2 protein level *(65)*.
– Exposure of human prostate cancer (DU145) and breast cancer (MCF-7 and MDA-MB-468) cell lines to MSeA, but not to selenite, led to a rapid and sustained decrease of cellular and secreted VEGF protein levels *(65)*. The concentration of monomethyl Se required for inhibiting endothelial expression of MMP-2 and cancer epithelial expression of VEGF was within the physiological range and much lower than that needed for apoptosis induction *(67)*.
– Sub-micromolar methylselenol (from seleno-L-methionine and methioninase) increased not only the enzyme activity of pro-MMP-2 (the active form of MMP-2) but also protein levels of anti-metastasic tissue inhibitor metalloproteinase (TIMP)-1 and TIMP-2 in HT1080 human fibrosarcoma cells giving a net effect of inhibition of pro-MMP-2 activation and carcinogenic potential *(64)*.

2.10. Activation of p53 Tumor-Suppressive Activity

p53 is a transcription factor that activates a number of downstream genes that function in cellular responses to DNA damage. p53 activation is common to Se compounds but specific mechanisms differ between Se chemical forms *(68)*. SeMet activates the DNA repair branch of the p53 pathway by redox regulation of key p53 cysteine residues *(13)*, while methyl seleninic acid and sodium selenite affect p53 phosphorylation in treated cells. Different Se chemical forms may differentially modify p53 for DNA repair or apoptosis in conjunction with a given level of endogenous or exogenous DNA damage *(68)*. Thus Se-enriched broccoli which is a rich source of *Se*-methyl-selenocysteine upregulates p53 and promotes apoptosis in Min mice *(69)*. There is some evidence that increase in p53 activity could also help to switch off angiogenesis in early lesions *(6)*.

2.11. Upregulation of Phase II Carcinogen-Detoxifying Enzymes

Sources of some Se compounds [e.g. Se-enriched garlic, mushrooms, selenite, selenate, 1,4-phenylenebis(methylene)selenocyanate (*p*-XSC)] have been shown to detoxify carcinogens and/or reduce DNA-adduct formation in rats and mice *(8)*. For example, prior feeding with a Se-garlic-containing diet (at 3 ppm Se, a source of *Se*-methylselenocysteine) for two weeks resulted in an elevation of glutathione *S*-transferase and uridine 5′-diphosphate-glucuronyltransferase activities to a maximum of 2- to 2.5-fold in liver and kidney *(70)*. There was a consistent reduction of all dimethylbenz[a]anthracene (DMBA) adducts in liver and mammary gland accompanied by a 40% increase in urinary excretion of DMBA metabolites over a 2-day period. These results are supported by microarray analysis that has shown that Se can upregulate genes related to phase II detoxification enzymes *(71)*.

2.12. Inactivation of PKC

PKC is a signalling receptor that plays a crucial role in tumour promotion by oxidants that can be inactivated by redox-active selenometabolites (see above) *(14)*. Thus Se-induced inactivation of PKC may, at least in part, be responsible for the Se-induced inhibition of tumor promotion, cell growth, invasion, metastasis and for the induction of apoptosis *(14)*. *Se*-methylselenocysteine, an effective chemopreventive agent against mammary cell growth in vivo and in vitro (mouse mammary epithelial tumor cell line), was shown to decrease PKC activity *(72)*. Thus PKC may be an upstream target for *Se*-methylselenocysteine that may trigger downstream events such as the decrease in cdk2 kinase activity and DNA synthesis, elevation of *gadd* gene expression and finally apoptosis *(72)*.

2.13. Androgen Receptor Down-regulation (Relevant to Prostate Cancer)

The prostate seems to be particularly sensitive to the anti-cancer effects of Se. The androgen receptor (AR) is a key mediator of prostate cancer progression. Androgen binding to the AR stimulates its translocation to the nucleus where it interacts with specific androgen-responsive elements (ARE) on the promoters of target genes. The interaction leads to the activation or repression of genes involved in the proliferation and differentiation of the prostate cells *(73)*. The inhibitory effect of Se on prostate cancer progression may be mediated through androgen receptor down-regulation *(73–75)*.

Se compounds have been shown to inhibit cell growth and induce apoptosis in both androgen-dependent and androgen-independent prostate cancer cells *(12)*. According to

Combs and Lü, sub-apoptotic concentrations of methylated Se reduce androgen receptor protein expression, inhibit androgen-stimulated PSA promoter transcription, reduce PSA expression and secretion and cause rapid PSA degradation *(76)*. Thus methylseleninic acid decreased the expression of androgen receptor and PSA in five human prostate cell lines *(73–75)*. Furthermore, methylseleninic acid inhibited the expression of a number of androgen-receptor-regulated genes that are consistently over-expressed in prostate cancer *(73)*: PSA, KLK2, ATP-binding cassette C4 (ABCC4, also known as MRP4), 24-dehydrocholesterol reductase (DHCR24, also known as seladin-1) and soluble guanylate cyclase 1 α3 (GUCY1A3).

Selenite has also been shown to inhibit AR expression and activity in LAPC-4 and LNCaP prostate cancer cells though by a different mechanism. Sp1 is a ubiquitously expressed transcription factor: its binding sequence is the major positive regulatory element in the AR promoter. Prostate cancer cells exposed to selenite had decreased Sp1 activity and reduced Sp1 expression in the nucleus whereas methylseleninic acid had no effect. The effect of selenite on Sp1 expression leading to inhibition of AR expression and activity was redox dependent, involving GSH and superoxide *(12)*.

2.14. Species of Se Responsible for Anti-cancer Effects

There has been fairly general acceptance that a Se metabolite, methyl selenol, is a proximal anti-carcinogen at supra-nutritional doses, despite the fact that the presence of methyl selenol is only inferred from reactions of its precursors, most notably the model compound, methylseleninic acid *(77)*. Se doses large enough to support high, steady-state concentrations of methyl selenol are likely to be required.

Despite the fact that selenoproteins can reduce oxidative stress and inflammation and limit DNA damage, all of which have been linked to cancer risk, it was at first thought that selenoenzymes were not involved in anti-cancer mechanisms. This was largely because their activity/concentration was already believed to be optimized in the US population that showed reduced cancer risk on supplementation with 200 μg Se/d in the Nutritional Prevention of Cancer Trial *(25)*. However, it has recently become clear that optimal expression of selenoprotein P, the carrier of Se in the plasma, requires a higher intake, as yet undetermined, of dietary Se than other selenoproteins *(78)*. Furthermore, a substantial number of individuals may have a higher than average requirement for Se for efficient selenoprotein synthesis. Effects of functional polymorphisms in selenoprotein genes and of hypermethylation of their promoter regions have shown that the selenoproteins/selenoenzymes do appear to affect cancer risk, particularly at nutritional levels of intake.

2.14.1. Polymorphisms in Selenoproteins/Selenoenzymes Show an Effect on Cancer Risk

People differ substantially in their ability to increase selenoprotein activity in response to additional dietary Se *(79)*. This inter-individual variation in selenoprotein expression levels may be accounted for by SNPs in selenoprotein genes that determine the efficiency with which individuals can incorporate selenium into selenoproteins *(80–83)*. Thus requirements for dietary selenium for optimal protection against cancer may be much higher in individuals carrying particular functional selenoprotein SNPs such as those described below in various selenoproteins.

2.14.2. CYTOSOLIC GLUTATHIONE PEROXIDASE, GPx1

Some recent studies have reported a link between cancer risk and polymorphisms in the cytosolic glutathione peroxidase selenoprotein (*GPx1*) gene at Pro198Leu (rs1050450). Such a link might be explained by a genotype effect on enzyme activity. GPx1 with the Leu-allele has been reported to be less responsive to stimulation of its enzyme activity by selenium supplementation than GPx1 with the Pro-allele *(81)*. There have also been reports of a difference in GPx activity between the genotypes, e.g. in Danish women, the catalytic activity of GPx1 was lowered 5% for each additional copy of the variant Leu-allele ($p = 0.0003$) *(84)* while in a Californian study, male Leu/Leu homozygotes had significantly lower GPx1 activity than other genotypes *(85)*. However, that same Californian study found no difference in GPx activity by genotype in women. By contrast, two much smaller studies, one in a Finnish/Swedish population and one in men from the Former Yugoslav Republic of Macedonia (FYROM) could not detect a difference in erythrocyte GPx activity between GPx1 genotypes *(86, 87)*. These disparities might be explained if the change in GPx activity were to be caused by another polymorphism that co-segregates with the studied polymorphism. There are several such candidate polymorphisms in GPx (http://egp.gs.washington.edu/directory.html) *(84)*.

Lung: Four studies have looked at the association between the Pro198Leu polymorphism and the risk of lung cancer *(83, 88–90)*. Compared to Pro homozygotes, two studies – in Finland and Korea – found a significantly increased risk of lung cancer in Leu hetero-/homozygotes *(83, 88)*, while a small US study found a significantly increased risk in never smoker Leu hetero-/homozygotes (only 13 cases), though a significantly decreased risk was found in elderly smokers *(89)*. The fourth study, carried out in Denmark, found that Leu/Leu homozygosity was associated with decreased risk *(90)*. The authors of the Danish study were themselves surprised by their result since they had previously shown that the variant Leu-allele was associated with a significant, although moderate, 5% lower erythrocyte GPx1 enzyme activity per allele *(84)*. They have suggested that the apparently protective effect of the Leu-allele of the GPx1 polymorphism may be caused by a co-segregating functional polymorphism in another gene in the same region of the genome and not by the GPx1 polymorphism *per se (90)*.

Breast: Five studies have investigated the effect of the Pro198Leu polymorphism on breast cancer risk with varying results. In a nested Danish case–control study of 377 cases and 377 controls, carriers of the variant Leu-allele had a 1.43 (95% CI 1.07–1.92) times higher risk of breast cancer compared with non-carriers *(84)*. Furthermore, the Leu/Leu genotype was found to be almost twice as common in DNA from breast cancer tissue from a tissue bank at the University of Illinois as in DNA from cancer-free individuals, while the Pro/Leu genotype was underrepresented, indicating loss of heterozygosity at this locus in breast tumour development *(81)*. The authors suggest that this may implicate GPx1 in the risk and development of breast tumours.

By contrast, in a Canadian case–control study of 399 cases of incident, invasive breast cancer and 372 controls, no association between breast cancer and GPx1 Pro198Leu was found *(91)*. Similarly, there was no evidence that the variant GPx1 genotype was associated with an increased risk of breast cancer in the Long Island Breast Cancer Study Project of 1,038 cases and 1,088 controls, except in nulliparous Leu homozygotes who had increased risk (OR 2.12, 95% CI 1.01–4.48) compared with parous Pro/Pro women *(92)*. Interestingly, though no association was observed between the polymorphism and breast cancer risk in the prospective Nurses' Health Study, where 1,323 women with breast cancer were compared with 1,910 controls *(93)*, an increased risk of breast cancer (OR 1.87, 95% CI 1.09–3.19) *was* observed in Leu homozygotes who were also homozygous for the Ala16 genotype of SOD2 (Val16Ala, as discussed above) *(94)*.

Bladder: Possession of the GPx1 Leu198 allele appears to confer an increased risk of bladder cancer and that risk is further raised in men that have one or two Ala alleles of the Val9Ala (more often described as Val16Ala, rs4880) MnSOD polymorphism *(95)*. In the 213 bladder cancer patients, the Pro/Leu genotype was significantly associated with advanced tumour stage: OR 2.58 (95% CI 1.07, 6.18, $p = 0.034$) for tumour stage T2–4 *vs.* Ta+1 when compared with the Pro/Pro genotype *(95)*.

Prostate: In the context of the above results, it is perhaps surprising that an overall protective effect of the variant GPx1 Leu-allele was found on prostate cancer risk in 82 prostate cancer cases and 123 control individuals in FYROM *(87)*. It is, however, somewhat suspicious that while heterozygous carriers of the variant Leu-allele had a significantly lower risk of prostate cancer compared with Pro homozygotes (OR 0.38, 95% CI 0.20–0.75, $p = 0.004$), Leu homozygotes had a non-significant and lesser reduction in risk. No significant differences in erythrocyte GPx activity by genotype were found in the healthy control group of 90 subjects.

Other cancers: No associations were found between the GPx Pro198Leu polymorphism and risk of basal-cell carcinoma or colorectal adenomas or carcinomas *(96, 97)*. However, loss of heterozygosity at GPx1 was found in a significant percentage of colorectal cancers (42%) *(98)* suggesting that loss of heterozygosity at the GPx1 locus is a common event in the development of colorectal cancer and that GPx1 or other tightly linked genes may be involved in the aetiology of this disease. Similarly DNA samples from head and neck tumours exhibited fewer heterozygotes and an increased frequency of the Leu/Leu genotype compared with DNA from the cancer-free population *(99)*.

2.14.3. 15 kDa SELENOPROTEIN, SEP15

The 15 kDa selenoprotein (Sep15) is expressed at high levels in normal liver and prostate but at reduced levels in the corresponding malignant organs *(100)*. The *Sep15* gene lies on chromosome 1p22.3 at a locus commonly deleted or mutated in human cancers *(4, 82)* giving rise to expectations that this selenoprotein might be important to cancer risk. Two SNPs at positions 811 (C/T) and 1,125 (G/A) that are in strong allelic association have been studied in the 3′-UTR of the *Sep15* gene: G/A1125 lies within a functional SECIS element *(82)*. The T811-A1125 variant was more effective in supporting UGA readthrough than the C811-G1125 variant, but was less responsive to the addition of Se to the culture medium *(80, 101)*. Individuals possessing one or other of these haplotypes may therefore differ in the efficiency with which they can make Sep15 and in how well they can use dietary Se *(82)*. Though the frequency of the T811/A1125 haplotype is 0.25 in Caucasians and 0.57 in African Americans, who have a higher incidence of prostate cancer *(80)*, no evidence of an effect of this polymorphism on prostate cancer risk has been reported nor found *(102)*. However, among African Americans (but not Caucasians), a difference in allele frequencies was seen in DNA from breast or head and neck tumours and that from cancer-free controls though the authors suggest that this difference is likely to be due largely to loss of heterozygosity at the *Sep15* locus *(80, 103)*.

The A1125 variant of Sep15 was found to be less responsive to the apoptotic and growth-inhibitory effects of Se than the G1125 variant *(104)*. In that study, the *Sep15* gene was shown to be down-regulated in 60% of malignant-mesothelioma cell lines and tumour specimens.

A Polish study of 325 lung cancer cases and 287 controls, all of whom were smokers, showed an effect of *Sep15* G/A1125 genotype that varied according to Se status *(105)*. Among individuals of lower Se status (below 50 μg/L), the risk was higher for those with the AA genotype compared to those with the GG genotype, whereas among those of higher Se status (above 50 μg/L), the opposite was the case. Though the effects on risk did not reach significance, there was a general significant association between Se concentration and lung cancer risk for the GG, GA and AA genotypes.

2.14.4. SELENOPROTEIN P

A number of SNPs have also been identified in selenoprotein P (e.g. SEPP1, Ala234Thr, rs3877899), a selenoprotein believed to be involved both in protection from reactive oxygen and nitrogen species and in the transport of Se to tissues. Normally, the *SEPP1* gene is highly expressed in prostatic epithelium but it is down-regulated in a subset of human prostate tumours, mouse tumours and the androgen-dependent (LNCaP) and androgen-independent (PC-3) prostate cancer cell lines *(106)*. Our own results *(102)* from genotyping some 5,000 prostate cancer cases/controls from the population-based Prostate Cancer in Sweden (CAPS) study implicate SEPP1 in prostate cancer risk in a low-Se population.

Genetic variants at or near the SEPP1 locus may also be associated with advanced colorectal adenoma, a cancer precursor. Cases with a left-sided advanced adenoma ($n = 772$) and matched controls ($n = 777$), screen negative for polyps, were randomly selected from participants in the Prostate, Lung, Colorectal, and Ovarian Cancer Screening Trial *(107)*. Three variants in SEPP1, one of which was very rare, were significantly associated with advanced adenoma risk and a significant overall association with adenoma risk was observed for SEPP1 (global $p = 0.02$).

2.14.5. THIOREDOXIN REDUCTASE 1

In the colorectal adenoma study described above *(107)* a significant 80% reduction for advanced colorectal adenoma risk was also seen for carriers of the variant allele at thioredoxin reductase 1 (TXNRD1) IVS1-181C>G (OR 0.20; 95% CI 0.07–0.55;

$p_{trend} = 0.004$). A significant overall association with adenoma risk for TXNRD1 (global $p = 0.008$) was observed.

2.14.6. PHOSPHOLIPID GLUTATHIONE PEROXIDASE, GPx4

GPx4 decreases lipid hydroperoxide levels. A GPx4 C718T polymorphism (rs713041) which is known to be functional *(108–110)* has been shown to be linked to colorectal cancer risk in a pilot study *(111)*. Carriage of the T allele appears to be protective. Though no effect of this polymorphism has been found on risk of breast cancer, carriage of the T allele was found to be associated with mortality in 4,470 breast cancer cases *(112)*.

2.14.7. SUMMARY OF THE EVIDENCE ON SELENOPROTEIN POLYMORPHISMS AND CANCER RISK

It is difficult to draw clear conclusions from the evidence, as summarised in Tables 1 and 2, on selenoprotein polymorphisms and cancer risk. The situation appears to have become more confused as more studies are published. With regard to the GPx1 Pro198Leu polymorphism, some studies have shown an allele effect on GPx activity while others have not. Some authors have suggested that these disparities might be explained if the change in GPx activity were to be caused by another polymorphism that co-segregates with the studied polymorphism *(84)*. Interestingly, though only one study showed a significant effect of carriage of the Leu-allele on breast cancer risk *(84)*, increased risk was observed in Leu homozygotes who were also homozygous for SOD2 16Ala *(93)*, implying that the risk associated with this polymorphism is affected by other genotypes and perhaps other environmental factors as well. This is an illustration of the fact that cancer is a multifactorial complex disease and a combination of factors – not just a single polymorphism – is generally required to cause disease. It is also possible that some of the discrepancies noted above may relate to differing Se status between populations investigated. The fact that development of colorectal, breast and head and neck tumours is linked with loss of heterozygosity at GPx1 suggests that loss of GPx1 activity may increase cancer risk. Loss of heterozygosity in Sep 15 also occurs in breast or head and neck tumours, again suggesting that ability to make this selenoprotein may be important in reducing risk.

Though there are many fewer studies that have investigated associations between polymorphisms in thioredoxin reductase (TXNRD1 IVS1-181C>G) and selenoprotein P, significant effects on risk have been associated with these polymorphisms, i.e. risk of advanced colorectal adenoma.

As a general comment, however, genetic variants in other genes at or near the loci of the selenoprotein polymorphisms under study might co-segregate, contributing to the effects observed. All of the genetic variants that might contribute to such an effect must therefore be identified before disease risk can be definitely attributed to a particular polymorphism.

Table 1

GPx1: Proline/Leucine SNP at codon 198, 3p21. Effect of 198 Leu allele on cancer risk

Cancer	No. Subjects		SNP genotype vs Pro/Pro	OR (95% CI) * = significant	Location	Comments	Reference
	Cases	Contr					
Lung	315	315	Pro/Leu Leu/Leu	1.8 (1.2 -2.8)* 2.3 (1.3 -3.8)*	Finland		RatnasingheD et al 2000
Lung	200	200	Pro/Leu & Leu/Leu	2.29	Korea	Article in Korean, no CIs in abstract	Lee C et al. 2006
Lung	432	798	Leu/Leu	0.60 (0.35 - 1.05)	Denmark		Raaschou-Nielsen O et al. 2007
Prostate	82	123	Pro/Leu Leu/Leu	0.38 (0.20-0.75)* 0.61 (0.27-1.40)	FYROM	Would expect stronger effect in Leu/Leu; small study	Arsova-Sarafinovska Z et al. 2008
Prostate	1433	780	Pro/Leu Leu/Leu	1.07 (0.89-1.29) 0.93 (0.69-1.26)	Sweden	CAPS study	Rayman M et al. unpublished
Breast	399	372	Pro/Leu Leu/Leu	0.92 (0.68 -1.24) 0.77 (0.46 -1.27)	Canada	Pre-and post-menopausal	Knight J et al 2004
Breast	377	377	Pro/Leu + Leu/Leu	1.43 (1.07 -1.92)*	Denmark	Postmenopausal	Ravn-Haren et al. 2006
Breast	1038	1088	Pro/Leu Leu/Leu	1.10 (0.92 -1.32) 1.06 (0.79 -1.42)	US	Long Island Breast Cancer Study	Ahn J et al 2005
Breast	1229	1629	Pro/Leu Leu/Leu	0.91 (0.77 -1.07) 1.07 (0.82 -1.40)	US	Nurses' Health Study	Cox D et al 2004
Breast	1262	1533	Pro/Leu + SOD2 A/A Leu/Leu +SOD2 A/A	1.01 (0.83 -1.23) 1.87 (1.09 -3.19)*	US	Nurses' Health Study	Cox D et al 2006
Bladder	213	209	Pro/Leu +SOD2 V/A+A/A	2.6 (1.5 -4.8)* 6.3 (1.3 -31.2)*	Japan	Pro/Leusignif. assoc. with advanced tumorstage	IchimuraY et al 2004

Table 2
Effect of Selenoprotein SNPs on Cancer Risk

Selenoprotein SNP	Cancer	No. Subjects		Comparison	OR (95% CI)	Location	Comments	Reference
		Cases	Contr					
GPx4 C718T rs713041	Breast	569 deaths	3901	T allele vs CC	**1.27 (1.13-1.43)*** per T allele carried	UK	Association of T allele with mortality in 4470 breast cancer cases	Udler M et al. 2007
	Colorectal	252	187	CT+ TT vs CC	**0.60 (0.37-0.96)***	UK	Carriage of T allele appears to be protective	Bermano G et al. 2007
	Prostate	1438	790	CT+TT vs CC	1.01 (0.91-1.32)	Sweden	CAPS study	Rayman M et al. unpublished
Sep15 G1125A linked C811T	Lung	325 smokers	287 smokers	GA vs GG AA vs GG	0.91 (0.64-1.32) 0.80 (0.39-1.65)	Poland	Above 80 μg/L Se, those carrying the G allele had increased risk	Jablonska E et al. 2008
G1125A linked C811T	Prostate	1419 318	781 **781**	CG/TA+TA/TA vs CG/CG	1.03(0.86-1.24) 1.38 (1.05-1.83)*	Sweden	CAPS study Men with PSA>100 Incr risk if TA homo/hererozygotes	Rayman M et al. unpublished
TRR TXNRD1 IVS1-181C->G rs35009941	Advanced colorectal adenoma	772	777	GC+GG vs CC	**0.20 (0.07-0.55)***	US	Prostate, Lung, Colorectal, and Ovarian Cancer Screening Trial Carriage of G allele protective	Peters U et al. 2008
SEPP1 rs3797310 rs2972994 -4166 rs3877899	Advanced colorectal adenoma	746 750 749 752	762 764 763 766	AA vs GG CT vs CC CG vs CC AG vs GG AA vs GG	**1.53 (1.05-2.22)*** **0.73 (0.57-0.92)*** **P trend = 0.002*** 0.99 (0.79-1.24) 0.98 (0.61-1.56)	US	Prostate, Lung, Colorectal, and Ovarian Cancer Screening Trial	Peters U et al. 2008
rs3877899	Prostate	2975	2149	AG vs GG AA vs GG	0.94 (0.82-1.07) 1.09 (0.83-1.42)	Sweden	CAPS study	Rayman et al. unpublished

2.14.8. HYPERMETHYLATION OF PROMOTOR REGIONS SILENCE SELENOPROTEIN GENES AND INCREASE CANCER RISK

Abnormal DNA methylation patterns are associated with neoplasia and inactivation of tumour-suppressor genes. Hypermethylation of promoter regions of selenoprotein genes can effectively silence the gene resulting in loss (or reduced amount) of the seleno-protein and increasing cancer risk. Examples of an effect of promoter methylation on cancer risk are found for GPx3 in prostate cancer and Barrett's oesophagus and for the selenoprotein, methionine sulphoxide reductase in breast cancer metastasis.

Down-regulation of GPx3 occurs widely in prostate cancer. GPx3 was shown to be hypermethylated in LnCAP (lymph node metastasis) and PC3 (bone metastasis) prostate cancer cell lines and in 93% of primary prostate cancer tumours (113). In a later study, the GPx3 promoter was found to be 90% methylated in prostate cancer tissue samples and its down-regulation was associated with higher rate of post-prostatectomy metastasis (114). Somewhat decreased expression of GPx3 can be detected in morphologically benign prostate tissues adjacent to cancer tissue, implying that such a decrease precedes the development of frank malignancy. Deletions of GPx3 occurred in 39% of samples suggesting that deletion, as well as methylation, probably plays a major role in down-regulating the expression of this gene (114). A reduction in mortality and tumour volume was observed when GPx3 was expressed in PC-3 xenograft mice suggesting that GPx3 has a tumour-suppressor role (114).

GPx3 was also shown to be hypermethylated in 62% of Barrett's metaplasia, 82% of dysplasia and in 88% Barrett's adenoma samples (115). Consistently reduced levels of GPx3 mRNA were seen in 91% of Barrett's adenoma samples. Monoallelic methylation was associated with partial loss of GPx3 expression in metaplasia while biallelic methylation and severe loss of GPx3 expression were most frequently seen in Barrett's adenoma samples ($p = 0.001$) (Table 3).

Table 3

Frequency of GPx3 Promoter Hypermethylation According to Histomorphologic Diagnosis [Lee et al. (115)]

GPx3 methylation status	Histologic diagnosis			
	Normal (n = 10)	Barrett's oesophagus (n = 21)	Barrett's dysplasia (n = 11)	Barrett's adenocarcinoma (n = 34)
No methylation (M⁻)	10 (83%)	8 (38%)	8 (38%)	4 (12%)
Monoallelic (M⁺/M⁻)	2 (17%)	7 (33%)	8 (73%)	14 (41%)
Biallelic (M⁺/M⁺)	0	6 (29%)	1 (9%)	16 (47%)*

M, methylation; (⁻) negative; (⁺) positive.
*Biallelic methylation was significantly more frequent in Barrett's adenocarcinoma ($P < 0.01$).

The last example of methylation affecting transcription of a selenoprotein relates to methionine sulfoxide reductase 1 (MsrB1), a selenoprotein linked with longer lifespan that is highly expressed in the weakly metastatic breast carcinoma cell line MCF7 but poorly expressed in the highly metastatic cell line MDA-MB231 *(116)*. The promoter of this selenoprotein is regulated by epigenetic modification as evidenced by the upregulation of the gene transcript after treatment with the demethylating agent, 5-aza-2′-deoxycytidine *(116)*. A CpG site within the Sp1 consensus site located 46 bp upstream of the transcription start site was found to be hypermethylated in the highly metastatic cell line suggesting a possible cause for the repression of transcription.

These examples clearly illustrate that functional *GPx3*, at least (and probably MsrB1), is important in reducing the risk of some cancers.

3. IN VITRO STUDIES AND ANIMAL EXPERIMENTS

Cell-culture studies have made a massive contribution to the understanding of the multiple mechanisms by which Se acts in the prevention of the incidence and spread of cancer. Such studies are too numerous to describe again here given that those that have made the most significant contribution to our current knowledge have already been covered under the appropriate mechanism sections.

There is similarly extensive experimental evidence from animal studies that indicates that Se supplementation reduces the incidence of cancer in animals, lowering the yield of tumours and reducing metastases *(25, 59, 62, 63, 76, 117)*. It is difficult, however, to generalize from such studies to the human situation, as animal studies have generally used doses at least ten times greater than those required to prevent clinical signs of deficiency, which, on a per unit body-weight basis, are considerably higher than most human Se intakes. In recent years, evidence from transgenic models has been most useful in demonstrating that selenoproteins are important for the cancer-protective effects of selenium as in the studies quoted below.

A unique mouse model was developed by inter-breeding transgenic mice with reduced selenoprotein levels because of the expression of an altered selenocysteine-tRNA (i6A-) with mice that develop prostate cancer because of the targeted expression of the SV40 large T and small t oncogenes to that organ (C3 (1)/Tag) to give bigenic animals (i6A-/Tag) *(118)*. The selenoprotein-deficient mice exhibited accelerated development of lesions associated with prostate cancer progression, suggesting that selenoproteins are important in reducing prostate cancer risk and development.

Transgenic mice with the same mutant selenocysteine-tRNA gene (i6A-) described above were fed selenium-deficient diets supplemented with 0, 0.1 or 2.0 μg Se (as selenite)/g diet *(119)*. Compared with wild-type mice, transgenic mice had more ($p < 0.05$) azoxymethane-induced aberrant crypt formation (a preneoplastic lesion for colon cancer). Se supplementation significantly decreased the number of aberrant crypts and aberrant crypt foci in both wild-type and transgenic mice. It is clear from this study that a lack of selenoprotein activity causes increased colon cancer susceptibility but furthermore that low molecular weight selenocompounds were able to reduce preneoplastic lesions in these animals. This important study thus provided evidence that *both* selenoproteins *and* low molecular weight selenocompounds are important for the cancer-protective effects of selenium (Irons et al. *(119)*).

4. EPIDEMIOLOGICAL STUDIES

Numerous cohort and nested case–control studies have shown that higher Se status is associated with a lower risk of malignancies or death from cancer (e.g. prostate, liver, lung, colon/rectum, oesophagus, gastric cardia, bladder, pancreas and thyroid) *(23, 24, 26, 28, 120–128)*.

Cancer mortality in relation to prediagnostic Se status was investigated in the large US Third National Health and Nutrition Examination Survey (NHNES III) *(120)*. Serum Se was measured at baseline in 13,887 adult participants who were then followed up for up to 12 years. Mean serum selenium concentration was 125.6 μg/L. The multivariate-adjusted hazard ratios (HR) comparing the highest (≥ 130.39 μg/L) with the lowest (< 117.31 μg/L) serum selenium tertile were 0.83 (95% confidence interval [CI] 0.72–0.96) for all-cause mortality and 0.69 (95% CI 0.53–0.90) for cancer mortality. The association between serum Se and all-cause and cancer mortality was nonlinear, showing an inverse association with total cancer mortality up to a serum Se concentration of around 130 μg/L (Fig. 4). While total cancer mortality began to rise again above a serum concentration of 150 μg/L, mortality from colorectal and prostate cancers continued to decline. Similar benefits of higher Se status on cancer mortality were seen in the smaller EVA study conducted among elderly French volunteers. There the risk of mortality from cancer was increased four-fold in volunteers in the bottom quartile of

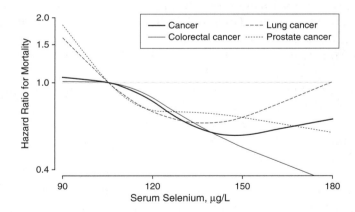

Fig. 4. Hazard ratios for all-cancer and colorectal, lung and prostate cancer mortality by serum Se concentration. The curves represent multivariate-adjusted hazard ratios based on restricted quadratic splines with knots at the 5th, 50th and 95th percentiles of the serum Se distribution. The reference value (hazard ratio, 1) was set at the 10th percentile of the serum Se level distribution (105.4 ng/ml). Hazard ratios were adjusted for age, sex, race/ethnicity, education, family income, menopausal status, cigarette smoking status, serum cotinine level, alcohol consumption, physical activity, body mass index and vitamin and/or mineral supplement use. The *p* values were 0.006 for all-cancer mortality, 0.72 for colorectal cancer mortality, 0.14 for lung cancer mortality and 0.77 for prostate cancer mortality. To convert Se to μmol/L, divide by 78.96. Reproduced with permission from reference *114*.

baseline plasma Se compared to those in the top quartile (relative risk, RR = 4.06; 95% CI 1.51–10.92, $p = 0.006$) *(129)*.

A few epidemiological studies have specifically investigated the association between Se and bladder cancer. Of seven prospective studies, five found a decreased risk of bladder cancer with high vs. low serum/toenail Se *(128)*. The largest of these prospective studies, carried out in the Netherlands, included 431 cases and 2,459 sub-cohort members. A significant inverse association between toenail Se concentrations and the risk of bladder cancer in the highest vs. lowest toenail Se quintile (RR 0.67; 95% CI 0.46–0.97) was reported *(121)*. The association was most pronounced in ex-smokers and in those with invasive transitional-cell carcinomas.

The relationship between baseline serum Se and the subsequent risk of death from oesophageal squamous cell carcinoma (ESCC) and gastric cardia cancer (GCC) was investigated over 15 years of follow-up of 1,103 subjects randomly selected from a larger trial cohort of all participants in the General Population Trial (the 5-year intervention did not involve Se) of Linxian, China. Compared with those in the lowest quartile of serum Se at baseline, those in the highest quartile had a 65% significant reduction in the risk of mortality from ESCC (RR: 0.35, 95% CI 0.16–0.81) and a 69% reduction in the risk of death from GCC (RR: 0.31, 95% CI 0.11–0.87) *(123)*.

The association between plasma Se concentration and subsequent risk of hepatocellular carcinoma (HCC) was investigated among chronic carriers of hepatitis-B and/or C virus in a cohort of 7,342 men in Taiwan *(24)*. Mean baseline Se concentration was significantly lower in the 69 men who developed HCC over 5.3 years of follow-up than in the 139 matched, healthy HBsAg-positive controls ($p = 0.01$). Adjusted odds ratios of HCC for subjects in increasing quintiles of plasma Se were 1.00, 0.52, 0.32, 0.19 and 0.62, respectively. The inverse association between plasma Se and HCC was most striking among cigarette smokers and among those with low plasma levels of retinol or various carotenoids.

Colorectal adenoma is closely associated with subsequent development of colorectal cancer. Peters and colleagues have tabulated observational studies of the effect of Se on colorectal tumours *(130)*. Such studies have generally supported a preventive role for selenium although not always with statistically significant effects. Jacobs and colleagues *(131)* carried out a pooled analysis of data from three studies that could be considered as prospective studies of Se and risk of colorectal adenoma. The Wheat Bran Fiber Trial, the Polyp Prevention Trial and the Polyp Prevention Study were 3–4-year interventions in subjects that had recently undergone adenoma removal, 1,763 of whom had baseline serum or plasma Se measured. None of the trials affected the risk of adenoma recurrence. Analysis of pooled data showed that those with baseline serum or plasma Se in the highest quartile (median 150 µg/L), when compared with those in the lowest quartile (median 113 µg/L), had significantly lower risk of adenoma recurrence (OR 0.66; 95% CI 0.50, 0.87). These results support previous findings that are suggestive of a beneficial effect of higher Se status on colorectal cancer risk.

In recent years, systematic reviews and meta-analyses have increasingly been used in an attempt to summarize the evidence for an effect of Se on the risk of some common cancers: a meta-analysis of 16 studies of Se and lung cancer showed that the summary relative risk (RR) for subjects with higher vs. lower Se exposures was 0.74 (95%

CI 0.57–0.97), suggesting a protective effect of Se against lung cancer *(124)*. Effects occurred primarily in populations with low-Se levels defined as serum Se < 100 mg/L or intake < 55 mg/d. Above a certain level, increasing Se intake had little further benefit, suggesting the existence of a threshold effect.

The strongest evidence for an effect of Se on a specific cancer site relates to its effect on prostate cancer. Large prospective studies of Se in prostate cancer are summarized in Table 4 *(21, 23, 26, 28, 125, 132–135)*. Most interestingly, many of these studies have examined the effect of Se separately on advanced prostate cancer (cancer that has spread beyond the prostate) and found the effect to be greater than on localized prostate cancer *(23, 26, 28, 125)*. Recent systematic reviews and meta-analyses have reinforced these findings. A systematic review and meta-analysis of 16 studies *(126)* found that the pooled relative risk of prostate cancer for any intake of Se (average between first and fourth quintile or first and third quartile, compared to the lowest

Table 4
Large Prospective Studies of Prostate Cancer/Advanced Prostate Cancer Using Tissue Indicators of Exposure

Study	Population	No. of cases	Indicator of exposure	Comparison High *vs.* low	RR[1]	95% confidence interval	P for trend
Knekt *et al.* 1990	Finland General population	51	Serum	Quintile	1.15	–	0.71
Yoshizawa *et al.* 1998	USA Health professionals	181	Toenails	Quintile	0.35[2]	0.16–0.78*	0.03
Nomura *et al.* 2000	USA Hawaii Japanese ancestry	249	Serum	Quartile	0.5	0.3–0.9*	0.02
	Non smoker	87			0.8	0.4–1.9	0.93
	Ex-smoker	86			0.5	0.2–1.1	0.03
	Current smoker	76			0.2	0.1–0.8	0.02
	Localised disease	120			0.8	0.4–1.8	0.76
	Advanced disease	64			0.3[2]	0.1–0.8	0.01
Helzlsouer *et al.* 2000	USA Washington County	117	Toenails	Quintile	0.58	0.29–1.18	0.27
					0.38[3]	0.17–0.85*	0.12
Goodman *et al.* 2001	USA CARET Trial asbestos workers/ current/ex-smokers	235	Serum	Quartile	1.02	0.7–1.6	0.69
	retinol/β-carotene arm	111			0.75	0.41–1.36	0.40
	placebo arm	124			1.52	0.78–2.79	0.12
Brooks *et al.* 2001	USA Baltimore	52	Plasma	Quartile	0.24	0.08–0.77*	0.01

Table 4
(Continued)

van den Brandt *et al.* 2003	Netherlands Cohort Study	540	Toenails	Quintile	0.69	0.48–0.99*	0.008
	Never smoker	72			1.19	0.48–2.92	
	Ex-smoker	300			0.46	0.27–0.79*	
	Current smoker	168			0.97	0.42–2.22	
	Localised disease	189			0.72	0.42–1.24	0.043
	Advanced disease	183			0.62[2]	0.37–1.05	0.020
Li *et al.* 2004	USA Physicians' Health Study	586	Plasma	Quintile	0.78	0.54–1.13	0.16
	Baseline PSA>4	228			0.49	0.28–0.86*	0.002
	Baseline PSA<4	293			0.77	0.48–1.22	0.59
	Localised disease	348			0.97	0.64–1.49	0.91
	Advanced disease	171			0.52[2]	0.28–0.98*	<0.05
Peters *et al.* 2006	USA PLCO Trial	724	Serum	Quartile	0.84	0.62–1.14	0.70
	High vitamin E intake (≥28 IU/d)	363			0.58	0.37–0.90*	0.05
	Multi-vitamin use	302			0.61	0.36–1.04	0.06

*denotes statistically-significant effect

[1]RR relative risk for highest versus lowest category

[2]Advanced disease

[3]Adjusted for BMI at age 21, education and hours since last meal

intake category) was 0.72 (95% CI 0.61–0.84) for cohort studies and 0.74 (0.61–1.39) for case–control studies. Sub-group analysis showed a stronger protective effect among those with advanced disease with a dose–response trend, though the results were not significant, probably because of small sample size. Brinkman and colleagues *(128)* carried out a meta-analysis of 20 studies in which the pooled standardized mean difference between serum/plasma/toenail Se in cases and controls was −0.23 (−0.40, −0.05; p = 0.01) indicating an inverse association between Se status and risk of prostate cancer.

The recent World Cancer Research Report *(136)* which systematically reviewed the available research on diet and cancer prevention concurred with the above findings, concluding that there is strong evidence from trials and cohort studies that Se probably protects against prostate cancer and limited evidence that it protects against lung, colorectal and stomach cancers.

5. INTERVENTION STUDIES

A Cochrane review of randomised trials comparing antioxidant supplements with placebo for prevention of gastrointestinal cancers *(137)* found that Se significantly decreased the risk (RR 0.49, 95% CI 0.36–0.67). Notably, Se administered vs. placebo to high-risk groups (i.e. carriers of hepatitis-B surface antigen and members of families with high incidence of liver cancer) for 2–4 years reduced the incidence of hepatocellular carcinoma by 50% (RR 0.50, 95% CI 0.35–0.71). The Bjelakovic Cochrane review concludes "Se alone (of antioxidant supplements) may have preventive effects on cancer. This finding, however, is based on trials with flaws in their design and needs confirmation in properly conducted randomised clinical trials."

Bardia and colleagues systematically reviewed the trial evidence for the effect of Se in primary cancer prevention (138). Se gave a pooled relative risk (RR) for cancer incidence of 0.88 (95% CI 0.77–1.00) from pooling four trials with considerable heterogeneity ($I^2 = 52$%). When the two trials that assessed Se in combination with beta-carotene and vitamin E were excluded, heterogeneity disappeared ($I^2 = 0$%) and benefit increased: for incidence RR 0.69 (95% CI 0.56–0.85) and death RR 0.61 (95% CI 0.42–0.89). The results of the Nutritional Prevention of Cancer (NPC) trial were the major driver of the benefits found in that analysis.

The NPC trial provided compelling evidence that Se can reduce cancer incidence and mortality (139). Of people with a history of non-melanoma skin cancer, 1,312 were randomised to 200 mcg Se/day (as high-Se yeast) vs. yeast placebo. After $4\frac{1}{2}$ years of treatment and $6\frac{1}{2}$ of follow-up, there was no effect on the primary end point of skin cancer but those receiving Se had 50% lower total cancer mortality (RR 0.50; 95% CI 0.31–0.80) and 63% lower cancer incidence (RR 0.63; 95% CI 0.47–0.85) with fewer cancers of the prostate (RR 0.37; 95% CI 0.18–0.71), colon/rectum (RR 0.42; 95% CI 0.18–0.95) and lung (RR 0.54; 95% CI 0.30–0.98). No effect on breast cancer was seen but there were only 332 women.

In follow-up analyses, though the effects of Se were attenuated, they remained significant for total cancer incidence (Cox proportional hazards model, HR 0.75; 95% CI 0.58–0.97) and prostate cancer incidence (HR 0.48; 95% CI 0.28–0.80) (140) but just missed significance for colorectal cancer incidence (HR 0.46; 95% CI 0.21–1.02; $p = 0.057$). Analysis by initial Se status showed that the strongest effect of Se was seen in those who fell into the bottom tertile (<105 μg/L) of plasma Se at baseline: HR total cancer 0.51, 95% CI 0.32–0.81 (140); HR lung cancer 0.42, 95% CI 0.18–0.96; odds ratio (OR) prevalent colorectal adenoma 0.27, 95% CI 0.09–0.77 (141, 142). Furthermore, when adjustment was made for the lower rate of PSA measurement in the Se-treated group, only those men with baseline plasma selenium <106 μg/L still showed a lower risk of prostate cancer on Se supplementation. By contrast, participants in the highest tertile (>122 μg/L) had a non-significant elevated incidence of total cancer incidence (HR 1.20, 95% CI 0.77–1.86) (140).

Although follow-up analyses confirmed initial findings that Se supplementation was not statistically significantly associated with the incidence of basal-cell carcinoma (HR 1.09; 95% CI 0.94–1.26), the extended treatment period raised the elevated risk of squamous cell carcinoma and total non-melanoma skin cancer to statistically significant levels (HR 1.25; 95% CI 1.03–1.51 and HR 1.17; 95% CI 1.02–1.34, respectively) (143). However, it must be remembered that the subjects in the NPC Trial were all skin cancer patients whose skin had sustained heavy sun-damage (143). In fact when subjects were divided into tertiles according to baseline Se status, those in the bottom tertile, whose status resembled that found in Europe, did not have an increased risk of squamous cell carcinoma (HR 0.87; 95% CI 0.62, 1.22). Of more concern is the fact that more recent analysis of NPC trial data showed an increased risk of self-reported type-2 diabetes in those supplemented with Se, though the effect was significant only in those in the top tertile of plasma Se at baseline *(144)*.

Overall, the trial showed that the protective effect of selenium was confined to males (HR 0.67; 95% CI 0.50–0.89) and was most pronounced in former smokers and in those in the bottom tertile of plasma Se at baseline *(140)*. It is notable that most of the population of Europe would fall into the bottom tertile of plasma Se, as defined in that study.

The later Selenium and Vitamin E Cancer Prevention Trial (SELECT) that investigated the effect of Se and vitamin E on prostate cancer risk showed that giving 200 µg Se/d (as selenomethionine) to a population of men of mean plasma Se 136 µg/L did not reduce the risk of localized prostate cancer *(145)*. In the light of NPC trial results, it is unfortunate that SELECT had no subjects within the range of Se status (i.e. <106 µg/L) that had previously shown benefit from Se supplementation on prostate cancer risk. In SELECT men, baseline serum Se ranged from 122.9 to 150.0 µg/L, which in fact, according to the NPC trial, put them into the category of non-significant increased risk from Se supplementation: in fact there were some potential indications of toxic effects in terms of alopecia and grades 1–2 dermatitis in the Se group.

Furthermore, SELECT supplemented with SeMet rather than Se-yeast as used in the NPC trial. As Se-yeast contains only some 60–70% of its total Se as SeMet *(146)*, it is possible that some other Se species than SeMet may have been responsible for the beneficial effects seen in the NPC trial.

Unfortunately SELECT results tell us nothing about the effect of Se on risk of advanced disease on which a number of studies have suggested a greater effect *(9, 102)* only 1.1% of cases were non-localised – nor on men of lower Se status. Clearly while at least one third of NPC men did not have optimal selenoprotein P or even GPx concentration/activity, this was not true of SELECT men, all of whose selenoproteins were likely to have been optimised *(147)*. Therefore if selenoproteins are important in cancer prevention, no effect would have been seen in SELECT, as was indeed the case. Such a trial conducted in Europe where Se status is substantially lower might have shown a very different outcome.

6. INTERVENTION WITH SELENIUM IN CANCER PATIENTS

A number of randomized controlled trials have been initiated in men with localized prostate cancer to see if supplementation with high-Se yeast can inhibit spread beyond the prostate. Thus the Watchful Waiting Trial *(148)* is being conducted in the Arizona Cancer Center in men with prostate cancer who have chosen watchful waiting rather than active intervention while my colleagues and I are conducting a double-blind, placebo-controlled, randomised phase II trial of Se supplementation in men with localised prostate cancer in men under active surveillance for prostate cancer at the Institute of Cancer Research, UK.

A few clinical trials have used Se supplementation in combination with DNA-damaging chemotherapeutic agents such as cisplatin, doxorubicin and irinotecan *(149)*.

These agents produce bulky DNA-adducts that are repaired by nucleotide excision repair (NER) of DNA. Se appears to be able to enhance DNA repair but only in cells with normal p53 *(13)*. Se supplementation elevates the expression of proteins responsible for recognition of DNA damage, selectively protecting genetically normal cells from DNA-damaging chemotherapeutic agents, while simultaneously offering no detectable protection to cells either completely lacking p53 or possessing only mutant p53 *(150)*. It is important to note that as many as 70% of tumours have a mutant p53 phenotype. Thus Se appears to be able to protect tissues from dose-limiting toxicity, reducing DNA damage, the frequency of chromosomal aberrations, the number of aberrant metaphases and the frequency of apoptotic cells and allowing delivery of higher chemotherapeutic doses without affording protection to cancer cells *(150, 151)*. Other mechanisms have also been implicated in the sensitization of cancer cells to chemotherapeutic agents by Se *(152, 153)*.

7. TISSUE SPECIFICITY AND TOTALITY OF THE EVIDENCE

Evidence from molecular biology (selenoprotein SNPs and methylation of promoter regions of selenoprotein genes) suggests that adequate Se intake may be able to affect favourably the risk of prostate, lung and bladder cancers, and oesophageal and colorectal adenomas.

Aside from that evidence, while it is safe to draw conclusions from well-run randomised controlled trials, the evidence from observational or case–control studies, even when nested within a prospective cohort study, is subject to some uncertainty owing to the effect of inflammation (or acute phase response) on blood/plasma/serum (or perhaps even toenail) Se concentration *(154, 155)*. The plasma concentration of Se decreases in proportion to the magnitude of the inflammatory response. Plasma selenoprotein concentration declines, most notably that of selenoprotein P, with inflammatory activity *(154, 156)*. Even the early stages of degenerative disease and cancer may have a subclinical inflammatory component *(154, 157, 158)*. Thus chronic low-level inflammation may long precede the appearance of symptoms. For instance, increasing age, smoking, symptoms of chronic bronchitis, Helicobacter pylori and Chlamydia pneumonia infections and body mass index were all associated with raised concentrations of C reactive protein, a recognised marker of inflammation, in UK men aged 50–69 years from general practice registers *(157)*. Hence when interpreting plasma selenium concentrations, a marker of the inflammatory response, such as CRP, should always be included to distinguish true nutritional depletion from the inherent effects of disease *(154)*.

Given the caveats referred to above, and therefore summarizing only the results found from trial evidence, for individual cancers the following conclusions can be drawn:

- Prostate cancer: There is evidence that Se probably protects against prostate cancer in men of relatively low-Se status (baseline plasma Se < 106 μg/L) *(140)*, but not in men of replete Se status (i.e. serum Se >123 μg/L) *(145)*. Se seems to have a specific role in down-regulation of the androgen receptor which may be a key factor in its effect.
- Liver cancer: There is a likely beneficial effect of Se on the risk of hepatocellular carcinoma in high-risk groups (i.e. carriers of hepatitis-B surface-antigen and members of families with high incidence of liver cancer). However, the relevant trials have flaws in

their design and the work needs confirmation in properly conducted randomised clinical trials *(137)*.

– Lung cancer: There is a trend towards a reduction in risk of incident lung cancer with Se supplementation though a significant reduction in risk occurred only in those with a plasma Se concentration less than 106 μg/L.

– Colorectal cancer and its precursor, colorectal adenoma: Se supplementation is associated with a trend towards a reduction in risk of incident colorectal cancer and a significant decrease in prevalent adenomatous polyps, particularly in current smokers and subjects with baseline plasma selenium <105.5 μg/L *(140–142)*.

– Squamous cell carcinoma: Se supplementation was associated with a higher risk of SCC in participants in the highest two tertiles of baseline plasma selenium, i.e. >105.6 μg/L though there was no increased risk in participants whose plasma Se was below 105.2 μg/L *(143)*.

In general, trial evidence for a protective effect of Se, which comes mainly from one study, relates only to men, is most pronounced in former smokers and in those with plasma Se <105 μg/L *(140)*. Indeed, there is a suggestion that those with plasma Se above 122 μg/L may have an elevated incidence of total cancer with selenium supplementation *(140)*. It is notable that data from the Third National Health and Nutrition Examination Survey (NHANES III) show that around half of the US population fall into this category and should probably *not* be exposed to additional Se *(159)*. On the other hand, plasma Se concentrations in Europe, New Zealand and many parts of China lie below 105 μg/L, and those populations might benefit from an increased Se intake to reduce cancer risk.

8. FUTURE RESEARCH DIRECTIONS

From the arguments presented above that show that chronic low-grade inflammation can effect measures of Se status long before the appearance of disease, it is clear that only intervention studies can give a truly reliable picture of the influence of Se on disease risk and so we need more trials, though it should be noted that these need to be in appropriate populations, i.e. those of low-Se status or in specific high-risk genotype groups. Unfortunately randomised controlled trials (RCTs) are extremely expensive.

Recent studies have implicated high serum Se or Se supplementation in increased risk of type-2 diabetes *(144, 160, 161)*. Furthermore, it appears that high serum Se concentrations may be associated with high total cholesterol, LDL-cholesterol, triglycerides, apo B and apo A1 levels *(162, 163)*. We must therefore work towards identifying a safe intake of Se which, while reducing cancer risk, will not increase the risk of other serious conditions.

Given these and other considerations, we badly need a large RCT of the effect of Se on all cancers which fulfils the following criteria:

– carried out in a population with a relatively low baseline Se intake, such as a European population;
– includes enough women to look at the effect on risk in females as there has been no sizeable trial of Se supplementation in women;

– uses a lower dose of Se, e.g. 100 μg/d, as if such a dose is effective in reducing cancer risk, it may avoid adverse effects that may appear at a higher daily dose. Furthermore, it will be easier to implement a public-health policy to achieve that level of intake.

Trials with *Se*-methylselenocysteine, particularly in early prostate cancer, are also needed and will no doubt follow on from the currently planned pharmacokinetic studies with this small molecular weight Se compound.

Most importantly, given the data summarised above that has appeared in the last 10 years showing that selenoprotein genotype can affect cancer risk, trials in subjects of known SNP genotype for selenoproteins (or genes in related pathways) must be initiated as we can no longer assume that each person's Se requirement to reduce cancer risk is the same.

Aside from trials, adjunctive therapy with Se in cancer chemotherapy has clear potential for a better prognosis from treatment as outlined above.

9. CONCLUSIONS AND RECOMMENDATIONS FOR INTAKE/DIETARY CHANGES

Given what we know about the effect of selenoprotein genotype on the ability to make selenoproteins and on cancer risk, there will be considerable individual variation in Se requirements for optimal health. To date, few epidemiological studies have taken genotype into account and so the recommendations that follow cannot be prescriptive for an individual.

From prospective studies, the mean/median level of plasma Se required for a significant reduction in cancer risk ranges from > 84 μg/L (e.g. for oesophageal and gastric cardia cancer in China) to 147 μg/L (e.g. for prostate cancer in Hawaii) according to the study, while from trial data, the minimum mean plasma Se for significant reduction in cancer risk in an Eastern US population in the NPC Trial ranged from 105 μg/L (all cancers) to 123 μg/L (prostate cancer) *(164)*. The minimum Se intake required to achieve these plasma concentrations ranges from just below the US RDA/UK RNI (55–75 μg/d) level to a total intake of around 140 μg/d from dietary Se [or Se-yeast, which is similarly absorbed and retained *(146)*. This assertion is based on results of a UK supplementation study in healthy volunteers with a baseline dietary intake of approximately 40 μg/d in which a further 100 μg Se/d as Se-enriched yeast raised plasma Se from 90.3 to 148.4 μg/L *(165)*. To date, no cancer trial has used a level of dose that would give a total intake of 140 μg Se/d as suggested above, all having opted for an additional 200 μg Se/d or more.

Trial evidence, which as explained above is more reliable, has only supplied information on a supplemental dose of 200 μg Se/d. While this appeared to benefit men of relatively low-Se status (plasma Se ≤ 105 μg/L), there was no benefit on the risk of prostate cancer for men of replete Se status (serum Se >123 μg/L) *(145)*. Those with plasma Se >122 μg/L, if given 200 μg Se/d, may run the risk of developing squamous cell carcinoma *(143)* and type-2 diabetes *(144)*. The advisability of supplementing individuals of already-replete status (say 125 μg/L or more) *(147)* with Se must be questioned. Certainly it should be apparent that in populations that already have a mean baseline intake at the level associated with reduced cancer risk, e.g. the Prostate, Lung, Colorectal and Ovarian Cancer Trial population, where mean plasma Se was 141.3 μg/L *(135)*, or SELECT, where mean serum Se was 136 μg/L, no significant benefit at higher intake/status should be expected, nor indeed was seen in the higher Se status individuals in those populations. Such populations should *not* be exposed to additional dietary Se or supplementation.

Additional Se may benefit those living in regions of low-to-moderate Se status (plasma Se ≤ 105 μg/L). Good food sources of Se in such regions are scarce but include the following:-

Brazil nuts, kidney, fish, liver and shellfish *(164)*. However, many people rarely eat such foods. Men in this category (e.g. Europeans), particularly if there is a family history of prostate cancer, should be able to take an additional daily dose of up to 200 μg Se/d without adverse effects. There appears to be no case for women of low-to-moderate Se status supplementing with a dose higher than 100 μg Se/d, as 100 μg/d should be able to raise plasma Se to near 150 μg/L, a level associated with decreased risk in a number of studies *(164)*.

Definitive guidelines on optimal intake await further research and, for individuals rather than populations, these must ultimately be genotype related.

REFERENCES

1. Berry, M.J., Banu, L., Chen, Y.Y., Mandel, S.J., Kieffer, J.D., Harney, J.W., and Larsen, P.R. (1991) Recognition of UGA as a selenocysteine codon in type I deiodinase requires sequences in the 3′ untranslated region. *Nature* **353**, 273–76.
2. Berry, M.J., Banu, L., Harney, J.W., and Larsen, P.R. (1993) Functional characterization of the eukaryotic SECIS elements which direct selenocysteine insertion at UGA codons. *Embo J* **12**, 3315–22.
3. Hatfield, D.L., and Gladyshev, V.N. (2002) How selenium has altered our understanding of the genetic code. *Mol Cell Biol* **22**, 3565–76.
4. Kryukov, G.V., Castellano, S., Novoselov, S.V., Lobanov, A.V., Zehtab, O., Guigó, R., and Gladyshev, V.N. (2003 May 30) Characterization of mammalian selenoproteomes. *Science* **300**(5624), 1439–43.
5. Rayman, M.P., Infante, H.G., and Sargent, M. (2008 Aug) Food-chain selenium and human health: Spotlight on speciation. *Br J Nutr* **100**(2), 238–53.
6. Combs, G.F., Jr (2006) Selenium as a cancer preventive agent. D.L. Hatfield, M.J. Bery, V.N. Gladyshev eds. In: *Selenium: Its Molecular Biology and Role in Human Health*. 249–64, NY, USA: Springer.
7. Lü, J., and Jiang, C. (2005 Nov-Dec) Selenium and cancer chemoprevention: Hypotheses integrating the actions of selenoproteins and selenium metabolites in epithelial and non-epithelial target cells. *Antioxid Redox Signal* **7**(11–12), 1715–27.
8. Davis, C.D., and Finley, J.W. (2003) Chemical versus food forms of selenium in cancer prevention. In: Ronald R.W. ed. *Functional foods and nutraceuticals in cancer prevention*. 55–85, Ames, IA: Iowa State Press.
9. Rayman, M.P. (2005 Nov) Selenium in cancer prevention: A review of the evidence and mechanism of action. *Proc Nutr Soc* **64**(4), 527–42.
10. Whanger, P.D. (2004) Selenium and its relationship to cancer: An update. *Br J Nutr* **91**, 11–28.
11. Ganther, H.E. (1999 Sep) Selenium metabolism, selenoproteins and mechanisms of cancer prevention: Complexities with thioredoxin reductase. *Carcinogenesis* **20**(9), 1657–66.
12. Husbeck, B., Bhattacharyya, R.S., Feldman, D., and Knox, S.J. (2006 Aug) Inhibition of androgen receptor signaling by selenite and methylseleninic acid in prostate cancer cells: Two distinct mechanisms of action. *Mol Cancer Ther* **5**(8), 2078–85.

13. Seo, Y.R., Kelley, M.R., and Smith, M.L. (2002 Oct 29) Selenomethionine regulation of p53 by a ref1-dependent redox mechanism. *Proc Natl Acad Sci U S A* **99**(22), 14548–53.

14. Gopalakrishna, R., and Gundimeda, U. (2001) Protein kinase C as a molecular target for cancer prevention by selenocompounds. *Nutr Cancer* **40**(1), 55–63.

15. Wu, Y., Zhang, H., Dong, Y., Park, Y.M., and Ip, C. (2005 Oct 1) Endoplasmic reticulum stress signal mediators are targets of selenium action. *Cancer Res* **65**(19), 9073–79.

16. Kim, K.H., Gao, Y., Walder, K., Collier, G.R., Skelton, J., and Kissebah, A.H. (2007 Mar 2) SEPS1 protects RAW264.7 cells from pharmacological ER stress agent-induced apoptosis. *Biochem Biophys Res Commun* **354**(1), 127–32. Epub 2007 Jan 2.

17. Rayman, M.P. (2000 Jul 15) The importance of selenium to human health. *Lancet* **356**(9225), 233–41.

18. Willett, W.C., Polk, B.F., Morris, J.S., Stampfer, M.J., Pressel, S., Rosner, B., Taylor, J.O., Schneider, K., and Hames, C.G. (1983) Prediagnostic serum selenium and risk of cancer. *The Lancet* **16**, 130–34.

19. Kok, F.J., de Bruijn, A.M., Hofman, A., Vermeeren, R., and Valkenburg, H.A. (1987) Is serum selenium a risk factor for cancer in men only?. *Am J Epidemiol* **125**, 12–16.

20. Salonen, J.T., Salonen, R., Lappetelainen, R., Maenpaa, P., Alfthan, G., and Puska, P. (1985) Risk of cancer in relation to serum concentrations of selenium and vitamins A and E: Matched case-control analysis of prospective data. *Br Med J* **290**, 417–20.

21. Knekt, P., Aromaa, A., Maatela, J., Alfthan, G., Aaran, R.K., Hakama, M., Hakulinen, T., Peto, R., and Tepo, L. (1990) Serum selenium and subsequent risk of cancer among Finnish men and women. *J Natl Cancer Inst* **82**, 864–68.

22. van den Brandt, P.A., Goldbohm, R.A., van't Veer, P., Bode, P., Dorant, E., Hermus, R.J., and Sturmans, F. (1993) A prospective cohort study on selenium status and the risk of lung cancer. *Cancer Res* **53**, 4860–65.

23. van den Brandt, P.A., Zeegers, M.P., Bode, P., and Goldbohm, R.A. (2003) Toenail selenium levels and the subsequent risk of prostate cancer: A prospective cohort study. *Cancer Epidemiol Biomark Prev* **12**, 866–71.

24. Yu, M.W., Horng, I.S., Hsu, K.H., Chiang, Y.C., Liaw, Y.F., and Chen, C.J. (1999) Plasma selenium levels and the risk of hepatocellular carcinoma among men with chronic hepatitis virus infection. *Am J Epidemiol* **150**, 367–74.

25. Combs, G.F., Jr., and Gray, W.P. (1998) Chemopreventive agents: Selenium. *Pharmacol Ther* **79**, 179–92.

26. Yoshizawa, K., Willett, W.C., Morris, S.J., Stampfer, M.J., Spiegelman, D., Rimm, E.B., and Giovanucci, E. (1998) Study of prediagnostic selenium levels in toenails and the risk of advanced prostate cancer. *J Natl Cancer Inst* **90**, 1219–24.

27. Duffield-Lillico, A.J., Reid, M.E., Turnbull, B.W., Combs, G.F., Jr, Slate, E.H., Fischbach, L.A., Marshall, J.R., and Clark, L.C. (2002 Jul) Baseline characteristics and the effect of selenium supplementation on cancer incidence in a randomized clinical trial: A summary report of the Nutritional Prevention of Cancer Trial. *Cancer Epidemiol Biomark Prev* **11**(7), 630–39.

28. Nomura, A.M., Lee, J., Stemmermann, G.N., and Combs, G.F., Jr. (2000 Sep) Serum selenium and subsequent risk of prostate cancer. *Cancer Epidemiol Biomarkers Prev* **9**(9), 883–87.

29. Sutton, A., Khoury, H., Prip-Buus, C., Cepanec, C., Pessayre, D., and Degoul, F. (2003) The Ala16Val genetic dimorphism modulates the import of human manganese superoxide dismutase into rat liver mitochondria. *Pharmacogenetics* **13**(3), 145–57.

30. Lim, S.D., Sun, C., Lambeth, J.D., Marshall, F., Amin, M., Chung, L. et al. (2005) Increased Nox1 and hydrogen peroxide in prostate cancer. *Prostate* **62**(2), 200–07.

31. Nelson, K.K., Ranganathan, A.C., Mansouri, J., Rodriguez, A.M., Providence, K.M., Rutter, J.L., Pumiglia, K., Bennett, J.A., and Melendez, J.A. (2003 Jan) Elevated sod2 activity augments matrix metalloproteinase expression: Evidence for the involvement of endogenous hydrogen peroxide in regulating metastasis. *Clin Cancer Res* **9**(1), 424–32.

32. Polytarchou, C., Hatziapostolou, M., and Papadimitriou, E. (2005) Hydrogen peroxide stimulates proliferation and migration of human prostate cancer cells through activation of activator protein-1 and up-regulation of the heparin affin regulatory peptide gene. *J Biol Chem* **280**(49), 40428–35.

33. Li, H., Kantoff, P.W., Giovannucci, E., Leitzmann, M.F., Gaziano, J.M., Stampfer, M.J., and Ma, J. (2005 Mar 15) Manganese superoxide dismutase polymorphism, prediagnostic antioxidant status, and risk of clinical significant prostate cancer. *Cancer Res* **65**(6), 2498–504.

34. Caruso, C., Lio, D., Cavallone, L., and Franceschi, C. (2004) Aging, longevity, inflammation, and cancer. *Ann N Y Acad Sci* **1028**, 1–13.

35. Porta, C., Subhra Kumar, B., Larghi, P., Rubino, L., Mancino, A., and Sica, A. (2007) Tumor promotion by tumor-associated macrophages. *Adv Exp Med Biol* **604**, 67–86.

36. Vunta, H., Davis, F., Palempalli, U.D., Bhat, D., Arner, R.J., Thompson, J.T., Peterson, D.G., Reddy, C.C., and Prabhu, K.S. (2007 Jun 22) The Anti-inflammatory Effects of Selenium Are Mediated through 15-Deoxy-{Delta}12,14-prostaglandin J2 in Macrophages. *J Biol Chem* **282**(25), 17964–73. Epub 2007 Apr 17.

37. Vunta, H., Belda, B.J., Arner, R.J., Channa Reddy, C., Vanden Heuvel, J.P., and Sandeep Prabhu, K. (2008, Nov) Selenium attenuates pro-inflammatory gene expression in macrophages. *Mol Nutr Food Res* **52**(11), 1316–23.

38. Ricote, M., Li, A.C., Willson, T.M., Kelly, C.J., and Glass, C.K. (1998 Jan 1) The peroxisome proliferator-activated receptor-gamma is a negative regulator of macrophage activation. *Nature* **391**(6662), 79–82.

39. Touyz, R.M., and Schiffrin, E.L. (2006 Jul) Peroxisome proliferator-activated receptors in vascular biology-molecular mechanisms and clinical implications. *Vascul Pharmacol* **45**(1), 19–28. Epub 2006 Jun 16.

40. Kirkby, K.A., and Adin, C.A. (2006 Mar) Products of heme oxygenase and their potential therapeutic applications. *Am J Physiol Renal Physiol* **290**(3), F563–F71.

41. Trigona, W.L., Mullarky, I.K., Cao, Y., and Sordillo, L.M. (2006 Feb 15) Thioredoxin reductase regulates the induction of haem oxygenase-1 expression in aortic endothelial cells. *Biochem J* **394** (Pt 1), 207–16.

42. Ejima, K., Layne, M.D., Carvajal, I.M., Nanri, H., Ith, B., Yet, S.F., and Perrella, M.A. (2002) Modulation of the thioredoxin system during inflammatory responses and its effect on heme oxygenase-1 expression. *Antioxid Redox Signal* **4**, 569–75.

43. Lee, T.S., Tsai, H.L., and Chau, L.Y. (2003) Induction of heme oxygenase-1 expression in murine macrophages is essential for the anti-inflammatory effect of low dose 15-deoxy-Delta-12, 14-prostaglandin J2. *J Biol Chem* **278**, 19325–30.

44. Krönke, G., Kadl, A., Ikonomu, E., Blüml, S., Fürnkranz, A., Sarembock, I.J., Bochkov, V.N., Exner, M., Binder, B.R., and Leitinger, N. (2007) Expression of heme oxygenase-1 in human vascular cells is regulated by peroxisome proliferator-activated receptors. *Arterioscler Thromb Vasc Biol* **27**, 1276–82. Epub 2007 Apr 5.

45. Gao, Y., Hannan, N.R., Wanyonyi, S., Konstantopolous, N., Pagnon, J., Feng, H.C., Jowett, J.B., Kim, K.H., Walder, K., and Collier, G.R. (2006 Mar 7) Activation of the selenoprotein SEPS1 gene expression by pro-inflammatory cytokines in HepG2 cells. *Cytokine* **33**(5), 246–51. Epub 2006 Mar 30.

46. Curran, J.E., Jowett, J.B., Elliott, K.S., Gao, Y., Gluschenko, K., Wang, J., Abel Azim, D.M., Cai, G., Mahaney, M.C., Comuzzie, A.G., Dyer, T.D., Walder, K.R., Zimmet, P., MacCluer, J.W., Collier, G.R., Kissebah, A.H., and Blangero, J. (2005 Nov) Genetic variation in selenoprotein S influences inflammatory response. *Nat Genet* **37**(11), 1234–41. Epub 2005 Oct 9.

47. Shrimali, R.K., Irons, R.D., Carlson, B.A., Sano, Y., Gladyshev, V.N., Park, J.M., and Hatfield, D.L. (2008 May 16) Selenoproteins mediate T cell immunity through an antioxidant mechanism. *J Biol Chem* **283**, 20181–5.

48. Kiremidjian-Schumacher, L., Roy, M., Wishe, H.I., Cohen, M.W., and Stotzky, G. (1994 Apr-May) Supplementation with selenium and human immune cell functions. II. Effect on cytotoxic lymphocytes and natural killer cells. *Biol Trace Elem Res* **41**(1–2), 115–27.

49. Kiremidjian-Schumacher, L., Roy, M., Glickman, R., Schneider, K., Rothstein, S., Cooper, J., Hochster, H., Kim, M., and Newman, R. (2000) Selenium and immunocompetence in patients with head and neck cancer. *Biol Trace Elem Res* **73**, 97–111.

50. Kiremidjian-Schumacher, L., and Roy, M. (2001) Effect of selenium on the immunocompetence of patients with head and neck cancer and on adoptive immunotherapy of early and established lesions. *Biofactors* **14**(1–4), 161–68.

51. Baliga, M.S., Wang, H., Zhuo, P., Schwartz, J.L., and Diamond, A.M. (2007 Mar) Selenium and GPx-1 overexpression protect mammalian cells against UV-induced DNA damage. *Biol Trace Elem Res* **115**(3), 227–42.

52. Fischer, J.L., Lancia, J.K., Mathur, A., and Smith, M.L. (2006 Mar-Apr) Selenium protection from DNA damage involves a Ref1/p53/Brca1 protein complex. *Anticancer Res* **26**(2A), 899–904.

53. Kowalska, E., Narod, S.A., Huzarski, T., Zajaczek, S., Huzarska, J., Gorski, B., and Lubinski, J. (2005) Increased rates of chromosome breakage in BRCA1 carriers are normalized by oral selenium supplementation. *Cancer Epidemiol Biomark Prev* **14**, 1302–06.

54. Karunasinghe, N., Ryan, J., Tuckey, J., Masters, J., Jamieson, M., Clarke, L.C., Marshall, J.R., and Ferguson, L.R. (2004) DNA stability and serum selenium levels in a high-risk group for prostate cancer. *Cancer Epidemiol Biomarkers Prev* **13**, 391–97.

55. Zeng, H., and Combs, G.F., Jr. (2008 Jan) Selenium as an anticancer nutrient: Roles in cell proliferation and tumor cell invasion. *J Nutr Biochem* **19**(1), 1–7. Epub 2007 Jun 27.

56. Lu, J., Pei, H., Ip, C., Lisk, D.J., Ganther, H., and Thompson, H.J. (1996) Effect on an aqueous extract of selenium-enriched garlic on in vitro markers and in vivo efficacy in cancer prevention. *Carcinogenesis* **17**, 1903–07.

57. Jiang, C., Wang, Z., Ganther, H., and Lü, J. (2002 Oct) Distinct effects of methylseleninic acid versus selenite on apoptosis, cell cycle, and protein kinase pathways in DU145 human prostate cancer cells. *Mol Cancer Ther* **1**(12), 1059–66.

58. Kaeck, M., Lu, J., Strange, R., Ip, C., Ganther, H.E., and Thompson, H.J. (1997 Apr 4) Differential induction of growth arrest inducible genes by selenium compounds. *Biochem Pharmacol* **53**(7), 921–26.

59. Ip, C. (1998 Nov) Lessons from basic research in selenium and cancer prevention. *J Nutr* **128**(11), 1845–54.

60. Wang, Z., Jiang, C., and Lu, J. (2002) Induction of caspase-mediated apoptosis and cell-cycle G1 arrest by selenium metabolite methylselenol. *Mol Carcinog* **34**, 113–20.

61. Yoon, S.O., Kim, M.M., and Chung, A.S. (2001 Jun 8) Inhibitory effect of selenite on invasion of HT1080 tumor cells. *J Biol Chem* **276**(23), 20085–92.

62. Yan, L., Yee, J.A., Li, D., McGuire, M.H., and Graef, G.L. (1999 Mar-Apr) Dietary supplementation of selenomethionine reduces metastasis of melanoma cells in mice. *Anticancer Res* **19**(2A), 1337–42.

63. Yan, L., Yee, J.A., McGuire, M.H., and Graef, G.L. (1997) Effect of dietary supplementation of selenite on pulmonary metastasis of melanoma cells in mice. *Nutr Cancer* **28**(2), 165–69.

64. Zeng, H., Briske-Anderson, M., Idso, J.P., and Hunt, C.D. (2006 Jun) The selenium metabolite methylselenol inhibits the migration and invasion potential of HT1080 tumor cells. *J Nutr* **136**(6), 1528–32.

65. Jiang, C., Ganther, H., and Lu, J. (2000 Dec) Monomethyl selenium–specific inhibition of MMP-2 and VEGF expression: Implications for angiogenic switch regulation. *Mol Carcinog* **29**(4), 236–50.

66. Jiang, C., Jiang, W., Ip, C., Ganther, H., and Lu, J. (1999 Dec) Selenium-induced inhibition of angiogenesis in mammary cancer at chemopreventive levels of intake. *Mol Carcinog* **26**(4), 213–25.

67. Lu, J., and Jiang, C. (2001) Antiangiogenic activity of selenium in cancer chemoprevention: Metabolite-specific effects. *Nutr Cancer* **40**(1), 64–73.

68. Smith, M.L., Lancia, J.K., Mercer, T.I., and Ip, C. (2004 May-Jun) Selenium compounds regulate p53 by common and distinctive mechanisms. *Anticancer Res* **24**(3a), 1401–08.

69. Zeng, H., Davis, C.D., and Finley, J.W. (2003 Apr) Effect of selenium-enriched broccoli diet on differential gene expression in min mouse liver. *J Nutr Biochem* **14**(4), 227–31.

70. Ip, C., and Lisk, D.J. (1997) Modulation of phase I and phase II xenobiotic-metabolizing enzymes by selenium-enriched garlic in rats. *Nutr Cancer* **28**, 184–88.

71. El-Bayoumy, K., and Sinha, R. (2005 Dec 11) Molecular chemoprevention by selenium: A genomic approach. *Mutat Res* **591**(1–2), 224–36. (or use Zeng&Combs).

72. Sinha, R., Kiley, S.C., Lu, J.X., Thompson, J.J., Moraes, R. et al. (1999) Effects of methylseleno-cysteine on PKC activity, cdk2 phosphorylation and *gad* gene expression in synchronized mouse mammary epithelial tumor cells. *Cancer Lett* **146**, 135–45.

73. Dong, Y., Zhang, H., Gao, A.C., Marshall, J.R., and Ip, C. (2005 Jul) Androgen receptor signaling intensity is a key factor in determining the sensitivity of prostate cancer cells to selenium inhibition of growth and cancer-specific biomarkers. *Mol Cancer Ther* **4**(7), 1047–55.

74. Dong, Y., Lee, S.O., Zhang, H., Marshall, J., Gao, A.C., and Ip, C. (2004) Prostate specific antigen expression is down-regulated by selenium through disruption of androgen receptor signaling. *Cancer Res* **64**, 19–22.

75. Cho, S.D., Jiang, C., Malewicz, B., Dong, Y., Young, C.Y., Kang, K.S., Lee, Y.S., Ip, C., and Lu, J. (2004 May) Methyl selenium metabolites decrease prostate-specific antigen expression by inducing protein degradation and suppressing androgen-stimulated transcription. *Mol Cancer Ther* **3**(5), 605–11.

76. Combs, G.F., Jr, and Lü, J. (2006) Selenium as a cancer preventive agent. In: D.L. Hatfield, M.J. Berry, V.N. Gladyshev eds. *Selenium: Its Molecular Biology and Role in Human Health.* 205–18, 2nd ed., NY, USA: Springer.

77. Ip, C., Thompson, H.J., Zhu, Z., and Ganther, H.E. (2000) In vitro and in vivo studies of methylse-leninic acid: Evidence that a monomethylated selenium metabolite is critical for cancer chemoprevention. *Cancer Res* **60**(11), 2882–86.

78. Xia, Y., Hill, K.E., Byrne, D.W., Xu, J., and Burk, R.F. (2005 Apr) Effectiveness of selenium supplements in a low-selenium area of China. *Am J Clin Nutr* **81**(4), 829–34.

79. Brown, K.M., Pickard, K., Nicol, F., Beckett, G.J., Duthie, G.G., and Arthur, J.R. (2000 May) Effects of organic and inorganic selenium supplementation on selenoenzyme activity in blood lymphocytes, granulocytes, platelets and erythrocytes. *Clin Sci (Lond)* **98**(5), 593–99.

80. Hu, Y.J., Korotkov, K.V., Mehta, R., Hatfield, D.L., Rotimi, C.N., Luke, A., Prewitt, T.E., Cooper, R.S., Stock, W., Vokes, E.E., Dolan, M.E., Gladyshev, V.N., and Diamond, A.M. (2001 Mar 1) Distribution and functional consequences of nucleotide polymorphisms in the 3′-untranslated region of the human Sep15 gene. *Cancer Res* **61**(5), 2307–10.

81. Hu, Y.J., and Diamond, A.M. (2003 Jun 15) Role of glutathione peroxidase 1 in breast cancer: Loss of heterozygosity and allelic differences in the response to selenium. *Cancer Res* **63**(12), 3347–51.

82. Kumaraswamy, E., Malykh, A., Korotkov, K.V., Kozyavkin, S., Hu, Y., Kwon, S.Y., Moustafa, M.E., Carlson, B.A., Berry, M.J., Lee, B.J., Hatfield, D.L., Diamond, A.M., and Gladyshev, V.N. (2000 Nov 10) Structure-expression relationships of the 15-kDa selenoprotein gene. Possible role of the protein in cancer etiology. *J Biol Chem* **275**(45), 35540–47.

83. Ratnasinghe, D., Tangrea, J.A., Andersen, M.R., Barrett, M.J., Virtamo, J., Taylor, P.R., and Albanes, D. (2000 Nov 15) Glutathione peroxidase codon 198 polymorphism variant increases lung cancer risk. *Cancer Res* **60**(22), 6381–83.

84. Ravn-Haren, G., Olsen, A., Tjønneland, A., Dragsted, L.O., Nexø, B.A., Wallin, H., Overvad, K., Raaschou-Nielsen, O., and Vogel, U. (2006 Apr) Associations between GPX1 Pro198Leu polymorphism, erythrocyte GPX activity, alcohol consumption and breast cancer risk in a prospective cohort study. *Carcinogenesis* **27**(4), 820–25.

85. Bastaki, M., Huen, K., Manzanillo, P., Chande, N., Chen, C., Balmes, J.R., Tager, I.B., and Holland, N. (2006 Apr) Genotype-activity relationship for Mn-superoxide dismutase, glutathione peroxidase 1 and catalase in humans. *Pharmacogenet Genomics* **16**(4), 279–86.

86. Forsberg, L., de Faire, U., Marklund, S.L., Andersson, P.M., Stegmayr, B., and Morgenstern, R. (2000 Oct) Phenotype determination of a common Pro-Leu polymorphism in human glutathione peroxidase 1. *Blood Cells Mol Dis* **26**(5), 423–26.

87. Arsova-Sarafinovska, Z., Matevska, N., Eken, A., Petrovski, D., Banev, S., Dzikova, S., Georgiev, V., Sikole, A., Erdem, O., Sayal, A., Aydin, A., and Dimovski, A.J. (2008 Jun 19) Glutathione peroxidase 1 (GPX1) genetic polymorphism, erythrocyte GPX activity, and prostate cancer risk. *Int Urol Nephrol* **41**, 63–70.

88. Lee, C.H., Lee, K.Y., Choe, K.H., Hong, Y.C., Noh, S.I., Eom, S.Y., Ko, Y.J., Zhang, Y.W., Yim, D.H., Kang, J.W., Kim, H., and Kim, Y.D. (2006) Effects of oxidative DNA damage and genetic polymorphism of the glutathione peroxidase 1 (GPX1) and 8-oxoguanine glycosylase 1 (hOGG1) on lung cancer. *J Prev Med Pub Health* **39**, 130–34.

89. Yang, P., Bamlet, W.R., Ebbert, J.O., Taylor, W.R., and de Andrade, M. (2004 Oct) Glutathione pathway genes and lung cancer risk in young and old populations. *Carcinogenesis* **25**(10), 1935–44.

90. Raaschou-Nielsen, O., Sørensen, M., Hansen, R.D., Frederiksen, K., Tjønneland, A., Overvad, K., and Vogel, U. (2007 Mar 18) GPX1 Pro198Leu polymorphism, interactions with smoking and alcohol consumption, and risk for lung cancer. *Cancer Lett* **247**(2), 293–300.

91. Knight, J.A., Onay, U.V., Wells, S., Li, H., Shi, E.J., Andrulis, I.L., and Ozcelik, H. (2004 Jan) Genetic variants of GPX1 and SOD2 and breast cancer risk at the Ontario site of the Breast Cancer Family Registry. *Cancer Epidemiol Biomarkers Prev* **13**(1), 146–49.

92. Ahn, J., Gammon, M.D., Santella, R.M., Gaudet, M.M., Britton, J.A., Teitelbaum, S.L., Terry, M.B., Neugut, A.I., and Ambrosone, C.B. (2005 Oct) No association between glutathione peroxidase Pro198Leu polymorphism and breast cancer risk. *Cancer Epidemiol Biomarkers Prev* **14**(10), 2459–61.

93. Cox, D.G., Hankinson, S.E., Kraft, P., and Hunter, D.J. (2004 Nov) No association between GPX1 Pro198Leu and breast cancer risk. *Cancer Epidemiol Biomarkers Prev* **13**(11 Pt 1), 1821–2.

94. Cox, D.G., Tamimi, R.M., and Hunter, D.J. (2006 Aug 31) Gene x Gene interaction between MnSOD and GPX-1 and breast cancer risk: A nested case-control study. *BMC Cancer* **6**, 217.

95. Ichimura, Y., Habuchi, T., Tsuchiya, N., Wang, L., Oyama, C., Sato, K., Nishiyama, H., Ogawa, O., and Kato, T. (2004 Aug) Increased risk of bladder cancer associated with a glutathione peroxidase 1 codon 198 variant. *J Urol* **172**(2), 728–32.

96. Hansen, R., Saebo, M., Skjelbred, C.F. et al. (2005) GPX Pro198Leu and OGG1 Ser326Cys polymorphisms and risk of development of colorectal adenomas and colorectal cancer. *Cancer Lett* **229**, 85–91.

97. Vogel, U., Olsen, A., Wallin, H., Overvad, K., Tjonneland, A., and Nexo, B.A. (2004) No association between GPX Pro198Leu and risk of basal cell carcinoma. *Cancer Epidemiol Biomark Prev* **13**, 1412–1413.

98. Hu, Y., Benya, R.V., Carroll, R.E., and Diamond, A.M. (2005 Dec) Allelic loss of the gene for the GPX1 selenium-containing protein is a common event in cancer. *J Nutr* **135**(12 Suppl), 3021S–3024S.

99. Hu, Y.J., Dolan, M.E., Bae, R., Yee, H., Roy, M., Glickman, R., Kiremidjian-Schumacher, L., and Diamond, A.M. (2004 Nov) Allelic loss at the GPx-1 locus in cancer of the head and neck. *Biol Trace Elem Res* **101**(2), 97–106.

100. Behne, D., Kyriakopoulos, A., Kalcklösch, M., Weiss-Nowak, C., Pfeifer, H., Gessner, H., and Hammel, C. (1997 Sep) Two new selenoproteins found in the prostatic glandular epithelium and in the spermatid nuclei. *Biomed Environ Sci* **10**(2–3), 340–45.

101. Kumaraswamy, E., Korotkov, K.V., Diamond, A.M., Gladyshev, V.N., and Hatfield, D.L. (2002) Genetic and functional analysis of mammalian Sep15 selenoprotein. *Methods Enzymol* **347**, 187–97.

102. Cooper, M.L., Adami, H.-O., Grönberg, H., Wiklund, F., Green, F.R., and Rayman, M.P. (2008 Dec 15) Interaction between SNPs in selenoprotein P and mitochondrial superoxide dismutase determines prostate cancer risk. *Cancer Res* **68**(24), 10171–77.

103. Diwadkar-Navsariwala, V., and Diamond, A.M. (2004 Nov) The link between selenium and chemoprevention: A case for selenoproteins. *J Nutr* **134**(11), 2899–902.

104. Apostolou, S., Klein, J.O., Mitsuuchi, Y., Shetler, J.N., Poulikakos, P.I., Jhanwar, S.C., Kruger, W.D., and Testa, J.R. (2004 Jun 24) Growth inhibition and induction of apoptosis in mesothelioma cells by selenium and dependence on selenoprotein SEP15 genotype. *Oncogene* **23**(29), 5032–40.

105. Jablonska, E., Gromadzinska, J., Sobala, W., Reszka, E., and Wasowicz, W. (2008 Feb) Lung cancer risk associated with selenium status is modified in smoking individuals by Sep15 polymorphism. *Eur J Nutr* **47**(1), 47–54.

106. Calvo, A., Xiao, N., Kang, J., Best, C.J., Leiva, I., Emmert-Buck, M.R. et al. (2002) Alterations in gene expression profiles during prostate cancer progression: Functional correlations to tumorigenicity and down-regulation of selenoprotein-P in mouse and human tumors. *Cancer Res* **62**(18), 5325–35.

107. Peters, U., Chatterjee, N., Hayes, R.B., Schoen, R.E., Wang, Y., Chanock, S.J., and Foster, C.B. (2008) Variation in the selenoenzyme genes and risk of advanced distal colorectal adenoma. *Cancer Epidemiol Biomarkers Prev* **17**, 1144–54.

108. Villette, S., Kyle, J.A., Brown, K.M. et al. (2002) A novel single nucleotide polymorphism in the 3′ untranslated region of human glutathione peroxidase 4 influences lipoxygenase metabolism. *Blood Cells Mol Dis* **29**, 174–78.

109. Méplan, C., Crosley, L.K., Nicol, F., Horgan, G.W., Mathers, J.C., Arthur, J.R., and Hesketh, J.E. (2008 Apr) Functional effects of a common single-nucleotide polymorphism (GPX4c718t) in the glutathione peroxidase 4 gene: Interaction with sex. *Am J Clin Nutr* **87**(4), 1019–27.

110. Méplan, C., Crosley, L.K., Nicol, F., Beckett, G.J., Howie, A.F., Hill, K.E. et al. (2007) Genetic polymorphisms in the human selenoprotein P gene determine the response of selenoprotein markers to selenium supplementation in a gender-specific manner (the SELGEN study). *Faseb J* **21**, 3063–74.

111. Bermano, G., Pagmantidis, V., Holloway, N., Kadri, S., Mowat, N.A.G., Shiel, R.S., Arthur, J.R., Mathers, J.C., Daly, A.K., Broom, J., and Hesketh, J.E. (2007) Evidence that a polymorphism within the 30UTR of glutathione peroxidase 4 is functional and is associated with susceptibility to colorectal cancer. *Genes Nutr* **2**, 225–32.

112. Udler, M., Maia, A.T., Cebrian, A., Brown, C., Greenberg, D., Shah, M., Caldas, C., Dunning, A., Easton, D., Ponder, B., and Pharoah, P. (2007 Jul 20) Common germline genetic variation in antioxidant defense genes and survival after diagnosis of breast cancer. *J Clin Oncol* **25**(21), 3015–23.

113. Lodygin, D., Epanchintsev, A., Menssen, A., Diebold, J., and Hermeking, H. (2005 May 15) Functional epigenomics identifies genes frequently silenced in prostate cancer. *Cancer Res* **65**(10), 4218–27.

114. Yu, Y.P., Yu, G., Tseng, G., Cieply, K., Nelson, J., Defrances, M., Zarnegar, R., Michalopoulos, G., and Luo, J.H. (2007 Sep 1) Glutathione peroxidase 3, deleted or methylated in prostate cancer, suppresses prostate cancer growth and metastasis. *Cancer Res* **67**(17), 8043–50.

115. Lee, O.J., Schneider-Stock, R., McChesney, P.A., Kuester, D., Roessner, A., Vieth, M., Moskaluk, C.A., and El-Rifai, W. (2005) Hypermethylation and loss of expression of glutathione peroxidase-3 in Barrett's tumorigenesis. *Neoplasia* **7**, 854 – 861.

116. De Luca, A., Sacchetta, P., Nieddu, M., Di Ilio, C., and Favaloro, B. (2007 May) Important roles of multiple Sp1 binding sites and epigenetic modifications in the regulation of the methionine sulfoxide reductase B1 (MsrB1) promoter. *BMC Mol Biol* **22**(8), 39.

117. Medina, D., and Morrison, D. (1988) Current ideas on selenium as a chemopreventive agent. *Pathol Immunopathol* **7**, 187–99.

118. Diwadkar-Navsariwala, V., Prins, G.S., Swanson, S.M., Birch, L.A., Ray, V.H., Hedayat, S., Lantvit, D.L., and Diamond, A.M. (2006 May 23) Selenoprotein deficiency accelerates prostate carcinogenesis in a transgenic model. *Proc Natl Acad Sci U S A* **103**(21), 8179–84.

119. Irons, R., Carlson, B.A., Hatfield, D.L., and Davis, C.D. (2006 May) Both selenoproteins and low molecular weight selenocompounds reduce colon cancer risk in mice with genetically impaired selenoprotein expression. *J Nutr* **136**(5), 1311–17.

120. Bleys, J., Navas-Acien, A., and Guallar, E. (2008 Feb 25) Serum selenium levels and all-cause, cancer, and cardiovascular mortality among US adults. *Arch Intern Med* **168**(4), 404–10.

121. Zeegers, M.P., Goldbohm, R.A., Bode, P., and van den Brandt, P.A. (2002 Nov) Prediagnostic toenail selenium and risk of bladder cancer. *Cancer Epidemiol Biomarkers Prev* **11**(11), 1292–97.

122. Glattre, E., Thomassen, Y., Thoresen, S.O., Haldorsen, T., Lund-Larsen, P.G., Theodorsen, L., and Aaseth, J. (1989 Mar) Prediagnostic serum selenium in a case-control study of thyroid cancer. *Int J Epidemiol* **18**(1), 45–49.

123. Wei, W.Q., Abnet, C.C., Qiao, Y.L., Dawsey, S.M., Dong, Z.W., Sun, X.D., Fan, J.H., Gunter, E.W., Taylor, P.R., and Mark, S.D. (2004) Prospective study of serum selenium concentrations and

esophageal and gastric cardia cancer, heart disease, stroke, and total death. *Am J Clin Nutr* **79**(1), 80–85.

124. Zhuo, H., Smith, A.H., and Steinmaus, C. (2004 May) Selenium and lung cancer: A quantitative analysis of heterogeneity in the current epidemiological literature. *Cancer Epidemiol Biomarkers Prev* **13**(5), 771–78.

125. Li, H., Stampfer, M.J., Giovannucci, E.L., Morris, J.S., Willett, W.C., Gaziano, J.M., and Ma, J. (2004 May 5) A prospective study of plasma selenium levels and prostate cancer risk. *J Natl Cancer Inst* **96**(9), 696–703.

126. Etminan, M., FitzGerald, J.M., Gleave, M., and Chambers, K. (2005 Nov) Intake of selenium in the prevention of prostate cancer: A systematic review and meta-analysis. *Cancer Causes Control* **16**(9), 1125–31.

127. Brinkman, M., Buntinx, F., Muls, E., Zeegers, M.P. (2006, Sept) Use of selenium in chemoprevention of bladder cancer. *Lancet Oncol* **7**(9), 766–74.

128. Brinkman, M., Reulen, R.C., Kellen, E., Buntinx, F., and Zeegers, M.P. (2006 Oct) Are men with low selenium levels at increased risk of prostate cancer?. *Eur J Cancer* **42**(15), 2463–71. Epub 2006 Sep 1.

129. Akbaraly, N.T., Arnaud, J., Hininger-Favier, I., Gourlet, V., Roussel, A.M., and Berr, C. (2005 Nov) Selenium and mortality in the elderly: Results from the EVA study. *Clin Chem* **51**(11), 2117–23. Epub 2005 Aug 25.

130. Peters, U., Chatterjee, N., Church, T.R., Mayo, C., Sturup, S., Foster, C.B., Schatzkin, A., and Hayes, R.B. (2006 Feb) High serum selenium and reduced risk of advanced colorectal adenoma in a colorectal cancer early detection program. *Cancer Epidemiol Biomarkers Prev* **15**(2), 315–20.

131. Jacobs, E.T., Jiang, R., Alberts, D.S., Greenberg, E.R., Gunter, E.W., Karagas, M.R., Lanza, E., Ratnasinghe, L., Reid, M.E., Schatzkin, A., Smith-Warner, S.A., Wallace, K., and Martinez, M.E. (2004) Selenium and colorectal adenoma: Results of a pooled analysis. *J Natl Cancer Inst* **96**, 1669–75.

132. Helzlsouer, K.J., Huang, H.-Y., Alberg, A.J., Hoffman, S., Burke, A., Norkus, E.P., Morris, J.S., and Comstock, G.W. (2000) Association between alpha-tocopherol, gamma-tocopherol, selenium, and subsequent prostate cancer. *J Natl Cancer Inst* **92**, 2018–23.

133. Goodman, G.E., Schaffer, S., Bankson, D.D., Hughes, M.P., and Omenn, G.S., and the Carotene and Retinol Efficacy Trial (CARET) Co-Investigators (2001) Predictors of serum in cigarette smokers and the lack of association with lung and prostate cancer risk. *Cancer Epidemiol Biomark Prev* **10**, 1069–76.

134. Brooks, J.D., Metter, E.J., Chan, D.W., Sokoll, L.J., Landis, P., Nelson, W.G., Muller, D., Andres, R., and Carter, H.B. (2001) Plasma selenium level before diagnosis and the risk of prostate cancer development. *J Urol* **166**, 2034–38.

135. Peters, U., Foster, C.B., Chatterjee, N., Schatzkin, A., Reding, D., Andriole, G.L., Crawford, E.D., Sturup, S., Chanock, S.J., and Hayes, R.B. (2007 Jan) Serum selenium and risk of prostate cancer-a nested case-control study. *Am J Clin Nutr* **85**(1), 209–17. Erratum in: Am J Clin Nutr. 2007 Sep; **86**(3), 808.

136. World Cancer Research Fund, American Institute for Cancer Research (2007) Food, Nutrition and the Prevention of Cancer: A Global Perspective. Washington, DC: AICR.

137. Bjelakovic, G., Nikolova, D., Simonetti, R.G., and Gluud, C. (2004 Oct 18) Antioxidant supplements for preventing gastrointestinal cancers. *Cochrane Database Syst Rev* **4**, CD004183.

138. Bardia, A., Tleyjeh, I.M., Cerhan, J.R., Sood, A.K., Limburg, P.J., Erwin, P.J., and Montori, V.M. (2008 Jan) Efficacy of antioxidant supplementation in reducing primary cancer incidence and mortality: Systematic review and meta-analysis. *Mayo Clin Proc* **83**(1), 23–34.

139. Clark, L.C., Combs, G.F., Jr, Turnbull, B.W., Slate, E.H., Chalker, D.K., Chow, J., Davis, L.S., Glover, R.A., Graham, G.F., Gross, E.G., Krongrad, A., Lesher, J.L., Jr, Park, H.K., Sanders, B.B., Jr, Smith, C.L., and Taylor, J.R. (1996) Effects of selenium supplementation for cancer prevention in patients with carcinoma of the skin. A randomized controlled trial. Nutritional Prevention of Cancer Study Group. *JAMA* **276**, 1957–63.

140. Duffield-Lillico, A.J., Dalkin, B.L., Reid, M.E. et al., Nutritional Prevention of Cancer Study Group (2003) Selenium supplementation, baseline plasma selenium status and incidence of prostate cancer: An analysis of the complete treatment period of the Nutritional Prevention of Cancer Trial. *BJU Int* **91**, 608–12.

141. Reid, M.E., Duffield-Lillico, A.J., Garland, L., Turnbull, B.W., Clark, L.C., and Marshall, J.R. (2002 Nov) Selenium supplementation and lung cancer incidence: An update of the nutritional prevention of cancer trial. *Cancer Epidemiol Biomarkers Prev* **11**(11), 1285–91.

142. Reid, M.E., Duffield-Lillico, A.J., Sunga, A., Fakih, M., Alberts, D.S., and Marshall, J.R. (2006) Selenium supplementation and colorectal adenomas: An analysis of the nutritional prevention of cancer trial. *Int J Cancer* **118**, 1777–81.

143. Duffield-Lillico, A.J., Slate, E.H., Reid, M.E. et al., Nutritional Prevention of Cancer Study Group (2003) Selenium supplementation and secondary prevention of nonmelanoma skin cancer in a randomized trial. *J Natl Cancer Inst* **95**, 1477–81.

144. Stranges, S., Marshall, J.R., Natarajan, R. et al. (2007) Effects of long-term selenium supplementation on the incidence of type 2 diabetes: A randomized trial. *Ann Intern Med* **147**, 217–23.

145. Lippman, S.M., Klein, E.A., Goodman, P.J. et al. (2009) Effect of selenium and vitamin E on risk of prostate cancer and other cancers: The Selenium and Vitamin E Cancer Prevention Trial (SELECT). *JAMA* **301**, 39–51.

146. Rayman, M.P. (2004 Oct) The use of high-selenium yeast to raise selenium status: How does it measure up?. *Br J Nutr* **92**(4), 557–73.

147. Burk, R.F., Norsworthy, B.K., Hill, K.E., Motley, A.K., and Byrne, D.W. (2006) Effects of chemical form of selenium on plasma biomarkers in a high-dose human supplementation trial. *Cancer Epidemiol Biomarkers Prev* **15**, 804–10.

148. Stratton, M.S., Reid, M.E., Schwartzberg, G., Minter, F.E., Monroe, B.K., Alberts, D.S., Marshall, J.R., and Ahmann, F.R. (2003b) Selenium and inhibition of disease progression in men diagnosed with prostate carcinoma: Study design and baseline characteristics of the 'Watchful Waiting' Study. *Anticancer Drugs* **14**, 595–600.

149. Fischer, J.L., Mihelc, E.M., Pollok, K.E., and Smith, M.L. (2007 Jan) Chemotherapeutic selectivity conferred by selenium: A role for p53-dependent DNA repair. *Mol Cancer Ther* **6**(1), 355–61.

150. Fischer, J.L., Lancia, J.K., Mathur, A., and Smith, M.L. (2006 Mar-Apr) Selenium protection from DNA damage involves a Ref1/p53/Brca1 protein complex. *Anticancer Res* **26**(2A), 899–904.

151. Santos, R.A., and Takahashi, C.S. (2008 Feb) Anticlastogenic and antigenotoxic effects of selenomethionine on doxorubicin-induced damage in vitro in human lymphocytes. *Food Chem Toxicol* **46**(2), 671–77.

152. Li, S., Zhou, Y., Wang, R., Zhang, H., Dong, Y., and Ip, C. (2007 Mar) Selenium sensitizes MCF-7 breast cancer cells to doxorubicin-induced apoptosis through modulation of phospho-Akt and its downstream substrates. *Mol Cancer Ther* **6**(3), 1031–38.

153. Jüliger, S., Goenaga-Infante, H., Lister, T.A., Fitzgibbon, J., and Joel, S.P. (2007) Chemosensitization of B-cell lymphomas by methylseleninic acid involves nuclear factor-kappaB inhibition and the rapid generation of other selenium species. *Cancer Res* **67**(22), 10984–92.

154. Nichol, C., Herdman, J., Sattar, N., O'Dwyer, P.J., St, J., O'Reilly, D., Littlejohn, D., and Fell, G. (1998 Aug) Changes in the concentrations of plasma selenium and selenoproteins after minor elective surgery: Further evidence for a negative acute phase response?. *Clin Chem* **44**(8 Pt 1), 1764–66.

155. Drain, P.K., Baeten, J.M., Overbaugh, J., Wener, M.H., Bankson, D.D., Lavreys, L., Mandaliya, K., Ndinya-Achola, J.O., and McClelland, R.S. (2006 May) Low serum albumin and the acute phase response predict low serum selenium in HIV-1 infected women. *BMC Infect Dis* **19**(6), 85.

156. Moschos, M.P. (2000) Selenoprotein, P. *Cell Mol Life Sci* **57**, 1836–45.

157. Mendall, M.A., Patel, P., Ballam, L., Strachan, D., and Northfield, T.C. (1996 Apr 27) C reactive protein and its relation to cardiovascular risk factors: A population based cross sectional study. *BMJ* **312**(7038), 1061–65.

158. Surh, Y.J., Chun, K.S., Cha, H.H., Han, S.S., Keum, Y.S., Park, K.K., and Lee, S.S. (2001) Molecular mechanisms underlying chemopreventive activities of anti-inflammatory phytochemicals:

Down-regulation of COX-2 and iNOS through suppression of NF-κB activation. *Mutat Res* **480**, 243–68.

159. Niskar, A.S., Paschal, D.C., Kieszak, S.M. et al. (2003) Serum selenium levels in the US population: Third National Health and Nutrition Examination Survey, 1988–1994. *Biol Trace Elem Res* **91**, 1–10.

160. Czernichow, S., Couthouis, A., Bertrais, S., Vergnaud, A.C., Dauchet, L., Galan, P., and Hercberg, S. (2006) Antioxidant supplementation does not affect fasting plasma glucose in the Supplementation with Antioxidant Vitamins and Minerals (SU.VI.MAX) study in France: Association with dietary intake and plasma concentrations. *Am J Clin Nutr* **84**, 395–99.

161. Bleys, J., Navas-Acien, A., and Guallar, E. (2007) Serum selenium and diabetes in US Adults. *Diabetes Care* **30**, 829–34.

162. Bleys, J., Navas-Acien, A., Stranges, S., Menke, A., Miller, E.R., 3rd, and Guallar, E. (2008 Aug) Serum selenium and serum lipids in US adults. *Am J Clin Nutr* **88**(2), 416–23.

163. Stranges, S., Laclaustra, M., Ji, C., Cappuccio, F.P., Navas-Acien, A., Ordovas, J.M., Rayman, M.P., and Guallar, E. (2010, Jan) Higher selenium status is associated with adverse blood lipid profile in British adults. *J Nutr* **140**(1), 81–87. Epub 2009 Nov 11.

164. Rayman, M.P. (2008) Food-chain selenium and human health: Emphasis on intake. *Br J Nutr* **100**, 254–58.

165. Rayman, M., Thompson, A., Warren-Perry, M., Galassini, R., Catterick, J., Hall, E., Lawrence, D., and Bliss, J. (2006) Impact of selenium on mood and quality of life: A randomized, controlled trial. *Biol Psychiatry* **59**, 147–54.

20 Calcium and Cancer

Joan M. Lappe

Key Points

1. The importance of calcium and vitamin D acting together has long been recognized for skeletal health. Evidence now suggests that calcium and vitamin D are important in the prevention of cancer.
2. Clinical studies suggest that optimal calcium and vitamin D nutrition can prevent from 30 to 77% of various types of cancer.
3. High calcium intake has shown to have a protective effect against colon cancer. Experiments show that unabsorbed calcium in the lumen of the colon can prevent the adverse effects of bile acids and free fatty acids on the epithelial cells.
4. Calcium is shown to have a positive effect against cancer through its regulation of cell division, proliferation, and differentiation. Increased calcium concentrations in cell and organ culture media show decrease in cell proliferation and stimulate cell differentiation in numerous types of cells.
5. Numerous studies have evaluated the association between breast cancer and calcium intake. Most of the case–control studies found an inverse association between dietary calcium intake and risk of breast cancer. At least four cohort studies have evaluated the effect of dietary calcium on incidence of breast cancer and found a significantly reduced risk of breast cancer associated with higher dietary calcium.

Key Words: Calcium; cancer; colon; breast

1. INTRODUCTION

Experimental studies suggest that calcium prevents colon cancer through two potential mechanisms. The classical hypothesis holds that high calcium intakes are protective for colon cancer because unabsorbed calcium complexes with free unconjugated bile acids and free fatty acids in the lumen of the colon *(1–5)*. These complexes of calcium fat soaps have been observed *(6, 7)*. The bile and fatty acids have been shown to have irritating effects and to stimulate cell proliferation, thereby promoting a variety of cell damaging effects in the colon. Subsequent repair mechanisms that involve inflammation and hyperproliferation of undifferentiated cells initiate the malignant process *(8)*. By complexing with these acids, unabsorbed calcium prevents the adverse effects on epithelial cells.

From: *Nutrition and Health: Bioactive Compounds and Cancer*
Edited by: J.A. Milner, D.F. Romagnolo, DOI 10.1007/978-1-60761-627-6_20,
© Springer Science+Business Media, LLC 2010

More recently, considerable attention has been given to a more complex mechanism whereby calcium may decrease the risk of colon cancer, as well as other types of cancer. This mechanism is based on the widely accepted view that calcium is a pivotal regulator of numerous cell functions and modulates cell properties *(9)*. Of particular importance is its role in regulation of cell division, proliferation, and differentiation *(9)*. It has been shown that low levels of intracellular ionized calcium play a role in cell proliferation and that increasing the calcium concentration in cell and organ culture media decreases cell proliferation and stimulates cell differentiation in numerous types of cells *(10–12)*. In this paradigm, persistent calcium malnutrition leads to a decrease in calcium concentration in extracellular fluid compartments, which is translated into modulation of cell functions that can lead to initiation of cancer.

It is well established that systemic calcium homeostasis is regulated by the effects of parathyroid hormone and 1,25 dihydroxyvitamin D (1,25(OH)$_2$D, calcitriol) on the intestine, kidney, and skeleton. Through this system, serum calcium is maintained within a narrow range such that even wide variations in calcium intake cause only slight changes in serum calcium levels. However, the concentration of calcium in other extracellular fluid compartments, for example, the intestine, depends on the kinetics of tissue-specific calcium fluxes and not on plasma calcium levels. The extracellular ionized calcium-sensing receptor (CaR) is thought to be a key step in the pathway through which calcium mediates a protective effect against cancer development *(13–17)*. Even minute variations in extracellular fluid calcium concentrations are able to affect cellular functions such as proliferation, differentiation, and apoptosis, via modulation of the CaR *(13, 18)*. Studies suggest that signaling pathways involved in cell growth and differentiation that are activated by calcium through the CaR include promotion of E-cadherin expression, suppression of β-catenin–T-cell factor activation, and activation of the p38 mitogen-activated protein kinase cascade *(14, 16, 19)*. Persistent calcium malnutrition leads to a decrease in calcium concentration in extracellular fluid that affects CaR activity.

The CaR, which is a G protein-coupled type plasma membrane receptor, modifies intracellular signaling in a cell-type-specific manner *(20)*. Several cell types are known to express the CaR, including osteoblasts, monocytes, and mammary, ovary, and colon epithelial cells, to name a few *(21–25)*. In addition to its presence on normal cells, the CaR has been found on several malignant cells: colon, breast, ovary, and prostate cancer cells *(21–23, 26)*. Studies of human colon carcinomas demonstrate that CaR-positive cells are found almost exclusively in differentiated areas within the malignant lesion *(15, 21)*.

Specifically, the numerous cellular effects of calcium on colonic epithelial cells suggest its role in colon carcinogenesis. The proliferative compartment of epithelial cells increases in size in colonic crypts of persons at risk for colon cancer *(27)*. In vitro and in vivo studies and randomized human trials have shown that calcium supplementation with calcium tablets or dairy foods decreases colonic epithelial cell proliferation *(27–34)*. Numerous preclinical experimental studies have demonstrated very consistent calcium effects on colon cancer development and on cellular processes associated with colon cancer. These include the following effects: (a) decreasing and normalizing excessive proliferation of colonic epithelial cells, thereby decreasing the susceptibility of proliferating epithelial cells to accumulation of abnormalities in DNA; (b) decreasing the cytotoxicity of fecal water; (c) increasing the maturation and differentiation of colonic epithelial cells; and (d) reducing the development of colon cancers in animal models *(35–39)*.

It has been shown that, mediated by calcium, vitamin D deficiency slows apoptosis of colonic epithelial cells at the mouths of the crypts, resulting in an abnormally long life span of these epithelial cells *(40)*. Thus, the resultant proliferative colonic epithelial cell population was unusually large. In a study of human colon adenocarcinoma cells, Cross et al. demonstrated that cell growth could be slowed by increasing the extracellular calcium concentration in the culture medium *(41, 42)*. Cell cycle analysis suggested that transition from the G1 into the S phase was a crucial step in the ionized calcium regulation of the colon cancer cell proliferation *(15)*.

Peterlik and Cross *(43)* have suggested that the development of tumors from the hyperproliferative foci of colonic adenomas into malignant lesions could be used as a paradigm for the role of CaR in modulating growth of ionized calcium-sensitive proliferating normal and malignant cells. Proliferation, differentiation, and apoptosis of colonic epithelial cells occur simultaneously along the axis of the colonic crypt. This is predicated on synchronization of cell division at the base with cell death at the mouth of the crypt. A calcium gradient might play a role in this synchronization, assuming there is a "calcium switch" in crypt cells that stimulates proliferation at low ionized calcium levels and promotes differentiation and apoptosis with increasing ionized calcium levels from the base to the mouth. The CaR, which is located at the base of the crypt, might serve as the "switch" by setting the rate of proliferation dependent on the ambient ionized calcium. In this paradigm, increasing ionized calcium would inhibit division of crypt base cells and ease their progression from the proliferating to the differentiating compartment in the upper part of the crypt. Thus in this scenario, calcium supplementation, which increases the ambient ionized calcium, could serve as an effective measure to prevent colon cancer.

The action of calcium on cells other than colon has not been as thoroughly studied. However, it has long been recognized that, in culture, normal human breast epithelial cells reduce growth and become terminally differentiated when ambient ionized calcium is increased within the physiological range *(11)*. Cheng et al. demonstrated that the CaR is present in normal as well as in malignant mammary epithelial cells *(22)*. Thus, it is likely that the existing clinical evidence of an inverse association between calcium intake and breast cancer eventually may be linked to a CaR-mediated inhibition of mammary cell growth by local ionized calcium. In vitro studies have shown that calcium slows the progression of breast cancer through inhibition of secretion of proteins, such as insulin-like growth factors and parathyroid hormone-related protein, responsible for advanced breast cancer *(44, 45)*. Studies by Xuet et al. have found that decreased dietary calcium and vitamin D in a high-fat diet induced hyperplasia and hyperproliferation in the mammary gland in a rodent model *(46)*. Furthermore, these adverse changes were reversed by increasing dietary calcium and vitamin D *(37, 47)*.

A cancer protective effect of calcium is likely connected to vitamin D status. Most cells in the body express vitamin D receptors (VDRs) and 1α-hydroxylase and are thus able to locally produce $1,25(OH)_2D$ *(48, 49)*. Evidence suggests that $1,25(OH)_2D$

within the cell stimulates vitamin D response elements (VDRE) to regulate transcription of genes whose protein products are involved in cell proliferation, differentiation, and apoptosis, activities that are necessary for initiation and promotion of cancer *(48, 50)*. VDREs are found in the promoter regions of the CaR, and this provides an intriguing link between calcium and vitamin D at the molecular level *(51)*. For more details on the effect of vitamin D on cancer, see Chapter 17.

2. EPIDEMIOLOGICAL STUDIES

2.1. Colon Cancer

The association between calcium intake and cancer prevention in humans has been reported more commonly with colon cancer than with other types of cancer. In 1980, Garland et al. suggested that calcium and vitamin D might reduce the risk of colon cancer *(52)*. This was based on the observation that age-adjusted death rates of colon cancer were nearly three times higher in males who lived in sunnier regions of the United States than in males who lived in regions with fewer days of sunshine *(52)*. The authors proposed that the effect of vitamin D was through its influence on calcium metabolism. To investigate the possibility that differences in endogenous vitamin D production and calcium absorption might decrease the risk of colon cancer, Garland et al. conducted a prospective study following 1,954 men for 19 years *(53)*. The subjects had completed detailed 28-day diet diaries between 1957 and 1959 and were followed to ascertain diagnosis of colon cancer. Indeed, incidence of colon cancer was inversely associated with dietary vitamin D and calcium. Those in the highest quartile of calcium intake showed a significantly lower risk of developing colon cancer than those in the lowest quartile ($P < 0.05$). Similarly, intake of vitamin D and a combined index of calcium and vitamin D were inversely associated with risk of colon cancer ($P < 0.05$). This was one of the first prospective studies to support the role of calcium intake in prevention of colon cancer.

In a 1998 review of more than 20 epidemiologic geographical studies of calcium and colorectal cancer, Martinez et al. *(54)* concluded that the epidemiologic evidence of a calcium effect is inconsistent and inconclusive. On the other hand, more recently, several large cohort studies and at least one case–control study from various parts of the world suggest that higher levels of calcium intake decrease the incidence of colorectal adenomas and cancer *(55–65)*.

For example, researchers conducting the Multiethnic Cohort study of 85,903 men and 105,108 women reported that total calcium intake was inversely associated with colorectal cancer risk in both men and women *(55)*. Men in the highest quintile of total calcium intake (from supplements and food) had a 30% lower risk than those in the lowest quintile (RR = 0.70, 95% CI 0.52–0.93; $p_{trend} = 0.006$). For women, the risk of colon cancer was reduced by 36% if they were in the highest quintile of intake (RR = 0.64, 95% CI 0.50–0.83; $p_{trend} = 0.003$) *(55)*. Likewise, intake of dairy food was protective for colon cancer, especially in persons who did not take supplemental calcium.

The Cancer Prevention Study II Nutrition followed a U.S. cohort of 60,866 men and 66,883 women for 4–5 years to examine the relationships between calcium, vitamin D, and dairy intake and the risk of incident colon cancer *(58)*. During follow-up,

683 cases of colorectal cancer were diagnosed. Calcium from supplements was associated with incident cancer (RR = 0.69, 95% CI 0.49–0.96 for ≥ 500 mg/day vs. none, p_{trend} = 0.03). Calcium intake from diet and supplements combined showed a marginal association (RR = 0.87, 95% CI 0.67–1.12, highest vs. lowest quintiles, p_{trend} = 0.02).

Thus, numerous large cohort studies support the preventive effect of calcium on colorectal cancer and suggest that risk is reduced by at least 30%.

2.2. Breast Cancer

Numerous studies have evaluated the association between breast cancer and calcium intake. Most of the case–control studies found an inverse association between dietary calcium intake and risk of breast cancer, although not all were statistically significant (66–75). At least four cohort studies have evaluated the effect of dietary calcium on incidence of breast cancer and found a significantly reduced risk of breast cancer associated with higher dietary calcium (76–79). One of these, the Nurses Health Study of 88,691 women, found breast cancer risk to be inversely related to total calcium intake and dietary calcium intake in premenopausal, but not postmenopausal, women (80). The relative risk for >1 serving/day of low-fat milk compared to ≤3 servings/month was 0.68 (95% CI 0.48–0.98). The researchers found similar associations for vitamin D and calcium, also in premenopausal women only. In contrast, the Cancer Prevention Study II studied only postmenopausal women and found inverse associations between breast cancer and total and dietary calcium intakes (77). Women who were in the highest quintile of total calcium intake (>1,250 mg/day) had a lower risk of incident breast cancer than women in the lowest quintile (≤500 mg/day) (RR 0.80, 95% CI 0.67–0.95, P_{trend} = 0.02). Similarly, dairy intake was inversely associated with breast cancer. Consuming ≥2 servings/day decreased the risk of breast cancer compared to intake of <0.05 servings/day (RR0.81, 95% CI 0.69–0.95, P_{trend} = 0.002). In an earlier analysis of this cohort, dairy food and calcium intake had an inverse association with breast cancer mortality with premenopausal and postmenopausal women pooled (81).

Of the cohort studies that evaluated the relationship of breast cancer with vitamin D intake as well as with calcium intake (76, 77, 82), two investigations reported an inverse association between vitamin D intake and breast cancer incidence (76, 82). Unfortunately, none of these studies reported serum levels of 25(OH)D, which is the functional indicator of vitamin D status. The cohort study by Levi et al. found a significant interaction between calcium and vitamin D intake and incidence of breast cancer in premenopausal women, suggesting that consuming high levels of calcium may lower risk of developing breast cancer when vitamin D consumption is also high (69).

Mammographic breast density is strongly correlated with the risk of breast cancer (83, 84). Furthermore, mammographic breast density is associated with the extent of epithelial and nonepithelial cells in the breast as well as epithelial and stromal proliferation, which may partially account for the breast density/cancer relationship (85, 86). Thus, mammographic density has been used as an intermediate marker for breast cancer risk in preventive studies of breast cancer. At least two cohort studies have found that calcium and vitamin D intake independently were negatively associated with mammographic breast density *(87, 88)*. However, the combined effect of calcium and vitamin D was greater than either of the independent effects. One study found an inverse relationship with total dairy intake *(89)*.

Thus, the preponderance of epidemiological evidence supports an effect of dietary calcium in reducing risk of breast cancer, although the relationship to menopausal status is not clearly elucidated by these observational studies.

2.3. Prostate

In contrast to reports about the benefits of calcium for preventing colon and breast cancer, some reports suggest that calcium may *increase* the risk of prostate cancer. Numerous epidemiologic studies, including both cohort and case–control studies, have evaluated the relationship between dairy products or calcium intake and prostate cancer. The results are somewhat inconsistent, with some studies documenting a positive association *(90–95)*, whereas others finding no association *(96–100)*. A few studies have found calcium and dairy intake to be associated with high-grade and advanced and fatal prostate cancer, but not with overall incident prostate cancer *(91, 92, 99, 101)*.

In 2005, Gao et al. reported a meta-analysis of prospective studies that examined the association between dairy product consumption and/or calcium intake and risk of prostate cancer *(102)*. They found that the estimated excess risk of prostate cancer in men with higher intake of dairy products compared with those with lower intakes was about 11%, while the estimated excess risk associated with calcium intake was about 38%. The meta-analysis found no significant association of either dairy or calcium intake with advanced prostate cancer *(102)*. Subsequent inclusion of a recent prospective study of 14,642 men in Australia *(103)*, slightly decreased the pooled relative risk from 1.11 to 1.09 ($P = 0.059$) for the highest to lowest dairy intake categories and from 1.38 to 1.32 ($P = 0.026$) for the highest vs. lowest calcium intake categories *(103)*. The conclusion drawn from the meta-analysis was that a high intake of dairy food and calcium may contribute to an increased risk of prostate cancer, but the increase is small.

More recently, Huncharek et al. reported a thorough meta-analysis and found that dairy products, dietary calcium, and vitamin D were not risk factors for prostate cancer *(104)*. Forty-five observational studies, both case–control and cohort, were included in the analyses.

The mechanism by which dietary calcium might be linked to prostate cancer is unclear. It has been hypothesized that relatively high calcium consumption promotes prostate cancer by reducing the production of $1,25(OH)_2D$ *(105)*. It is well accepted that many types of cells, including prostate epithelial cells, produce $1,25(OH)_2D$ from its physiological precursor $25(OH)D$ and that $1,25(OH)_2D$ directly affects these cells and tissues through its autocrine function *(106)*. Among these effects of $1,25(OH)_2D$ are reducing cell proliferation and enhancing cell differentiation *(107, 108)*. In vitro studies show that $1,25(OH)_2D$ reduces prostate cell proliferative activity by 50–65% *(109)*, and in vivo studies confirm that $1,25(OH)_2D$ increases prostate epithelial differentiation and inhibits growth of cancer cells *(110, 111)*. Additionally, some clinical studies show an inverse association between prostate cancer and sunlight exposure or serum $25(OH)D$, which is a critical substrate for production of $1,25(OH)_2D$ *(112, 113)*.

However, of studies that evaluated the serum $1,25(OH)_2D$ in relation to prostate cancer, most found no reduced levels in patients with prostate cancer *(114–120)*.

It is also well accepted that calcium suppresses serum parathyroid hormone (PTH) and decreases renal 1-α-hydroxylase to result in lower renal production of serum $1,25(OH)_2D$. However, large variations in dietary calcium induce only minor fluctuations in serum $1,25(OH)_2D$ *(113, 115, 121)*. Furthermore, studies show that in normal prostatic tissue, PTH and calcium do not influence 1-α-hydroxylase and thus do not affect local production of $1,25(OH)_2D$ *(122)*. Finally, there is no evidence that a high-calcium diet results in decreased production of $1,25(OH)_2D$ at the cellular level. Thus, the hypothesis that dietary calcium is positively associated with risk of prostate cancer has weak support in the epidemiological data, and the mechanisms of such a relationship have not been clearly elucidated.

3. INTERVENTION STUDIES – INDIVIDUALIZED PREVENTION AND/OR TREATMENT?

Preventive intervention studies with colorectal cancer as an endpoint are difficult to conduct due to the long follow-up that is required. Because most colorectal cancers originate in adenomatous polyps and about 5% of all adenomas progress into a malignant lesion *(123)*, colorectal adenomas are often used as surrogate endpoints in chemopreventive trials. In addition, adenomas are much more common than colorectal cancer and can, therefore, be studied using smaller sample sizes. Adenomas are also a valuable endpoint because they offer a logical target for prevention developing over a 20–30 year period and evolving through many phases of abnormal cell development to malignant colon tumors *(4)*.

Strong evidence exists for the effect of calcium supplementation in preventing colorectal adenomas. Two large randomized clinical trials have demonstrated that calcium supplementation reduces the incidence of recurrent colorectal adenomas, consistent with a role of calcium in early stages of carcinogenesis *(57, 124)*. In the Calcium Polyp Prevention Study (CPPS), 930 men and women with at least one previous adenoma were randomly assigned to either 1,200 mg of elemental calcium carbonate or placebo and followed for 4 years *(57)*. Baseline calcium intake for the treatment and placebo groups were 889 ± 451 and 865 ± 423 mg/day, respectively. The adjusted risk ratio of having a recurrent adenoma in the calcium group compared to placebo was 0.81 (95% CI = 0.67–0.99; $P = 0.04$). In subsequent analyses, risk ratios for adenoma recurrence were determined for calcium supplementation in serum 25(OH)D subgroups *(125)*. Calcium supplementation decreased the risk of recurrent adenoma in the subjects who had baseline 25(OH)D levels above the median of 29.1 ng/ml (RR = 0.71; CI = 0.57–0.89; P for interaction 0.012). However, no association was seen in persons with 25(OH)D levels at or below the median. Serum 25(OH)D levels were associated with a significantly lower risk of adenoma only in subjects in the calcium supplemented group (RR per 12 ng/ml increase of 25(OH)D = 0.88; CI = 0.77–0.99, P for interaction = 0.006).

A recent follow-up analysis of this study found that 5 years after the end of the intervention, subjects in the calcium group continued to have a lower risk of colorectal adenoma than those in the placebo group (31.5 and 43.2% respectively; RR = 0.63;

CI = 0.46–0.87; $P = 0.005$). In fact, 5 years after the end of supplementation (RR = 0.63) the relative risk was lower than at the end of 4 years of intervention (RR = 0.81). However, 10 years after the end of the intervention, the protective effect of calcium was not detected. This study provides strong support for the long-term effects of calcium supplementation, along with adequate vitamin D levels, on prevention of colorectal adenomas.

The European Cancer Prevention (ECP) Intervention Study, a randomized double-blind clinical trial *(126)* of 665 persons found a nonsignificant reduction in risk of recurrent adenomas for subjects given 2,000 mg elemental calcium for 3 years compared to placebo (adjusted odds ratio = 0.66; CI = 0.38–1.17; $P = 0.16$). Subjects ranged in age from 35 to 75 years, with a mean of 59 years. The mean baseline calcium intake was 918 mg/day. The findings were consistent with the Calcium Polyp Prevention Study, and the reduction in risk was actually greater than in the CPPS (RR = 0.66 vs. 0.81, respectively). However, the sample size in the ECP study was most likely too small to find statistically significant effect. Furthermore, the intervention time was 3 years compared to 4 years in the CPPS. When the results of the CPPS and the ECP were combined in a Cochrane review *(127)*, a reduction in recurrent adenomas of about 26% was found (OR 0.74, CI 0.58–0.95) for doses of calcium supplementation ranging from 1,200 to 2,000 mg/day.

Only one calcium clinical trial was found that had colon cancer endpoints or reported cancer outcomes. The Women's Health Initiative (WHI) study of more than 36,000 women assigned calcium and vitamin D supplementation for an average of 7 years found no effect on incidence of colorectal cancer *(128)*. However, there were several limitations to the study: (1) the WHI did not perform colonoscopies to determine presence of adenomas or cancer; (2) participants had high calcium intake at enrollment; (3) a large number of persons in the placebo group reported supplement use; and (4) the dose of calcium (1,000 mg/d) was lower than many trials using calcium to decrease the incidence of adenomas. Thus, the only trial of calcium supplementation with colon cancer as an endpoint does not provide a definitive answer.

Intervention studies of calcium with mammographic breast density or breast cancer outcomes are sparse. Very recently, an analysis from the WHI found that calcium and vitamin D supplementation did not reduce the risk of invasive breast cancer in post-menopausal women *(129)*. The sample included 36,282 women who were randomly assigned to 1,000 mg of calcium and 400 IU of vitamin D3. Breast cancer was a secondary outcome. Although there were fewer cases of breast cancer in the supplemented ($N = 528$) vs. the placebo ($N = 546$) group after 7 years of follow-up, the difference was not statistically significant.

Although this was a very large study, the results need to be considered in light of several limitations. Baseline calcium intake levels were high in the cohort, 1,150 mg/day *(130)*. Thus, supplemental calcium may have provided no additional benefit to cancer prevention. Adherence to the supplementation was less than optimal. At the end of the trial, only 59% of the subjects were taking at least 80% of the study pills *(129)*. Personal use of calcium and vitamin D was allowed, and 15% of placebo subjects "dropped in" to the active group. In addition, 58% of the participants in the supplement study were also assigned to hormone replacement therapy (HRT). In fact, the study was stopped early because in an interim analysis the combination of estrogen and progesterone was found to increase the risk of breast cancer (http://www.nhibi.nih.gov/whi/pr-02-7-9). It was not clear from this recent report how many women in each supplement group were also on HRT. Another limitation is that the 400 IU/day vitamin D3 dose given in this study is low. Recent evidence suggests that doses of vitamin D as high as 1,100–2,000 IU/day may be required to prevent cancer *(131, 132)*.

The effect of calcium alone was not assessed in any of the WHI analyses. However, the researchers did attempt to address the independent effect of vitamin D. To that end, baseline 25(OH)D levels were obtained for a nested case–control study that included 895 cases and 898 matched controls who were breast cancer free. The mean baseline level of 25(OH)D in the cases was 50.0 ± 21.0 nmol/l, while the level in the controls was 52.0 ± 21.1 nmol/l (NS). Thus, both groups were, on average, vitamin D insufficient. However, in a multivariate analysis that included hormone therapy as one of several independent variables, higher baseline 25(OH)D was significantly associated with lower risk of breast cancer ($P = 0.04$). Furthermore, among women in the lowest baseline quartile of vitamin D intake (from diet and supplement), fewer cancers occurred in the supplemented group (HR $= 0.79$, 95% CI $= 0.65$–0.97, $P_{\text{interaction}} = 0.003$). Unfortunately, 25(OH)D levels were not obtained during the study to ascertain the effects of supplement on raising serum 25(OH)D levels.

Recently, another double-blind, placebo-controlled, randomized trial of calcium and vitamin D supplementation found that supplementation decreased the risk of all-type cancer by 60% in a population-based sample of postmenopausal women *(132)*. Furthermore, a sub-analysis suggested that the combination of supplements reduced the risk of breast cancer (unpublished data). In that study, 1,179 participants were randomly assigned to one of three interventions: (1) placebo; (2) 1,400–1,500 mg/day of calcium (Ca group); and (3) 1,100 IU/day of calcium plus vitamin D_3 (Ca plus D group) and were followed for 4 years. Median baseline calcium intake was 1,072 mg/day (interquartile range 697–1,530 mg/day), and mean baseline 25(OH)D level was 71.8 ± 20.3 nmol/l with no statistically significant differences among groups. Serum 25(OH)D was measured annually.

Of 1,179 women enrolled, 1,024 (86.9%) completed the 4 years of study. Mean adherence to supplements (defined as $\geq 80\%$ of assigned doses) was 85.7% for the vitamin D component of the combined regimen and 74.4% for the calcium component. The effect of treatment on vitamin D status was reflected in the induced change in serum 25(OH)D. The 1,100 IU/d dose of vitamin D produced an elevation in serum 25(OH)D in the Ca plus D group of 23.9 ± 17.8 nmol/l, whereas the placebo and Ca-only groups had no significant change. Within the Ca plus D group, the rise in serum 25(OH)D was directly related to recorded compliance with vitamin D supplements ($P < 0.01$).

Fifty women developed non-skin cancer over the course of the study, 13 in the first year and 37 thereafter. The RR of developing cancer for the Ca plus D group was 0.402 (CI 0.20–0.82, $P = 0.013$), and for the Ca-only group 0.532 (CI 0.27–1.03; $P = 0.063$). Both treatment assignment and either 12-month 25(OH)D or baseline 25(OH)D concentration were significant, independent determinants of cancer risk ($P < 0.002$ and $P < 0.03$, respectively, for the two serum 25(OH)D values).

In a subsequent analysis for the group free of cancer at 1 year, the RR of all-type cancer for the Ca plus D group dropped to 0.232 (CI 0.09–0.60; $P < 0.005$). However, for the Ca-only group, RR was essentially unchanged, at 0.587 (CI 0.29–1.21; $P = 0.147$). In an analysis of specific types of cancer, the RR of developing breast cancer for the Ca plus D group compared to placebo was 0.22 (CI 0.043–1.079, $P = 0.062$) (unpublished data). Thus, this study suggests that calcium and vitamin D combined may decrease the risk of breast cancer, while the WHI study did not find an effect. There were several differences between the Lappe et al. and the WHI studies that possibly accounted for different findings: (1) Lappe et al. randomly sampled the population, which better represented the true population than a convenience sample; (2) the dose of vitamin D3 supplementation was nearly three times as high in Lappe et al. as in WHI; (3) adherence to supplementation was considerably higher in the Lappe et al. study; (4) in the WHI, some women in each group were randomly assigned to a trial of HRT. In the Lappe et al. study, 46% of the subjects received estrogen on prescription from their personal physicians for ≥ 6 mo during the study, but the three treatment groups did not differ significantly in estrogen use; (5) on the other hand, the WHI was much larger than the Lappe study, 36,282 women vs. 1,179, respectively. However, the effect of supplementation in the Lappe study was large enough to be detected with their sample size. In both studies, cancer was an a priori secondary outcome. In the Lappe et al. study, calcium supplementation decreased the risk of all-type cancer by nearly 50%, but the decrease did not quite reach statistical significance. Nonetheless, the results are intriguing and warrant further study.

Only one study has reported an intervention with prostate cancer as an outcome. That recent randomized trial found that, as a secondary outcome, calcium supplementation did not increase the risk of prostate cancer and suggested that the risk might be *decreased* by approximately half *(121)*. In this study, 672 men were randomly assigned to receive 1,200 mg of calcium carbonate or placebo daily for 4 years to determine the effect on the incidence of colorectal adenomas. At baseline, there was no significant difference between calcium intake in the supplemented and the placebo groups (919 and 902 mg/day, respectively). Subjects were followed for up to 12 years. Cancer diagnoses were ascertained and confirmed with medical records.

After 10.3 years of follow-up, there were 33 cases of prostate cancer in the calcium group and 37 in the placebo group (R.R. 0.83, 95% CI 0.52–1.32). Although this difference was not statistically significant after 10 years, there was a significantly lower risk of prostate cancer after 6 years of follow-up in the calcium group compared to placebo (R.R. 0.52, 95% CI 0.28–0.98). The cumulative incidence curves for prostate cancer show a reduced risk in the calcium group starting about 2 years after the beginning of treatment and continuing until about 2 years after treatment stopped.

In a subset who had serum vitamin D concentrations measured at baseline and at the end of 4 years of treatment ($N = 483$), serum $1,25(OH)_2D$ decreased slightly in the calcium group (42.9–41.2 pg/ml) and increased a small amount in the placebo group (43.4–44.8 pg/ml). There was no significant association between baseline $1,25(OH)_2D$ or $25(OH)D$ and prostate cancer risk. Calcium supplementation did not result in increased risk of prostate-specific antigen (PSA) conversion, which is considered a marker of preclinical cancer. This study, which provides the most rigorous test to date, does not support a dietary calcium and prostate cancer connection. Thus, the existence of a pathophysiological connection between higher calcium intake and reduced levels of circulating 1,25(OH)$_2$D that might result in prostate cancer remains a hypothesis for which there is weak support in the clinical data.

Considerable clinical evidence shows that vitamin D and calcium work together to decrease cancer risk. For example, a study by Grau et al. found that vitamin D and calcium supplementation reduced recurrence of colorectal adenomas only in persons with normal 25(OH)D levels *(125)*. On the other hand, high 25(OH)D levels reduced the risk of adenomas only in persons receiving calcium supplementation. More recently, Mizoue et al. reported a case–control study of 836 cases of colorectal cancer and 861 sex-matched and age-matched controls in an Asian population *(56)*. A lower risk of colorectal cancer associated with a high-calcium diet was seen in those who had higher levels of vitamin D intake or greater daily sunlight exposure. However, this association with calcium intake was not seen in those with medium or low intake of vitamin D or in those with decreased sunlight exposure. In another study, high intake of vitamin D-fortified milk was associated with lower incidence of breast cancer in premenopausal women *(76)*. As mentioned earlier, the cohort study by Levi et al. found a significant interaction between calcium and vitamin D intake and incidence of breast cancer *(69)*.

The intervention studies reviewed in this chapter support the effects of calcium on *prevention* of cancer. In fact, no studies were found that reported the effect of calcium on treatment of existing malignancy. However, based on preclinical data, a treatment effect is highly possible.

4. TISSUE SPECIFICITY AND TOTALITY OF THE EVIDENCE

Studies of the relationship between calcium and cancer have progressed from epidemiologic observations to clinical trials. In vitro studies have shown that increasing levels of calcium decrease proliferation of epithelial cells and induce cell differentiation and apoptosis. Studies in animal models have demonstrated that calcium decreases carcinogen-induced colon tumor formation. Several large cohort studies also link increased dietary calcium with a decreased risk of colon cancer. The only clinical trial that has been conducted with colon cancer as an outcome found no effect. However, several major limitations of that randomized trial render the findings questionable. Several large clinical trials have found that calcium supplementation lowers risk of recurrent colonic adenomas. The preponderance of evidence strongly supports the effect of adequate dietary calcium in decreasing risk of colon cancer. Estimates are that calcium supplementation ranging from about 1,200–2,000 mg/day reduces the risk of recurrent adenomas by about 26%.

Regarding breast cancer, supplemental calcium decreases mammary epithelial cell hyperplasia and hyperproliferation in vitro as well as in vivo. Most, but not all, epidemiological studies have found a significantly reduced risk of breast cancer associated with higher dietary calcium. No studies were found that reported a positive association. Three cohort studies reported that higher levels of dietary calcium or dairy food are negatively associated with mammographic breast density, a surrogate for breast cancer. The two clinical trials that evaluated the effect of calcium and vitamin D supplementation together on breast cancer had contrasting findings. Although the evidence for an effect of dietary calcium in reducing breast cancer is not as compelling as the evidence for a colon cancer effect, preclinical and clinical studies do strongly suggest that optimal dietary calcium decreases risk of breast cancer.

Numerous epidemiologic studies have assessed the relationship between dietary calcium and prostate cancer with conflicting results. A recent thorough meta-analysis found no relationship between dairy food or dietary calcium and prostate cancer. Furthermore, the only randomized trial of calcium and prostate cancer found no increased risk, and, in fact, suggested that calcium may be protective of prostate cancer. The major limitation of that trial was that prostate cancer was a secondary outcome. Interestingly, black men in the USA have the highest prostate cancer incidence in the country but the lowest calcium and dairy intakes. Taken together, a large body of research is building that strongly suggests a combined effect of calcium and vitamin D on decreasing cancer risk, although this chapter only briefly addressed some of those studies.

5. FUTURE RESEARCH DIRECTIONS

A large study funded by the National Cancer Institute currently is underway to determine the effect of vitamin D3 and calcium supplementation on prevention of large bowel adenomas (http://clinicaltrials.gov/ct/show/NCT00153816?order=1). The study, which started in 2004, is a double-blind, placebo-controlled trial of vitamin D3 1,000 IU/day and calcium carbonate 1,200 mg/day given to four groups: (1) placebo; (2) calcium only; (3) vitamin D3 only; and (4) calcium plus vitamin D3. Subjects will include men and women ranging from 45 to 77 years of age and who have had at least one large bowel adenoma removed in the 4 months prior to study entry. The estimated study completion date is December 2017. Successful completion of this well-designed study will provide strong evidence for the efficacy (or non-efficacy) of calcium and vitamin D3 supplementation in prevention of colon adenomas, which are precursors of colon cancer.

It is critical that future studies address the effects of calcium and vitamin D in combination on cancer prevention. Well-established understanding of their interactive physiologic role points out clearly that it is virtually impossible to study the effects of one of these nutrients without the results being confounded by the other. Studies need to address the optimal levels of intake and the variations in mean levels for different segments of the population.

Robert Heaney (133) has pointed out eloquently the challenges of studying the effects of nutrients on chronic diseases, such as cancer, that have long latency and multifactorial causation. The challenge of determining efficacy in the context of long latency is not solved by randomized clinical trials. It is virtually impossible to randomize individuals to a pure placebo-controlled calcium intervention, since calcium is found in drinking water and many natural and fortified foods. Furthermore, researchers cannot ethically expose research participants to inadequate intakes based on well-established nutrient needs (e.g., skeletal needs for calcium). Another problem is the long latency of many cancers. For example, colon cancer develops over the course of 20–30 years, while it is an exceptional randomized trial that continues for more than 5–10 years.

Heaney has admonished the scientific community to "confront the difficulty of designing investigative approaches that are sufficient to demonstrate and quantify benefit from altered nutrient input at a population level." *(133, p. 298)*

6. CONCLUSIONS AND RECOMMENDATIONS FOR INTAKE/DIETARY CHANGES

It is well established that calcium nutrition is essential for optimal skeletal development and for maintenance of bone health. Since excess calcium cannot be stored, adequate intake of this nutrient is required to avoid calcium being taken from the skeleton to support plasma calcium homeostasis. Accordingly, recommendations have been made for levels of daily calcium intake in various age groups. The most recent Dietary Reference Intakes (DRIs) established in 1997 by the U.S. Institute of Medicine recommend that adults of 70 years of age and under ingest at least 1,000 mg/day of calcium and those over 70 years of age take in 1,200 mg/day *(134)*. These are levels determined to assure optimal whole-body calcium retention and adequate development and maintenance of bone mass. The recommendations were not based on evidence that calcium may decrease the risk of cancer.

Surveys indicate that calcium intake is below recommended levels in many segments of the population. According to 2005–2006 data concerning US males ranging from 20 to 49 years of age, calcium intake averages more than 1,000 mg/day. Calcium intake for women in the same age bracket averages only 900 mg/day compared to the 1,000 mg/day recommendation. However, men and women over 50 years of age average less than 800 mg/day or about 66% of the Adequate Intake (AI).

Clinical studies suggest that optimal calcium and vitamin D nutrition can prevent from 30 to 77% of various types of cancer. Furthermore, knowledge is increasing about the mechanisms responsible for the cancer preventative effects of calcium. Waiting for results of long, expensive randomized trials to make recommendations about the importance of calcium intake for cancer prevention is not prudent. It may be causing us to miss a window of opportunity to obliterate cancer in a large segment of the population. Although the optimal levels of calcium intake for prevention of cancer have not yet been determined, it has been shown that the levels are likely at least 1,200 mg/day, at or near the currently recommended levels. Public policy officials could do the public a great service by emphasizing the importance of obtaining at least the currently recommended levels of dietary calcium daily for prevention of breast and colon cancer. Considering the lack of solid evidence for a prostate cancer–dietary calcium connection and the profound benefits of adequate calcium intake for prevention of osteoporosis, encouraging currently recommended levels of calcium intake for men seems reasonable.

Scientists are currently working within a shifting paradigm, one in which evidence supports the effect of optimal nutrition on preventing many cancers. Less than a century ago, scientists scoffed at the notion that not eating something could result in illness *(135)*. Since then, it has been accepted that nutritional deficiencies do result in short latency diseases, such as rickets, pellagra, and beriberi. Perhaps before the end of this century, we will be able to establish the role of calcium and vitamin D in preventing the long latency disease of cancer.

REFERENCES

1. Garland, C., Garland, F., and Gorham, E. (1991) Can colon cancer incidence and death rates be reduced with calcium and vitamin D? *Am J Clin Nutr* **54**, 193S–201S.
2. Slattery, M., Sorenson, A., and Ford, M. (1988) Dietary calcium intake as a mitigating factor in colon cancer. *Am J Epidemiol* **128**, 504–14.
3. Newmark, H.L., Wargovich, M.J., and Bruce, W.R. (1984) Colon cancer and dietary fat, phosphate, and calcium: A hypothesis. *J Natl Cancer Inst* **72**, 1323–25.
4. Lipkin, M.,, and Newmark, H. (1995) Calcium and the prevention of colon cancer. *J Cell Biochem* **22**(Supp) 65–73.
5. Van der Meer, R., Lapra, J.A., Govers, M.J., and Kleibeuker, J.H. (1997) Mechanisms of the intestinal effects of dietary fats and milk products on colon carcinogenesis. *Cancer Lett* **114**, 75–83.
6. Pence, B. (1993) Role of calcium in colon cancer prevention: Experimental and clinical studies. *Mutat Res* **290**, 87–95.
7. Appleton, G., Owen, R., Wheeler, E., Challacombe, D., and Williamson, R. (1991) Effect of dietary calcium on the colonic luminal environment. *Gut* **32**, 1374–77.
8. Peterlik, M. (2008) Role of bile acid secretion in human colorectal cancer. *Wien Med Wochenschr* **158**, 539–41.
9. Rasmussen, H. (1986) The calcium messenger system (2). *New Engl J Med* **314**, 1164–70.
10. Hennings, H., Michael, D., Cheng, C., Steinert, P., Holbrook, K., and Yuspa, S.H. (1980) Calcium regulation of growth and differentiation of mouse epidermal cells in culture. *Cell* **19**, 245–54.
11. McGrath, C.M., and Soule, H.D. (1984) Calcium regulation of normal human mammary epithelial cell growth in culture. *In Vitro* **20**, 652–62.
12. Babcock, M.S., Marino, M.R., Gunning, W.T., III, and Stoner, G.D. (1983) Clonal growth and serial propagation of rat esophageal epithelial cells. *In Vitro* **19**, 403–15.
13. Brown, E.M., Gamba, G., Riccardi, D., Lombardi, M., Butters, R., Kifor, O. et al. (1993) Cloning and characterization of an extracellular Ca(2+)-sensing receptor from bovine parathyroid. *Nature* **366**, 575–80.
14. Chakrabarty, S., Radjendirane, V., Appelman, H., and Varani, J. (2003) Extracellular calcium and calcium sensing receptor function in human colon carcinomas: Promotion of E-cadherin expression and suppression of beta-catenin/TCF activation. *Cancer Res* **63**, 67–71.
15. Kallay, E., Bajna, E., Wrba, F., Kriwanek, S., Peterlik, M., and Cross, H.S. (2000) Dietary calcium and growth modulation of human colon cancer cells: Role of the extracellular calcium-sensing receptor. *Cancer Detect Prev* **24**, 127–36.
16. Lamprecht, S.A., and Lipkin, M. (2003) Chemoprevention of colon cancer by calcium, vitamin D and folate: Molecular mechanisms. *Nat Rev Cancer* **3**, 601–14.
17. Brown, E.M., and MacLeod, R.J. (2001) Extracellular calcium sensing and extracellular calcium signaling. *Physiol Rev* **81**, 239–97.
18. Orrenius, S., Zhivotovsky, B., and Nicotera, P. (2003) Regulation of cell death: The calcium-apoptosis link. *Nat Rev Mol Cell Biol* **4**, 552–65.
19. Hobson, S. (2003) Activation of the MAP kinase cascade by exogenous calcium-sensing receptor. *Mol Cell Endocrinol* **200**, 189–98.
20. Kallay, E., Bonner, E., Wrba, F., Thakker, R.V., Peterlik, M., and Cross, H.S. (2003) Molecular and functional characterization of the extracellular calcium-sensing receptor in human colon cancer cells. *Oncol Res* **13**, 551–59.
21. Sheinin, Y., Kallay, E., Wrba, F., Kriwanek, S., Peterlik, M., and Cross, H.S. (2000) Immunocyto-chemical localization of the extracellular calcium-sensing receptor in normal and malignant human large intestinal mucosa. *J Histochem Cytochem* **48**, 595–602.
22. Cheng, I., Klingensmith, M.E., Chattopadhyay, N., Kifor, O., Butters, R.R., Soybel, D.I. et al. (1998) Identification and localization of the extracellular calcium-sensing receptor in human breast. *J Clin Endocrinol Metab* **83**, 703–07.
23. McNeil, L., Hobson, S., Nipper, V., and Rodland, K.D. (1998) Functional calcium-sensing receptor expression in ovarian surface epithelial cells. *Am J Obstet Gynecol* **178**, 305–13.

24. Yamaguchi, T., Kifor, O., Chattopadhyay, N., and Brown, E.M. (1998) Expression of extracellular calcium (Ca2 + o)-sensing receptor in the clonal osteoblast-like cell lines, UMR-106 and SAOS-2. *Biochem Biophys Res Commun* **243**, 753–57.

25. Yamaguchi, T., Olozak, I., Chattopadhyay, N., Butters, R.R., Kifor, O., Scadden, D.T. et al. (1998) Expression of extracellular calcium (Ca2+o)-sensing receptor in human peripheral blood monocytes. *Biochem Biophys Res Commun* **246**, 501–06.

26. Sanders, J.L., Chattopadhyay, N., Kifor, O., Yamaguchi, T., and Brown, E.M. (2001) Ca(2+)-sensing receptor expression and PTHrP secretion in PC-3 human prostate cancer cells. *Am J Physiol Endocrinol Metab* **281**, E1267–E74.

27. Lipkin, M. (1988) Biomarkers of increased susceptibility to gastrointestinal cancer: New application to studies of cancer prevention in human subjects. *Cancer Res* **48**, 235–45.

28. Wargovich, M.J., Isbell, G., Shabot, M., Winn, R., Lanza, F., Hochman, L. et al. (1992) Calcium supplementation decreases rectal epithelial cell proliferation in subjects with sporadic adenoma. *Gastroenterology* **103**, 92–97.

29. Barsoum, G.H., Hendrickse, C., Winslet, M.C., Youngs, D., Donovan, I.A., Neoptolemos, J.P. et al. (1992) Reduction of mucosal crypt cell proliferation in patients with colorectal adenomatous polyps by dietary calcium supplementation. *Br J Surg* **79**, 581–83.

30. Holt, P.R., Wolper, C., Moss, S.F., Yang, K., and Lipkin, M. (2001) Comparison of calcium supplementation or low-fat dairy foods on epithelial cell proliferation and differentiation. *Nutr Cancer* **41**, 150–55.

31. Holt, P.R., Atillasoy, E.O., Gilman, J., Guss, J., Moss, S.F., Newmark, H. et al. (1998) Modulation of abnormal colonic epithelial cell proliferation and differentiation by low-fat dairy foods: A randomized controlled trial. *JAMA* **280**, 1074–79.

32. Lipkin, M., and Newmark, H. (1985) Effect of added dietary calcium on colonic epithelial-cell proliferation in subjects at high risk for familial colonic cancer. *N Engl J Med* **313**, 1381–84.

33. Sinotte, M., Rousseau, F., Ayotte, P., Dewailly, E., Diorio, C., Giguere, Y. et al. (2008) Vitamin D receptor polymorphisms (FokI, BsmI) and breast cancer risk: Association replication in two case-control studies within French Canadian population. *Endocr Relat Cancer* **15**(4), 975–83.

34. Lipkin, M., Newmark, H., and Kelloff, G. (1990) Calcium, Vitamin D, and Prevention of Colon Cancer. Bethesda, MD: National Cancer Institute and CRC Press.

35. Lipkin, M. (1999) Preclinical and early human studies of calcium and colon cancer prevention. *Ann N Y Acad Sci* **889**, 120–27.

36. Govers, M.J., Termont, D.S., and Van der Meer, R. (1994) Mechanism of the antiproliferative effect of milk mineral and other calcium supplements on colonic epithelium. *Cancer Res* **54**, 95–100.

37. Xue, L., Lipkin, M., Newmark, H., and Wang, J. (1999) Influence of dietary calcium and vitamin D on diet-induced epithelial cell hyperproliferation in mice. *J Natl Cancer Inst* **91**, 176–81.

38. Risio, M., Lipkin, M., Newmark, H., Yang, K., Rossini, F.P., Steele, V.E. et al. (1996) Apoptosis, cell replication, and Western-style diet-induced tumorigenesis in mouse colon. *Cancer Res* **56**, 4910–16.

39. Guo, Y.S., Draviam, E., Townsend, C.M., Jr., and Singh, P. (1990) Differential effects of Ca2+ on proliferation of stomach, colonic, and pancreatic cancer cell lines in vitro. *Nutr Cancer* **14**, 149–57.

40. Brenner, B.M., Russell, N., Albrecht, S., and Davies, R.J. (1998) The effect of dietary vitamin D3 on the intracellular calcium gradient in mammalian colonic crypts. *Cancer Lett* **127**, 43–53.

41. Cross, H.S., Pavelka, M., Slavik, J., and Peterlik, M. (1992) Growth control of human colon cancer cells by vitamin D and calcium in vitro. *J Natl Cancer Inst* **84**, 1355–57.

42. Cross, H.S., Huber, C., and Peterlik, M. (1991) Antiproliferative effect of 1,25-dihydroxyvitamin D3 and its analogs on human colon adenocarcinoma cells (CaCo-2): Influence of extracellular calcium. *Biochem Biophys Res Commun* **179**, 57–62.

43. Peterlik, M., and Cross, H.S. (2005) Vitamin D and calcium deficits predispose for multiple chronic diseases. *Eur J Clin Invest* **35**, 290–304.

44. Luparello, C., Santamaria, F., and Schilling, T. (2000) Regulation of PTHrP and PTH/PTHrP receptor by extracellular Ca2+ concentration and hormones in the breast cancer cell line 8701-BC. *Biol Chem* **381**, 303–08.

45. Xie, S.P., James, S.Y., and Colston, K.W. (1997) Vitamin D derivatives inhibit the mitogenic effects of IGF-I on MCF-7 human breast cancer cells. *J Endocrinol* **154**, 495–504.

46. Xue, L., Newmark, H., Yang, K., and Lipkin, M. (1996) Model of mouse mammary gland hyperproliferation and hyperplasia induced by a western-style diet. *Nutr Cancer* **26**, 281–87.

47. Jacobsen, E., James, K., Newmark, H., and Carroll, K. (1989) Effects of dietary fat, caclium and vitamin D on growth and mammary tumorigenesis induced by 7,12-dimethyl(a)anthracene in female Sprague-Dawley rats. *Cancer Res* **49**, 6300–03.

48. Holick, M. (2003) Vitamin D: A millenium perspective. *J Cell Biochem* **88**, 296–307.

49. DeLuca, H. (2004) Overview of general physiologic features and functions of vitamin D. *Am J Clin Nutr* **80**(supp), 1689S–96S.

50. Rachez, C.,, and Freedman, L.P. (2000) Mechanisms of gene regulation by vitamin D(3) receptor: A network of coactivator interactions. *Gene* **246**, 9–21.

51. Canaff, L.,, and Hendy, G.N. (2002) Human calcium-sensing receptor gene. Vitamin D response elements in promoters P1 and P2 confer transcriptional responsiveness to 1,25-dihydroxyvitamin D. *J Biol Chem* **277**, 30337–50.

52. Garland, C., and Garland, F. (1980) Do sunlight and Vitamin D reduce the likelihood of colon cancer? *Int J Epidemiol* **9**, 227–31.

53. Garland, C., Shekelle, R., and Barrett-Connor, E. (1985) Dietary vitamin D and calcium and risk of colorectal cancer: A 19-year prospective study in men. *Lancet* **1**, 307–09.

54. Martinez, M.E., and Willett, W.C. (1998) Calcium, vitamin D, and colorectal cancer: A review of the epidemiologic evidence. *Cancer Epidemiol Biomarkers Prev* **7**, 163–68.

55. Park, S.Y., Murphy, S.P., Wilkens, L.R., Nomura, A.M., Henderson, B.E., and Kolonel, L.N. (2007) Calcium and vitamin D intake and risk of colorectal cancer: The Multiethnic Cohort Study. *Am J Epidemiol* **165**, 784–93.

56. Mizoue, T., Kimura, Y., Toyomura, K., Nagano, J., Kono, S., Mibu, R. et al. (2008) Calcium, dairy foods, vitamin D and colorectal cancer risk: The Fukuoka Colorectal Cancer Study. *Cancer Epidemiol Biomarkers Prev* **17**, 2800–07.

57. Baron, J., Mandell, J., Beach, M., Van Stolk, R., Haile, R., Sandler, R. et al. (1999) Calcium supplements for the prevention of colorectal adenomas. *New Engl J Med* **340**, 101–07.

58. McCullough, M.L., Robertson, A.S., Rodriguez, C., Jacobs, E.J., Chao, A., Carolyn, J. et al. (2003) Calcium, vitamin D, dairy products, and risk of colorectal cancer in the Cancer Prevention Study II Nutrition Cohort (United States). *Cancer Causes Control* **14**, 1–12.

59. Kampman, E., Slattery, M.L., Caan, B., and Potter, J.D. (2000) Calcium, vitamin D, sunshine exposure, dairy products and colon cancer risk (United States). *Cancer Causes Control* **11**, 459–66.

60. Wu, K., Willett, W.C., Fuchs, C.S., Colditz, G.A., and Giovannucci, E.L. (2002) Calcium intake and risk of colon cancer in women and men. *J Natl Cancer Inst* **94**, 437–46.

61. Terry, P., Baron, J.A., Bergkvist, L., Holmberg, L., and Wolk, A. (2002) Dietary calcium and vitamin D intake and risk of colorectal cancer: A prospective cohort study in women. *Nutr Cancer* **43**, 39–46.

62. Flood, A., Peters, U., Chatterjee, N., Lacey, J., Schairer, C., and Schatzkin, A. (2005) Calcium from diet and supplements is associated with reduced risk of colorectal cancer in a prospective cohort of women. *Cancer Epidemiol Biomarkers Prev* **14**, 126–32.

63. Kesse, E., Boutron-Ruault, M.C., Norat, T., Riboli, E., and Clavel-Chapelon, F. (2005) Dietary calcium, phosphorus, vitamin D, dairy products and the risk of colorectal adenoma and cancer among French women of the E3N-EPIC prospective study. *Int J Cancer* **117**, 137–44.

64. Larsson, S.C., Bergkvist, L., Rutegard, J., Giovannucci, E., and Wolk, A. (2006) Calcium and dairy food intakes are inversely associated with colorectal cancer risk in the Cohort of Swedish Men. *Am J Clin Nutr* **83**, 667.

65. Miller, E.A., Keku, T.O., Satia, J.A., Martin, C.F., Galanko, J.A., and Sandler, R.S. (2005) Calcium, vitamin D, and apoptosis in the rectal epithelium. *Cancer Epidemiol Biomarkers Prev* **14**, 525–28.

66. Landa, M.C., Frago, N., and Tres, A. (1994) Diet and the risk of breast cancer in Spain. *Eur J Cancer Prev* **3**, 313–20.

67. Zaridze, D., Lifanova, Y., Maximovitch, D., Day, N.E., and Duffy, S.W. (1991) Diet, alcohol consumption and reproductive factors in a case-control study of breast cancer in Moscow. *Int J Cancer* **48**, 493–501.

68. Katsouyanni, K., Willett, W., Trichopoulos, D., Boyle, P., Trichopoulou, A., Vasilaros, S. et al. (1988) Risk of breast cancer among Greek women in relation to nutrient intake. *Cancer* **61**, 181–85.

69. Levi, F., Pasche, C., Lucchini, F., and La Vecchia, C. (2001) Dietary intake of selected micronutrients and breast-cancer risk. *Int J Cancer* **91**, 260–63.

70. Braga, C., La Vecchia, C., Negri, E., Franceschi, S., and Parpinel, M. (1997) Intake of selected foods and nutrients and breast cancer risk: An age- and menopause-specific analysis. *Nutr Cancer* **28**, 258–63.

71. Franceschi, S., Favero, A., Decarli, A., Negri, E., La Vecchia, C., Ferraroni, M. et al. (1996) Intake of macronutrients and risk of breast cancer. *Lancet* **347**, 1351–56.

72. Boyapati, S.M., Shu, X.O., Jin, F., Dai, Q., Ruan, Z., Gao, Y.T. et al. (2003) Dietary calcium intake and breast cancer risk among Chinese women in Shanghai. *Nutr Cancer* **46**, 38–43.

73. Adzersen, K.H., Jess, P., Freivogel, K.W., Gerhard, I., and Bastert, G. (2003) Raw and cooked vegetables, fruits, selected micronutrients, and breast cancer risk: A case-control study in Germany. *Nutr Cancer* **46**, 131–37.

74. Witte, J.S., Ursin, G., Siemiatycki, J., Thompson, W.D., Paganini-Hill, A., and Haile, R.W. (1997) Diet and premenopausal bilateral breast cancer: A case-control study. *Breast Cancer Res Treat* **42**, 243–51.

75. Van der Veer, P., van Leer, E.M., Rietdijk, A., Kok, F.J., Schouten, E.G., Hermus, R.J. et al. (1991) Combination of dietary factors in relation to breast-cancer occurrence. *Int J Cancer* **47**, 649–53.

76. Shin, M., Holmes, M., Hankinson, S., Wu, K., Colditz, G., and Willett, W. (2002) Intake of dairy products, calcium, and vitamin D and risk of breast cancer. *J Natl Cancer Inst* **94**, 1301–11.

77. McCullough, M.L., Rodriguez, C., Diver, W.R., Feigelson, H.S., Stevens, V.L., Thun, M.J. et al. (2005) Dairy, calcium, and vitamin D intake and postmenopausal breast cancer risk in the Cancer Prevention Study II Nutrition Cohort. *Cancer Epidemiol Biomarkers Prev* **14**, 2898–904.

78. Knekt, P., Jarvinen, R., Seppañnen, R., Pukkala, E., and Aromaa, A. (1996) Intake of dairy products and the risk of breast cancer. *Br J Cancer* **73**, 687–91.

79. Kesse-Guyot, E., Bertrais, S., Duperray, B., Arnault, N., Bar-Hen, A., Galan, P. et al. (2007) Dairy products, calcium and the risk of breast cancer: Results of the French SU.VI.MAX prospective study. *Ann Nutr Metab* **51**, 139–45.

80. Speers, C., and Brown, P. (2008) Breast cancer prevention using calcium and vitamin D: A bright future? *J Natl Cancer Inst* **100**, 1562–64.

81. Holmes, M.D., Stampfer, M.J., Colditz, G.A., Rosner, B., Hunter, D.J., and Willett, W.C. (1999) Dietary factors and the survival of women with breast carcinoma. *Cancer* **86**, 826–35.

82. Lin, J., Manson, J.E., Lee, I.M., Cook, N.R., Buring, J.E., and Zhang, S.M. (2007) Intakes of calcium and vitamin d and breast cancer risk in women. *Arch Intern Med* **167**, 1050–59.

83. Saftlas, A.F., Hoover, R.N., Brinton, L.A., Szklo, M., Olson, D.R., Salane, M. et al. (1991) Mammographic densities and risk of breast cancer. *Cancer* **67**, 2833–38.

84. Brisson, J., Diorio, C., and Maósse, B. (2003) Wolfe's parenchymal pattern and percentage of the breast with mammographic densities: Redundant or complementary classifications? *Cancer Epidemiol Biomarkers Prev* **12**, 728–32.

85. Li, T., Sun, L., Miller, N., Nicklee, T., Woo, J., Hulse-Smith, L. et al. (2005) The association of measured breast tissue characteristics with mammographic density and other risk factors for breast cancer. *Cancer Epidemiol Biomarkers Prev* **14**, 343–49.

86. Boyd, N.F., Lockwood, G.A., Byng, J.W., Tritchler, D.L., and Yaffe, M.J. (1998) Mammographic densities and breast cancer risk. *Cancer Epidemiol Biomarkers Prev* **7**, 1133–44.

87. Berube, S., Diorio, C., Maósse, B.T., Hebert-Croteau, N., Byrne, C., Cote, G. et al. (2005) Vitamin D and calcium intakes from food or supplements and mammographic breast density. *Cancer Epidemiol Biomarkers Prev* **14**, 1653–59.

88. Berube, S., Diorio, C., Verhoek-Oftedahl, W., and Brisson, J. (2004) Vitamin D, calcium, and mammographic breast densities. *Cancer Epidemiol Biomarkers Prev* **13**, 1466–72.

89. Vachon, C.M., Kushi, L.H., Cerhan, J.R., Kuni, C.C., and Sellers, T.A. (2000) Association of diet and mammographic breast density in the Minnesota breast cancer family cohort. *Cancer Epidemiol Biomarkers Prev* **9**, 151–60.

90. Rodriguez, C., McCullough, M.L., Mondul, A.M., Jacobs, E.J., Fakhrabadi-Shokoohi, D., Giovan-nucci, E.L. et al. (2003) Calcium, dairy products, and risk of prostate cancer in a prospective cohort of United States men. *Cancer Epidemiol Biomarkers Prev* **12**, 597–603.

91. Giovannucci, E., Liu, Y., Stampfer, M.J., and Willett, W.C. (2006) A prospective study of calcium intake and incident and fatal prostate cancer. *Cancer Epidemiol Biomarkers Prev* **15**, 203–10.

92. Giovannucci, E., Liu, Y., Platz, E.A., Stampfer, M.J., and Willett, W.C. (2007) Risk factors for prostate cancer incidence and progression in the health professionals follow-up study. *Int J Cancer* **121**, 1571–78.

93. Tseng, M., Breslow, R., Graubard, B., and Ziegler, R. (2005) Dairy, calcium, and vitamin D intakes and prostate cancer risk in the National Health and Nutrition Examination Epidemiologic Follow-up Study cohort. *Am J Clin Nutr* **81**, 1147–54.

94. Kurahashi, N., Inoue, M., Iwasaki, M., Sasazuki, S., and Tsugane, A.S. (2008) Dairy product, sat-urated fatty acid, and calcium intake and prostate cancer in a prospective cohort of Japanese men. *Cancer Epidemiol Biomarkers Prev* **17**, 930–37.

95. Mitrou, P., Albanes, D., Weinstein, S., Pietinen, P., Taylor, P., Virtamo, J. et al. (2007) A prospective study of dietary calcium, dairy products and prostate cancer risk. *Int J Cancer* **120**, 2466–73.

96. Hayes, R.B., Ziegler, R.G., Gridley, G., Swanson, C., Greenberg, R.S., Swanson, G.M. et al. (1999) Dietary factors and risks for prostate cancer among blacks and whites in the United States. *Cancer Epidemiol Biomarkers Prev* **8**, 25–34.

97. Berndt, S.I., Carter, H.B., Landis, P.K., Tucker, K.L., Hsieh, L.J., Metter, E.J. et al. (2002) Calcium intake and prostate cancer risk in a long-term aging study: The Baltimore Longitudinal Study of Aging. *Urology* **60**, 1118–23.

98. Tavani, A., Bertuccio, P., Bosetti, C., Talamini, R., Negri, E., Franceschi, S. et al. (2005) Dietary intake of calcium, vitamin D, phosphorus and the risk of prostate cancer. *Eur Urol* **48**, 27–33.

99. Kristal, A.R., Cohen, J.H., Qu, P., and Stanford, J.L. (2002) Associations of energy, fat, calcium, and vitamin D with prostate cancer risk. *Cancer Epidemiol Biomarkers Prev* **11**, 719–25.

100. Chan, J.M., Pietinen, P., VCancer Epidemiol Biomarkers Previrtanen, M., Malila, N., Tangrea, J., Albanes, D. et al. (2000) Diet and prostate cancer risk in a cohort of smokers, with a specific focus on calcium and phosphorus (Finland). *Cancer Causes Control* **11**, 859–67.

101. Chan, J.M., Stampfer, M.J., Ma, J., Gann, P.H., Gaziano, J.M., and Giovannucci, E.L. (2001) Dairy products, calcium, and prostate cancer risk in the Physicians' Health Study. *Am J Clin Nutr* **74**, 549–54.

102. Gao, X., LaValley, M.P., and Tucker, K.L. (2005) Prospective studies of dairy product and calcium intakes and prostate cancer risk: A meta-analysis. *J Natl Cancer Inst* **97**, 1768–77.

103. Severi, G., English, D.R., Hopper, J.L., and Giles, G.G. (2006) Re: Prospective studies of dairy prod-uct and calcium intakes and prostate cancer risk: A meta-analysis. *J Natl Cancer Inst* **98**, 794.

104. Huncharek, M. (2008) Dairy products, dietary calcium and vitamin D intake as risk factors for prostate cancer: A meta-analysis of 26,769 cases from observational studies. *Nutr Cancer* **60**, 421–41.

105. Giovannucci, E. (1998) Dietary influences of 1,25(OH)2 vitamin D in relation to prostate cancer: A hypothesis. *Cancer Causes Control* **9**, 567–82.

106. Lips, P. (2006) Vitamin D physiology. *Prog Biophysics Mol Biol* **92**, 4–8.

107. Reichel, H., Koeffler, H.P., and Norman, A.W. (1989) The role of the vitamin D endocrine system in health and disease. *New Engl J Med* **320**, 980–91.

108. Schwartz, G., Whitlatch, L., Chen, T., Lokeshwar, B., and Holick, M. (1998) Human prostate cells synthesize 1, 25-dihydroxyvitamin D3 from 25-hydroxyvitamin D3. *Cancer Epidemiol Biomarkers Prev* **7**, 391–95.

109. Hsieh, T., Ng, C., Mallouh, C., Tazaki, H., and Wu, J. (1996) Regulation of growth, PSA/PAP and androgen receptor expression by 1 alpha, 25-dihydroxyvitamin D3 in androgen-dependent LNCaP cells. *Biochem Biophys Res Commun* **223**, 141–46.

110. Konety, B., Schwartz, G., Acierno, J., Becich, M., and Getzenberg, R. (1996) The role of vitamin D in normal prostate growth and differentiation. *Cell Growth Differ* **7**, 1563–70.

111. Lucia, M., Anzano, M., Slayter, M., Anver, M., Green, D., Shrader, M. et al. (1995) Chemo-preventive activity of tamoxifen, N-(4-hydroxyphenyl)retinamide, and the vitamin D analogue

Ro24-5531 for androgen-promoted carcinomas of the rat seminal vesicle and prostate. *Cancer Res* **55**, 5621–27.

112. Ahonen, M., Tenkanen, L., and Teppo, L. (2000) Prostate cancer risk and prediagnostic serum 25-hydroxyvitamin D levels (Finland). *Cancer Causes Control* **11**, 847–52.

113. Luscombe, C.J., Fryer, A.A., French, M.E., Liu, S., Saxby, M.F., Jones, P.W. et al. (2001) Exposure to ultraviolet radiation: Association with susceptibility and age at presentation with prostate cancer. *Lancet* **358**, 641–2.

114. Gann, P., Ma, J., and Hennekens, C. (1996) Circulating vitamin D metabolites in relation to subsequent development of prostate cancer. *Cancer Epidemiol Biomarkers Prev* **5**, 121–26.

115. Gallagher, J.C., Riggs, B.L., Eisman, J., Hamstra, A., Arnaud, S.B., and DeLuca, H.F. (1979) Intestinal calcium absorption and serum vitamin D metabolites in normal subjects and osteoporotic patients: Effect of age and dietary calcium. *J Clin Invest* **64**, 729–36.

116. Ferrari, S.L., Bonjour, J.P., and Rizzoli, R. (2005) Fibroblast growth factor-23 relationship to dietary phosphate and renal phosphate handling in healthy young men. *J Clin Endocrinol Metab* **90**, 1519–24.

117. Braun, M.M., Helzlsouer, K.J., Hollis, B.W., and Comstock, G.W. (1995) Prostate cancer and prediagnostic levels of serum vitamin D metabolites (Maryland, United States). *Cancer Causes Control* **6**, 235–39.

118. Nomura, A.M., Stemmermann, G.N., Lee, J., Kolonel, L.N., Chen, T.C., Turner, A. et al. (1998) Serum vitamin D metabolite levels and the subsequent development of prostate cancer (Hawaii, United States). *Cancer Causes Control* **9**, 425–32.

119. Jacobs, E.T., Giuliano, A.R., Martinez, M.E., Hollis, B.W., Reid, M.E., and Marshall, J.R. (2004) Plasma levels of 25-hydroxyvitamin D, 1,25-dihydroxyvitamin D and the risk of prostate cancer. *J Steroid Biochem Mol Biol* **89–90**, 533–37.

120. Platz, E.A., Leitzmann, M.F., Hollis, B.W., Willett, W.C., and Giovannucci, E. (2004) Plasma 1,25-dihydroxy- and 25-hydroxyvitamin D and subsequent risk of prostate cancer. *Cancer Causes Control* **15**, 255–65.

121. Baron, J., Beach, M., Wallace, K., Grau, M., Sandler, R., Mandeli, J. et al. (2005) Risk of prostate cancer in a randomized clinical trial of calcium supplementation. *Cancer Epidemiol Biomarkers Prev* **14**, 586–89.

122. Young, M.V., Schwartz, G.G., Wang, L., Jamieson, D.P., Whitlatch, L.W., Flanagan, J.N. et al. (2004) The prostate 25-hydroxyvitamin D-1 alpha-hydroxylase is not influenced by parathyroid hormone and calcium: Implications for prostate cancer chemoprevention by vitamin D. *Carcinogenesis* **25**, 967–71.

123. Midgeley, R., and Kerr, D. (1999) Colorectal cancer. *Lancet* **353**, 391–99.

124. Wallace, K., Baron, J.A., Cole, B.F., Sandler, R.S., Karagas, M.R., Beach, M.A. et al. (2004) Effect of calcium supplementation on the risk of large bowel polyps. *J Natl Cancer Inst* **96**, 921–25.

125. Grau, M., Baron, J., Sandler, R., Haile, R., Beach, M., Church, T. et al. (2003) Vitamin D, calcium supplementation, and colorectal adenomas: Results of a randomized trial. *J Natl Cancer Inst* **95**, 1765–71.

126. Bonithon-Kopp, C., Kronborg, O., Giacosa, A., Rath, U., and Faivre, J. (2000) Calcium and fibre supplementation in prevention of colorectal adenoma recurrence: A randomised intervention trial. European Cancer Prevention Organisation Study Group. *Lancet* **356**, 1300–06.

127. Weingarten, M., Zalmanovici, A., and Yaphe, J.. (2008) Dietary calcium supplementation for preventing colorectal cancer and adenomatous polyps (Review). Cochrane.Database.Syst.Rev. 1–16. John Wiley & Sons.

128. Wactawski Wende, J., Kotchen, J.M., Anderson, G.L., Assaf, A.R., Brunner, R.L., O'Sullivan, M.J. et al. (2006) Calcium plus vitamin D supplementation and the risk of colorectal cancer. *N Engl J Med* **354**, 684–96.

129. Chlebowski, R., Johnson, K., Kooperberg, C., Pettinger, M., Wactawski-Wende, J., Rohan, T. et al. (2008) Calcium plus vitamin D supplementation and the risk of breast cancer. *J Natl Cancer Inst* **100**, 1581–91.

130. Jackson, R.D., LaCroix, A.Z., Gass, M., Wallace, R.B., Robbins, J., Lewis, C.E. et al. (2006) Calcium plus vitamin D supplementation and the risk of fractures. *N Engl J Med* **354**, 669–83.
131. Gorham, E.D., Garland, C.F., Garland, F.C., Grant, W.B., Mohr, S.B., Lipkin, M. et al. (2007) Optimal vitamin D status for colorectal cancer prevention: A quantitative meta analysis. *Am J Prev Med* **32**, 210–16.
132. Lappe, J.M., Travers Gustafson, D., Davies, K.M., Recker, R.R., and Heaney, R.P. (2007) Vitamin D and calcium supplementation reduces cancer risk: Results of a randomized trial. *Am J Clin Nutr* **85**, 1586–91.
133. Heaney, R. (2006) Nutrition and chronic disease. *Mayo Clin Proc* **81**, 297–99.
134. National Academy of Science (1999) Dietary Reference Intakes for Calcium, Magnesium, Phosphorus, Vitamin D, and Fluoride. Washington, DC: Food and Nutrition Board, Institute of Medicine. National Academy Press.
135. Heaney, R. (2008) Nutrients, endpoints, and the problem of proof. *J Nutr* **138**, 1591–95.

21 Iron and Cancer

James R. Connor and Sang Y. Lee

Key Points

1. As a transition element, iron is essential for reducing oxygen for the production of ATP by mitochondria. It is therefore critical for normal cell function. At the same time, because of its ability to reduce oxygen, iron is the most potent inducer of free radicals in most biological systems.
2. Excess iron accumulation in the body can lead to increased risk of cancer, but excess accumulation and storage of iron is usually associated with a genetic mutation or mutations.
3. Because iron is required for many normal cellular functions, an overall recommendation that people limit iron intake due to cancer risks cannot be formulated based on available experimental data.
4. Hemochromatosis is the disease resulting from significant iron overload in tissue, especially in the liver. Therefore, liver cancer (hepatocellular carcinoma) is the primary cancer associated with iron overload. There is compelling evidence, however, that carrying the HFE gene variants without the clinical disease of hereditary hemochromatosis is associated with breast cancer, colorectal cancer, acute lymphoblastic leukemia, and may predict outcomes in brain tumors.
5. The FDA recommended dietary allowance for iron varies with age and gender, ranging from 6 mg/d for adult men 19–70+ years of age to 18 mg/d of iron for menstruating women 19–50 years of age. The recommended dietary allowance of iron for infants (7–12 months), children, adolescents, and teens is in this range. A recommended dietary allowance has not been set for infants 0–6 months of age.

Key Words: Iron; free radicals; iron intake; cancer risk; HFE gene variants

Abbreviations

DFO	desferrioxamine
DMT1	divalent metal transporter 1
IRE	iron-responsive element
IRP	iron regulatory protein
TfR	transferrin receptor

From: *Nutrition and Health: Bioactive Compounds and Cancer*
Edited by: J.A. Milner, D.F. Romagnolo, DOI 10.1007/978-1-60761-627-6_21,
© Springer Science+Business Media, LLC 2010

1. INTRODUCTION

As a transition element, iron is essential for reducing oxygen for the production of ATP by mitochondria. It is therefore critical for normal cell function. At the same time, because of its ability to reduce oxygen, iron is the most potent inducer of free radicals in most biological systems. Free radicals are well known to cause DNA damage that can lead to mutations that result in a cell becoming cancerous. Once a cell becomes cancerous its iron requirement can increase dramatically because of the characteristic elevated metabolism observed in cancer cells. The mitotic activity of the tumor itself can also drive iron requirements higher because enzymes such as ribonucleotide reductase, the rate-limiting step in DNA synthesis, require iron as a co-factor. The increased iron requirements for tumors often contribute to the anemia of chronic disease seen in cancer patients *(1)*. Iron also has essential functions in the immune system and normal functioning of the immune system is critical to cancer biology. A detailed review of the role of iron in the immune system and cancer is beyond the scope of this review. In brief, iron also modulates immune cell proliferation and host immune surveillance. Cancer cells disrupt the immune system through iron deficiency environment in the immune cells *(2)*. Inflammation also promotes tumor development *(3)*. The host immune system reacts against tumor-specific antigens or tumor-associated antigens. This leads to the use of antibodies and T cells in cancer immunotherapy, immunosuppression therapy, and cancer vaccine development *(4)*.

1.1. Iron Consumption

Certainly, excess iron accumulation in the body can lead to increased risk of cancer, but excess accumulation and storage of iron is usually associated with a genetic mutation or mutations and will be discussed later in this chapter. The average amount of iron in the human body is 2.3 g for women and 3.8 g for men. The majority of iron in the body is absorbed from the diet. Not only is there a wide variety of the amount of iron in food, but the amount of absorbable iron is different among different foods. This latter point has made a direct analysis of iron consumption in foods and cancer risk difficult to prove. Furthermore, humans absorb heme iron better than any other form of iron *(5)*. Foods that are enriched in heme iron include meat, pork, and fish. Foods with high iron content in a non-heme form include breakfast cereals, cooked beans, pumpkin seeds, and blackstrap molasses. Rice, beans, and green vegetables contain a relatively high iron concentration; however, only 1–6% of the iron in these foods is absorbed into the body compared to the 10–20% of iron in fish and meat. Milk and milk products are low in iron content.

1.2. Dietary Iron Intake and Cancer

Nutritional epidemiologic studies seeking to establish a relationship between food consumption and cancer have been inconclusive, and it is difficult to compare these studies. In general, dietary intake of iron from food sources has been associated with risks of colorectal, lung, and other cancers. Red and processed meat consumption has been associated with increased risk of colorectal cancer *(6, 7)*. In a contrasting study on Canadian women, no association was found between intake of iron, heme iron, or iron from meat with overall risk of colorectal cancer *(8)*. However, individuals who were classified as having a diet high in red meat had significantly increased nitrosyl iron and nitrosothiols compared to individuals on a vegetarian diet. This increased uptake of nitrosyl iron via red or processed meat is associated with colorectal cancer *(9)*. In the heme supplemented diet of a randomized crossover human study, there was a twofold increase in 1,4-dihydroxynonane mercapturic acid (DHN-MA), the major urinary metabolite of 4-hydroxynonenal, indicating that the heme supplemented diet puts a person at risk for colon cancer *(10)*. Another study suggested that the elevated risk of colon cancer observed with heme iron intake can be decreased by chlorophyll intake *(11)*.

The risk of other cancers that have been associated with dietary iron intake include hepatocellular carcinoma, breast, lung, rectal, and prostate cancer. Iron intake via the diet was associated with increased hepatocellular carcinoma risk in an Italian population, but this association was considerably reduced by wine *(12)*. In Chinese women, heme iron intake was positively associated with breast cancer risk *(13)*. However, there has been no association of iron or heme iron intake with overall risk of breast cancer in Canadian women consuming ≥ 30 g of alcohol per day or in women who have used hormone replacement therapy *(8)*. Dietary iron may play an important role in the development of lung cancer, especially among current smokers based on a study of 923 patients with lung cancer and 1,125 healthy controls in Massachusetts *(14)*. At increased transferrin saturation levels, a daily intake of dietary iron more than 18 mg is associated with an increased risk of lung cancer *(15)*. Consumption of fresh red and processed meat maybe associated with an increased risk of rectal cancer in an Australian population *(16)*. A recent study on prostate cancer did not find an association between iron intake and overall risk, but there was a suggestion of increased risk of clinically aggressive prostate cancer with higher iron intake *(17)*. As mentioned before, not all studies found an association between dietary iron intake and cancer risk. For example, some investigations found no association between iron intake in meat or any of the other dietary iron-related sources with risk of cancers such as endometrial cancer *(18)* or childhood acute lymphoblastic leukemia *(19)*.

Vegetarian diets have been described as being deficient in several nutrients including iron, but they do not have a higher prevalence of iron-deficient anemia than control groups *(20–22)*. In an English study that involved a 17-year follow-up of 11,000 vegetarians, there was reduced mortality from all combined cancers of malignant neoplasms, lung cancer, colorectal cancer, and breast cancer *(23)*, but the findings did not translate to a broader population *(24)*. The positive findings in the initial study were attributed to the high levels of fresh fruits consumed by this population as opposed to the decreased amount of iron in the diet. From that standpoint, most researchers believe that fresh vegetables are beneficial for cancer prevention. One vegetable with relatively high iron is perilla. Perilla also has anti-cancer and anti-bacterial properties thought to result from its high vitamin and anti-oxidant content *(25)*. Furthermore, the phytol and methyl 11,14,17-eicosatrienoic acid of perilla leaves inhibited the growth of human colon, osteosarcoma, and gastric cancer cells as well as decreased DNA synthesis in these cells. Other chapters in this book will review the subject of cancer and antioxidants.

An additional confounding variable when trying to determine iron consumption and cancer is that the amount of iron absorbed from food is affected by what is being consumed at the same time. Uptake of iron in the body is increased when it is consumed with vitamin C and other acidic substances like tomatoes, but uptake is decreased when accompanied by food containing tannins like red wine, phytin acid of grain flours, and phytol from plants. The amount of iron absorbed is also affected by the iron-need in the body. Low iron status will increase iron absorption.

The amount of iron uptake from food is tightly regulated at the level of the gut. Excessive iron absorption can lead to a disease known as hemochromatosis. However, even without the full blown disease of hemochromatosis, a number of studies have shown that higher amounts of iron in the blood are associated with an increased risk of cancer.

1.3. Measurement of Body Iron

Measurements of serum iron status are thought to reflect total body iron status, although serum iron itself is probably a poor indicator of total body iron *(26)*. Thus, measurement of transferrin (the iron mobilization protein) saturation has been used to determine the iron status in the body. Under normal physiological conditions, transferrin in the serum is about 30% saturated with iron, but the levels of saturation can increase with iron overload or decrease with iron deficiency. The total amounts of transferrin in the blood are not a good indicator of body iron status and measurements of transferrin saturation for clinical use are not practical. The amount of ferritin, normally considered an iron storage protein, but clearly released into the serum in significant amounts has also been used to report on body iron stores. The concentration of this protein in the blood can vary significantly under conditions of inflammation and normal values range dramatically. Ferritin in the serum, as discussed later, may also be a prognostic indicator for cancer. The most recent protein to be used as a serum marker to reflect body iron stores is the soluble (cleaved extracellular portion) transferrin receptor. To date, this measurement has proven the most reliable with increased soluble receptor indicating low iron *(27, 28)*. There is a fairly large body of literature on the use of blood markers to determine iron status and cancer risk. Studies evaluating the relationship between serum iron, iron proteins in the serum, and elevated iron in cancer have been summarized in Table 1.

1.4. Iron Metabolism and Regulation in Cancer Tissue

In addition to serum iron levels, cancerous tissue itself has higher than normal iron levels. For example, biopsies of breast cancer have shown significantly higher levels of iron and other metals (nickel, zinc, etc.) compared to normal tissues *(29)*. Liver iron overload is associated with hepatocellular carcinoma in patients with end-stage liver disease *(30)*. Hepatocellular carcinoma was also associated with patients with hepatitis B, hepatitis C, and hereditary hemochromatosis. The cellular relationship between iron and cancer is thought to stem from the effects of iron accumulation on enhancing oxidative stress and subsequent damage to DNA *(31–33)*. Compared to normal cells, cancer cells have higher iron requirements *(34–36)* and exhibit greater sensitivity to iron chelators *(37, 38)*. This higher iron demand of cancer cells has been exploited in studies that used

Table 1
Body Iron is a Predictor of Cancer Risk

Iron measure	Tumor type	Found a relationship with elevated iron	References
Serum iron	Colorectal cancer	Yes. Transferrin saturation is also significantly higher	Wurzelmann et al. (131)
Serum iron	Lung cancer	No. Serum copper was markedly elevated but serum zinc was significantly reduced	el-Ahmady et al. (132)
Serum iron	Lung cancer	Yes. Very low density lipoprotein cholesterol was also associated with an increased risk	Mainous et al. (133)
Serum iron	Oral leukoplakia and squamous cell carcinoma	No. Copper was significantly increased. In carcinomas, serum iron was significantly decreased	Jayadeep et al. (134)
Serum ferritin	Breast cancer	Yes. Auxiliary lymph node metastases rate was also increased, but serum iron, transferrin, and transferrin receptor were not increased	Ulbrich et al. (135)
Serum ferritin	Colon cancer, breast cancer, and prostate cancer	Yes. Iron status was not related to cancer risk in men, but women with serum ferritin concentrations > 160 µg/l had an increased risk of cancer. Serum transferrin was not related to the risk of cancer in either men or women	Hercberg et al. (136)
Serum ferritin	Colorectal cancer	No. Inverse association between serum ferritin and colorectal cancer risk	Cross et al. (137)
Total iron or heme iron	Breast cancer	No. Alcohol was associated with increased risk of breast cancer	Kabat et al. (8)
Serum ferritin, transferrin saturation	Prostate cancer	No. Body iron is inversely associated in men with prostate cancer compared to healthy controls	Kuvibidila et al. (138)
Serum transferrin saturation	Cirrhosis or liver cancer	Yes. Effect is greater with elevated alcohol consumption	Ioannou et al. (139)
Total iron	Malignant lymphoma	No. Soluble transferrin receptor levels in serum were increased	Bjerner et al. (140)

antisense ferritin oligonucleotides to limit tumor growth *(39)* or target the iron uptake mechanism of tumors to deliver cytotoxins *(40)*.

The regulation of cellular iron uptake and storage depends on several proteins. Transferrin carries iron to a cell and binds to a transferrin receptor. The transferrin receptor can bind to two transferrin molecules at one time. Transferrin carries two atoms of iron when it binds to the receptor so a single binding event can deliver four atoms of iron. There are two types of transferrin receptor (TfR). The TfR1 is a primary cellular iron homeostasis protein, and the TfR2 is an emerging key player in the regulation of iron homeostasis. For example, mutations in TfR2 are responsible for type 3 hereditary hemochromatosis. The Tf-Fe and TfR complex is internalized via receptor-mediated endocytosis *(41)*. Iron is released from the endosome through a transport protein known as divalent metal transporter 1 (DMT1) and joins the labile iron pool *(42)*. Once inside the cell, if not immediately required in the myriad of metabolic processes in which it plays a role, iron is stored in ferritin. Ferritin is a dynamic protein made of differing ratios of two subunits; H and L-ferritin. The H subunit contains ferroxidase activity and is responsible for converting soluble ferrous (Fe^{+2}) iron to the storable (Fe^{+3}) form. The L subunit does not have ferroxidase activity, and thus stores iron at a very low rate compared with the H subunit *(43)*.

Another protein responsible for the maintenance of cellular iron homeostasis is the iron-regulatory protein (IRP), which coordinates ferritin and Tf receptor translation in response to iron availability. The IRP1 coordinately controls the expression of transferrin receptor 1 (TfR1) and ferritin by binding to iron-responsive elements (IREs) within their mRNAs. A second isoform of IRP, IRP2, is a mammalian cytosolic iron sensing protein that regulates expression of iron metabolism proteins *(44)*.

Recently a new iron regulatory protein has been discovered known as hepcidin *(45)*. Hepcidin is up-regulated in response to increased iron or inflammatory stimuli and reduces serum iron by promoting iron retention in the reticuloendothelial macrophages. Iron sequestration in macrophages is used as a defense mechanism against infection, and it also has a beneficial effect on the control of cancer *(46)*.

Another key protein in maintaining cellular iron homeostasis is HFE. This protein also plays a key role in iron absorption from the gut, and variations in the gene for this protein are associated with the iron overload disorder known as hemochromatosis as discussed above. Normally, HFE negatively regulates transferrin receptor-mediated iron uptake. Increased HFE expression is associated with decreased iron uptake and can result in iron deficiency anemia *(47)*. The two most common HFE gene variants are H63D and C282Y. These gene variants are the most common in Caucasians. A single mutation of G to A at nucleotide 845 results in the substitution of tyrosine for cysteine at amino acid 282 resulting in the Cys282Tyr or C282Y polymorphism. A second mutation of C to G at nucleotide 187 results in a substitution of aspartate for histidine at amino acid 63. This His63Asp or H63D polymorphism does not, except in very rare instances, occur on the same allele as C282Y *(48)*. When the H63D allele is present, the HFE protein will migrate to the surface, but will not sterically hinder the interaction of Tf with the TfR. The C282Y allele causes the HFE protein to remain within the cytosol and not migrate to the membrane (for a review see *(49)*). The binding of Tf to the TfR requires that Tf be loaded with iron. Therefore, when HFE is not present or functional the uptake of iron into cells can not be limited once iron is bound to Tf. Consequently, more iron will enter the cell because transferrin binds to both sites of the transferrin receptor *(50)*. All functions of the above discussed iron metabolism proteins have been summarized in Table 2.

1.5. Expression of Iron Metabolism Genes and Proteins in Cancer

Because of the tight cellular regulation of iron, mutations or significant changes in expression patterns in proteins responsible for regulation of iron uptake from the gut and storage at the cellular level may be expected to have an impact on cancer risk. Studies that have examined these associations are summarized in Table 3.

1.5.1. FERRITIN

Tumor initiation and/or progression can be closely associated with over-expression of ferritin during tumor development in a number of cancers. Levels of H-ferritin mRNA increased in a rat tumor model of hepatocellular carcinoma and were more than 10-fold over-expressed as the tumor progressed. Thus, it was suggested that ferritin expression level is a useful early marker for hepatocellular carcinoma *(51)*. In addition, H-ferritin gene expression is amplified in breast cancer patients *(52)*. The L-ferritin gene and protein were also over-expressed in human metastatic melanoma cells and melanoma tissues *(53)*. In addition, the expression of ferritin in cancer cells correlates with their status as migratory versus core proliferating cells *(54)*. Furthermore, cancer cells expressed H-ferritin in the cell nucleus *(55)*. Although the role of nuclear H-ferritin has not been clearly elucidated, studies have suggested it may enhance tumor cell growth. Therefore, some studies have targeted ferritin to reduced tumor growth. For example, antisense to both H- and L-ferritin oligodeoxynucleotides specifically inhibited MCF-7 breast carcinoma cell growth through increased apoptosis as well as inhibition of DNA synthesis and gene expression *(39)*. In a human metastatic melanoma cell line, down-regulation of L-ferritin by antisense mRNA inhibited cell proliferation in vitro and cell growth in vivo *(53)*. This study also found that down-regulation of L-ferritin in human metastatic melanoma cells enhanced sensitivity to oxidative stress and to apoptosis. We also observed that silencing of the H-ferritin gene using small interfering RNA (siRNA) increased sensitivity of chemotherapeutic agents in a glioma cell line *(56)* and limited tumor growth *(57)*.

1.5.2. TRANSFERRIN RECEPTOR

Transferrin receptor (TfR) is the primary mechanism for cellular iron acquisition; thus, it is not surprising that this protein is up-regulated in diverse cancer cells including pancreatic cancer, chronic lymphocytic leukemia, carcinomas, and sarcomas *(52, 58–60)*. In addition, a relationship between the expression of TfR1 and the grade of cancer was also observed in colorectal carcinoma *(61)* and malignant epithelial cells *(59)*. Although different levels of TfR mRNA expression have been reported in lymphocytic leukemia samples, protein expression levels appear to be nearly similar. This finding is consistent with the evidence that the expression of TfR is post-transcriptionally controlled *(58)*.

Table 2
Iron Metabolism Proteins and Their Functions

Gene name	Gene symbol	Protein name	Protein symbol	Functions
Cytochrome B reductase 1	*CYBRD1*	Duodenal cytochrome B	DCYTB	Ferric reductase activity, dietary iron absorption
Solute carrier family 11 (proton coupled divalent metal ion transporters), member 2	*SLC11A2*	Divalent metal ion transporter 1	DMT1	Ferrous ion membrane transport
Solute carrier family 40 (iron-regulated transporters), member 1	*SLC40A1*	Ferroportin	FPN	Involved iron export from duodenal epithelial cells
Hepcidin antimicrobial peptide	*HAMP*	Hepcidin	HEPC	Maintenance of iron homeostasis, regulation of iron storage in macrophage, intestinal iron absorption
Hemochromatosis	*HFE*	HFE	HFE	Regulate iron absorption
Ferritin, heavy polypeptide 1	*FTH1*	H-ferritin	FTH	Storage of iron in a soluble uptake and nontoxic state
Aconitase 1, soluble	*ACO1*	Iron regulatory protein 1	IRP1	Cellular iron homeostasis
Iron-responsive element binding protein 2	*IRPB2*	Iron regulatory protein 2	IRP2	Cellular iron homeostasis
Ferritin, light polypeptide 1	*FTL*	L-ferritin	FTL	Storage of iron in a soluble uptake and nontoxic state
Transferrin receptor (p90, CD71)	*TFRC*	Transferrin receptor 1	TfR1	Cellular uptake of transferrin-bound iron
Transferrin receptor 2	*TFR2*	Transferrin receptor 2	TfR2	Cellular uptake of transferrin-bound iron
Transferrin	*TF*	Transferrin	Tf	Iron carrier

Table 3
Over-Expression of Iron Metabolism Genes and Proteins in Cancer Cells and Patients

Protein	Expression level	Key findings	References
Ferritin	Over-expression	Ferritin was found in 88% of endometrial carcinoma, but absent in normal and hyperplastic endometria	Tsionou et al. (141)
Ferritin	Over-expression	High expression of ferritin was found in renal cell carcinoma and expression level was significantly related to tumor stage	Yu et al. (142)
Ferritin	Over-expression	Infants at 3 weeks screening, 4 of 44 neuroblastoma had elevated serum ferritin. At 6 months screening, 14 of 54 neuroblastoma patients had elevated ferritin	Brodeur et al. (143)
Ferritin	Over-expression	High mRNA levels in migratory F98 cells and also showed higher protein expression in the infiltrating edge of human gliomas	Holtkamp et al. (54)
H-Ferritin	Over-expression	Over-expression of H-ferritin during tumor development is correlated with tumor initiation and/or progression	Wu et al. (51)
L-ferritin	Over-expression	L-ferritin over-expression in human metastatic melanoma cells	Maresca et al. (144)
TfR	Over-expression	TfR is not expressed in normal lung tissue but expressed in the majority of lung cancers	Whitney et al. (145)
TfR, H-ferritin	Over-expression	TfR mRNA levels were positively correlated with the ferritin H-chain mRNA levels in 42 breast cancer patients	Yang et al. (52)

(Continued)

Table 3
(Continued)

Protein	Expression level	Key findings	References
TfR	Over-expression	Over-expression of TfR1 and TfR2 in chronic lymphocytic leukemia	Smilevska et al. (58)
DCYTB, DMT1, TfR1	Over-expression	Progression to colorectal cancer is associated with increased expression in iron import proteins (DCYTB, DMT1, TfR1) and a block in iron export due to decreased expression and aberrant localization of hephaestin and ferroportin in 11 human colorectal cancers	Brookes et al. (65)
DCYTB, DMT1, TfR1	Over-expression	Progression to adenocarcinoma is associated with increased expression of iron import proteins	Boult et al. (146)
TfR2	Over-expression	TfR2 was frequently expressed in ovarian cancer, colon cancer, and glioblastoma cell lines	Calzolari et al. (63)
IRP1	Over-expression	Over-expression of IRP1 is associated with an apparent tumor suppressor phenotype	Chen et al. (67)
Hepcidin	Over-expression	Hepcidin induction by p53 might be involved in the pathogenesis of anemia accompanying cancer	Weizer-Stern et al. (46)

DCYTB, duodenal cytochrome b; DMT1, divalent metal transporter 1; IRP1, iron regulatory protein 1; TfR1, transferrin receptor 1; TfR2, transferrin receptor 2

An additional transferrin receptor protein, transferrin receptor 2 (TfR2), is expressed in tumor cell lines. TfR2 is normally found in liver cells, but not in normal erythroid cells *(62)*. It is weakly expressed in leukemia and melanoma cell lines, but more strongly present in other types of cancer cells such as ovarian, colon, and glioblastoma *(63)*. In these different tumor cells, TfR2 expression was inversely related to that of TfR1 *(63)*. However, significant correlations were noted between the transcription levels of both TfR1 and TfR2-α (membrane form) and TfR1 and TfR2-β (non-membrane form) in acute myeloid leukemia *(42)*. Whereas TfR2 is mainly associated with the plasma membrane where it promotes activation of ERK1/ERK2 and p38 MAP kinases, TfR1 is largely distributed to intracellular organelles and spontaneously undergoes endocytosis and recycling *(64)*.

1.5.3. OTHER IRON PROTEINS

A few studies have examined the involvement of other proteins in iron metabolism and reported distinct patterns of expression. For example, increased expression of the duodenal cytochrome b (DCYTB) and divalent metal transporter 1 (DMT1) were reported in colorectal cancers. These results would be consistent with increased cellular iron uptake. In contrast, the total expression level of iron efflux proteins such as ferroportin (also known as MTP1) were decreased in colorectal tumors and closely associated with cancer progress *(65)*.

Increased iron deposition along with over-expression of DMT1, TfR1, DCYTB, ferroportin, and H-ferritin were observed in adenocarcinoma. Over-expression of DMT1 was further associated with metastatic adenocarcinoma. Like nuclear ferritin, the IRE form of DMT1 was found in the nucleus in astrocytomas and primary and neoplastic glial cells *(66)*. These data support the concept that cancer cells may have unique nuclear requirements for iron and offer potential novel targets for interference gene therapy.

Iron regulatory protein 1 (IRP1) is the protein responsible for post-transcriptional regulation of the transferrin receptor and ferritin, and it controls the expression of TfR1 and ferritin by binding to iron-responsive elements (IREs) within their mRNAs. Experimental induction of IRP1 did not affect the proliferation of the H1299 lung cancer cells. In a solid tumor xenograft in nude mice tumor model, tumors derived from IRP1-transfectants were 80% smaller compared to those from parent cells. The expression of ferritin and ferroportin was not suppressed by IRP1 in tumor xenografts in nude mice *(67)*. These data suggest that increased expression of IRP1 could limit tumor growth.

Hepcidin, an antimicrobial and iron regulatory peptide, is over-expressed in colorectal cancer, but the hepcidin expression level is not the cause of the systemic anemia associated with colorectal cancer *(68)*. The hepcidin level is also increased after radiation therapy in prostate cancer *(69)*. These data indicate that hepcidin level is associated with inflammation but not cancer risk.

1.6. HFE and Cancer

The relationship between HFE gene variants and cancer has received relatively more attention than any of the other iron-related genes. As mentioned, HFE gene variants occur in Caucasians more frequently than any other gene variant and also occur in many other races. Early work focused on the relationship between the iron overload disorder hemochromatosis and cancer. In particular, the focus was on hepatocarcinoma because the liver was found to accumulate high quantities of iron. A strong connection between the liver iron concentration and hepatocarcinoma was found in a number of studies (70, 71). For some time, the paradigm was that the liver accumulated iron as a result of the altered HFE protein and high iron in the liver was associated with DNA damage. There was little attempt until more recently to consider that the HFE gene variants were themselves a risk factor for cancer, perhaps associated with "subclinical" iron loading. Studies that have looked for an association of HFE gene variants and cancer without hemochromatosis have found a positive relationship (see Table 4). Results of human studies in this area are discussed in Section 1.8. Below, we review the limited in vitro literature on the cellular mechanisms of HFE regulation and related cancer phenotype.

Most of the laboratory-based studies have focused on the relationship between HFE expression and iron metabolism (72, 73). The expression of HFE in cancer cells has not been studied except in the context of transfecting HFE and looking at the effect on iron metabolism. In general, the expression of wild-type HFE is linked to down-regulation of iron uptake by cells (47, 74–79). The expression of wild-type HFE in human H1299 lung cancer cells induced an apparent iron-deficient phenotype, characterized by activation of iron regulatory protein, increased Tf receptor levels, and decreased ferritin expression (80). In MCF-7 breast cancer cells, transfection with wild-type HFE decreased the growth inhibitory effects of doxorubicin (81) suggesting that iron status, and indirectly HFE genotype, could influence treatment strategy. In the human neuroblastoma study, we observed that the expression of HFE or the common mutant forms of HFE had a significant, but varied impact, on the cells (82). The effect of wild-type HFE on Tf receptor and ferritin in the neuroblastoma cells was consistent with those reported for HeLa cells, but was not consistent with the changes reported for IRP activity (74, 83, 84). The decrease in ferritin expression observed in neuroblastoma cells is consistent with that documented in HEK293 cells (77, 85), although expression of TfR was unchanged in the HEK293 cells, indicating the existence of cell-type specific differences. A unique aspect of the neuroblastoma cell studies was the absence of endogenous HFE expression in these cell lines providing the opportunity to study the effect of HFE gene variants without the confounding variable of endogenous wildtype HFE. Of particular note was that the cells carrying the C282Y allelic variant had a distinct cancer phenotype (increased proliferation, failure to respond to differentiating agents) that included resistance to treatment strategies currently in effect (86). This cancer phenotype, including resistance to treatment, was present in commercially available human astrocytoma cell lines (86). This prompted us to examine the effect of C282Y alleles on patient outcomes in our brain tumor population. We found that those individuals carrying C2824 alleles tend to have worse tumors on presentation and worse outcomes (86).

1.7. Preclinical Studies

A consistent observation in cell culture models is that iron chelation will limit proliferation of a variety of tumor cell lines in culture. In addition to limiting proliferation,

Table 4
Epidermiology of Iron Metabolism Genes in Cancer

Protein	Subject/location	Found a relationship with gene variant	References
HFE	12 hepatocellular carcinoma with no clinical signs of hereditary hemochromatosis/130 normal subject/Italy	No	Racchi et al. (147)
HFE (C282Y)	35 patients with hepatocellular carcinoma developed in non-cirrhotic liver/France	Yes. May be related to iron overload	Blanc et al. (101)
HFE (C282Y)	137 patients with hepatocellular carcinoma and no history of hemochromatosis/107 patients with cirrhosis without hepatocellular carcinoma/126 healthy controls/Germany	Yes. Cancer is associated with significantly increased intrahepatic iron deposition and systemic iron stores	Hellerbrand et al. (100)
HFE	303 cirrhotic patients who developed hepatocellular carcinoma/Italy	Yes. Association of HBV infection to male C282Y carrier and HCV infection to female H63D heterozygous	Fracanzani et al. (102)
HFE (C282Y)	301 consecutive cirrhotic patients (162 alcoholics and 139 HCV-infected patients)/France	Yes. Cancer risk is increased with alcohol but not Hepatitis C virus-related cirrhosis. Related to iron overload	Nahon et al. (103)
HFE (H63D)	196 hepatocellular carcinoma patients/181 healthy controls/Spain	Yes. H63D frequency was higher in hepatocellular carcinoma than healthy controls. No significant variation in the frequency of HFE gene variants in relation with sex, age at diagnosis, status for antiHCV and antiHBc, and excessive ethanol use	Ropero et al. (104)

(Continued)

Table 4
(Continued)

Protein	Subject/location	Found a relationship with gene variant	References
HFE, TfR, Ferroportin	688 breast cancer/724 controls/Germany	No	Abraham et al. (105)
HFE	116 male breast cancer/843 prostate cancer/480 controls/Finland	No	Syrjakoski et al. (107)
HFE (H63D)	88 women breast cancer/100 woman controls/Turkey	Yes. H63D has a positive association with breast cancer	Gunel-Ozcan et al. (106)
HFE	475 colon cancer patients/833 control subjects/North Carolina	Yes. Cancer risk is greatest in mutation carriers who are older or consume high quantities of iron	Shaheen et al. (108)
HFE	327 colorectal cancer/322 controls/England	Yes. Cancer risk is increased by compound heterozygosity for the HFE mutations	Robinson et al. (148)
HFE	527 women with colorectal adenoma/527 matched control subjects/Boston	No	Chan et al. (109)
HFE (C282Y)	78 childhood acute lymphoblastic leukemia/415 controls/South Wales; 102 childhood acute lymphoblastic leukemia/238 controls/West Scotland	Yes. Effect is greater in males	Dorak et al. (149)
HFE, TfR2	82 adult acute leukemia/Italy	No	Veneri et al. (112)
HFE (H63D)	154 adult acute leukemia/230 control/Italy	Yes. H63D mutation is significantly more frequent in acute lymphoblastic leukemia than controls	Viola et al. (114)

HFE (H63D)	174 high-grade gliomas and 29 low-grade gliomas/144 controls/Italy	Yes. The frequency of H63D variant was increased in malignant gliomas	Martinez di Montemuros et al. (115)
HFE (C282Y)	201 women with cervical neoplasia/146 control women/Portugal	Yes. But H63D mutation is a significantly lower risk of development and time-to-onset of women cervical neoplasia	Cardoso et al. (116)
HFE	49 multiple myeloma patients/61 myelodysplastic syndrome patients/Hungary	Yes. May be related to iron overload	Varkonyi et al. (117)
HFE	36 non-small cell lung cancer/California	No	Muller et al. (150)

some tumor cells are exquisitely sensitive to the iron chelator desferrioxamine (DFO), especially neuroblastoma and leukemia cells *(87, 88)*. The mechanisms by which iron chelation can be toxic to tumor cells reportedly involves enhanced caspase-3-mediated apoptosis in human lymphocytes *(89)* and apoptosis by DNA fragmentation in the MCF-7 human breast cancer cell line *(90)*.

Presumably, the antiproliferative effects of iron chelators on cancer cells are mediated by depletion of the intracellular labile iron pool that is necessary for metabolic activity. Iron chelators have also been shown to arrest cells in the G1/S phase of the cell cycle in a human neuronal tumor cell line *(91)* and in the S phase in hematopoietic cells *(92)*. The growth arrest by iron chelation may be mediated by cell cycle regulatory proteins such as p53 in the breast cancer cells *(93)*, human lymphocytes *(89)*, and oral cancer *(94)*. In astrocytoma cells, iron chelation decreased energy production along with cell cycle arrest *(95)*.

We have shown that the neuroblastoma cells with the different HFE alleles also differ in their sensitivity to iron chelators *(82)*. At equimolar concentrations, the iron chelator DFO had no effect on the wild-type HFE cells, provoked a modest but significant increase in the number of H63D cells, and was toxic to C282Y cells. In addition, DFO protected the wild-type HFE and H63D carrying cell lines from exposure to 100 μM hydrogen peroxide but not the C282Y cell line, suggesting the genotype may impact sensitivity to iron chelation *(82)*.

The anti-tumor effects of iron chelation have been extended to in vivo animal studies. DFO inhibited tumor growth and tumor size in a hepatocellular carcinoma athymic nude mouse tumor model *(96)*. Because significant side effects have limited the clinical use of DFO, efforts have been made to develop other novel iron chelators. Nevertheless, the development of an effective iron chelator has been severely hampered by trying to differentiate between a chelator strong enough to limit the iron requirements for the tumor cells without limiting the daily iron requirements of normal cells. One example of a novel iron chelator that was tested against cancer is diethylene triamine penta-acetic acid (DTPA), which had strong anti-tumor activity against neuroblastoma cells while DFO showed moderate toxic effects to neuroblastoma cells *(97)*.

Given some of the laboratory and clinical success of iron chelators, studies have examined the impact of limiting the availability of dietary iron. Although this could be a problematic approach because it may interfere with the normal body's requirements for iron, in the 13762NF rat mammary adenocarcinoma model, in situ TUNEL assays showed that both a low iron diet or intravenous injection of deferoxamine mesylate produced an increase in apoptotic cells in the tumor compared to rats maintained on a normal diet *(90)*. Combination therapies have also been attempted using monoclonal antibodies against TfRs and the iron chelator DFO. This combination of chelator and antibodies inhibited lymphoid tumor growth in vitro, prevented initial tumor outgrowth, and caused regression of established tumors in the 38C13 murine lymphoma model *(98)*.

1.8. Epidemiological Studies

In Table 4, we summarized the epidemiological studies that have addressed the role of gene variants in iron metabolic pathways on cancer incidence. Most of the studies in this area have focused on the association between HFE gene variants, hemochromatosis, and cancer. Compelling evidence supports the idea that the HFE gene variants themselves, without evidence of clinically defined iron overload, can increase the risk of cancer. Most of the HFE-related cancers are reportedly associated with the HFE C282Y variant. HFE gene variants have been associated with a variety of cancers such as hepatocellular carcinoma, breast cancer, colorectal cancer, childhood acute lymphoblastic leukemia, and cervical neoplasia.

1.8.1. HFE POLYMORPHISMS AND CANCER

HFE polymorphism is associated with hereditary hemochromatosis. Hereditary hemochromatosis patients have a higher probability of developing hepatocellular cancer (99) based on the finding that increased frequency of C282Y is observed in hepatocellular carcinoma patients (100, 101). These C282Y heterozygote hepatocellular carcinoma patients also had significantly higher levels of serum ferritin, transferrin saturation, and iron deposition than wild-type HFE hepatocellular carcinoma patients. These data support the concept that high levels of iron enhance hepatocellular development. In contrast, the association between HFE polymorphisms and hepatocellular carcinoma in cirrhotic patients has not been demonstrated (102–104).

In addition to hepatocellular carcinoma, a study involving German women with breast cancer revealed that the C282Y HFE gene variant was associated with increased prevalence in a number of effected lymph nodes, suggesting that the HFE gene variant may effect tumor progression and prognosis (105). The H63D allelic frequencies were increased in Turkish women with breast cancer (106). However, no association was found between HFE gene variants and male breast cancer patients in Finland (107).

The relationship between HFE gene variants and colorectal cancer is not consistent. Among colon cancer patients with HFE H63D and C282Y variations, cancer risk increased with increasing age and total iron intake (108). In a study conducted in Boston, women with either HFE gene variant had higher total body iron stores and higher transferrin saturations than women with wild-type HFE; however, the HFE gene variants were not associated with colorectal adenoma (109). A gender (male)-specific effect of the C282Y HFE gene variant was shown to be risk factor for hematopoietic malignancies (110) and childhood acute lymphoblastic leukemia in Celtic populations (111). In adult acute lymphoblastic leukemia, the association of HFE gene variants with the disease was not evident (112, 113), even though one study found an association with the H63D variant (114).

Very few studies have examined the relationship between HFE gene variants and brain tumors. A study conducted at the University of Milan reported that individuals carrying the H63D allele had a high frequency of malignant gliomas (115). We are currently examining the frequency of HFE allelic variants in brain tumors. Our preliminary results suggest an apparent trend of higher frequency of H63D alleles in brain tumor patients than in normal subjects. In addition, it appears that the C282Y allele may be associated with a poor outcome.

In cervical neoplasia there was a difference in the C282Y allelic frequency between cervical neoplasia and the controls. The H63D HFE gene variant frequency was lower in women cervical neoplasia compared to control women. The age of onset of cervical lesion was also significantly different between H63D carrier and non-carrier *(116)*. A higher rate of HFE gene variants has been reported in myelodysplastic syndrome compared to multiple myeloma patients *(117)*. Patients with myelodysplastic syndrome also had higher iron and transferrin saturation levels than multiple myeloma patients.

Taken together, these studies strongly suggest that HFE polymorphisms, and specifically the C282Y and possibly the H63D gene variants, could be a risk factor for cancer. This conclusion is not surprising given the increase in potential for cellular oxidative stress in the presence of these gene variants and the likelihood that tumor cells that carry these variants would acquire more iron than tumor cells with wild-type HFE. Based on the prevalence of these gene variants in the Caucasian population, additional studies that examine the contribution of these variants to cancer risk and outcome are clearly warranted.

1.8.2. TRANSFERRIN RECEPTOR VARIANTS AND CANCER

Although the majority of the genetic studies on iron proteins is focused on the role of HFE, some investigations have examined the contribution of the TfR, which is over-expressed in some cancers. Three studies examined the relationship between expression of the TfR S142G allele and incidence of colorectal, lung, ovarian, and breast cancer, but none of these studies reported an association *(105, 118, 119)*.

Given the potential role of iron as a risk factor in the cancer process, it is surprising that only a few genetic analyses have examined the links between cancer risk and genes involved in regulation of iron metabolism. Clearly, this is an area requiring further development.

1.9. Clinical Studies

Although many experimental chelators have been shown to be effective as anti-cancer agents, only a few compounds , e.g., dexrazoxane, deferoxamine (DFO), and triapine, have reached the stage of clinical testing or application *(120)*. Desferal® (Deferoxamine mesylate USP) and more recently Exjade (deferasirox; ICL670) of Novartis are the only drugs available in US to treat iron overload disease.

Treating cancer with iron chelation therapy was attempted almost 20 years ago in patients with acute leukemia *(87, 121–123)*. The intravenous administration of desferal for 48 h led to immature cells that no longer expressed lymphoid antigens and became strongly positive for myelomonocytic markers. An identical outcome was observed in a cell culture study *(121)*. Other chemicals have been used in combination with DFO to increase its efficacy. For example, the effect of DFO was enhanced with low-dose cytosine arabinoside in leukemic cancer patients *(121)*. In another study, DFO treatment caused dose- dependent and time-dependent cytotoxic effects on human bone marrow neuroblastoma cells in two otherwise untreated children with stage IV Evans disease. In the latter study, the cytotoxic effects of DFO on neuroblastoma cells were prevented by addition of iron salts *(122)*. In a study on recurrent neuroblastoma, DFO treatment at a dose of 150 mg/kg/day for five consecutive days had an anti-tumor activity without any serious side effects *(124)*.

Although the results of clinical studies for treating cancer with the iron chelator DFO appear promising, the efficacy of DFO is severely limited due to its poor ability to permeate cell membranes and directly access intracellular iron pools. DFO also has a very short half-life (20 min) and requires continuous infusion for 8–12 h/d to be effective *(125, 126)*. Finally, iron chelation by DFO is not selective to iron associated with tumors and can limit iron availability to the immune system and other functions important for normal oxidative metabolism.

These limitations have accelerated the development of novel and more effective iron chelators. Desferri-exochelins, siderophores secreted by *Mycobacterium tuberculosis*, are both lipid-soluble and water-soluble and have a high binding affinity for iron. Desferri-exochelins can enter cells rapidly and access intracellular iron *(127)*. Exjade (deferasirox; ICL670), another iron chelator, is the first orally administered medication for chronic iron overload due to multiple blood transfusions. It was approved by the U.S. Food and Drug Administration in 2005. To our knowledge, there are no clinical trial data available on the use of this pharmaceutical agent in cancer therapeutics.

Triapine (3-AP or 3-Aminopyridine-2-carboxaldehyde thiosemicarbazone) is an iron chelator and a potent inhibitor of ribonucleotide reductase *(128)*. In combination with high-dose cytarabine, advanced myeloid leukemia patients had some possible benefits in a phase 1 trial *(129)*. In a phase 2 consortium trial in advanced pancreatic cancer, however, there were observed toxicities of Triapine and no clinical benefit *(130)*.Therefore, it is clear that an area for future development is an effective and perhaps tumor selective iron chelator. Because of the high iron requirements for cancerous cells and the strong cell culture data suggesting that iron chelators could be effective in cancer treatment if they were more selective for tumors, it can be argued that limiting iron utilization by tumor cells may be an effective treatment option. The possibility of limiting iron in the diet as a means of limiting cancer growth is addressed later.

1.10. Cancers Associated with Iron Overload

Hemochromatosis is the disease resulting from significant iron overload in tissue, especially in the liver. Therefore, liver cancer (hepatocellular carcinoma) is the primary cancer associated with iron overload. There is compelling evidence, however, that carrying the HFE gene variants without the clinical disease of hereditary hemochromatosis is associated with breast cancer, colorectal cancer, acute lymphoblastic leukemia, and may predict outcomes in brain tumors. The current paradigm in which HFE is researched and the data interpreted is that HFE gene variants have too low of a penetrability for the iron overload to reach clinical disease. However, the cell culture data *(82)* show that fundamental differences in cell phenotype relate to expression of different HFE gene variants. That is the variants have the same effect on cell iron status but different effects in terms of gene expression profiles including response to cytotoxins and radiation *(86)*. Perhaps, given the evidence reviewed in Table 4 as well as cell culture data this paradigm should be re-evaluated.

2. FUTURE RESEARCH DIRECTIONS

Perhaps, the two most promising areas for future research related to iron nutrition and cancer are to understand the impact of HFE polymorphisms and the development of treatment strategies that limit iron availability to cancer cells. Because HFE gene variants are the most common genetic alterations in Caucasian subjects, understanding how the mutant HFE protein impacts the cancer phenotype and treatment response would be considerable in these populations. Due to the increased requirement for iron by cancer cells, treatments aimed at limiting iron availability to tumors should be expanded. Although this approach appears promising, a concern is that treatment with iron chelators or the consumption of diets with minimal iron can be associated with undesired effects in cancer patients including depression of the immune system and decreased iron available for hemoglobin synthesis. Methods that target cancer cells to specifically disrupt iron metabolism are clearly needed.

3. CONCLUSIONS AND RECOMMENDATIONS FOR INTAKE/DIETARY CHANGES

Because iron is required for many normal cellular functions, an overall recommendation that people limit iron intake due to cancer risks cannot be formulated based on available experimental data. Nevertheless, it is becoming increasingly clear that carriers of HFE gene variants associated with increased iron uptake may be at higher risk for cancer. For these individuals, limiting iron intake or frequent blood donations may be useful strategies. The FDA recommended dietary allowance for iron varies with age and gender, ranging from 6 mg/d for adult men 19–70+ years of age to 18 mg/d of iron for menstruating women 19–50 years of age. The recommended dietary allowance of iron for infants (7–12 months), children, adolescents, and teens are in this range. A recommended dietary allowance has not been set for infants 0–6 months of age. The absorption rates for iron differ among individuals and iron absorption from foods is affected not only by the type of iron consumed, but also by interactions among foods consumed in concert. For example, vitamin C increases absorption of non-heme iron, whereas tannins found in red wines may decrease iron absorption. Any recommendation for limiting dietary iron consumption should bear in mind that iron is required for a healthy immune system, brain functions, growth and development, and oxidative metabolism in general. Nevertheless, oxidative stress related to iron metabolism may damage DNA and proteins and promote cancer. Thus, the recommendation would be to monitor the intake of iron-rich foods while supplementing the diet with antioxidants. The literature indicates the beneficial effect of vegetables, fruits, and grain against many types of cancer. Many nutrition societies also recommend the daily consumption of 375 g of vegetables, about 250–300 g of fruit, as well as decreased consumption of red meat.

REFERENCES

1. Schwartz, R.N. (2007) Anemia in patients with cancer: Incidence, causes, impact, management, and use of treatment guidelines and protocols. *Am J Health Syst Pharm* **64**, S5–S13, quiz S28–30.
2. Grotto, H.Z. (2008) Anaemia of cancer: An overview of mechanisms involved in its pathogenesis. *Med Oncol* **25**, 12–21.

3. Mantovani, A., Allavena, P., Sica, A., and Balkwill, F. (2008) Cancer-related inflammation. *Nature* **454**, 436–44.

4. Finn, O.J. (2008) Cancer immunology. *N Engl J Med* **358**, 2704–15.

5. Miret, S., Simpson, R.J., and McKie, A.T. (2003) Physiology and molecular biology of dietary iron absorption. *Annu Rev Nutr* **23**, 283–301.

6. Norat, T., Bingham, S., Ferrari, P., Slimani, N., Jenab, M., Mazuir, M., Overvad, K., Olsen, A., Tjonneland, A., Clavel, F., Boutron-Ruault, M.C., Kesse, E., Boeing, H., Bergmann, M.M., Nieters, A. et al. (2005) Meat, fish, and colorectal cancer risk: The European Prospective Investigation into cancer and nutrition. *J Natl Cancer Inst* **97**, 906–16.

7. Larsson, S.C., and Wolk, A. (2006) Meat consumption and risk of colorectal cancer: A meta-analysis of prospective studies. *Int J Cancer* **119**, 2657–64.

8. Kabat, G.C., Miller, A.B., Jain, M., and Rohan, T.E. (2007) Dietary iron and heme iron intake and risk of breast cancer: A prospective cohort study. *Cancer Epidemiol Biomarkers Prev* **16**, 1306–08.

9. Kuhnle, G.G., Story, G.W., Reda, T., Mani, A.R., Moore, K.P., Lunn, J.C., and Bingham, S.A. (2007) Diet-induced endogenous formation of nitroso compounds in the GI tract. *Free Radic Biol Med* **43**, 1040–47.

10. Pierre, F., Peiro, G., Tache, S., Cross, A.J., Bingham, S.A., Gasc, N., Gottardi, G., Corpet, D.E., and Gueraud, F. (2006) New marker of colon cancer risk associated with heme intake: 1,4-dihydroxynonane mercapturic acid. *Cancer Epidemiol Biomarkers Prev* **15**, 2274–79.

11. Balder, H.F., Vogel, J., Jansen, M.C., Weijenberg, M.P., van den Brandt, P.A., Westenbrink, S., van der Meer, R., and Goldbohm, R.A. (2006) Heme and chlorophyll intake and risk of colorectal cancer in the Netherlands cohort study. *Cancer Epidemiol Biomarkers Prev* **15**, 717–25.

12. Polesel, J., Talamini, R., Montella, M., Maso, L.D., Crovatto, M., Parpinel, M., Izzo, F., Tommasi, L.G., Serraino, D., La Vecchia, C., and Franceschi, S. (2007) Nutrients intake and the risk of hepatocellular carcinoma in Italy. *Eur J Cancer* **43**, 2381–87.

13. Kallianpur, A.R., Lee, S.A., Gao, Y.T., Lu, W., Zheng, Y., Ruan, Z.X., Dai, Q., Gu, K., Shu, X.O., and Zheng, W. (2008) Dietary animal-derived iron and fat intake and breast cancer risk in the Shanghai Breast Cancer Study. *Breast Cancer Res Treat* **107**, 123–32.

14. Zhou, W., Park, S., Liu, G., Miller, D.P., Wang, L.I., Pothier, L., Wain, J.C., Lynch, T.J., Giovannucci, E., and Christiani, D.C. (2005) Dietary iron, zinc, and calcium and the risk of lung cancer. *Epidemiology* **16**, 772–79.

15. Mainous, A.G., 3rd., Gill, J.M., and Everett, C.J. (2005) Transferrin saturation, dietary iron intake, and risk of cancer. *Ann Fam Med* **3**, 131–37.

16. English, D.R., MacInnis, R.J., Hodge, A.M., Hopper, J.L., Haydon, A.M., and Giles, G.G. (2004) Red meat, chicken, and fish consumption and risk of colorectal cancer. *Cancer Epidemiol Biomarkers Prev* **13**, 1509–14.

17. Choi, J.Y., Neuhouser, M.L., Barnett, M.J., Hong, C.C., Kristal, A.R., Thornquist, M.D., King, I.B., Goodman, G.E., and Ambrosone, C.B. (2008) Iron intake, oxidative stress-related genes (MnSOD and MPO) and prostate cancer risk in CARET cohort. *Carcinogenesis* **29**, 964–70.

18. Kabat, G.C., Miller, A.B., Jain, M., and Rohan, T.E. (2008) Dietary iron and haem iron intake and risk of endometrial cancer: A prospective cohort study. *Br J Cancer* **98**, 194–98.

19. Dockerty, J.D., Herbison, P., Skegg, D.C., and Elwood, M. (2007) Vitamin and mineral supplements in pregnancy and the risk of childhood acute lymphoblastic leukaemia: A case-control study. *BMC Public Health* **7**, 136.

20. Craig, W.J. (1994) Iron status of vegetarians. *Am J Clin Nutr* **59**, 1233S–1237S.

21. Haddad, E.H., Berk, L.S., Kettering, J.D., Hubbard, R.W., and Peters, W.R. (1999) Dietary intake and biochemical, hematologic, and immune status of vegans compared with nonvegetarians. *Am J Clin Nutr* **70**, 586S–593S.

22. Ball, M.J., and Bartlett, M.A. (1999) Dietary intake and iron status of Australian vegetarian women. *Am J Clin Nutr* **70**, 353–58.

23. Key, T.J., Thorogood, M., Appleby, P.N., and Burr, M.L. (1996) Dietary habits and mortality in 11,000 vegetarians and health conscious people: Results of a 17 year follow up. *BMJ* **313**, 775–79.

24. Key, T.J., Fraser, G.E., Thorogood, M., Appleby, P.N., Beral, V., Reeves, G., Burr, M.L., Chang-Claude, J., Frentzel-Beyme, R., Kuzma, J.W., Mann, J., and McPherson, K. (1998) Mortality in vegetarians and non-vegetarians: A collaborative analysis of 8300 deaths among 76,000 men and women in five prospective studies. *Public Health Nutr* **1**, 33–41.

25. Lee, K.I., Rhee, S.H., and Park, K.Y. (1999) Anticancer activity of phytol and eicosatrienoic acid identified from perilla leaves. *J Korean Soc Food Sci Nutr* **28**, 1107–12.

26. Beard, J.L., Murray-Kolb, L.E., Rosales, F.J., Solomons, N.W., and Angelilli, M.L. (2006) Interpretation of serum ferritin concentrations as indicators of total-body iron stores in survey populations: The role of biomarkers for the acute phase response. *Am J Clin Nutr* **84**, 1498–505.

27. Bohmer, F., Fruhwald, T., and Lapin, A. (2003) Soluble transferrin receptor and iron status in elderly patients. *Wien Med Wochenschr* **153**, 232–36.

28. Akesson, A., Bjellerup, P., Berglund, M., Bremme, K., and Vahter, M. (1998) Serum transferrin receptor: A specific marker of iron deficiency in pregnancy. *Am J Clin Nutr* **68**, 1241–46.

29. Ionescu, J.G., Novotny, J., Stejskal, V.D., Latsch, A., Blaurock-Busch, E., and Eisenmann-Klein, M. (2006) Increased levels of transition metals in breast cancer tissue. *Neuro Endocrinol Lett* **27**, 36–39.

30. Ko, C., Siddaiah, N., Berger, J., Gish, R., Brandhagen, D., Sterling, R.K., Cotler, S.J., Fontana, R.J., McCashland, T.M., Han, S.H., Gordon, F.D., Schilsky, M.L., and Kowdley, K.V. (2007) Prevalence of hepatic iron overload and association with hepatocellular cancer in end-stage liver disease: Results from the National Hemochromatosis Transplant Registry. *Liver Int* **27**, 1394–401.

31. Jungst, C., Cheng, B., Gehrke, R., Schmitz, V., Nischalke, H.D., Ramakers, J., Schramel, P., Schirmacher, P., Sauerbruch, T., and Caselmann, W.H. (2004) Oxidative damage is increased in human liver tissue adjacent to hepatocellular carcinoma. *Hepatology* **39**, 1663–72.

32. Valko, M., Izakovic, M., Mazur, M., Rhodes, C.J., and Telser, J. (2004) Role of oxygen radicals in DNA damage and cancer incidence. *Mol Cell Biochem* **266**, 37–56.

33. Habel, M.E., and Jung, D. (2006) Free radicals act as effectors in the growth inhibition and apoptosis of iron-treated Burkitt's lymphoma cells. *Free Radic Res* **40**, 789–97.

34. Freitas, I., Boncompagni, E., Vaccarone, R., Fenoglio, C., Barni, S., and Baronzio, G.F. (2007) Iron accumulation in mammary tumor suggests a tug of war between tumor and host for the microelement. *Anticancer Res* **27**, 3059–65.

35. Toyokuni, S. (1996) Iron-induced carcinogenesis: The role of redox regulation. *Free Radic Biol Med* **20**, 553–66.

36. Weinberg, E.D. (1992) Roles of iron in neoplasia. Promotion, prevention, and therapy. *Biol Trace Elem Res* **34**, 123–40.

37. Lovejoy, D.B., and Richardson, D.R. (2002) Novel "hybrid" iron chelators derived from aroylhydrazones and thiosemicarbazones demonstrate selective antiproliferative activity against tumor cells. *Blood* **100**, 666–76.

38. Turner, J., Koumenis, C., Kute, T.E., Planalp, R.P., Brechbiel, M.W., Beardsley, D., Cody, B., Brown, K.D., Torti, F.M., and Torti, S.V. (2005) Tachpyridine, a metal chelator, induces G2 cell-cycle arrest, activates checkpoint kinases, and sensitizes cells to ionizing radiation. *Blood* **106**, 3191–99.

39. Yang, D.C., Jiang, X., Elliott, R.L., and Head, J.F. (2002) Antisense ferritin oligonucleotides inhibit growth and induce apoptosis in human breast carcinoma cells. *Anticancer Res* **22**, 1513–24.

40. Li, Y.Q., Liu, B., Zhao, C.G., Zhang, W., and Yang, B.S. (2006) Characterization of transferrin receptor-dependent GaC-Tf-FeN transport in human leukemic HL60 cells. *Clin Chim Acta* **366**, 225–32.

41. Dautry-Varsat, A. (1986) Receptor-mediated endocytosis: The intracellular journey of transferrin and its receptor. *Biochimie* **68**, 375–81.

42. Nakamaki, T., Kawabata, H., Saito, B., Matsunawa, M., Suzuki, J., Adachi, D., Tomoyasu, S., and Phillip Koeffler, H. (2004) Elevated levels of transferrin receptor 2 mRNA, not transferrin receptor 1 mRNA, are associated with increased survival in acute myeloid leukaemia. *Br J Haematol* **125**, 42–49.

43. Levi, S., Yewdall, S.J., Harrison, P.M., Santambrogio, P., Cozzi, A., Rovida, E., Albertini, A., and Arosio, P. (1992) Evidence of H- and L-chains have co-operative roles in the iron-uptake mechanism of human ferritin. *Biochem J* **288**(Pt 2), 591–96.

44. Rouault, T.A. (2006) The role of iron regulatory proteins in mammalian iron homeostasis and disease. *Nat Chem Biol* **2**, 406–14.

45. Pigeon, C., Ilyin, G., Courselaud, B., Leroyer, P., Turlin, B., Brissot, P., and Loreal, O. (2001) A new mouse liver-specific gene, encoding a protein homologous to human antimicrobial peptide hepcidin, is overexpressed during iron overload. *J Biol Chem* **276**, 7811–19.

46. Weizer-Stern, O., Adamsky, K., Margalit, O., Ashur-Fabian, O., Givol, D., Amariglio, N., and Rechavi, G. (2007) Hepcidin, a key regulator of iron metabolism, is transcriptionally activated by p53. *Br J Haematol* **138**, 253–62.

47. Carlson, H., Zhang, A.S., Fleming, W.H., and Enns, C.A. (2005) The hereditary hemochromatosis protein, HFE, lowers intracellular iron levels independently of transferrin receptor 1 in TRVb cells. *Blood* **105**, 2564–70.

48. Best, L.G., Harris, P.E., and Spriggs, E.L. (2001) Hemochromatosis mutations C282Y and H63D in 'cis' phase. *Clin Genet* **60**, 68–72.

49. Eisenstein, R.S. (1998) Interaction of the hemochromatosis gene product HFE with transferrin receptor modulates cellular iron metabolism. *Nutr Rev* **56**, 356–58.

50. Lebron, J.A., West, A.P., Jr., and Bjorkman, P.J. (1999) The hemochromatosis protein HFE competes with transferrin for binding to the transferrin receptor. *J Mol Biol* **294**, 239–45.

51. Wu, C.G., Groenink, M., Bosma, A., Reitsma, P.H., van Deventer, S.J., and Chamuleau, R.A. (1997) Rat ferritin-H: cDNA cloning, differential expression and localization during hepatocarcinogenesis. *Carcinogenesis* **18**, 47–52.

52. Yang, D.C., Wang, F., Elliott, R.L., and Head, J.F. (2001) Expression of transferrin receptor and ferritin H-chain mRNA are associated with clinical and histopathological prognostic indicators in breast cancer. *Anticancer Res* **21**, 541–49.

53. Baldi, A., Lombardi, D., Russo, P., Palescandolo, E., De Luca, A., Santini, D., Baldi, F., Rossiello, L., Dell'Anna, M.L., Mastrofrancesco, A., Maresca, V., Flori, E., Natali, P.G., Picardo, M., and Paggi, M.G. (2005) Ferritin contributes to melanoma progression by modulating cell growth and sensitivity to oxidative stress. *Clin Cancer Res* **11**, 3175–83.

54. Holtkamp, N., Afanasieva, A., Elstner, A., van Landeghem, F.K., Konneker, M., Kuhn, S.A., Kettenmann, H., and von Deimling, A. (2005) Brain slice invasion model reveals genes differentially regulated in glioma invasion. *Biochem Biophys Res Commun* **336**, 1227–33.

55. Surguladze, N., Patton, S., Cozzi, A., Fried, M.G., and Connor, J.R. (2005) Characterization of nuclear ferritin and mechanism of translocation. *Biochem J* **388**, 731–40.

56. Liu, X., Madhankumar, A.B., Sheehan, J., Slagle-Webb, B., McCauley, M., Yang, Q.X., and Connor, J.R. (2007) H-Ferritin siRNA delivered by cationic liposome increases the efficacy of chemotherapy for treating glioma. In 12 th Annual Meeting of the Society for Neuro-Oncology pp. 484 (ET-411)

57. Liu, X., Madhankumar, A.B., Surguladze, N., Sheehan, J., Slagle-Webb, B., Yang, Q.X., and Connor, J.R. (2008) H-Ferritin plays a role in glioma cell progression. In 13 th Annual Meeting of the Society for Neuro-Oncology pp. 761 (CB-705)

58. Smilevska, T., Stamatopoulos, K., Samara, M., Belessi, C., Tsompanakou, A., Paterakis, G., Stavroyianni, N., Athanasiadou, I., Chiotoglou, I., Hadzidimitriou, A., Athanasiadou, A., Douka, V., Saloum, R., Laoutaris, N., Anagnostopoulos, A., Fassas, A., Stathakis, N., and Kollia, P. (2006) Transferrin receptor-1 and 2 expression in chronic lymphocytic leukemia. *Leuk Res* **30**, 183–89.

59. Ryschich, E., Huszty, G., Knaebel, H.P., Hartel, M., Buchler, M.W., and Schmidt, J. (2004) Transferrin receptor is a marker of malignant phenotype in human pancreatic cancer and in neuroendocrine carcinoma of the pancreas. *Eur J Cancer* **40**, 1418–22.

60. Singh, S., Singh, M., Kalra, R., Marwah, N., Chhabra, S., and Arora, B. (2007) Transferrin receptor expression in reactive and neoplastic lesions of lymph nodes. *Indian J Pathol Microbiol* **50**, 433–36.

61. Prutki, M., Poljak-Blazi, M., Jakopovic, M., Tomas, D., Stipancic, I., and Zarkovic, N. (2006) Altered iron metabolism, transferrin receptor 1 and ferritin in patients with colon cancer. *Cancer Lett* **238**, 188–96.

62. Calzolari, A., Deaglio, S., Sposi, N.M., Petrucci, E., Morsilli, O., Gabbianelli, M., Malavasi, F., Peschle, C., and Testa, U. (2004) Transferrin receptor 2 protein is not expressed in normal erythroid cells. *Biochem J* **381**, 629–34.

63. Calzolari, A., Oliviero, I., Deaglio, S., Mariani, G., Biffoni, M., Sposi, N.M., Malavasi, F., Peschle, C., and Testa, U. (2007) Transferrin receptor 2 is frequently expressed in human cancer cell lines. *Blood Cells Mol Dis* **39**, 82–91.

64. Calzolari, A., Raggi, C., Deaglio, S., Sposi, N.M., Stafsnes, M., Fecchi, K., Parolini, I., Malavasi, F., Peschle, C., Sargiacomo, M., and Testa, U. (2006) TfR2 localizes in lipid raft domains and is released in exosomes to activate signal transduction along the MAPK pathway. *J Cell Sci* **119**, 4486–98.

65. Brookes, M.J., Hughes, S., Turner, F.E., Reynolds, G., Sharma, N., Ismail, T., Berx, G., McKie, A.T., Hotchin, N., Anderson, G.J., Iqbal, T., and Tselepis, C. (2006) Modulation of iron transport proteins in human colorectal carcinogenesis. *Gut* **55**, 1449–60.

66. Lis, A., Barone, T.A., Paradkar, P.N., Plunkett, R.J., and Roth, J.A. (2004) Expression and localization of different forms of DMT1 in normal and tumor astroglial cells. *Brain Res Mol Brain Res* **122**, 62–70.

67. Chen, G., Fillebeen, C., Wang, J., and Pantopoulos, K. (2007) Overexpression of iron regulatory protein 1 suppresses growth of tumor xenografts. *Carcinogenesis* **28**, 785–91.

68. Ward, D.G., Roberts, K., Brookes, M.J., Joy, H., Martin, A., Ismail, T., Spychal, R., Iqbal, T., and Tselepis, C. (2008) Increased hepcidin expression in colorectal carcinogenesis. *World J Gastroenterol* **14**, 1339–45.

69. Christiansen, H., Saile, B., Hermann, R.M., Rave-Frank, M., Hille, A., Schmidberger, H., Hess, C.F., and Ramadori, G. (2007) Increase of hepcidin plasma and urine levels is associated with acute proctitis and changes in hemoglobin levels in primary radiotherapy for prostate cancer. *J Cancer Res Clin Oncol* **133**, 297–304.

70. Turlin, B., Juguet, F., Moirand, R., Le Quilleuc, D., Loreal, O., Campion, J.P., Launois, B., Ramee, M.P., Brissot, P., and Deugnier, Y. (1995) Increased liver iron stores in patients with hepatocellular carcinoma developed on a noncirrhotic liver. *Hepatology* **22**, 446–50.

71. Kim, M.J., Mitchell, D.G., Ito, K., Hann, H.W., Park, Y.N., and Kim, P.N. (2001) Hepatic iron deposition on MR imaging in patients with chronic liver disease: Correlation with serial serum ferritin concentration. *Abdom Imaging* **26**, 149–56.

72. Enns, C.A. (2006) Possible roles of the hereditary hemochromatosis protein, HFE, in regulating cellular iron homeostasis. *Biol Res* **39**, 105–11.

73. Parkkila, S., Niemela, O., Britton, R.S., Fleming, R.E., Waheed, A., Bacon, B.R., and Sly, W.S. (2001) Molecular aspects of iron absorption and HFE expression. *Gastroenterology* **121**, 1489–96.

74. Riedel, H.D., Muckenthaler, M.U., Gehrke, S.G., Mohr, I., Brennan, K., Herrmann, T., Fitscher, B.A., Hentze, M.W., and Stremmel, W. (1999) HFE downregulates iron uptake from transferrin and induces iron-regulatory protein activity in stably transfected cells. *Blood* **94**, 3915–21.

75. Enns, C.A. (2001) Pumping iron: The strange partnership of the hemochromatosis protein, a class I MHC homolog, with the transferrin receptor. *Traffic* **2**, 167–74.

76. Arredondo, M., Munoz, P., Mura, C.V., and Nunez, M.T. (2001) HFE inhibits apical iron uptake by intestinal epithelial (Caco-2) cells. *Faseb J* **15**, 1276–78.

77. Feeney, G.P., and Worwood, M. (2001) The effects of wild-type and mutant HFE expression upon cellular iron uptake in transfected human embryonic kidney cells. *Biochim Biophys Acta* **1538**, 242–51.

78. Fergelot, P., Orhant, M., Thenie, A., Loyer, P., Ropert-Bouchet, M., Lohyer, S., Le Gall, J.Y., and Mosser, J. (2003) Over-expression of wild-type and mutant HFE in a human melanocytic cell line reveals an intracellular bridge between MHC class I pathway and transferrin iron uptake. *Biol Cell* **95**, 243–55.

79. Arredondo, M., Tapia, V., Rojas, A., Aguirre, P., Reyes, F., Marzolo, M.P., and Nunez, M.T. (2006) Apical distribution of HFE-beta2-microglobulin is associated with inhibition of apical iron uptake in intestinal epithelia cells. *Biometals* **19**, 379–88.

80. Wang, J., Chen, G., and Pantopoulos, K. (2003) The haemochromatosis protein HFE induces an apparent iron-deficient phenotype in H1299 cells that is not corrected by co-expression of beta 2-microglobulin. *Biochem J* **370**, 891–99.

81. Chitambar, C.R., Kotamraju, S., and Wereley, J.P. (2006) Expression of the hemochromatosis gene modulates the cytotoxicity of doxorubicin in breast cancer cells. *Int J Cancer* **119**, 2200–04.

82. Lee, S.Y., Patton, S.M., Henderson, R.J., and Connor, J.R. (2007) Consequences of expressing mutants of the hemochromatosis gene (HFE) into a human neuronal cell line lacking endogenous HFE. *FASEB J* **21**, 564–76.

83. Gross, C.N., Irrinki, A., Feder, J.N., and Enns, C.A. (1998) Co-trafficking of HFE, a nonclassical major histocompatibility complex class I protein, with the transferrin receptor implies a role in intracellular iron regulation. *J Biol Chem* **273**, 22068–74.

84. Corsi, B., Levi, S., Cozzi, A., Corti, A., Altimare, D., Albertini, A., and Arosio, P. (1999) Overexpression of the hereditary hemochromatosis protein, HFE, in HeLa cells induces and iron-deficient phenotype. *FEBS Lett* **460**, 149–52.

85. Roy, C.N., Carlson, E.J., Anderson, E.L., Basava, A., Starnes, S.M., Feder, J.N., and Enns, C.A. (2000) Interactions of the ectodomain of HFE with the transferrin receptor are critical for iron homeostasis in cells. *FEBS Lett* **484**, 271–74.

86. Lee, S.Y., Slagle-Webb, B., Farace, E., Sheehan, J.M., and Connor, J.R. (2007) HFE genetic variants are a risk factor for brain tumors and increase resistance to therapy. In 12th Annual Meeting of the Society for Neuro-Oncology pp. 497 (GE-401)

87. Brodie, C., Siriwardana, G., Lucas, J., Schleicher, R., Terada, N., Szepesi, A., Gelfand, E., and Seligman, P. (1993) Neuroblastoma sensitivity to growth inhibition by deferrioxamine: Evidence for a block in G1 phase of the cell cycle. *Cancer Res* **53**, 3968–75.

88. Fukuchi, K., Tomoyasu, S., Tsuruoka, N., and Gomi, K. (1994) Iron deprivation-induced apoptosis in HL-60 cells. *FEBS Lett* **350**, 139–42.

89. Kim, B.M., Choi, J.Y., Kim, Y.J., Woo, H.D., and Chung, H.W. (2007) Desferrioxamine (DFX) has genotoxic effects on cultured human lymphocytes and induces the p53-mediated damage response. *Toxicology* **229**, 226–35.

90. Jiang, X.P., Wang, F., Yang, D.C., Elliott, R.L., and Head, J.F. (2002) Induction of apoptosis by iron depletion in the human breast cancer MCF-7 cell line and the 13762NF rat mammary adenocarcinoma in vivo. *Anticancer Res* **22**, 2685–92.

91. Renton, F.J., and Jeitner, T.M. (1996) Cell cycle-dependent inhibition of the proliferation of human neural tumor cell lines by iron chelators. *Biochem Pharmacol* **51**, 1553–61.

92. Gazitt, Y., Reddy, S.V., Alcantara, O., Yang, J., and Boldt, D.H. (2001) A new molecular role for iron in regulation of cell cycling and differentiation of HL-60 human leukemia cells: Iron is required for transcription of p21(WAF1/CIP1) in cells induced by phorbol myristate acetate. *J Cell Physiol* **187**, 124–35.

93. Pahl, P.M., Reese, S.M., and Horwitz, L.D. (2007) A lipid-soluble iron chelator alters cell cycle regulatory protein binding in breast cancer cells compared to normal breast cells. *J Exp Ther Oncol* **6**, 193–200.

94. Lee, S.K., Lee, J.J., Lee, H.J., Lee, J., Jeon, B.H., Jun, C.D., Lee, S.K., and Kim, E.C. (2006) Iron chelator-induced growth arrest and cytochrome c-dependent apoptosis in immortalized and malignant oral keratinocytes. *J Oral Pathol Med* **35**, 218–26.

95. Ye, Z., and Connor, J.R. (1999) Screening of transcriptionally regulated genes following iron chelation in human astrocytoma cells. *Biochem Biophys Res Commun* **264**, 709–13.

96. Hann, H.W., Stahlhut, M.W., Rubin, R., and Maddrey, W.C. (1992) Antitumor effect of deferoxamine on human hepatocellular carcinoma growing in athymic nude mice. *Cancer* **70**, 2051–56.

97. Shen, L., Zhao, H.Y., Du, J., and Wang, F. (2005) Anti-tumor activities of four chelating agents against human neuroblastoma cells. *In Vivo* **19**, 233–36.

98. Kemp, J.D. (1997) Iron deprivation and cancer: A view beginning with studies of monoclonal antibodies against the transferrin receptor. *Histol Histopathol* **12**, 291–96.

99. Niederau, C., Fischer, R., Sonnenberg, A., Stremmel, W., Trampisch, H.J., and Strohmeyer, G. (1985) Survival and causes of death in cirrhotic and in noncirrhotic patients with primary hemochromatosis. *N Engl J Med* **313**, 1256–62.

100. Hellerbrand, C., Poppl, A., Hartmann, A., Scholmerich, J., and Lock, G. (2003) HFE C282Y heterozygosity in hepatocellular carcinoma: Evidence for an increased prevalence. *Clin Gastroenterol Hepatol* **1**, 279–84.

101. Blanc, J.F., De Ledinghen, V., Bernard, P.H., de Verneuil, H., Winnock, M., Le Bail, B., Carles, J., Saric, J., Balabaud, C., and Bioulac-Sage, P. (2000) Increased incidence of HFE C282Y mutations in patients with iron overload and hepatocellular carcinoma developed in non-cirrhotic liver. *J Hepatol* **32**, 805–11.

102. Fracanzani, A.L., Fargion, S., Stazi, M.A., Valenti, L., Amoroso, P., Cariani, E., Sangiovanni, A., Tommasini, M., Rossini, A., Bertelli, C., Fatta, E., Patriarca, V., Brescianini, S., and Stroffolini, T. (2005) Association between heterozygosity for HFE gene mutations and hepatitis viruses in hepatocellular carcinoma. *Blood Cells Mol Dis* **35**, 27–32.

103. Nahon, P., Sutton, A., Rufat, P., Ziol, M., Thabut, G., Schischmanoff, P.O., Vidaud, D., Charnaux, N., Couvert, P., Ganne-Carrie, N., Trinchet, J.C., Gattegno, L., and Beaugrand, M. (2008) Liver iron, HFE gene mutations, and hepatocellular carcinoma occurrence in patients with cirrhosis. *Gastroenterology* **134**, 102–10.

104. Ropero, P., Briceno, O., Lopez-Alonso, G., Agundez, J.A., Gonzalez Fernandez, F.A., Garcia-Hoz, F., Villegas Martinez, A., Diaz-Rubio, M., and Ladero, J.M. (2007) The H63D mutation in the HFE gene is related to the risk of hepatocellular carcinoma. *Rev Esp Enferm Dig* **99**, 376–81.

105. Abraham, B.K., Justenhoven, C., Pesch, B., Harth, V., Weirich, G., Baisch, C., Rabstein, S., Ko, Y.D., Bruning, T., Fischer, H.P., Haas, S., Brod, S., Oberkanins, C., Hamann, U., and Brauch, H. (2005) Investigation of genetic variants of genes of the hemochromatosis pathway and their role in breast cancer. *Cancer Epidemiol Biomarkers Prev* **14**, 1102–07.

106. Gunel-Ozcan, A., Alyilmaz-Bekmez, S., Guler, E.N., and Guc, D. (2006) HFE H63D mutation frequency shows an increase in Turkish women with breast cancer. *BMC Cancer* **6**, 37.

107. Syrjakoski, K., Fredriksson, H., Ikonen, T., Kuukasjarvi, T., Autio, V., Matikainen, M.P., Tammela, T.L., Koivisto, P.A., and Schleutker, J. (2006) Hemochromatosis gene mutations among Finnish male breast and prostate cancer patients. *Int J Cancer* **118**, 518–20.

108. Shaheen, N.J., Silverman, L.M., Keku, T., Lawrence, L.B., Rohlfs, E.M., Martin, C.F., Galanko, J., and Sandler, R.S. (2003) Association between hemochromatosis (HFE) gene mutation carrier status and the risk of colon cancer. *J Natl Cancer Inst* **95**, 154–59.

109. Chan, A.T., Ma, J., Tranah, G.J., Giovannucci, E.L., Rifai, N., Hunter, D.J., and Fuchs, C.S. (2005) Hemochromatosis gene mutations, body iron stores, dietary iron, and risk of colorectal adenoma in women. *J Natl Cancer Inst* **97**, 917–26.

110. Nelson, R.L., Davis, F.G., Persky, V., and Becker, E. (1995) Risk of neoplastic and other diseases among people with heterozygosity for hereditary hemochromatosis. *Cancer* **76**, 875–79.

111. Dorak, M.T., Lawson, T., Machulla, H.K., Darke, C., Mills, K.I., and Burnett, A.K. (1999) Unravelling an HLA-DR association in childhood acute lymphoblastic leukemia. *Blood* **94**, 694–700.

112. Veneri, D., Franchini, M., Krampera, M., de Matteis, G., Solero, P., and Pizzolo, G. (2005) Analysis of HFE and TFR2 gene mutations in patients with acute leukemia. *Leuk Res* **29**, 661–64.

113. Hannuksela, J., Savolainen, E.R., Koistinen, P., and Parkkila, S. (2002) Prevalence of HFE genotypes, C282Y and H63D, in patients with hematologic disorders. *Haematologica* **87**, 131–35.

114. Viola, A., Pagano, L., Laudati, D., D'Elia, R., D'Amico, M.R., Ammirabile, M., Palmieri, S., Prossomariti, L., and Ferrara, F. (2006) HFE gene mutations in patients with acute leukemia. *Leuk Lymphoma* **47**, 2331–34.

115. Martinez di Montemuros, F., Tavazzi, D., Salsano, E., Piepoli, T., Pollo, B., Fiorelli, G.,, and Finocchiaro, G. (2001) High frequency of the H63D mutation of the hemochromatosis gene (HFE) in malignant gliomas. *Neurology* **57**, 1342.

116. Cardoso, C.S., Araujo, H.C., Cruz, E., Afonso, A., Mascarenhas, C., Almeida, S., Moutinho, J., Lopes, C., and Medeiros, R. (2006) Haemochromatosis gene (HFE) mutations in viral-associated neoplasia: Linkage to cervical cancer. *Biochem Biophys Res Commun* **341**, 232–38.

117. Varkonyi, J., Demeter, J., Tordai, A., and Andrikovics, H. (2006) The significance of the hemochromatosis genetic variants in multiple myeloma in comparison to that of myelodysplastic syndrome. *Ann Hematol* **85**, 869–71.

118. Sikstrom, C., and Beckman, L. (1994) RsaI and BclI polymorphism of the transferrin receptor gene. *Hum Hered* **44**, 312–15.

119. McGlynn, K.A., Sakoda, L.C., Hu, Y., Schoen, R.E., Bresalier, R.S., Yeager, M., Chanock, S., Hayes, R.B., and Buetow, K.H. (2005) Hemochromatosis gene mutations and distal adenomatous colorectal polyps. *Cancer Epidemiol Biomarkers Prev* **14**, 158–63.

120. Kontoghiorghes, G.J., Efstathiou, A., Ioannou-Loucaides, S., and Kolnagou, A. (2008) Chelators controlling metal metabolism and toxicity pathways: Applications in cancer prevention, diagnosis and treatment. *Hemoglobin* **32**, 217–27.

121. Estrov, Z., Tawa, A., Wang, X.H., Dube, I.D., Sulh, H., Cohen, A., Gelfand, E.W., and Freedman, M.H. (1987) In vitro and in vivo effects of deferoxamine in neonatal acute leukemia. *Blood* **69**, 757–61.

122. Becton, D.L., and Bryles, P. (1988) Deferoxamine inhibition of human neuroblastoma viability and proliferation. *Cancer Res* **48**, 7189–92.

123. Oblender, M., and Carpentieri, U. (1991) Growth, ribonucleotide reductase and metals in murine leukemic lymphocytes. *J Cancer Res Clin Oncol* **117**, 444–48.

124. Donfrancesco, A., Deb, G., Dominici, C., Pileggi, D., Castello, M.A., and Helson, L. (1990) Effects of a single course of deferoxamine in neuroblastoma patients. *Cancer Res* **50**, 4929–4930.

125. Porter, J.B., and Huehns, E.R. (1989) The toxic effects of desferrioxamine. *Baillieres Clin Haematol* **2**, 459–74.

126. Treadwell, M.J., Law, A.W., Sung, J., Hackney-Stephens, E., Quirolo, K., Murray, E., Glendenning, G.A., and Vichinsky, E. (2005) Barriers to adherence of deferoxamine usage in sickle cell disease. *Pediatr Blood Cancer* **44**, 500–07.

127. Hodges, Y.K., Antholine, W.E., and Horwitz, L.D. (2004) Effect on ribonucleotide reductase of novel lipophilic iron chelators: The desferri-exochelins. *Biochem Biophys Res Commun* **315**, 595–98.

128. Cory, J.G., Cory, A.H., Rappa, G., Lorico, A., Liu, M.C., Lin, T.S., and Sartorelli, A.C. (1994) Inhibitors of ribonucleotide reductase. Comparative effects of amino- and hydroxy-substituted pyridine-2-carboxaldehyde thiosemicarbazones. *Biochem Pharmacol* **48**, 335–44.

129. Odenike, O.M., Larson, R.A., Gajria, D., Dolan, M.E., Delaney, S.M., Karrison, T.G., Ratain, M.J., and Stock, W. (2008) Phase I study of the ribonucleotide reductase inhibitor 3-aminopyridine-2-carboxaldehyde-thiosemicarbazone (3-AP) in combination with high dose cytarabine in patients with advanced myeloid leukemia. *Invest New Drugs* **26**, 233–39.

130. Attia, S., Kolesar, J., Mahoney, M.R., Pitot, H.C., Laheru, D., Heun, J., Huang, W., Eickhoff, J., Erlichman, C., and Holen, K.D. (2008) A phase 2 consortium (P2C) trial of 3-aminopyridine-2-carboxaldehyde thiosemicarbazone (3-AP) for advanced adenocarcinoma of the pancreas. *Invest New Drugs* **26**, 369–79.

131. Wurzelmann, J.I., Silver, A., Schreinemachers, D.M., Sandler, R.S., and Everson, R.B. (1996) Iron intake and the risk of colorectal cancer. *Cancer Epidemiol Biomarkers Prev* **5**, 503–07.

132. el-Ahmady, O., el-Maraghy, A., Ibrahim, A., and Ramzy, S. (1995) Serum copper, zinc, and iron in patients with malignant and benign pulmonary diseases. *Nutrition* **11**, 498–501.

133. Mainous, A.G., 3rd, Wells, B.J., Koopman, R.J., Everett, C.J., and Gill, J.M. (2005) Iron, lipids, and risk of cancer in the Framingham Offspring cohort. *Am J Epidemiol* **161**, 1115–22.

134. Jayadeep, A., Raveendran Pillai, K., Kannan, S., Nalinakumari, K.R., Mathew, B., Krishnan Nair, M., and Menon, V.P. (1997) Serum levels of copper, zinc, iron and ceruloplasmin in oral leukoplakia and squamous cell carcinoma. *J Exp Clin Cancer Res* **16**, 295–300.

135. Ulbrich, E.J., Lebrecht, A., Schneider, I., Ludwig, E., Koelbl, H., and Hefler, L.A. (2003) Serum parameters of iron metabolism in patients with breast cancer. *Anticancer Res* **23**, 5107–09.

136. Hercberg, S., Estaquio, C., Czernichow, S., Mennen, L., Noisette, N., Bertrais, S., Renversez, J.C., Briancon, S., Favier, A., and Galan, P. (2005) Iron status and risk of cancers in the SU.VI.MAX cohort. *J Nutr* **135**, 2664–68.

137. Cross, A.J., Gunter, M.J., Wood, R.J., Pietinen, P., Taylor, P.R., Virtamo, J., Albanes, D., and Sinha, R. (2006) Iron and colorectal cancer risk in the alpha-tocopherol, beta-carotene cancer prevention study. *Int J Cancer* **118**, 3147–52.

138. Kuvibidila, S.R., Gauthier, T., and Rayford, W. (2004) Serum ferritin levels and transferrin saturation in men with prostate cancer. *J Natl Med Assoc* **96**, 641–49.

139. Ioannou, G.N., Weiss, N.S., and Kowdley, K.V. (2007) Relationship between transferrin-iron saturation, alcohol consumption, and the incidence of cirrhosis and liver cancer. *Clin Gastroenterol Hepatol* **5**, 624–29.

140. Bjerner, J., Amlie, L.M., Rusten, L.S., and Jakobsen, E. (2002) Serum levels of soluble transferrin receptor correlate with severity of disease but not with iron stores in patients with malignant lymphomas. *Tumour Biol* **23**, 146–53.

141. Tsionou, C., Minaretzis, D., Papageorgiou, I., Nakopoulou, L., Michalas, S., and Aravantinos, D. (1991) Expression of carcinoembryonic antigen and ferritin in normal, hyperplastic, and neoplastic endometrium. *Gynecol Oncol* **41**, 193–98.

142. Yu, D.S., Yueh, K.C., Chang, S.Y., Yang, T.H., and Ma, C.P. (1995) The expression of ferritin on renal cancers and its relationship with cellular differentiation and tumour stage. *Br J Urol* **75**, 733–35.

143. Brodeur, G.M., Look, A.T., Shimada, H., Hamilton, V.M., Maris, J.M., Hann, H.W., Leclerc, J.M., Bernstein, M., Brisson, L.C., Brossard, J., Lemieux, B., Tuchman, M., and Woods, W.G. (2001) Biological aspects of neuroblastomas identified by mass screening in Quebec. *Med Pediatr Oncol* **36**, 157–59.

144. Maresca, V., Flori, E., Cardinali, G., Briganti, S., Lombardi, D., Mileo, A.M., Paggi, M.G., and Picardo, M. (2006) Ferritin light chain down-modulation generates depigmentation in human metastatic melanoma cells by influencing tyrosinase maturation. *J Cell Physiol* **206**, 843–48.

145. Whitney, J.F., Clark, J.M., Griffin, T.W., Gautam, S., and Leslie, K.O. (1995) Transferrin receptor expression in nonsmall cell lung cancer. Histopathologic and clinical correlates. *Cancer* **76**, 20–25.

146. Boult, J., Roberts, K., Brookes, M.J., Hughes, S., Bury, J.P., Cross, S.S., Anderson, G.J., Spychal, R., Iqbal, T., and Tselepis, C. (2008) Overexpression of cellular iron import proteins is associated with malignant progression of esophageal adenocarcinoma. *Clin Cancer Res* **14**, 379–87.

147. Racchi, O., Mangerini, R., Rapezzi, D., Gaetani, G.F., Nobile, M.T., Picciotto, A., and Ferraris, A.M. (1999) Mutations of the HFE gene and the risk of hepatocellular carcinoma. *Blood Cells Mol Dis* **25**, 350–53.

148. Robinson, J.P., Johnson, V.L., Rogers, P.A., Houlston, R.S., Maher, E.R., Bishop, D.T., Evans, D.G., Thomas, H.J., Tomlinson, I.P., and Silver, A.R. (2005) Evidence for an association between compound heterozygosity for germ line mutations in the hemochromatosis (HFE) gene and increased risk of colorectal cancer. *Cancer Epidemiol Biomarkers Prev* **14**, 1460–63.

149. Dorak, M.T., Burnett, A.K., Worwood, M., Sproul, A.M., and Gibson, B.E. (1999) The C282Y mutation of HFE is another male-specific risk factor for childhood acute lymphoblastic leukemia. *Blood* **94**, 3957.

150. Muller, C.I., Miller, C.W., Kawabata, H., McKenna, R.J., Jr., Marchevsky, A.M., and Koeffler, H.P. (2005) Do cancer cells selectively mutate HFE to increase their intracellular iron? *Oncol Rep* **14**, 299–303.

22 Zinc in Cancer Development and Prevention

Louise Y.Y. Fong

Key Points

1. Zinc is an essential trace element required for maintaining enzyme activity, the immune system, and the conformation of many transcription factors that control cell proliferation, apoptosis, and signaling pathways. The role of zinc in cancer development and prevention is gaining attention.
2. Compelling evidence from epidemiological, clinical, and rodent studies shows that dietary zinc deficiency is associated with an increased risk of developing esophageal and oral cancer.
3. Zinc has similar tumor suppressor effects in esophageal and oral tumors as well as several other types of tumor. Additionally, zinc supplementation has beneficial effects in several diseases in the elderly who are zinc deficiency-prone, including diseases related to dysregulation of the inflammatory/immune response.
4. The concept of zinc as a tumor suppressor agent in cancer prevention is supported by abundant experimental and clinical studies in esophageal, lingual, prostate, and colon cancer. Recent data from gene profiling and immunohistochemical analyses, showing that zinc regulates the proinflammation mediator S100A8 expression, its interaction with RAGE, and the downstream NF-κB-COX-2 signaling pathway, provide the first evidence for an inflammation-modulating role of zinc in early esophageal carcinogenesis and its reversal.
5. Given the recent reignited interest of researchers in the concept of an association of inflammation and the genesis and perpetuation of cancer, the finding that zinc regulates a key inflammation pathway and modulates miRNA expression in esophageal preneoplasia offers opportunities to conduct studies to more precisely define the role of zinc in cancer initiation, progression, and prevention and also to explore the possible link between microRNA expression and inflammation.
6. The finding that targeting only the COX-2 pathway in zinc-deficient animals does not prevent UADT tumor progression strongly suggests that correcting nutritional deficiencies is necessary in a more successful cancer treatment protocol.

Key Words: Zinc deficiency; zinc supplementation; esophageal and oral cancer; cancer prevention; antitumor effects of zinc; gene and microRNA expression profiling; apoptosis; cell proliferation

From: *Nutrition and Health: Bioactive Compounds and Cancer*
Edited by: J.A. Milner, D.F. Romagnolo, DOI 10.1007/978-1-60761-627-6_22,
© Springer Science+Business Media, LLC 2010

1. INTRODUCTION

Zinc is an essential nutrient. It has diverse biological functions due to its role in a multitude of cellular components. As a constituent of more than 300 enzymes, zinc acts as a catalytic, structural, or regulatory ion *(1)*. As a key structural component of more than 2,000 proteins that are mainly nuclear transcription factors, zinc ions contribute through regulation of gene expression to control of cell proliferation, differentiation, and apoptosis *(2)*. In addition, zinc is capable of undergoing rapid ligand exchange reactions. Consequently, alterations in zinc status are translated into changes in gene expression *(3)*. In vivo zinc levels can be used in an information-carrying role, as calcium is, in a variety of signal transduction pathways *(3)*. Thus zinc plays an important role in maintaining the activities of many enzymes, signaling pathways, transcription factors, as well as the immune system *(4)*. On the other hand, failure to maintain and regulate a normal cellular concentration of zinc has complex implications in a number of organs and can contribute to the onset of many diseases and cancers *(5, 6)*. In recent years, the role of zinc deficiency as a cause of disease and determinant in the progression of disease is drawing attention *(7)*. This review examines the mechanistic role of zinc in the pathogenesis and prevention of esophageal and oral cancer, which has been the research focus of the author.

2. HUMAN ZINC DEFICIENCY

In 1869, Raulin first demonstrated in *Aspergillus niger* that zinc was essential for the growth of living organisms *(8)*. It took more than six decades before it was recognized that zinc was necessary for the growth of animals *(9)*. A zinc-inadequate diet in the rat resulted in anorexia, retarded growth, definite foci of alopecia, and testicular atrophy. Finally in the early 1960s, Prasad et al. reported the discovery of primary zinc deficiency in humans in Egypt and Iran *(10, 11)*. Patients afflicted by zinc deficiency showed clinical features of dwarfism, hypogonadism in males, rough and dry skin, and mental lethargy, which are reminiscent of the gross anatomy of severe zinc deficiency in the rat. These patients had negligible intake of animal protein and consumed a very restricted diet mainly comprised of wheat flour bread. Importantly, all of these clinical signs were corrected by zinc supplementation. At present, severe zinc deficiency is rare in human populations, although mild to moderate deficiency is estimated to be prevalent worldwide *(12)*.

Except for red meat and seafood, zinc is present at low concentrations in a large variety of foods. Whole grain and most vegetables are poor sources of zinc because of the presence of phytates that bind zinc and inhibit its absorption. The Recommended Daily Allowance for zinc is approximately 12–15 mg, an amount that can be obtained in a balanced diet by consuming meat and other animal proteins. A person subsisting on a cereal and vegetarian diet is likely to have a low intake of zinc. The elderly are also vulnerable to zinc deficiency owing to inadequate diets and/or intestinal malabsorption, and as a result, they are susceptible to age-related diseases such as infections and cancer *(13)*. Moreover, conditioned zinc deficiency can occur in individuals with diseases associated with impaired intestinal absorption, chronic inflammatory bowel diseases, rheumatoid arthritis, diabetes, alcoholism, stress, and cancer *(7)*. Thus, zinc deficiency is more widespread than is often assumed *(14)*. In the United States, it is estimated that the intake of zinc is less than 50% of the recommended daily allowance in about 10% of the population *(15)*. In the developing world, dietary zinc deficiency may affect more than 2 billion people *(16)*.

3. ZINC DEFICIENCY AND UADT CANCER: EPIDEMIOLOGICAL STUDIES

Upper aerodigestive tract (UADT) cancer, including esophageal and oral cancer, is an important cause of morbidity and mortality worldwide *(17)*. The two main types of esophageal cancer are esophageal squamous cell carcinoma (ESCC) and esophageal adenocarcinoma (EAC). ESCC is the more common type. According to the American Cancer Society statistics, 16,470 new cases of esophageal cancer were diagnosed in the United States in 2008, and 14,280 deaths were attributed to this malignancy *(18)*. Subjects diagnosed with esophageal cancers have a 5-year survival of ~10%. The prognosis of oral cancer, the major site being the tongue, is equally dismal. The incidence of oral cancer is increasing worldwide, even among young adults and individuals without the documented risk factors of tobacco and alcohol use *(19)*. Patients with oral cancer have a high mortality rate because of field cancerization effects that result in second primary tumors, particularly in the esophagus *(20, 21)*. Thus, new chemopreventive and therapeutic approaches are much needed to prevent and treat these deadly cancers.

Chronic alcohol consumption and tobacco use are the major risk factors for UADT cancer in western countries. Nevertheless, epidemiological and clinical studies have long implicated exposure to carcinogenic nitrosamines such as *N*-nitrosomethylbenzylamine (NMBA) *(22)*, and nutritional deficiencies, in particular, zinc deficiency, as causative factors for esophageal and oral cancer in several high incidence areas, including northern China, Iran, India, central Asia, and the Transkei region of South Africa *(23, 24, 25, 26, 27)*. Since alcohol consumption is associated with a general poor nutrition, zinc deficiency is thus a likely risk factor for UADT cancer in western countries *(28)*.

In 2005, Abnet et al. *(29)* provided the first evidence in humans of an association between zinc deficiency and ESCC. Using x-ray fluorescence spectroscopy, these investigators measured zinc, copper, iron, nickel, and sulfur levels in paraffin-embedded sections of esophageal biopsy samples from a high ESCC incidence area in China. Subjects were matched on baseline histology and followed for 16 years. Overall, 90% of the subjects in the highest zinc quartile were alive and cancer-free after 16 years as compared to only 65% of the subjects in the lowest quartile. There were no consistent associations with cancer risk for any of the other trace elements studied. This study unequivocally established that low tissue zinc concentrations are strongly associated with an increased risk of developing ESCC.

4. BIOLOGICAL ROLES OF ZINC

4.1. Zinc Homeostasis

The maintenance of normal cellular concentrations of zinc is crucial to the function, growth, proliferation, differentiation, and survival of cells. Recent advances in the study of zinc transporters and the involvement of metallothioneins (MTs) in intracellular zinc homeostasis have provided a new understanding of how zinc levels might be maintained in tissues under normal and cancer conditions (6).

MTs are low molecular weight proteins with high cysteine content that bind zinc as well as other metal ions. MTs are very sensitive to dietary zinc supply and are involved in intracellular zinc homeostasis. It is thought that MT synthesis, mediated by the metal-responsive transcription factor 1 (MTF-1), is responsible for the intracellular regulation of zinc concentration and detoxification of harmful heavy metals (30). In addition, MTs act as antioxidants. The zinc–sulfur ligand is sensitive to changes of cellular redox state and the oxidizing sites in MT induce the transfer of zinc from its binding sites in MT to those of lower affinity in other proteins (31).

Two main families of cellular zinc transporter proteins have been identified in mammals: the ZnT (CDF, cation diffusion facilitator, in eukaryotes) (SLC30) and the ZIP (SLC39) (32, 33). These transporter proteins appear to have opposite roles in cellular zinc homeostasis. While the ZnT transporters remove zinc from the cytoplasm by either transporting it out of the cell or trafficking it into cellular organelles, the ZIP transporters act by bringing zinc into the cytoplasm from the extracellular space. To date, 24 zinc transporters (10 ZnT and 14 ZIP) have been identified through mammalian genome analyses, and 15 have been functionally characterized (ZnT1-8 and Zip 1-7). The zinc transporters maintain intracellular zinc concentrations in a narrow physiologic range and their mode of action is tissue- and cell-type specific.

Several studies have shown a correlation of zinc levels and zinc transporter protein expression with cancer risk. For example, human breast cancer is marked by low zinc levels in serum and scalp hair (34), but elevated zinc concentrations in cancer tissue (35, 36). The increased zinc levels are found to be associated with high expression levels of zinc transporters ZIP6, ZIP10, and ZIP7 (6). While ZIP6 overexpression is thought to be a possible marker for a low-grade, non-aggressive cancer (37), elevated expression levels of ZIP10 and ZIP7 indicate the presence of a more aggressive cancer with increased risk of metatasis (38). In human pancreatic cancer, ZIP4 overexpression and zinc accumulation significantly contribute to the pathogenesis and progression of this malignancy (39). On the other hand, malignant prostate cells exhibit silencing of ZIP1 gene expression, which is accompanied by depletion of cellular zinc (40).

In animal experiments, zinc accumulation in N-methyl-N-nitrosourea-induced rat mammary tumors is attended by reduced expression of ZnT-1 and overexpression of MT (41). Additionally, acute inflammation in ZD mouse lungs is accompanied by alterations in zinc transporter expression, including increases in ZIP1 and ZIP14, but decreases in ZIP4 and ZnT4 (42). Thus, alterations in zinc transporter gene expression during inflammation are directed toward increasing zinc uptake as a means to counteract the local loss of zinc in the airway and to meet an increased demand for zinc-dependent proteins. Intriguingly, zinc supplementation restored ZIP1 and ZIP14 expression (42).

To date, there are no published reports about the role of zinc transporter proteins in the maintenance of zinc homeostasis in UADT cancer. Although ZnT1 protein is abundantly expressed in the squamous epithelium of the normal mouse esophagus *(43)*, it remains to be determined whether dysregulation of zinc transporter protein expression can lead to a reduced zinc level in the esophagus *(44)* and increase the susceptibility to carcinogenesis *(29, 45)*.

4.2. Zinc as an Antioxidant

Oxidative stress, which results from an imbalance between formation and neutralization of free radicals, is now recognized as an important contributing factor in many diseases, including cancer, atherosclerosis, neurodegeneration, immunologic disorders, and the aging process *(46)*. A free radical is defined as any species that has one or more unpaired electrons. How zinc acts as an antioxidant is unclear. Its antioxidant role, however, is influenced by several factors *(47)*. For instance, zinc competes with pro-oxidant iron for binding to the membrane, thus decreasing the production of reactive oxygen species *(48)*. Zinc is important in maintaining an adequate level of the zinc-binding protein MTs, which are also free radical scavengers *(13)*. Zinc may also act as an antioxidant by protecting protein sulfhydryl groups against oxidation *(49)*.

Multiple studies have shown that zinc deficit has a negative impact on the antioxidant capacity of the cell. In vitro low intracellular zinc induces DNA damage and affects DNA repair in a rat glioma cell line *(15)*. In vivo, zinc deficiency causes oxidative damage to proteins, lipids, and DNA in rat testis *(50)* and stimulates the production of endogenous free radicals in rat lung microsomes by an NADPH- and cytochrome P-450-dependent system *(51)*. In contrast, zinc supplementation protects human cutaneous fibroblasts from DNA strand breakage and apoptosis, suggesting that zinc could have beneficial effects for skin cell protection against UVA1 irradiation *(52)*. Additionally, zinc supplementation in humans slows the progression of age-related macular degeneration, a disease associated with increased free radical production *(53)*.

4.3. Zinc and Immune Response

It has been long established that zinc is essential for the immune system and zinc deficiency has profound effects on immune functions *(4, 54, 55)*. Young adult mice on a zinc-deficient diet showed thymic atrophy, reductions in the number of splenocytes, and depressed responses to both thymic T-cell-dependent and T-cell-independent antigens *(56, 57)*. In addition, zinc deficiency reduces the activities of serum thymulin (a thymic hormone) and natural killer (NK) cells and affects the functions of T cells by causing a shift of the T helper (Th) cell response that leads to a decreased Th_1 cell and a Th_2 cell predominance *(58)*.

Zinc deficiency in humans leads to complex deregulated immune functions, presenting in its most severe form in acrodermatitis enteropathica (AE). This zinc malabsorption syndrome is an autosomal recessive disorder characterized by dermatitis, alopecia, and diarrhea. AE is caused by mutations in ZIP4 *(59)*, a zinc importer required for the absorption of dietary zinc by enterocytes and other cell types *(60)*. The clinical symptoms of AE are corrected by treatment with zinc *(61)*. In addition to AE, oral zinc has been used to treat, with varying degrees of success, diseases such as diarrhea, chronic hepatitis C, leprosy, tuberculosis, and pneumonia. The clear beneficial effects of zinc supplementation on numerous immune parameters, including proinflammatory cytokines and T lymphocytes, probably contribute to the positive results observed in supplementation trials for these diseases (62).

4.4. Zinc and Intracellular Signaling in Cancer

In vivo zinc is known to undergo rapid ligand exchange reactions and thus it can be used as an information carrier like calcium in signal transduction pathways (3). This labile or loosely bound zinc has the potential to modulate cellular functions and influence signaling pathways. Moreover, labile zinc shows intracellular fluctuations after stimulation, yielding a complex interaction between zinc homeostasis and signaling (63). Bruinsma et al. (64) reported that in *Caenorhabditis elegans*, CDF proteins positively regulated Ras signaling by reducing the concentration of cytosolic Zn^{2+}, and Zn^{2+} inhibited Ras signaling. Since lowering the concentration of Zn^{2+} enhances signaling and raising the concentration of Zn^{2+} diminishes signaling, Zn^{2+} is therefore dynamically regulated to control the activity of the Ras-mediated signaling pathway. This function of zinc is conserved because homologous mammalian ZnT1 and non-mammalian CDF-1 zinc transporters also activate Ras by decreasing intracellular zinc levels. As Ras is a pivotal signaling protein that regulates many cellular processes, and mutations that activate Ras are a common cause of human cancers (65), it is likely that zinc ions are involved in intracellular signaling in cancer. Consistent with this idea, our recent data in an animal model of esophageal preneoplasia initiation and reversal show that zinc deficiency enhances tumor initiation by increasing S100A8–RAGE interaction and nuclear factor κB (NF-κB) signaling, and zinc replenishment reverses preneoplasia by reducing this interaction and inhibiting NF-κB signaling (66). In prostate cancer cells, zinc is reported to inhibit TNF-α-induced activation of NF-κB (67). Taken together, these studies show that zinc affects divergent signaling pathways during cancer development.

5. ZINC-DEFICIENT RODENT CANCER MODELS

In 1941, Follis et al. (68) first reported the histological findings of tissues from rats fed a diet low in zinc content. The most pronounced pathological changes were found in the esophagus and to a lesser extent in the buccal cavity and skin, and in the cornea. The esophagus displayed hyperkeratosis, parakeratosis, and an increase in the number of epithelial cell layers (68). These early reports from epidemiological (23, 24, 25, 26, 27, 29) and animal (68) studies suggest that zinc deficiency might play a role in esophageal carcinogenesis. In 1978, the author and her colleagues first reported that zinc deficiency increased the incidence and reduced the induction time of esophageal tumors in rats exposed to NMBA (69). Similar findings were later published by other workers (44, 70) and extended to experiments in which the precursor amine and nitrite were simultaneously administered (71).

The zinc-deficient rodent tumor models reproduce features of human UADT cancer and have many attractions for the study of the molecular mechanisms by which zinc, a risk factor for UADT cancer, influences cancer development and prevention. In this model, a deficient diet containing 3 ppm and 1.5 ppm zinc is used to induce and maintain a sustained, increased cellular proliferation in the rat and mouse, respectively. NMBA and 4-nitroquinoline 1-oxide (NQO) are used to induce esophageal and lingual tumors, respectively. NMBA methylates rat esophageal DNA with a concomitant accumulation of the promutagenic adduct O^6-methylguanine *(72)*. Interestingly, elevated levels of O^6-methyldeoxyguanosine were found in human esophageal mucosal DNA in areas associated with a high risk for esophageal cancer *(73)*. Both NMBA- and NQO-induced esophageal and tongue tumors are morphologically similar to human ESCC and lingual SCC, showing a histopathologic progression from hyperplasia, to mild and severe dysplasia, carcinoma in situ, and, finally, to invasive carcinoma *(74)*.

5.1. Initiation and Reversal of Protumorigenic Environment

Dietary zinc deficiency induces a protumorigenic environment in the rat esophagus and tongue by causing a sustained, uncontrolled cell proliferation *(45, 75)* and extensive changes in gene expression in the squamous epithelium (reviewed in Sections 5.6 and 5.7) *(66, 76, 77)*. Conversely, zinc replenishment (ZR) rapidly reverses cell proliferation, stimulates apoptosis, corrects abnormal gene expression, and inhibits esophageal and lingual tumorigenesis *(66, 75, 77, 78, 79)*. As an example, Fig. 1 shows the zinc modulatory effects on lingual cell proliferation, as assessed by proliferating cell nuclear antigen (PCNA) immunohistochemistry. PCNA is an endogenous cell proliferation marker that identifies cells in S phase *(80)*. Tongues from pair-fed zinc-sufficient (ZS) control rats showed very mild proliferation, with PCNA-positive nuclei largely restricted to the basal cell layers (Fig. 1, A, D, and G). In contrast, ZD lingual epithelia displayed abundant PCNA-positive nuclei in many cell layers and in focal hyperplastic lesions (Fig. 1, B, E, and H). ZR reduced cell proliferation, as assayed by PCNA staining, within hours. By 48 h, PCNA-positive nuclei were mostly found in the basal cell layers of a thinned lingual epithelium (Fig. 1, C, F, and I). In a similar manner, within hours after ZR the hyperplastic ZD esophagus is also thinned *(77, 78)*. As increased cell proliferation is a hallmark of cancer, the hyperplastic protumorigenic phenotype in ZD esophagus and tongue is highly relevant to cancer development *(81)*.

5.2. Zinc Deficiency and Animal Tumorigenesis Studies

5.2.1. ESOPHAGEAL SQUAMOUS CELL TUMORS

Esophageal tumor induction by NMBA is very rapid in ZD esophagus. A single, otherwise non-tumorigenic dose of NMBA in nutritionally complete rats *(82)* elicits a rapid tumorigenic response in ZD esophagus as early as 3 weeks *(83)* and a greater than 80% tumor incidence 14 weeks after carcinogen treatment *(78, 83, 84)*. As early as 24 h after a single NMBA treatment, the expanded focal hyperplastic lesions in the esophageal epithelium showed overexpression of cyclin D1, cyclin-dependent kinase-4 (cdk4), and the retinoblastoma protein, but lack of expression of p16ink4a *(83)*. Thus,

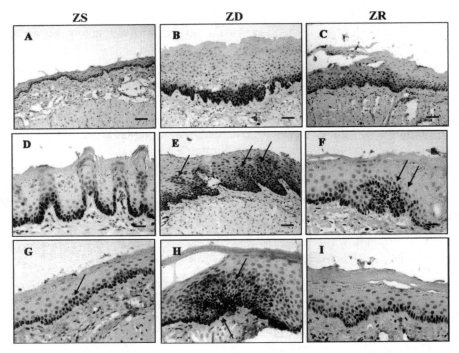

Fig. 1. Effects of zinc deficiency (ZD) and zinc replenishment (ZR) on lingual cell proliferation. Immunohistochemistry for proliferating cell nuclear antigen (PCNA) was used to identify proliferating cells. Representative pictures of tongue sections from individual rats are shown. (**A, D, G**) In zinc-sufficient (ZS) control epithelia, PCNA-positive cells occurred mainly in the basal cell layer, with occasional staining in the suprabasal layer (*arrow*, **G**). (**B, E, H**) In ZD epithelia, PCNA staining was abundant in many cell layers and focal hyperplastic lesions (*arrows*) (**E, H**). (**C, F, I**) ZR epithelia had fewer cell layers and fewer PCNA-positive nuclei in the still-hyperplastic epithelium 8 h after zinc replenishment (ZR8, **C**) and in focal hyperplastic lesions 12 h after replenishment (ZR12, **F**). After 48 h, ZR48 epithelium resembled that of ZS rats, with PCNA-positive nuclei largely restricted to the basal cell layer (**I**). Scale bars: 50 μm (in **A–C**) and 25 μm (in **D–F**). (Reproduced from *J Natl Cancer Inst* 2005; 97:40–50).

the rapid tumor initiation is associated with an early deregulation of the p16ink4a-cyclin D1/Cdk4-Rb pathway.

5.2.2. Lingual Tumors

Continuous exposure of ZD rats to NQO resulted in the development of tumors at multiple sites in the UADT, including lingual SCC (74%), esophageal (39%), and forestomach (considered a dilation of the lower esophagus, 61%) tumors. In contrast, ZS control rats showed a substantially lower incidence of lingual SCC (22%; $P = 0.015$) and no macroscopic abnormalities in the esophagus or the forestomach (*75*). These findings provide the first evidence that ZD causes substantial cell proliferation in the squamous epithelium of the UADT, thereby producing a "field cancerization" effect *(21)* and a fertile environment for the genetic events that culminate in the development of malignant lesions at multiple sites after continuous exposure to NQO *(75)*.

The mechanism by which zinc deficiency increases esophageal and lingual cancer risk is unclear. It is possible that it acts by inducing the activity of cyclooxygenase-2 (COX-2), an enzyme that catalyzes the formation of various proinflammatory prostaglandins from arachidonic acid. COX-2 is overexpressed in a variety of human premalignant and malignant lesions, including esophageal and oral cancers *(85, 86)*. Overexpression of COX-2 enhances cell proliferation, inhibits apoptosis *(87)*, modulates cell adhesion and angiogenesis *(88)*, and increases metastatic potential *(89)*, thereby contributing to carcinogenesis *(90)*. Our earlier data *(75)* showed that esophageal and lingual hyperplasia in ZD rats is accompanied by overexpression of COX-2 protein and mRNA. Within hours, ZR reduced COX-2 overexpression to near control levels in ZS animals and reversed the hyperplastic phenotypes. In addition, oral treatments with the COX-2 inhibitors celecoxib or indomethacin led to a reduction in COX-2 activity and cell proliferation. These data demonstrate a direct role for overexpression of COX-2 in the increased susceptibility to esophageal carcinogenesis seen in ZD rats. Such a conclusion is supported by the known roles of COX-2 in carcinogenesis *(90)*.

5.2.3. ESOPHAGEAL ADENOCARCINOMA

Guy et al. demonstrated that dietary zinc deficiency together with an increased intake of hydrophobic bile acids led to the development of esophagitis, and Barrett's esophagus (BE) in C56BL/6 mice *(91)*. BE is a premalignant lesion of EAC in which columnar epithelium replaces esophageal squamous cells. This mouse model of esophagitis and BE is expected to contribute to a deeper understanding of the role of zinc deficiency in BE pathogenesis and prevention of BE progression to cancer.

5.2.4. COLON TUMORS

In vivo zinc deprivation promotes progression of 1,2-dimethylhydrazine (DMH)-induced colon tumors but reduces malignant invasion in mice, *(92)* and zinc supplementation has a positive beneficial effect against chemically induced colonic preneoplastic progression in rats induced by DMH-induced colon carcinogenesis *(93)*.

5.3. Zinc Deficiency and Tumorigenesis Studies in Knockout/Transgenic Models

The mouse esophagus and tongue are not sensitive to chemical carcinogenesis *(94, 95)*. In 1999, the development of a zinc-deficient mouse forestomach cancer model opened the door to using transgenic and knockout mouse models to understand nutrient–gene interactions in carcinogenesis *(94)*. The interactions between zinc deficiency and loss of *TP53 (96, 97)*, overexpression of *cyclin D1 (98)*, loss of Testin gene (*TES*) *(99)*, overexpression of antizyme (*AZ*) gene *(100)*, and loss of expression of *COX-2* gene *(101)* were explored in transgenic/knockout mice fed a ZD diet.

Loss of function of the *TP53* tumor suppressor gene occurs in more than 50% of all human cancers, including ESCC, EAC, and oral cancer *(102)*. Combined deficiency of zinc and loss of function of p53 in mice led to speedy development and progression of esophageal and forestomach tumors by NMBA *(96)*, as well as lingual and esophageal tumors by NQO *(97)*. In zinc-deprived p53$^{-/-}$ mice, the balance of cell proliferation and apoptosis, two critical factors that influence the course of carcinogenesis, is tipped toward cell proliferation, thereby unleashing a cascade of events that culminate in cancer development with progression to malignancy in just 30 days after a single NMBA treatment. Thus, it is possible that the genetic changes that lead to the rapid appearance of cancers in the zinc- and p53-deficient mice may recapitulate those that may occur in the same human cancers.

Cyclin D1 overexpression due to gene amplification is a critical genetic alteration in human ESCC *(103)*. In the rat model, overexpression of cyclin D1 was found in esophageal papillomas and carcinomas induced by NMBA *(104)*. Transgenic mice overexpressing cyclin D1 fed a diet low in zinc had a high rate of cell proliferation in target tissues, setting the stage for rapid development and progression of esophageal and forestomach tumors by NMBA *(98)*. Without the added proliferation provided by ZD, however, NMBA was unable to initiate esophageal tumorigenesis or to mount a vigorous tumorigenic response in the forestomach of transgenic mice overexpressing cyclin D1 *(98)*.

AZ is a multifunctional regulator of polyamine metabolism that inhibits ornithine decarboxylase activity and restricts polyamine levels *(105)* and thereby inhibiting cell proliferation *(106)*. In contrast to cyclin D1 overexpressing mice, the inhibition of tumor development in ZD mice by AZ overexpression was associated with suppression of cell proliferation and stimulation of apoptosis *(100)*. Consistent with this finding, in AZ overexpressing mice, α-difluoromethylornithine, the irreversible ODC inhibitor and an anticancer agent, reverses zinc deficiency-induced esophageal cell proliferation by stimulation of apoptosis, and thereby inhibiting esophageal tumor induction by NMBA *(107, 108)*.

Deletion of the *COX-2* gene in *Apc* knockout mice greatly reduces intestinal polyp formation, a result that provides the genetic evidence that COX-2 plays a key role in tumorigenesis *(109)*. Consistent with the intestinal and skin tumor studies *(109, 110)*, COX-2-deficient mice on a ZS diet had a lower incidence of forestomach tumors than wild-type controls *(101)*. Instead of being protected, zinc-deficient COX-2-null mice developed significantly greater tumor multiplicity and forestomach carcinoma incidence than wild-type controls. Additionally, zinc-deficient COX-2$^{-/-}$ forestomach displayed strong leukotriene A$_4$ hydrolase (LTA$_4$H) immunostaining, indicating that alternative pathways such as the 5-LOX/LTA$_4$H pathway may be stimulated under ZD conditions when the COX-2 pathway is blocked *(101)*.

Together, these studies in transgenic/knockout mouse models highlight the divergent tumorigenic outcome brought about by the cooperativity between zinc deficiency and loss of function or overexpression of various genes, and at the same time, demonstrate the influence of zinc deficiency on the stimulation and repression of these different carcinogenic pathways.

5.4. Prevention of Esophageal Carcinogenesis by Replenishing Zinc

Nutritional zinc deficiency in rats increases esophageal cell proliferation and the incidence of NMBA-induced esophageal tumors. Replenishing zinc with a zinc-sufficient diet reduces these effects in ZD rats (79). Importantly, zinc replenishment initiated within hours rather than days after NMBA treatment is more effective in preventing the development of esophageal tumors by stimulating apoptosis in the esophageal epithelium (78). Thus, replenishment initiated at 1 (ZR_1), 24 (ZR_{24}), 72 (ZR_{72}), and 432 h (ZR_{432}) after NMBA treatment reduced esophageal tumor incidence from 93% in ZD rats, to 8, 14, 19, and 48%, respectively. Figure 2 illustrates events of apoptosis in the ZR_1 rat esophageal epithelia at 24 and 30 h after NMBA treatment and zinc replenishment. About 10% of cells in the ZR_1 esophagi were undergoing apoptosis as compared with ~2.9% in ZD esophagus (Fig. 2, E and F vs. A and B; M and N vs. I and J). There was a surge in Bax expression (Fig. 2, G vs. C and O vs. K) and a reduction in Bcl-2 expression (Fig. 2, H vs. D and P vs. L) in cells undergoing apoptosis, compared with ZD esophagi at similar times after NMBA treatment. Within 48 h, the ZR_1 epithelium was 3–5 cell layers thick compared with 10–20 layers before zinc replenishment, with PCNA-positive nuclei mostly found in the basal cell layer (24 h: Fig. 2, R vs. Q; 48 h: Fig. 2, T vs. S). These findings identify a cell death program that is dependent on members of the Bcl-2 gene family (111, 112). In the highly proliferative ZD esophagus, the Bax/Bcl-2 immunoreactive ratio was 0.5 and remained at this level throughout the experiment. In contrast, the Bax/Bcl-2 ratio increased to 1.3 at 24 h after zinc replenishment in ZR_1 esophagus and remained at an elevated level throughout the experiment. Thus, zinc replenishment increases Bax expression and reduces Bcl-2 expression, which increases the Bax/Bcl-2 ratio. This in vivo study demonstrates for the first time that apoptosis is triggered in the esophageal epithelium shortly after NMBA-treated ZD rats are given a zinc-sufficient diet and, as a result, NMBA-induced esophageal tumor formation is stopped in the very early stages of the tumorigenesis pathway.

5.5. Inefficacy of Molecular Targeting of COX-2 in Cancer Prevention in Zinc-Deficient Rodents

Targeted molecular intervention and therapies have been used in attempts to prevent or cure cancer. The rationale for targeting the COX-2 pathway for cancer prevention is supported by numerous preclinical and human studies, culminating in use of the selective COX-2 inhibitor celecoxib with Food and Drug Administration approval for cancer prevention in patients with familial adenomatous polyposis (113). COX-2 selective inhibitors are actively being tested in clinical trials for the prevention of several cancers, including colorectal, esophageal adenocarcinoma, and head and neck SCC (114, 115, 116).

Results from two ZD rodent cancer models show that without correcting nutritional zinc deficiency targeted disruption of the COX-2 pathway by the celecoxib or by genetic deletion does not prevent UADT carcinogenesis (101). First, tongue cancer prevention studies were conducted in ZD rats previously exposed to the tongue carcinogen NQO by celecoxib treatment with or without ZR, or by ZR alone. Celecoxib alone at 500 ppm

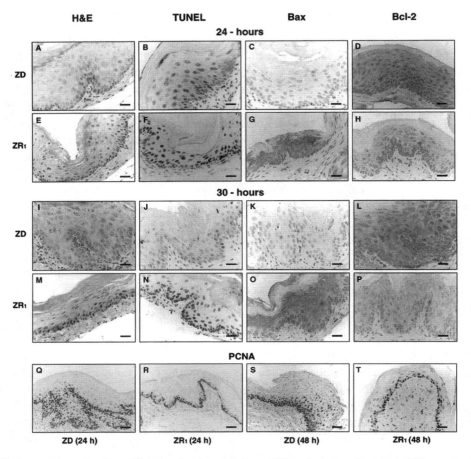

Fig. 2. Apoptosis and cell proliferation in zinc-deficient (ZD) and zinc-replenished (ZR) esophagi at 24 (**A–H, Q,** and **R**), 30 (**I–P**), and 48 (**S** and **T**) H after treatment with *N*-nitrosomethylbenzylamine (NMBA). Hematoxylin–eosin (**H&E**) staining, terminal deoxynucleotidyltransferase-mediated deoxyuridine triphosphate end labeling (TUNEL) analyses, and immunohistochemistry for Bax, Bcl-2, and proliferating cell nuclear antigen (PCNA) were used. *Panels* **A–D, I–L, Q,** and **S**: rats in the ZD group. *Panels* **E–H, M–P, R,** and **T**: rats in the ZR group (ZR1, replenished 1 h after NMBA treatment). **H&E**-stained esophageal sections from ZD rats (**A** and **I**) show hyperplastic epithelium with mature differentiated suprabasal cells. ZR1 esophagi (**E** and **M**) had suprabasal cells undergoing apoptosis. TUNEL analysis shows sporadic apoptotic cells in the proliferative ZD esophageal epithelia (**B** and **J**), but numerous apoptotic cells in the basal and suprabasal layers in ZR1 esophagi (**F** and **N**). Apoptotic bodies are intensely stained by 3,3′-diaminobenzidine tetrahydrochloride and counterstained with methyl green. Bax in a ZD esophagus showing hyperplasia is weakly detected in the cytoplasm (**C** and **K**), but strongly detected (3,3′-diaminobenzidine tetrahydrochloride) in suprabasal cells of ZR1 esophagus, showing apoptotic activities (**G** and **O**). Bcl-2 in the ZD esophagus with hyperplasia is strongly detected in the cytoplasm (**D** and **L**), but Bcl-2 in the ZR1 esophagi is weakly and diffusely detected in suprabasal cells (**H** and **P**). *Panels* **Q–T**: PCNA immunohistochemistry detects many cells in S phase and G1–S/G2 phase in the basal and suprabasal layers of the proliferative esophagus from rats in the ZD group (24 h: **Q**; 48 h: **S**), but detects few of these cells, mainly in basal layer of the restored esophageal epithelium, in the ZR1 group (24 h: **R**; 48 h: **T**). PCNA-positive nuclei were stained by 3-amino-9-ethylcarbazole substrate-chromogen and counterstained with hematoxylin. Panels **A–P** and **T**: scale bar = 25 μm; panels **Q–S**: scale bar = 50 μm. (Reproduced from *J Natl Cancer Inst* 2001; 93:1525–33).

levels significantly decreased lingual tumor multiplicity by 25% ($P < 0.001$), but had no effect on the incidence of large tumors or carcinomas. Nevertheless, zinc replenishment significantly reduced tumor multiplicity by 58%, incidence of large tumors by 40%, and squamous cell carcinoma by 32%. Combination of celecoxib plus ZR had an additive effect over ZR alone, but the result was not statistically significant. In addition, celecoxib alone slightly reduced overexpression of the three biomarkers COX-2, NF-κB p65, and LTA$_4$H in tumors, compared with intervention with ZR. Thus, the data document the similar ability of ZR to inhibit esophageal carcinogenesis in ZD animals *(78, 79)*. The lack of efficacy of celecoxib in curbing lingual cancer progression indicates its inability to block other cancer pathways that may be stimulated under nutritional ZD conditions. In this regard, in animals with complete nutrition the COX-2-specific inhibitors, nimesulide, etodolac, and celecoxib, inhibited NQO-induced lingual SCC development in rats *(117, 118)*. Second, instead of being protected, zinc-deficient COX-2-null mice developed significantly greater tumor multiplicity and forestomach carcinoma incidence than wild-type controls. Additionally, zinc-deficient COX-2$^{-/-}$ forestomachs displayed strong LTA$_4$H immunostaining, indicating activation of an alternative pathway under zinc deficiency when the COX-2 pathway is blocked.

Given that zinc deficiency causes extensive alterations in gene expression in the pro-tumorigenic esophagus and tongue (reviewed in Sections 5.6 and 5.7) *(66, 76, 77)*, it is not surprising that genetic deletion or pharmacological inhibition of COX-2 alone does not lead to cancer prevention in zinc-deficient animals. In contrast, zinc prevents both esophageal and lingual carcinogenesis in ZD animals. This finding strongly supports that zinc supplementation should be more thoroughly explored in human clinical trials for cancer prevention. Interestingly, in vivo zinc supplementation in humans led to downregulation of inflammatory cytokines and inhibition of induced NF-κB activation *(119)*. In vitro zinc supplementation inhibited NF-κB activation and suppressed the tumorigenic potential of human prostate cancer cells *(120)*. Since many cancer patients present symptoms of nutritional zinc deficiency at the time of diagnosis *(121)*, it might prove to be beneficial to include zinc in combination therapy.

5.6. *Modulation of Gene Expression*

DNA microarray analysis provides a powerful tool to understand how bioactive compounds modify genetic events in the onset, progression, and prevention of cancer. To date, several array studies have investigated the effects of zinc deficit and supplementation on gene expression in cells and rodent tissues. These studies were performed in cell lines such as human prostate epithelial cells *(122)*, THP-1 mononuclear cells *(123)*, colon adenocarcinoma cell line *(124)*, and leukocyte subsets *(125)*, and in vivo in rodent tissues such as esophagus *(66, 77)*, small intestine *(126)*, liver *(127, 128, 129)*, jejunum *(129)*, and thymus *(130)*. These array analyses show that alterations in cellular zinc status can affect hundreds of different target genes and that the effects of zinc on gene expression are tissue and cell-type specific.

Blanchard et al. *(126)* first reported in vivo in rat intestine the effectiveness of using cDNA array to compare the global changes in expression of genes during the early stages of dietary zinc deficiency. The genes that were expressed differentially in ZD rat intestine included those that influence growth, redox, and energy utilization. On the other hand, liver from ZD rat showed a set of differentially expressed genes that participate in growth, signal transduction, and in metabolism of xenobiotics, nitrogen, and lipid *(127, 128, 129)*.

Our earlier study using bioarray chips with ~8,000 genes identified 33 differentially expressed genes in hyperplastic ZD vs. control ZS esophagus, including upregulation of the zinc-sensitive gene metallothionein MT-1 and the esophageal tumorigenesis biomarker keratin 14 (KRT 14) *(77)*. This profile in the hyperplastic ZD rat esophagus is different from those reported for the small intestine or the liver, which are not known to become hyperplastic during dietary ZD *(126, 127, 128, 129)*. In particular, the cysteine-rich metal-binding protein MT expression that is upregulated in ZD esophagus was reported to be downregulated in liver and kidney from growing and adult rats under conditions of dietary zinc deprivation *(126, 128, 129, 131)*. High MT levels can arise from the inability of MT to release zinc, resulting in low intracellular free zinc ion availability for other biological functions *(13)*. This concept provides an explanation for the observed MT overexpression under conditions of inflammation and cancer, including precancerous ZD rat esophagus *(77)*, ZD rat lungs with pulmonary edema and inflammation *(42, 132)*, aged human liver and brain *(13)*, human inflammatory bowel disease *(133)*, as well as a variety of human cancers such as ESCC *(134)* and tongue SCC *(135)*. Additionally, MT overexpression in ESCC is often positively correlated with the metastatic and proliferative activities of the cancer *(134)*.

Our recent global transcriptome profiling analysis *(66)*, using an expanded rat genome array (Affymetrix Rat Genome 230 2.0 GeneChip) containing >30,000 transcripts and variants from ~28,000 rat genes, has discovered novel candidate genes involved in the pathogenesis of esophageal preneoplasia that were not previously reported *(77)*. The hyperplastic ZD rat esophagus has a distinct molecular signature of 103 differentially expressed genes with ≥4-fold differences in expression levels as compared with ZS esophagus (Fig. 3). This signature of preneoplasia included upregulated genes such as *S100A8, SERPINB3, AREG, DNMT3A, CDKN1A, BIRCA, EGF, GADD45A, S100A9, JUNB, ZFP36*, and *PTGES*, as well as downregulated genes *P2RX2, TPM1, G0S2*, and *TRDN*. Within hours after ZR the altered expression of 29 genes, including the proinflammation gene S100A8 (up 57-fold) and its heterodimer S100A9 (up 5-fold) reverted to control ZS levels, accompanied by the reversal of the hyperplastic phenotype. Importantly, S100A8 is a member of the seven genes that belong to the only significantly overrepresented pathway "response to external stimulus" among the upregulated genes (EASE score = 0.02), as identified by the Expression Analysis Systematic Explorer (EASE) pathway analysis. This finding strongly suggests that S100A8 is a relevant marker belonging to a causal pathway that drives esophageal preneoplasia rather than simply an epiphenomenon of esophageal preneoplasia or of nutritional zinc deficit. Consistent with this conclusion, a positive correlation was found between *S100A8* and *S100A9* mRNA expression and esophageal tumor incidence/burden in NMBA-induced carcinogenesis in ZD and ZR rats. The respective increase and decrease in expression of these two proteins are associated with the high and low tumorigenic outcome in ZD and ZR rats. Together, these data demonstrate that S100A8/A9 plays an important role in ZD-driven esophageal tumorigenesis *(66)*.

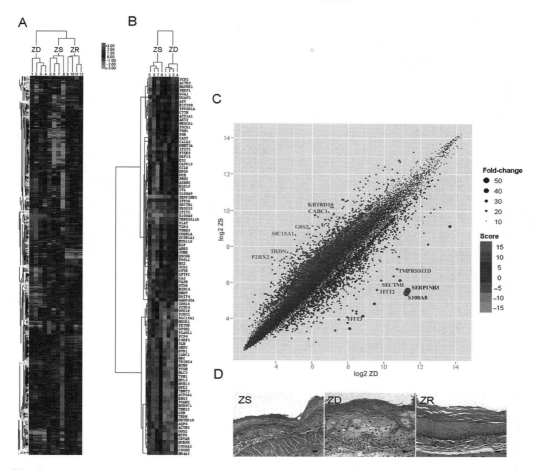

Fig. 3. Expression profiling of zinc-modulated rat esophageal mucosa. **A** and **B**, Dendrogram and color plot illustrating clustering of genes in zinc-modulated rat esophageal mucosa. Average linkage clustering was performed by uncentered correlation metric after log2 transformation and normalization. Columns represent four individual esophageal epithelial samples from zinc-deficient (ZD, no. 1–4), control zinc-sufficient (ZS, no. 5–8), and zinc-replenished (ZR, no. 9–12) rats. *Rows* represent genes with upregulated (*black*), or downregulated (*gray*) expression. **A**, Dendrogram and *color plot* illustrating clustering of 30,000 transcripts in 4 ZD, 4 ZR, and 4 ZS esophagi. **B**, Dendrogram and *black-gray plot* illustrating clustering of 103 genes that were differentially expressed in 4 ZD vs. 4 ZS esophagi (cutoff: q value <5% and expression fold changes ≥4). Gene symbols are presented; details including gene symbol, title, and function are presented in Table 1. **C**, Scatter plot. The data points show the expression mean (log 2 scale) on the variable ZS samples plotted against ZD samples. The size of each point represents the fold changes (ZD vs. ZS), whereas the *gray scale* shows the score (t-value) correlated with significance of a gene (q-value). The most upregulated and downregulated genes are shown in *black* and *dark gray*, respectively. **D**, Hematoxylin and eosin-stained esophageal tissue sections that show a normal ZS epithelium with 2–3 cells thick, a hyperplastic ZD epithelium, and a restored ZR epithelium at 48 h after oral zinc replenishment. Scale bar: 25 μm. (Reproduced from *Gastroenterology*, 2009; 136:953–66).

Table 1
Gene expression signature in precancerous zinc-deficient rat esophagus

Affymetrix id	Gene Symbol	Gene Title	Fold-Change ZD versus ZS	Score	q-value (%)	Function
Sixty-one up-regulated genes associated with dietary ZD						
1368494_at	S100A8	S100 calcium binding protein A8 (calgranulin A)	57	8.7	0	chemotaxis
1384973_at	SERPINB3	serine protease inhibitor B3	56	8.0	0	serine-type endopeptidase inhibitor activity
1379568_at	IFIT2	interferon-induced protein with tetratricopeptide repeats 2	16	8.6	0	binding
1387620_a_at	TMPRSS11D	transmembrane protease, serine 11d	16	8.9	0	proteolysis
1376908_at	IFIT3	interferon-induced protein with tetratricopeptide repeats 3	15	3.9	0.6	binding
1376976_at	SECTM1	secreted and transmembrane 1B	13	7.9	0	immune response
1379747_at	PRSS35	Protease, serine, 35	12	8.9	0	proteolysis
1367800_at	PLAT	plasminogen activator, tissue	10	5.7	0.1	protein modification process
1367733_at	CA2	carbonic anhydrase 2	9.5	7.4	0	kidney development
1369202_at	MX2	myxovirus (influenza virus) resistance 2	8.7	3.0	2.0	defense response
1386889_at	SCD2	stearoyl-Coenzyme A desaturase 2	8.4	3.6	0.9	lipid metabolic process
1369871_at	AREG	amphiregulin	8.3	5.4	0.2	epidermal growth factor receptor signaling pathway
1367566_at	SCGB1A1	secretoglobin, family 1A, member 1 (uteroglobin)	8.2	4.9	0.3	signal transduction
1371100_at	ES2	esterase 2	7.8	2.9	2.4	carboxylesterase activity
1370355_at	SCD1	stearoyl-Coenzyme A desaturase 1	7.6	6.8	0	lipid metabolic process
1384960_at	CFTR	cystic fibrosis transmembrane conductance regulator homolog	7.4	8.6	0	transport

Probe ID	Symbol	Gene				Function
1392678_a_at	DNMT3A	DNA methyltransferase 3A	7.2	3.1	2.0	DNA methylation
1369640_at	GJA1	gap junction membrane channel protein alpha 1	6.7	4.4	0.5	in utero embryonic development
1387391_at	CDKN1A	cyclin-dependent kinase inhibitor 1A	6.6	5.3	0.2	regulation of progression through cell cycle
1380083_at	KLK10	kallikrein 10	6.5	4.8	0.3	proteolysis
1381024_at	PPP2R1A	protein phosphatase 2 (formerly 2A)	6.4	5.3	0.2	protein phosphatase type 2A activity
1395886_at	ACTR3	ARP3 actin-related protein 3 homolog	6.3	3.4	1.2	structural constituent of cytoskeleton
1391481_at	CAST	Calpastatin	6.2	6.0	0.1	myoblast fusion
1380533_at	APP	amyloid beta (A4) precursor protein	6.2	3.0	2.0	G2 phase of mitotic cell cycle
1369248_a_at	BIRC4	baculoviral IAP repeat-containing 4	6.2	6.5	0	apoptosis
1368025_at	DDIT4	DNA-damage-inducible transcript 4	6.2	9.4	0	response to hypoxia
1368325_at	EGF	epidermal growth factor	6.1	5.7	0.1	activation of MAPKK activity
1397675_at	WBSCR1	Williams-Beuren syndrome chromosome region 1 homolog	5.8	4.7	0.4	translation
1370153_at	GDF15	growth differentiation factor 15	5.6	3.5	1.1	signal transduction
1384784_at	CLCA2	chloride channel calcium activated 2	5.5	4.2	0.5	translation
1369846_at	IVL	involucrin	5.3	3.5	1.1	keratinocyte differentiation
1398143_at	PRKX	protein kinase, X-linked	5.2	3.7	0.7	protein amino acid phosphorylation
1370627_at	RHOV	ras homolog gene family, member V	5.1	6.6	0	signal transduction
1387982_at	TLR4	toll-like receptor 4	5.1	3.8	0.7	inflammatory response
1368213_at	POR	P450 (cytochrome) oxidoreductase	5.0	7.0	0	electron transport
1369517_at	PSCD1	pleckstrin homology, Sec7 and coiled-coil domains 1	5.0	4.9	0.3	Golgi to secretory vesicle transport
1387125_at	S100A9	S100 calcium binding protein A9 (calgranulin B)	5.0	4.5	0.4	inflammatory response

Table 1
(Continued)

Affymetrix id	Gene Symbol	Gene Title	Fold-Change ZD versus ZS	Score	q-value (%)	Function
1397674_at	EIF3S8	eukaryotic translation initiation factor 3, subunit 8, 110kDa	4.9	4.0	0.6	translational initiation
1368489_at	FOSL1	fos-like antigen 1	4.9	6.3	0.1	regulation of transcription, DNA-dependent
1369568_at	STX6	syntaxin 6	4.9	12	0	transport
1370255_at	SFTPC	surfactant associated protein C	4.8	9.0	0	respiratory gaseous exchange
1370792_at	MAPRE1	microtubule-associated protein, RP/EB family, member 1	4.7	3.4	1.2	cell cycle
1387605_at	CASP12	caspase 12	4.6	4.0	0.6	proteolysis
1371108_a_at	ATP1A1	ATPase, Na+/K+ transporting, alpha 1 polypeptide	4.6	3.5	1.1	ATP catabolic process
1369406_at	ASAH2	N-acylsphingosine amidohydrolase 2	4.6	3.1	1.7	lipid metabolic process
1387631_at	HPGD	hydroxyprostaglandin dehydrogenase 15 (NAD)	4.4	3.1	1.7	lipid metabolic process
1371618_s_at	TUBB3	tubulin, beta 3	4.3	5.5	0.2	microtubule-based process
1387788_at	JUNB	Jun-B oncogene	4.3	9.8	0	regulation of progression through cell cycle
1370174_at	MYD116	myeloid differentiation primary response gene 116	4.3	5.5	0.2	myeloid differentiation primary response gene 116
1369597_at	VAPB	vesicle-associated membrane protein, associated protein B and C	4.3	5.6	0.1	protein complex assembly
1370123_a_at	CTTN	cortactin	4.3	5.5	0.2	receptor-mediated endocytosis
1396262_at	PBEF1	pre-B-cell colony enhancing factor 1	4.3	4.5	0.4	cell cycle

Probe ID	Symbol	Gene name				Process
1368024_at	QSCN6	quiescin Q6	4.2	7.2	0	regulation of progression through cell cycle
1370477_at	OCM	oncomodulin	4.2	3.5	1.1	calcium ion binding
1389123_at	CCL	chemokine (C-C motif) ligand 6	4.2	2.6	3.4	apoptosis
1384328_at	TOM1	target of myb1 homolog (chicken)	4.2	6.0	0.1	intracellular protein transport
1368947_at	GADD45A	growth arrest and DNA-damage-inducible 45 alpha	4.2	3.9	0.6	regulation of progression through cell cycle
1387353_at	AKT2	thymoma viral proto-oncogene 2	4.2	7.2	0	protein amino acid phosphorylation
1395614_at	U2AF2	U2 small nuclear ribonucleoprotein auxiliary factor (U2AF) 2	4.1	2.8	2.4	nuclear mRNA splicing, via spliceosome
1387870_at	ZFP36	zinc finger protein 36	4.1	6.7	0	mRNA catabolic process
1368014_at	PTGES	prostaglandin E synthase	4.1	4.2	0.5	prostaglandin biosynthetic process

Forty-two down-regulated genes associated with dietary ZD

Probe ID	Symbol	Gene name				Process
1387578_a_at	P2RX2	purinergic receptor P2X, ligand-gated ion channel, 2	0.08	−6.3	0.1	transport
1369381_a_at	SLC15A1	solute carrier family 15 (oligopeptide transporter), member 1	0.09	−3.8	0.5	transport
1388395_at	G0S2	G0/G1 switch gene 2	0.11	−3.4	0.7	integral to membrane
1370198_at	TRDN	triadin	0.12	−2.4	2.8	calcium ion homeostasis
1368252_at	KBTBD10	kelch repeat and BTB (POZ) domain containing 10	0.13	−2.8	1.7	cell motility
1372536_at	CABC1	chaperone, ABC1 activity of bc1 complex like	0.13	−4.2	0.4	protein folding
1398243_at	CSRP3	cysteine and glycine-rich protein 3	0.13	−2.1	4.6	blood vessel remodeling
1371247_at	TNNT3	troponin T3, skeletal, fast	0.14	−2.9	1.7	muscle contraction
1383875_at	UPK1B	uroplakin 1B	0.14	−3.5	0.7	epithelial cell differentiation

Table 1
(Continued)

Affymetrix id	Gene Symbol	Gene Title	Fold-Change ZD versus ZS	Score	q-value (%)	Function
1387181_at	MYF6	myogenic factor 6	0.14	−2.6	2.4	somitogenesis
1374248_at	MYBPC1	myosin binding protein C, slow type	0.14	−2.9	1.5	muscle contraction
1367572_at	MYL3	myosin, light polypeptide 3	0.14	−2.9	1.5	muscle contraction
1371053_at	MYH8	myosin, heavy polypeptide 8, skeletal muscle, perinatal	0.14	−3.8	0.6	striated muscle contraction
1374391_at	SLN	sarcolipin	0.14	−3.2	1.1	transport
1370165_at	SMPX	small muscle protein, X-linked	0.15	−2.7	2.0	striated muscle contraction
1368108_at	ATP2A1	ATPase, Ca++ transporting, cardiac muscle, fast twitch 1	0.16	−2.7	2.0	ATP catabolic process
1368145_at	PCP4	Purkinje cell protein 4	0.16	−4.9	0.3	central nervous system development
1370026_at	CRYAB	crystallin, alpha B	0.16	−3.6	0.6	glucose metabolic process
1372639_at	TRIM54	tripartite motif-containing 54	0.16	−3.8	0.6	negative regulation of microtubule
1370982_at	PYGM	muscle glycogen phosphorylase	0.16	−3.4	0.7	response to hypoxia
1391429_at	HFE2	hemochromatosis type 2 (juvenile) homolog (human)	0.16	−2.9	1.5	GPI anchor binding
1367782_at	COX6A2	cytochrome c oxidase, subunit VIa, polypeptide 2	0.17	−2.9	1.5	electron transport
1378430_at	MOXD1	monooxygenase, DBH-like 1	0.17	−8.2	0	catecholamine metabolic process
1367626_at	CKM	creatine kinase, muscle	0.17	−2.3	4.0	phosphocreatine metabolic process
1387082_at	FETUB	fetuin beta	0.17	−5.9	0.1	cysteine protease inhibitor activity
1390355_at	RYR1	ryanodine receptor 1, skeletal muscle	0.17	−3.7	0.6	transport

Probe ID	Symbol	Gene name	q-value	Score		Function
1387122_at	PLAGL1	pleiomorphic adenoma gene-like 1	0.17	−8.3	0	induction of apoptosis
1367962_at	ACTN3	actinin alpha 3	0.18	−4.2	0.4	muscle contraction
1372383_at	GPSM1	G-protein signalling modulator 1	0.18	−6.2	0.1	signal transduction
1372190_at	AQP4	Aquaporin 4	0.18	−4.8	0.3	transport
1367964_at	TNNI2	troponin I type 2 (skeletal, fast)	0.18	−2.8	1.7	hydrogen transport
1368724_a_at	TPM1	tropomyosin 1, alpha	0.18	−3.1	1.2	cell motility
1386907_at	ENO3	enolase 3, beta	0.18	−2.8	1.7	glycolysis
1387092_at	FXYD4	FXYD domain-containing ion transport regulator 4	0.19	−2.6	2.4	transport
1377499_a_at	HRC	histidine rich calcium binding protein	0.19	−3.8	0.6	structural molecule activity
1369067_at	NR4A3	nuclear receptor subfamily 4, group A, member 3	0.20	−2.3	4.0	mesoderm formation
1367951_at	PGAM2	phosphoglycerate mutase 2	0.20	−2.4	2.8	glycolysis
1370033_at	MLC3	myosin, light polypeptide 1	0.21	−3.1	1.2	cardiac muscle contraction
1378698_at	MYH13	myosin, heavy polypeptide 8, skeletal muscle, perinatal	0.21	−2.3	4.0	striated muscle contraction
1368966_at	MYBPH	myosin binding protein H	0.21	−2.2	4.6	striated muscle contraction
1367739_at	COX8H	Cytochrome c oxidase subunit VIII-H (heart/muscle)	0.22	−2.5	2.8	electron transport
1390822_at	CDH16	cadherin 16	0.22	−2.5	2.8	tRNA aminoacylation for protein translation

A group of 103 differentially expressed genes were identified, using a cutpoint of q value <5% and fold-change ≥4.0. Score is the T-statistic value; q-value is the lowest False Discovery Rate at which the gene is considered significant. ZD = zinc-deficient; ZS = zinc-sufficient (Reproduced from *Gastroenterology*, 2009; 136, 953–66).

S100A8 and S100A9 have emerged as important mediators in inflammation and may play a key role in inflammation-associated cancers *(136)*. They encode the S100 family member of calcium and zinc-binding proteins. S100A8/A9 form heterodimers and are frequently co-expressed. Overexpression of these two proteins occurs in a variety of human cancers *(136)*, including skin SCC *(137)*, ESCC *(138)*, and Barrett's esophagus, a precancerous condition of EAC *(139)*. RAGE (the receptor for advanced glycation endproducts) is the putative receptor of these two proteins. In vitro engagement of the receptor RAGE by S100A8/A9 activates NF-κB signaling in various tumor cells *(140, 141)*. In a multistage mouse skin carcinogenesis model, Gebhardt et al.*(142)* provided direct genetic evidence that S100A8/A9 binds to RAGE and the RAGE–S100A8/9 signaling mediates sustained skin inflammation and promotes tumor development. Additionally, blockade of RAGE suppresses tumor growth and metastasis *(142, 143)*.

The immunohistochemical data on archived near serial sections of esophageal sections (Fig. 4) further showed that RAGE and S100A8 proteins were overexpressed in the hyperplastic ZD rat esophagus that evidenced overexpression of NF-κB p65 and COX-2 proteins *(101)*. In addition, ZR reduced the overexpression of all four proteins, thereby suppressing RAGE/S100A8 signaling, and reversed esophageal preneoplasia (Fig. 4). The data demonstrate for the first time that zinc regulates S100A8 mRNA and protein expression in vivo, providing evidence for an inflammation-modulating role of zinc in esophageal preneoplasia initiation and its reversal. Moreover, the data establish a link between zinc and RAGE/S100A8 interaction and NF-κB COX-2 activation in early esophageal carcinogenesis and prevention. Most importantly, our unpublished data on global transcriptome profiling of mouse forestomach mucosa showed that S100A8 and S100A9 are highly upregulated in COX-2-null mice on a ZD diet as compared with COX-2-null mice on a ZS diet. This finding demonstrates that in the presence of genetic COX-2 deletion zinc deficiency activates the S100A8 signaling pathway, thereby enhancing instead of reducing NMBA-induced forestomach tumorigenesis in zinc-deficient COX-2-null mice.

5.7. Modulation of MicroRNA Expression

MicroRNAs (miRNAs) are short non-coding RNAs of ∼21 nucleotides that regulate the translation of many genes through imperfect pairing with target mRNA of protein-coding genes or by destroying messenger RNA *(144, 145, 146)*. The predicted number of miRNA in humans is ∼1,000 and each of these miRNAs is thought to have hundreds of targets, regulating a variety of cellular processes, including cell proliferation, differentiation, and apoptosis *(147)*. Recent data have shown that miRNAs expression levels were altered in most tumor types *(148)* and led to the conclusion that miRNAs may play a causal role in carcinogenesis. In tumors, miRNAs may play significant roles as oncogenes or tumor suppressors *(149, 150, 151)*.

To date, there are only two reports that link altered expression of miRNA in cancer with nutritional deficiencies. The overexpression of miR-222 was identified in vitro in human lymphoblastoid cells grown under folate-deficient conditions and confirmed in

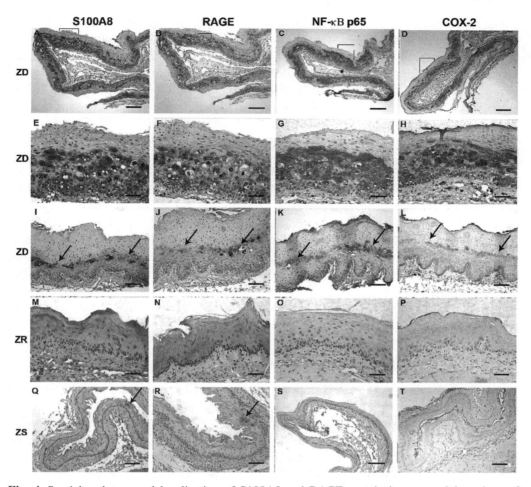

Fig. 4. Spatial and temporal localization of S100A8 and RAGE protein in near serial sections of archived formalin-fixed, paraffin-embedded esophageal tissues from zinc-modulated rats that overexpressed NF-κB p65 and COX-2. S100A8 (**A**, **E**, and **I**) and the putative receptor of S100A8, RAGE (**B**, **F**, and **J**), were intensely and abundantly co-expressed in near serial sections of zinc-deficient (ZD) esophagus and occurred in similar spatial patterns as those of NF-κB p65 (**C**, **G**, and **K**: reproduced from *Int J Cancer* 2007) and COX-2 (**D**, **H**, and **L**: reproduced from 2005, *J Natl Cancer Inst* 97, 40–50). 100A8 (**M**) and RAGE (**N**) expression was greatly reduced at 48 h after zinc replenishment, as was NF-κB p65 (**O**) and COX-2 (**P**). Zinc-sufficient (ZS) esophagi showed sporadic and moderate expression (*arrows*) of 100A8 (**Q**) and RAGE (**R**) and weak or absent staining of NF-κB p65 (**S**) and COX-2 (**T**). S100A8 and RAGE localization was visualized by incubation with 3-amino-9-ethylcarbazole substrate-chromogen. Expression of NF-κB p65 proteins was localized by incubation with 3,3′-diaminobenzidine tetrahydrochloride. Scale bars: 100 μm (in **A–D** and **Q–T**); 50 μm (in **I–P**); 25 μm (in **E–H**, higher magnification of bracketed area in **A–D**). (Reproduced from *Gastroenterology*, 2009; 136:953–66)

vivo in human peripheral blood from individuals with low folate intake *(152)*. miR-122, an abundant liver-specific miRNA, was reported to be downregulated in liver tumors from rats fed a folic acid-methionine-choline deficient diet *(153)*.

Our unpublished data show that miRNAs expression levels in rat esophagus and tongue are modulated by dietary zinc *(76)*. The precancerous ZD esophagus has a distinct miRNA expression signature as compared with control ZS esophagus, including upregulation of miR-31 (up ∼ 6-fold) and miR-183 (up 4-fold) and downregulation of miR-100 (down 2-fold). Interestingly, upregulation of miR-31 was also found in the hyperplastic tongue mucosa, *(75)* but not in liver, kidney, spleen, brain, prostate, or lung from ZD rats. In human cancers, miR-31 upregulation was reported in human colorectal cancer *(154)* and squamous cell carcinoma of tongue *(155)* and miR-100 downregulation in ESCC *(156)*.

While ZR rapidly reversed the abnormal expression of many genes within hours *(77)*, it is less effective in reversing the abnormal expression of miR-31. After 5 weeks of zinc treatment, miR-31 overexpression in ZD esophagus was reduced by approximately 50%. Importantly, miR-31 overexpression was sustained during NMBA-induced esophageal carcinogenesis in ZD rats with a high tumorigenic outcome but it was suppressed in NMBA-treated ZR rats with a low tumorigenic outcome. These data demonstrate that zinc regulates miR-31 expression in vivo in esophageal carcinogenesis and prevention. The influence of zinc on miR expression provides a novel mechanism by which zinc elicits its protumorigenic and antitumorigenic effects in cancer development and prevention.

6. ANTITUMOR EFFECTS IN OTHER TUMOR CELLS

In addition to esophageal and oral cancer, zinc exhibits antitumor effects in other types of tumor, in particular, prostate cancer. The pathogenesis of prostate cancer involves transformation of normal prostate epithelial cells that accumulate zinc to malignant prostate cells that do not accumulate zinc *(157)*. The inability to accumulate zinc is, at least in part, probably due to the downregulation of the zinc uptake transporter ZIP1 in malignant prostate cells *(40)*. Although the precise role of zinc in the prostate is unclear, numerous studies support the concept that zinc has antitumor effects in prostate cancer *(157)*. Yan et al. *(122)* showed that zinc deficiency in prostate epithelial cells resulted in DNA damage and altered expression of genes involved in cell cycle, apoptosis, DNA damage, and repair and transcription, thus compromising DNA integrity in the prostate. Uzzo et al. *(120)* demonstrate that physiological levels of zinc inhibit activation of the transcription factor NF-κB in human prostate cancer cells, thereby suppressing the tumorigenic potential of these cells and sensitizing malignant cells to apoptosis induced by the chemotherapeutic agent paclitaxel. Conversely, paclitaxel-induced apoptosis was reduced in prostate cancer cells from zinc-deficient compared to zinc-replete conditions *(158)*.

One of the major antitumor effects of zinc is its inhibition of cancer cell growth by inducing apoptosis. In this regard, several studies have reported inhibitory effects of zinc on apoptosis when high concentrations of zinc (500–1,000 μM) were used and stimulatory effects of zinc with zinc being depleted by metal chelators *(159, 160)*. With lower or more physiologic concentrations of zinc, however, Fraker and Telford *(54)* demonstrated that zinc could actually induce death in such cell types. In prostate cancer cells, Feng et al. *(161)* reported that physiological levels of zinc-induced apoptosis by facilitating a Bax-associated pore formation process, providing evidence that Bax is implicated in the zinc induction of mitochondrial apoptosis and prevention of prostate cell growth *(162, 163)*.

Finally, zinc also elicits apoptotic antitumor effects in human epithelial ovarian cancer *(164)*, choriocarcinoma *(165)*, and human hepatocellular carcinoma HEP-2 cells *(166)*, and inhibits cell proliferation in colon cancer cells *(167)*. Together, these reports lend support to the idea of zinc as a tumor suppressor agent in cancer therapeutic strategies and prevention.

7. HUMAN INTERVENTION STUDIES

7.1. Esophageal Cancer

To date, only a limited number of nutrition intervention trials have been conducted in populations with a high incidence of esophageal cancer to determine whether combined nutrient treatments that include zinc could lower the prevalence of lesions of the esophagus. The Chinese Linxian trials *(168, 169, 170, 171)* were conducted in populations that were nutritionally inadequate, whereas the SU.VI.MAX French trial *(172)* was performed in an apparently healthy population.

A randomized double-blind intervention trial in Huixian showed that a once-a-week treatment with retinol, riboflavin, and zinc (50 mg) for 1 year had no effect on the prevalence of precancerous lesions of the esophagus *(169)*. However, a statistically significant reduction ($P = 0.04$) in the prevalence of micronuclei in esophageal cells was observed in the treatment group as compared to the placebo *(168)*. In a Linxian intervention study, subjects who were given supplemental multiple vitamins and minerals, including zinc, for 30 months to prevent the progression of esophageal dysplasia to cancer appeared to have reduced esophageal proliferation *(171)*. In the randomized, placebo-controlled Linxian nutrition intervention trial, no significant reductions in the prevalence of esophageal or gastric dysplasia or cancer were seen with any of the four vitamin and mineral supplement groups taken for 5.25 years at daily supplement levels that ranged from one to two times the United States Recommended Daily Allowance (retinol and zinc (22 mg); riboflavin and niacin; vitamin C and molybdenum; and B-carotene, vitamin, and selenium). However, the prevalence of gastric cancer among participants receiving retinol and zinc was 62% ($P = 0.09$) lower than those subjects not receiving supplements, a finding that suggested the potential benefits of such an intervention *(170)*.

The SU.VI.MAX French study was designed to determine the efficacy of a daily supplement of antioxidants (vitamin C, vitamin E, β-carotene, selenium, and zinc (22 mg)) for the primary prevention of cancer. The French trial found that the supplement reduced the rate of total cancer incidence and all-cause mortality by 31% in men but not in women who had higher serum levels of antioxidants *(172)*.

On the other hand, Limberg et al. *(173)* reported a possible beneficial effect for selenomethionine (a synthetic form of organic selenium) against ESCC in a randomized controlled trial among residents in Linxian China. In the latter trial, subjects with histologically confirmed mild or moderate esophageal squamous dysplasia at baseline received selenomethionine (200 µg daily) and/or celecoxib (200 mg twice daily for

10 months). Neither selenomethionine nor celecoxib inhibited ESCC carcinogenesis for high-risk subjects, but selenomethionine showed a protective effect among subjects with mild esophageal squamous dysplasia. This study represents the first report of a possible beneficial effect for any candidate chemopreventive agent.

In summary, data from intervention studies with multivitamin/mineral supplements that included zinc indicate that such interventions may prevent cancer in persons with poor nutritional status *(172, 174)*. To date, there are no studies that report controlled clinical trials of the efficacy of zinc treatment against cancer. Results of animal studies support the use in humans of zinc as a potential chemopreventive agent for esophageal and oral cancer prevention *(78, 101)*, particularly among subjects with preexisting nutritional zinc deficit. The requirement for zinc replenishment in chemoprevention of tongue tumors in ZD rats suggests that the nutritional status of patients should be considered in cancer treatment protocols *(101)*.

7.2. *Prostate Cancer*

Despite evidence from experimental studies pointing to a protective effect of zinc against prostate cancer development and progression *(120, 122, 158)*, epidemiological reports have produced conflicting and divergent results. The efficacy of zinc supplement against prostate cancer ranged from no effect of zinc *(175, 176)*, a protective effect of zinc *(177, 178)*, to a moderate increased risk with high doses of zinc supplement prescribed over a long period *(179)*. The increased risk of prostate cancer associated with high doses of zinc supplement might be due to possible contaminants such as cadmium in commercial zinc supplement products *(180)*. In view of these conflicting data, further epidemiological studies are necessary to resolve the issue of whether zinc has efficacy against prostate cancer *(157)*.

7.3. *Colon Cancer*

In 2004, the Iowa Women's Health Study provided epidemiological evidence that a high dietary zinc intake is associated with a decreased risk of both proximal and distal colon cancer *(181)*.

8. CONCLUSIONS

Based on the myriad of biological functions of zinc and its tumorigenic effects in rodent cancer models, the role of zinc deficiency as a causative factor for cancer and a deciding factor in the progression of cancer is beginning to take root. Of equal importance, the concept of zinc as a tumor suppressor agent in cancer prevention is supported by abundant experimental and clinical studies in esophageal, lingual, prostate, and colon cancer. Recent data from gene profiling and immunohistochemical analyses, showing that zinc regulates the proinflammation mediator S100A8 expression, its interaction with RAGE, and the downstream NF-κB-COX-2 signaling pathway, provide the first evidence for an inflammation-modulating role of zinc in early esophageal carcinogenesis and its reversal. Consistent with this notion, NF-κB is recognized as a link between inflammation/immunity and cancer development and progression. The

IkB kinase/NF-κB activation pathway is a target for cancer prevention *(182)*. Thus, zinc supplementation might have important implications in cancer prevention, predominantly through suppression of S100A8–RAGE interactions and downstream NF-κB signaling.

Given the recent reignited interest of researchers in the concept of an association of inflammation and the genesis and perpetuation of cancer *(183, 184)*, the finding that zinc regulates a key inflammation pathway and modulates miRNA expression in esophageal preneoplasia offers opportunities to conduct studies to more precisely define the role of zinc in cancer initiation, progression, and prevention and also to explore the possible link between miR expression and inflammation *(183)*.

Despite convincing experimental evidence, limited effort has been directed toward clinical investigations to determine efficacy of zinc for the prevention of human cancers. In particular, the finding that targeting only the COX-2 pathway in zinc-deficient animals does not prevent UADT tumor progression strongly suggests that correcting nutritional deficiencies is necessary in a more successful cancer treatment protocol. More broadly, zinc supplementation should be thoroughly explored in human clinical trials for the prevention of UADT cancer, especially in the aged *(185)* and people with zinc deficiency in high-risk populations.

REFERENCES

1. Vallee, B.L., and Falchuk, K.H. (1993) The biochemical basis of zinc physiology. *Physiol Rev* **73**, 79–118.
2. Berg, J.M., and Shi, Y. (1996) The galvanization of biology: A growing appreciation for the roles of zinc. *Science* **271**, 1081–85.
3. O'Halloran, T.V. (1993) Transition metals in control of gene expression. *Science* **261**, 715–25.
4. Shankar, A.H., and Prasad, A.S. (1998) Zinc and immune function: The biological basis of altered resistance to infection. *Am J Clin Nutr* **68**, 447S–63S.
5. Devirgiliis, C., Zalewski, P.D., Perozzi, G., and Murgia, C. (2007) Zinc fluxes and zinc transporter genes in chronic diseases. *Mutat Res* **622**, 84–93.
6. Levenson, C.W., and Somers, R.C. (2008) Nutritionally regulated biomarkers for breast cancer. *Nutr Rev* **66**, 163–66.
7. Maret, W., and Sandstead, H.H. (2006) Zinc requirements and the risks and benefits of zinc supplementation. *J Trace Elem Med Biol* **20**, 3–18.
8. Raulin, J. (1869) Etudes cliniques sur la vegetation. *Ann Sci Nat Bot Biol Veg* **11**, 93–229.
9. Todd, W.R., Elvehjem, C.A., and Hart, E.B. (1934) Zinc in the nutrition of the rat. *Am J Physiol* **107**, 146–56.
10. Prasad, A.S., Halsted, J.A., and Nadimi, M. (1961) Syndrome of iron deficiency anemia, hepatosplenomegaly, hypogonadism, dwarfism and geophagia. *Am J Med* **31**, 532–46.
11. Prasad, A.S., Miale, A., Jr., Farid, Z., Sandstead, H.H., and Schulert, A.R. (1963) Zinc metabolism in patients with the syndrome of iron deficiency anemia, hepatosplenomegaly, dwarfism, and hypogonadism. *J Lab Clin Med* **61**, 537–49.
12. Brown, K.H., Wuehler, S.E., and Peerson, J.M. (2001) The importance of zinc in human nutrition and estimation of the global prevalence of zinc deficiency. *Food and Nutrition Bulletin* **22**, 113–25.
13. Mocchegiani, E., Giacconi, R., Cipriano, C. et al. (2007) Zinc, metallothioneins, and longevity—effect of zinc supplementation: Zincage study. *Ann N Y Acad Sci* **1119**, 129–46.
14. Sandstead, H.H. (1973) Zinc nutrition in the United States. *Am J Clin Nutr* **26**, 1251–60.
15. Ho, E., and Ames, B.N. (2002) Low intracellular zinc induces oxidative DNA damage, disrupts p53, NFkappa B, and AP1 DNA binding, and affects DNA repair in a rat glioma cell line. *Proc Natl Acad Sci USA* **99**, 16770–75.

16. Prasad, A.S., and Kucuk, O. (2002) Zinc in cancer prevention. *Cancer Metastasis Rev* **21**, 291–95.
17. Parkin, D.M., Bray, F., Ferlay, J., and Pisani, P. (2001) Estimating the world cancer burden: Globocan 2000. *Int J Cancer* **94**, 153–56.
18. American Cancer Society (2008) Cancer Facts and Figures. Atlanta, GA: American Cancer Society.
19. Moore, S.R., Johnson, N.W., Pierce, A.M., and Wilson, D.F. (2000) The epidemiology of tongue cancer: A review of global incidence. *Oral Dis* **6**, 75–84.
20. Makuuchi, H., Machimura, T., Shimada, H. et al. (1996) Endoscopic screening for esophageal cancer in 788 patients with head and neck cancers. *Tokai J Exp Clin Med* **21**, 139–45.
21. Slaughter, D.P., Southwick, H.W., and Smejkal, W. (1953) Field cancerization in oral stratified squamous epithelium; clinical implications of multicentric origin. *Cancer* **6**, 963–68.
22. Magee, P.N. (1989) The experimental basis for the role of nitroso compounds in human cancer. *Cancer Surv* **8**, 207–39.
23. Yang, C.S. (1980) Research on esophageal cancer in China: A review. *Cancer Res* **40**, 2633–44.
24. van Rensburg, S.J. (1981) Epidemiologic and dietary evidence for a specific nutritional predisposition to esophageal cancer. *J Natl Cancer Inst* **67**, 243–51.
25. Gupta, P.C., Hebert, J.R., Bhonsle, R.B., Murti, P.R., Mehta, H., and Mehta, F.S. (1999) Influence of dietary factors on oral precancerous lesions in a population-based case-control study in Kerala, India. *Cancer* **85**, 1885–93.
26. Iran-IARC study group (1977) Esophageal cancer studies in the Caspian littoral of Iran: Results of population studies—a prodrome. Joint Iran-International Agency for Research on Cancer Study Group. *J Natl Cancer Inst* **59**, 1127–38.
27. Hebert, J.R., Gupta, P.C., Bhonsle, R.B. et al. (2002) Dietary exposures and oral precancerous lesions in Srikakulam District, Andhra Pradesh, India. *Public Health Nutr* **5**, 303–12.
28. Poschl, G., and Seitz, H.K. (2004) Alcohol and cancer. *Alcohol Alcohol* **39**, 155–65.
29. Abnet, C.C., Lai, B., Qiao, Y.L. et al. (2005) Zinc concentration in esophageal biopsy specimens measured by x-ray fluorescence and esophageal cancer risk. *J Natl Cancer Inst* **97**, 301–06.
30. Davis, S.R., and Cousins, R.J. (2000) Metallothionein expression in animals: A physiological perspective on function. *J Nutr* **130**, 1085–88.
31. Maret, W., and Vallee, B.L. (1998) Thiolate ligands in metallothionein confer redox activity on zinc clusters. *Proc Natl Acad Sci USA* **95**, 3478–82.
32. Eide, D.J. (2004) The SLC39 family of metal ion transporters. *Pflugers Arch* **447**, 796–800.
33. Palmiter, R.D., and Huang, L. (2004) Efflux and compartmentalization of zinc by members of the SLC30 family of solute carriers. *Pflugers Arch* **447**, 744–51.
34. Memon, A.U., Kazi, T.G., Afridi, H.I. et al. (2007) Evaluation of zinc status in whole blood and scalp hair of female cancer patients. *Clin Chim Acta* **379**, 66–70.
35. Margalioth, E.J., Schenker, J.G., and Chevion, M. (1983) Copper and zinc levels in normal and malignant tissues. *Cancer* **52**, 868–72.
36. Cui, Y., Vogt, S., Olson, N., Glass, A.G., and Rohan, T.E. (2007) Levels of zinc, selenium, calcium, and iron in benign breast tissue and risk of subsequent breast cancer. *Cancer Epidemiol Biomarkers Prev* **16**, 1682–85.
37. Kasper, G., Weiser, A.A., Rump, A. et al. (2005) Expression levels of the putative zinc transporter LIV-1 are associated with a better outcome of breast cancer patients. *Int J Cancer* **117**, 961–73.
38. Kagara, N., Tanaka, N., Noguchi, S., and Hirano, T. (2007) Zinc and its transporter ZIP10 are involved in invasive behavior of breast cancer cells. *Cancer Sci* **98**, 692–97.
39. Li, M., Zhang, Y., Liu, Z. et al. (2007) Aberrant expression of zinc transporter ZIP4 (SLC39A4) significantly contributes to human pancreatic cancer pathogenesis and progression. *Proc Natl Acad Sci USA* **104**, 18636–41.
40. Franklin, R.B., Feng, P., Milon, B. et al. (2005) hZIP1 zinc uptake transporter down regulation and zinc depletion in prostate cancer. *Mol Cancer* **4**, 32.
41. Lee, R., Woo, W., Wu, B., Kummer, A., Duminy, H., and Xu, Z. (2003) Zinc accumulation in N-methyl-N-nitrosourea-induced rat mammary tumors is accompanied by an altered expression of ZnT-1 and metallothionein. *Exp Biol Med (Maywood)* **228**, 689–96.

42. Lang, C., Murgia, C., Leong, M. et al. (2007) Anti-inflammatory effects of zinc and alterations in zinc transporter mRNA in mouse models of allergic inflammation. *Am J Physiol Lung Cell Mol Physiol* **292**, L577–L84.

43. Yu, Y.Y., Kirschke, C.P., and Huang, L. (2007) Immunohistochemical analysis of ZnT1, 4, 5, 6, and 7 in the mouse gastrointestinal tract. *J Histochem Cytochem* **55**, 223–34.

44. Barch, D.H., Kuemmerle, S.C., Hollenberg, P.F., and Iannaccone, P.M. (1984) Esophageal microsomal metabolism of N-nitrosomethylbenzylamine in the zinc-deficient rat. *Cancer Res* **44**, 5629–33.

45. Fong, L.Y., Li, J.X., Farber, J.L., and Magee, P.N. (1996) Cell proliferation and esophageal carcinogenesis in the zinc-deficient rat. *Carcinogenesis* **17**, 1841–48.

46. Castro, L., and Freeman, B.A. (2001) Reactive oxygen species in human health and disease. *Nutrition* **17**(161), 3–5.

47. Ho, E. (2004) Zinc deficiency, DNA damage and cancer risk. *J Nutr Biochem* **15**, 572–78.

48. Conte, D., Narindrasorasak, S., and Sarkar, B. (1996) In vivo and in vitro iron-replaced zinc finger generates free radicals and causes DNA damage. *J Biol Chem* **271**, 5125–30.

49. Bray, T.M., and Bettger, W.J. (1990) The physiological role of zinc as an antioxidant. *Free Radic Biol Med* **8**, 281–91.

50. Oteiza, P.I., Olin, K.L., Fraga, C.G., and Keen, C.L. (1995) Zinc deficiency causes oxidative damage to proteins, lipids and DNA in rat testes. *J Nutr* **125**, 823–29.

51. Bray, T.M., Kubow, S., and Bettger, W.J. (1986) Effect of dietary zinc on endogenous free radical production in rat lung microsomes. *J Nutr* **116**, 1054–60.

52. Leccia, M.T., Richard, M.J., Favier, A., and Beani, J.C. (1999) Zinc protects against ultraviolet A1-induced DNA damage and apoptosis in cultured human fibroblasts. *Biol Trace Elem Res* **69**, 177–90.

53. Age Related Eye Disease Study Research Group (2001) A randomized, placebo-controlled, clinical trial of high-dose supplementation with vitamins C and E, beta carotene, and zinc for age-related macular degeneration and vision loss: AREDS report no. 8. *Arch Ophthalmol* **119**, 1417–36.

54. Fraker, P.J., and Telford, W.G. (1997) A reappraisal of the role of zinc in life and death decisions of cells. *Proc Soc Exp Biol Med* **215**, 229–36.

55. Rink, L., and Haase, H. (2007) Zinc homeostasis and immunity. *Trends Immunol* **28**, 1–4.

56. Fernandes, G., Nair, M., Onoe, K., Tanaka, T., Floyd, R., and Good, R.A. (1979) Impairment of cell-mediated immunity functions by dietary zinc deficiency in mice. *Proc Natl Acad Sci USA* **76**, 457–61.

57. Fraker, P.J. (1983) Zinc deficiency: A common immunodeficiency state. *Surv Immunol Res* **2**, 155–63.

58. Ibs, K.H., and Rink, L. (2003) Zinc-altered immune function. *J Nutr* **133**, 1452S–6S.

59. Kury, S., Dreno, B., Bezieau, S. et al. (2002) Identification of SLC39A4, a gene involved in acrodermatitis enteropathica. *Nat Genet* **31**, 239–40.

60. Liuzzi, J.P., Bobo, J.A., Lichten, L.A., Samuelson, D.A., and Cousins, R.J. (2004) Responsive transporter genes within the murine intestinal-pancreatic axis form a basis of zinc homeostasis. *Proc Natl Acad Sci USA* **101**, 14355–60.

61. Gartside, J.M., and Allen, B.R. (1975) Treatment of acrodermatitis enteropathica with zinc sulphate. *Br Med J* **3**, 521–2.

62. Overbeck, S., Rink, L., and Haase, H. (2008) Modulating the immune response by oral zinc supplementation: A single approach for multiple diseases. *Arch Immunol Ther Exp (Warsz)* **56**, 15–30.

63. Haase, H., Hebel, S., Engelhardt, G., and Rink, L. (2006) Flow cytometric measurement of labile zinc in peripheral blood mononuclear cells. *Anal Biochem* **352**, 222–30.

64. Bruinsma, J.J., Jirakulaporn, T., Muslin, A.J., and Kornfeld, K. (2002) Zinc ions and cation diffusion facilitator proteins regulate Ras-mediated signaling. *Dev Cell* **2**, 567–78.

65. Barbacid, M. (1987) ras genes. *Annu Rev Biochem* **56**, 779–827.

66. Taccioli, C., Wan, S.G., Liu, C.G. et al. (2009) Zinc replenishment reverses overexpression of the proinflammatory mediator S100A8 and esophageal preneoplasia in the rat. *Gastroenterology*, **136**, 953–66.

67. Uzzo, R.G., Leavis, P., Hatch, W. et al. (2002) Zinc inhibits nuclear factor-kappa B activation and sensitizes prostate cancer cells to cytotoxic agents. *Clin Cancer Res* **8**, 3579–83.

68. Follis, R., Day, H., and McCollum, E. (1941) Histological studies of the tissues of rats fed a diet extremely low in zinc. *J Nutr* **22**, 223–37.

69. Fong, L.Y., Sivak, A., and Newberne, P.M. (1978) Zinc deficiency and methylbenzylnitrosamine-induced esophageal cancer in rats. *J Natl Cancer Inst* **61**, 145–50.

70. Gabrial, G.N., Schrager, T.F., and Newberne, P.M. (1982) Zinc deficiency, alcohol, and retinoid: Association with esophageal cancer in rats. *J Natl Cancer Inst* **68**, 785–89.

71. Fong, L.Y., Lee, J.S., Chan, W.C., and Newberne, P.M. (1984) Zinc deficiency and the development of esophageal and forestomach tumors in Sprague-Dawley rats fed precursors of N-nitroso-N-benzylmethylamine. *J Natl Cancer Inst* **72**, 419–25.

72. Fong, L.Y., Lin, H.J., and Lee, C.L. (1979) Methylation of DNA in target and non-target organs of the rat with methylbenzylnitrosamine and dimethylnitrosamine. *Int J Cancer* **23**, 679–82.

73. Umbenhauer, D., Wild, C.P., Montesano, R. et al. (1985) O(6)-methyldeoxyguanosine in oesophageal DNA among individuals at high risk of oesophageal cancer. *Int J Cancer* **36**, 661–65.

74. Stinson, S.F., Squire, R.A., and Sporn, M.B. (1978) Pathology of esophageal neoplasms and associated proliferative lesions induced in rats by N-methyl-N-benzylnitrosamine. *J Natl Cancer Inst* **61**, 1471–75.

75. Fong, L.Y., Zhang, L., Jiang, Y., and Farber, J.L. (2005) Dietary zinc modulation of COX-2 expression and lingual and esophageal carcinogenesis in rats. *J Natl Cancer Inst* **97**, 40–50.

76. Taccioli, C., Liu, C.G., Wan, S.G. et al. (2008) Dietary Zinc Modulation of miR-31 Expression in Precancerous Esophagus and Tongue in Rats. San Diego, CA: American Association for Cancer Research, p. abstract # 5028.

77. Liu, C.G., Zhang, L., Jiang, Y. et al. (2005) Modulation of gene expression in precancerous rat esophagus by dietary zinc deficit and replenishment. *Cancer Res* **65**, 7790–99.

78. Fong, L.Y., Nguyen, V.T., and Farber, J.L. (2001) Esophageal cancer prevention in zinc-deficient rats: Rapid induction of apoptosis by replenishing zinc. *J Natl Cancer Inst* **93**, 1525–33.

79. Fong, L.Y., Farber, J.L., and Magee, P.N. (1998) Zinc replenishment reduces esophageal cell proliferation and N-nitrosomethylbenzylamine (NMBA)-induced esophageal tumor incidence in zinc-deficient rats. *Carcinogenesis* **19**, 1591–96.

80. Dietrich, D.R. (1993) Toxicological and pathological applications of proliferating cell nuclear antigen (PCNA), a novel endogenous marker for cell proliferation. *Crit Rev Toxicol* **23**, 77–109.

81. Hanahan, D., and Weinberg, R.A. (2000) The hallmarks of cancer. *Cell* **100**, 57–70.

82. Siglin, J.C., Khare, L., and Stoner, G.D. (1995) Evaluation of dose and treatment duration on the esophageal tumorigenicity of N-nitrosomethylbenzylamine in rats. *Carcinogenesis* **16**, 259–65.

83. Fong, L.Y., Nguyen, V.T., Farber, J.L., Huebner, K., and Magee, P.N. (2000) Early deregulation of the p16ink4a-cyclin D1/cyclin-dependent kinase 4-retinoblastoma pathway in cell proliferation-driven esophageal tumorigenesis in zinc-deficient rats. *Cancer Res* **60**, 4589–95.

84. Fong, L.Y., Lau, K.M., Huebner, K., and Magee, P.N. (1997) Induction of esophageal tumors in zinc-deficient rats by single low doses of N-nitrosomethylbenzylamine (NMBA): Analysis of cell proliferation, and mutations in H-ras and p53 genes. *Carcinogenesis* **18**, 1477–84.

85. Zimmermann, K.C., Sarbia, M., Weber, A.A., Borchard, F., Gabbert, H.E., and Schror, K. (1999) Cyclooxygenase-2 expression in human esophageal carcinoma. *Cancer Res* **59**, 198–204.

86. Maaser, K., Daubler, P., Barthel, B. et al. (2003) Oesophageal squamous cell neoplasia in head and neck cancer patients: Upregulation of COX-2 during carcinogenesis. *Br J Cancer* **88**, 1217–22.

87. Tsujii, M., and DuBois, R.N. (1995) Alterations in cellular adhesion and apoptosis in epithelial cells overexpressing prostaglandin endoperoxide synthase 2. *Cell* **83**, 493–501.

88. Tsujii, M., Kawano, S., Tsuji, S., Sawaoka, H., Hori, M., and DuBois, R.N. (1998) Cyclooxygenase regulates angiogenesis induced by colon cancer cells. *Cell* **93**, 705–16.

89. Tsujii, M., Kawano, S., and DuBois, R.N. (1997) Cyclooxygenase-2 expression in human colon cancer cells increases metastatic potential. *Proc Natl Acad Sci USA* **94**, 3336–40.

90. Smith, W.L., DeWitt, D.L., and Garavito, R.M. (2000) Cyclooxygenases: Structural, cellular, and molecular biology. *Annu Rev Biochem* **69**, 145–82.

91. Guy, N.C., Garewal, H., Holubec, H. et al. (2007) A novel dietary-related model of esophagitis and Barrett's esophagus, a premalignant lesion. *Nutr Cancer* **59**, 217–27.

92. Carter, J.W., Lancaster, H., Hardman, W.E., and Cameron, I.L. (1997) Zinc deprivation promotes progression of 1,2-dimethylhydrazine-induced colon tumors but reduces malignant invasion in mice. *Nutr Cancer* **27**, 217–21.

93. Dani, V., Goel, A., Vaiphei, K., and Dhawan, D.K. (2007) Chemopreventive potential of zinc in experimentally induced colon carcinogenesis. *Toxicol Lett* **171**, 10–18.

94. Fong, L.Y., and Magee, P.N. (1999) Dietary zinc deficiency enhances esophageal cell proliferation and N-nitrosomethylbenzylamine (NMBA)-induced esophageal tumor incidence in C57BL/6 mouse. *Cancer Lett* **143**, 63–69.

95. Tang, X.H., Knudsen, B., Bemis, D., Tickoo, S., and Gudas, L.J. (2004) Oral cavity and esophageal carcinogenesis modeled in carcinogen-treated mice. *Clin Cancer Res* **10**, 301–13.

96. Fong, L.Y., Ishii, H., Nguyen, V.T. et al. (2003) p53 deficiency accelerates induction and progression of esophageal and forestomach tumors in zinc-deficient mice. *Cancer Res* **63**, 186–95.

97. Fong, L.Y., Jiang, Y., and Farber, J.L. (2006) Zinc deficiency potentiates induction and progression of lingual and esophageal tumors in p53-deficient mice. *Carcinogenesis* **27**, 1489–96.

98. Fong, L.Y., Mancini, R., Nakagawa, H., Rustgi, A.K., and Huebner, K. (2003) Combined cyclin D1 overexpression and zinc deficiency disrupts cell cycle and accelerates mouse forestomach carcinogenesis. *Cancer Res* **63**, 4244–52.

99. Drusco, A., Zanesi, N., Roldo, C. et al. (2005) Knockout mice reveal a tumor suppressor function for Testin. *Proc Natl Acad Sci USA* **102**, 10947–51.

100. Fong, L.Y., Feith, D.J., and Pegg, A.E. (2003) Antizyme overexpression in transgenic mice reduces cell proliferation, increases apoptosis, and reduces N-nitrosomethylbenzylamine-induced forestomach carcinogenesis. *Cancer Res* **63**, 3945–54.

101. Fong, L.Y., Jiang, Y., Riley, M. et al. (2008) Prevention of upper aerodigestive tract cancer in zinc-deficient rodents: Inefficacy of genetic or pharmacological disruption of COX-2. *Int J Cancer* **122**, 978–89.

102. Greenblatt, M.S., Bennett, W.P., Hollstein, M., and Harris, C.C. (1994) Mutations in the p53 tumor suppressor gene: Clues to cancer etiology and molecular pathogenesis. *Cancer Res* **54**, 4855–78.

103. Jiang, W., Zhang, Y.J., Kahn, S.M. et al. (1993) Altered expression of the cyclin D1 and retinoblastoma genes in human esophageal cancer. *Proc Natl Acad Sci USA* **90**, 9026–30.

104. Wang, Q.S., Sabourin, C.L., Wang, H., and Stoner, G.D. (1996) Overexpression of cyclin D1 and cyclin E in N-nitrosomethylbenzylamine-induced rat esophageal tumorigenesis. *Carcinogenesis* **17**, 1583–88.

105. Feith, D.J., Shantz, L.M., and Pegg, A.E. (2001) Targeted antizyme expression in the skin of transgenic mice reduces tumor promoter induction of ornithine decarboxylase and decreases sensitivity to chemical carcinogenesis. *Cancer Res* **61**, 6073–81.

106. Mitchell, J.L., Leyser, A., Holtorff, M.S. et al. (2002) Antizyme induction by polyamine analogues as a factor of cell growth inhibition. *Biochem J* **366**, 663–71.

107. Fong, L.Y., Nguyen, V.T., Pegg, A.E., and Magee, P.N. (2001) Alpha-difluoromethylornithine induction of apoptosis: A mechanism which reverses pre-established cell proliferation and cancer initiation in esophageal carcinogenesis in zinc-deficient rats. *Cancer Epidemiol Biomarkers Prev* **10**, 191–99.

108. Fong, L.Y., Pegg, A.E., and Magee, P.N. (1998) Alpha-difluoromethylornithine inhibits N-nitrosomethylbenzylamine-induced esophageal carcinogenesis in zinc-deficient rats: Effects on esophageal cell proliferation and apoptosis. *Cancer Res* **58**, 5380–88.

109. Oshima, M., Dinchuk, J.E., Kargman, S.L. et al. (1996) Suppression of intestinal polyposis in Apc delta716 knockout mice by inhibition of cyclooxygenase 2 (COX-2). *Cell* **87**, 803–09.

110. Tiano, H.F., Loftin, C.D., Akunda, J. et al. (2002) Deficiency of either cyclooxygenase (COX)-1 or COX-2 alters epidermal differentiation and reduces mouse skin tumorigenesis. *Cancer Res* **62**, 3395–401.

111. Korsmeyer, S.J., Shutter, J.R., Veis, D.J., Merry, D.E., and Oltvai, Z.N. (1993) Bcl-2/Bax: A rheostat that regulates an anti-oxidant pathway and cell death. *Semin Cancer Biol* **4**, 327–32.

112. Reed, J.C. (1995) Regulation of apoptosis by bcl-2 family proteins and its role in cancer and chemoresistance. *Curr Opin Oncol* **7**, 541–46.
113. Altorki, N.K., Subbaramaiah, K., and Dannenberg, A.J. (2004) COX-2 inhibition in upper aerodigestive tract tumors. *Semin Oncol* **31**, 30–36.
114. Greenwald, P. (2002) Cancer prevention clinical trials. *J Clin Oncol* **20**, 14S–22S.
115. Wirth, L.J., Haddad, R.I., Lindeman, N.I. et al. (2005) Phase I study of gefitinib plus celecoxib in recurrent or metastatic squamous cell carcinoma of the head and neck. *J Clin Oncol* **23**, 6976–81.
116. Heath, E.I., Canto, M.I., Piantadosi, S. et al. (2007) Secondary chemoprevention of Barrett's esophagus with celecoxib: Results of a randomized trial. *J Natl Cancer Inst* **99**, 545–57.
117. Shiotani, H., Denda, A., Yamamoto, K. et al. (2001) Increased expression of cyclooxygenase-2 protein in 4-nitroquinoline-1-oxide-induced rat tongue carcinomas and chemopreventive efficacy of a specific inhibitor, nimesulide. *Cancer Res* **61**, 1451–56.
118. Yamamoto, K., Kitayama, W., Denda, A., Morisaki, A., Kuniyasu, H., and Kirita, T. (2003) Inhibitory effects of selective cyclooxygenase-2 inhibitors, nimesulide and etodolac, on the development of squamous cell dysplasias and carcinomas of the tongue in rats initiated with 4-nitroquinoline 1-oxide. *Cancer Lett* **199**, 121–29.
119. Prasad, A.S., Bao, B., Beck, F.W., Kucuk, O., and Sarkar, F.H. (2004) Antioxidant effect of zinc in humans. *Free Radic Biol Med* **37**, 1182–90.
120. Uzzo, R.G., Crispen, P.L., Golovine, K., Makhov, P., Horwitz, E.M., and Kolenko, V.M. (2006) Diverse effects of zinc on NF-kappaB and AP-1 transcription factors: Implications for prostate cancer progression. *Carcinogenesis* **27**, 1980–90.
121. Doerr, T.D., Prasad, A.S., Marks, S.C. et al. (1997) Zinc deficiency in head and neck cancer patients. *J Am Coll Nutr* **16**, 418–22.
122. Yan, M., Song, Y., Wong, C.P., Hardin, K., and Ho, E. (2008) Zinc deficiency alters DNA damage response genes in normal human prostate epithelial cells. *J Nutr* **138**, 667–73.
123. Cousins, R.J., Blanchard, R.K., Popp, M.P. et al. (2003) A global view of the selectivity of zinc deprivation and excess on genes expressed in human THP-1 mononuclear cells. *Proc Natl Acad Sci USA* **100**, 6952–57.
124. Kindermann, B., Doring, F., Pfaffl, M., and Daniel, H. (2004) Identification of genes responsive to intracellular zinc depletion in the human colon adenocarcinoma cell line HT-29. *J Nutr* **134**, 57–62.
125. Haase, H., Mazzatti, D.J., White, A. et al. (2007) Differential gene expression after zinc supplementation and deprivation in human leukocyte subsets. *Mol Med* **13**, 362–70.
126. Blanchard, R.K., Moore, J.B., Green, C.L., and Cousins, R.J. (2001) Modulation of intestinal gene expression by dietary zinc status: Effectiveness of cDNA arrays for expression profiling of a single nutrient deficiency. *Proc Natl Acad Sci USA* **98**, 13507–13.
127. tom Dieck, H., Doring, F., Fuchs, D., Roth, H.P., and Daniel, H. (2005) Transcriptome and proteome analysis identifies the pathways that increase hepatic lipid accumulation in zinc-deficient rats. *J Nutr* **135**, 199–205.
128. tom Dieck, H., Doring, F., Roth, H.P., and Daniel, H. (2003) Changes in rat hepatic gene expression in response to zinc deficiency as assessed by DNA arrays. *J Nutr* **133**, 1004–10.
129. Pfaffl, M.W., Gerstmayer, B., Bosio, A., and Windisch, W. (2003) Effect of zinc deficiency on the mRNA expression pattern in liver and jejunum of adult rats: Monitoring gene expression using cDNA microarrays combined with real-time RT-PCR. *J Nutr Biochem* **14**, 691–702.
130. Moore, J.B., Blanchard, R.K., McCormack, W.T., and Cousins, R.J. (2001) cDNA array analysis identifies thymic LCK as upregulated in moderate murine zinc deficiency before T-lymphocyte population changes. *J Nutr* **131**, 3189–96.
131. Moore, J.B., Blanchard, R.K., and Cousins, R.J. (2003) Dietary zinc modulates gene expression in murine thymus: Results from a comprehensive differential display screening. *Proc Natl Acad Sci USA* **100**, 3883–88.
132. Gomez, N.N., Davicino, R.C., Biaggio, V.S. et al. (2006) Overexpression of inducible nitric oxide synthase and cyclooxygenase-2 in rat zinc-deficient lung: Involvement of a NF-kappaB dependent pathway. *Nitric Oxide* **14**, 30–38.

133. Bruwer, M., Schmid, K.W., Metz, K.A., Krieglstein, C.F., Senninger, N., and Schurmann, G. (2001) Increased expression of metallothionein in inflammatory bowel disease. *Inflamm Res* **50**, 289–93.

134. Hishikawa, Y., Koji, T., Dhar, D.K., Kinugasa, S., Yamaguchi, M., and Nagasue, N. (1999) Metallothionein expression correlates with metastatic and proliferative potential in squamous cell carcinoma of the oesophagus. *Br J Cancer* **81**, 712–20.

135. Sundelin, K., Jadner, M., Norberg-Spaak, L., Davidsson, A., and Hellquist, H.B. (1997) Metallothionein and Fas (CD95) are expressed in squamous cell carcinoma of the tongue. *Eur J Cancer* **33**, 1860–64.

136. Gebhardt, C., Nemeth, J., Angel, P., and Hess, J. (2006) S100A8 and S100A9 in inflammation and cancer. *Biochem Pharmacol* **72**, 1622–31.

137. Hummerich, L., Muller, R., Hess, J. et al. (2006) Identification of novel tumour-associated genes differentially expressed in the process of squamous cell cancer development. *Oncogene* **25**, 111–21.

138. Kumar, A., Chatopadhyay, T., Raziuddin, M., and Ralhan, R. (2007) Discovery of deregulation of zinc homeostasis and its associated genes in esophageal squamous cell carcinoma using cDNA microarray. *Int J Cancer* **120**, 230–42.

139. Bax, D.A., Siersema, P.D., Haringsma, J. et al. (2007) High-grade dysplasia in Barrett's esophagus is associated with increased expression of calgranulin A and B. *Scand J Gastroenterol* **42**, 902–10.

140. Hermani, A., De Servi, B., Medunjanin, S., Tessier, P.A., and Mayer, D. (2006) S100A8 and S100A9 activate MAP kinase and NF-kappaB signaling pathways and trigger translocation of RAGE in human prostate cancer cells. *Exp Cell Res* **312**, 184–97.

141. Ghavami, S., Rashedi, I., Dattilo, B.M. et al. (2008) S100A8/A9 at low concentration promotes tumor cell growth via RAGE ligation and MAP kinase-dependent pathway. *J Leukoc Biol* **83**, 1484–92

142. Gebhardt, C., Riehl, A., Durchdewald, M. et al. (2008) RAGE signaling sustains inflammation and promotes tumor development. *J Exp Med* **205**, 275–85.

143. Taguchi, A., Blood, D.C., del Toro, G. et al. (2000) Blockade of RAGE-amphoterin signalling suppresses tumour growth and metastases. *Nature* **405**, 354–60.

144. Lagos-Quintana, M., Rauhut, R., Lendeckel, W., and Tuschl, T. (2001) Identification of novel genes coding for small expressed RNAs. *Science* **294**, 853–58.

145. Lau, N.C., Lim, L.P., Weinstein, E.G., and Bartel, D.P. (2001) An abundant class of tiny RNAs with probable regulatory roles in Caenorhabditis elegans. *Science* **294**, 858–62.

146. Lee, R.C., and Ambros, V. (2001) An extensive class of small RNAs in Caenorhabditis elegans. *Science* **294**, 862–64.

147. Ambros, V. (2003) MicroRNA pathways in flies and worms: Growth, death, fat, stress, and timing. *Cell* **113**, 673–76.

148. Calin, G.A., and Croce, C.M. (2006) MicroRNA signatures in human cancers. *Nat Rev Cancer* **6**, 857–66.

149. Costinean, S., Zanesi, N., Pekarsky, Y. et al. (2006) Pre-B cell proliferation and lymphoblastic leukemia/high-grade lymphoma in E(mu)-miR155 transgenic mice. *Proc Natl Acad Sci USA* **103**, 7024–29.

150. He, L., Thomson, J.M., Hemann, M.T. et al. (2005) A microRNA polycistron as a potential human oncogene. *Nature* **435**, 828–33.

151. Lu, J., Getz, G., Miska, E.A. et al. (2005) MicroRNA expression profiles classify human cancers. *Nature* **435**, 834–38.

152. Marsit, C.J., Eddy, K., and Kelsey, K.T. (2006) MicroRNA responses to cellular stress. *Cancer Res* **66**, 10843–48.

153. Kutay, H., Bai, S., Datta, J. et al. (2006) Downregulation of miR-122 in the rodent and human hepatocellular carcinomas. *J Cell Biochem* **99**, 671–78.

154. Bandres, E., Cubedo, E., Agirre, X. et al. (2006) Identification by Real-time PCR of 13 mature microRNAs differentially expressed in colorectal cancer and non-tumoral tissues. *Mol Cancer* **5**, 29.

155. Wong, T.S., Liu, X.B., Wong, B.Y., Ng, R.W., Yuen, A.P., and Wei, W.I. (2008) Mature miR-184 as Potential Oncogenic microRNA of Squamous Cell Carcinoma of Tongue. *Clin Cancer Res* **14**, 2588–92.

156. Guo, Y., Chen, Z., Zhang, L. et al. (2008) Distinctive microRNA profiles relating to patient survival in esophageal squamous cell carcinoma. *Cancer Res* **68**, 26–33.

157. Costello, L.C., Franklin, R.B., Feng, P., Tan, M., and Bagasra, O. (2005) Zinc and prostate cancer: A critical scientific, medical, and public interest issue (United States). *Cancer Causes Control* **16**, 901–15.

158. Killilea, A.N., Downing, K.H., and Killilea, D.W. (2007) Zinc deficiency reduces paclitaxel efficacy in LNCaP prostate cancer cells. *Cancer Lett* **258**, 70–79.

159. Sunderman, F.W., Jr. (1995) The influence of zinc on apoptosis. *Ann Clin Lab Sci* **25**, 134–42.

160. Donadelli, M., Dalla Pozza, E., Costanzo, C., Scupoli, M.T., Scarpa, A., and Palmieri, M. (2008) Zinc depletion efficiently inhibits pancreatic cancer cell growth by increasing the ratio of antiproliferative/proliferative genes. *J Cell Biochem* **104**, 202–12.

161. Feng, P., Li, T., Guan, Z., Franklin, R.B., and Costello, L.C. (2008) The involvement of Bax in zinc-induced mitochondrial apoptogenesis in malignant prostate cells. *Mol Cancer* **7**, 25.

162. Liang, J.Y., Liu, Y.Y., Zou, J., Franklin, R.B., Costello, L.C., and Feng, P. (1999) Inhibitory effect of zinc on human prostatic carcinoma cell growth. *Prostate* **40**, 200–07.

163. Feng, P., Liang, J.Y., Li, T.L. et al. (2000) Zinc induces mitochondria apoptogenesis in prostate cells. *Mol Urol* **4**, 31–36.

164. Bae, S.N., Lee, Y.S., Kim, M.Y., Kim, J.D., and Park, L.O. (2006) Antiproliferative and apoptotic effects of zinc-citrate compound (CIZAR(R)) on human epithelial ovarian cancer cell line, OVCAR-3. *Gynecol Oncol* **103**, 127–36.

165. Bae, S.N., Kim, J., Lee, Y.S., Kim, J.D., Kim, M.Y., and Park, L.O. (2007) Cytotoxic effect of zinc-citrate compound on choriocarcinoma cell lines. *Placenta* **28**, 22–30.

166. Rudolf, E., Rudolf, K., and Cervinka, M. (2005) Zinc induced apoptosis in HEP-2 cancer cells: The role of oxidative stress and mitochondria. *Biofactors* **23**, 107–20.

167. Jaiswal, A.S., and Narayan, S. (2004) Zinc stabilizes adenomatous polyposis coli (APC) protein levels and induces cell cycle arrest in colon cancer cells. *J Cell Biochem* **93**, 345–57.

168. Munoz, N., Hayashi, M., Bang, L.J., Wahrendorf, J., Crespi, M., and Bosch, F.X. (1987) Effect of riboflavin, retinol, and zinc on micronuclei of buccal mucosa and of esophagus: A randomized double-blind intervention study in China. *J Natl Cancer Inst* **79**, 687–91.

169. Munoz, N., Wahrendorf, J., Bang, L.J. et al. (1985) No effect of riboflavine, retinol, and zinc on prevalence of precancerous lesions of oesophagus. Randomised double-blind intervention study in high-risk population of China. *Lancet* **2**, 111–14.

170. Taylor, P.R., Li, B., Dawsey, S.M. et al. (1994) Prevention of esophageal cancer: The nutrition intervention trials in Linxian, China. Linxian Nutrition Intervention Trials Study Group. *Cancer Res* **54**, 2029s–31s.

171. Rao, M., Liu, F.S., Dawsey, S.M. et al. (1994) Effects of vitamin/mineral supplementation on the proliferation of esophageal squamous epithelium in Linxian, China. *Cancer Epidemiol Biomarkers Prev* **3**, 277–79.

172. Hercberg, S., Galan, P., Preziosi, P. et al. (2004) The SU.VI.MAX study: A randomized, placebo-controlled trial of the health effects of antioxidant vitamins and minerals. *Arch Intern Med* **164**, 2335–42.

173. Limburg, P.J., Wei, W., Ahnen, D.J. et al. (2005) Randomized, placebo-controlled, esophageal squamous cell cancer chemoprevention trial of selenomethionine and celecoxib. *Gastroenterology* **129**, 863–73.

174. Huang, H.Y., Caballero, B., Chang, S. et al. (2006) The efficacy and safety of multivitamin and mineral supplement use to prevent cancer and chronic disease in adults: A systematic review for a National Institutes of Health state-of-the-science conference. *Ann Intern Med* **145**, 372–85.

175. Andersson, S.O., Wolk, A., Bergstrom, R. et al. (1996) Energy, nutrient intake and prostate cancer risk: A population-based case-control study in Sweden. *Int J Cancer* **68**, 716–22.

176. Vlajinac, H.D., Marinkovic, J.M., Ilic, M.D., and Kocev, N.I. (1997) Diet and prostate cancer: A case-control study. *Eur J Cancer* **33**, 101–07.

177. Kristal, A.R., Stanford, J.L., Cohen, J.H., Wicklund, K., and Patterson, R.E. (1999) Vitamin and mineral supplement use is associated with reduced risk of prostate cancer. *Cancer Epidemiol Biomarkers Prev* **8**, 887–92.

178. Key, T.J., Silcocks, P.B., Davey, G.K., Appleby, P.N., and Bishop, D.T. (1997) A case-control study of diet and prostate cancer. *Br J Cancer* **76**, 678–87.

179. Leitzmann, M.F., Stampfer, M.J., Wu, K., Colditz, G.A., Willett, W.C., and Giovannucci, E.L. (2003) Zinc supplement use and risk of prostate cancer. *J Natl Cancer Inst* **95**, 1004–07.

180. Krone, C.A., and Harms, L.C. (2003) Re: Zinc supplement use and risk of prostate cancer. *J Natl Cancer Inst* **95**, 1556.

181. Lee, D.H., Anderson, K.E., Harnack, L.J., Folsom, A.R., and Jacobs, D.R., Jr. (2004) Heme iron, zinc, alcohol consumption, and colon cancer: Iowa Women's Health Study. *J Natl Cancer Inst* **96**, 403–07.

182. Greten, F.R., and Karin, M. (2004) The IKK/NF-kappaB activation pathway-a target for prevention and treatment of cancer. *Cancer Lett* **206**, 193–99.

183. Perwez Hussain, S., and Harris, C.C. (2007) Inflammation and cancer: An ancient link with novel potentials. *Int J Cancer* **121**, 2373–80.

184. Balkwill, F., Charles, K.A., and Mantovani, A. (2005) Smoldering and polarized inflammation in the initiation and promotion of malignant disease. *Cancer Cell* **7**, 211–17.

185. Moroni, F., Di Paolo, M.L., Rigo, A. et al. (2005) Interrelationship among neutrophil efficiency, inflammation, antioxidant activity and zinc pool in very old age. *Biogerontology* **6**, 271–81.

IV ROLE OF DIETARY BIOACTIVE COMPONENTS IN CANCER PREVENTION AND/OR TREATMENT: OTHER BIOACTIVE FOOD COMPONENTS

23 Cruciferous Vegetables, Isothiocyanates, Indoles, and Cancer Prevention

Cynthia A. Thomson, Sally Dickinson, and G. Tim Bowden

Key Points

1. Recent studies have shown that vegetables of the *Brassica* species can contribute to the prevention of cancer. The *Brassica* vegetables include broccoli, bok choy, cabbage, and Brussels sprouts, to name a few.
2. *Brassica*-derived compounds tend to induce the expression of batteries of genes involved in cytoprotection, repress the expression of genes involved in carcinogenesis, improve access to DNA, and induce apoptosis.
3. Cruciferous vegetables are known to contain bioactive compounds that activate Nrf2, a possible tumor suppressor, in various cellular models.
4. Isothiocyanates have been found to inhibit the activity of oncogenic transcription factors such as activator protein-1 (AP-1) and nuclear factor kappa B (NFκB). AP-1 is a protein dimer consisting of either Jun-related proteins or heterodimers of Jun and Fos-related proteins. In its active state, AP-1 can bind to the TPA-response element (TRE). Once bound to the TRE, AP-1 recruits factors to regulate the transcription of genes involved in proliferation, differentiation, apoptosis, and angiogenesis.
5. Researchers have started to explore the ability of isothiocyanates and indoles to inhibit COX-2 activity and inflammation in general. In particular, sulforaphane (SUL) has been noted to block inflammatory responses in both cultured RAW 264.7 macrophages (via NFκB inhibition) and mouse BV-2 microglial cells.
6. Cruciferous vegetables intake appears to reduce the risk for colorectal, prostate and possibly renal cancers. To date the available evidence is not as strong for lung, breast, and oral cancers.

Key Words: Cruciferous; isothiocyanates; AP-1; NFκB; cancer

From: *Nutrition and Health: Bioactive Compounds and Cancer*
Edited by: J.A. Milner, D.F. Romagnolo, DOI 10.1007/978-1-60761-627-6_23,
© Springer Science+Business Media, LLC 2010

1. INTRODUCTION

One class of vegetables that is of particular importance in the prevention of cancer is the vegetables of the *Brassica* species. *Brassica* vegetables are a group of vegetables from the mustard family, Cruciferae, and includes numerous vegetables ranging from broccoli to bok choy to condiments such as wasabi. Recently, other varieties including broccolini and broccoli sprouts have also been cultivated, largely in an effort to enhance the concentration of health-promoting bioactive food components in the human diet. Table 1 lists the most commonly consumed cruciferous vegetables by genus and species. Although there is a paucity of human intervention trials focusing on the chemopreventive effects of cruciferous vegetables consumed as whole foods, cell culture models, animal studies, and small feeding studies with select bioactive components found in these plants, such as indole-3-carbinol (I3C) and diindolylmethane (DIM), suggest there is significant potential to favorably modify cancer risk through increased consumption. This chapter will begin by describing our current understanding of the molecular effects of *Brassica*-derived compounds, isothiocyanates, and indoles on the cell, as well as recent work with animal models using these compounds to prevent or delay various forms of cancer. We will then describe intake patterns as well as intake levels associated with reduced cancer risk, discuss exposure estimates, and review the current epidemiological data, which examine the hypothesis that constituents of cruciferous vegetables protect against cancer.

2. MOLECULAR MECHANISMS OF CANCER PREVENTION BY ISOTHIOCYANATES AND INDOLES: CELL CULTURE MODELS

Numerous studies have investigated the effects of *Brassica*-derived compounds on models of cancer in cell culture (Fig. 1). These studies often find that there are differences in dose–response and specific reactivity when using the same natural product on different cancer cell lines. However, there are definite trends of response, which have been noted between the various compounds tested: *Brassica*-derived compounds tend to induce the expression of batteries of genes involved in cytoprotection, repress the expression of genes involved in carcinogenesis, improve access to DNA, and induce apoptosis. These and other effects of cruciferous vegetable-derived chemicals will be described in detail below.

2.1. Cytoprotection via the Keap1/Nrf2 Pathway

One transcription factor that has been under recent scrutiny as a possible tumor suppressor is *n*uclear E2-factor *r*elated *f*actor 2 (Nrf2). To date, three members of the Nrf family have been identified. Nrf1 is ubiquitously expressed and is essential for embryonal development *(1)*. Nrf3 is primarily active in placental tissue *(2)*. Nrf2 is also ubiquitously expressed, but is induced significantly when cells are exposed to stimuli such as oxidative stress, electrophiles, or xenobiotics *(3) (4)*. Nrf2 is normally held in the cytoplasm by its repressor, Keap-1, which recruits a Cul3 ubiquitin ligase to ubiquitinate Nrf2 and present it to the proteasome for degradation. Thus, low steady-state levels of Nrf2 are maintained via continual turnover of the protein. Certain stimuli,

Table 1
Cruciferous Vegetables Consumed in the Human Diet

Brassicaceae/Cruciferae family	Genus	Species	Plant
Brassicaceae	Brassica	Oleracea	Broccoli, Brussels sprouts, cabbage, savoy cabbage, red cabbage, cauliflower, collards, kale, Chinese kale, Italian broccoli, asparagus broccoli, sea kale, wild cabbage, kohlrabi
Brassicaceae	Brassica	Rapa	Chinese cabbage, celery, cabbage, spinach mustard, turnip, turnip tops, turnip broccoli, toria
Brassicaceae	Brassica	Napus	Rape, colza, Siberian kale, rutabaga
Brassicaceae	Brassica	Japonica	Wasabi
Brassicaceae	Brassica	Juncea	Chinese mustards, mustard greens, curled mustard, Pak Choi, Bok celery, brown mustard
Brassicaceae	Brassica	Negra	Black mustard oil, black mustard seeds
	Nasturtium	Amoracia	Horseradish
Cruciferae	Nasturtium	Officinale	Watercress
Brassicaceae	Raphanus	Sativus	Radish

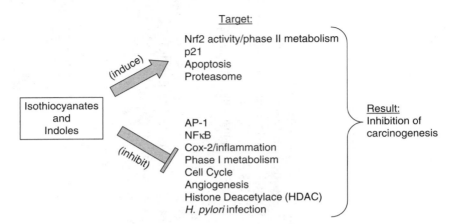

Fig. 1. Schematic representation of the chemopreventive actions of isothiocyanates and indoles. Molecular activities of each compound are unique depending upon the dose and cell type.

such as electrophiles, sulfhydryl-modifying agents, and activated protein kinases cause an inhibition of the degradation of Nrf2, either through release of Keap-bound protein or through inhibiting the degradation of the currently bound substrate (5). Free or newly translated Nrf2 may then translocate to the nucleus, heterodimerize with binding partners (traditionally small Maf proteins), and bind to the Antioxidant Response Element (ARE, consensus sequence: 5'-G/ATGAG/CnnnGCG/A-3'). The ARE is a *cis*-acting element present in many phase II metabolism antioxidant and detoxification-related genes, such as hemeoxygenase-1 (HO-1), glutathione *S*-transferases (GSTs), and NAD(P)H quinone oxidoreductase-1 (NQO1). Nrf2 activation has, therefore, been linked to cytoprotective events, especially as relates to protection from oxidative stress. Nrf2 knockout mice are viable, but cannot induce expression of certain phase II enzymes when challenged with acetaminophen and carcinogens (6, 7). Functional Nrf2 has been implicated in many physiological functions including protecting neurons from oxidative stress, fighting *Helicobacter pylori* infections in the stomach, and regulating the defenses that protect against cellular and DNA damage that lead to cancer (4). Although the exact mechanism is not clear, it is thought that by increasing GST activity, and boosting levels of enzymes such as NQO1 and SOD1(8), Nrf2 provides increased defenses against oxidants and xenobiotics that would normally damage the cell or play a role in carcinogenesis. It is therefore apparent that agents that activate Nrf2 (without harming the cell) may prove useful in preventing human cancer. Many agents (bioactives) found in cruciferous vegetables, such as sulforaphane (SUL), phenethylisothiocyanate (PEITC), benzylisothiocyanate (BITC), and indole-3-carbinol (I3C), have been found to activate Nrf2 in various cellular models (9, 10, 11). However, it should be noted that overactivation of Nrf2 in certain tumor types may, in fact, lead to decreased sensitivity to anti-tumorigenic agents. Nrf2 activity has, therefore, been labeled a "double-edged sword," which can protect against carcinogenesis in many cases, but may also offer selective advantages in others (12, 13).

2.2. Inhibition of AP-1 and NFκB Transcription Factors

In addition to activation of cytoprotective transcription factors, isothiocyanates have been found to inhibit the activity of oncogenic transcription factors such as activator protein-1 (AP-1) and nuclear factor kappa B (NFκB). AP-1 is a protein dimer consisting of either Jun-related proteins (c-Jun, JunB, or JunD) or heterodimers of Jun and Fos-related proteins (c-Fos, FosB, Fra1, or Fra2). In its active state, AP-1 can bind to the TPA-response element (TRE), a *cis*-acting element with a consensus sequence of TGA(G or C)TCA. Once bound to the TRE, AP-1 recruits factors to regulate the transcription of genes involved in proliferation, differentiation, apoptosis, and angiogenesis *(14)*. Therefore, overactivity of AP-1 may lead to a differential growth advantage in precancerous cells *(15)*. The upstream signaling pathways involved in AP-1 activation have been well studied, and include the mitogen-activated protein kinases (MAPKinases) p38, c-Jun N-terminal kinase (JNK), and extracellular signal-regulated kinase (ERK), as well as the phosphoinositol-3 (PI3) kinase/Akt pathway. Due to these diverse signaling mechanisms, AP-1 can be activated by a variety of extracellular stimuli, including UV light, cytokines, growth factors, stress, and various tumor promoters *(16)*. The effect of isothiocyanates on AP-1 activity appears to depend upon both the cell type and the dose of the compound. For example, SUL inhibits AP-1 luciferase activity and in vitro DNA binding in HaCaT human keratinocytes after UVB stimulation *(17)*. However, when tested in HT-29 human colon cancer cells, SUL slightly induced AP-1 luciferase when stimulated by TPA treatment, while high doses of PEITC inhibited this activity *(18)*. The mechanism of AP-1 activity by these compounds is also quite diverse. SUL may inhibit AP-1 directly by binding to a key cysteine residue in its DNA-binding domain, or may also inhibit AP-1 by changing the redox status of the cell through Nrf2 activation *(17)*. Paradoxically, isothiocyanates are often found to increase the activity of MAPKinases upstream of AP-1 (reviewed in *(19)*).

As was mentioned above, NFκB is also a frequent target of isothiocyanates and indoles. The NFκB transcription factor is made up of combinations of members from either the Rel or NFκB families. There are three Rel proteins (RelA/p65, RelB, and c-Rel) and two NFκB proteins (NFκB1/p50 and NFκB2/p52). All family members may form homo or heterodimers and bind to DNA, although only Rel proteins contain transcription activation domains. The most common dimer found in activated cells contains p65/p50 (RelA/NFκB1). The transcription factors are typically retained in the cytoplasm by inhibitor IκBalpha proteins. Stimulation of resting cells by various agents (UV light, cytokines, oxidative stress) results in phosphorylation of IκBalpha, resulting in its subsequent ubiquitination and degradation by the proteasome. The removal of IκBalpha exposes a nuclear localization sequence in NFκB, which results in transit into the nucleus and activation of target genes. In general, activation of the NFκB signaling pathway is associated with inhibition of apoptosis (reviewed in *(20)*). Several human cancer cell lines, from prostate *(21)*, breast *(22)*, pancreas *(23)*, to leukemia donors *(24)*, have been shown to constitutively express NFκB. Thus, NFκB has been flagged as a potential chemopreventive target, and certain studies have found that inhibiting this pathway can sensitize tumors to further treatments with chemotherapeutic drugs, presumably through the activation of apoptotic signaling *(25)*.

Compounds found in cruciferous vegetables have been found to inhibit NFκB signaling in several ways. SUL and PEITC were found to dose-dependently inhibit NFκB–luciferase reporter activity when exposed to LPS-induced HT-29 human colon cancer cells *(26)*. SUL was shown to reduce the ability of LPS-stimulated NFκB to bind to DNA in macrophages *(27)*. The inhibition of NFκB/DNA binding by SUL was postulated to be a result of SUL interacting with redox-sensitive cysteine groups in the DNA-binding domain of the transcription factor, or the result of modulations of activity of redox effectors such as Ref1 or thioredoxin. This postulated mechanism of action for SUL on NFκB is remarkably similar to that proposed for the activity of SUL on AP-1 DNA binding *(17)*. SUL has also been shown to reduce NFκB expression in malignant glioblastoma *(28)*. The indole I3C has also been extensively studied for its effects on NFκB. I3C-related inhibition of NFκB was noted in multiple cell lines, and after activation with multiple inducers *(29)*. In contrast, others have found that the isothiocyanate BITC-enhanced binding of NFκB to DNA in unstimulated HT-29 cells *(30)*, suggesting that differences in NFκB activity may be influenced by cell type, dose, and type of bioactive compound.

2.3. Inhibition of COX-2 and the Inflammatory Response

Cyclooxygenase-2 (COX-2) is the inducible form of the two known cyclooxygenase enzymes in the cell. Also known as prostaglandin H synthases, COX enzymes catalyze the oxidation of arachidonic acid to prostaglandin H_2 (PGH_2). Signaling events initiated by the formation of prostaglandins can lead to inflammatory responses, epithelial cell growth and invasion, and survival responses, thus linking COX activity to overstimulation of the immune response and tumor promotion *(31–33)*. Such overactivity has been linked to cancer promotion in several model systems *(34, 35)*. It should be noted as well that COX-2 levels are regulated in part by NFκB and AP-1 transcription factors *(36)*. Although COX-1 is constitutively expressed, COX-2 expression is induced by several types of stimuli, including UVA/UVB irradiation, oxidative stress, TPA, and cytokines. COX-2 has been found to be overexpressed in human colon adenomas and colon cancer, and COX-2 knockout mice have a reduced incidence of UV-induced skin cancer *(37)*. In fact, inhibition of COX-2 has been shown to protect against several forms of cancer in both rodents and humans *(38–41)*.

Only recently have researchers started to explore the ability of isothiocyanates and indoles to inhibit COX-2 activity and inflammation in general. In particular, SUL has been noted to block inflammatory responses in both cultured RAW 264.7 macrophages (via NFκB inhibition) and mouse BV-2 microglial cells *(27, 42)*. Another recent study examined the response of mouse peritoneal macrophages to immune stimulation and determined that Nrf2 activity was required for SUL to inhibit COX-2 and other inflammatory responses in these cells *(43)*. In rats, diet containing PEITC was found to inhibit the activation of COX-2 after inhalation of the tobacco-specific lung carcinogen 4-(methylnitrosamino)-1-(3-pyridyl)-1-butanone (NNK), and also to significantly inhibit lung carcinogenesis after NNK exposure *(44)*. BITC was also found to suppress COX-2 activation in macrophages, via stabilization of IκB, thus preventing the accumulation of NFκB after stimulation *(45)*. To date, there have been no studies regarding the direct action of the indole I3C on COX-2 activity or inflammation, although one group fed I3C to Apc(Min+) mice and reported significant reduction in the number of aberrant crypt foci *(46)*.

2.4. Regulation of Apoptosis and Cell Cycle Arrest

The regulation of apoptosis (programmed cell death) is one of the key factors determining the fate of a cancer cell. In brief, there are two primary means of activating apoptosis. First, the intrinsic pathway in which activation of mitochondrial factors leads to cytochrome c release and activation of caspase 9. Second, the extrinsic pathway in which binding of external factors to cell surface receptors results in activation of caspase 8. The stimulation of the initiator caspases (8 and 9) ultimately leads to the activation of executer caspases (3, 6, 7) which will cleave specific targets leading to the irreversible initiation of cell suicide. Therefore, as initiated cells divide and progress toward forming tumors, they must develop mechanisms to help to evade the normal apoptotic signals, which would typically result in their death. Many effective chemopreventive agents have a direct or net effect of re-sensitizing tumor cells to apoptosis, or of blocking the cell cycle. Both of these effects would have the overall result of slowing clonal expansion of initiated cells and inhibiting promotion.

Isothiocyanates, and SUL in particular, have been shown to induce apoptosis through multiple pathways in multiple cell types. Studies have found that SUL induces mitochondrial-based activation of apoptotic cascades, in some cases by increasing the ratio of Bad and Bax proteins relative to Bcl-2 and activation of p53 (reviewed in *(19, 47, 48)*). SUL treatment often results in release of cytochrome c from the mitochondrial membrane and activation of caspase 3 *(48)*. Recently, Singh et al. *(49)* reported that SUL treatment also resulted in caspase 8 cleavage, thus indicating that the extrinsic pathway had been activated. The same authors reported that the apoptotic death and cell cycle arrest noted after SUL treatment in prostate cancer cells were strongly linked to the production of reactive oxygen species (ROS). They suggested that SUL could act in three ways to inhibit prostate cancer in their system: (1) ROS generation causing the release of cytochrome c, resulting in apoptosis; (2) triggering of a signaling cascade that leads to the phosphorylation and inhibition of cyclin-dependent kinase 1 (Cdk1); and (3) by conjugation and, therefore, depletion of the baseline cellular levels of glutathione (GSH). It was postulated that reductions of free GSH could sensitize the cell to other apoptotic signals *(49, 50)*. ROS production has also been linked to apoptosis after SUL treatment in colon cancer cells *(51)*. Other work with colon cancer cells revealed that treatment with SUL induced cell cycle arrest and several markers of apoptosis *(48)*. NFκB may act upstream of some inducers of apoptosis. Therefore, the treatment with SUL may work through regulation of this transcription factor, as well as through the MAPKinase and AP-1 signaling pathways. It should be noted, however, that SUL treatment is also linked to protection against ROS due to induction of the Nrf2 transcription factor/phase II response *(52, 53)*. There is evidence that cells may switch their responses from protective (Nrf2/phase II induction) to apoptotic depending on the dose of SUL used in human hepatoma cells *(54)*. SUL treatment has also been shown to induce apoptosis in many other cell lines, including human MCF-7 breast cancer cells, lymphoblastoid cells, medulloblastoma cells, and pancreatic cancer cells (reviewed in *(55)*).

PEITC, BITC, and I3C have all also been linked with induction of apoptosis, and exerted similar dose- and tissue-specific effects. I3C has been shown to induce caspase 3, down-regulate Bcl-2, and up-regulate/redistribute Bax in Her-2/neu overexpressing breast cancer cells *(56)*. The latter study reported that growth inhibition through induction of apoptosis was apparent in tumorigenic breast cancer models treated with I3C, but not in non-tumorigenic breast cell lines *(57)*. Some researchers have found that the apoptosis-stimulating ability of PEITC is linked to its ability to activate the JNK MAPKinase *(58, 59)*. This activation has been linked to the ability of PEITC to block JNK-specific phosphatases in prostate cancer cell lines *(60)*. Also, PEITC was found to induce apoptosis through activation of caspase 8 (extrinsic pathway) in leukemia cells *(61)*, but through the intrinsic pathway in Hela cells *(62)*. BITC was also found to induce JNK, which in this case was linked to phosphorylation and inactivation of Bcl-2, thus contributing to apoptosis *(63)*. Mitochondrial cytochrome c release and apoptosis after BITC treatment was also shown in rat hepatocytes. This was postulated to be due to ROS-related mechanisms *(64)*. Recently, it has been shown in breast cancer cells that the induction of ROS after BITC treatment was due to inhibition of complex III of the mitochondrial respiratory chain. In addition, it was documented that BITC caused JNK and p38 MAPKinase activation, and that a normal human mammary epithelial cell line did not produce ROS as it underwent apoptosis after exposure to BITC *(65)*.

2.5. Additional Molecular Methods of Chemoprevention

As may be apparent from above, the chemopreventive activity of isothiocyanates and indoles is multifaceted. Each of the above compounds hits multiple targets in the cell, with specificity depending upon dose and cell type involved. Additional effects of SUL, PEITC, BITC and I3C include inhibition of histone deacetylases, leading to opening of the chromatin structure and increased expression of p21, which in turn, can block progression through the cell cycle *(66, 67)*; inhibition of microtubule formation, thus halting the cell cycle *(68, 69)*; inhibition of phase I enzymes, therefore reducing the rate of conversion of xenobiotics to carcinogens and protecting cells from DNA damage *(70)*; eradication of *H. pylori* infections *(71, 72)*; and possibly stimulation of proteasome activity *(73, 74)*. Excellent reviews are available on the molecular effects of isothiocyanates and indoles in cancer cells *(19, 47, 55, 75–78)*.

2.6. Effects in Animal Models

Isothiocyanates and indoles have been shown to exert preventive effects in various animal models. The specific effects of I3C have been examined in HPV16-transgenic mice, which are prone to developing cervical cancer after treatment with estradiol. Studies documented that dietary I3C increased the rate of apoptosis in the cervical epithelium. Rahman et al. *(79)* found that I3C blocked breast cancer cells from metastasizing into bone in a SCID mouse model. Other studies have examined the effects of intraperitoneal (I.P.) injection of I3C (20 mg/kg) on the growth of subdermally injected mouse prostate cancer cells *(80)*. The latter treatment significantly inhibited the growth of tumors, activated apoptosis, and reduced proliferation and angiogenesis. The supplementation with I3C has also been shown to significantly inhibit UV-induced skin carcinogenesis in hairless mice *(81)*. Feeding a diet containing 0.05% PEITC to Apc(Min/+) mice for 3 weeks resulted in significant reductions in size and number of polyps when compared to mice on a standard diet *(82)*. The same group reported a similar effect in Apc (Min/+) mice fed SUL at 300 or 600 ppm for 3 weeks *(83)*. Studies have examined the preventive efficacy of *N*-acetyl cysteine (NAC) conjugated forms of BITC and PEITC against lung tumors initiated by feeding A/J mice a carcinogenic dose of benzo(*a*)pyrene [B(a)P]. Both NAC-conjugated forms of BITC and PEITC significantly reduced lung tumor multiplicity 140 days after dosing with B(a)P. In the isothiocyanate-treated groups, the tumor inhibition was linked to increased MAPKinase activity, especially JNK, as well as to marked activation of AP-1 and increased markers of apoptosis *(84)*. The same group reported that SUL and PEITC reduced the incidence of lung adenocarcinomas, but not adenomas, in mice exposed to tobacco carcinogens *(85)*. The effects of BITC have been examined in mouse skin after treatment with TPA. The treatment with BITC reduced both the oxidative damage caused by the carcinogen and subsequent infiltration by leukocytes *(86)*. SUL has been shown to inhibit skin carcinogenesis in mice when used against both UV-induced and chemically induced cancer models *(87, 88)*. The chemically induced skin carcinogenesis response to SUL was linked to the activity of Nrf2 *(88)*. Experimental evidence from in vivo models suggests isothiocyanates and indoles may inhibit carcinogenesis and be effective cancer prevention agents.

Finally, recent studies have explored whether combinations of natural products may exert synergistic effects against cancer. For example, one group reported that the combination of SUL+PEITC or SUL+curcumin led to a more efficient inhibition of inflammation compared to individual treatments *(89)*. The same study indicated that the combined treatment with SUL+EGCG synergistically activated AP-1 in human colon cancer cells, and that SUL+DBM (dibenzoylmethane, from licorice) completely blocked colon adenocarcinomas in Apc/Min+ mice. The latter inhibition was more pronounced and seen following treatment with SUL or DBM alone *(90, 91)*. Therefore, strategies based on combinations of two or more isothiocyanates and/or indoles may prove more powerful in the fight against cancer.

3. INTAKE ESTIMATES

Using data from the USDA 1994–1996 Continuing Survey of Food Intake (CSFII), cruciferous vegetable intake among US adults is estimated to be 0.2 servings or 18–20 g/day or just over a single serving per week. An estimated 20% of Americans were reported to consume any cruciferous vegetable during a 2-day diet reporting period *(92)*. Intake estimates from case–control and cohort studies vary widely depending on the population studied and the dietary assessment approach employed. In fact, food frequency questionnaires, the standard dietary instrument used in collecting dietary data for epidemiological studies, are limited in terms of the number of cruciferous vegetables listed. Table 2 lists the cruciferous vegetable items included in the most commonly employed FFQ used in the USA for epidemiological research.

Table 2
Cruciferous Vegetable Items Included in Food Frequency Questionnaires Commonly Used in the USA

Block Food Frequency Questionnaire (brief) (Block 2000 Brief; ©2000; BDDS)
- Broccoli
- Spinach or greens like collard
- Coleslaw, cabbage

Block Food Frequency Questionnaire (Standard) (Block 98.2; ©1998; BDDS)
- Broccoli
- Mustard greens, turnip greens, collards
- Coleslaw, cabbage
- Chinese food, Thai, or Asian food

Brigham and Women's Food Frequency Questionnaire (©1991; Brigham and Women's Hospital)
- Broccoli
- Cabbage, cauliflower, Brussels sprouts
- Spinach or collard greens

Fred Hutchinson Cancer Center Food Frequency Questionnaire
- Broccoli
- Cauliflower, cabbage, Brussels sprouts
- Cooked greens (spinach, mustard greens, collards)
- Coleslaw

University of Hawaii Food Frequency Questionnaire (©1998; Epidemiology Program, Cancer Research Center of Hawaii, University of Hawaii)
- Stir fried beef or pork and vegetables or fajitas
- Stir fried vegetables
- Pork and greens
- Coleslaw
- Broccoli
- Cabbage
- Mustard
- Cauliflower
- Dark green leafy vegetables (spinach, collards, mustard greens, turnip greens, bok choy, watercress, chard)
- Oriental salad or pickled vegetable

National Cancer Institute (NCI) Diet History Questionnaire (ver. EW-213950-3-654321; National Institutes of Health)
- Broccoli (fresh or frozen)
- Cooked greens (spinach, turnip greens, collard greens, mustard greens, chard, kale)
- Raw greens (spinach, turnip greens, collard greens, mustard greens, chard, kale)
- Coleslaw
- Sauerkraut or cabbage
- Cauliflower or Brussels sprouts (fresh or frozen)

Willet Food Frequency Questionnaire (©1996; President and Fellows of Harvard College)
- Broccoli
- Cabbage or coleslaw
- Cauliflower
- Brussels sprouts
- Kale, mustard greens, chard

Reprinted with permission, *J Amer Diet Assoc*, 2007.

The majority of these questionnaires include the most commonly consumed cruciferous vegetables. In the USA, broccoli is the most commonly consumed cruciferous vegetable, intake is threefold greater than cauliflower and cabbage, followed by mustard, kale, related greens, sauerkraut, and Brussels sprouts. In contrast, other sources are infrequently consumed. However, select foods such as wasabi or horseradish may contribute significantly to cancer prevention due to the higher concentration of isothiocyanate and indole compounds. The intake is also variable across ethnic groups. For example, Seow et al. estimated daily cruciferous vegetable intake among Singapore Chinese adults ($N = 246$) to be 40.6 g or approximately one-half serving/day with choi sum, bok choi, and cabbage contributing greater than 50% of the daily intake *(93)*. Evidence from the European Prospective Investigation of Cancer (EPIC) – Spain estimated intakes even lower than the USA averaging 11.3 g/day. In this population, the intake of cruciferous vegetables was also associated with body mass index, physical activity, and education level achieved *(94)*.

3.1. Assessment of Intake and Exposure

Food frequency questionnaires (FFQ) are the primary tool used to assess the relationship between dietary intake and the relative risk or odds ratio for cancer. Repeated 24 h recalls are an additional approach to improve intake assessments. A report comparing intake estimates for cruciferous vegetables using both FFQ and repeat recalls suggested significantly correlated intake of broccoli, cauliflower, and cabbage/sauerkraut/coleslaw, but poor correlations for intake of greens *(95)*. However, no data are currently available to estimate the number of days of recall required to have a valid assessment of usual exposure in a population. Moreover, recalls are also more costly and time-intensive to collect and analyze than FFQ. An option may be to utilize a focused FFQ that specifically assesses the intake of a comprehensive list of cruciferous vegetables with information on preparation/cooking methods, which may alter the efficacy of specific bioactive food components of cruciferous vegetables. A cruciferous vegetable FFQ (CVFFQ) has been developed and validated at the University of Arizona *(95)* for this purpose.

Metabolism of cruciferous vegetables generates several intermediate and end products depending on the specific vegetable consumed. Figure 2 illustrates common bioactive metabolic products of cruciferous vegetables that are of interest in relation to cancer prevention. Broccoli and broccoli sprouts are a source of both SUL and I3C. Both compounds exert significant anticancer activity in cell culture models. Brussels sprouts also contain I3C. Watercress is a primary food source of PEITC, which has been investigated for its apoptotic activity.

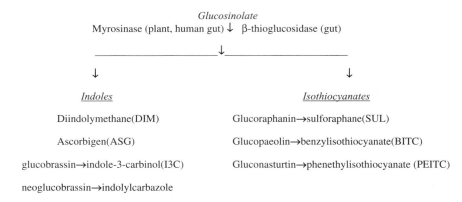

Fig. 2. Bioactive metabolic end products of cruciferous vegetables.

Paired-ion chromatography *(96)* and cyclocondensation reaction assays can be used to reliably quantitate glucosinolates in cruciferous vegetables *(97)*. Although an international database has been developed, there is a lack of information in the form of a well-described USDA database for glucosinolates or isothiocyanates content of specific cruciferous vegetable *(98)*. Applying such a database to more accurately estimate dietary exposure to glucosinolates will allow for more precise assessment of glucosinolate–cancer associations in population studies. Even with improved estimates of cruciferous vegetables and glucosinolates exposure, the true concentration of bioactive food components in the actual plant foods consumed may be variable depending on plant age *(99, 100)*, variety in relation to accessions *(101, 102)*, and preparation and storage *(103, 104)*. The distribution of glucosinolates within the *Brassica* plant also varies widely across plant organs (seeds, stems, sprouts, roots, and leaves). For a comprehensive review of the topic, readers are referred to Fahey, 1999 *(100)*. An additional limitation is the lack of specific information on the plant variety consumed, which introduces significant variations in the content of bioactive food components and may account for some of the variability in glucosinolates exposure observed among different ethnic groups and geographical regions *(98)*. Furthermore, the specific varieties available for purchase frequently differ by geographic region of sale as well as season of purchase. While USDA-sampling approaches reduce this error for foods listed in the USDA database, other data sources would not.

The anticancer activity of bioactive compounds found in cruciferous vegetables is influenced by cooking procedures and/or myrosinase activity. Myrosinase is the enzyme required for metabolism of glucosinolates in cruciferous vegetables to their bioactive isothiocyanates. Myrosinase is activated within the plant food matrix when cell membranes are severed either during food preparation or during the mastication process. Although cooking has been shown to destroy myrosinase, human feeding studies have demonstrated some, although less, cancer-preventive biological activity even for cooked cruciferous vegetables *(105–107)* likely due to β-thioglucosidase in the gut microflora, which serves as an alternative source of enzymatic activity associated with hydrolyzation of glucosinolates *(108, 109)*. Even with ample hydrolysis, glucosinolates are predominantly hydrophilic and as such are lost in cooking water during boiling or steaming *(110)*. Defrosting of frozen vegetables *(111)* and ascorbic acid *(104)* has been postulated to release myrosinase leading to an enhancement of the bioavailability of glucosinolates *(111)*. Exposure estimates have been improved through the development and validation of reliable biomarkers of dietary intake. A valid and reliable HPLC-based assay has been developed to quantify total isothiocyanates and dithiocarbamates in human urine using a cyclocondensation reaction that generates 1,3-benzodithiole-2-thione *(97, 108)*. In general, peak urinary excretion of the majority of isothiocyanates is within 8 h of intake and excretion is 80% complete within 24 h *(112)*. The half-life of isothiocyanates found in cruciferous vegetables has been estimated to range from 2.1 to 3.9 h *(113)*. At minimum, in studies designed to assess the relationship between urinary metabolites and disease outcomes urine samples should be collected overnight since the highest intake of cruciferous vegetables in humans occurs during lunch and evening meals. Laboratory assays have been developed to quantify phenethyl *(114)*, allyl isothiocyanate *(115)*. More recently, a liquid chromatography–tandem mass spectrometry assay has been used to quantify PEITC in human plasma and urine after intake of a standard dose of watercress *(116)*. The cyclocondensation assay also has been applied in quantifying plasma ITC and dithiocarbamates pre-post exposure to Cruciferous vegetables *(117)*. More recently a controlled feeding trial with two doses of cruciferous vegetables (80 g vs. 320 g) following a 4-day washout suggested that the HPLC cyclocondensation assay quantifying 1,2-bezenedithiol could recover 69–74% of isothiocyanates consumed with correlations between diet and metabolic measures of 0.9 *(118)*. These biomarkers have also been employed in epidemiological research. Measures of isothiocyanates in stored urine collected from Chinese elderly living in Singapore were shown to correlate significantly with reported dietary intake *(93)*. Further, Fowke and colleagues demonstrated that measurement of cyclocondensation products from isocyanates was effective in subjects who regularly consumed approximately 100 g/day (one serving) of cruciferous vegetables. Interestingly, isothiocyanates analysis was shown to be less accurate during periods of very low or sporadic intake and when intake was greater than 200 g/day *(119)*. Raw vegetable intake was more strongly associated with urinary isothiocyanates than cooked vegetable intake ($r = 0.23$ vs. 0.07, respectively). Similar correlations were shown in healthy US adults consuming, on average, 50 g/day of cruciferous vegetables. However, US estimates were similar for raw ($r = 0.27$) and cooked ($r = 0.23$) cruciferous vegetables possibly related to duration of cooking and/or the use (or non-use) of water-based cooking *(95)*.

4. EPIDEMIOLOGICAL EVIDENCE FOR CANCER PREVENTIVE ROLE OF CRUCIFEROUS VEGETABLES

The 2007 AICR/WCRF report suggests that an inverse, protective relationship exists between cruciferous vegetable intake and cancer risk *(120)* although for several cancer sites the evidence is inconsistent and may vary depending on the study design (case–control vs. cohort). Although a few intervention trials on cruciferous vegetables are available, no specific intervention trials have targeted increased cruciferous vegetables intake with cancer outcomes (Table 3). Epidemiological evidence limited to

Table 3

Summary of Epidemiological Evidence Since 2000: Cruciferous Vegetable Intake and Cancer Risk

Lead author, year (geographic location) Sample size	Assessment measure	Average intake of CV	Odds ratio or relative risk (95% confidence interval)[a]
Bladder			
Tang, 2008 (USA) (121) Hospital-based, cases = 275; controls = 825	Total, raw, and cooked cruciferous vegetables	Cases total cruciferous vegetables = 13.5 servings/month; raw = 4.5 servings/month Controls 15.8 –servings/month; raw = 5.9 servings/month	Total 0.81 (0.53–1.24) Raw 0.64 (0.46–0.97) Raw broccoli 0.57 (0.40–0.81)
Breast			
Adebamowo, 2005 (USA) (122) Nurses Health Study II N = 90,638 (740 cases)	Broccoli	<1/month vs. 5–6/week	RR, 0.99 (0.50–1.65)
Frazier, 2003 (USA) (123) Nurses' Health Study n = 843 case–control pairs	Cabbage, broccoli	Adolescent consumption (median ½ cup servings/day): Cabbage: 0.14; Broccoli: 0.07	RR, 1.00 (0.64–1.57) RR, 0.74 (0.39–1.41)
Ambrosone, 2004 (USA) (124) Cases, 740 (301 pre- and 396 post-menopausal); controls = 810	Broccoli, Brussels sprouts, sauerkraut, coleslaw, cauliflower, cabbage	Mean intake – premenopausal cases, 1,531 g/month; controls, 1,650 g/month postmenopausal cases, 1,368 g/month; controls, 1,479 g/month	Premenopausal OR, 0.7 (0.5–1.2) Broccoli – 0.6 (0.4–1.0) Postmenopausal OR, 0.8 (0.6–1.2) Broccoli – 1.0 (0.7–1.4)

Study	Cruciferous vegetables	Intake	Results
Colon/colorectal			
Seow, 2002 (China) (125)	9 commonly consumed cruciferous vegetables	Greater or less than median Cases, 26 g/1,000 kcal; controls, 28.9 g/1,000 kcals	OR, 0.81 (0.59–1.12) Colon 0.83(0.56–1.22) Rectal 0.76 (0.46–1.25)
Moy, 2008 (China) (126) Cases = 225; Matched controls = 1,119	Urinary ITC	<0.45 μmol/g creatinine vs. >2.95 μmol/g creatinine	Highest quartile; urine collected 10 years prior to diagnosis: OR, 0.46 (0.25–0.83)
Hara, 2003 (Japan) (127) Cases = 115; controls = 230	Cabbage, Komatsuna, Japanese radish, broccoli, Chinese cabbage,	Quartiles overall Broccoli < 1 servings/week vs. > 3 Cabbage < 2 servings/week vs. > 5	OR, 0.64 (0.25–1.63) Strongest for well differentiated 0.18 (0.06–0.58) 0.42 (0.17–1.03)
Hu, 2007 (Canada) (128) Rectal Cases only = 1,380; controls = 3,097	Broccoli, cabbage, cauliflower, Brussels sprouts, other greens	Mean intake 2.5 servings/week for cases and controls	NS, overall Females only OR, 0.6 (0.4–0.8)
Lung			
Feskanich, 2000 (USA) (129) Cases = 519; total study sample = 77,283 Nurses' Health Study (NHS) and 47,778 Health Professionals Follow-up Study (HPFS)	Broccoli, cabbage, cauliflower, coleslaw, Brussels sprouts, sauerkraut, kale, mustard or chard greens	NHS, 1.4–2.2 servings/week vs. > 4.8 HPFS 1.4–2.1 vs. > 5 servings/week	NHS, 0.74 (0.55–0.99) HPFS, 1.11 (0.76–1.64)

(Continued)

Table 3
(Continued)

Lead author, year (geographic location) Sample size	Assessment measure	Average intake of CV	Odds ratio or relative risk (95% confidence interval)[a]
Smith-Warner, 2003 (130) (pooled International) Cases = 3,206; total sample population = 430,281	Variable	No servings/week vs. > ½ serving daily Cabbage	Broccoli – RR, 1.05 (0.89–1.24); Cabbage – RR, 1.01 (0.88–1.17)
Voorrips, 2000 (131) (Netherlands) Cases = 1,010; Subcohort/Controls = 1,456 males and 1,497 females	Brussels sprouts, cauliflower, cabbage, kale	< 1 serving/month vs. > 3 servings/week Mean intake Males – cases = 31.1 g/day, Subcohort = 32.7 g/day Females – cases = 32.4 g/day, Subcohort = 31.6 g/day	Brassicas-RR, 0.7 (0.5–1.0) highest vs. lowest quintiles
Neuhouser, 2003 (USA) (132) Cases = 742; study sample population = 14,120 (β-Carotene and Retinol Efficacy Trial – CARET)	Broccoli, Brussels sprouts, cauliflower, coleslaw, cabbage, sauerkraut, mustard greens, turnip greens, collards	< 0.5 servings/week vs. > 3.5 servings/week	RR, Intervention arm, 0.91 (0.65–1.23); Placebo arm, 0.68 (0.45–1.04)
Miller, 2004 (Europe) (133) Cases = 1,074; total sample population = 478,021 in the European Prospective in Cancer Investigation (EPIC) Multiple myeloma	Variable by country	Quintiles of intake	RR, 1.21 (0.92–1.60) Southern Europe RR, 1.81 (1.09–3.03) Northern Europe RR, 1.01 (0.73–1.42)

Hosgood, 2007 (USA) (134) 179 cases; 691 controls	Broccoli, cauliflower, cabbage, Brussels sprouts	< 1 serving per week vs. > 2 per week	OR, 0.5, CI – 0.3–0.8
Non-Hodgkins lymphoma			
Kelemen, 2006 (USA) (135) Cases = 466; controls = 391 (w/diet data)	Broccoli, Brussels sprouts, cauliflower, mustard greens, coleslaw, radish	Mean intake Cases – 1.2 serving/week vs. controls 1.6 servings/week	OR, 0.62 (0.39–1.00)
Oral			
Rajkumar, 2002 (India) (136) Cases = 591; controls = 582	Not specified	< 1 serving/week vs. > 2/week	OR, 0.47 (0.32–0.70)
Ovarian			
Fairfield, 2001 (USA) (137) Cases = 301; total subjects = 80,326 Nurses' Health Study	Broccoli, cabbage, Brussels sprouts, coleslaw, greens	≤ 1 serving/week vs. > 3 servings/week	RR, 1.04 (0.69–1.57)
Pan, 2004 (Canada) (138) Cases = 442; controls = 2,135	Not specified	Mean intake 0.5 cup/week; quartiles of intake	OR, 0.76 (0.56–0.99)
Pancreas			
Chan, 2005 (USA, San Francisco) (139) Cases = 532; controls = 1,701	Broccoli, cabbage, coleslaw, cauliflower, and Brussels sprouts	Quartiles of intake	OR, 0.76 (0.56–1.0)

(Continued)

Table 3
(Continued)

Lead author, year (geographic location) Sample size	Assessment measure	Average intake of CV	Odds ratio or relative risk (95% confidence interval)[a]
Larsson, 2006 (Sweden) (140) Cases = 135; total study population = 81,922 in Swedish mammography cohort and cohort of Swedish men	All cabbages, cauliflower, broccoli, Brussels sprouts	< 1 serving/week vs. > 3 servings/week	RR, 0.70 (90.43–1.13)
Nothlings, 2006 (USA) (141) Cases = 529; total subjects = 183,522 in multi-ethnic cohort	Broccoli, cauliflower, head cabbage, won bok, Brussels sprouts, etc.	20.2 g/1,000 kcals vs. 98.1 g/1,000 kcals	RR, 0.83(0.62–1.10)
Prostate Kolonel, 2000 (USA) (142) Cases = 1,619; controls = 1,618	Coleslaw, broccoli, cabbage, mustard, cauliflower, collards, mustard greens, turnip greens, bok choy, watercress, chard, oriental salad, or pickled vegetable	< 8.8 g/day vs. > 72.9 g/day	OR, 0.78 (0.61–1.00) Advanced cases, 0.61 (0.42–0.88)
Giovannucci, 2003 (USA) (143) 2,969 cases; 47,365 controls	Broccoli, cabbage, coleslaw, sauerkraut, cauliflower, Brussels sprouts, kale/mustard, or chard greens	< 1 serving/week vs. > 5 servings/week	Moderate protection only among men < 65 years RR, 0.81 (0.64–1.02)

Kirsh, 2007 (USA) (144) 1,338 cases/520 with aggressive disease; 29,361 controls	Broccoli, cauliflower, coleslaw, cabbage, sauerkraut, mustard and turnip greens, kale	>1 serving/week vs. <1 serving/month	NS with total cases; significant with aggressive disease incidence: Total CV – RR, 0.60, 95% CI, 0.36–0.98; Broccoli – RR, 0.55, 95% CI, 0.34–0.89; Cauliflower – RR, 0.48, 0.25–0.89
Key, 2004 (Europe) (145) 972 cases; 130,544 controls EPIC	Variable by country	Mean intake ranged from 9.7 to 29.2 g/day	NS
Renal Hsu, 2007 (Russia, Romania, Poland, Czech Republic) (146) Cases = 1,065; controls = 1,509	Cabbage, broccoli, Brussels sprouts	Tertiles of intake 53.5 and 46.0% cases eat cabbage > 1/week; very low intake of broccoli and Brussels sprouts	OR, 0.68 (0.55–0.84) Cabbage 0.76 (0.58–0.99)
Hu, 2003 (Canada) (147) Cases = 1,279; controls = 5,370	Broccoli, cabbage, cauliflower, Brussels sprouts, greens	Not provided	OR, 0.6 (0.4–0.8) for females; NS in males

(Continued)

Table 3
(Continued)

Lead author, year (geographic location) Sample size	Assessment measure	Average intake of CV	Odds ratio or relative risk (95% confidence interval)[a]
Thyroid			
Bosetti, 2002 (USA, Asia, Europe – pooled analysis) (148) Cases = 2,241; controls = 3,716	Variable across studies: cabbages, broccoli, Brussels sprouts, cauliflower, etc.	Variable across studies Never-sometimes; 1/month vs. > 3/months; < 2/among vs. > 6/month	Significant inverse association: Connecticut – OR, 0.49 (0.29–0.84) (also cabbage or broccoli alone); Hawaii – OR, 0.57 (0.37–0.90) broccoli alone Significant increase risk: Japan – OR, 1.56 (1.07–2.31) w/o Japan – 0.71 (0.58–0.86)
Memon, 2002 (Kuwait) (149) Cases = 313;Controls = 313	Cabbage, cauliflower, broccoli, and Brussels sprouts	Never/seldom vs. > 2 servings/week	Not analyzed for total Cabbage OR, 1.9 (1.1–3.3) Cauliflower 1.8 (1.0–3.2)

[a] All OR and RR are adjusted for confounders found to be significant in the selected statistical models applied.

case–control studies is generally strongest for prostate (aggressive disease), colorectal, and renal cancers. Based on the paucity of studies available, cruciferous vegetables intake appears to reduce the risk for less common cancers including multiple myeloma and non-Hodgkins lymphoma. To date the available evidence is not as strong for lung, breast, and oral cancers. Effect modifiers that have been identified include raw vs. cooked vegetables and specific type of cruciferous vegetables consumed. For example, a recent case–control study identified a protective association between raw, but not total cruciferous vegetables intake and bladder cancer (OR 0.64, 95% confidence interval, 0.42–0.97) *(121)*. Another study suggested a reduced risk for thyroid cancer related to cruciferous vegetables intake in the USA, but elevated disease risk for high consumers in Japan possibly related to the common practice of pickling these vegetables in Asian countries, thus increasing exposure to carcinogens *(148)*. These studies support the need to collect more detailed information regarding cruciferous vegetables preparation and intake for future epidemiological research. Confounders that have been identified include age, gender, and menopausal status.

Polymorphisms in glutathione-*S*-transferase genes also influence associations between cruciferous vegetables intake and cancer outcomes. Using breast cancer as an example, it has been postulated that among those women carrying deletions in GSTM1, GSTT1, or both, exposure to isothiocyanates may be prolonged due to reduced phase II enzyme induction, increasing availability of isothiocyanates in target tissue and reducing breast cancer risk. In a case–control study among 337 breast cancer cases and 337 controls residing in Shanghai, China, urinary measures of isothiocyanates were inversely associated with breast cancer risk (OR, 0.5, 95% CI, 0.3–0.8) when comparing the lowest to the highest quartile of isothiocyanates exposure. This association persisted regardless of menopausal status; it may be modified by GST genotype since women with the GSTP1 val/val genotype who also reported low cruciferous vegetables intake had a significant elevation in breast cancer risk (OR, 1.74, 95% CI, 1.13–2.67). Conversely, risk was not elevated in women with Ile/Ile or heterozygous genotype *(150)*. A case–control analysis by Ambrosone et al. among 740 breast cancer cases and 810 controls showed that GST genotype did not modulate breast cancer risk nor was there a significant interaction between cruciferous vegetables intake and GST genotype and breast cancer risk *(124)*. A case–control report of renal cancer suggested that low intake of cruciferous vegetables was associated with an increase in risk among individuals null for GSTT1 (OR, 1.86, 95% CI, 1.07–3.23) or GSTT1 and GSTM1 (OR, 2.49, 95% CI, 1.08–5.77). A controlled broccoli feeding study among healthy adults documented that the "protective" polymorphism in terms of enhancing exposure to bioactive compounds found in broccoli may actually be the GSTM1 present genotype and that there may be variability in the "responsive" genotype across ethnic groups *(151)*.

Finally, data are very limited as to the role of cruciferous vegetables in modulating the risk for cancer recurrence. One prospective cohort study conducted among 609 women diagnosed and treated for invasive epithelial ovarian cancer in Australia *(152)* suggested greater intake of CV was associated with a 25% reduction in the adjusted hazards ratio for recurrent disease (HR, 0.75, 95% CI, 0.58–1.01). Breast cancer patients taking tamoxifen have also demonstrated a significant survival advantage when consuming, on average, 1 serving of cruciferous vegetables daily *(153)*. In this study, the protective association for cruciferous vegetables was found for a population of over 3,000 breast cancer survivors, but was most pronounced among those women taking tamoxifen. These findings suggested that bioactive compounds in cruciferous vegetables may synergize with tamoxifen reducing the risk of estrogen-associated recurrent disease.

5. CLINICAL STUDIES OF CRUCIFEROUS VEGETABLES AND RELATED BAFC

Few intervention trials with cruciferous vegetables or bioactive constituents of cruciferous vegetables have been completed and those available are pilot in nature enrolling less than 50 subjects (Table 4). Further, no intervention trials have assessed cancer endpoints. Generally, outcome measures include biomarkers of plausible chemopreventive activity such as modulation of oxidative stress or lowering of estrogen levels in subjects at risk for hormone-related cancers. A study of 20 healthy adults randomized to a *Brassica*-rich diet vs. vitamin–mineral–fiber supplement used a cross-over design with 4-week interventions separated by a 2-week washout period. The *Brassica* intervention was associated with a 22% reduction in lipid peroxidation as assessed by urinary F2-isoprostane levels *(154)*. Similar reductions (28%) in oxidative stress (urinary 8-oxo-7,8-dihydroxy-2′-deoxyguanosine) were demonstrated among healthy males assigned to cruciferous vegetable free diet vs. 300 g/day of cooked Brussels sprouts for a 3 week intervention period *(106)*. Cruciferous vegetables have also been shown to enhance urinary mutant excretion among subjects exposed to fried meat ($n = 4$ fried meat with cruciferous vegetables; $n = 4$ with fried meat and non-cruciferous vegetables intake daily for 6 weeks) *(155)*. Furthermore, a larger study among 200 healthy adults residing in China showed that randomization to glucoraphanin beverages (broccoli sprouts) nightly for 2 weeks, while not associated with lower aflatoxin–DNA adduct formation overall, did demonstrate significantly higher excretion of these adducts among subject concurrently demonstrating high urinary dithiocarbamate levels. These results suggest that the protective effects are likely related to the ability of cruciferous vegetables to induce phase I/II enzymes including NAT and GST. One study with heavy smokers documented a significant reduction in DNA adducts in exfoliated bladder cells after 12 months of a high Cruciferous vegetables diet ($P = 0.02$), with cauliflower and cabbage as the major food sources of BAFC *(156)*.

6. CONCLUSIONS

There is significant and compelling mechanistic evidence that cruciferous vegetables and the component bioactive food compounds therein can modulate human risk for cancer. The epidemiological evidence, while inconsistent, also supports a protective role for cruciferous vegetables for several cancer types. Current dietary intake of cruciferous vegetables in the US population is well below estimates thought to be associated with reduced cancer risk. While intake levels associated with protection vary, broccoli and cabbage may afford unique protection, possibly related to the presence of specific BAFCs. Well-designed, prospective cohort studies and even more relevant, clinical tri-

Table 4
Select Clinical Trials Testing the Efficacy of Cruciferous Vegetables, Indole-3-carbinol, and/or Diindolylmethane in Disease Prevention

Author, year	Sample population	Study design	Dose/duration	Findings
Cruciferous vegetables				
Fowke et al., 2006 (154)	20 healthy adults	Randomized, controlled	Brassica-rich diet vs. fiber/multivitamin supplement 4 weeks	225 reduction in lipid peroxidation
Verhagen et al., 1995 (106)	Healthy males	Randomized, controlled	Cruciferous vegetables-free vs. 300 g Brussels sprouts diet for 3 weeks	28% reduction in 8-OHdG
Greenlee et al., 2007 (157)	40 healthy premenopausal women (n = 10 randomized to diet change)	Placebo-controlled, parallel arm	3 crucifers or 3 dark green leafy vs. botanical mix vs. placebo pill – all with 30 g fiber/day	2OHE:16α-OHE decreased by a non-significant 5.88% in diet group. Unknown average cruciferous vegetables vs. green leafy vegetable intake
Talaska et al., 2006 (156)	Healthy male heavy smokers	Blind, randomized controlled trial	High cruciferous vegetables diet – cauliflower and cabbage – for 12 months	Significant reduction in ^{32}P-postlabeling DNA adducts in exfoliated bladder cells

(*Continued*)

Table 4
(Continued)

Author, year	Sample population	Study design	Dose/duration	Findings
Kensler et al., 2005 (158)	200 Healthy adults	Randomized, placebo-controlled	Glucoraphanin-rich juice (400 μmol) or placebo juice for 2 weeks	No significant difference in urinary aflatoxin-N^7-guanine; significant inverse association between DNA adduct levels and urinary dithiocarbamate levels
Indole-3-carbinol				
Reed et al., 2005 (159)	Healthy pre and post-menopausal women	Controlled, dose-escalating phase I–II trials	400 and 800 mg/day for 4 weeks/dose	Significant reduction in 2-OHE:16-α-OHE ratio
Bradlow et al., 1994 (160)	60 pre-menopausal women with increased cancer risk	Randomized, 3-arm clinical trial	400 mg I3C/day for 3 months; 20 g α-cellulose; placebo	Increase in 2-OHE-estriol ratio with I3C; statistical differences across groups not reported
Wong et al., 1997 (161)	57 Women at increased risk for breast cancer	Placebo-controlled, double-blind, dose-ranging phase I-II trials	I3C:50 escalating to 200 mg vs. 300 escalating to 400 mg for 4 weeks vs. placebo	Significant reduction in 2-OHE:16-α-OHE ratio with ≥300 mg/day vs. placebo or lower dose
3,3′-Diindolylmethane				
Dalessandri, 2004 (162)	19 women with previous diagnosis of early stage, post-menopausal breast cancer	Randomized, controlled trial	BioResponse-DIM 108 mg/day for 1 month vs. placebo	2-OHE:16-α-OHE ratio increased from 1.79 to 1.82 in the placebo group and from 1.46 to 2.14 (47%, non-significant) in DIM group

als, are needed to advance our understanding of the role of Cruciferous vegetables in cancer prevention.

REFERENCES

1. Leung, L., Kwong, M., Hou, S. et al. (2003) Deficiency of the Nrf1 and Nrf2 transcription factors results in early embryonic lethality and severe oxidative stress. *J Biol Chem* **278**, 48021–9.
2. Kobayashi, A., Ito, E., Toki, T. et al. (1999) Molecular cloning and functional characterization of a new Cap'n' collar family transcription factor Nrf3. *J Biol Chem* **274**, 6443–52.
3. Cho, H.Y., Reddy, S.P., and Kleeberger, S.R. (2006) Nrf2 defends the lung from oxidative stress. *Antioxid Redox Signal* **8**, 76–87.
4. Lee, J.M., Li, J., Johnson, D.A. et al. (2005) Nrf2, a multi-organ protector? *Faseb J* **19**, 1061–6.
5. Zhang, D.D. (2006) Mechanistic studies of the Nrf2-Keap1 signaling pathway. *Drug Metab Rev* **38**, 769–89.
6. Enomoto, A., Itoh, K., Nagayoshi, E. et al. (2001) High sensitivity of Nrf2 knockout mice to acetaminophen hepatotoxicity associated with decreased expression of ARE-regulated drug metabolizing enzymes and antioxidant genes. *Toxicol Sci* **59**, 169–77.
7. Ramos-Gomez, M., Kwak, M.K., Dolan, P.M. et al. (2001) Sensitivity to carcinogenesis is increased and chemoprotective efficacy of enzyme inducers is lost in nrf2 transcription factor-deficient mice. *Proc Natl Acad Sci USA* **98**, 3410–5.
8. Park, E.Y., and Rho, H.M. (2002) The transcriptional activation of the human copper/zinc superoxide dismutase gene by 2,3,7,8-tetrachlorodibenzo-p-dioxin through two different regulator sites, the antioxidant responsive element and xenobiotic responsive element. *Mol Cell Biochem* **240**, 47–55.
9. Xu, C., Yuan, X., Pan, Z. et al. (2006) Mechanism of action of isothiocyanates: The induction of ARE-regulated genes is associated with activation of ERK and JNK and the phosphorylation and nuclear translocation of Nrf2. *Mol Cancer Ther* **5**, 1918–26.
10. Jakubikova, J., Sedlak, J., Bod'o, J. et al. (2006) Effect of isothiocyanates on nuclear accumulation of NF-kappaB, Nrf2, and thioredoxin in caco-2 cells. *J Agric Food Chem* **54**, 1656–62.
11. Jeong, W.S., Keum, Y.S., Chen, C. et al. (2005) Differential expression and stability of endogenous nuclear factor E2-related factor 2 (Nrf2) by natural chemopreventive compounds in HepG2 human hepatoma cells. *J Biochem Mol Biol* **38**, 167–76.
12. Hayes, J.D., and McMahon, M. (2006) The double-edged sword of Nrf2: Subversion of redox homeostasis during the evolution of cancer. *Mol Cell* **21**, 732–4.
13. Padmanabhan, B., Tong, K.I., Ohta, T. et al. (2006) Structural basis for defects of Keap1 activity provoked by its point mutations in lung cancer. *Mol Cell* **21**, 689–700.
14. Eferl, R., and Wagner, E.F. (2003) AP-1: A double-edged sword in tumorigenesis. *Nat Rev Cancer* **3**, 859–68.
15. Domann, F.E., Jr., Levy, J.P., Finch, J.S. et al. (1994) Constitutive AP-1 DNA binding and transactivating ability of malignant but not benign mouse epidermal cells. *Mol Carcinog* **9**, 61–66.
16. Shaulian, E., and Karin, M. (2001) AP-1 in cell proliferation and survival. *Oncogene* **20**, 2390–400.
17. Zhu, M., Zhang, Y., Cooper, S. et al. (2004) Phase II enzyme inducer, sulforaphane, inhibits UVB-induced AP-1 activation in human keratinocytes by a novel mechanism. *Mol Carcinog* **41**, 179–86.
18. Jeong, W.S., Kim, I.W., Hu, R. et al. (2004) Modulation of AP-1 by natural chemopreventive compounds in human colon HT-29 cancer cell line. *Pharm Res* **21**, 649–60.
19. Juge, N., Mithen, R.F., and Traka, M. (2007) Molecular basis for chemoprevention by sulforaphane: A comprehensive review. *Cell Mol Life Sci* **64**, 1105–27.
20. Shen, G., Jeong, W.S., Hu, R. et al. (2005) Regulation of Nrf2, NF-kappaB, and AP-1 signaling pathways by chemopreventive agents. *Antioxid Redox Signal* **7**, 1648–63.
21. Huang, S., Pettaway, C.A., Uehara, H. et al. (2001) Blockade of NF-kappaB activity in human prostate cancer cells is associated with suppression of angiogenesis, invasion, and metastasis. *Oncogene* **20**, 4188–97.

22. Kim, D.W., Sovak, M.A., Zanieski, G. et al. (2000) Activation of NF-kappaB/Rel occurs early during neoplastic transformation of mammary cells. *Carcinogenesis* **21**, 871–9.

23. Wang, W., Abbruzzese, J.L., Evans, D.B. et al. (1999) The nuclear factor-kappa B RelA transcription factor is constitutively activated in human pancreatic adenocarcinoma cells. *Clin Cancer Res* **5**, 119–27.

24. Hatta, Y., Arima, N., Machino, T. et al. (2003) Mutational analysis of IkappaBalpha in hematologic malignancies. *Int J Mol Med* **11**, 239–42.

25. Bharti, A.C., and Aggarwal, B.B. (2002) Nuclear factor-kappa B and cancer: Its role in prevention and therapy. *Biochem Pharmacol* **64**, 883–8.

26. Jeong, W.S., Kim, I.W., Hu, R. et al. (2004) Modulatory properties of various natural chemopreventive agents on the activation of NF-kappaB signaling pathway. *Pharm Res* **21**, 661–70.

27. Heiss, E., Herhaus, C., Klimo, K. et al. (2001) Nuclear factor kappa B is a molecular target for sulforaphane-mediated anti-inflammatory mechanisms. *J Biol Chem* **276**, 32008–15.

28. Karmakar, S., Weinberg, M.S., Banik, N.L. et al. (2006) Activation of multiple molecular mechanisms for apoptosis in human malignant glioblastoma T98G and U87MG cells treated with sulforaphane. *Neuroscience* **141**, 1265–80.

29. Aggarwal, B.B., and Ichikawa, H. (2005) Molecular targets and anticancer potential of indole-3-carbinol and its derivatives. *Cell Cycle* **4**, 1201–5.

30. Patten, E.J., and DeLong, M.J. (1999) Temporal effects of the detoxification enzyme inducer, benzyl isothiocyanate: Activation of c-Jun N-terminal kinase prior to the transcription factors AP-1 and NFkappaB. *Biochem Biophys Res Commun* **257**, 149–55.

31. Krysan, K., Reckamp, K.L., Dalwadi, H. et al. (2005) Prostaglandin E2 activates mitogen-activated protein kinase/Erk pathway signaling and cell proliferation in non-small cell lung cancer cells in an epidermal growth factor receptor-independent manner. *Cancer Res* **65**, 6275–81.

32. Riedl, K., Krysan, K., Pold, M. et al. (2004) Multifaceted roles of cyclooxygenase-2 in lung cancer. *Drug Resist Updat* **7**, 169–84.

33. Tsujii, M., and DuBois, R.N. (1995) Alterations in cellular adhesion and apoptosis in epithelial cells overexpressing prostaglandin endoperoxide synthase 2. *Cell* **83**, 493–501.

34. Kundu, J.K., and Surh, Y.J. (2008) Inflammation: Gearing the journey to cancer. *Mutat Res* **659**, 15–30.

35. Surh, Y.J., and Kundu, J.K. (2007) Cancer preventive phytochemicals as speed breakers in inflammatory signaling involved in aberrant COX-2 expression. *Curr Cancer Drug Targets* **7**, 447–58.

36. Woo, K.J., and Kwon, T.K. (2007) Sulforaphane suppresses lipopolysaccharide-induced cyclooxygenase-2 (COX-2) expression through the modulation of multiple targets in COX-2 gene promoter. *Int Immunopharmacol* **7**, 1776–83.

37. Fischer, S.M., Pavone, A., Mikulec, C. et al. (2007) Cyclooxygenase-2 expression is critical for chronic UV-induced murine skin carcinogenesis. *Mol Carcinog* **46**, 363–71.

38. Agrawal, A., and Fentiman, I.S. (2008) NSAIDs and breast cancer: A possible prevention and treatment strategy. *Int J Clin Pract* **62**, 444–9.

39. Bair, W.B., 3rd, Hart, N., Einspahr, J. et al. (2002) Inhibitory effects of sodium salicylate and acetylsalicylic acid on UVB-induced mouse skin carcinogenesis. *Cancer Epidemiol Biomarkers Prev* **11**, 1645–52.

40. Liu, J.F., Zhang, S.W., Jamieson, G.G. et al. (2008) The effects of a COX-2 inhibitor meloxicam on squamous cell carcinoma of the esophagus in vivo. *Int J Cancer* **122**, 1639–44.

41. Xin, B., Yokoyama, Y., Shigeto, T. et al. (2007) Anti-tumor effect of non-steroidal anti-inflammatory drugs on human ovarian cancers. *Pathol Oncol Res* **13**, 365–9.

42. Konwinski, R.R., Haddad, R., Chun, J.A. et al. (2004) Oltipraz, 3H-1,2-dithiole-3-thione, and sulforaphane induce overlapping and protective antioxidant responses in murine microglial cells. *Toxicol Lett* **153**, 343–55.

43. Lin, W., Wu, R.T., Wu, T. et al. (2008) Sulforaphane suppressed LPS-induced inflammation in mouse peritoneal macrophages through Nrf2 dependent pathway. *Biochem Pharmacol* **76**(8), 967–73.

44. Ye, B., Zhang, Y.X., Yang, F. et al. (2007) Induction of lung lesions in Wistar rats by 4-(methylnitrosamino)-1-(3-pyridyl)-1-butanone and its inhibition by aspirin and phenethyl isothiocyanate. *BMC Cancer* **7**, 90.

45. Murakami, A., Matsumoto, K., Koshimizu, K. et al. (2003) Effects of selected food factors with chemopreventive properties on combined lipopolysaccharide- and interferon-gamma-induced IkappaB degradation in RAW264.7 macrophages. *Cancer Lett* **195**, 17–25.
46. Kim, D.J., Shin, D.H., Ahn, B. et al. (2003) Chemoprevention of colon cancer by Korean food plant components. *Mutat Res* **523–524**, 99–107.
47. Fimognari, C., and Hrelia, P. (2007) Sulforaphane as a promising molecule for fighting cancer. *Mutat Res* **635**, 90–104.
48. Gamet-Payrastre, L., Li, P., Lumeau, S. et al. (2000) Sulforaphane, a naturally occurring isothiocyanate, induces cell cycle arrest and apoptosis in HT29 human colon cancer cells. *Cancer Res* **60**, 1426–33.
49. Singh, S.V., Srivastava, S.K., Choi, S. et al. (2005) Sulforaphane-induced cell death in human prostate cancer cells is initiated by reactive oxygen species. *J Biol Chem* **280**, 19911–24.
50. Singh, S.V., Herman-Antosiewicz, A., Singh, A.V. et al. (2004) Sulforaphane-induced G2/M phase cell cycle arrest involves checkpoint kinase 2-mediated phosphorylation of cell division cycle 25C. *J Biol Chem* **279**, 25813–22.
51. Shen, G., Xu, C., Chen, C. et al. (2006) p53-independent G1 cell cycle arrest of human colon carcinoma cells HT-29 by sulforaphane is associated with induction of p21CIP1 and inhibition of expression of cyclin D1. *Cancer Chemother Pharmacol* **57**, 317–27.
52. Gao, X., Dinkova-Kostova, A.T., and Talalay, P. (2001) Powerful and prolonged protection of human retinal pigment epithelial cells, keratinocytes, and mouse leukemia cells against oxidative damage: The indirect antioxidant effects of sulforaphane. *Proc Natl Acad Sci USA* **98**, 15221–6.
53. Gao, X., and Talalay, P. (2004) Induction of phase 2 genes by sulforaphane protects retinal pigment epithelial cells against photooxidative damage. *Proc Natl Acad Sci USA* **101**, 10446–51.
54. Kim, B.R., Hu, R., Keum, Y.S. et al. (2003) Effects of glutathione on antioxidant response element-mediated gene expression and apoptosis elicited by sulforaphane. *Cancer Res* **63**, 7520–5.
55. Myzak, M.C., and Dashwood, R.H. (2006) Chemoprotection by sulforaphane: Keep one eye beyond Keap1. *Cancer Lett* **233**, 208–18.
56. Rahman, K.M., Aranha, O., Glazyrin, A. et al. (2000) Translocation of Bax to mitochondria induces apoptotic cell death in indole-3-carbinol (I3C) treated breast cancer cells. *Oncogene* **19**, 5764–71.
57. Rahman, K.M., Aranha, O., and Sarkar, F.H. (2003) Indole-3-carbinol (I3C) induces apoptosis in tumorigenic but not in nontumorigenic breast epithelial cells. *Nutr Cancer* **45**, 101–12.
58. Chen, Y.R., Wang, W., Kong, A.N. et al. (1998) Molecular mechanisms of c-Jun N-terminal kinase-mediated apoptosis induced by anticarcinogenic isothiocyanates. *J Biol Chem* **273**, 1769–75.
59. Yu, R., Jiao, J.J., Duh, J.L. et al. (1996) Phenethyl isothiocyanate, a natural chemopreventive agent, activates c-Jun N-terminal kinase 1. *Cancer Res* **56**, 2954–9.
60. Chen, Y.R., Han, J., Kori, R. et al. (2002) Phenylethyl isothiocyanate induces apoptotic signaling via suppressing phosphatase activity against c-Jun N-terminal kinase. *J Biol Chem* **277**, 39334–42.
61. Xu, K., and Thornalley, P.J. (2000) Studies on the mechanism of the inhibition of human leukaemia cell growth by dietary isothiocyanates and their cysteine adducts in vitro. *Biochem Pharmacol* **60**, 221–31.
62. Yu, R., Mandlekar, S., Harvey, K.J. et al. (1998) Chemopreventive isothiocyanates induce apoptosis and caspase-3-like protease activity. *Cancer Res* **58**, 402–08.
63. Miyoshi, N., Uchida, K., Osawa, T. et al. (2004) A link between benzyl isothiocyanate-induced cell cycle arrest and apoptosis: Involvement of mitogen-activated protein kinases in the Bcl-2 phosphorylation. *Cancer Res* **64**, 2134–42.
64. Nakamura, Y., Kawakami, M., Yoshihiro, A. et al. (2002) Involvement of the mitochondrial death pathway in chemopreventive benzyl isothiocyanate-induced apoptosis. *J Biol Chem* **277**, 8492–9.
65. Xiao, D., Powolny, A.A., and Singh, S.V. (2008) Benzyl isothiocyanate targets mitochondrial respiratory chain to trigger ros-dependent apoptosis in human breast cancer cells. *J Biol Chem* **283**(44), 30151–63.
66. Myzak, M.C., Hardin, K., Wang, R. et al. (2006) Sulforaphane inhibits histone deacetylase activity in BPH-1, LnCaP and PC-3 prostate epithelial cells. *Carcinogenesis* **27**, 811–9.

67. Myzak, M.C., Karplus, P.A., Chung, F.L. et al. (2004) A novel mechanism of chemoprotection by sulforaphane: Inhibition of histone deacetylase. *Cancer Res* **64**, 5767–74.

68. Jackson, S.J., and Singletary, K.W. (2004) Sulforaphane inhibits human MCF-7 mammary cancer cell mitotic progression and tubulin polymerization. *J Nutr* **134**, 2229–36.

69. Mi, L., Xiao, Z., Hood, B.L. et al. (2008) Covalent binding to tubulin by isothiocyanates. A mechanism of cell growth arrest and apoptosis. *J Biol Chem* **283**, 22136–46.

70. Maheo, K., Morel, F., Langouet, S. et al. (1997) Inhibition of cytochromes P-450 and induction of glutathione S-transferases by sulforaphane in primary human and rat hepatocytes. *Cancer Res* **57**, 3649–52.

71. Fahey, J.W., Haristoy, X., Dolan, P.M. et al. (2002) Sulforaphane inhibits extracellular, intracellular, and antibiotic-resistant strains of Helicobacter pylori and prevents benzo[a]pyrene-induced stomach tumors. *Proc Natl Acad Sci USA* **99**, 7610–5.

72. Haristoy, X., Angioi-Duprez, K., Duprez, A. et al. (2003) Efficacy of sulforaphane in eradicating Helicobacter pylori in human gastric xenografts implanted in nude mice. *Antimicrob Agents Chemother* **47**, 3982–4.

73. Hu, R., Xu, C., Shen, G. et al. (2006) Gene expression profiles induced by cancer chemopreventive isothiocyanate sulforaphane in the liver of C57BL/6 J mice and C57BL/6 J/Nrf2 (–/–) mice. *Cancer Lett* **243**, 170–92.

74. Kwak, M.K., Wakabayashi, N., Greenlaw, J.L. et al. (2003) Antioxidants enhance mammalian proteasome expression through the Keap1-Nrf2 signaling pathway. *Mol Cell Biol* **23**, 8786–94.

75. Clarke, J.D., Dashwood, R.H., and Ho, E. (2008) Multi-targeted prevention of cancer by sulforaphane. *Cancer Lett* **269**, 291–304.

76. Hayes, J.D., Kelleher, M.O., and Eggleston, I.M. (2008) The cancer chemopreventive actions of phytochemicals derived from glucosinolates. *Eur J Nutr* **47**(Suppl 2), 73–88.

77. Nakamura, Y., and Miyoshi, N. (2006) Cell death induction by isothiocyanates and their underlying molecular mechanisms. *Biofactors* **26**, 123–34.

78. Thornalley, P.J. (2002) Isothiocyanates: Mechanism of cancer chemopreventive action. *Anticancer Drugs* **13**, 331–8.

79. Rahman, K.M., Sarkar, F.H., Banerjee, S. et al. (2006) Therapeutic intervention of experimental breast cancer bone metastasis by indole-3-carbinol in SCID-human mouse model. *Mol Cancer Ther* **5**, 2747–56.

80. Souli, E., Machluf, M., Morgenstern, A. et al. (2008) Indole-3-carbinol (I3C) exhibits inhibitory and preventive effects on prostate tumors in mice. *Food Chem Toxicol* **46**, 863–70.

81. Cope, R.B., Loehr, C., Dashwood, R. et al. (2006) Ultraviolet radiation-induced non-melanoma skin cancer in the Crl:SKH1:hr-BR hairless mouse: Augmentation of tumor multiplicity by chlorophyllin and protection by indole-3-carbinol. *Photochem Photobiol Sci* **5**, 499–507.

82. Khor, T.O., Cheung, W.K., Prawan, A. et al. (2008) Chemoprevention of familial adenomatous polyposis in Apc(Min/+) mice by phenethyl isothiocyanate (PEITC). *Mol Carcinog* **47**, 321–5.

83. Hu, R., Khor, T.O., Shen, G. et al. (2006) Cancer chemoprevention of intestinal polyposis in ApcMin/+ mice by sulforaphane, a natural product derived from cruciferous vegetable. *Carcinogenesis* **27**, 2038–46.

84. Yang, Y.M., Conaway, C.C., Chiao, J.W. et al. (2002) Inhibition of benzo(a)pyrene-induced lung tumorigenesis in A/J mice by dietary N-acetylcysteine conjugates of benzyl and phenethyl isothiocyanates during the postinitiation phase is associated with activation of mitogen-activated protein kinases and p53 activity and induction of apoptosis. *Cancer Res* **62**, 2–7.

85. Conaway, C.C., Wang, C.X., Pittman, B. et al. (2005) Phenethyl isothiocyanate and sulforaphane and their N-acetylcysteine conjugates inhibit malignant progression of lung adenomas induced by tobacco carcinogens in A/J mice. *Cancer Res* **65**, 8548–57.

86. Nakamura, Y., Miyoshi, N., Takabayashi, S. et al. (2004) Benzyl isothiocyanate inhibits oxidative stress in mouse skin: Involvement of attenuation of leukocyte infiltration. *Biofactors* **21**, 255–7.

87. Dinkova-Kostova, A.T., Jenkins, S.N., Fahey, J.W. et al. (2006) Protection against UV-light-induced skin carcinogenesis in SKH-1 high-risk mice by sulforaphane-containing broccoli sprout extracts. *Cancer Lett* **240**, 243–52.

88. Xu, C., Huang, M.T., Shen, G. et al. (2006) Inhibition of 7,12-dimethylbenz(a)anthracene-induced skin tumorigenesis in C57BL/6 mice by sulforaphane is mediated by nuclear factor E2-related factor 2. *Cancer Res* **66**, 8293–6.
89. Cheung, K.L., Khor, T.O., and Kong, A.N. (2008) Synergistic Effect of Combination of Phenethyl Isothiocyanate and Sulforaphane or Curcumin and Sulforaphane in the Inhibition of Inflammation. *Pharm Res* **26**(1), 224–31.
90. Nair, S., Hebbar, V., Shen, G. et al. (2008) Synergistic effects of a combination of dietary factors sulforaphane and (–) epigallocatechin-3-gallate in HT-29 AP-1 human colon carcinoma cells. *Pharm Res* **25**, 387–99.
91. Shen, G., Khor, T.O., Hu, R. et al. (2007) Chemoprevention of familial adenomatous polyposis by natural dietary compounds sulforaphane and dibenzoylmethane alone and in combination in ApcMin/+ mouse. *Cancer Res* **67**, 9937–44.
92. Johnston, C.S., Taylor, C.A., and Hampl, J.S. (2000) More Americans are eating "5 a day" but intakes of dark green and cruciferous vegetables remain low. *J Nutr* **130**, 3063–7.
93. Seow, A., Shi, C.Y., Chung, F.L. et al. (1998) Urinary total isothiocyanate (ITC) in a population-based sample of middle-aged and older Chinese in Singapore: Relationship with dietary total ITC and glutathione S-transferase M1/T1/P1 genotypes. *Cancer Epidemiol Biomarkers Prev* **7**, 775–81.
94. Agudo, A., Ibanez, R., Amiano, P. et al. (2008) Consumption of cruciferous vegetables and glucosinolates in a Spanish adult population. *Eur J Clin Nutr* **62**, 324–31.
95. Thomson, C.A., Newton, T.R., Graver, E.J. et al. (2007) Cruciferous vegetable intake questionnaire improves cruciferous vegetable intake estimates. *J Am Diet Assoc* **107**, 631–43.
96. Prestera, T., Fahey, J.W., Holtzclaw, W.D. et al. (1996) Comprehensive chromatographic and spectroscopic methods for the separation and identification of intact glucosinolates. *Anal Biochem* **239**, 168–79.
97. Zhang, Y., Wade, K.L., Prestera, T. et al. (1996) Quantitative determination of isothiocyanates, dithiocarbamates, carbon disulfide, and related thiocarbonyl compounds by cyclocondensation with 1,2-benzenedithiol. *Anal Biochem* **239**, 160–7.
98. McNaughton, S.A., and Marks, G.C. (2003) Development of a food composition database for the estimation of dietary intakes of glucosinolates, the biologically active constituents of cruciferous vegetables. *Br J Nutr* **90**, 687–97.
99. Fahey, J.W., Zhang, Y., and Talalay, P. (1997) Broccoli sprouts: An exceptionally rich source of inducers of enzymes that protect against chemical carcinogens. *Proc Natl Acad Sci USA* **94**, 10367–72.
100. Fahey, J.W., and Stephenson, K.K. (1999) Cancer chemoprotective effects of cruciferous vegetables. *Hortscience* **34**, 4–8.
101. Fenwick, G.R., Heaney, R.K., and Mullin, W.J. (1983) Glucosinolates and their breakdown products in food and food plants. *Crit Rev Food Sci Nutr* **18**, 123–201.
102. Kushad, M.M., Brown, A.F., Kurlich, A.C. et al. (1999) Variation of glucosinolation in vegetable crops Brassica Oleracea. *J Agric Food Chem* **47**, 1541–8.
103. Johnson, I.T. (2002) Glucosinolates: Bioavailability and importance to health. *Int J Vitam Nutr Res* **72**, 26–31.
104. Verkerk, R., van der Gaag, M.S., Dekker, M. et al. (1997) Effects of processing conditions on glucosinolates in cruciferous vegetables. *Cancer Lett* **114**, 193–4.
105. Pantuck, E.J., Pantuck, C.B., Garland, W.A. et al. (1979) Stimulatory effect of Brussels sprouts and cabbage on human drug metabolism. *Clin Pharmacol Ther* **25**, 88–95.
106. Verhaggen, H., Poulsen, H.E., Loft, S. et al. (1995) Reduction of oxidative DNA-damage in humans by Brussels sprouts. *Carcinogenesis* **16**, 969–70.
107. Vitisen, K., Poulsen, L.S., and Cytochrome, H.E. (1991) P4501A2 activity in man measured by caffeine metabolism: Effect of smoking, broccoli and exercise. *Advanced Exp Med Biol* **283**, 407–11.
108. Chung, F.L., Jiao, D., Getahun, S.M. et al. (1998) A urinary biomarker for uptake of dietary isothiocyanates in humans. *Cancer Epidemiol Biomarkers Prev* **7**, 103–8.

109. Rabot, S., Nugon-Baudon, L., Raibaud, P. et al. (1993) Rape-seed meal toxicity in gnotobiotic rats: Influence of a whole human faecal flora or single human strains of Escherichia coli and Bacteroides vulgatus. *Br J Nutr* **70**, 323–31.

110. Rosa, E.A.S., Heaney, R.K., Fenwick, G.R., and Portal, C.A.M. (1997) Glucosinolates in crop plants. *Horticul Rev* **19**, 99–215.

111. McDannell, R., Hanley, A.B. et al. (1987) Differential induction of mixed-function oxidase (MFO) activity in rat liver and intestine by diets containing processed cabbage: Correlation with cabbage levels of glucosinolates and glucosinolate hydrolysis products. *Food Chem Toxicol* **25**, 363–8.

112. Shapiro, T.A., Fahey, J.W., Wade, K.L. et al. (1998) Human metabolism and excretion of cancer chemoprotective glucosinolates and isothiocyanates of cruciferous vegetables. *Cancer Epidemiol Biomarkers Prev* **7**, 1091–100.

113. Vermeulen, M., van den Berg, R., Freidig, A.P. et al. (2006) Association between consumption of cruciferous vegetables and condiments and excretion in urine of isothiocyanate mercapturic acids. *J Agric Food Chem* **54**, 5350–8.

114. Chung, F.L., Morse, M.A., Eklind, K.I. et al. (1992) Quantitation of human uptake of the anticarcinogen phenethyl isothiocyanate after a watercress meal. *Cancer Epidemiol Biomarkers Prev* **1**, 383–8.

115. Jaio, D., Ho, C.T., Foiles, P., and Chung, F.L. (1994) Identification and quantification of N-acetylcysteine conjugate of allyl isothiocyanate in human urine after ingestion of mustard. *Cancer Epidemiol Biomarkers Prev* **3**, 487–92.

116. Ji, Y., and Morris, M.E. (2003) Determination of phenethyl isothiocyanate in human plasma and urine by ammonia derivatization and liquid chromatography-tandem mass spectrometry. *Anal Biochem* **323**, 39–47.

117. Liebes, L., Conaway, C.C., Hochster, H. et al. (2001) High-performance liquid chromatography-based determination of total isothiocyanate levels in human plasma: Application to studies with 2-phenethyl isothiocyanate. *Anal Biochem* **291**, 279–89.

118. Kristensen, M., Krogholm, K.S., Frederiksen, H. et al. (2007) Urinary excretion of total isothiocyanates from cruciferous vegetables shows high dose-response relationship and may be a useful biomarker for isothiocyanate exposure. *Eur J Nutr* **46**, 377–82.

119. Fowke, J.H., Fahey, J.W., Stephenson, K.K. et al. (2001) Using isothiocyanate excretion as a biological marker of Brassica vegetable consumption in epidemiological studies: Evaluating the sources of variability. *Public Health Nutr* **4**, 837–46.

120. AICR/WCRF, *Food, Nutrition, Physical Activity, and the Prevention of Cancer: A Global Perspective* 2007.

121. Tang, L., Zirpoli, G.R., Guru, K. et al. (2008) Consumption of raw cruciferous vegetables is inversely associated with bladder cancer risk. *Cancer Epidemiol Biomarkers Prev* **17**, 938–44.

122. Adebamowo, C.A., Cho, E., Sampson, L. et al. (2005) Dietary flavonols and flavonol-rich foods intake and the risk of breast cancer. *Int J Cancer* **114**, 628–33.

123. Frazier, A.L., Ryan, C.T., Rockett, H., Willett, W.C., and Colditz, G.A. (2003) Adolescent diet and risk of breast cancer. *Breast Cancer Res* **5**, R59–R64.

124. Ambrosone, C.B., McCann, S.E., Freudenheim, J.L. et al. (2004) Breast cancer risk in premenopausal women is inversely associated with consumption of broccoli, a source of isothiocyanates, but is not modified by GST genotype. *J Nutr* **134**, 1134–8.

125. Seow, A., Yuan, J.M., Sun, C.L. et al. (2002) Dietary isothiocyanates, glutathione S-transferase polymorphisms and colorectal cancer risk in the Singapore Chinese Health Study. *Carcinogenesis* **23**, 2055–61.

126. Moy, K.A., Yuan, J.M., Chung, F.L. et al. (2008) Urinary total isothiocyanates and colorectal cancer: A prospective study of men in Shanghai, China. *Cancer Epidemiol Biomarkers Prev* **17**, 1354–9.

127. Hara, M., Hanaoka, T., Kobayashi, M. et al. (2003) Cruciferous vegetables, mushrooms, and gastrointestinal cancer risks in a multicenter, hospital-based case–control study in Japan. *Nutr Cancer* **46**, 138–47.

128. Hu, J., Mery, L., Desmeules, M. et al. (2007) Diet and vitamin or mineral supplementation and risk of rectal cancer in Canada. *Acta Oncol* **46**, 342–54.

129. Feskanich, D., Ziegler, R.G., Michaud, D.S. et al. (2000) Prospective study of fruit and vegetable consumption and risk of lung cancer among men and women. *J Natl Cancer Inst* **92**, 1812–23.

130. Smith-Warner, S.A., Spiegelman, D., Yaun, S.S. et al. (2003) Fruits, vegetables and lung cancer: A pooled analysis of cohort studies. *Int J Cancer* **107**, 1001–11.

131. Voorrips, L.E., Goldbohm, R.A., Verhoeven, D.T. et al. (2000) Vegetable and fruit consumption and lung cancer risk in the Netherlands Cohort Study on diet and cancer. *Cancer Causes Control* **11**, 101–15.

132. Neuhouser, M.L., Patterson, R.E., Thornquist, M.D. et al. (2003) Fruits and vegetables are associated with lower lung cancer risk only in the placebo arm of the beta-carotene and retinol efficacy trial (CARET). *Cancer Epidemiol Biomarkers Prev* **12**, 350–8.

133. Miller, A.B., Altenburg, H.P., Bueno-De-Mesquita, B. et al. (2004) Fruits and vegetables and lung cancer: Findings from the European Prospective Investigation into cancer and nutrition. *Int J Cancer* **108**, 269–70.

134. Hosgood, H.D., 3rd, Baris, D., Zahm, S.H. et al. (2007) Diet and risk of multiple myeloma in Connecticut women. *Cancer Causes Control* **18**, 1065–76.

135. Kelemen, L.E., Cerhan, J.R., Lim, U. et al. (2006) Vegetables, fruit, and antioxidant-related nutrients and risk of non-Hodgkin lymphoma: A National Cancer Institute-Surveillance, epidemiology, and end results population-based case–control study. *Am J Clin Nutr* **83**, 1401–10.

136. Rajkumar, T., Sridhar, H., Balaram, P. et al. (2003) Oral cancer in Southern India: The influence of body size, diet, infections and sexual practices. *Eur J Cancer Prev* **12**, 135–43.

137. Fairfield, K.M., Hankinson, S.E., Rosner, B.A. et al. (2001) Risk of ovarian carcinoma and consumption of vitamins A, C, and E and specific carotenoids: A prospective analysis. *Cancer* **92**, 2318–26.

138. Pan, S.Y., Ugnat, A.M., Mao, Y. et al. (2004) A case–control study of diet and the risk of ovarian cancer. *Cancer Epidemiol Biomarkers Prev* **13**, 1521–7.

139. Chan, J.M., Wang, F., and Holly, E.A. (2005) Vegetable and fruit intake and pancreatic cancer in a population-based case–control study in the San Francisco bay area. *Cancer Epidemiol Biomarkers Prev* **14**, 2093–7.

140. Larsson, S.C., Hakansson, N., Naslund, I. et al. (2006) Fruit and vegetable consumption in relation to pancreatic cancer risk: A prospective study. *Cancer Epidemiol Biomarkers Prev* **15**, 301–5.

141. Nothlings, U., Wilkens, L.R., Murphy, S.P. et al. (2007) Vegetable intake and pancreatic cancer risk: The multiethnic cohort study. *Am J Epidemiol* **165**, 138–47.

142. Kolonel, L.N., Hankin, J.H., Whittemore, A.S. et al. (2000) Vegetables, fruits, legumes and prostate cancer: A multiethnic case–control study. *Cancer Epidemiol Biomarkers Prev* **9**, 795–804.

143. Giovannucci, E., Rimm, E.B., Liu, Y. et al. (2003) A prospective study of cruciferous vegetables and prostate cancer. *Cancer Epidemiol Biomarkers Prev* **12**, 1403–9.

144. Kirsh, V.A., Peters, U., Mayne, S.T. et al. (2007) Prospective study of fruit and vegetable intake and risk of prostate cancer. *J Natl Cancer Inst* **99**, 1200–9.

145. Key, T.J., Allen, N., Appleby, P. et al. (2004) Fruits and vegetables and prostate cancer: No association among 1,104 cases in a prospective study of 130,544 men in the European Prospective Investigation into Cancer and Nutrition (EPIC). *Int J Cancer* **109**, 119–24.

146. Hsu, C.C., Chow, W.H., Boffetta, P. et al. (2007) Dietary risk factors for kidney cancer in Eastern and Central Europe. *Am J Epidemiol* **166**, 62–70.

147. Hu, J., Mao, Y., and White, K. (2003) Diet and vitamin or mineral supplements and risk of renal cell carcinoma in Canada. *Cancer Causes Control* **14**, 705–14.

148. Bosetti, C., Negri, E., Kolonel, L. et al. (2002) A pooled analysis of case–control studies of thyroid cancer. VII. Cruciferous and other vegetables (International). *Cancer Causes Control* **13**, 765–75.

149. Memon, A., Varghese, A., and Suresh, A. (2002) Benign thyroid disease and dietary factors in thyroid cancer: A case–control study in Kuwait. *Br J Cancer* **86**, 1745–50.

150. Lee, S.A., Fowke, J.H., Lu, W. et al. (2008) Cruciferous vegetables, the GSTP1 Ile105Val genetic polymorphism, and breast cancer risk. *Am J Clin Nutr* **87**, 753–60.

151. Steck, S.E., Gammon, M.D., Hebert, J.R. et al. (2007) GSTM1, GSTT1, GSTP1, and GSTA1 polymorphisms and urinary isothiocyanate metabolites following broccoli consumption in humans. *J Nutr* **137**, 904–9.

152. Nagle, C.M., Purdie, D.M., Webb, P.M. et al. (2003) Dietary influences on survival after ovarian cancer. *Int J Cancer* **106**, 264–9.

153. Thomson, C.A., Rock, C.L., Thompson, P.A., Caan, B.I., Cussler, E., Flatt, S.W., Pierce, J.P. Vegetable intake associated with reduced breast cancer recurrence in tamoxifen users. *Canc Prev Res* (under review)

154. Fowke, J.H., Morrow, J.D., Motley, S. et al. (2006) Brassica vegetable consumption reduces urinary F2-isoprostane levels independent of micronutrient intake. *Carcinogenesis* **27**, 2096–102.

155. DeMarini, D.M., Hastings, S.B., Brooks, L.R. et al. (1997) Pilot study of free and conjugated urinary mutagenicity during consumption of pan-fried meats: Possible modulation by cruciferous vegetables, glutathione S-transferase-M1, and N-acetyltransferase-2. *Mutat Res* **381**, 83–96.

156. Talaska, G., Al-Zoughool, M., Malaveille, C. et al. (2006) Randomized controlled trial: Effects of diet on DNA damage in heavy smokers. *Mutagenesis* **21**, 179–83.

157. Greenlee, H., Atkinson, C., Stanczyk, F.Z. et al. (2007) A pilot and feasibility study on the effects of naturopathic botanical and dietary interventions on sex steroid hormone metabolism in premenopausal women. *Cancer Epidemiol Biomarkers Prev* **16**, 1601–9.

158. Kensler, T.W., Chen, J.G., Egner, P.A. et al. (2005) Effects of glucosinolate-rich broccoli sprouts on urinary levels of aflatoxin-DNA adducts and phenanthrene tetraols in a randomized clinical trial in He Zuo township, Qidong, People's Republic of China. *Cancer Epidemiol Biomarkers Prev* **14**, 2605–13.

159. Reed, G.A., Peterson, K.S., Smith, H.J. et al. (2005) A phase I study of indole-3-carbinol in women: Tolerability and effects. *Cancer Epidemiol Biomarkers Prev* **14**, 1953–60.

160. Bradlow, H.L., Michnovicz, J.J., Halper, M. et al. (1994) Long-term responses of women to indole-3-carbinol or a high fiber diet. *Cancer Epidemiol Biomarkers Prev* **3**, 591–5.

161. Wong, G.Y., Bradlow, L., Sepkovic, D. et al. (1997) Dose-ranging study of indole-3-carbinol for breast cancer prevention. *J Cell Biochem Suppl* **28–29**, 111–6.

162. Dalessandri, K.M., Firestone, G.L., Fitch, M.D. et al. (2004) Pilot study: Effect of 3,3′-diindolylmethane supplements on urinary hormone metabolites in postmenopausal women with a history of early-stage breast cancer. *Nutr Cancer* **50**, 161–7.

24 Garlic and Cancer Prevention

John A. Milner

Key Points

1. Research during the past decade has provided a wealth of evidence that links garlic intake and its associated sulfur compounds as an important deterrent to cancer.
2. Both water- and lipid-sulfur allyl sulfur compounds appear to account for much of garlic's anticarcinogenic and antitumorigenic properties.
3. Some of the strongest evidence comes from preclinical models where garlic and its constituents have been found to retard chemically induced cancer at multiple sites as well as to inhibit proliferation and induce apoptosis of established human and murine cell lines.
4. The molecular site of action of the active allyl sulfur compounds accounting for the reduction in cancer risk and/or a change in tumor behavior remains an area of active investigation but clearly multiple cellular processes are likely being modified simultaneously.
5. Evidence exists that the response is related to garlic's ability to influence carcinogen bioactivation, DNA repair, cell division, apoptosis, angiogenesis, and immunocompetence.

Key Words: Garlic; allyl sulfur; antioxidant; carcinogenesis; proliferation; apoptosis; angiogenesis

1. INTRODUCTION

Garlic (*Allium sativum*) is cherished worldwide as for its savory characteristics and for its possible medicinal benefits. Historically, it has surfaced in many parts of the world as an intriguing functional food with the potential to reduce the risk of an array of diseases, admittedly with varying degrees of support *(1–6)*. Regardless, similarities in belief emphasize that folk wisdom should not always be ignored since it can provide important clues about dietary habits that can maintain or improve health.

Evidence continues to point to garlic and associated sulfur constituents to modify several physiological processes that may influence heart disease and cancer risk *(7–10)*. Overall, this information serves as a solid foundation for considering garlic and its constituents as a dietary factor with pleiotropic characteristics; however, the magnitude of the response appears to vary from individual to individual. The potential usefulness of garlic, yet variability in response in the scientific literature, continues to fascinate, intrigue, and confuse scientists, legislators, and consumers worldwide.

From: *Nutrition and Health: Bioactive Compounds and Cancer*
Edited by: J.A. Milner, D.F. Romagnolo, DOI 10.1007/978-1-60761-627-6_24,
© Springer Science+Business Media, LLC 2010

2. GARLIC: A COMPLEX FOOD

Garlic is not simply a spice, herb, or vegetable, but a combination thereof. It along with onions, shallots, leeks, and chives constitutes the major *Allium* foods that are consumed by humans. The garlic bulb consists of several individual pieces, also known as bulblets or cloves, each weighting about 3 g. The unique flavor and odor characteristics of garlic come from its sulfur constituents. Since about 1% of its dry weight is sulfur it is certainly unique in its composition *(11–13)*. While it does not generally serve as a major source of essential nutrients, garlic can contribute to a variety of different dietary factors that may influence health including selenium, arginine, and fructo-oligosaccharides *(14)*. Fructo-oligosaccharides and its content of arginine-rich protein may be particularly important as modifiers of gastrointestinal flora and/or gastrointestinal function including immunocompetence *(15–17)* and may account for some of garlic's health benefits. Admittedly, the influence of arginine can be positive or negative depending on multiple circumstances *(17)*. Likewise, the presence of selenium and flavonoids may influence the magnitude of the response to garlic *(6)*.

The principal sulfur-containing constituents in garlic bulbs are γ-glutamyl-*S*-alk(en)yl-L-cysteines and *S*-alk(en)yl-L-cysteine sulfoxides. The range of *S*-alk(en)ylcysteine sulfoxide content in garlic varies between 0.53 and 1.3%, with alliin (*S*-allylcysteine sulfoxide) the largest contributor *(18)*. Alliin concentrations can increase during storage as a result of γ-glutamylcysteine transformation. In addition to alliin, garlic bulbs contain small amounts of (+)-*S*-metyl-L-cysteine sulfoxide (methiin) and (+)-*S*-(*trans*-1-propenyl)-L-cysteine sulfoxide, *S*-(2-carboxypropyl)glutathione, γ-glutamyl-*S*-allyl-L-cysteine, γ-glutamyl-*S*-(trans-1-propenyl)-L-cysteine, and γ-glutamyl-*S*-allyl-mercapto-L-cysteine *(11, 12)*.

The method used to process garlic can also influence the sulfur compounds that predominate *(19, 14, 13)*. Table 1 provides a list of some of the allyl sulfur compounds in commercially available garlic preparations. Allicin is the major thiosulfinate compound (allyl 2-propenethiosulfinate or diallyl thiosulfinate) occurring in garlic and several of

Table 1
Sulfur Compounds in Garlic with Potential Health Benefit Properties

E-Ajoene
Z-Ajoene
Allicin
Allixin
Allyl mercaptan
Allyl methyl sulfide
Diallyl disulfide
Diallyl sulfide
Diallyl trisulfide
S-Allyl cysteine
S-Allylmercaptocysteine

its extracts *(20)*. The characteristic odor of garlic arises from allicin (thio-2-propene-1-sulfinic acid *S*-allyl ester) and oil-soluble sulfur compounds formed when the bulb is crushed or damaged. Crushing or chopping garlic releases allinase, an enzyme in the outer membrane, which converts alliin to form the odiferous alkyl alkane-thiosulfinates, including allicin. Allicin is unstable and further decomposes to sulfides, ajoene, and dithiins *(21, 22)*. Tamaki and Sonoki *(22)* reported that strong garlic flavor and scent were linked to a higher content of volatile sulfur. Heating garlic is associated with a denaturing of allinase and a reduction in allyl mercaptan, methyl mercaptan, and allyl methyl sulfide and a reduction in smell *(22)*.

Processing, including steam-distillation, of garlic can produce garlic oil which also has several different allyl sulfur constituents *(20)*. Garlic oils can contain about 26% diallyl disulfide (DADS), 19% in the trisulfide form (DATS), 15% as the allyl methyl trisulfide, 13% allyl methyl disulfide, 8% diallyl tetrasulfide, 6% allyl methyl tetrasulfide, 3% dimethyl trisulfide, 4% penta sulfide, and 1% hexa sulfide. The oil-macerated garlic oil contains the vinyl-dithiins and ajoenes. Storage of garlic in ethanol for several months produces aged garlic extract (AGE). This process substantially reduces the amount of allicin and increases the occurrence of *S*-allyl cysteine (SAC), *S*-allylmercaptocysteine, and allixin *(14)*.

The pharmacodynamics of allyl sulfur compounds remains largely unexplored. Nevertheless, allicin likely does not occur to any significant extent once garlic is processed and consumed. If it does exist, it would be rapidly transformed in liver to diallyl disulfide (DADS) and allyl mercaptan as suggested by studies of Egen-Schwind et al. *(23)*. Teyssier et al. *(24)* concluded diallyl disulfide might be reconverted to diallyl thiosulfinate (allicin) in tissues by oxidation via cytochrome P450 monooxygenases and to a limited extent by flavin-containing monooxygenases. Liver monooxygenases are also probably responsible for the oxidization of *S*-allyl cysteine (SAC), among many other sulfur compounds *(25)*. The importance of this conversion of allyl sulfur compounds in humans remains unknown. Since DADS is recognized to cause an autocatalytic destruction of this cytochrome P450 IIE1, it is unclear to what extent allicin would be formed by this process under conditions of physiological relevant exposures. Recently, Germain et al. *(26)* provided evidence that DADS is absorbed and transformed into allyl mercaptan, allyl methyl sulfide, allyl methyl sulfoxide (AMSO), and allyl methyl sulfone (AMSO$_2$). Allyl methyl sulfone predominated in tissues. Both the sulfoxide and sulfone have been found in urine.

3. GARLIC EXPOSURES – RANGE AND SAFETY

The intake of garlic has been reported to vary from region to region and from individual to individual. Unfortunately, absolute intakes are not known with any degree of certainty because of the lack of compositional analysis of foods and the dearth of information collected as part of eating behavior surveys. The USDA reports that on any typical day, about 18% of Americans consume at least one food containing garlic. There is some evidence that average intakes in the United States are approximately 0.6 g/week or less *(27)*, while intakes in some areas of China reach 20 g/day *(28)*. In a recent usage patterns evaluation published by Block et al. *(29)*, about 50% of the long-term multiple dietary supplement users, both men and women, were daily taking 1 g supplemental garlic. As might be expected, garlic supplements were being taken to reduce the risk of various diseases. Unfortunately, the amounts needed to produce a desired effect appear to vary widely and thus many inconsistencies exist in the literature.

It is unclear if a response to garlic increases proportionally with intakes and at what point that a threshold is reached. Hsing et al. *(30)* provided evidence that 10 g/day was more protective against prostate cancer risk than 2.2 g/day or less, suggesting that the threshold response may be rather large. While the intake may depend on several factors, it is not clear that intakes above 3 g/day are typically required to influence a physiological process and therefore a disease outcome; admitted considered debate surrounds this topic *(6)*.

Exaggerated intakes, such as those occurring in many parts of China, appear to occur basically without ill consequences. However, not all individuals consuming large amount are without some complication. Case reports have highlighted the possibility that garlic use may cause allergic reactions (allergic contact dermatitis, generalized urticaria, angiedema, pemphigus, anaphylaxis, and photoallergy) and burns (when fresh garlic is applied on the skin, particularly under occlusive dressings) *(31, 32)*. The incidence of the spectrum of adverse allergic reactions is very low *(33)*. In a recent study involving 132 children, garlic was linked with only 1 case (3%) *(34)*. Excessive garlic may also cause bleeding abnormalities depending on the quantity consumed and blood clotting homeostasis. Alterations in platelet function and the process of coagulation may account for the bleeding problems *(32)*. While this may not be a significant problem in most circumstances *(35)*, it may be more of an issue postoperatively *(36)*. Animal studies provide additional evidence that some of the allyl sulfides can foster hemolysis by enhanced free radical generation *(37)*. Although there appear to be few, if any reports of hemolysis in humans following consumption of *Allium* vegetables, the potent hemolytic activity of the trisulfides and tetrasulfides in rodents indicates that caution should be given if garlic is to be given in large quantities.

Tyrosinase-related protein-1 (TRPA1) is an excitatory ion channel targeted by pungent irritants including mustard and garlic. It has been proposed to function in diverse sensory processes, including thermal (cold) nociception, hearing, and inflammatory pain. Using TRPA1-deficient mice, Bautisa et al. *(7)* concluded that this enzyme was a primary target for garlic. DADS and allicin are able to excite an allyl isothiocyanate-sensitive subpopulation of sensory neurons and induce vasodilation by activating capsaicin-sensitive perivascular sensory nerve endings (Bautisa et al. 2008). It remains to be established whether this mechanism contributes to the systemic hypotensive activity that has been reported for some consuming garlic. It is also unclear if ill consequences might arise because of interactions with hypotensive drugs and garlic.

Garlic may enhance the pharmacological effect of anticoagulants (e.g., warfarin, fluindione) and reduce the efficacy of anti-AIDS drugs (i.e., saquinavir) *(38, 32)*. Case reports suggest the combination of garlic and warfarin leads to episodes of bleeding. However, in vitro and in vivo evidence is less compelling. In a recent study by Mohammed Abdul et al. *(39)*, garlic supplied as Garliplex 2000 enteric-coated garlic tablets and containing the equivalent to 3.71 mg of allicin per tablet, and given one tablet twice daily, had no effect on warfarin pharmacokinetics or pharmacodynamics and no effect on platelet aggregation induced by ADP, arachidonic acid, collagen, or ristocetin. These results are consistent with a randomized, placebo-controlled study by Macan et al. *(40)* using an aged garlic extract preparation. It should be noted that the significance of the proposed adverse effects of garlic on saquinavir efficacy also has been challenged *(41)*. Again the quantity and type of garlic used as well as the genetics of the individuals may determine the magnitude of any interaction.

4. IMPLICATIONS IN CANCER PREVENTION

The literature contains numerous studies that showcase the ability of garlic and several associated allyl sulfur compounds to alter cellular processes that are associated with cancer prevention and therapy (Fig. 1). While long-term intervention studies are lacking, a variety of preclinical and epidemiological investigations support that key molecular targets involved with cancer risk and tumor behavior are modified by garlic or its active constituents.

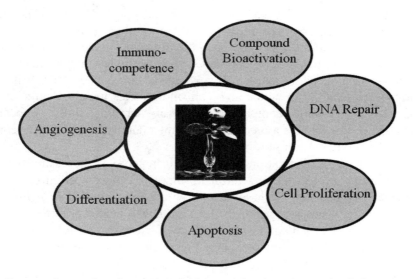

Fig. 1. Garlic, sometimes referred to as the stinking rose, has been reported to influence a number of cellular processes associated with cancer prevention and therapy. It is likely that more than one of these cellular events are being influenced simultaneously. The amount of garlic or allyl surfur component required to bring about a change in these processes remains an active area of investigation.

Scientists and consumers are becoming increasingly aware that several foods, including garlic, may be involved in reducing cancer risk *(42–48, 6)*. Although major limitations exist in defining the precise role that garlic has in the cancer process, the likelihood of its significance is underscored by a relatively large number of epidemiological and preclinical studies *(49–52)*.

Undeniably, preclinical studies employing a variety of models provide some of the most compelling evidence that garlic and its related sulfur components are able to suppress cancer risk and tumor behavior. Below is a brief account of some of the current beliefs about possible mechanisms by which this protection occurs.

4.1. Antimicrobial Response

Garlic is one of several plants with bioactive components which can serve as antimicrobial agents. Garlic has been historically recognized for its antimicrobial activity against several spoilage and pathogenic bacteria (53, 54). A range of Gram-negative and Gram-positive bacteria can be inhibited by garlic extracts (55, 56). Addition of garlic to butter enhanced the rates of inactivation of three pathogens (*Salmonella*, *Escherichia coli o157 H7*, and *Listeria monocytogenes*) when incubated at 21 and 37°C (56). Friedman et al. (57) have recently reported the antimicrobial benefits of wine marinades containing garlic and thus a reduction in foodborne illnesses.

The antimicrobial properties associated with garlic arise from several of its allyl sulfur components. In addition to allicin, compounds including diallyl sulfide (DAS), DADS, *E*-ajoene, *Z*-ajoene, *E*-4,5,9-trithiadeca-1,6-diene-9-oxide (*E*-10-devinylajoene, *E*-10-DA), and *E*-4,5,9-trithiadeca-1,7-diene-9-oxide (iso-*E*-10-devinylajoene, iso-*E*-10-DA) have been suggested to contribute to these antimicrobial properties. Although differences in efficacy among these compounds exist, relatively small amounts appear to be effective microbial growth deterrents (54, 58). Nevertheless, not all microorganisms are equally sensitive to garlic extracts or allyl sulfur compounds (56). It is unclear if rates of uptake or metabolism within an organism may determine to degree of the overall response to the allyl sulfur compounds. However, membrane fluidity appears to be a site of action and thus may be a predictor about the quantity of allyl sulfur compounds needed to bring about a response (58).

Helicobacter pylori colonization of the gastric mucosa is increasingly recognized as a factor leading to gastritis, and ultimately gastric cancer. Cellini et al. (59) provided evidence that aqueous garlic extracts (2–5 mg/ml) inhibited *H. pylori* proliferation. Reduced effectiveness occurred when the garlic was heated prior to extraction (59) suggesting that allicin or a breakdown product was likely responsible for the response. Since both DAS and DADS are recognized to elicit a dose-dependent depression in *H. pylori* proliferation in cultured (60), a reduction in their formation may have accounted for this heat-induced loss of effectiveness. Canizares et al. (61) examined water, acetone, ethanol, and hexane extracts of garlic to inhibit *Helicobacter*. While all were protective, acetone and ethanol were the most effective. The efficacy of various garlic preparations to inhibit *H. pylori* in humans was predicted since the minimum inhibitory concentration occurred between 10 and 17.5 mg/ml raw garlic extracts and with three commercially available garlic tablets (62). The recent report by the World Cancer Research Fund identified garlic as a potentially important modifier of gastric cancers, possibly by altering the proliferation of *Helicobacter*. While it is clear that *Helicobacter* is a risk factor it is only one since gastric cancer is rather low in infected individuals. Overall, it is becoming increasing apparent that significant interactions exist between diet, microflora, and gastrointestinal genomics (63).

Unfortunately, few clinical studies have been undertaken with garlic or specific allyl sulfides to examine its antimicrobial benefits. Until this is accomplished the physiological important will remain an area of considerable debate and controversy. The strongest evidence about benefits comes from the ability of several garlic preparations to serve as antifungal agents in humans and can reduce otitis *(64, 65)*.

The antimicrobial response to allyl sulfurs may reflect fluctuations in thiols in various enzymes and/or a change in the cell's overall redox state. A change in thiol homeostasis has been proposed as one mechanism by which garlic and related sulfur compounds may suppress tumor proliferation *(6, 66)*. Both alliin and allicin have antioxidant properties in a Fenton oxygen-radical generating system [H_2O_2–Fe(II)] *(67)*. DADS, but not diallyl sulfide, dipropyl sulfide or dipropyl disulfide, also has been found to inhibit liver microsomal lipid peroxidation induced by NADPH, ascorbate, and doxorubicin *(68)*. Water-soluble SAC has also been shown to possess antioxidant activity *(69, 70)*. Thus multiple compounds arising from processed garlic may contribute to its antimicrobial properties. While a change in redox status is a logical explanation, the data to prove this mechanism of action are inadequate.

4.2. Multiple Cancer Risk Processes Are Influenced

Animal models provide rather compelling evidence that garlic and its associated sulfur components can reduce the incidence of breast, colon, skin, uterine, esophagus, and lung cancers *(6, 47, 71)*. The ability to inhibit tumors arising from different inducing agents and in different tissues suggests the mechanism of action may be a general cellular response rather that tissue-specific change. Collectively, the protection appears to relate to fluctuations in several processes associated with cancer including suppressed carcinogen formation and bioactivation, enhanced DNA repair, depressed tumor cell proliferation, increased apoptosis and possible retarded angiogenesis. It is likely that several of these cellular changes are occurring simultaneously. The quantity of allyl sulfur needed and temporality relationships remain an area of active investigation.

Carcinogen Formation and Bioactivation. Suppressed nitrosamine formation continues to surface as a likely mechanism by which garlic may reduce cancer risk. Allyl sulfur compounds are recognized for their ability to retard the spontaneous and bacterial mediated formation of nitrosamines *(72)*. Since most nitrosamines are carcinogens in a variety of biological systems this particular response likely has physiological importance. Chung et al. *(73)* noted that a garlic extract was more effective in blocking in vitro chemical nitrozation than was strawberry or kale extracts. Dion et al. *(74)* demonstrated that all allyl sulfur compounds were not equal in retarding nitrosamine formation. The ability of *S*-allyl cysteine (SAC) and its nonallyl analog *S*-propyl cysteine to retard NOC formation, but not diallyl disulfide (DADS), dipropyl disulfide, and diallyl sulfide reveal the critical role that the cysteine residue has in the inhibition. The reduction in the formation of nitrosamines may actually arise secondarily to increase formation of nitrosothiols. Williams *(75)* proposed about 25 years ago that several sulfur compounds may reduce nitrite availability for nitrosamine formation by enhancing the formation of nitrosothiols. Since it is known that the allyl sulfur content can vary among garlic preparations, it is reasonable to assume that all commercial preparation will not be equivalent in their ability to retard nitrosamine formation.

Some of the most compelling evidence that garlic depresses nitrosamine formation in humans comes from studies conducted by Mei et al. *(76).* Their studies demonstrated that providing 5 g garlic/day completely blocked the enhanced urinary excretion of nitrosoproline resulting from exaggerated nitrate and proline intakes. Since nitrosoproline is predictive of the capacity to form all nitrosamines these findings may be particularly important *(77).* Evidence that garlic inhibits the formation of multiple nitrosamines comes from data of Lin et al. *(78)* and *(74).*

Garlic's anticancer attributes are also associated with its ability to suppress nitrosamine bioactivation. Evidence from multiple sources points to the effectiveness of garlic to block DNA alkylation, an initial step in nitrosamine carcinogenesis *(79–81).* Consistent with this reduction in bioactivation both water-soluble *S*-allyl sulfide and lipid-soluble diallyl disulfide retarded nitrosomorpholine mutagenicity in *Salmonella typhimurium* TA100 *(74).*

A block in nitrosamine bioactivation possibly arises from changes in phase I enzymatic activity. In particular cytochrome P450 2E1 (CYP2E1) appears to be involved with this depression *(82, 48).* An autocatalytic destruction of CYP2E1 may account for some of the chemoprotective effects of diallyl sulfide and possible other allyl sulfur compounds *(83, 48).* Diallylsulfide and allylmethylsulfide are the most significant modifiers of activity *(48).* Hernandez and Forkert *(84)* suggest that garlic may also be effective in blocking vinyl carbamate-induced mutagenicity by inhibiting CYP2E1. Variation in the content and overall activity of P450 2E1 may be an important variable in the degree of protection provided by garlic and associated allyl sulfur components. To date only one study appears to have examined gene polymorphisms in CYP2E1 as a factor in the response to garlic. According to data from Gao et al. *(85)* the *Rsa*I polymorphism of CYP2E1 did not appear to influence the response to garlic in terms of changing the impact of garlic on esophageal or stomach cancer.

Bioactivation and Response to Other Carcinogens. Garlic and several of its allyl sulfur compounds are also effective blockers of the bioactivation and carcinogenicity of a host of carcinogenic compounds (Table 2). This protection which traverses a diverse array of compounds and in cancers occurring in multiple sites suggests an overarching biological response. Since metabolic activation is required for many of these carcinogens used in these studies there is likelihood that phase I and II enzymes are involved *(48).* Cytochromes P450 1A1 and 1A2 (CYP1A1 and CYP1A2) are phase I enzymes considered to be important in establishing human cancer risk. Specifically these enzymes are responsible for the metabolic activation of heterocyclic amines and polycyclic aromatic hydrocarbons. Interestingly, little change in cytochrome P-450 1A1, 1A2, 2B1, or 3A4 activities have been observed following treatment with garlic or related sulfur compounds *(86, 87).* However, this lack of response may relate to the quantity and duration of exposure, the quantity of carcinogen administered, or the methods used to assess cytochrome content or activity. Wu et al. *(88)* using immunoblot assays found that the protein content of cytochrome P450 1A1, 2B1, and 3A1 was increased by garlic oil and each of several isolated disulfide compounds. Their data demonstrated as the number of sulfur atoms in the allyl compound was inversely related to the depression in these cytochromes. Davenport and Wargovish *(89)* reported that some but not all allyl sulfur compounds were effective in stimulating P450 1A1 and 1A2.

Table 2
Garlic and Allyl Sulfur Compounds Influence the Response to Multiple Carcinogens[a]

Compound	Site	Host
1,2-Dimethylhydrazine	Colon	Rat
2-Amino-3,8-dimethylimidazo[4,5-f] quinoxaline	Liver	Rat
3-Methylcholanthrene	Cervix	Mouse
4-(Methylnitrosamino)-1-(3-pyridyl)-1-butanone	Nasal	Rat
7,12-Dimethylbenz(a)anthracene	Mammary	Rat
7,12-Dimethylbenz(a)anthracene	Skin	Mouse
7,12-Dimethylbenz[a]anthracene	Forestomach	Hamster
7,12-Dimethylbenz[a]anthracene	Buccal pouch	Hamster
Aflatoxin B1	Liver	Toad, rat
Azoxymethane	Colon	Rat
Benzo(a)pyrene	Forestomach	Mouse
Benzo(a)pyrene	Lung	Mouse
Benzo(a)pyrene	Skin	Mouse
Benzo[a]pyrene	Bone marrow	Mouse.
Methylnitronitrosoguanidine	Gastric	Rat
N-methyl-N-nitrosourea	Mammary	Rat
N-nitrosodiethylamine	Colon	Rat
N-nitrosodiethylamine	Nasal	Rat
N-nitrosodimethylamine	Liver	Rat
N-nitrosodimethylamine	Nasal	Rat
N-nitrosodimethylamine	Skin	Mouse
N-nitrosomethylbenzylamine	Esophagus	Rat
Vinyl carbamate	Skin	Mouse

[a]The overall response to garlic and/or specific allyl sulfur components depends on the quantity provided and the amount of carcinogen administered.

CYP3A enzymes are the most abundant in mammalian liver and intestines, and since they metabolize such a large number of xenobiotics, maybe very important in carcinogenesis and determining the response to drugs. Davenport and Wargovich (89) reported that several allyl sulfur compounds were effective in stimulating CYP3A2 activity. Overall, change in phase I enzyme activity changes may account for some of the anticancer properties attributed to garlic, however, additional studies are needed to clarify their overall importance in modifying cancer risk.

Changes in bioactivation resulting from a block in cyclooxygenase and lipoxygenase may also partially account for the reduction in tumors following treatment with some carcinogens (90, 91). Ajoene has also been demonstrated to interfere with the COX-2 pathway by using lipopolysaccharide (LPS)-activated RAW 264.7 cells as in vitro mode (92). Ajoene lead to a dose-dependent inhibition of the release of LPS (1 μg/ml)-induced prostaglandin E(2) in RAW 264.7 macrophages (IC(50) value: 2.4 μM). The response was thought to be linked to an inhibition of COX-2 enzyme activity by ajoene. Ajoene did not reduce COX-2 expression, but rather increased LPS-induced COX-2 protein and mRNA expression compared to LPS-stimulated cells only. In the absence of LPS, however, ajoene was unable to induce COX-2. The nonsteroidal anti-inflammatory drug indomethacin behaved similarly. These data suggest that ajoene works by a mechanism of action similar to that attributed to nonsteroidal anti-inflammatory drugs. Youn et al. *(93)* recently reported that an ethyl acetate garlic extract directly inhibits the toll-like receptors (TLRs) by blocking dimerization of TLR4, which resulted in the inhibition of NF-kappaB activation and the expression of cyclooxygenase 2 and nitric oxide synthase.

While limited, there is some evidence that garlic and associated sulfur components can inhibit lipoxygenase activity *(94)*. Fifteen lipoxygenase activity has been implicated in the biotransformation of DMBA and probably several other carcinogens *(95)*. Camargo et al. *(96)* provided a set of models to describe why different organosulfur compounds may inhibit soy lipoxygenase based on bulkiness, hydrophobicity, and electronic features. Collectively, these intriguing studies pose interesting questions about the role of both cyclooxygenase and lipoxygenase in explaining not only forming prostaglandins, but also their involvement in the bioactivation of carcinogens. Clearly, additional attention is need to clarify what role, if any, these bioactivation enzymes have in determine the biological response to dietary garlic and its allyl sulfur components.

Enhanced removal of carcinogenic metabolites may also be key to the protection offered by garlic. Singh et al. *(97)* provided evidence that a suppression in NAD(P)H:quinone oxido-reductase activity is correlated with the ability of garlic preparations to inhibit benzo(a)pyrene tumorigenesis. Subsequent studies suggest the activation of the antioxidant responsive element and Nrf2 protein accumulation correlated with phase II gene expression induction *(98)*.

Garlic or its constituents do not appear to influence estradiol metabolism. However, a change in the biological response to diethylstilbestrol (DES), a synthetic estrogen known to increase mammary cancer in animal models, has been demonstrated *(99)*. Part of the effects of DES may stem from its ability to increase lipid hydroperoxides in mammary tissue. Recent studies demonstrate that this increase in ROS can be attenuated by providing DAS in the diet. This reduction was also related to a depression in DNA adducts *(99)*.

Changes in glutathione concentration and the activity of specific glutathione-*S*-transferase, both factors involved in phase II detoxification, may be important in the protection provided by garlic *(48)*. Garlic powder feeding increases both rat liver and mammary GST activity *(86, 100)*. Hu et al. *(101)* provided evidence that the induction of glutathione (GSH) *S*-transferase pi (mGSTP1-1) may be particularly important in the anticarcinogenic properties associated with garlic and allyl sulfur components. The allyl portion of the DADS molecular may be particularly important in GST induction since Bose et al. *(102)* demonstrated that mGSTP1 mRNA expression was either unaltered in liver or moderately increased in forestomach following treatment with dipropyl disulfide (DPDS).

4.3. Antitumorigenic Response to Garlic

Several of the lipid- and water-soluble organosulfur compounds have been examined for their antiproliferative efficacy *(103–108)*. Some of the more frequently tested lipid-soluble allyl sulfur compounds include ajoene, diallyl sulfide (DAS), diallyl disulfide (DADS), and diallyl trisulfide (DATS). A breakdown of allicin appears to be necessary for achieving maximum tumor inhibition but there is considerable confusion in the literature. A host of tumor cells, both human and murine, have been shown to be inhibited by one or more allyl sulfur compounds during the past 5 years (Table 3).

Table 3

Neoplasms that Are Reported to Be Inhibited by Garlic or Its Allyl Sulfur Components During the Past 5 Years[a]

Tumor cell line
I. Human
Bladder – T24 cells
Breast – MCF-7 and MCF-7ras, MDA-MB-231, MDA-MB-435
Intestinal – Caco-2, Colo 205, Colo 320 DM, HCT-15 HT 29, HCT-116, HT29, SW480, SW620
Esophageal – CE 81T/VGH
Gastric – MGC803, BGC823, SNU-1
Glioblastoma – T98G, U87MG
Leukemic – HL60
Liver – J5, HepG2
Lung – A549
Lymphatic leukemia – CCRF CEM
Neuroblastoma – SH-SY5Y cells
Prostate cancer – LNCaP, LNCaP-C81, LNCaP-C4-2, PC-3, and DU145
II. Murine
Leukemia – WEHI-3
Mammary – Ehrlich ascites tumor cell
Melanoma cells – B16/BL6
Myeloma cells – Sp2/O-Ag14-
Skin – NIH3T3 fibroblasts

[a]Information obtained from Medline search from 2003 to 2008.

Previous studies reported that lipid-soluble DAS, DADS, and DATS (100 μM) were more effective in suppressing canine tumor cell proliferation than isomolar water-soluble SAC, *S*-ethyl cysteine, and *S*-propyl cysteine *(109)*. However, some water-extracted preparations also appear to be effective in retarding tumor proliferation *(107, 110)*. Sundaram and Milner *(109)* reported SAC was ineffective in altering the proliferation of canine mammary or human colon cells; others have demonstrated that it inhibits the growth of melanoma, prostatic, and neuroblastoma cells *(111, 112)*. Whether these differences in efficacy are related to cell type or the amount of agent added needs to be resolved. Tissue culture studies provide evidence that allyl sulfur compounds, in particular S-allylmercaptocysteine (SAMC), enhance testosterone disappearance from the medium and presumably account for part of the antitumorigenic properties (113). Collectively, SAMC treatment causes a response similar to androgen deprivation. The importance of the diminished effects of testosterone in accounting for the ability of allyl sulfur compounds to inhibit tumors remains uncertain.

Evidence exists that these allyl sulfur compounds preferentially suppress neoplastic over nonneoplastic cells (114, 115). Adding DATS (10 µM) in vitro to cultures of A549 lung tumor cells inhibited their proliferation by 47%, whereas it did not influence nonneoplastic MRC-5 lung cells (115). Likewise, normal prostate cells do not appear to respond like neoplastic prostatic cells (116). The antiproliferative effects of allyl sulfides are generally reversible assuming that apoptosis is not extensive (104, 115).

Allyl sulfur compounds from garlic largely increase the percentage of cells blocked within the G_2/M phase (117, 104). The ability of garlic to block the G_2/M phase is not limited to in vitro studies. Kimuray and Yamamoto (118) observed an increased number of metaphase-arrested tumor cells in MTK-sarcoma III xenographs in rats receiving an aqueous extract of garlic (1–10 mg/100 g body wt) for 4 day compared to those not receiving the extract.

$p34^{cdc2}$ kinase is a complex that governs the progression of cells from the G_2 into the M phase of the cell cycle (119, 120). This complex is controlled by the association of the $p34^{cdc2}$ catalytic unit with the cyclin B_1 regulatory unit. Activation is governed both by the cyclin B_1 protein synthesis and degradation and by the phosphorylation and dephosphorylation of threonine and tyrosine residues on the $p34^{cdc2}$ subunit. DADS causes a doubling in cyclin B_1 protein expression in cultured HCT-15 cells after a 12-h exposure to DADS (104). Overall, the ability of DADS to inhibit p34(cdc2) kinase activation appears to occur as a result of a decreased p34(cdc2)/cyclin B(1) complex formation and a change in p34(cdc2) hyperphosphorylation (104). Singh and colleagues reported that DATS inhibited the proliferation of PC-3 and DU145 human prostate cancer cells by causing G(2)-M phase cell cycle arrest in association with inhibition of cyclin-dependent kinase 1 activity and hyperphosphorylation of Cdc25C at Ser(216) (121). Similar types of results were obtained using human promyelocytic leukemia cells (HL-60) and with Z-ajoene as the modifying agent (122).

One of the mechanisms by which allyl sulfur compounds may cause apoptosis is by inducing free radical generation, rather than serving as an antioxidant. These reactive oxygen species trigger signal transduction culminating in cell cycle arrest and/or apoptosis. These investigations suggest that the source of the increased radical formation is via a release of iron from ferritin (70, 123). Interestingly the ability of allyl sulfur compounds to induce radicals appears to be tumor cell specific since it is not observed in normal cells (123). Sriram et al. (124) have reported that apoptosis of Colo 320 DM human colon cancer cells caused by DAS may also relate to increased radical formation.

Recent studies using cellular and animal models indicate that garlic and its components can influence tumor angiogenesis and metastasis. Taylor et al. (125) provided evidence that injecting ajoene (5–25 µg/g body weight) inhibited pulmonary metastasis in C57BL/6 mice injected with B16/BL6 melanoma cells. Another compound, SAMC, administration (300 mg/kg) to CB-17 SCID/SCID mice orthotopically implanted with PC-3 cells caused a 90% reduction in lung metastasis without toxicity (126). However, there was no effect on local metastasis *(126)*. DAS administered to C57BL/6 mice injected with B16F-10 melanoma cells increased circulating levels of anti-angiogenic factors, tissue inhibitor of metalloproteinase, and interleukin-2 levels compared with the untreated animals *(127)*. DATS has also been reported to reduce the migration of human umbilical vein endothelial cell in vitro and that this was accompanied by suppression of vascular endothelial growth factor (VEGF) secretion, down-regulation of VEGF-receptor 2 expression, inactivation of Akt, and activation of ERK $\frac{1}{2}$ *(128)*. Water-soluble allyl sulfur compounds also appear effective in retarding angiogenesis since Matsuura et al. *(110)* reported aged garlic extract (AGE) reduced the invasiveness of the endothelial cells by about 20–30% as assessed by the Matrigel chemoinvasion assay. Thejass and Kuttan *(127)* suggest that the response to DADS and DAS might occur as a result of a reduction in matrix metalloproteinases 2 and 9. While these findings are intriguing, it remains less clear if the response will occur through dietary treatment or if this is a pharmacological response.

5. GENETIC AND EPIGENETIC EVENTS INFLUENCE GARLIC RESPONSE

Genetic polymorphisms appear to influence to response to at least some foods and their components. Unfortunately a dearth of information exists about the role of specific genetic polymorphisms in determining the response to garlic. However, given findings about the importance of gene polymorphisms in determining drug metabolism and tumor proliferation an association with garlic is likely. A search of the current literature only revealed one publication that focused on the *Rsa*I polymorphism of CYP2E1 and the risk of esophageal and stomach cancers, which was not influenced by garlic intake *(85)*.

Cancer progression is also dependent on epigenetic changes *(129)*. Two extensively examined mechanisms for epigenetic gene regulation are (i) patterns of DNA methylation and (ii) histone acetylations/deacetylations. Lea et al. *(130)* reported that at least part of the ability of DADS to induce differentiation in DS19 mouse erythroleukemic cells might relate to its ability to increased histone acetylation. The depression in acetylation likely arises from a depression in histone deacetylase (HDAC) activity, possibly by the transformation of DADS to *S*-allylmercaptocysteine and related intermediates which would then provide a spacer ending with a carboxylic acid functional group as a necessary inhibitor of this enzyme *(131)*. Diallyl disulfide caused a marked increase in the acetylation of H4 and H3 histones in DS19 and K562 human leukemic cells. Similar results were also obtained with rat hepatoma and human breast cancer cells. In 2001, Lea and Randolph provided evidence DADS administered to rats could also increase histone acetylation in liver and a transplanted hepatoma cell line. The evidence suggested an increase in the acetylation of core mucosomal histones and enhanced differentiation. More recently, Druesne-Pecollo et al. *(132)* provided evidence that intracaecal perfusion or gavage with DADS increased histone H4 and H3 acetylation in rat colonocytes. Moreover, they provided evidence this may have resulted in the modulation of the expression of a subset of genes. These findings need to be confirmed through controlled intervention studies with appropriate dietary intakes of garlic or its intermediates to truly assess their physiological importance.

The anticarcinogenic and antitumorigenic response to garlic likely is manifested by changes in gene expression patterns. DADS treatment has been reported to down-regulated the expression of aggrecan 1, tenascin R, vitronectin, and cadherin 5, whereas it up-regulated 40S ribosomal protein stubarista protein (SA), platelet-derived growth factor-associated protein, and glia-derived neurite-promoting factor levels *(133)*. Changes in matrix expression of protein may reflect the ability of garlic and related sulfur compounds to suppress adhesion. Franz et al. *(134)* reported that the increase in HT-29 cell detachment by aqueous garlic extracts is related to an increase in epidermal growth factor receptor and integrin-α6 mRNA expression. Additional studies are needed to characterize in greater detail which changes in patterns of gene expression are critical to explaining the likely multiple targets involved with the anticancer and antitumorigenic properties attributed to garlic and its related sulfur constituents. Zhou et al. *(135)* found that adding DATS to HepG2 cells up-regulated peroxisome proliferator-activated receptor alpha (PPAR-alpha) and hepatocyte nuclear factor 4alpha (HNF-4alpha) and down-regulated CYP7A1.

6. DIETARY MODIFIERS

The influence of garlic on the cancer process cannot be considered in isolation since many dietary components may influence the response. Among the factors recognized to influence the response to garlic are total fat, selenium, methionine, and vitamin A *(136)*. Amagase et al. *(136)* and Ip et al. *(137)* reported that selenium supplied either as a component of the diet or as a constituent of the garlic supplement, respectively, enhanced the protection against 7,12 dimethylbenz(a)anthracene (DMBA) mammary carcinogenesis over that provided by garlic alone.

Combination prevention approaches using multiple diet-derived agents may offer advantages. Part of the benefits of a combined approach may arise from the lower quantity that is needed to provide a positive response as suggested by Davis and Hord *(138)*. There is suggestive evidence that several foods can influence the response to garlic. Velmurugan and Nagini *(139)* examined the combined effects of SAC and lycopene, a major carotenoid present in tomatoes, against N-methyl-N'-nitro-N-nitrosoguanidine (MNNG) and saturated sodium chloride (*S*-NaCl)-induced gastric carcinogenesis in Wistar rats. Although SAC and lycopene alone significantly suppressed the development of gastric cancer, administration of SAC and lycopene in combination was more effective in inhibiting MNNG-induced stomach tumors and modulating the redox status in the tumor and host tissues. In similar types of studies using azoxymethane induced aberrant crypt foci in the colon, Sengupta et al. *(140)* found benefits of combining garlic and tomatoes. They proposed that part of the synergistic benefits arose from a reduction in cyclooxygenase 2 activity.

Dietary fatty acid supply can also influence the bioactivation of DMBA to metabolites capable of binding to rat mammary cell DNA. Chen et al. *(141)* provided evidence that garlic oil and fish oil modulated the antioxidant and drug-metabolizing capacity of rats and that the combined effects of both on drug-metabolizing enzymes were additive.

Interestingly, co-administration of garlic with fish oil was found to be well tolerated in humans and had a beneficial effect on serum lipid and lipoprotein concentrations by providing a combined lowering of total cholesterol, LDL-C, and triglyceride concentrations, as well as the ratios of total cholesterol to HDL-C and LDL-C to HDL-C *(142)*.

Tsuchiya and Nagayama *(58)* recently proposed a novel action of garlic, namely that it interacts with membrane lipids to modify the membrane fluidity. Allyl derivatives were found to influence the rigidity of tumor cell and platelet model membranes consisting of unsaturated phospholipids and cholesterol at 20–500 nM with the potency being diallyl trisulfide (DATS) > diallyl disulfide (DADS) by preferentially acting on the hydrocarbon cores of lipid bilayers.

7. CONCLUSIONS

Garlic may well have significance in promoting personal health. Since it has relatively few side effects there are few disadvantages associated with its expanded use, except for its lingering odor. However, odor does not appear to be an absolute prerequisite for its anticancer benefits since preclinical studies with chemical carcinogenesis models indicate water-soluble *S*-allyl cysteine provides comparable benefits to those compounds that are linked to odor. It is probable that garlic and its associated sulfur compounds influence several key molecular targets involved with cancer prevention. Interestingly, these compounds appear to have both antioxidant and oxidative potential depending on the quantity provided. While most can savor the culinary experiences identified with garlic, some individual because of their gene profile and/or environmental exposures may be particularly responsive to more exaggerated intakes. While a wealth of evidence points to the anticancer benefits of garlic, there is a crying need for controlled intervention studies to truly assess its physiological importance for specific individuals.

REFERENCES

1. Benavides, G.A., Squadrito, G.L., Mills, R.W., Patel, H.D., Isbell, T.S., Patel, R.P., Darley-Usmar, V.M., Doeller, J.E., and Kraus, D.W. (2007) Hydrogen sulfide mediates the vasoactivity of garlic. *Proc Natl Acad Sci USA* **104**(46), 17977–82.
2. Borek, C. (2006) Garlic reduces dementia and heart-disease risk. *J Nutr* **136**(3 Suppl), 810S–812S.
3. Gardner, C.D., Lawson, L.D., Block, E., Chatterjee, L.M., Kiazand, A., Balise, R.R., and Kraemer, H.C. (2007) Effect of raw garlic vs commercial garlic supplements on plasma lipid concentrations in adults with moderate hypercholesterolemia: A randomized clinical trial. *Arch Intern Med* **167**(4), 346–53.
4. Gorinstein, S., Jastrzebski, Z., Namiesnik, J., Leontowicz, H., Leontowicz, M., and Trakhtenberg, S. (2007) The atherosclerotic heart disease and protecting properties of garlic: Contemporary data. *Mol Nutr Food Res* **51**(11), 1365–81.
5. Liu, C.T., Sheen, L.Y., and Lii, C.K. (2007) Does garlic have a role as an antidiabetic agent? *Mol Nutr Food Res* **51**(11), 1353–64.
6. Milner, J.A. (2006) Preclinical perspectives on garlic and cancer. *J Nutr* **136**(3 Suppl), 827S–31S.
7. Bautista, D.M., Jordt, S.E., Nikai, T., Tsuruda, P.R., Read, A.J., Poblete, J., Yamoah, E.N., Basbaum, A.I., and Julius, D. (2006) TRPA1 mediates the inflammatory actions of environmental irritants and proalgesic agents. *Cell* **124**(6), 1269–82.
8. Durak, I., Aytaç, B., Atmaca, Y., Devrim, E., Avci, A., Erol, C., and Oral, D. (2004) Effects of garlic extract consumption on plasma and erythrocyte antioxidant parameters in atherosclerotic patients. *Life Sci* **75**(16), 1959–66.

9. Ross, S.A., Finley, J.W., and Milner, J.A. (2006) Allyl sulfur compounds from garlic modulate aberrant crypt formation. *J Nutr* **136**(3 Suppl), 852S–4S.

10. Yang, J.S., Kok, L.F., Lin, Y.H., Kuo, T.C., Yang, J.L., Lin, C.C., Chen, G.W., Huang, W.W., Ho, H.C., and Chung, J.G. (2006) Diallyl disulfide inhibits WEHI-3 leukemia cells in vivo. *Anticancer Res* **26**(1A), 219–25.

11. Fenwick, G.R., and Hanley, A.B. (1985a) The genus Allium – Part 2. *Crit Rev Food Sci Nutr* **22**(4), 273–7.

12. Fenwick, G.R., and Hanley, A.B. (1985b) The genus Allium – Part 3. *Crit Rev Food Sci Nutr* **23**(1), 1–73.

13. Arnault, I., Christides, J.P., Mandon, N., Haffner, T., Kahane, R., and Auger, J. (2003) High-performance ion-pair chromatography method for simultaneous analysis of alliin, deoxyalliin, allicin and dipeptide precursors in garlic products using multiple mass spectrometry and UV detection. *J Chromatogr A* **991**(1), 69–75.

14. Amagase, H. (2006) Clarifying the real bioactive constituents of garlic. *J Nutr* **136**(3 Suppl), 716S–725S.

15. Bornet, F.R., and Brouns, F. (2002) Immune-stimulating and gut health-promoting properties of short-chain fructo-oligosaccharides. *Nutr Rev* **60**(10 Pt 1), 326–34.

16. Foster, M.W., McMahon, T.J., and Stamler, J.S. (2003) S-nitrosylation in health and disease. *Trends Mol Med* **9**(4), 160–8.

17. Peranzoni, E., Marigo, I., Dolcetti, L., Ugel, S., Sonda, N., Taschin, E., Mantelli, B., Bronte, V., and Zanovello, P. (2007) Role of arginine metabolism in immunity and immunopathology. *Immunobiology* **212**(9–10), 795–812.

18. Kubec, R., Svobodova, M., and Velisek, J. (1999) A Gas chromatographic determination of S-alk(en)ylcysteine sulfoxides. *J Chromatogr* **862**(1), 85–94.

19. Li, L., Hu, D., Jiang, Y., Chen, F., Hu, X., and Zhao, G. (2008) Relationship between gamma-glutamyl transpeptidase activity and garlic greening, as controlled by temperature. *J Agric Food Chem* **56**(3), 941–5.

20. Lawson, L.D., and Gardner, C.D. (2005) Composition, stability, and bioavailability of garlic products used in a clinical trial. *J Agric Food Chem* **53**(16), 6254–61.

21. Lawson, L.D. (1994) Bioactive organosulfur compounds of garlic and garlic products. In: Kinghorn A.D., Balandrin, M.F. eds. Human Medicinal Agents from Plants. 306–30, Washington, DC: *American Chemical Society.*

22. Tamaki, T., and Sonoki, S. (1999) Volatile sulfur compounds in human expiration after eating raw or heat-treated garlic. *J Nutr Sci Vitaminol (Tokyo)* **45**(2), 213–22.

23. Egen-Schwind, C., Eckard, R., and Kemper, F.H. (1992) Metabolism of garlic constituents in the isolated perfused rat liver. *Planta Med* **58**(4), 301–5.

24. Teyssier, C., Guenot, L., Suschetet, M., and Siess, M.H. (1999) Metabolism of diallyl disulfide by human liver microsomal cytochromes P-450 and flavin-containing monooxygenases. *Drug Metab Dispos* **27**(7), 835–41.

25. Ripp, S.L., Overby, L.H., Philpot, R.M., and Elfarra, A.A. (1997) Oxidation of cysteine S-conjugates by rabbit liver microsomes and cDNA-expressed flavin-containing mono-oxygenases: Studies with S-(1,2-dichlorovinyl)-L-cysteine, S-(1,2,2 trichlorovinyl)-L-cysteine, S-allyl-L-cysteine, and S-benzyl-L-cysteine. *Mol Pharmacol* **51**(3), 507–15.

26. Germain, E., Auger, J., Ginies, C., Siess, M.H., and Teyssier, C. (2002) In vivo metabolism of diallyl disulphide in the rat: Identification of two new metabolites. *Xenobiotica* **32**(12), 1127–38.

27. Steinmetz, K.A., Kushi, L.H., Bostick, R.M., Folsom, A.R., and Potter, J.D. (1994) Vegetables, fruit, and colon cancer in the Iowa Women's Health Study. *Amer J Epid* **139**, 1–15.

28. Mei, X., Wang, M.L., and Pan, X.Y. (1982) Garlic and gastric cancer 1. The influence of garlic on the level of nitrate and nitrite in gastric juice. *Acta Nuti Sin* **4**, 53–56.

29. Block, G., Jensen, C.D., Norkus, E.P., Dalvi, T.B., Wong, L.G., McManus, J.F., and Hudes, M.L. (2007) Usage patterns, health, and nutritional status of long-term multiple dietary supplement users: A cross-sectional study. *Nutr J* **6**, 30.

30. Hsing, A.W., Chokkalingam, A.P., Gao, Y.T., Madigan, M.P., Deng, J., Gridley, G., and Fraumeni, J.F., Jr. (2002) Allium vegetables and risk of prostate cancer: A population-based study. *J Natl Cancer Inst* **94**(21), 1648–51.

31. Ekeowa-Anderson, A.L., Shergill, B., and Goldsmith, P. (2007) Allergic contact cheilitis to garlic. *Contact Dermatitis* **56**(3), 174–5.

32. Borrelli, F., Capasso, R., and Izzo, A.A. (2007) Garlic (Allium sativum L.): Adverse effects and drug interactions in humans. *Mol Nutr Food Res* **51**(11), 1386–97.

33. Jappe, U., Bonnekoh, B., Hausen, B.M., and Gollnick, H. (1999) Garlic-related dermatoses: Case report and review of the literature. *Am J Contact Dermat* **10**(1), 37–39.

34. Nowak-Wegrzyn, A., Conover-Walker, M.K., and Wood, R.A. (2001) Food-allergic reactions in schools and preschools. *Arch Pediatr Adolesc Med* **155**(7), 790–5.

35. Scharbert, G., Kalb, M.L., Duris, M., Marschalek, C., and Kozek-Langenecker, S.A. (2007) Garlic at dietary doses does not impair platelet function. *Anesth Analg* **105**(5), 1214–8.

36. Burnham, B.E. (1995) Garlic as a possible risk for postoperative bleeding. *Plast Reconstr Surg* **95**(1), 213.

37. Munday, R., Munday, C.M., and Munday, J.S. (2005) Hemolytic anemia and induction of phase II detoxification enzymes by diprop-1-enyl sulfide in rats: Dose-response study. *J Agric Food Chem* **53**(25), 9695–700.

38. Piscitelli, S.C., Burstein, A.H., Welden, N., Gallicano, K.D., and Falloon, J. (2002) The effect of garlic supplements on the pharmacokinetics of saquinavir. *Clin Infect Dis* **34**, 234–8.

39. Mohammed Abdul, M.I., Jiang, X., Williams, K.M., Day, R.O., Roufogalis, B.D., Liauw, W.S., Xu, H., and McLachlan, A.J. (2008) Pharmacodynamic interaction of warfarin with cranberry but not with garlic in healthy subjects. *Br J Pharmacol* **154**(8), 1691–700.

40. Macan, H., Uykimpang, R., Alconcel, M., Takasu, J., Razon, R., Amagase, H., and Niihara, Y. (2006) Aged garlic extract may be safe for patients on warfarin therapy. *J Nutr* **136**(3 Suppl), 793S–5S.

41. Borek, C. (2002) Garlic supplements and saquinavir. *Clin Infect Dis* **35**(3), 343.

42. Nagini, S. (2008) Cancer chemoprevention by garlic and its organosulfur compounds-panacea or promise? *Anticancer Agents Med Chem* **8**(3), 313–21.

43. Devrim, E., and Durak, I. (2007) Is garlic a promising food for benign prostatic hyperplasia and prostate cancer? *Mol Nutr Food Res* **51**(11), 1319–23.

44. Ngo, S.N., Williams, D.B., Cobiac, L., and Head, R.J. (2007) Does garlic reduce risk of colorectal cancer? A systematic review. *J Nutr* **137**(10), 2264–9.

45. Shukla, Y., and Kalra, N. (2007) Cancer chemoprevention with garlic and its constituents. *Cancer Lett* **247**(2), 167–81.

46. El-Bayoumy, K., Sinha, R., Pinto, J.T., and Rivlin, R.S. (2006) Cancer chemoprevention by garlic and garlic-containing sulfur and selenium compounds. *J Nutr* **136**(3 Suppl), 864S–9S.

47. Pinto, J.T., Krasnikov, B.F., and Cooper, A.J. (2006) Redox-sensitive proteins are potential targets of garlic-derived mercaptocysteine derivatives. *J Nutr* **136**(3 Suppl), 835S–41S.

48. Wargovich, M.J. (2006) Diallylsulfide and allylmethylsulfide are uniquely effective among organosulfur compounds in inhibiting CYP2E1 protein in animal models. *J Nutr* **136**(3 Suppl), 832S–4S.

49. Fleischauer, A.T., and Arab, L. (2001) Garlic and cancer: A critical review of the epidemiologic literature. *J Nutr* **131**(3s), 1032S–40S.

50. González, C.A., Pera, G., Agudo, A., Bueno-de-Mesquita, H.B., Ceroti, M., Boeing, H., Schulz, M., Del Giudice, G., Plebani, M., Carneiro, F., Berrino, F., Sacerdote, C., Tumino, R., Panico, S., Berglund, G., Simán, H., Hallmans, G., Stenling, R., Martinez, C., Dorronsoro, M., Barricarte, A., Navarro, C., Quiros, J.R., Allen, N., Key, T.J., Bingham, S., Day, N.E., Linseisen, J., Nagel, G., Overvad, K., Jensen, M.K., Olsen, A., Tjønneland, A., Büchner, F.L., Peeters, P.H., Numans, M.E., Clavel-Chapelon, F., Boutron-Ruault, M.C., Roukos, D., Trichopoulou, A., Psaltopoulou, T., Lund, E., Casagrande, C., Slimani, N., Jenab, M., and Riboli, E. (2006) Fruit and vegetable intake and the risk of stomach and oesophagus adenocarcinoma in the European Prospective Investigation into Cancer and Nutrition (EPIC-EURGAST). *Int J Cancer* **118**(10), 2559–66.

51. Schulz, M., Lahmann, P.H., Boeing, H., Hoffmann, K., Allen, N., Key, T.J., Bingham, S., Wirfält, E., Berglund, G., Lundin, E., Hallmans, G., Lukanova, A., Martínez Garcia, C., González, C.A., Tormo,

M.J., Quirós, J.R., Ardanaz, E., Larrañaga, N., Lund, E., Gram, I.T., Skeie, G., Peeters, P.H., van Gils, C.H., Bueno-de-Mesquita, H.B., Büchner, F.L., Pasanisi, P., Galasso, R., Palli, D., Tumino, R., Vineis, P., Trichopoulou, A., Kalapothaki, V., Trichopoulos, D., Chang-Claude, J., Linseisen, J., Boutron-Ruault, M.C., Touillaud, M., Clavel-Chapelon, F., Olsen, A., Tjønneland, A., Overvad, K., Tetsche, M., Jenab, M., Norat, T., Kaaks, R., and Riboli, E. (2005) Fruit and vegetable consumption and risk of epithelial ovarian cancer: The European Prospective Investigation into Cancer and Nutrition. *Cancer Epidemiol Biomarkers Prev* **14**(11 Pt 1), 2531–5.

52. World Cancer Research Fund and American Institute for Cancer Research (2007) Food, Nutrition, Physical Activity and the Prevention of Cancer: A Global Perspective http://www.dietandcancerreport.org .

53. Harris, J.C., Cottrell, S.L., Plummer, S., and Lloyd, D. (2001) Antimicrobial properties of Allium sativum (garlic). *Appl Microbiol Biotechnol* **57**(3), 282–6.

54. Konaklieva, M.I., and Plotkin, B.J. (2006) Antimicrobial properties of organosulfur anti-infectives: A review of patent literature 1999–2005. *Recent Patents Anti-Infect Drug Disc* **1**(2), 177–80.

55. Arora, D.S., and Kaur, J. (1999) Antimicrobial activity of spices. *Int J Antimicrob Agents* **12**(3), 257–62.

56. Adler, B.B., and Beuchat, L.R. (2002) Death of Salmonella, Escherichia coli O157:H7, and Listeria monocytogenes in garlic butter as affected by storage temperature. *J Food Prot* **65**(12), 1976–80.

57. Friedman, M., Henika, P.R., Levin, C.E., and Mandrell, R.E. (2007) Recipes for antimicrobial wine marinades against Bacillus cereus, Escherichia coli O157:H7, Listeria monocytogenes, and Salmonella enterica. *J Food Sci* **72**(6), M207–M13.

58. Tsuchiya, H., and Nagayama, M. (2008) Garlic allyl derivatives interact with membrane lipids to modify the membrane fluidity. *J Biomed Sci* **15**(5), 653–60.

59. Cellini, L., Di Campli, E., Masulli, M., Di Bartolomeo, S., and Allocati, N. (1996) Inhibition of Helicobacter pylori by garlic extract (Allium sativum). *FEMS Immunol Med Microbiol* **13**(4), 273–7.

60. Chung, J.G., Chen, G.W., Wu, L.T., Chang, H.L., Lin, J.G., Yeh, C.C., and Wang, T.F. (1998) Effects of garlic compounds diallyl sulfide and diallyl disulfide on arylamine N-acetyltransferase activity in strains of Helicobacter pylori from peptic ulcer patients. *Am J Chin Med* **26**(3–4), 353–64.

61. Canizares, P., Gracia, I., Gomez, L.A., Martin de Argila, C., de Rafael, L., and Garcia, A. (2002) Optimization of Allium sativum solvent extraction for the inhibition of in vitro growth of Helicobacter pylori. *Biotechnol Prog* **18**(6), 1227–32.

62. Jonkers, D., van den Broek, E., van Dooren, I., Thijs, C., Dorant, E., Hageman, G., and Stobberingh, E. (1999) Antibacterial effect of garlic and omeprazole on Helicobacter pylori. *J Antimicrob Chemother* **43**(6), 837–9.

63. Vaughan, E.E., de Vries, M.C., Zoetendal, E.G., Ben-Amor, K., Akkermans, A.D., and de Vos, W.M. (2002) The intestinal LABs. *Antonie Van Leeuwenhoek* **82**(1–4), 341–52.

64. Pai, S.T., and Platt, M.W. (1995) Antifungal effects of Allium sativum (garlic) extract against the Aspergillus species involved in otomycosis. *Lett Appl Microbiol* **20**(1), 14–18.

65. Davis, S.R. (2005) An overview of the antifungal properties of allicin and its breakdown products-the possibility of a safe and effective antifungal prophylactic. *Mycoses* **48**(2), 95–100.

66. Jakubíková, J., and Sedlák, J. (2006) Garlic-derived organosulfides induce cytotoxicity, apoptosis, cell cycle arrest and oxidative stress in human colon carcinoma cell lines. *Neoplasma* **53**(3), 191–9.

67. Banerjee, S.K., Mukherjee, P.K., and Maulik, S.K. (2003) Garlic as an antioxidant: The good, the bad and the ugly. *Phytother Res* **17**(2), 97–106.

68. Dwivedi, C., John, L.M., Schmidt, D.S., and Engineer, F.N. (1998) Effects of oil-soluble organosulfur compounds from garlic on doxorubicin-induced lipid peroxidation. *Anticancer Drugs* **9**, 291–94.

69. Ide, N., and Lau, B.H. (1999) S-allylcysteine attenuates oxidative stress in endothelial cells. *Drug Dev Ind Pharm* **25**(5), 619–24.

70. Dillon, S.A., Burmi, R.S., Lowe, G.M., Billington, D., and Rahman, K. (2003) Antioxidant properties of aged garlic extract: An in vitro study incorporating human low density lipoprotein. *Life Sci* **72**(14), 1583–94.

71. Antosiewicz, J., Ziolkowski, W., Kar, S., Powolny, A.A., and Singh, S.V. (2008, Jul 31) Role of reactive oxygen intermediates in cellular responses to dietary cancer chemopreventive agents. *Planta Med* **74**(13), 1570–9.

72. Milner, J.A. (2001) Mechanisms by which garlic and allyl sulfur compounds suppress carcinogen bioactivation. Garlic and carcinogenesis. *Adv Exp Med Biol* **492**, 69–81.

73. Chung, M.J., Lee, S.H., and Sung, N.J. (2002) Inhibitory effect of whole strawberries, garlic juice or kale juice on endogenous formation of N-nitrosodimethylamine in humans. *Cancer Lett* **182**(1), 1–10.

74. Dion, M.E., Agler, M., and Milner, J.A. (1997) S-allyl cysteine inhibits nitrosomorpholine formation and bioactivation. *Nutr Cancer* **28**(1), 1–6.

75. Williams, D.H. (1983) S-Nitrosation and the reactions of S-Nitroso compounds. *Chem Soc Rev* **15**, 171–96.

76. Mei, X., Lin, X., Liu, J., Lin, X.Y., Song, P.J., Hu, J.F., and Liang, X.J. (1989) The blocking effect of garlic on the formation of N-nitrosoproline in humans. *Acta Nutrimenta Sinica* **11**, 141–5.

77. Ohshima, H., and Bartsch, H. (1999) Quantitative estimation of endogenous N-nitrosation in humans by monitoring N-nitrosoproline in urine. *Methods Enzymol* **301**, 40–49.

78. Lin, X.-Y., Liu, J.Z., and Milner, J.A. (1994) Dietary garlic suppresses DNA adducts caused by N-nitroso compounds. *Carcinogenesis* **15**(2), 349–52.

79. Sundaresan, S., and Subramanian, P. (2008) Prevention of N-nitrosodiethylamine-induced hepatocarcinogenesis by S-allylcysteine. *Mol Cell Biochem* **310**(1–2), 209–14.

80. Singh, V., Belloir, C., Siess, M.H., and Le Bon, A.M. (2006) Inhibition of carcinogen-induced DNA damage in rat liver and colon by garlic powders with varying alliin content. *Nutr Cancer* **55**(2), 178–84.

81. Zhou, L., and Mirvish, S.S. (2005) Inhibition by allyl sulfides and crushed garlic of O6-methylguanine formation in liver DNA of dimethylnitrosamine-treated rats. *Nutr Cancer* **51**(1), 68–77.

82. Yang, C.S., Chhabra, S.K., Hong, J.Y., and Smith, T.J. (2001) Mechanisms of inhibition of chemical toxicity and carcinogenesis by diallyl sulfide (DAS) and related compounds from garlic. *J Nutr* **131**(3s), 1041S–5S.

83. Jin, L., and Baillie, T.A. (1997) Metabolism of the chemoprotective agent diallyl sulfide to glutathione conjugates in rats. *Chem Res Toxicol* **10**(3), 318–27.

84. Hernandez, L.G., and Forkert, P.G. (2007) Inhibition of vinyl carbamate-induced mutagenicity and clastogenicity by the garlic constituent diallyl sulfone in F1 (Big Blue x A/J) transgenic mice. *Carcinogenesis* **28**(8), 1824–30.

85. Gao, C., Takezaki, T., Wu, J., Li, Z., Wang, J., Ding, J., Liu, Y., Hu, X., Xu, T., Tajima, K., and Sugimura, H. (2002) Interaction between cytochrome P-450 2E1 polymorphisms and environmental factors with risk of esophageal and stomach cancers in Chinese. *Cancer Epidemiol Biomarkers Prev* **11**(1), 29–34.

86. Manson, M.M., Ball, H.W., Barrett, M.C., Clark, H.L., Judah, D.J., Williamson, G., and Neal, G.E. (1997) Mechanism of action of dietary chemoprotective agents in rat liver: Induction of phase I and II drug metabolizing enzymes and aflatoxin B1 metabolism. *Carcinogenesis* **18**(9), 1729–38.

87. Wang, B.H., Zuzel, K.A., Rahman, K., and Billington, D. (1999) Treatment with aged garlic extract protects against bromobenzene toxicity to precision cut rat liver slices. *Toxicology* **132**(2–3), 215–25.

88. Wu, C.C., Sheen, L.Y., Chen, H.W., Kuo, W.W., Tsai, S.J., and Lii, C.K. (2002) Differential effects of garlic oil and its three major organosulfur components on the hepatic detoxification system in rats. *J Agric Food Chem* **50**(2), 378–83.

89. Davenport, D.M., and Wargovich, M.J. (2005) Modulation of cytochrome P450 enzymes by organosulfur compounds from garlic. *Food Chem Toxicol* **43**(12), 1753–62.

90. Ali, M. (1995) Mechanism by which garlic (Allium sativum) inhibits cyclooxygenase activity. Effect of raw versus boiled garlic extract on the synthesis of prostanoids. *Prostaglandins Leukot Essent Fatty Acids* **53**(6), 397–400.

91. Rioux, N., and Castonguay, A. (1998) Inhibitors of lipoxygenase: A new class of cancer chemopreventive agents. *Carcinogenesis* **19**(8), 1393–400.

92. Dirsch, V.M., and Vollmar, A.M. (2001) Ajoene, a natural product with non-steroidal anti-inflammatory drug (NSAID)-like properties? *Biochem Pharmacol* **61**(5), 587–93.

93. Youn, H.S., Lim, H.J., Lee, H.J., Hwang, D., Yang, M., Jeon, R., and Ryu, J.H. (2008) Garlic (Allium sativum) extract inhibits lipopolysaccharide-induced Toll-like receptor 4 dimerization. *Biosci Biotechnol Biochem* **72**(2), 368–75.

94. Belman, S., Solomon, J., Segal, A., Block, E., and Barany, G. (1989) Inhibition of soybean lipoxygenase and mouse skin tumor promotion by onion and garlic components. *J Biochem Toxicol* **4**(3), 151–60.

95. Sun, Z., Sood, S., Li, N., Ramji, D., Yang, P., Newman, R.A., Yang, C.S., and Chen, X. (2005) Overexpression of 5-lipoxygenase and cyclooxygenase 2 in hamster and human oral cancer and chemopreventive effects of zileuton and celecoxib. *Clin Cancer Res* **11**(5), 2089–96.

96. Camargo, A.B., Marchevsky, E., and Luco, J.M. (2007) QSAR study for the soybean 15-lipoxygenase inhibitory activity of organosulfur compounds derived from the essential oil of garlic. *J Agric Food Chem* **55**(8), 3096–103.

97. Singh, S.V., Pan, S.S., Srivastava, S.K., Xia, H., Hu, X., Zaren, H.A., and Orchard, J.L. (1998) Differential induction of NAD(P)H: Quinone oxidoreductase by anti-carcinogenic organosulfides from garlic. *Biochem Biophys Res Commun* **244**(3), 917–20.

98. Chen, C., Pung, D., Leong, V., Hebbar, V., Shen, G., Nair, S., Li, W., and Kong, A.N. (2004) Induction of detoxifying enzymes by garlic organosulfur compounds through transcription factor Nrf2: Effect of chemical structure and stress signals. *Free Radic Biol Med* **37**(10), 1578–90.

99. Green, M., Thomas, R., Gued, L., and Sadrud-Din, S. (2003) Inhibition of DES-induced DNA adducts by diallyl sulfide: Implications in liver cancer prevention. *Oncol Rep* **10**(3), 767–71.

100. Singh, A., and Singh, S.P. (1997) Modulatory potential of smokeless tobacco on the garlic, mace or black mustard-altered hepatic detoxication system enzymes, sulfhydryl content and lipid peroxidation in murine system. *Cancer Lett* **118**(1), 109–14.

101. Hu, X., Benson, P.J., Srivastava, S.K., Xia, H., Bleicher, R.J., Zaren, H.A., Awasthi, S., Awasthi, Y.C., and Singh, S.V. (1997) Induction of glutathione S-transferase pi as a bioassay for the evaluation of potency of inhibitors of benzo(a)pyrene-induced cancer in a murine model. *Int J Cancer* **73**(6), 897–902.

102. Bose, C., Guo, J., Zimniak, L., Srivastava, S.K., Singh, S.P., Zimniak, P., and Singh, S.V. (2002) Critical role of allyl groups and disulfide chain in induction of Pi class glutathione transferase in mouse tissues in vivo by diallyl disulfide, a naturally occurring chemopreventive agent in garlic. *Carcinogenesis* **23**(10), 1661–5.

103. Sundaram, S.G., and Milner, J.A. (1996) Diallyl disulfide inhibits the proliferation of human tumor cells in culture. *Biochim Biophys Acta* **1315**, 15–20.

104. Knowles, L.M., and Milner, J.A. (2000) Diallyl disulfide inhibits p34(cdc2) kinase activity through changes in complex formation and phosphorylation. *Carcinogenesis* **21**(6), 1129–34.

105. Miron, T., Wilchek, M., Sharp, A., Nakagawa, Y., Naoi, M., Nozawa, Y., and Akao, Y. (2008) Allicin inhibits cell growth and induces apoptosis through the mitochondrial pathway in HL60 and U937 cells. *J Nutr Biochem* **19**(8), 524–35.

106. Arunkumar, A., Vijayababu, M.R., Gunadharini, N., Krishnamoorthy, G., and Arunakaran, J. (2007) Induction of apoptosis and histone hyperacetylation by diallyl disulfide in prostate cancer cell line PC-3. *Cancer Lett* **251**(1), 59–67.

107. De Martino, A., Filomeni, G., Aquilano, K., Ciriolo, M.R., and Rotilio, G. (2006) Effects of water garlic extracts on cell cycle and viability of HepG2 hepatoma cells. *J Nutr Biochem* **17**(11), 742–9.

108. Matsuura, N., Miyamae, Y., Yamane, K., Nagao, Y., Hamada, Y., Kawaguchi, N., Katsuki, T., Hirata, K., Sumi, S., and Ishikawa, H. (2006) Aged garlic extract inhibits angiogenesis and proliferation of colorectal carcinoma cells. *J Nutr* **136**(3 Suppl), 842S–6S.

109. Sundaram, S.G., and Milner, J.A. (1993) Impact of organosulfur compounds in garlic on canine mammary tumor cells in culture. *Cancer Lett* **74**(1–2), 85–90.

110. Matsuura, N., Miyamae, Y., Yamane, K., Nagao, Y., Hamada, Y., Kawaguchi, N., Katsuki, T., Hirata, K., Sumi, S., and Ishikawa, H. (2006) Aged garlic extract inhibits angiogenesis and proliferation of colorectal carcinoma cells. *J Nutr* **136**(3 Suppl), 842S–6S.

111. Pinto, J.T., Qiao, C., Xing, J., Rivlin, R.S., Protomastro, M.L., Weissler, M.L., Tao, Y., Thaler, H., and Heston, W.D. (1997) Effects of garlic thioallyl derivatives on growth, glutathione concentration, and polyamine formation of human prostate carcinoma cells in culture. *Am J Clin Nutr* **66**, 398–405.

112. Welch, C., Wuarin, L., and Sidell, N. (1992) Antiproliferative effect of the garlic compound S-allyl cysteine on human neuroblastoma cells in vitro. *Cancer Lett* **63**(3), 211–9.

113. Pinto, J.T., Qiao, C., Xing, J., Suffoletto, B.P., Schubert, K.B., Rivlin, R.S., Huryk, R.F., Bacich, D.J., and Heston, W.D. (2000) Alterations of prostate biomarker expression and testosterone utilization in human LNCaP prostatic carcinoma cells by garlic-derived S-allylmercaptocysteine. *Prostate* **45**(4), 304–14.

114. Scharfenberg, K., Wagner, R., and Wagner, K.G. (1990) The cytotoxic effect of ajoene, a natural product from garlic, investigated with different cell lines. *Cancer Lett* **53**, 103–8.

115. Sakamoto, K., Lawson, L.D., and Milner, J. (1997) Allyl sulfides from garlic suppress the in vitro proliferation of human A549 lung tumor cells. *Nutr Cancer* **29**(2), 152–6.

116. Kim, Y.A., Xiao, D., Xiao, H., Powolny, A.A., Lew, K.L., Reilly, M.L., Zeng, Y., Wang, Z., and Singh, S.V. (2007) Mitochondria-mediated apoptosis by diallyl trisulfide in human prostate cancer cells is associated with generation of reactive oxygen species and regulated by Bax/Bak. *Mol Cancer Ther* **6**(5), 1599–609.

117. Zheng, S., Yang, H., Zhang, S., Wang, X., Yu, L., Lu, J., and Li, J. (1997) Initial study on naturally occurring products from traditional Chinese herbs and vegetables for chemoprevention. *J Cell Biochem Suppl* **27**, 106–12.

118. Kimuray, Y., and Yamamoto, K. (1964) Cytological effect of chemicals in tumors. Influence of crude extracts from garlic and some related species on MTK-sarcoma 3. *Gann* **55**, 325–9.

119. Nurse, P. (1991) The Florey Lecture, 1990. How is the cell division cycle regulated? *Philos Trans R Soc Lond B Biol Sci* **332**(1264), 271–6.

120. Knowles, L.M., and Milner, J.A. (1998) Depressed p34cdc2 kinase activity and G2/M phase arrest induced by diallyl disulfide in HCT-15 cells. *Nutr Cancer* **30**(3), 169–74.

121. Herman-Antosiewicz, A., and Singh, S.V. (2005) Checkpoint kinase 1 regulates diallyl trisulfide-induced mitotic arrest in human prostate cancer cells. *J Biol Chem* **280**(31), 28519–28.

122. Ye, Y., Yang, H.Y., Wu, J., Li, M., Min, J.M., and Cui, J.R. (2005) Z-ajoene causes cell cycle arrest at G2/M and decrease of telomerase activity in HL-60 cells. *Zhonghua Zhong Liu Za Zhi* **27**(9), 516–20.

123. Powolny, A.A., and Singh, S.V. (2008, Jun 23) Multitargeted prevention and therapy of cancer by diallyl trisulfide and related Allium vegetable-derived organosulfur compounds. *Cancer Lett* **269**(2), 305–14.

124. Sriram, N., Kalayarasan, S., Ashokkumar, P., Sureshkumar, A., and Sudhandiran, G. (2008) Diallyl sulfide induces apoptosis in Colo 320 DM human colon cancer cells: Involvement of caspase-3, NF-kappaB, and ERK-2. *Mol Cell Biochem* **311**(1–2), 157–65.

125. Taylor, P., Noriega, R., Farah, C., Abad, M.J., Arsenak, M., and Apitz, R. (2006) Ajoene inhibits both primary tumor growth and metastasis of B16/BL6 melanoma cells in C57BL/6 mice. *Cancer Lett* **239**(2), 298–304.

126. Howard, E.W., Ling, M.T., Chua, C.W., Cheung, H.W., Wang, X., and Wong, Y.C. (2007) Garlic-derived S-allylmercaptocysteine is a novel in vivo antimetastatic agent for androgen-independent prostate cancer. *Clin Cancer Res* **13**(6), 1847–56.

127. Thejass, P., and Kuttan, G. (2007) Inhibition of angiogenic differentiation of human umbilical vein endothelial cells by diallyl disulfide (DADS). *Life Sci* **80**(6), 515–21.

128. Xiao, D., Li, M., Herman-Antosiewicz, A., Antosiewicz, J., Xiao, H., Lew, K.L., Zeng, Y., Marynowski, S.W., and Singh, S.V. (2006) Diallyl trisulfide inhibits angiogenic features of human umbilical vein endothelial cells by causing Akt inactivation and down-regulation of VEGF and VEGF-R2. *Nutr Cancer* **55**(1), 94–107.

129. Ross, S.A. (2007) Nutritional genomic approaches to cancer prevention research. *Exp Oncol* **29**(4), 250–6.

130. Lea, M.A., Randolph, V.M., and Patel, M. (1999) Increased acetylation of histones induced by diallyl disulfide and structurally related molecules. *Int J Oncol* **15**(2), 347–52.

131. Dashwood, R.H., and Ho, E. (2007) Dietary histone deacetylase inhibitors: From cells to mice to man. *Semin Cancer Biol* **17**(5), 363–9.

132. Druesne-Pecollo, N., Chaumontet, C., Pagniez, A., Vaugelade, P., Bruneau, A., Thomas, M., Cherbuy, C., Duée, P.H., and Martel, P. (2007) In vivo treatment by diallyl disulfide increases histone acetylation in rat colonocytes. *Biochem Biophys Res Commun* **354**(1), 140–7.

133. Knowles, L.M., and Milner, J.A. (2003) Diallyl disulfide induces ERK phosphorylation and alters gene expression profiles in human colon tumor cells. *J Nutr* **133**(9), 2901–6.

134. Frantz, D.J., Hughes, B.G., Nelson, D.R., Murray, B.K., and Christensen, M.J. (2000) Cell cycle arrest and differential gene expression in HT-29 cells exposed to an aqueous garlic extract. *Nutr Cancer* **38**(2), 255–64.

135. Zhou, Z., Tan, H.L., Xu, B.X., Ma, Z.C., Gao, Y., and Wang, S.Q. (2005) Microarray analysis of altered gene expression in diallyl trisulfide-treated HepG2 cells. *Pharmacol Rep* **57**(6), 818–23.

136. Amagase, H., Schaffer, E.M., and Milner, J.A. (1996) Dietary components modify garlic's ability to suppress 7,12-dimethylbenz(a)anthracene induced mammary DNA adducts. *J. Nutr* **126**(4), 817–24.

137. Ip, C., Lisk, D.J., and Stoewsand, G.S. (1992) Mammary cancer prevention by regular garlic and selenium-enriched garlic. *Nutr Cancer* **17**(3), 279–86.

138. Davis, C.D., and Hord, N.G. (2005) Nutritional "omics" technologies for elucidating the role(s) of bioactive food components in colon cancer prevention. *J Nutr* **135**(11), 2694–7.

139. Velmurugan, B., and Nagini, S. (2005) Combination chemoprevention of experimental gastric carcinogenesis by s-allylcysteine and lycopene: Modulatory effects on glutathione redox cycle antioxidants. *J Med Food* **8**(4), 494–501.

140. Sengupta, A., Ghosh, S., and Das, S. (2006) Modulatory influence of garlic and tomato on cyclooxygenase-2 activity, cell proliferation and apoptosis during azoxymethane induced colon carcinogenesis in rat. *Eur J Cancer Prev* **15**(4), 301–5.

141. Chen, H.W., Tsai, C.W., Yang, J.J., Liu, C.T., Kuo, W.W., and Lii, C.K. (2003) The combined effects of garlic oil and fish oil on the hepatic antioxidant and drug-metabolizing enzymes of rats. *Br J Nutr* **89**(2), 189–200.

142. Adler, A.J., and Holub, B.J. (1997) Effect of garlic and fish-oil supplementation on serum lipid. *Am J Clin Nutr* **65**(2), 445–50.

25 Mammary and Prostate Cancer Chemoprevention and Mechanisms of Action of Resveratrol and Genistein in Rodent Models

Timothy G. Whitsett, Leah M. Cook, Brijesh B. Patel, Curt E. Harper, Jun Wang, and Coral A. Lamartiniere

Key Points

1. Almost 200,000 men and women in the United States will be diagnosed with prostate and breast cancers, respectively, this year alone. It has become increasingly clear that environmental exposures, including diet, influence the risk of both breast and prostate cancers.
2. Two natural polyphenols that have received much interest in the field of cancer prevention are genistein, an isoflavone component of soy, and resveratrol, a phytoalexin found in red grapes and red wine. Epidemiological and in vitro laboratory data suggest that these polyphenols may protect against breast and prostate cancers.
3. Using in vivo rodent models of breast and prostate cancers, our lab and others have shown that genistein and resveratrol, administered alone or in combination, can suppress both breast and prostate carcinogenesis.
4. Genistein, at concentrations resulting in serum levels comparable to humans on a high soy diet, suppressed mammary tumor multiplicity through enhanced mammary gland maturation and a reduction in the targets of mammary carcinogens. Genistein also reduced the incidence of aggressive prostate tumors in a transgenic mouse model of prostate cancer.
5. Resveratrol, administered in the diet, suppressed mammary tumor multiplicity and increased tumor latency. Reductions in mammary epithelial cell proliferation and increased apoptosis help to explain these mammary protective effects. Resveratrol was also able to reduce the incidence of poorly differentiated prostate tumors through modulation of cell proliferation and critical growth factor pathways in the rodent prostate.
6. Chemoprevention of both breast and prostate cancers with combinational genistein and resveratrol treatments was also demonstrated. Both resveratrol and genistein, alone and in combination, were effective at suppressing breast and prostate carcinogenesis using in vivo models.

Key Words: Chemoprevention; genistein; resveratrol; breast cancer; prostate cancer

From: *Nutrition and Health: Bioactive Compounds and Cancer*
Edited by: J.A. Milner, D.F. Romagnolo, DOI 10.1007/978-1-60761-627-6_25,
© Springer Science+Business Media, LLC 2010

1. INTRODUCTION

Cancers of the breast and prostate are two of the most prevalent types of malignancies in the United States and throughout the world. It is estimated that this year in the United States, there will be more than 184,000 new cases of breast cancer and 186,000 new cases of prostate cancer (*1*). There will also be more than 41,000 and 28,000 deaths attributed to breast and prostate cancers, respectively. Interestingly, genetic factors such as BRCA mutations in breast cancer account for a small percentage (5–10%) of the overall incidence. Genetic factors that play a major role in prostate cancer have not been well defined to date. It has become increasingly clear that environmental factors, especially dietary exposures, can have a significant impact on one's risk of breast or prostate cancer.

Despite significant advances in novel therapies and screening methods, breast and prostate cancers remain widespread in the United States and throughout the world. Both breast and prostate cancers are considered diseases of the aging and cancers that can take up to decades to develop. Often times, even with a prolonged tumor latency, cancers are not detected until late stages, at a point when the tumors are aggressive, motile, and can be resistant to commonly used cancer therapeutics, which themselves are highly toxic to the body. An attractive alternative to treating an aggressive cancer is to begin the fight before tumor onset and advancement. With the slow growth of some breast and prostate tumors, delaying tumor onset or tumor progression could have significant clinical impact in terms of morbidity (quality of life) and mortality. Chemoprevention involves the administration of natural or synthetic agents designed to suppress the development or progression of cancer. Over the past 25 years, the National Cancer Institute's chemoprevention program has tested hundreds of compounds and currently has approximately 60 ongoing clinical trials testing agents for differing types of cancers. Thus, preclinical testing of agents that can prevent breast and prostate cancers can lead to human trials, which ultimately could lead to a reduction in the incidence and mortality of these deadly cancers.

As stated above, hundreds of agents, both natural and synthetic, have and are being tested for cancer chemopreventive activities. In this chapter, we will focus on two natural polyphenols that have shown promise in preventing cancer, including cancers of the breast and prostate. Genistein (a major isoflavone found in soy) and resveratrol (a phytoalexin found in red grape skins and red wine) have both attracted interest in the fields of breast and prostate cancer chemoprevention. Our aim is to discuss epidemiological data, in vitro, and in vivo chemoprevention experiments using these polyphenols, alone and in combination to suppress development of cancers of the breast and prostate.

2. GENISTEIN

Genistein (4,5,7-trihydroxyisoflavone) is a naturally occurring isoflavone found in soy (Fig. 1), which has attracted a lot of attention in the cancer chemoprevention field. It is a planar molecule with an aromatic A-ring, a second oxygen atom 11.5 Å from the one in the A-ring, and a molecular weight similar to that of steroidal estrogens. Genistein has shown promise in preventing breast and prostate cancers in both in vitro and in vivo

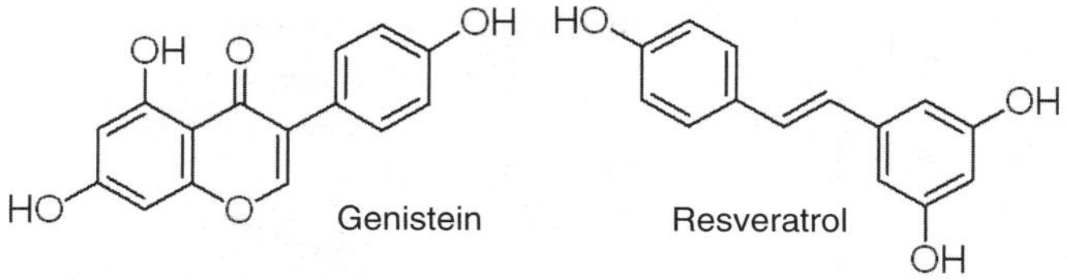

Fig. 1. Chemical structures of genistein and resveratrol.

experiments. There is also epidemiology data supporting the idea that soy consumption can inversely affect one's risk of developing breast or prostate cancers, with an emphasis placed on the timing of exposure.

2.1. Genistein and Breast Cancer: In Vitro Results

It has been demonstrated that genistein binds to the estrogen receptor-alpha (ERα) and beta (ERβ), with a higher affinity for the latter (2). The biochemical mechanisms of genistein and the inhibition of carcinogenesis in vitro have been thoroughly reviewed in the literature (3–5). Genistein is reported to be an in vitro inhibitor of protein tyrosine kinases, topoisomerases I and II, and 5-alpha reductase. The inhibition of tyrosine kinases may help to explain the inhibition of growth in many cancer cell lines, including breast and prostate. Genistein can also induce cell cycle arrest and apoptosis in cancer cell lines, including breast cancer cells, as well as inhibit the activation of transcription factors such as NF-κB and growth stimulating pathways such as the Akt and MAP kinase pathways. Drawbacks to these in vitro studies have been the use of high polyphenol concentrations (~50 μM) and conflicting data with the use of low and high concentrations of genistein. The plasma level of genistein in people on a soy-rich diet was reported to be ~276 nM (6). Differences derived from in vitro experiments created the need for in vivo experimentation with nutritionally relevant doses of soy and genistein.

2.2. Genistein and Breast Cancer: In Vivo Chemoprevention

In 1990, dietary soy was reported to protect against chemically induced mammary cancers (7, 8). In 1995, pure genistein isolated from soy and administered via subcutaneous injections to Sprague-Dawley rats was shown to suppress dimethylbenz(a)anthracene (DMBA)-induced mammary tumorigenesis (9). In later studies that used a physiologically relevant protocol, dietary supplementation with chemically synthesized genistein was also shown to be protective against DMBA-induced mammary cancer (10). In these experiments, rats were exposed to increasing concentrations of genistein in the diet from conception to 21 days postpartum. Then, the offspring were treated with 80 mg DMBA/kg body weight at 50 days postpartum to induce mammary cancer. With dietary concentrations of 0, 25, and 250 mg genistein/kg AIN-76A diet (phytoestrogen-free), there was a dose-dependent protection against mammary tumor multiplicity, as measured by the number of tumors per rat (Fig. 2). These mammary chemoprotective effects of genistein administered in the diet have since been confirmed by other labs (11, 12).

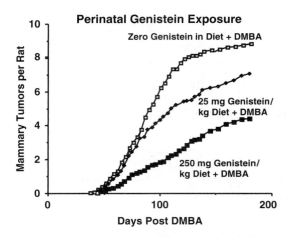

Fig. 2. Ontogeny of palpable mammary tumors in female Sprague-Dawley CD rats exposed perinatally to genistein in the diet from conception until 21 days postpartum. After weaning, the offspring were fed AIN-76A only. On day 50 postpartum, all animals were treated with 80 mg DMBA/kg body weight. Adapted from (*10*) with permission.

Serum total genistein concentrations in lactating dams fed 25 and 250 mg genistein/kg AIN-76A diet were 40 and 418 pmol/ml, respectively (*10*). In 7-day-old rats, serum genistein concentrations were 86 and 726 pmol/ml. In 21-day-old female rats, serum genistein concentrations were 54 and 1,810 pmol/ml. It is important to note that the 25 and 250 mg genistein/kg diet resulted in serum genistein concentrations similar to those found in Asian men (276 pmol/ml) eating a traditional diet high in soy (*6*).

Several other developmental periods have been tested for mammary cancer protection (Table 1). In utero only administration of 250 mg genistein/kg diet failed to protect the female offspring against chemically induced cancer, but importantly it did not enhance DMBA-induced mammary tumorigenesis in the adult offspring (*13, 14*). The effects of genistein on tumor promotion were also investigated. Female rats were gavaged with DMBA at 50 days postpartum. Starting at 7 weeks after exposure to the carcinogen (about the time to first palpable tumor), animals were fed 250 mg genistein/kg diet. There were no observed differences in tumor formation or adenocarcinoma development compared to animals that did not receive genistein. These results suggested that in this cancer model, genistein ingested after tumor development did not promote mammary cancer. These data are consistent with epidemiology data demonstrating that Asians eating a traditional diet high in soy have a reduced incidence of breast cancer.

Another experiment looked at exposure to genistein in the diet both prepubertally and in adults. Rats that received genistein at both time points were protected further than those that only received genistein before puberty (Table 1). Based on these results, we concluded that early prepubertal exposure to genistein was the critical time for the initial mammary protective effects. Furthermore, it appears that genistein exposure early in life sets the biochemical blueprint for which the ensuing adult responds to future carcinogen exposure whereby it is less susceptible for cancer.

Table 1

Dietary Genistein, Timing of Exposure, and Mammary Cancer Chemoprevention. All Exposures to Genistein Were at 250 mg/kg AIN-76A Diet. At 50 Days Postpartum, All Female Offspring Were Treated with DMBA (80 mg/kg of Body Weight) to Induce Mammary Tumorigenesis. Adapted from (*14*) with Permission from the American Society for Nutrition Sciences

Exposure period	Relative mammary tumor multiplicity
No genistein	8.9
Prenatal (in utero) genistein (throughout gestation)	8.8
Adult genistein (starting at 100 days postpartum)	8.2
Prepubertal genistein (days 1–21 postpartum)	4.3
Prepubertal + adult genistein (days 1–21 and 100+)	2.8

A few studies have reported no effect or a stimulating effect of genistein on mammary tumorigenesis (*15*). The majority of these studies looked at adult exposures or exposures after the induction of tumorigenesis to soy or genistein. However, the animals were not treated prepubertally with genistein, an important aspect of this novel approach to chemoprevention. Studies have also been carried out in ovariectomized mice that were immuno-compromised and implanted with transformed human breast cancer cells. Giving genistein to this model has resulted in a promotional effect on cancer cell growth (*16–19*). On the other hand, in another mouse model of breast cancer in which the ovaries were left intact, genistein prevented the appearance of mammary tumors (*20*) or increased the latency period before tumors appeared (*21*). These studies highlight the importance of the model system and timing of exposure to soy or genistein.

Another area of investigation with soy isoflavone exposure is protection against cancer metastasis. The spread of malignant cells to distant organs that results in secondary tumors is a devastating aspect of cancer and responsible for many deaths. Soybean isoflavones including genistein have been reported to reduce metastasis. Vantyghem et al. demonstrated that genistein administration in the diet could reduce metastatic burden to the lungs by 10-fold after implantation of the human breast cancer cells, MDA-MB-435/HAL (*22*). Soy isoflavones, including genistein, have also shown protection against the spread of other primary tumors in rodent models such as melanoma (*23*), bladder cancer (*24*), and prostate cancer (*25*).

2.3. Genistein and Breast Cancer: Mechanisms of Action

Our lab and others have clearly shown that genistein administered prepubertally in the diet can protect against chemically induced mammary cancer. We have looked at mammary gland maturation as a potential mechanism for chemoprevention. Rats treated prepubertally with genistein in the diet were killed at 50 days postpartum (time of carcinogen administration in the tumorigenesis studies) to observe changes in mammary maturation and architecture. At 50 days postpartum, there was a significant decrease in the number of terminal end buds (TEB) present in mammary gland whole mounts, consistent with a more mature mammary gland (*10*). Prepubertal injections of genistein resulted in significantly fewer terminal end buds and more mature lobule structures at 50 days postpartum (Fig. 3) (*26*). Russo et al. have previously shown that mammary TEB contain highly proliferative cells that are the most susceptible to carcinogenic insult, while the more mature lobules are less susceptible terminal ductal structures (*27*). Thus, with pharmacologic or dietary genistein treatments there are fewer structures that may be susceptible to a carcinogen such as DMBA. This is akin to an explanation by which early pregnancy may protect a woman against breast cancer later in life (*28*). The maturation associated with pregnancy and lactation results in a gland that is biologically more mature (different genomic signature and different ability to respond to insult) than that of a nulliparous woman.

Also, cell proliferation was inhibited in the mammary terminal ductal structures and there was a significant decrease in the protein expression of the epidermal growth factor receptor (EGFR), which could help to explain the decreased cell proliferation (*29*). Increased apoptosis in mammary glands of rats exposed to genistein early in life has been reported with a significant increase in the tumor suppressor protein PTEN (phosphatase and tensin homolog deleted in chromosome 10) (*30*). Cabanes et al. demonstrated that prepubertal exposure to genistein or estradiol (both via subcutaneous injection) up-regulated the mRNA expression of BRCA-1, a known tumor suppressor gene (*31*). Thus, prepubertal exposure to genistein may protect against mammary cancer by a host of mechanisms including enhanced mammary maturation, decreased cell proliferation, increased apoptosis, and increased expression of tumor suppressors such as PTEN and BRCA1.

More recently, our lab has used proteomic technologies to investigate novel mechanisms of genistein chemoprevention (*32*). Rats were treated with or without genistein

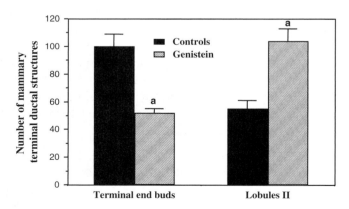

Fig. 3. Terminal ductal structures in mammary glands of 50-day-old female rats treated prepubertally with genistein or DMSO. Values for terminal end buds from DMSO-treated rats were set at 100. Numbers represent terminal end buds or lobules in the outer fringe of the abdominal mammary gland. [a] represents statistical significance ($p < 0.05$) compared to DMSO-treated rats. Adapted from (*26*) with permission.

at days 16, 18, and 20 postpartum. At 21 days postpartum, mammary glands were subjected to 2D polyacrylamide gel electrophoresis. This discovery technique allows a system-wide resolution of proteins that are differentially expressed between groups. Six proteins were differentially expressed, with one, GTP-cyclohydrolase 1 (GTP-CH1), confirmed by immunoblot analysis. Further investigation of the downstream pathway of GTP-CH1 revealed that tyrosine hydroxylase was up-regulated and vascular endothelial growth factor receptor 2 (VEGFR2) was down-regulated in the mammary glands of 50-day-old rats treated with genistein in the prepubertal period. This result was consistent with, and could help to explain, the mammary gland maturation and cell proliferation data that had been observed previously. This report demonstrated the importance of using new, "systems biology", approaches to look for novel mechanisms of action after treatment with phytochemicals.

2.4. Genistein and Prostate Cancer: In Vitro Results

In vitro prostate cancer studies have demonstrated the anti-proliferative and pro-apoptotic properties of genistein (*14, 33–35*). Genistein inhibits topoisomerases I and II (*36*), 5 alpha-reductase (*37*), and the NF-κB and AKT signaling pathways (*38, 39*) in cell culture. It can act as an antioxidant (*35*) and inhibit angiogenesis (*40*) and metastasis (*41*). Using LNCap prostate cancer cells, genistein was able to limit prostate cancer growth by trans-differentiating neuroendocrine cells (*42*).

2.5. Genistein and Prostate Cancer: In Vivo Chemoprevention

Pollard and Luckert showed that high-isoflavone-supplemented soy diet fed to Lobund-Wistar rats reduced the incidence of *N*-methyl-*N*-nitrosourea (NMU)-induced prostate-related cancer and the disease-free period was prolonged by 27% compared with rats fed the same diet, but low in isoflavones (*43*). Soy has been found to have a protective effect against prostatic dysplasia (*44*) and to inhibit the growth of transplantable human prostate carcinomas and tumor angiogenesis in mice (*45*). Our lab has shown that genistein suppresses NMU-induced prostate cancer in Lobund-Wistar rats (*46*), reduces the incidence of poorly differentiated prostatic adenocarcinomas in *t*ransgenic *a*denocarcinoma of the *m*ouse *p*rostate (TRAMP) mice (*47, 48*). Wang et al. have shown that dietary genistein suppresses the formation and progression of poorly differentiated prostate cancer by a 35% decrease compared with the control group in castrated TRAMP mice (*48*). This is related to down-regulation of proliferation of cell nuclear antigen and SV40 Tag protein expressions in dietary genistein exposure. All tumors that developed in castrated TRAMP mice were poorly differentiated in contrast to the 37% of noncastrated TRAMP mice that developed poorly differentiated tumors. The percentage of transgenic males that developed poorly differentiated tumors was reduced in both intact and castrated models by dietary genistein, demonstrating that it can be a promising chemopreventive agent.

2.6. Genistein and Prostate Cancer: Mechanisms of Action

Dalu et al. showed that genistein inhibited the expression of the epidermal growth factor (EGF) and ErbB2/Neu receptors, while Fritz et al. reported that genistein down-regulated androgen (AR) and ER expression in the rat dorsolateral prostate (49, 50). In nontransgenic C57/BL6 mice, the progesterone receptor as well as the AR and ER were down-regulated (48). In another study, genistein treatment resulted in a dose-dependent, significant inhibitory effect on osteopontin, an extracellular matrix protein secreted by macrophages infiltrating prostate tumors, in TRAMP mice with poorly differentiated tumors (51). Likewise, genistein given in the diet significantly down-regulated cell proliferation, EGFR, insulin-like growth factor receptor (IGF-1R), and extracellular regulating kinases (ERKs-1/2) restoration of GSK-3β activation, and maintenance of cadherin-1 expression via down-regulation of snail-1 in TRAMP mice (52).

2.7. Genistein: Breast and Prostate Cancer Epidemiology

An important consideration of any cancer causation and prevention study is the correlation between animal studies and human health. Asian countries, with soybeans as a dietary staple, have historically had very low incidences of breast and prostate cancers. Epidemiological studies have indicated an inverse correlation between dietary soy intake and breast cancer incidence (53, 54). Interestingly, immigration from Asian countries to the United States negates the protection against breast cancer, especially when immigration occurs early in life (55). Following our reports of prepubertal genistein suppressing mammary tumor development in rats, epidemiology studies were conducted and the results supported the concept of timing of exposure to genistein providing a protective effect. These epidemiology reports show the importance of early exposure (13–15 years old) demonstrating a significant reduction of breast cancer risk with consumption of soy (56). It appears that the most sensitive period for mammary cancer chemoprevention in the rat is the prepubertal period, and in the human probably the adolescent period. Adult exposure following prepubertal exposure may also contribute to protection.

It is known that prostate cancer incidence is less prevalent among Asian men who have a diet high in soy (57). However, Asians who move to the United States and adopt the Western diet are no longer protected against prostate cancer (58–61). Animal studies with soy and genistein support the reports of soy consumers having a lower incidence of clinically manifested prostate cancer.

3. RESVERATROL

Resveratrol (trans-3,4′,5-trihydroxystilbene) (Fig. 1), a phytoalexin found in red grape skins and red wine, has received a lot of attention for health-beneficial properties. Resveratrol is a polyphenol and a member of the stilbene family. It has also been detected in a host of other sources, including peanuts, berries, and several traditional oriental medicine plants (62). Resveratrol has recently been associated with a number of beneficial health effects that range from antioxidant to cardiovascular benefits and protection against the deleterious effects of high fat diets and cancers of many organs.

Over the last 10 years, there has been a host of reports on the anti-cancer effects of resveratrol in cell culture systems, animal models and a few epidemiological reports. Seminal work by Jang et al. demonstrated that resveratrol could inhibit the three major stages of carcinogenesis, specifically, initiation, promotion, and progression (*63*). Resveratrol was found to function as an antioxidant and anti-mutagen that could induce phase II enzymes, all of which could play a role in blocking cancer initiation. Resveratrol also mediated anti-inflammatory responses, including blocking cyclooxygenase enzymes. All of these properties could play a role against the progression of cancer. Also, resveratrol induced human promyelocytic leukemia cell differentiation, a demonstration that resveratrol could inhibit progression. Resveratrol has also been reported to inhibit metastasis, the mechanism responsible for the majority of deaths due to cancer (*64*). Resveratrol has shown promise against a number of tumor types including breast and prostate cancers.

3.1. Resveratrol and Breast Cancer: In Vitro Results

Over the past 10 years, there has been a wealth of studies investigating the anti-tumor effects of resveratrol against breast cancer. In a review of the literature, Bhat and Pezzuto highlighted several mechanisms responsible for the cancer chemopreventive activities of resveratrol (*65*). Resveratrol has antioxidant effects and can inhibit chemically-induced free radical formation. Inhibition of the cytochrome P450 enzymes was a proposed mechanism. Resveratrol has been shown to inhibit CYP1A1, 2A6, and 3A4, all of which are involved in the metabolism of carcinogens. Resveratrol also inhibited cell cycle progression and induced apoptosis in a number of breast cancer cell lines. Effects on apoptosis have implicated the Bcl-2 family of proteins. Resveratrol was also reported to suppress NF-κB, which is known to play a role in inflammation and oncogenesis.

A recent review by Le Corre et al. points out features of resveratrol that may be associated with inhibition of cancer development (*66*). Suppression of CYP 1A1 is again highlighted in breast cancer cells. Some phase II carcinogen activators such as *O*-acetyltransferase and sulfotransferase are inhibited by resveratrol in breast cancer cells. In human breast cancer cells, resveratrol suppressed the induction of prostaglandins and the activity of cyclooxygenase-2 (COX-2), known inflammatory mediators that can play a role in cancer progression. As for cell cycle inhibition in breast cancer cells, resveratrol inhibited D-type cyclins and increased mRNA levels of p21 and p53. Another pathway highlighted in this review was the PI3K signaling pathway, postulated to play a role in cell survival. High concentrations of resveratrol inhibited PI3K signaling. Unique to breast cancer cells, resveratrol increased the expression of BRCA-1 and -2, which are factors that play a role in the repair of DNA. Germ-line mutations in BRCA-1 and -2 are well known for conferring a high risk of breast and ovarian cancers (*67*). It is clear that resveratrol is an effective agent against breast cancer cells in vitro. Nevertheless, studies investigating the anti-cancer effects and mechanisms of action of resveratrol in vivo are warranted.

3.2. *Resveratrol and Breast Cancer: In Vivo Chemoprevention*

Several groups have reported that resveratrol can effectively suppress mammary tumorigenesis in rodent models. Resveratrol administered by oral gavage at 10 and 100 mg/kg body weight 1 week prior to mammary tumor induction by the direct acting carcinogen, NMU, was studied (*68*). The higher dose of resveratrol was able to suppress mammary tumorigenesis, decreasing mammary tumor incidence and multiplicity while increasing tumor latency in this model. Banerjee et al. then showed that resveratrol could suppress DMBA-induced mammary carcinogenesis in rats (*69*). Resveratrol again reduced incidence and tumor multiplicity while extending the latency period. As for mechanisms, resveratrol inhibited protein levels of COX-2 and matrix metalloprotease-9 in the breast tumors. A drawback to this study was the small number of animals (*n* = 12) used and the use of a sub-optimal dose of DMBA, which resulted in a mix of tumor types. It has also been demonstrated that resveratrol is effective at suppressing spontaneous mammary carcinogenesis (*64*). Resveratrol supplementation delayed the development of spontaneous mammary tumors, reduced tumor number and size, and inhibited the number of lung metastases in Her-2/neu-transgenic mice. Decreased gene expression of Her-2/neu and increased tumor apoptosis are mechanisms of action for resveratrol.

Our lab has since reported that resveratrol is an effective chemopreventive agent against DMBA-induced mammary tumors (*70*). Using a dose of DMBA that caused 100% tumor incidence (adenocarcinomas) and at least 30 animals per group, we showed that resveratrol administered in the diet at 1 g/kg diet could significantly reduce mammary tumor multiplicity (Fig. 4) and increase tumor latency (Fig. 5) (*71*).

To our knowledge, only one report on resveratrol has shown an increased incidence of chemically induced mammary tumors. Sato et al. injected resveratrol for 5 days prior to puberty (postnatal days 15–19) and then induced mammary tumors with NMU (*72*). Rats prepubertally treated with 100 mg resveratrol/kg body weight showed a signifi-

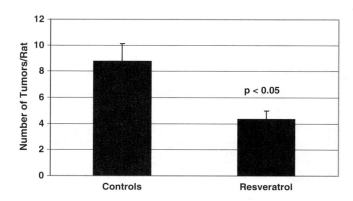

Fig. 4. Resveratrol chemoprevention in a chemically induced rat model of mammary cancer. Animals were exposed to 1 g resveratrol/kg AIN-76A diet or AIN-76A diet only starting at birth. On day 50 postpartum, all rats were treated with 60 mg DMBA/kg body weight. Values represent mean number of tumors per rat ±2 standard errors. A *p*-value <0.05 was considered statistically significant. Adapted from (*71*) with permission.

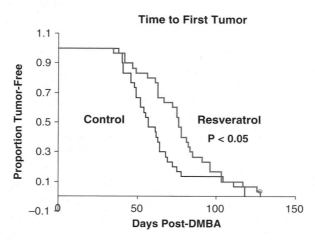

Fig. 5. Effects of resveratrol on mammary tumor latency. Animals were exposed to 1 g resveratrol/kg AIN-76A diet or AIN-76A diet starting at birth. On day 50 postpartum, all rats were treated with 60 mg DMBA/kg body weight. Kaplan–Meier estimates of tumor-free survival were plotted. A p-value <0.05 was considered statistically significant. Adapted from (*71*) with permission.

cant increase in the incidence of rats with tumors ≥1 cm. This contrasting result may be due to the route of administration (subcutaneous injection). By not being ingested orally, as with human exposure to resveratrol, the differing metabolism of resveratrol may compromise its effectiveness as an anti-tumor agent.

3.3. Resveratrol and Breast Cancer: Mechanisms of Action

The mechanisms through which resveratrol can suppress breast cancer in animal models are just beginning to be elucidated. Recently, our lab looked at the effects of resveratrol on mammary gland architecture, epithelial cell proliferation, and epithelial cell apoptosis in Sprague-Dawley rats. We have shown that a mechanism through which genistein can protect against mammary carcinogenesis is an enhancement of the maturation of the mammary gland, which serves to increase the number of lobular structures (least susceptible terminal ductal structures to carcinogenesis) and decrease the number of terminal end buds, the most susceptible mammary structure to carcinogenesis (*10*, *13*, *73*). Hence, our lab determined the effects of resveratrol administered in the diet on mammary architecture and differentiation (*72*). Female Sprague-Dawley rats exposed to 1 g resveratrol/kg AIN-76A diet from birth onward were killed at 50 days postpartum (the time of carcinogen exposure in the tumorigenesis study). The number 4 abdominal mammary glands were dissected, mounted on glass slides, and stained with alum carmine. The predominant mammary terminal ductal structures found in 50-day-old rats were terminal end buds (37%), terminal ducts (31%), lobules type I (23%), and lobules type II (9%). Treatment with resveratrol in the diet had no effect on the number of terminal end buds at 50 days postpartum. While resveratrol in the diet did not significantly alter the numbers of individual structures, the combined lobules types I and II were significantly increased compared to the control group. This increase in lobules, the most mature structures found in the mammary gland, may explain the protection observed against chemically induced mammary cancers.

With only a modest increase in mammary gland maturation, turnover of the cells in the differing terminal ductal structures of the mammary gland was determined. Bromodeoxyuridine (BrdU) incorporation was used as an index of cell proliferation. Female Sprague-Dawley rats exposed to 1 g resveratrol/kg diet were sacrificed at 50 days postpartum. BrdU was administered 2 h prior to sacrificing, injected i.p., with each rat receiving 100 mg BrdU/kg body weight. One of the number 4 abdominal mammary glands was dissected, fixed in 10% neutral buffered formalin, and blocked in paraffin. Five-micrometer sections were cut onto slides for immunohistochemical analysis of BrdU. In the mammary glands of 50-day-old control rats, the labeling indices were ~5% in terminal end buds and terminal ducts and ~2% in lobules type I. The supplementation with resveratrol in the diet significantly reduced cell proliferation in terminal ducts, terminal end buds, and lobules I to ~1, 2.5, and ~1%, respectively (Table 2). This reduction in epithelial cell proliferation helps to explain the protection observed against DMBA-induced mammary cancer.

Table 2

Cell Proliferation in Mammary Terminal Ductal Structures of Rats Fed Resveratrol in the Diet. Female Sprague-Dawley Rats Were Exposed to Resveratrol (1 g/kg AIN-76A Diet) or AIN-76A Diet Alone from Birth to 50 Days Postpartum. Two hours Prior to Killing, Rats Were Injected with 100 mg BrdU/kg Body Weight. BrdU Incorporation Was Measured by Immunohistochemistry for Terminal Ductal Structures. Values Represent Means ± SEM for At least Seven Rats/Treatment Group

	Control (AIN-76A)	Resveratrol (1 g/kg AIN-76A)
Terminal ducts	5.03 ± 1.07	0.79 ± 0.27*
Terminal end buds	4.83 ± 0.61	2.50 ± 0.75*
Lobules	1.75 ± 0.22	0.90 ± 0.14*

*p-value ≤ 0.05 and was considered statistically significant. Adapted from (71) with permission.

Using a DNA fragmentation assay, rate of apoptosis was investigated in mammary terminal end buds and lobules (combined type I and II) from 50-day-old rats. Rats supplemented with dietary resveratrol showed a significant increase (~25%) in apoptotic index in the mammary epithelial cells in terminal end buds and a slight, though not statistically significant, increased apoptosis in lobules as compared to control rats (Table 3). Importantly, we observed a significant decrease in epithelial cell proliferation and a significant increase in epithelial cell apoptosis in terminal end buds, which are immature structures susceptible to mammary carcinogens. The ratio of cells proliferating to those dying via apoptosis in the terminal end buds was 0.136 for rats on a control diet compared to 0.056 for rats administered resveratrol in the diet.

Besides effects on mammary gland architecture and epithelial cell proliferation and apoptosis, other molecular mechanisms for resveratrol mammary protection have been suggested. Banerjee et al. demonstrated that resveratrol inhibited protein levels of COX-2 and matrix metalloprotease-9 in breast tumors (69). In a Her-2/neu mouse model of

Table 3

Apoptotic Index in Mammary Terminal Ductal Structures of Rats Fed Resveratrol in the Diet. Female Sprague-Dawley Rats Were Exposed to Resveratrol (1 g/kg AIN-76A Diet) or AIN-76A Diet Alone from Birth to 50 Days Postpartum. Apoptotic Indices Were Determined in Terminal Ductal Structures from the Fourth Abdominal Mammary Gland. Values Represent Means ± SEM for Atleast Seven Rats Per Treatment Group

	Control	*Resveratrol*
Terminal end buds	35.43 ± 1.37	$44.18 \pm 1.84^*$
Lobules	39.39 ± 2.67	41.24 ± 2.38

*p-value ≤ 0.05 and was considered statistically significant. Adapted from (71) with permission.

breast cancer, resveratrol suppressed gene expression of Her-2/neu and increased tumor cell apoptosis (64). There is still much to be elucidated as to the mechanisms through which resveratrol can suppress mammary carcinogenesis.

3.4. Resveratrol and Prostate Cancer: In Vitro results

In vitro studies have demonstrated a reduction in cell proliferation and an increase in apoptosis in both androgen-dependent and androgen-independent prostate cancer cell lines (74–78). Resveratrol activates the tumor suppressor gene p53 (76), decreases COX-2 expression, abates NF-κB activation (79), and inhibits protein tyrosine kinase activity (80) in cell culture. In PC-12 cells, resveratrol also acts as an anti-inflammatory (81) and antioxidant (82) agent.

Resveratrol down-regulates the expression and function of the AR and a number of androgen-regulated genes including prostate-specific antigen, cyclin-dependent kinase inhibitor p21, and AR-coactivator ARA70 in androgen-dependent LNCaP prostate cancer cells (83). In contrast, a 4-day treatment with resveratrol resulted in an 80% reduction in PSA via an AR-independent mechanism in LNCaP prostate cancer cells (84). Moreover, Gao et al. (85) demonstrated that resveratrol modulated the AR by way of the Raf-MEK-ERK signaling pathway (85). In addition, it has been recently shown that resveratrol inhibits ER-α in androgen-independent PC-3 prostate tumor cells. These studies implicate resveratrol as an attractive candidate for prostate cancer chemoprevention.

3.5. Resveratrol and Prostate Cancer: In Vivo Chemoprevention

By 28 weeks of age, TRAMP mice fed control diet developed high-grade prostatic intraepithelial neoplasia (PIN) (grade 3) and prostate cancer (grades 4–6) at a frequency of 34 and 67%, respectively (Table 4). None of the TRAMP mice demonstrated normal (grade 1) or low-grade PIN (grade 2) in resveratrol-free diet. Dietary supplementation with resveratrol (625 mg/kg) significantly reduced the incidence of poorly differentiated prostatic adenocarcinoma (grade 6 lesions) from 23 to 3% (7.7-fold) and delayed the

Table 4
Histopathological Analysis of the Urogenital Tract of 28-Week-Old TRAMP
Mice Fed Control AIN-76A Diet or AIN-76A Diet Supplemented with 625 mg
Resveratrol/kg Diet Starting at 5 Weeks of Age. Samples Were Given a
Score of 1 (No Tumor), 2 (Low-Grade PIN), 3 (High-Grade PIN), 4 (Well-
Differentiated Tumor), 5 (Moderately Differentiated Tumor), and 6 (Poorly
Differentiated Tumor) Depending on the Presence and Progression of Lesions.
Results are the Percentage of Mice as a Function of the Pathological Score

| Treatment | n | *Grade level* | | | | | |
		1 (%)	*2 (%)*	*3 (%)*	*4 (%)*	*5 (%)*	*6 (%)*
Control	53	0	0	34	42	2	23
Resveratrol	29	0	0	31	62	3	3*

*$p = 0.027$ compared to control treatment. Adapted from (86) with permission.

progression of well-differentiated lesions (grade 4) from 42% in controls to 62% in
resveratrol-treated mice. There was no statistical change in latency, number of tumors
per animal, tumor weight, or number of liver, kidney, lung, or lymph node metastases
between control and resveratrol-treated animals.

3.6. Resveratrol and Prostate Cancer: Mechanisms of Action

In the dorsolateral prostate (DLP) of TRAMP mice, resveratrol significantly inhibited
cell proliferation, increased expression of AR, ER-β, and insulin-like growth factor-
1 receptor (IGF-1R), and significantly decreased the levels of IGF-1 and phospho-
extracellular regulating kinase 1 (phospho-ERK 1) (86). In the ventral prostate (VP),
resveratrol significantly reduced cell proliferation and phospho-ERK 1 and 2, but did
not significantly alter the levels of IGF-1R and IGF-1. Serum total testosterone, free
testosterone, estradiol, dihydrotestosterone (DHT), and sex hormone-binding globulin
(SHBG) concentrations and SV-40 Tag expression in the prostate were not altered in
resveratrol-treated mice. Taken together, the decrease in cell proliferation and levels of
the potent growth factor, IGF-1, the down-regulation of downstream effectors, phospho-
ERK 1 and 2, and the increased expression of the putative tumor suppressor, ER-β,
provide a biochemical basis to explain how resveratrol may antagonize prostate cancer
development.

A postulated mechanism of elevated AR is that it functions as a tumor suppressor
prior to the development of prostate cancer by inhibiting uncontrolled proliferation in
normal prostate epithelium (87–89). Then, upon malignant conversion, AR undergoes
a molecular switch to act as an oncogene and stimulate the growth of prostate cancer
cells. The up-regulation of AR as tumor suppressor at 12 weeks of age during the transition between high-grade PIN and well-differentiated prostate adenocarcinoma supports
the decreased cell proliferation observed in the prostate of resveratrol-treated TRAMP
mice (87).

3.7. *Resveratrol: Breast and Prostate Cancer Epidemiology*

Besides cancer, resveratrol consumption has been linked to another important health benefit. Resveratrol contained in red wine is a leading candidate in explaining the "French Paradox," a strikingly low incidence of coronary heart disease in a region with a high intake of fats (*90–92*). These reports highlight resveratrol as possessing antioxidant properties as well as the ability to inhibit platelet aggregation. These observations provided the basis for studies investigating the benefits of resveratrol in other organs and against other diseases. These epidemiological reports along with the work of Jang et al. (*63*) triggered a series of investigations examining the mechanisms of resveratrol protection against breast and prostate cancers.

Levi et al. showed a relationship between the intake of resveratrol and breast cancer risk in a Swiss cohort of 971 women, of whom 369 had histologically confirmed breast cancer (*93*). Total resveratrol consumption from both grapes and wine was inversely correlated with risk of breast cancer. The highest tertile of resveratrol consumption had a 0.39 odds ratio compared to the lowest tertile. One previous study had shown inconclusive results when searching for an association between consumption of red wine and breast cancer risk (*94*).

It is important to note that alcohol consumption is generally thought of as a risk factor for breast cancer. The association of alcohol consumption with increased risk for breast cancer has been a consistent finding in epidemiological studies over the past 20 years (*95–97*). While heavy alcohol consumption was generally associated with increased risk, moderate or low consumption has shown weak or no associations. In postmenopausal women, moderate alcohol intake reduces cardiac risk and increases life expectancy. Thus, level of consumption and age appear to play a role in the risk conferred by alcohol. It is also unclear whether solely consuming red wine acts similarly to any other form of alcohol consumption. Future studies should examine how the moderate consumption of red wine influences the risk for breast cancer. It is also important to note that exposure to resveratrol may occur through consumption of grapes or pharmaceutical supplements.

While there is limited epidemiological information concerning the effects of resveratrol on prostate cancer, there are suggestions that red wine may suppress prostate cancer development. It has been reported that drinking a glass of red wine a day may cut a man's risk of prostate cancer in half. The protective effect appears to be strongest against the most aggressive forms of the disease (*98*).

4. COMBINATIONAL CHEMOPREVENTION

The idea of combining treatments in breast and prostate cancers for a more efficacious outcome is not a new idea, although it is in its infancy in the chemoprevention field. This strategy is already used in the therapeutic regimens against these cancers, with multiple chemotherapy drugs targeting different mechanisms to improve efficacy of treatment while minimizing toxicity. This strategy of combining agents has been effective using soy and green tea extract. For example, the combined supplementation with green tea plus soy phytochemicals reduced tumor weight in an in vivo mammary cancer model beyond the reduction seen with only green tea (*99*). Combinations of protective bioactive compounds may improve the ability to suppress tumorigenesis by targeting multiple pathways, allowing lower doses to be effective and reducing possible toxicities. Our lab has begun to look at combinations of resveratrol and genistein in suppressing mammary and prostate cancers.

4.1. Combinational Breast Cancer Chemoprevention with Genistein and Resveratrol

To evaluate the combined effectiveness of genistein and resveratrol against mammary carcinogenesis in a rat model, we administered from birth throughout life single doses of 250 mg genistein/kg diet and 1,000 mg resveratrol/kg diet (*10, 71*) or lower doses of genistein and resveratrol (83 and 333 mg/kg diet, respectively) alone or in combination (83 mg genistein + 100 mg resveratrol or 333 mg resveratrol + 25 mg genistein/kg diet) (*70*). At the lower doses, both genistein and resveratrol protected against DMBA-induced mammary tumors with a reduction in multiplicity and an increase in tumor latency (Table 5). When 25 mg genistein/kg diet was added to the 333 mg resveratrol/kg diet treatment, a further, albeit not significant, reduction in tumor multiplicity was observed. However, we detected a trend toward increased maturation of the mammary gland at 50 days postpartum and a significant reduction in epithelial cell proliferation in the TEB with the lower doses of genistein and resveratrol.

Table 5
Mammary Tumor Multiplicity and Latency in a Chemically Induced Rat Model of Mammary Cancer Exposed to Genistein, Resveratrol, or Combinations of Genistein Plus Resveratrol in the Diet. Female Sprague-Dawley Rats Were Exposed from Birth Throughout Life to Genistein (Gen), Resveratrol (Resv), Combinations of Gen + Resv, or Control (AIN-76A) in the Diet. All Rats Were Exposed to DMBA (60 mg/kg Body Weight) at 50 Days Postpartum to Induce Tumorigenesis. A *p*-Value <0.05 was Considered Significant. Adapted from (*70*) with Permission

	Tumors per rat (multiplicity)	Reduction compared to control (%)	p-Value compared to control	Time to first tumor (days)	p-Value compared to control
Control	8.27	–	–	44	–
83 mg gen/kg diet	3.43	58	<0.0001	63.5	<0.0001
333 mg resv/kg diet	6.31	24	0.034	51	0.008
333 mg resv + 25 mg gen/kg diet	5.29	36	<0.001	52	0.006
100 mg resv + 83 mg gen/kg diet	5.50	33	<0.01	49.5	0.0024

Future research in this promising area of nutrition and cancer should investigate optimal dosing regimens for maximal prevention, the impact of sequential administration of genistein during puberty and resveratrol later in life, and test other bioactive compounds that could augment the effects of genistein and/or resveratrol. Progress in these areas requires a thorough understanding of the in vivo mechanisms through which these agents may suppress mammary tumorigenesis.

4.2. Combinational Prevention of Prostate Cancer with Genistein and Resveratrol

We have evaluated the potential of combinational genistein and resveratrol as chemopreventive agents against prostate cancer in TRAMP mice. In this study, we used a low dose of 125 mg genistein and 313 mg resveratrol per kg diet and a high dose of 250 mg genistein plus 625 mg resveratrol per kg diet and a control group devoid of genistein and resveratrol. At time of necropsy, we found that the high genistein and resveratrol dose resulted in a 5.3-fold decrease in poorly differentiated prostate tumors (grade 6) compared to the control group (Table 6). The low dose did not significantly alter grade 6 tumors.

Table 6

Histopathological Analysis of Prostates from 28-Week-Old TRAMP Mice Provided Genistein and Resveratrol in Combination Via the Diet Starting at 5 Weeks of Age. Tissue Sections Were Given Histopathological Scores of 1 (No Tumor), 2 (Low-Grade PIN), 3 (High-Grade PIN), 4 (Well-Differentiated Tumor), 5 (Moderately Differentiated Tumor), and 6 (Poorly Differentiated Tumor) Depending on the Presence and Progression of Lesions. Results Are the Percentage of Mice as a Function of the Pathological Score

		Grade level					
Treatment	n	1 (%)	2 (%)	3 (%)	4 (%)	5 (%)	6 (%)
Control (AIN-76A diet)	25	5.8	10.7	69.5	3.4	2.6	7.9
125 mg gen/kg diet + 313 mg resveratrol/kg diet	25	2.2	11.1	67.7	4.9	5.6	8.5
250 mg gen/kg diet + 625 mg resveratrol/kg diet	22	0.2	26.6	63.3	4.5	3.8	1.5*

*$p < 0.05$ When compared to control treatment by Fisher's Exact Test.

We subsequently examined cell proliferation and apoptosis in TRAMP mice fed the high dose of genistein and resveratrol. The experimental design included a group of nontransgenic mice (C57BL/6 mice) as background control. Measurements were made at 12 weeks, at the time TRAMP mice develop premalignant lesions. We found that DLP and VP of C57BL/6 mice had low proliferation index (Table 7). In contrast, DLP and VP of TRAMP mice had 19- and 16-fold more cell proliferation than the C57BL/6 DLP and VP, respectively. These results were not surprising since the SV-40 Tag antigen is known to suppress p53 and Rb expressions. On the other hand, TRAMP mice fed combinational genistein and resveratrol diet had significantly decreased cell proliferation in the DLP, but not in the VP compared to TRAMP mice fed control diet. The specific effect on the

Table 7
Prostate Cell Proliferation and Apoptosis in 12-Week-Old Mice. Cell Proliferation Was Measured by Immunohistochemical Staining of Ki-67 and Apoptosis Was Determined Using ApopTag® Plus Peroxidase In Situ Apoptosis Detection Kit in the Dorsolateral and Ventral Prostates of Mice

	Cell proliferation		Apoptosis	
Treatment	DLP	VP	DLP	VP
C57BL/6 mice	1.0 ± 0.2	0.8 ± 0.1	1.9 ± 0.3	1.8 ± 0.4
TRAMP controls	19.2 ± 4.2	12.7 ± 0.8	$0.4 \pm 0.1*$	$0.8 \pm 0.2*$
250 mg gen/kg diet + 625 mg resveratrol/kg diet	13.5 ± 1.7	12.7 ± 2.9	1.2 ± 0.2	1.9 ± 0.4

*$p < 0.05$ when compared to C57BL/6 and TRAMP mice receiving resveratrol and genistein in the diet by Fisher's Exact Test.

DLP is important because this site is first affected with cancerous lesions in the TRAMP model.

Apoptosis was significantly decreased in both the DLP and the VP by five- and two-fold, respectively, in TRAMP mice compared to C57BL/6 mice (Table 7). Interestingly, the combination of dietary supplementation with genistein and resveratrol reversed apoptosis in TRAMP mice by 3- and 2.4-fold in DLP and VP, respectively. These data demonstrate that cell turnover in the TRAMP prostate is significantly regulated by combinational diets supplemented with genistein and resveratrol.

5. CONCLUSIONS

Cancers of the breast and prostate remain two of the most common and deadly cancers. There is a strong need to evaluate agents that can suppress the initiation and progression of these cancers. Our lab and others have shown that the natural polyphenols genistein and resveratrol can be effective in the prevention of breast and prostate cancers.

Asian populations on high soy diets have decreased incidences of both breast and prostate cancers. Our lab has shown that genistein, a major soy component, can suppress chemically induced mammary cancer multiplicity by enhancing mammary gland differentiation. We have also shown that genistein suppresses NMU-induced prostate cancer in Lobund-Wistar rats, reduces the incidence of poorly differentiated prostatic adenocarcinomas in TRAMP mice, and decreases DMBA-induced mammary adenocarcinomas in Sprague-Dawley rats.

Our lab and others have shown that resveratrol, a phytoalexin found in red wine, can suppress both breast and prostate cancers in animal models. Resveratrol suppresses the incidence of mammary tumors while extending the tumor latency in rats. Down-regulation of mammary epithelial cell proliferation and increased apoptosis may help explain the protective effects of resveratrol against mammary tumorigenesis. Resveratrol administered in the diet also inhibits the progression of prostate cancer in TRAMP mice, significantly reducing the incidence of aggressive grade 6 tumors. The regulation of cell proliferation through modulation of critical sex steroid and growth factor pathways may help to explain the observed protection.

The combined use of genistein and resveratrol in the diet also suppresses mammary and prostate cancer development in animal models, suggesting that combining certain aspects of the Asian diet (genistein derived from soy) and Western world propensity to consume resveratrol (via red wine or supplements) can provide opportunity for better breast and prostate health.

There is a significant need to fully understand the mechanisms through which genistein and resveratrol protect the breast and prostate against carcinogenesis. A better understanding of the mechanisms of action of these agents will lead to more effective combinational prevention regimens and add to the preclinical testing necessary to design clinical trials with these polyphenols. Suppressing the incidence and progression of breast and prostate carcinogenesis through natural, dietary polyphenols may have a major impact in the fight against cancers afflicting men and women.

REFERENCES

1. American Cancer Society. (2008) Cancer Facts & Figures. Atlanta: American Cancer Society.
2. Kuiper, G.G., Lemmen, J.G., Carlsson, B. et al. (1998) Interaction of estrogenic chemicals and phytoestrogens with estrogen receptor beta. *Endocrinology* **139**, 4252–63.
3. Adlercreutz, H., and Mazur, W. (1997) Phyto-oestrogens and Western diseases. *Ann Med* **29**, 95–120.
4. Barnes, S., and Lamartiniere, C.A. (2003) The role of phytoestrogens as cancer prevention agents. In: Kelloff G.J., Hawk E.T., Sigman C.C. eds. Cancer Chemoprevention. 359–69, NJ, USA: Humana Press Inc.
5. Sarkar, F.H., and Li, Y. (2002) Mechanisms of cancer chemoprevention by soy isoflavone genistein. *Cancer Metastasis Rev* **21**, 265–80.
6. Adlercreutz, H., Markkanen, H., and Watanabe, S. (1993) Plasma concentrations of phyto-oestrogens in Japanese men. *Lancet* **342**, 1209–10.
7. Baggott, J.E., Ha, T., Vaughn, W.H., Juliana, M.M., Hardin, J.M., and Grubbs, C.J. (1990) Effect of miso (Japanese soybean paste) and NaCl on DMBA-induced rat mammary tumors. *Nutr Cancer* **14**, 103–9.
8. Barnes, S., Grubbs, C.J., Setchell, K.D.R., and Carlson, J. Soybeans Inhibit Mammary Tumors in Models of Breast Cancer. Wiley Liss: New York, USA; 1990.
9. Lamartiniere, C.A., Moore, J.B., Brown, N.M., Thompson, R., Hardin, M.J., and Barnes, S. (1995) Genistein suppresses mammary cancer in rats. *Carcinogenesis* **16**, 2833–40.
10. Fritz, W.A., Coward, L., Wang, J., and Lamartiniere, C.A. (1998) Dietary genistein: Perinatal mammary cancer prevention, bioavailability and toxicity testing in the rat. *Carcinogenesis* **19**, 2151–8.
11. Badger, T.M., Ronis, M.J., Hakkak, R., Rowlands, J.C., and Korourian, S. (2002) The health consequences of early soy consumption. *J Nutr* **132**, 559S–65S.
12. Hilakivi-Clarke, L., Onojafe, I., Raygada, M. et al. (1999) Prepubertal exposure to zearalenone or genistein reduces mammary tumorigenesis. *Br J Cancer* **80**, 1682–8.
13. Lamartiniere, C.A. (2002) Timing of exposure and mammary cancer risk. *J Mammary Gland Biol Neoplasia* **7**, 67–76.
14. Lamartiniere, C.A., Cotroneo, M.S., Fritz, W.A., Wang, J., Mentor-Marcel, R., and Elgavish, A. (2002) Genistein chemoprevention: Timing and mechanisms of action in murine mammary and prostate. *J Nutr* **132**, 552S–8S.
15. Anderson, J.J.B., Anthony, M., Messina, M., and Garner, S.C. (1999) Effects of phyto-oestrogens on tissues. *Nutr Res Rev* **12**, 75–116.

16. Allred, C.D., Allred, K.F., Ju, Y.H., Virant, S.M., and Helferich, W.G. (2001) Soy diets containing vary-ing amounts of genistein stimulate growth of estrogen-dependent (MCF-7) tumors in a dose-dependent manner. *Cancer Res* **61**, 5045–50.

17. Hsieh, C.Y., Santell, R.C., Haslam, S.Z., and Helferich, W.G. (1998) Estrogenic effects of genistein on the growth of estrogen receptor-positive human breast cancer (MCF-7) cells in vitro and in vivo. *Cancer Res* **58**, 3833–8.

18. Ju, Y.H., Allred, C.D., Allred, K.F., Karko, K.L., Doerge, D.R., and Helferich, W.G. (2001) Physio-logical concentrations of dietary genistein dose-dependently stimulate growth of estrogen-dependent human breast cancer (MCF-7) tumors implanted in athymic nude mice. *J Nutr* **131**, 2957–62.

19. Zava, D.T., and Duwe, G. (1997) Estrogenic and antiproliferative properties of genistein and other flavonoids in human breast cancer cells in vitro. *Nutr Cancer* **27**, 31–40.

20. Mizunuma, H., Kanazawa, K., Ogura, S., Otsuka, S., and Nagai, H. (2002) Anticarcinogenic effects of isoflavones may be mediated by genistein in mouse mammary tumor virus-induced breast cancer. *Oncology* **62**, 78–84.

21. Jin, Z., and MacDonald, R.S. (2002) Soy isoflavones increase latency of spontaneous mammary tumors in mice. *J Nutr* **132**, 3186–90.

22. Vantyghem, S.A., Wilson, S.M., Postenka, C.O., Al-Katib, W., Tuck, A.B., and Chambers, A.F. (2005) Dietary genistein reduces metastasis in a postsurgical orthotopic breast cancer model. *Cancer Res* **65**, 3396–403.

23. Li, D., Yee, J.A., McGuire, M.H., Murphy, P.A., and Yan, L. (1999) Soybean isoflavones reduce exper-imental metastasis in mice. *J Nutr* **129**, 1075–8.

24. Singh, A.V., Franke, A.A., Blackburn, G.L., and Zhou, J.R. (2006) Soy phytochemicals prevent ortho-topic growth and metastasis of bladder cancer in mice by alterations of cancer cell proliferation and apoptosis and tumor angiogenesis. *Cancer Res* **66**, 1851–8.

25. Raffoul, J.J., Banerjee, S., Che, M. et al. (2007) Soy isoflavones enhance radiotherapy in a metastatic prostate cancer model. *Int J Cancer* **120**, 2491–8.

26. Murrill, W.B., Brown, N.M., Zhang, J.X., Manzolillo, P.A., Barnes, S., and Lamartiniere, C.A. (1996) Prepubertal genistein exposure suppresses mammary cancer and enhances gland differentiation in rats. *Carcinogenesis* **17**, 1451–7.

27. Russo, J., and Russo, I.H. (1978) DNA labeling index and structure of the rat mammary gland as determinants of its susceptibility to carcinogenesis. *J Natl Cancer Inst* **61**, 1451–9.

28. Russo, J., Moral, R., Balogh, G.A., Mailo, D., and Russo, I.H. (2005) The protective role of pregnancy in breast cancer. *Breast Cancer Res* **7**, 131–42.

29. Brown, N.M., Wang, J., Cotroneo, M.S., Zhao, Y.X., and Lamartiniere, C.A. (1998) Prepubertal genis-tein treatment modulates TGF-alpha, EGF and EGF-receptor mRNAs and proteins in the rat mammary gland. *Mol Cell Endocrinol* **144**, 149–65.

30. Dave, B., Eason, R.R., Till, S.R. et al. (2005) The soy isoflavone genistein promotes apopto-sis in mammary epithelial cells by inducing the tumor suppressor PTEN. *Carcinogenesis* **26**, 1793–803.

31. Cabanes, A., Wang, M., Olivo, S. et al. (2004) Prepubertal estradiol and genistein exposures up-regulate BRCA1 mRNA and reduce mammary tumorigenesis. *Carcinogenesis* **25**, 741–8.

32. Rowell, C., Carpenter, D.M., and Lamartiniere, C.A. (2005) Chemoprevention of breast cancer, pro-teomic discovery of genistein action in the rat mammary gland. *J Nutr* **135**, 2953S–9S.

33. Fotsis, T., Pepper, M.S., Aktas, E. et al. (1997) Flavonoids, dietary-derived inhibitors of cell prolifera-tion and in vitro angiogenesis. *Cancer Res* **57**, 2916–21.

34. Kyle, E., Neckers, L., Takimoto, C., Curt, G., and Bergan, R. (1997) Genistein-induced apoptosis of prostate cancer cells is preceded by a specific decrease in focal adhesion kinase activity. *Mol Pharma-col* **51**, 193–200.

35. Suzuki, K., Koike, H., Matsui, H. et al. (2002) Genistein, a soy isoflavone, induces glutathione perox-idase in the human prostate cancer cell lines LNCaP and PC-3. *Int J Cancer* **99**, 846–52.

36. Okura, A., Arakawa, H., Oka, H., Yoshinari, T., and Monden, Y. (1988) Effect of genistein on topoi-somerase activity and on the growth of [Val 12]Ha-ras-transformed NIH 3T3 cells. *Biochem Biophys Res Commun* **157**, 183–9.

37. Evans, B.A., Griffiths, K., and Morton, M.S. (1995) Inhibition of 5 alpha-reductase in genital skin fibroblasts and prostate tissue by dietary lignans and isoflavonoids. *J Endocrinol* **147**, 295–302.

38. Davis, J.N., Kucuk, O., and Sarkar, F.H. (1999) Genistein inhibits NF-kappa B activation in prostate cancer cells. *Nutr Cancer* **35**, 167–74.

39. Gong, L., Li, Y., Nedeljkovic-Kurepa, A., and Sarkar, F.H. (2003) Inactivation of NF-kappaB by genistein is mediated via Akt signaling pathway in breast cancer cells. *Oncogene* **22**, 4702–9.

40. Fotsis, T., Pepper, M., Adlercreutz, H. et al. (1993) Genistein, a dietary-derived inhibitor of in vitro angiogenesis. *Proc Natl Acad Sci USA* **90**, 2690–4.

41. Li, Y., Che, M., Bhagat, S. et al. (2004) Regulation of gene expression and inhibition of experimental prostate cancer bone metastasis by dietary genistein. *Neoplasia (New York)* **6**, 354–63.

42. Pinski, J., Wang, Q., Quek, M.L. et al. (2006) Genistein-induced neuroendocrine differentiation of prostate cancer cells. *Prostate* **66**, 1136–43.

43. Pollard, M., and Luckert, P.H. (1997) Influence of isoflavones in soy protein isolates on development of induced prostate-related cancers in L-W rats. *Nutr Cancer* **28**, 41–45.

44. Pylkkanen, L., Makela, S., and Santti, R. (1996) Animal models for the preneoplastic lesions of the prostate. *Eur Urol* **30**, 243–8.

45. Zhou, J.R., Gugger, E.T., Tanaka, T., Guo, Y., Blackburn, G.L., and Clinton, S.K. (1999) Soybean phytochemicals inhibit the growth of transplantable human prostate carcinoma and tumor angiogenesis in mice. *J Nutr* **129**, 1628–35.

46. Wang, J., Eltoum, I.E., and Lamartiniere, C.A. (2002) Dietary genistein suppresses chemically induced prostate cancer in Lobund-Wistar rats. *Cancer Lett* **186**, 11–18.

47. Mentor-Marcel, R., Lamartiniere, C.A., Eltoum, I.E., Greenberg, N.M., and Elgavish, A. (2001) Genistein in the diet reduces the incidence of poorly differentiated prostatic adenocarcinoma in transgenic mice (TRAMP). *Cancer Res* **61**, 6777–82.

48. Wang, J., Eltoum, I.E., and Lamartiniere, C.A. (2007) Genistein chemoprevention of prostate cancer in TRAMP mice. *J Carcinog* **6**, 3. doi: 10.1186/1477-3163-6-3.

49. Dalu, A., Haskell, J.F., Coward, L., and Lamartiniere, C.A. (1998) Genistein, a component of soy, inhibits the expression of the EGF and ErbB2/Neu receptors in the rat dorsolateral prostate. *Prostate* **37**, 36–43.

50. Fritz, W.A., Wang, J., Eltoum, I.E., and Lamartiniere, C.A. (2002) Dietary genistein downregulates androgen and estrogen receptor expression in the rat prostate. *Mol Cell Endocrinol* **186**, 89–99.

51. Mentor-Marcel, R., Lamartiniere, C.A., Eltoum, I.A., Greenberg, N.M., and Elgavish, A. (2005) Dietary genistein improves survival and reduces expression of osteopontin in the prostate of transgenic mice with prostatic adenocarcinoma (TRAMP). *J Nutr* **135**, 989–95.

52. El Touny, L.H., and Banerjee, P.P. (2007) Akt/GSK3 pathway as a target in genistein-induced inhibition of TRAMP prostate cancer progression towards a poorly differentiated phenotype. *Carcinogenesis* **28**, 1710–7.

53. Adlercreutz, H., Honjo, H., Higashi, A. et al. (1991) Urinary excretion of lignans and isoflavonoid phytoestrogens in Japanese men and women consuming a traditional Japanese diet. *Amer J Clin Nutr* **54**, 1093–100.

54. Lee, H.P., Gourley, L., Duffy, S.W., Esteve, J., Lee, J., and Day, N.E. (1991) Dietary effects on breast-cancer risk in Singapore. *Lancet* **337**, 1197–200.

55. Ziegler, R.G., Hoover, R.N., Pike, M.C. et al. (1993) Migration patterns and breast cancer risk in Asian-American women. *J Nat Cancer Inst* **85**, 1819–27.

56. Shu, X.O., Jin, F., Dai, Q. et al. (2001) Soyfood intake during adolescence and subsequent risk of breast cancer among Chinese women. *Cancer Epidemiol Biomarkers Prev* **10**, 483–8.

57. Parkin, D.M., Pisani, P., and Ferlay, J. (1999) Global cancer statistics. *CA Cancer J Clin* **49**, 33–64.

58. Cook, L.S., Goldoft, M., Schwartz, S.M., and Weiss, N.S. (1999) Incidence of adenocarcinoma of the prostate in Asian immigrants to the United States and their descendants. *J Urol* **161**, 152–5.

59. Haenszel, W., and Kurihara, M. (1968) Studies of Japanese migrants. I. Mortality from cancer and other diseases among Japanese in the United States. *J Nat Cancer Inst* **40**, 43–68.

60. Shimizu, H., Ross, R.K., Bernstein, L., Yatani, R., Henderson, B.E., and Mack, T.M. (1991) Cancers of the prostate and breast among Japanese and white immigrants in Los Angeles County. *Br J Cancer* **63**, 963–6.

61. Whittemore, A.S., Kolonel, L.N., Wu, A.H. et al. (1995) Prostate cancer in relation to diet, physical activity, and body size in blacks, whites, and Asians in the United States and Canada. *J Natl Cancer Inst* **87**, 652–61.

62. Burns, J., Yokota, T., Ashihara, H., Lean, M.E., and Crozier, A. (2002) Plant foods and herbal sources of resveratrol. *J Agri Food Chem* **50**, 3337–40.

63. Jang, M., Cai, L., Udeani, G.O. et al. (1997) Cancer chemopreventive activity of resveratrol, a natural product derived from grapes. *Science* **275**, 218–20.

64. Provinciali, M., Re, F., Donnini, A. et al. (2005) Effect of resveratrol on the development of sponta-neous mammary tumors in HER-2/neu transgenic mice. *Int J Cancer* **115**, 36–45.

65. Bhat, K.P., and Pezzuto, J.M. (2002) Cancer chemopreventive activity of resveratrol. *Ann N Y Acad Sci* **957**, 210–29.

66. Le Corre, L., Chalabi, N., Delort, L., Bignon, Y.J., and Bernard-Gallon, D.J. (2005) Resveratrol and breast cancer chemoprevention: Molecular mechanisms. *Mol Nutr Food Res* **49**, 462–71.

67. Levy-Lahad, E., and Friedman, E. (2007) Cancer risks among BRCA1 and BRCA2 mutation carriers. *Br J Cancer* **96**, 11–15.

68. Bhat, K.P., Lantvit, D., Christov, K., Mehta, R.G., Moon, R.C., and Pezzuto, J.M. (2001) Estrogenic and antiestrogenic properties of resveratrol in mammary tumor models. *Cancer Res* **61**, 7456–63.

69. Banerjee, S., Bueso-Ramos, C., and Aggarwal, B.B. (2002) Suppression of 7,12-dimethylbenz(a) anthracene-induced mammary carcinogenesis in rats by resveratrol: Role of nuclear factor-kappaB, cyclooxygenase 2, and matrix metalloprotease 9. *Cancer Res* **62**, 4945–54.

70. Whitsett, T.G., Jr., and Lamartiniere, C.A. (2006) Genistein and resveratrol: Mammary cancer chemo-prevention and mechanisms of action in the rat. *Expert Rev Anticancer Ther* **6**, 1699–706.

71. Whitsett, T., Carpenter, M., and Lamartiniere, C.A. (2006) Resveratrol, but not EGCG, in the diet suppresses DMBA-induced mammary cancer in rats. *J Carcinog* **5**, 15. doi: 10.1186/1477-3163-5-15.

72. Sato, M., Pei, R.J., Yuri, T., Danbara, N., Nakane, Y., and Tsubura, A. (2003) Prepubertal resvera-trol exposure accelerates N-methyl-N-nitrosourea-induced mammary carcinoma in female Sprague-Dawley rats. *Cancer Lett* **202**, 137–45.

73. Russo, J., Wilgus, G., and Russo, I.H. (1979) Susceptibility of the mammary gland to carcinogenesis: I Differentiation of the mammary gland as determinant of tumor incidence and type of lesion. *Am J Pathol* **96**, 721–36.

74. Aziz, M.H., Nihal, M., Fu, V.X., Jarrard, D.F., and Ahmad, N. (2006) Resveratrol-caused apoptosis of human prostate carcinoma LNCaP cells is mediated via modulation of phosphatidylinositol 3'-kinase/Akt pathway and Bcl-2 family proteins. *Mol Cancer Ther* **5**, 1335–41.

75. Kim, Y.A., Rhee, S.H., Park, K.Y., and Choi, Y.H. (2003) Antiproliferative effect of resveratrol in human prostate carcinoma cells. *J Med Food* **6**, 273–80.

76. Lin, H.Y., Shih, A., Davis, F.B. et al. (2002) Resveratrol induced serine phosphorylation of p53 causes apoptosis in a mutant p53 prostate cancer cell line. *J Urol* **168**, 748–55.

77. Morris, G.Z., Williams, R.L., Elliott, M.S., and Beebe, S.J. (2002) Resveratrol induces apoptosis in LNCaP cells and requires hydroxyl groups to decrease viability in LNCaP and DU 145 cells. *Prostate* **52**, 319–29.

78. Sgambato, A., Ardito, R., Faraglia, B., Boninsegna, A., Wolf, F.I., and Cittadini, A. (2001) Resveratrol, a natural phenolic compound, inhibits cell proliferation and prevents oxidative DNA damage. *Mut Res* **496**, 171–80.

79. Manna, S.K., Mukhopadhyay, A., and Aggarwal, B.B. (2000) Resveratrol suppresses TNF-induced activation of nuclear transcription factors NF-kappa B, activator protein-1, and apoptosis: Potential role of reactive oxygen intermediates and lipid peroxidation. *J Immunol* **164**, 6509–19.

80. Jayatilake, G.S., Jayasuriya, H., Lee, E.S. et al. (1993) Kinase inhibitors from Polygonum cuspidatum. *J Nat Prod* **56**, 1805–10.

81. Kimura, Y., Okuda, H., and Arichi, S. (1985) Effects of stilbene derivatives on arachidonate metabolism in leukocytes. *Biochim Biophys Acta* **837**, 209–12.

82. Chanvitayapongs, S., Draczynska-Lusiak, B., and Sun, A.Y. (1997) Amelioration of oxidative stress by antioxidants and resveratrol in PC12 cells. *Neuroreport* **8**, 1499–502.

83. Mitchell, S.H., Zhu, W., and Young, C.Y. (1999) Resveratrol inhibits the expression and function of the androgen receptor in LNCaP prostate cancer cells. *Cancer Res* **59**, 5892–5.

84. Hsieh, T.C., and Wu, J.M. (2000) Grape-derived chemopreventive agent resveratrol decreases prostate-specific antigen (PSA) expression in LNCaP cells by an androgen receptor (AR)-independent mechanism. *Anticancer Res* **20**, 225–8.

85. Gao, S., Liu, G.Z., and Wang, Z. (2004) Modulation of androgen receptor-dependent transcription by resveratrol and genistein in prostate cancer cells. *Prostate* **59**, 214–25.

86. Harper, C.E., Patel, B.B., Wang, J., Arabshahi, A., Eltoum, I.A., and Lamartiniere, C.A. (2007) Resveratrol suppresses prostate cancer progression in transgenic mice. *Carcinogenesis* **28**, 1946–53.

87. Litvinov, I.V., De Marzo, A.M., and Isaacs, J.T. (2003) Is the Achilles' heel for prostate cancer therapy a gain of function in androgen receptor signaling? *J Clin Endocrinol Metab* **88**, 2972–82.

88. Litvinov, I.V., Vander Griend, D.J., Antony, L. et al. (2006) Androgen receptor as a licensing factor for DNA replication in androgen-sensitive prostate cancer cells. *Proc Natl Acad Sci USA* **103**, 15085–90.

89. Litvinov, I.V., Antony, L., Dalrymple, S.L., Becker, R., Cheng, L., and Isaacs, J.T. (2006) PC3, but not DU145, human prostate cancer cells retain the coregulators required for tumor suppressor ability of androgen receptor. *Prostate* **66**, 1329–38.

90. Kopp, P. (1998) Resveratrol, a phytoestrogen found in red wine. A possible explanation for the conundrum of the 'French paradox'? *Eur J Endocrinol* **138**, 619–20.

91. Renaud, S., and de Lorgeril, M. (1992) Wine, alcohol, platelets, and the French paradox for coronary heart disease. *Lancet* **339**, 1523–6.

92. Sun, A.Y., Simonyi, A., and Sun, G.Y. (2002) The "French Paradox" and beyond: Neuroprotective effects of polyphenols. *Free Radic Biol Med* **32**, 314–8.

93. Levi, F., Pasche, C., Lucchini, F., Ghidoni, R., Ferraroni, M., and La Vecchia, C. (2005) Resveratrol and breast cancer risk. *Eur J Cancer Prev* **14**, 139–42.

94. Bianchini, F., and Vainio, H. (2003) Wine and resveratrol: Mechanisms of cancer prevention? *Eur J Cancer Prev* **12**, 417–25.

95. Hanf, V., and Gonder, U. (2005) Nutrition and primary prevention of breast cancer: Foods, nutrients and breast cancer risk. *Eur J Obstet Gynecol Reprod Biol* **123**, 139–49.

96. Singletary, K.W., and Gapstur, S.M. (2001) Alcohol and breast cancer: Review of epidemiologic and experimental evidence and potential mechanisms. *JAMA* **286**, 2143–51.

97. Steinberg, J., and Goodwin, P.J. (1991) Alcohol and breast cancer risk – putting the current controversy into perspective. *Br Cancer Res Treat* **19**, 221–31.

98. Schoonen, W.M., Salinas, C.A., Kiemeney, L.A., and Stanford, J.L. (2005) Alcohol consumption and risk of prostate cancer in middle-aged men. *Int J Cancer* **113**, 133–40.

99. Zhou, J.R., Yu, L., Mai, Z., and Blackburn, G.L. (2004) Combined inhibition of estrogen-dependent human breast carcinoma by soy and tea bioactive components in mice. *Int J Cancer* **108**, 8–14.

26 Cancer Prevention by Catechins, Flavonols, and Procyanidins

Joshua D. Lambert and Chung S. Yang

Key Points

1. Dietary catechins, flavonols, and procyandins (PC) are found in a large variety of fruits, vegetables, tea, and other foods. Epidemiological studies have shown that the intake of a variety of fruits and vegetables has been supported by a lower risk of developing cancer.
2. Chemical studies have shown that these compounds have strong antioxidative activity in vitro and are capable of scavenging free radicals and chelating metal ions involved in the generation of free radicals. Given the proposed role of free radicals in aging and the development of many diseases, including cancer, it was hypothesized that compounds that prevent the development of free radicals might also prevent the development of related diseases.
3. Cancer prevention by dietary catechins, flavonols, and PC has been studied in many different animal models of carcinogenesis. These compounds have been shown to inhibit the development of cancer in animal models of oral, esophageal, forestomach, stomach, intestinal, colon, liver, prostate, skin, and breast cancers.
4. Tea catechins have been the most widely studied for cancer preventive activity and have been subjected to laboratory, epidemiological, and controlled clinical investigations. The results of studies in animal models of cancer suggest that tea catechins have cancer preventive activities against a broad range of cancer types.
5. Dietary flavonoids have a long history of safe dietary use, and human trials with higher doses of purified compounds have been conducted without serious adverse effects. However, several reports have recently suggested that these compounds may be potentially toxic. Therefore, caution should be exercised when recommending doses for human consumption, especially when considering concentrated or purified products.

Key Words: Catechins; flavonols; procyandins; free radicals; cancer

1. INTRODUCTION

Dietary catechins, flavonols, and procyandins (PC) are present in large amounts in many fruits, vegetables, tea, and other foodstuffs. The chemical structures of some representative catechins, flavonols, and PC are shown in Fig. 1. The rationale underlying

From: *Nutrition and Health: Bioactive Compounds and Cancer*
Edited by: J.A. Milner, D.F. Romagnolo, DOI 10.1007/978-1-60761-627-6_26,
© Springer Science+Business Media, LLC 2010

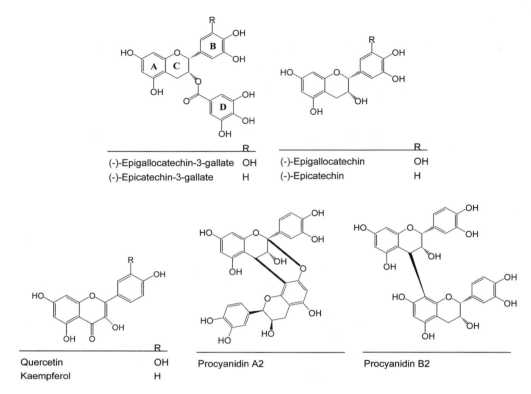

Fig. 1. Structures of biologically important catechins, flavonols, and procyanidins.

the potential efficacy of dietary catechins, flavonols, and PC as cancer preventive agents is based in part on epidemiological data linking intake of fruits and vegetables with lower risk of developing cancer *(1–3)*. Furthermore, chemical studies have shown that these compounds have strong antioxidative activity in vitro and are capable of scavenging free radicals and chelating metal ions involved in the generation of free radicals *(4, 5)*. Given the proposed role of free radicals in aging and the development of many diseases, including cancer, it was hypothesized that compounds that prevent the development of free radicals might also prevent the development of related diseases *(6–8)*. Based on these initial hypotheses, many epidemiological and laboratory studies have been conducted to determine the potential cancer preventive effects of dietary catechins, flavonols, and PC. We review these data herein.

2. ANIMAL AND IN VITRO EXPERIMENTS

2.1. Studies in Animal Models of Carcinogenesis

Cancer prevention by dietary catechins, flavonols, and PC has been studied in many different animal models of carcinogenesis (reviewed in *(9, 10)*). These compounds have been shown to inhibit the development of cancer in animal models of oral, esophageal, forestomach, stomach, intestinal, colon, liver, prostate, skin, and breast cancers.

Table 1
Animal Studies on the Cancer Preventive Effect of Tea
and Tea Polyphenols[a]

Organ site	Positive outcome	Negative outcome
Oral cavity	3	0
Esophagus	4	0
Stomach	7	0
Small intestine	8	0
Colon	10	5
Liver	7	1
Pancreas	3	0
Bladder	3	0
Lung	20	2
Skin	25	0
Breast	13	4
Prostate	6	0
Thyroid	1	0

[a]Studies reported for the years 1991–2008.

Table 1 summarizes the results of studies on tea and tea polyphenols in animal models of cancer.

Recent studies highlighted the inhibitory activity of tea preparations in animal models of tumorigenesis and provided some mechanistic data related to inhibitory effects. For example, our laboratory has extensively studied the anti-tumorigenic activities of tea polyphenols in the $APC^{min/+}$ mouse model of intestinal tumorigenesis. We have reported that EGCG, as the sole source of drinking fluid, dose-dependently (0.02–0.32% w/v) inhibited small intestinal tumorigenesis in this model (11). Inhibition of tumor multiplicity was associated with increased expression of E-cadherin and decreased levels of nuclear β-catenin, c-Myc, phospho-Akt, and phospho-extracellular regulated kinase (Erk) 1/2.

We directly compared the effectiveness of EGCG as pure compound with a defined catechin mixture, polyphenon E (PPE), containing 65% EGCG (12). Total tumor multiplicity was decreased by both dietary PPE (0.12%) and the corresponding amount of dietary EGCG (0.08%). Although there was a trend suggesting PPE was more effective than EGCG in reducing total tumor multiplicity (70 vs. 51% decrease, respectively), the difference was not statistically significant. Further studies are required to more fully elucidate whether PPE or other green tea catechin preparations are more effective than EGCG in the $APC^{min/+}$ mouse. Additional studies should also examine whether combinations of various catechins influence their cancer preventive properties.

We and others have examined the effect of PPE and EGCG on the development of aberrant crypt foci and adenomas in carcinogen-treated rats. Treatment of rats with PPE (0.12–0.24%) in the diet for 8 weeks following injection with azoxymethane (AOM) dose-dependently decreased the total number of aberrant crypt foci (ACF) per rat by 16.3 and 36.9% at 0.12 and 0.24% PPE, respectively (13). Decreases in ACF multiplicity were associated with decreased nuclear β-catenin, cyclin D_1, and retinoid X receptor α staining. The direct target of EGCG, however, remains to be investigated.

Carter et al. examined the effects of EGCG on 2-amino-1-methyl-6-pheny limidazo[4,5-*b*]pyridine (PhIP)-induced ACF in a rat model. EGCG was given during the post-initiation phase *(14)*. The treatment with EGCG for 15 weeks reduced ACF by 71% compared to water-treated controls. This decrease in ACF was associated with a 40% decrease in bromodeoxyuridine labeling in the crypt, suggesting that EGCG inhibited aberrant cell proliferation. However, the underlying mechanisms contributing to these responses remain unclear.

The treatment of TAg mice, which spontaneously develop mammary tumors, with 0.05% green tea catechins for 25 weeks has been shown to increase mean survival time (151 days compared to 144 days for controls) as well as induce a 25% reduction in tumor burden *(15)*. Inhibition of tumorigenesis was associated with increased apoptosis as well as decreased malonyldialdehyde-adducted DNA compared to water-treated controls. The authors propose that the antioxidative activity of tea catechins may play a role in the prevention of mammary carcinogenesis, although other mechanisms are also likely involved.

Studies with animal models of carcinogenesis have yielded mixed results concerning the cancer preventive activity of quercetin. For example, it was reported that 2% dietary quercetin inhibited AOM-induced hyperproliferation and focal dysplasia in mice *(16)*. Quercetin also reduced tumor incidence by 76% and tumor multiplicity by 48%. However, no inhibitory effects were observed in APC$^{min/+}$ mice treated with quercetin *(17)*. Similarly, although quercetin inhibited local, ultraviolet light B (UVB)-induced immunosuppression in SKH-1 hairless mice, it had no effect on skin tumorigenesis *(18)*. The administration of quercetin (9 μg/ml in the drinking fluid) during the initiation phase was shown to inhibit by 42% *N*-nitrosodiethylamine-induced lung tumor incidence in mice *(19)*. Tumor burden, however, was not affected. Quercetin has also been shown to inhibit dimethylbenzanthrene (DMBA)/phorbol 12-myristate 13-acetate (TPA)-induced skin tumorigenesis in mice. Topical application of 1–25 μmol quercetin inhibited tumor burden by 75–100% compared to acetone-treated controls *(20)*.

Recent studies have examined the effectiveness of parenterally-administered quercetin (i.e., either intraperitoneal or intravenous treatment). Administration of 50 mg/kg, i.v., liposomal quercetin every 3 days for 21 days inhibited the growth of subcutaneously-implanted LL/2 lung cancer tumors, CT26 colon cancer tumors, and H22 hepatoma tumors in mice by 40, 64, and 60%, respectively, compared to treatment with PBS *(21)*. Similarly, Piantelli et al. have reported that compared to controls daily dosing with 50 mg/kg, i.p., quercetin inhibited by 40% the development of B16 melanoma metastasis in C57bl/6 N mice *(22)*. The latter effects of quercetin were attributed to inhibition of expression of vascular cell adhesion molecule-1 and reduced tumor cell–endothelial cell interactions. These studies have generated interesting results regarding the antitumor activity of quercetin, but no clear recommendations for dietary supplementation with this compound can be extrapolated from these experimental data. Pharmacokinetic parameters including peak plasma and tissue levels are expected to be quite different depending on route of administration. For example, quercetin in the diet is present largely as glycoside conjugates, whereas these studies have used pure quercetin aglycone.

Procyandins have been studied in a number of different animal models of carcinogenesis. Work by Katiyar et al. demonstrated the potential efficacy and mechanisms of action of grape seed PC against UVB-induced skin tumorigenesis. In a study that examined the effects of photocarcinogenesis induced by UVB, the dietary administration of 0.2–0.5% grape seed PC reduced in a dose-dependent fashion tumor incidence, multiplicity, and size by 20–95, 46–95, and 29–94%, respectively, compared to controls *(23)*. In addition, the treatment with grape seed PC inhibited the transformation of tumors from papilloma to carcinoma. Compared to controls, the treatment with 0.5% PC for 21 weeks decreased by 64% the conversion to carcinoma. There was an association between inhibition of tumorigenesis and decreased body fat without change in overall body mass. Later studies by the same group suggested that the inhibition of skin tumorigenesis by PC was related to antioxidative and immunostimulatory effects. The treatment with UVB lowered skin levels of reduced glutathione (GSH), glutathione peroxidase (GPx), and catalase *(24)*. The treatment with 0.2 and 0.5% PC attenuated these decreases and prevented the formation of UVB-induced reactive oxygen species (ROS) in the skin *(24)*. One interesting possible mechanism of action is related to the cytokine interleukin (IL)-12, which is associated with response to DNA damage. UVB treatment induces immune suppression, which is abrogated by treatment with PC *(25)*. This abrogation is related to induction of IL-12 expression by PC. This prevention of immune suppression may lead to better immune surveillance of pre-cancerous cells and enhanced DNA repair.

PC have been shown to inhibit ACF in rat models of colon tumorigenesis. Treatment of AOM-pretreated rats with 0.025% PCB_2 significantly inhibited the formation of ACF *(26)*. This inhibition was associated with increased apoptosis and decreased cell proliferation. The administration of 0.01% PC in the drinking fluid of 1,7-dimethylhydrazine (DMH)-treated rats for 6 weeks inhibited by 50% the formation of ACF compared to water-treated control rats *(27)*. Based on results obtained with cell culture models, it has been suggested that PC may inhibit carcinogen-induced upregulation of ornithine decarboxylase (ODC) and polyamine biosynthesis. Previous work by Singletary and Meline had shown that the treatment of AOM-treated rats with 0.1–1% PC decreased ODC levels in the distal colon, which correlated with decreased ACF formation *(28)*.

Because of their large molecular weight and potential poor bioavailability, it remains unclear whether PC may exert protective effects against mammary tumorigenesis. The treatment for 48 weeks with 0.25% cacao PC did not significantly inhibit PhIP-induced mammary tumors in rats *(29)*. Likewise, PC did not inhibit the development of DMBA-induced mammary tumors in rats *(28)*. Currently, data pertaining to the effects of PC on prostate cancer in vivo are lacking.

2.2. In Vitro Studies

Based on the results of studies with human cancer cell lines, several mechanisms have been proposed to explain the cancer preventive activity of dietary catechins, flavonols, and PC (Fig. 2). This work has been extensively reviewed and important potential

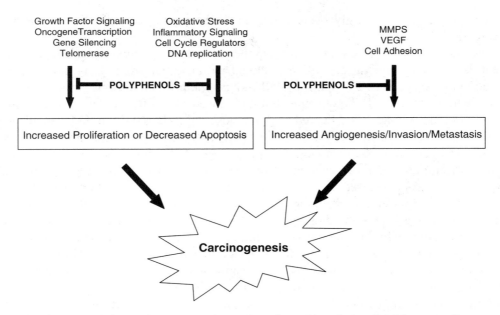

Fig. 2. Potential cancer chemopreventive targets of catechins, flavonols, and procyandins.

mechanisms include inhibition of key cellular enzymes (e.g., mitogen-activated protein (MAP) kinases, topoisomerase, and DNA methyltransferase), growth factor signaling (e.g., epidermal growth factor (EGF) and insulin-like growth factor (IGF)), transcription factors (e.g., nuclear factor kappa B (NFκB) and activator protein 1 (AP-1)), and induction of oxidative stress and DNA damage (reviewed in *(6, 10, 30–35))*. The end results of these effects could be the induction of apoptosis, inhibition of tumor cell growth, and/or the inhibition of angiogenesis *(30, 32, 33, 36)*. Most of these effects are observed at concentrations of the test compound greater than 10 μM. However, for many dietary polyphenols, especially higher molecular weight PC, such concentrations are not typically achievable in human plasma and tissues following consumption of normal dietary doses. This raises questions about the relevance of many of these mechanisms to cancer prevention in humans

In some experimental systems, so-called high-affinity targets have been identified for tea catechins including EGCG. These include 20S proteasome chymotryptic activity, the 67-kDa laminin receptor, vimentin, and Bcl-2, which are inhibited in the submicromolar concentration range *(37–40)*. Although these data are exciting, such potency has only been observed in cell-free systems and subsequent experiments in whole cells required much higher concentrations to achieve the same effect as well as cell death. This loss of potency is likely due to the non-specific binding of EGCG to cellular macromolecules and would be expected to increase in vivo. Furthermore, the general applicability of these mechanisms for cancer prevention remains unknown.

Discrepancies between effective concentrations used in cell line studies and those tested in animal studies (which are typically much lower) suggest that results of in vitro studies may be irrelevant for cancer prevention in vivo. Whereas no clear cut answer is currently available, one may argue that animals and humans ingest chronic levels of dietary polyphenols. Therefore, though concentrations of dietary polyphenols may be lower than those achievable experimentally, the prolonged exposure may produce significant preventive effects. This contention seems consistent with the observation that treatment of cancer cells with EGCG for longer periods of time (3 or 4 days) has stronger inhibitory effects compared to treatment for 1 or 2 days *(41)*. There is, however, no quantitative model that correlates the effective concentration of certain compounds used in vitro to the plasma and tissue concentrations observed in animals or humans. We thus believe that the mechanisms of cancer prevention for many bioactive food compounds should be demonstrated in vivo before inferences can be made about the development of preventive dietary strategies.

3. EPIDEMIOLOGICAL STUDIES

Although both animal model and cell culture studies have demonstrated the cancer preventive potential of dietary catechins, flavonols, and PC, epidemiological data on such activities are lacking or inconsistent *(9, 42–45)*. We have summarized the available epidemiological data for green tea in Table 2.

Table 2
Epidemiological Studies on the Cancer Preventive Effects of Green Tea

	Cohort studies				*Case–control studies*			
	Reduced risk	No association	Increased risk	Total	Reduced risk	No association	Increased risk	Total
Esophagus	0	0	2	2	3	2	2	7
Stomach	2	6	0	8	7	7	1	15
Colon	1	4	0	5	4	2	1	7
Pancreas	0	1	0	1	1	0	0	1
Kidney/ bladder	0	1	0	1	0	1	2	3
Lung	0	2	0	2	2	3	1	6
Prostate	1	0	0	1	1	0	0	1
Breast	2	4	0	6	3	0	0	3
Ovarian	1	0	0	1	1	0	0	1
Other	2	3	0	5	1	2	0	3

3.1. Tea Consumption and Cancer

Many case–control studies have shown that subjects who consume large amounts of tea had lower cancer risk. In particular, the risk of gastric and esophageal cancers was lower in green tea consumers in Japan and China. For example, Gao et al. reported in 1994 that green tea consumption was associated with a reduced risk of esophageal cancer *(46)*. From the Shanghai Cancer Registry, 1,016 eligible cases of esophageal cancer were identified and control subject records were selected by frequency matching in accordance with the age–sex distribution. Patient interviews were then conducted using a structured, standardized questionnaire to obtain information on demographic characteristics, residential history, height and weight, diet, smoking, alcohol and tea drinking, medical history, family history of cancer, occupation, physical activity, and reproductive history. After adjustment for known confounders, a protective effect for green tea was observed in women. For women consuming 1–14.9 g of dry green tea leaves per month (one cup of tea typically contains 2 g tea leaves), the odds ratio (OR) was 0.77 (95% CI: 0.39–1.53) whereas for those consuming ≥ 15 g tea/month, the OR was 0.34 (95% CI: 0.17–0.69). Among men, the OR was 0.80, although not statistically significant. In another study, green tea drinking was found to be inversely associated with the risk of stomach cancer, with OR of 0.77 (95% CI: 0.52–1.13) among female and 0.76 (CI: 55–1.27) among male heavy tea drinkers *(47)*.

In a more recent study, our group investigated the association between pre-diagnostic urinary tea polyphenols, their metabolites, and the risk of developing gastric and esophageal cancers. Using a nested case–control design, we compared 190 incident cases of gastric cancer and 46 cases of esophageal cancer with 772 control subjects from the Shanghai cohort (18,244 men aged 45–64 years at recruitment). Urinary tea polyphenols, including (–)-epigallocatechin (EGC) and (–)-epicatechin (EC), and their respective metabolites (–)-5-(3′,4′,5′-trihydroxyphenyl)-γ-valerolactone (M4) and (–)-5-(3′,4′-dihydroxyphenyl)-γ-valerolactone (M6), were measured in all study subjects by high performance liquid chromatography *(48)*. Urinary EGC positivity showed a statistically significant inverse association with gastric cancer (OR = 0.52, 95% CI = 0.28–0.97) after adjustment for confounders such as *Helicobactor pylori* seropositivity, smoking, alcohol consumption, and level of serum carotenoids. The protective effect was primarily seen among subjects with low (below population median) serum carotenoids. Similar tea polyphenol–cancer risk associations were observed for combined risk of gastric cancer and esophageal cancer *(49)*.

A population-based case–control study was conducted in Yangzhong, China, that included 133 stomach cancer cases, 166 chronic gastritis cases, and 433 healthy controls. An inverse association was observed between green tea drinking and chronic gastritis and stomach cancer risks. After adjusting for age, gender, education, body mass index, pack-years of smoking, and alcohol consumption, the OR of green tea consumption was 0.52 (95% CI: 0.29–0.94) and 0.49 (95% CI: 0.31–0.77) for stomach cancer and chronic gastritis, respectively. In addition, there were dose–response relationships between years of green tea drinking and both diseases. This was the first report documenting that green tea drinking was found to be protective against chronic gastritis. These results may be important when designing intervention strategies for stomach cancer and its pre-malignant lesions in high-risk populations *(50)*.

Tea consumption has been associated with reduced risk of cancer at sites other than the gastrointestinal tract. For example, a population-based case–control study of breast cancer was conducted among women of Asian descent living in Los Angeles to investigate the effect of green and black tea *(51)*. Green tea drinkers had a significantly reduced risk of breast cancer that was dose-dependent (OR = 0.71 and 0.53 for consumption of 0–85.7 ml and >85.7 ml of tea/day, respectively). Among women who carried at least one low-activity catechol-*O*-methyltransferase (COMT) allele, the effect was even stronger, and black tea was also found to reduce risk *(52)*. The effect of black tea had not been observed in the original study *(51)*. The authors concluded that women with a low-activity COMT allele may have a reduced risk of breast cancer because they metabolize tea polyphenols less efficiently and, therefore, have prolonged exposure to these compounds compared to women with normal COMT activity.

Recently, the Japanese Public Health Center-Based Prospective Study (JPHC) reported an association between green tea consumption and decreased risk of advanced prostate cancer *(53)*. In a cohort of 49,920 men (aged 40–69), a dose-dependent decrease in risk of advanced prostate cancer was observed (p for trend = 0.01). The OR for men consuming greater than five cups/day was 0.52. There was no association between tea consumption and risk of localized prostate cancer.

Although these studies demonstrate an association between tea consumption and decreased risk of cancer, other studies have not observed this protective effect. For example, a review of 21 epidemiological investigations of gastrointestinal cancer or pre-cancerous lesions suggested a protective effect of green tea on adenomatous polyps and chronic atrophic gastritis formation, but no clear support for the preventive role of green tea against stomach and intestinal cancer *(54)*. In two prospective Japanese studies, green tea was not associated with decreased breast cancer risk even in women drinking five or more cups of tea per day *(55)*. In the Ohsaki National Health Insurance Cohort Study conducted in Japan, after an 11-year follow-up, green tea consumption was associated with decreased mortality due to cardiovascular diseases, but no association was observed with cancer deaths *(56)*.

One possible explanation for the conflicting results of epidemiological studies related to tea consumption may be study design. In general, case–control studies are considered less powerful than prospective studies, because of the many confounding factors associated with the case–control design. As discussed by Tsubono et al. individuals with stomach conditions that predispose to gastric cancer may refrain from drinking green tea because of stomach irritation *(57)*. However, in the two nested case–control studies based on the Shanghai cohort, lower incidence of gastric and colon cancers was associated with green tea consumption *(49, 58)*. The protective effects of green tea against gastric cancer were only observed in individuals that had been followed for 4 years or longer.

The population selected may play a critical role in demonstrating the possible beneficial effects of tea consumption. As discussed above, a greater protective effect of tea against breast cancer was observed in women with at least one low-activity allele of COMT. In collaboration with Dr. Mimi C. Yu, we have also demonstrated the importance of nutritional status *(49)*. In particular, we have reported that the protective effects of tea against colon cancer was more clearly seen in subjects with lower serum levels of carotenoids, suggesting that the benefits of tea may be more readily manifested in subjects with low antioxidative nutritional status.

An important issue in epidemiological studies on tea is the quantity and quality of the tea consumed and accurate determination of tea consumption. Questions have been raised as to whether the lack of protective effects observed in prospective studies in Japan was due to insufficient amounts of tea consumed or the possible lower levels of effective constituents (presumably polyphenols) present in the green tea consumed by the cohort. Reliance on questions of "number of cups of tea consumed per day" represents a potential weakness in many epidemiological studies. In future studies, it will be important to report more precise quantitative and qualitative information of tea consumption. To report in "grams of tea consumed per month" is a good approach, especially when loose tea leaves are consumed and the habit of making tea is known. Likewise objective measurements of exposure biomarkers, such as the catechins and their metabolites, in the urine or in the plasma could be very useful and should be further utilized in epidemiological studies.

3.2. Dietary Flavonols, PC, and Cancer

The possible association between dietary flavonols, including quercetin, has been reviewed previously *(59–61)*. These reports have generally found an inverse correlation between intake of dietary flavonols and risk of cancers of the gastrointestinal (GI) tract, the lung, the breast, and other sites. Here, we will discuss some of the more recent studies and focus on associations between the structurally related compounds, quercetin and kaempferol.

Studies conducted in the United States and Finland have reported on an inverse relationship between flavonol consumption and risk of pancreatic cancer. A prospective study of the multiethnic cohort in Hawaii and California ($n = 183,518$) found a strong, dose-dependent decrease in relative risk (RR) of pancreatic cancer with increasing consumption of total dietary flavonols (RR $= 0.77$ in the highest quintile, $p = 0.046$ for trend) and dietary kaempferol (RR $= 0.78$ in the highest quintile, $p = 0.017$) *(62)*. When data were stratified by sex or smoking status, strong effects were observed for kaempferol in women (RR $= 0.72$ in the highest quartile) and kaempferol and quercetin in current smokers (RR $= 0.27$ and 0.55 in the highest quartile for kaempferol and quercetin, respectively).

In the Finnish study, a prospective analysis of the relationship between pancreatic cancer and flavonol intake was conducted in the α-tocopherol, β-carotene Cancer Prevention Study cohort ($n = 27,111$ healthy male smokers) *(44)*. In subjects that were not supplemented with α-tocopherol and β-carotene as part of the original intervention study, there was a significant dose-dependent inverse correlation between intake of total dietary flavonols ($p = 0.04$ for trend) and kaempferol ($p = 0.009$ for trend) and cancer risk. There was an inverse trend between dietary quercetin and risk of pancreatic cancer, but the effect was not significant ($p = 0.06$ for trend). Importantly, in subjects supplemented with α-tocopherol and β-carotene, the protective effects were not observed. This difference in outcomes suggests that antioxidant vitamin status may be a confounding factor as previously suggested for tea polyphenols.

A population-based case–control study was conducted in Los Angeles county, California, to study the relationship between flavonoid intake and lung cancer risk. Lung cancer cases ($n = 558$) were age and sex matched with controls ($n = 837$). A significant dose-dependent inverse relationship was observed between lung cancer and quercetin ($p = 0.025$ for trend) and kaempferol ($p = 0.0079$ for trend) intake *(63)*. This trend was observed only among current smokers whereas no protective effects were observed in non-smokers. Surprisingly, there was no significant association between total flavonoids and lung cancer risk.

A large prospective case–control study ($n = 1,456$ for both cases and control) of colon cancer found a significant inverse relationship between dietary quercetin intake (OR = 0.68, $p = 0.001$ for trend) and PC intake (OR = 0.78, $p = 0.031$ for trend) *(64)*. The study, conducted in Scotland, also included an analysis of food frequency questionnaires. This analysis revealed that tea, onions, and soups accounted for 52.1, 13.7, and 9.2% of quercetin intake, respectively. Tea, apples, and red wine accounted for 74.2, 11.2, and 8.4% of PC intake.

One epidemiological study that reported on the cancer preventive effects of PC is the Iowa Women's Heath Study *(43)*. In this prospective cohort study of 34,708 post-menopausal women, the authors found a strong, dose-dependent inverse relationship between PC intake and risk of lung cancer ($p < 0.01$ for trend). When data were stratified by smoking status, the protective effect was found in smokers ($p = 0.04$ for trend) but not in non-smokers ($p = 0.44$ for trend).

4. INTERVENTION STUDIES IN HUMANS

Several human studies have been conducted examining the effects of dietary cate-chins, flavonols, and PC on surrogate biomarkers of cancer such as effects on oxidative stress markers and carcinogen metabolism. For example, Hakim et al. found that supple-mentation of heavy smokers (>10 cigarettes/day) with four cups of decaffeinated green tea (73.5 mg catechins/cup) per day for 4 months reduced by 31% urinary 8-OHdG levels compared to control *(65)*. In a recent study in China, the treatment with 500 or 1,000 mg/day green tea polyphenols for 3 months increased by 10- and 8.4-fold, respectively, the urinary excretion of the mercapturic acid conjugated of aflatoxin B_1 (AFB_1) compared to baseline *(66)*. Similarly, in a pilot study by Schwartz et al. heavy smokers treated with green tea (400–500 mg green tea powder/cup) five times/day for 4 weeks had 50% lower levels of benzo[a]pyrene-DNA adducts and 8-hydroxy-2′-deoxyguanosine (8-OHdG) compared to control subjects *(67)*.

A recent double-blind study by Bettuzzi et al. followed 200 individuals with high-grade prostate intraepithelial neoplasia (PIN) receiving either 600 mg of green tea cat-echins daily or placebo (100 individuals in each group) for 12 months. Only 3% of the patients in the catechin treatment group developed prostate cancer, whereas the rate of cancer development on the placebo group was 30% *(68)*. No adverse effects were asso-ciated with the treatment. The impact of these results would be tremendous if they could be reproduced in similar trials with a larger number of subjects.

Previously, a Phase I study of green tea extract in patients with advanced lung cancer found that a dose of up to 3 g/m^2/day for 16 weeks was well tolerated, but produced no objective response in tumor volume *(69)*. Although the results of this study were negative, the study size was small ($n = 17$) and the disease stage was likely inappro-priate since most dietary components lack sufficient potency to affect late-stage cancer of any type. More interesting data are likely to be generated from an ongoing Phase II chemoprevention trial is currently being conducted by a consortium of cancer centers and universities in Canada and in the United States in former heavy smokers using PPE.

The effects of dietary flavonols and PC on antioxidant status in human volun-teers have been studied by multiple investigators (reviewed in *(70)*). Pure compounds, extracts, and foods have been examined. Although these compounds affected some markers, they had no effect on others. For example, supplementation with a "phenol-rich" diet, containing 21 mg quercetin and 9 mg kaempferol, for 6 days increased erythrocyte superoxide dismutase activity and decreased lymphocyte DNA damage, but had no effect on plasma α-tocopherol and β-carotene *(71)*. Another study of stable diabetic patients treated for 14 days with onion and tea (76–110 mg quercetin) found a decrease in oxidative damage to lymphocytes, but reported no effects on superoxide dismutase activity, GPx, plasma ascorbic acid, or α-tocopherol *(72)*. Several studies of PC-containing preparations have shown that treatment of human volunteers improved plasma antioxidant activity and decreased markers of oxidative stress including thiobarbituric acid reactive substances and nitrosylated plasma proteins *(70)*. Further human intervention studies are needed to more accurately assess the cancer chemopreventive effects of flavonols and PC.

5. TISSUE SPECIFICITY AND TOTALITY OF EVIDENCE

No significant tissue specificities have been identified for the potential cancer preventive activities of dietary catechins, flavonols, or PC. The lack of tissue specificity may be due to the low number of human intervention studies on the efficacy of these compounds against tumorigenesis at various sites. One potential factor, which may result in tissue-specific chemopreventive efficacy, is the bioavailability of many dietary catechins, flavonols, and PC *(73, 74)*.

Many of these compounds are predicted to have moderate to poor absorption based on physical and chemical characteristics including large number of hydrogen bond donors (four or more phenolic hydroxyl groups), relatively high molecular weights (>400 g/mol), the presence of hydrogen bond acceptors (ketone groups), and the formation of a large hydration shell due to hydrogen bonding with water *(75, 76)*. Additionally, both catechins and flavonols have been shown to undergo extensive biotransformation including methylation, glucuronidation, sulfation, and ring-fission metabolism *(74, 77–79)*. These properties will all work to limit the bioavailability of these compounds and may lead to preferential efficacy in GI tract and on the skin, where direct contact with high doses of test compounds is possible. This seems to be supported by the available animal model data, which show that catechins and PC have inhibitory activity against colon cancer, but are less efficacious against mammary tumorigenesis *(28)*. Similarly, the majority of epidemiological studies of tea catechins which have shown an inverse correlation between tea consumption and cancer risk involve prevention of cancers of the GI tract *(80)*.

The totality of the evidence regarding cancer prevention by dietary catechins, flavonols, and PC suggests that these compounds have cancer preventive efficacy. Tea catechins have been the most widely studied for cancer preventive activity and have been subjected to laboratory, epidemiological, and controlled clinical investigations. The results of studies in animal models of cancer (Table 1) suggest that tea catechins have cancer preventive activities against a broad range of cancer types. The number of intervention studies with modulation of cancer or cancer biomarkers has been more limited, but the results are mostly positive in terms of the potential efficacy of tea catechins.

The mechanisms of action of dietary catechins, flavonols, and PC remain unclear. All of these compounds bind extensively and non-specifically to a large number of proteins possibly leading to partial inhibition of multiple, likely overlapping, pathways. These combined effects of polyphenols may be responsible for the observed cell growth inhibition and apoptosis in vitro and cancer prevention in vivo.

6. FUTURE RESEARCH

The effects of dietary catechins, flavonols, and PC on cancer development are important public health issues. In order to gain a better understanding of the potential benefits associated with dietary intake of these compounds, the following lines of research should be developed:

(1) *To firmly establish the efficacy of dietary catechins, flavonols, and PC as cancer preventive compounds in humans.* In the case of dietary catechins and flavonols, there is a significant body of epidemiological and animal model data to suggest efficacy as cancer preventive agents (reviewed in the preceding sections). In order to clearly establish efficacy in humans, carefully controlled intervention studies in at risk populations are needed. For dietary PC, which have not been studied as extensively, further animal and epidemiological studies are needed. Care should be exercised in the design of animal studies to select models and doses that are physiologically relevant to humans. Epidemiological studies should include accurate exposure biomarkers for these polyphenols to reduce potential confounders such as recall bias.

(2) *To determine the mechanisms responsible for the cancer preventive activities of these compounds in vivo.* As mentioned above, the interpretation and extrapolation of in vitro mechanistic data to explain in vivo cancer chemopreventive activity remains a problematic area. We believe that carefully designed animal model studies, including short-term investigations, with mechanism-based endpoints represent powerful means to define the mechanisms of action of dietary catechins, flavonols, and PC. Furthermore, the robustness of data derived from in vitro studies could be improved by knowledge of the bioavailability of the test compound.

(3) *To clearly define safe levels of intake for these compounds in order to avoid adverse effects.* Consumption of dietary catechins, flavonols, and PC has generally been regarded as safe. Nevertheless, the potential adverse effects of these compounds given at high doses in pharmacological preparations remain largely unknown and represent an area for future investigation.

7. CONCLUSIONS AND RECOMMENDATIONS FOR INTAKE

Dietary flavonoids have a long history of safe dietary use, and human trials with higher doses of purified compounds have been conducted without serious adverse effects. However, several reports have recently suggested that these compounds may be potentially toxic. Therefore, caution should be exercised when recommending doses for human consumption, especially when considering concentrated or purified products. For example, several cases of hepatotoxicity have been associated with consumption of high doses of green tea-containing dietary supplements (10–29 mg/kg/day p.o.) *(81)*. Patients presented with elevated serum alanine aminotransferase and bilirubin levels, and a minority of patients exhibited periportal and portal inflammations. After cessation of supplement use, these symptoms were eliminated. In at least one case, re-injury was observed following re-challenge with the same preparations *(81)*. This phenomenon supports a causative role for the supplement in the observed hepatotoxicity.

These case reports are supported by studies in laboratory animals. Oral administration of Teavigo (a green tea polyphenol preparation containing 90% EGCG) or polyphenon E for 13 or 9 weeks, respectively, to Beagle dogs resulted in dose-dependent toxicity and death *(82)*. Vomiting and diarrhea were observed throughout both studies. In addition, 500 mg/kg, p.o., Teavigo caused proximal tubule necrosis and elevated serum bilirubin in all dogs treated. Elevated serum aspartate aminotransferase levels and liver necrosis were observed in some dogs. Oral administration of 2,000 mg/kg, i.g., Teavigo to rats resulted in lethality in 80% of animals treated *(82)*. Death was due to hemorrhagic lesions in both the stomach and the intestine.

These data suggest that high doses of EGCG can induce toxicity in the liver, kidneys, and intestine. Toxicity, especially in the liver and kidney, appears to be correlated with the bioavailability of EGCG. In the rat, where bioavailability is low ($F = 1.6\%$), toxicity is confined to the GI tract following oral administration *(83)*. In the dog, where bioavailability is much higher, hepatotoxicity and nephrotoxicity, as well as intestinal toxicity, were observed. Toxicity was greater in fasted, than in pre-fed, dogs *(82)*.

Although there are limited in vivo data concerning the potential toxicities of flavonols, they can be predicted to have similar effects at high doses. Possible areas of concern have been suggested by epidemiological and in vitro studies. For example, an epidemiological study suggested a link between maternal intake of dietary topoisomerase inhibitors II, including flavonoids, and development of acute myeloid leukemia (AML) in the offspring ($p = 0.04$ for trend with OR = 9.8 (95% CI: 1.1–84.8) and 10.2 (95% CI = 1.1–96.4) for medium and high consumption, respectively) *(84)*. Cell line studies with purified flavonoids (including quercetin, luteolin, and kaempferol) have suggested that the mechanistic basis for this increased risk is inhibition of topoisomerase II activity in the fetus, which results in chromosomal translocation at chromosome 11q23 involving the mixed-lineage leukemia *(MLL)* gene *(85)*. The most potent inhibitors were quercetin (25 μM) and fisetin (25 μM). Although studies have shown that administration of higher doses of purified flavonoids could result in serum levels equivalent to or higher than those necessary to cause chromosomal translocation in cell line studies, it is not clear whether such concentrations are achieved in fetal tissues at normal, dietary flavonoid consumption *(85)*.

Finally, in vivo studies with animal models and surveillance in human intervention studies are needed to establish the increased risk, if any, of adverse effects due to treatment with high levels of catechins, flavonols, and PC.

ACKNOWLEDGMENTS

This work was supported by AICR Grant 05A047 (to JDL), NIH grants CA125780 and AT004678 (to JDL), and NIH grants CA120915, CA122474 and CA133021 (to CSY).

REFERENCES

1. Block, G., Patterson, B., and Subar, A. (1992) Fruit, vegetables, and cancer prevention: A review of the epidemiological evidence. *Nutr Cancer* **18**, 1–29.
2. Kobayashi, M., Tsubono, Y., Sasazuki, S., Sasaki, S., and Tsugane, S. (2002) Vegetables, fruit and risk of gastric cancer in Japan: A 10-year follow-up of the JPHC Study Cohort I. *Int J Cancer* **102**, 39–44.
3. Steinmetz, K.A., and Potter, J.D. (1991) Vegetables, fruit, and cancer. I. Epidemiology. *Cancer Causes Control* **2**, 325–57.
4. Morel, I., Lescoat, G., Cogrel, P., Sergent, O., Pasdeloup, N., Brissot, P., Cillard, P., and Cillard, J. (1993) Antioxidant and iron-chelating activities of the flavonoids catechin, quercetin and diosmetin on iron-loaded rat hepatocyte cultures. *Biochem Pharmacol* **45**, 13–19.
5. Russo, A., Acquaviva, R., Campisi, A., Sorrenti, V., Di Giacomo, C., Virgata, G., Barcellona, M.L., and Vanella, A. (2000) Bioflavonoids as antiradicals, antioxidants and DNA cleavage protectors. *Cell Biol Toxicol* **16**, 91–98.
6. Valko, M., Rhodes, C.J., Moncol, J., Izakovic, M., and Mazur, M. (2006) Free radicals, metals and antioxidants in oxidative stress-induced cancer. *Chem Biol Interact* **160**, 1–40.
7. Alvarez-Gonzalez, R. (1999) Free radicals, oxidative stress, and DNA metabolism in human cancer. *Cancer Invest* **17**, 376–7.
8. Dreher, D., and Junod, A.F. (1996) Role of oxygen free radicals in cancer development. *Eur J Cancer* **32A**, 30–38.
9. Yang, C.S., Maliakal, P., and Meng, X. (2002) Inhibition of carcinogenesis by tea. *Annu Rev Pharmacol Toxicol* **42**, 25–54.
10. Lambert, J.D., Hong, J., Yang, G.Y., Liao, J., and Yang, C.S. (2005) Inhibition of carcinogenesis by polyphenols: Evidence from laboratory investigations. *Am J Clin Nutr* **81**, 284S–91S.
11. Ju, J., Hong, J., Zhou, J.N., Pan, Z., Bose, M., Liao, J., Yang, G.Y., Liu, Y.Y., Hou, Z., Lin, Y., Ma, J., Shih, W.J., Carothers, A.M., and Yang, C.S. (2005) Inhibition of intestinal tumorigenesis in Apcmin/+ mice by (–)-epigallocatechin-3-gallate, the major catechin in green tea. *Cancer Res* **65**, 10623–31.
12. Hao, X., Bose, M., Lambert, J.D., Ju, J., Lu, G., Lee, M.J., Park, S., Husain, A., Wang, S., Sun, Y., and Yang, C.S. (2007) Inhibition of intestinal tumorigenesis in Apc(min/+) mice by green tea polyphenols (polyphenon E) and individual catechins. *Nutr Cancer* **59**, 62–69.
13. Xiao, H., Hao, X., Simi, B., Ju, J., Jiang, H., Reddy, B.S., and Yang, C.S. (2008) Green tea polyphenols inhibit colorectal aberrant crypt foci (ACF) formation and prevent oncogenic changes in dysplastic ACF in azoxymethane-treated F344 rats. *Carcinogenesis* **29**, 113–9.
14. Carter, O., Dashwood, R.H., Wang, R., Dashwood, W.M., Orner, G.A., Fischer, K.A., Lohr, C.V., Pereira, C.B., Bailey, G.S., and Williams, D.E. (2007) Comparison of white tea, green tea, epigallocatechin-3-gallate, and caffeine as inhibitors of PhIP-induced colonic aberrant crypts. *Nutr Cancer* **58**, 60–65.
15. Kaur, S., Greaves, P., Cooke, D.N., Edwards, R., Steward, W.P., Gescher, A.J., and Marczylo, T.H. (2007) Breast cancer prevention by green tea catechins and black tea theaflavins in the C3(1) SV40 T, t antigen transgenic mouse model is accompanied by increased apoptosis and a decrease in oxidative DNA adducts. *J Agric Food Chem* **55**, 3378–85.
16. Deschner, E.E., Ruperto, J., Wong, G., and Newmark, H.L. (1991) Quercetin and rutin as inhibitors of azoxymethanol-induced colonic neoplasia. *Carcinogenesis* **12**, 1193–6.
17. Mahmoud, N.N., Carothers, A.M., Grunberger, D., Bilinski, R.T., Churchill, M.R., Martucci, C., Newmark, H.L., and Bertagnolli, M.M. (2000) Plant phenolics decrease intestinal tumors in an animal model of familial adenomatous polyposis. *Carcinogenesis* **21**, 921–7.
18. Steerenberg, P.A., Garssen, J., Dortant, P.M., van der Vliet, H., Geerse, E., Verlaan, A.P., Goettsch, W.G., Sontag, Y., Bueno-de-Mesquita, H.B., and Van Loveren, H. (1997) The effect of oral quercetin on UVB-induced tumor growth and local immunosuppression in SKH-1. *Cancer Lett* **114**, 187–9.
19. Khanduja, K.L., Gandhi, R.K., Pathania, V., and Syal, N. (1999) Prevention of N-nitrosodiethylamine-induced lung tumorigenesis by ellagic acid and quercetin in mice. *Food Chem Toxicol* **37**, 313–8.
20. Soleas, G.J., Grass, L., Josephy, P.D., Goldberg, D.M., and Diamandis, E.P. (2002) A comparison of the anticarcinogenic properties of four red wine polyphenols. *Clin Biochem* **35**, 119–24.

21. Yuan, Z.P., Chen, L.J., Fan, L.Y., Tang, M.H., Yang, G.L., Yang, H.S., Du, X.B., Wang, G.Q., Yao, W.X., Zhao, Q.M., Ye, B., Wang, R., Diao, P., Zhang, W., Wu, H.B., Zhao, X., and Wei, Y.Q. (2006) Liposomal quercetin efficiently suppresses growth of solid tumors in murine models. *Clin Cancer Res* **12**, 3193–9.

22. Piantelli, M., Rossi, C., Iezzi, M., La Sorda, R., Iacobelli, S., Alberti, S., and Natali, P.G. (2006) Flavonoids inhibit melanoma lung metastasis by impairing tumor cells endothelium interactions. *J Cell Physiol* **207**, 23–29.

23. Mittal, A., Elmets, C.A., and Katiyar, S.K. (2003) Dietary feeding of proanthocyanidins from grape seeds prevents photocarcinogenesis in SKH-1 hairless mice: Relationship to decreased fat and lipid peroxidation. *Carcinogenesis* **24**, 1379–88.

24. Sharma, S.D., Meeran, S.M., and Katiyar, S.K. (2007) Dietary grape seed proanthocyanidins inhibit UVB-induced oxidative stress and activation of mitogen-activated protein kinases and nuclear factor-kappaB signaling in in vivo SKH-1 hairless mice. *Mol Cancer Ther* **6**, 995–1005.

25. Sharma, S.D., and Katiyar, S.K. (2006) Dietary grape-seed proanthocyanidin inhibition of ultraviolet B-induced immune suppression is associated with induction of IL-12. *Carcinogenesis* **27**, 95–102.

26. Nomoto, H., Iigo, M., Hamada, H., Kojima, S., and Tsuda, H. (2004) Chemoprevention of colorectal cancer by grape seed proanthocyanidin is accompanied by a decrease in proliferation and increase in apoptosis. *Nutr Cancer* **49**, 81–88.

27. Gosse, F., Guyot, S., Roussi, S., Lobstein, A., Fischer, B., Seiler, N., and Raul, F. (2005) Chemopreventive properties of apple procyanidins on human colon cancer-derived metastatic SW620 cells and in a rat model of colon carcinogenesis. *Carcinogenesis* **26**, 1291–5.

28. Singletary, K.W., and Meline, B. (2001) Effect of grape seed proanthocyanidins on colon aberrant crypts and breast tumors in a rat dual-organ tumor model. *Nutr Cancer* **39**, 252–8.

29. Yamagishi, M., Natsume, M., Osakabe, N., Nakamura, H., Furukawa, F., Imazawa, T., Nishikawa, A., and Hirose, M. (2002) Effects of cacao liquor proanthocyanidins on PhIP-induced mutagenesis in vitro, and in vivo mammary and pancreatic tumorigenesis in female Sprague-Dawley rats. *Cancer Lett* **185**, 123–30.

30. Hou, Z., Lambert, J.D., Chin, K.V., and Yang, C.S. (2004) Effects of tea polyphenols on signal transduction pathways related to cancer chemoprevention. *Mutat Res* **555**, 3–19.

31. Yang, C.S., Lambert, J.D., Hou, Z., Ju, J., Lu, G., and Hao, X. (2006) Molecular targets for the cancer preventive activity of tea polyphenols. *Mol Carcinog* **45**, 431–5.

32. Nichenametla, S.N., Taruscio, T.G., Barney, D.L., and Exon, J.H. (2006) A review of the effects and mechanisms of polyphenolics in cancer. *Crit Rev Food Sci Nutr* **46**, 161–83.

33. Yang, C.S., Landau, J.M., Huang, M.T., and Newmark, H.L. (2001) Inhibition of carcinogenesis by dietary polyphenolic compounds. *Annu Rev Nutr* **21**, 381–406.

34. Khan, N., Afaq, F., Saleem, M., Ahmad, N., and Mukhtar, H. (2006) Targeting multiple signaling pathways by green tea polyphenol (–)-epigallocatechin-3-gallate. *Cancer Res* **66**, 2500–5.

35. Brownson, D.M., Azios, N.G., Fuqua, B.K., Dharmawardhane, S.F., and Mabry, T.J. (2002) Flavonoid effects relevant to cancer. *J Nutr* **132**, 3482S–9S.

36. Gupta, S., Hastak, K., Ahmad, N., Lewin, J.S., and Mukhtar, H. (2001) Inhibition of prostate carcinogenesis in TRAMP mice by oral infusion of green tea polyphenols. *Proc Natl Acad Sci USA* **98**, 10350–5.

37. Nam, S., Smith, D.M., and Dou, Q.P. (2001) Ester bond-containing tea polyphenols potently inhibit proteasome activity in vitro and in vivo. *J Biol Chem* **276**, 13322–30.

38. Tachibana, H., Koga, K., Fujimura, Y., and Yamada, K. (2004) A receptor for green tea polyphenol EGCG. *Nat Struct Mol Biol* **11**, 380–1.

39. Ermakova, S., Choi, B.Y., Choi, H.S., Kang, B.S., Bode, A.M., and Dong, Z. (2005) The intermediate filament protein vimentin is a new target for epigallocatechin gallate. *J Biol Chem* **280**, 16882–90.

40. Leone, M., Zhai, D., Sareth, S., Kitada, S., Reed, J.C., and Pellecchia, M. (2003) Cancer prevention by tea polyphenols is linked to their direct inhibition of antiapoptotic Bcl-2-family proteins. *Cancer Res* **63**, 8118–21.

41. Shimizu, M., Deguchi, A., Lim, J.T., Moriwaki, H., Kopelovich, L., and Weinstein, I.B. (2005) (–)-Epigallocatechin gallate and polyphenon E inhibit growth and activation of the epidermal growth

factor receptor and human epidermal growth factor receptor-2 signaling pathways in human colon cancer cells. *Clin Cancer Res* **11**, 2735–46.

42. Higdon, J.V., and Frei, B. (2003) Tea catechins and polyphenols: Health effects, metabolism, and antioxidant functions. *Crit Rev Food Sci Nutr* **43**, 89–143.

43. Cutler, G.J., Nettleton, J.A., Ross, J.A., Harnack, L.J., Jacobs, D.R., Jr., Scrafford, C.G., Barraj, L.M., Mink, P.J., and Robien, K. (2008) Dietary flavonoid intake and risk of cancer in postmenopausal women: The Iowa Women's Health Study. *Int J Cancer* **123**(3), 664–71.

44. Bobe, G., Weinstein, S.J., Albanes, D., Hirvonen, T., Ashby, J., Taylor, P.R., Virtamo, J., and Stolzenberg-Solomon, R.Z. (2008) Flavonoid intake and risk of pancreatic cancer in male smokers (Finland). *Cancer Epidemiol Biomarkers Prev* **17**, 553–62.

45. Fink, B.N., Steck, S.E., Wolff, M.S., Britton, J.A., Kabat, G.C., Gaudet, M.M., Abrahamson, P.E., Bell, P., Schroeder, J.C., Teitelbaum, S.L., Neugut, A.I., and Gammon, M.D. (2007) Dietary flavonoid intake and breast cancer survival among women on Long Island. *Cancer Epidemiol Biomarkers Prev* **16**, 2285–92.

46. Gao, Y.T., McLaughlin, J.K., Blot, W.J., Ji, B.T., Dai, Q., and Fraumeni, J.F., Jr. (1994) Reduced risk of esophageal cancer associated with green tea consumption. *J Natl Cancer Inst* **86**, 855–8.

47. Ji, B.T., Chow, W.H., Yang, G., McLaughlin, J.K., Gao, R.N., Zheng, W., Shu, X.O., Jin, F., Fraumeni, J.F., Jr., and Gao, Y.T. (1996) The influence of cigarette smoking, alcohol, and green tea consumption on the risk of carcinoma of the cardia and distal stomach in Shanghai, China. *Cancer* **77**, 2449–57.

48. Lee, M.J., Wang, Z.Y., Li, H., Chen, L., Sun, Y., Gobbo, S., Balentine, D.A., and Yang, C.S. (1995) Analysis of plasma and urinary tea polyphenols in human subjects. *Cancer Epidemiol Biomarkers Prev* **4**, 393–9.

49. Sun, C.L., Yuan, J.M., Lee, M.J., Yang, C.S., Gao, Y.T., Ross, R.K., and Yu, M.C. (2002) Urinary tea polyphenols in relation to gastric and esophageal cancers: A prospective study of men in Shanghai, China. *Carcinogenesis* **23**, 1497–503.

50. Setiawan, V.W., Zhang, Z.F., Yu, G.P., Lu, Q.Y., Li, Y.L., Lu, M.L., Wang, M.R., Guo, C.H., Yu, S.Z., Kurtz, R.C., and Hsieh, C.C. (2001) Protective effect of green tea on the risks of chronic gastritis and stomach cancer. *Int J Cancer* **92**, 600–4.

51. Wu, A.H., Yu, M.C., Tseng, C.C., Hankin, J., and Pike, M.C. (2003) Green tea and risk of breast cancer in Asian Americans. *Int J Cancer* **106**, 574–9.

52. Wu, A.H., Tseng, C.C., Van Den Berg, D., and Yu, M.C. (2003) Tea intake, COMT genotype, and breast cancer in Asian-American women. *Cancer Res* **63**, 7526–9.

53. Kurahashi, N., Sasazuki, S., Iwasaki, M., Inoue, M., and Tsugane, S. (2008) Green tea consumption and prostate cancer risk in Japanese men: A prospective study. *Am J Epidemiol* **167**, 71–77.

54. Borrelli, F., Capasso, R., Russo, A., and Ernst, E. (2004) Systematic review: Green tea and gastrointestinal cancer risk. *Aliment Pharmacol Ther* **19**, 497–510.

55. Suzuki, Y., Tsubono, Y., Nakaya, N., Koizumi, Y., and Tsuji, I. (2004) Green tea and the risk of breast cancer: Pooled analysis of two prospective studies in Japan. *Br J Cancer* **90**, 1361–3.

56. Kuriyama, S., Shimazu, T., Ohmori, K., Kikuchi, N., Nakaya, N., Nishino, Y., Tsubono, Y., and Tsuji, I. (2006) Green tea consumption and mortality due to cardiovascular disease, cancer, and all causes in Japan: The Ohsaki study. *Jama* **296**, 1255–65.

57. Tsubono, Y., Nishino, Y., Komatsu, S., Hsieh, C.C., Kanemura, S., Tsuji, I., Nakatsuka, H., Fukao, A., Satoh, H., and Hisamichi, S. (2001) Green tea and the risk of gastric cancer in Japan. *N Engl J Med* **344**, 632–6.

58. Yuan, J.H., Li, Y.Q., and Yang, X.Y. (2007) Inhibition of epigallocatechin gallate on orthotopic colon cancer by upregulating the Nrf2-UGT1A signal pathway in nude mice. *Pharmacology* **80**, 269–78.

59. Graf, B.A., Milbury, P.E., and Blumberg, J.B. (2005) Flavonols, flavones, flavanones, and human health: Epidemiological evidence. *J Med Food* **8**, 281–90.

60. Arts, I.C., and Hollman, P.C. (2005) Polyphenols and disease risk in epidemiologic studies. *Am J Clin Nutr* **81**, 317S–25S.

61. Knekt, P., Kumpulainen, J., Jarvinen, R., Rissanen, H., Heliovaara, M., Reunanen, A., Hakulinen, T., and Aromaa, A. (2002) Flavonoid intake and risk of chronic diseases. *Am J Clin Nutr* **76**, 560–8.

62. Nothlings, U., Murphy, S.P., Wilkens, L.R., Henderson, B.E., and Kolonel, L.N. (2007) Flavonols and pancreatic cancer risk: The multiethnic cohort study. *Am J Epidemiol* **166**, 924–31.

63. Cui, Y., Morgenstern, H., Greenland, S., Tashkin, D.P., Mao, J.T., Cai, L., Cozen, W., Mack, T.M., Lu, Q.Y., and Zhang, Z.F. (2008) Dietary flavonoid intake and lung cancer – a population-based case-control study. *Cancer* **112**, 2241–8.

64. Theodoratou, E., Kyle, J., Cetnarskyj, R., Farrington, S.M., Tenesa, A., Barnetson, R., Porteous, M., Dunlop, M., and Campbell, H. (2007) Dietary flavonoids and the risk of colorectal cancer. *Cancer Epidemiol Biomarkers Prev* **16**, 684–93.

65. Hakim, I.A., Harris, R.B., Brown, S., Chow, H.H., Wiseman, S., Agarwal, S., and Talbot, W. (2003) Effect of increased tea consumption on oxidative DNA damage among smokers: A randomized controlled study. *J Nutr* **133**, 3303S–9S.

66. Tang, L., Tang, M., Xu, L., Luo, H., Huang, T., Yu, J., Zhang, L., Gao, W., Cox, S.B., and Wang, J.S. (2008) Modulation of aflatoxin biomarkers in human blood and urine by green tea polyphenols intervention. *Carcinogenesis* **29**, 411–7.

67. Schwartz, J.L., Baker, V., Larios, E., and Chung, F.L. (2005) Molecular and cellular effects of green tea on oral cells of smokers: A pilot study. *Mol Nutr Food Res* **49**, 43–51.

68. Bettuzzi, S., Brausi, M., Rizzi, F., Castagnetti, G., Peracchia, G., and Corti, A. (2006) Chemoprevention of human prostate cancer by oral administration of green tea catechins in volunteers with high-grade prostate intraepithelial neoplasia: A preliminary report from a one-year proof-of-principle study. *Cancer Res* **66**, 1234–40.

69. Laurie, S.A., Miller, V.A., Grant, S.C., Kris, M.G., and Ng, K.K. (2005) Phase I study of green tea extract in patients with advanced lung cancer. *Cancer Chemother Pharmacol* **55**, 33–38.

70. Williamson, G., and Manach, C. (2005) Bioavailability and bioefficacy of polyphenols in humans. II. Review of 93 intervention studies. *Am J Clin Nutr* **81**, 243S–55S.

71. Kim, H.Y., Kim, O.H., and Sung, M.K. (2003) Effects of phenol-depleted and phenol-rich diets on blood markers of oxidative stress, and urinary excretion of quercetin and kaempferol in healthy volunteers. *J Am Coll Nutr* **22**, 217–23.

72. Lean, M.E., Noroozi, M., Kelly, I., Burns, J., Talwar, D., Sattar, N., and Crozier, A. (1999) Dietary flavonols protect diabetic human lymphocytes against oxidative damage to DNA. *Diabetes* **48**, 176–81.

73. Manach, C., Williamson, G., Morand, C., Scalbert, A., and Remesy, C. (2005) Bioavailability and bioefficacy of polyphenols in humans. I. Review of 97 bioavailability studies. *Am J Clin Nutr* **81**, 230S–42S.

74. Lambert, J.D., and Yang, C.S. (2003) Cancer chemopreventive activity and bioavailability of tea and tea polyphenols. *Mutat Res* **523–524**, 201–8.

75. Clark, D.E. (1999) Rapid calculation of polar molecular surface area and its application to the prediction of transport phenomena. 1. Prediction of intestinal absorption. *J Pharm Sci* **88**, 807–14.

76. Lipinski, C.A., Lombardo, F., Dominy, B.W., and Feeney, P.J. (2001) Experimental and computational approaches to estimate solubility and permeability in drug discovery and development settings. *Adv Drug Deliv Rev* **46**, 3–26.

77. van der Woude, H., Boersma, M.G., Vervoort, J., and Rietjens, I.M. (2004) Identification of 14 quercetin phase II mono- and mixed conjugates and their formation by rat and human phase II in vitro model systems. *Chem Res Toxicol* **17**, 1520–30.

78. Justino, G.C., Santos, M.R., Canario, S., Borges, C., Florencio, M.H., and Mira, L. (2004) Plasma quercetin metabolites: Structure-antioxidant activity relationships. *Arch Biochem Biophys* **432**, 109–21.

79. Day, A.J., Bao, Y., Morgan, M.R., and Williamson, G. (2000) Conjugation position of quercetin glucuronides and effect on biological activity. *Free Radic Biol Med* **29**, 1234–43.

80. Ju, J., Lu, G., Lambert, J.D., and Yang, C.S. (2007) Inhibition of carcinogenesis by tea constituents. *Semin Cancer Biol* **17**, 395–402.

81. Bonkovsky, H.L. (2006) Hepatotoxicity associated with supplements containing Chinese green tea (Camellia sinensis). *Ann Intern Med* **144**, 68–71.

82. Isbrucker, R.A., Edwards, J.A., Wolz, E., Davidovich, A., and Bausch, J. (2005) Safety studies on epigallocatechin gallate (EGCG) preparations. Part 2: Dermal, acute and short-term toxicity studies. *Food Chem Toxicol* **44**, 636–50.

83. Chen, L., Lee, M.J., Li, H., and Yang, C.S. (1997) Absorption, distribution, elimination of tea polyphenols in rats. *Drug Metab Dispos* **25**, 1045–50.

84. Ross, J.A., Potter, J.D., Reaman, G.H., Pendergrass, T.W., and Robison, L.L. (1996) Maternal exposure to potential inhibitors of DNA topoisomerase II and infant leukemia (United States): A report from the Children's Cancer Group. *Cancer Causes Control* **7**, 581–90.

85. Strick, R., Strissel, P.L., Borgers, S., Smith, S.L., and Rowley, J.D. (2000) Dietary bioflavonoids induce cleavage in the MLL gene and may contribute to infant leukemia. *Proc Natl Acad Sci USA* **97**, 4790–5.

27 Mechanisms of Action of Isoflavones in Cancer Prevention

Stephen Barnes

Key Points

1. Isoflavones are plant polyphenols and form part of the diet in regions of the world where the incidence of and death from some, but not all, cancers are much lower than in the United States and other Western countries. Isoflavones also have structural similarities to physiologic estrogens.
2. The amounts of isoflavones consumed in the diet vary considerably. Okinawans consuming traditional diets have intakes as much as 100 mg of the isoflavones genistein and daidzein per day. In contrast, at most Americans isoflavone intake is only 1–3 mg/day.
3. The soy isoflavone genistein in cellular and pre-clinical animal models has been shown to have estrogen-like effects, causing some concern about its safety. However, genistein and other common isoflavones have many other demonstrable mechanisms that may offset the estrogen-like effects, albeit that most occur at higher concentrations/doses.
4. The mechanisms of action of isoflavones over the past 40 years have been found to be as antioxidants, estrogen agonists, topoisomerase inhibitors, metastasis, and inhibitors of tyrosine kinases. Many of these mechanisms focus on targets that are relevant to anti-cancer therapy and may not be important for prevention.
5. Isoflavones have been used as chemopreventive agents in animal models of breast, endometrial, lung, and prostate cancer. In the case of breast cancer, preventive effects of soy (containing isoflavones) were observed in radiation and chemical carcinogen-induced mammary carcinogenesis in rats. Lamartiniere's group then showed that rats exposed briefly to genistein (500 μg daily by injection) in the perinatal and pre-pubertal periods had a 50% reduction in the number of mammary tumors compared to animals on a control (soy-free) diet.

Key Words: Isoflavones; polyphenols; estrogens; genistein; cancer prevention

1. INTRODUCTION

Isoflavones are bioflavonoids that belong to the much larger polyphenol family, i.e., they contain more than one phenolic group. As will be discussed later in this chapter, they have a plethora of potential mechanisms of action. There has been a considerable debate on whether they prevent or promote hormone-dependent cancers. The latter view

From: *Nutrition and Health: Bioactive Compounds and Cancer*
Edited by: J.A. Milner, D.F. Romagnolo, DOI 10.1007/978-1-60761-627-6_27,
© Springer Science+Business Media, LLC 2010

comes from their properties as ligands for estrogen receptor alpha (ERα) and beta (ERβ). But isoflavones are much more than that *(1)* and this may explain why the world's largest consumers of isoflavones are also those with the lowest risks of the hormone-dependent cancers (breast, endometrial, ovarian, and prostate cancer). The reader is referred to a previous summary of a more detailed background on the origins of soy isoflavones and their involvement in cancer research published in 2006 *(2)*.

2. ORIGINS

Isoflavones are synthesized in plants from the conversion of phenylalanine to cinnamoyl CoA and subsequent condensation with three molecules of malonyl CoA catalyzed by chalcone synthetase to form the flavanone naringenin. This compound has a phenyl ring substitution at the 2-position. Migration of the phenyl ring to the 3-position requires the (2S)-flavanone enantiomer, molecular oxygen and NADPH, and is catalyzed by the microsomal cytochrome P450 enzyme 2-hydroxyisoflavanone synthase *(3)*. The 2-hydroxyisoflavanone undergoes dehydration either spontaneously or via enzymatic reaction by 2-hydroxyisoflavanone dehydratase to form either genistein (4′,5,7-trihydroxyisoflavone) or daidzein (4′,7-dihydroxyisoflavone). The most common isoflavones in the diet are those in soybeans (daidzein, genistein, and glycitein; 7,4′-dihydroxy-6-methoxy-isoflavone) (Fig. 1).

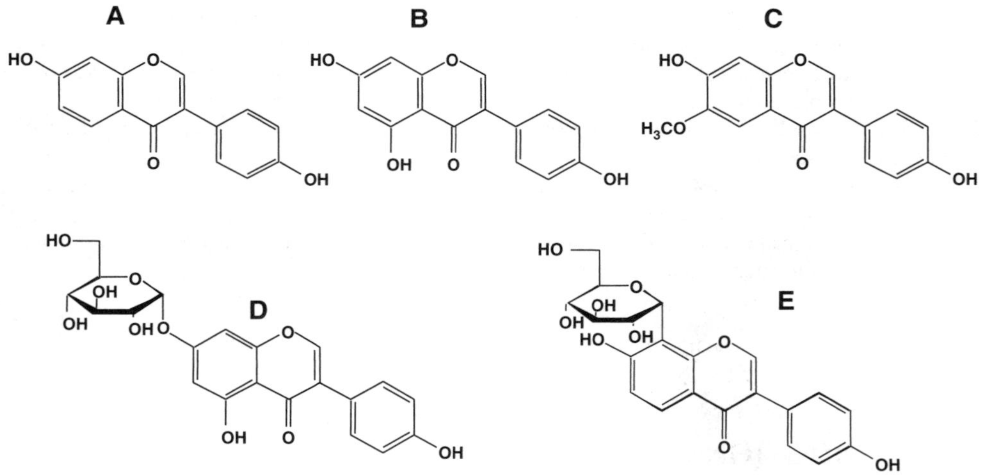

Fig. 1. Chemical structure of several isoflavones. Daidzein (**a**), genistein (**b**), glycitein (**c**), and daidzin (**d**) are all from soybeans. Puerarin (**e**) is a 8-*C*-glycoside of daidzein and is an isomer of daidzin (7-*O*-glycoside of daidzein).

Isoflavones are found in vacuoles in plants and are largely present as β-glycosides, which are also esterified with malonic acid in the 6″-position of the glucose moiety *(4)*. In the kudzu vine (*Pueraria lobata*), many of the isoflavones are C-glycosides (Fig. 1). These glycosides are metabolically stable in man and experimental animals *(5)*. In certain medicinal plants, the isoflavones are prenylated with isoprene groups *(6)*.

Prenylated flavonoids such 8-prenylnaringenin are strongly estrogenic *(7)*; a similar increase in estrogenicity is predicted for prenylated isoflavones.

The principal sources of isoflavones in the modern diet are from soybeans *(8)*, mung beans *(9, 10)*, and chick peas *(11)*. However, in traditional medicine practice in South East Asia, the root of kudzu vine, rich in the isoflavone C-glycoside puerarin, is used to treat fever, pain, diabetes, measles, diarrhea, and cardiovascular diseases *(12)*. Also, the Eastern native American Indians have a long tradition of consuming the American groundnut *(Apios americana)* *(13)*, a particularly rich source of the isoflavone genistein (as its 7-glucosylglucoside) *(14)*. *A. americana* is popular vegetable in markets on the West coast of the United States.

3. ISOFLAVONE INTAKE

The amounts of isoflavones consumed in the diet vary considerably. Okinawans consuming traditional diets have intakes as much as 100 mg of the isoflavones genistein and daidzein per day *(15)*. In contrast, in most Americans isoflavone intake is only 1–3 mg/day *(16)*. It's noteworthy to mention that it is rare in 2008 to find a subject/patient where isoflavones are unmeasurable in their blood. There is a low level of soy protein in food items sold in most supermarkets and groceries. Isolated soy protein is added to many canned meat products to improve the visual esthetics of the food when the can is opened. Occasionally, soy is found in the most unlikely places, e.g., in certain brands of canned tuna where the fish is in a protein (soy) broth *(17)*. At Thanksgiving and Christmas many Americans unwittingly consume soy isoflavones when they eat turkey that was injected with a soy broth to ensure that a good gravy can result during its cooking.

The nature of the isoflavones in soy food products also varies. In Asian countries, much of the soy is in the form of fermented foodstuffs such as miso (Japan), soy paste (Korea), and tempeh (Indonesia) *(18)*. In these foods, the isoflavones are mostly unconjugated and thereby easily absorbed by passive diffusion in the upper small intestine. In contrast, Americans consume processed soy foods such as isolated soy protein, soy protein concentrates, soy flour, and soy milk products. The isoflavones in these protein-enriched soy foods are largely glycosides. The simple β-glycosides are hydrolyzed by lactose-phlorizin hydrolase, an enzyme in enterocytes, before they can be absorbed *(19)*. Complex isoflavone glycosides (the malonylglycoside esters and their decarboxylated products, the acetylglycosides, formed during toasting of soy) are not readily hydrolyzed until they reach the microorganism-rich large bowel *(2)*.

4. ISOFLAVONE METABOLISM

Isoflavones undergo considerable metabolism once they are hydrolyzed. In the enterocyte, they are converted to β-glucuronides by UDP-glucuronyltransferases expressed in these cells *(20)*. A similar process occurs in the liver *(21)*. However, this means that isoflavones consumed by mouth (as a food or in a dietary supplement) circulate mostly as phase II metabolites. The proportion that is unconjugated and thereby easily taken up by peripheral tissues is low and rarely exceeds 5%. In contrast, isoflavones administered peripherally by subcutaneous or intramuscular injection or via a skin cream or patch will enter the peripheral blood in the unconjugated form and have to be transported to the liver before phase II metabolism can occur. These latter methods of administration should be expected to have very different physiological effects compared to the oral route. In many cases, the disparate results obtained by different investigators for isoflavones may have their explanations in the dosing regime that has been used.

5. MECHANISMS OF ACTION OF ISOFLAVONES

In the last few years there have been many excellent reviews on the mechanisms of action of phytochemicals (22–31), as well as those that have specifically addressed isoflavones (2, 32–43). The most frequently invoked mechanisms of action of isoflavones over the past 40 years have been as antioxidants (32, 44), estrogen agonists (45, 46), topoisomerase inhibitors (47), metastasis (48), and inhibitors of tyrosine kinases (49). Many of these mechanisms focus on targets that are relevant to anti-cancer therapy and may not be important for prevention. Also, since the plasma concentrations of unconjugated isoflavones rarely exceed a few hundred nM in the systemic circulation (they are mostly β-glucuronide conjugates) (50), studies carried out in cell culture at μM concentrations to determine the mechanisms of action are not necessarily significant. Indeed, this has led many to assume that the only relevant mechanism of action of isoflavones is as estrogen agonists since the equilibrium binding constant (K_d) of ERβ for genistein is in the low nM range (51). Nonetheless, other potential mechanisms of action have been described and the purpose of this chapter is to review those published over the past 4–5 years.

Table 1
Cellular Targets of Genistein

Apoptosis	Transcription factors	Cell cycle	Others
↑Bax	↓NF-κB	↓Cyclin B1	↓Akt
↓Bcl-2	↑Nrf1	↓Cyclin D1	↓AR
↓Bcl-xL	↑Nrf2	↑p21 WAF1	↓PSA
↑PARP	↓STAT-3	↑p27 KIP1	↓COX-2
↓Survivin	↓STAT-5	↑p16 INK4a	↓MMP-9
↓IAP	↓IGF-1R	↑Myt-1	↓MMP-2
↓XIAP	↓Ape-1/Ref	↓Wee-1	↓p38 MAPK
↑BAD	↓Wnt	↓CDK-1	↓ERK-1/2
↑Active caspases	↓Notch-2		↑GPx
↑ER stress regulators	↓AP-1		↑kangai-1
	↓CREB		↑Endoglin
	↑GADD 153		
	↓RANK/RANK-L		
	↓HIF-1α		↓PTEN

Reproduced with permission from Banerjee et al. (52).

In order to put a perspective on the value of mechanistic studies, it is first important to consider how such studies fit with what is known from human epidemiological data, pre-clinical animal models, and clinical intervention studies. Specific mechanisms – effects on aromatase, protein kinases and signaling pathways, apoptosis, metastasis, proteinases, exosomes, and epigenetics – are then reviewed in more detail. A collection of specific cellular targets of genistein are listed in Table 1, from a recent review by Banerjee et al. *(52)*.

6. EPIDEMIOLOGY OF SOY AND CANCER

Much of the work being carried out on nutritionally bioactive substances and cancer prevention has arisen from the comparison of cancer risk and cancer death rates in populations around the world. Very distinct differences are observed, with a high incidence of hormone-dependent cancers in the United States and much of Western Europe compared with much of SE Asia *(53, 54)*. In contrast, the incidence of gastric and liver cancer is high in Asian countries *(55)*. Interestingly, 70 years ago the incidence of gastric cancer in the United States was just as high as it is in Asia today (higher than present day breast, prostate, and lung cancer) *(56)*. This changed when refrigeration became part of Americana; the gastric cancer incidence in the United States has fallen by 90% since then *(56)*. This reveals that public health changes can have major effects on the cancer burden of a society.

The extensive immigration that occurred in the second half of the twentieth century revealed another aspect of cancer risk – that it is principally environmental and behavioral in nature. Immigrants to the United States adopt the cancer risk patterns associated with US-born Americans. In the case of prostate cancer, this occurs after the immigrant arrives in the United States *(57)*. Environment is important – there is a higher incidence of prostatic intraepithelial neoplasias (PIN) in Japanese men living in Hawaii than in Japan *(58)*. Thus, the diet–environment has a strong influence with regard to whether PIN lesions emerge into a clinical tumor. For breast cancer, the change over to the Western cancer risk occurs in the second-generation daughters of Asian immigrants *(59)*. This suggests that epigenetic events that occur early in life (prior to immigration) determine adult rates of breast cancer. Interestingly, the age-related breast cancer incidence in Singapore women is similar to Swedish women up to the menopause *(60)*. However, post-menopausally the breast cancer incidence does not increase in SE Asians, whereas it quickly accelerates in Swedish women. Although there are many possible nutritional factors that could account for these different patterns of cancer risk between countries, soy and its isoflavones have been frequently hypothesized to contribute to a lowered breast cancer risk. However, epidemiological data from cohort and case–control studies reveal only a modest benefit, albeit stronger in studies conducted in SE Asia or Asian populations in the United States *(61, 62)*. However, such studies did not take into account the intake of soy at critical times in development. In concert with pre-clinical data presented in the next section, data from the Shanghai Cancer Registry revealed that adolescent intake of soy is essential for an adult benefit of soy *(63)*. Messina and Woods *(64)* have carefully reviewed the use of soy in cancer patients and concluded that soy could be safely used in this group. However, many physicians take a more prudent view and limit the use of soy in those patients undergoing anti-estrogen therapy.

7. CHEMOPREVENTION MODELS

The role of diet in cancer prevention is described in many chapters in this volume. Isoflavones have been used as chemopreventive agents in animal models of breast, endometrial, lung, and prostate cancer. In the case of breast cancer, preventive effects of soy (containing isoflavones) were observed in radiation (65) and chemical carcinogen-induced mammary carcinogenesis (66, 67) in rats. Lamartiniere's group then showed that rats exposed briefly to genistein (500 μg daily by injection) in the perinatal (68) and pre-pubertal periods (69) had a 50% reduction in the number of mammary tumors compared to animals on a control (soy-free) diet. Importantly, this group went on to show that feeding a genistein diet (250 ppm in the diet) to the mother rat during the pre-weaning period also led to fewer mammary tumors in the pups when the latter were challenged with carcinogen (70). This postnatal effect of genistein has been confirmed (71), as has the use of biochanin A in a similar design (72). Another relevant result was that rats exposed to genistein (73) or soy (74) pre-pubertally and then restarted on dietary genistein 50 days after the administration of the carcinogen had a 75% reduction in mammary tumors. In contrast, rats that were not exposed pre-pubertally to genistein did not respond to the genistein administered in later life (74). A similar lack of effect was obtained when genistein or isolated soy protein was added to the diet of rats 1 week prior to administration of DMBA (75). This is an important result since it suggests that genistein may have little or no benefits in lowering breast cancer risk to the typical American consumer who starts using it in midlife.

8. NUDE MOUSE MODELS

Athymic nude mice models have been extensively used to evaluate the anti-cancer effect of compounds on human cancer cell lines in biological setting. Helferich and his colleagues have pursued a variation of this model in which the mice are ovariec-tomized (OVEX) to attempt to create the low estrogen environment that occurs post-natally. Human MCF-7 breast cancer cells were implanted into these animals. They were placed on diets containing differing amounts of genistein (0–500 ppm) or given 10 μg/day 17β-estradiol by injection. The physiological estrogen caused rapid growth of the tumor whereas no treatment led to a gradual reduction in tumor growth. Genistein reversed the decline in tumor cell growth in the OVEX animals and at the higher doses increased the size of the tumor (76). They extended their initial results by examining isoflavone-rich extracts of soy protein preparations in this model (77); the results were variable – soy flour did not increase tumor growth, whereas isolated soy protein did. This suggests that other components in soy are part of its chemoprevention properties (78). The other major soy isoflavone daidzein and its bacterial metabolite equol had only a small effect on MCF-7 cell growth in this model (79). A criticism of this OVEX nude mouse model is that ovariectomy ablates rather than lowers plasma 17β-estradiol levels. This led to a redesign in which low levels of 17β-estradiol were created in the

OVEX nude mouse model *(80)*. As in the simpler OVEX nude mouse model, dietary genistein increased tumor cell growth. Of course, one can still argue that the estrogen-supplemented OVEX nude mouse model is an incomplete model in that it lacks progesterone and other ovarian steroids. Nonetheless, what is clear from these data is that genistein in the absence of an immune system acts as an estrogen and stimulates cell proliferation of tumor cells containing ER. Furthermore, genistein opposes the anti-cancer effects of the anti-estrogen tamoxifen *(81)* and the aromatase inhibitor letrozole *(82)*.

In nude mice that have not undergone ovariectomy, subcutaneously injected genistein (up to 0.5 mg/kg BW) has anti-cancer effects on ER-positive MCF-7 cells and ER-negative MDA-MB-231 cells *(83)*. It downregulates matrix metalloproteinase-9 and upregulates an inhibitor of metalloproteinase-1, as well upregulating $p21_{(WAF1/CIP1)}$. It also had effects on angiogenesis and lowers vascular endothelial growth factor (VEGF) and transforming growth factor-β1 (TGFβ1). Genistein administered prior to implantation of MCF-7 or MDA-MB-468 cells prevented tumorigenesis *(84)*. Subcutaneously administered biochanin A (4′-methoxygenistein) also inhibits growth of MCF-7 cells in nude mice *(85)*. In contrast, Santell et al. found no anti-tumor effect of genistein on MDA-MB-231 cells when it was administered at 750 ppm in the diet *(86)*.

In contrast to breast cancer, genistein and isoflavones suppress tumor cell growth in other cancer models using nude mice. Genistein reduces the growth of tumor cells derived from renal cell carcinoma *(87)*, bladder cancer *(88)*, pancreatic cancer *(89)*, and prostate cancer *(90–92)*.

9. ESTROGEN-LIKE PROPERTIES OF ISOFLAVONES

The realization that isoflavones had estrogen-like properties preceded the discovery of ER. Farmers in Western Australia knew that clover isoflavones (biochanin A- and formononetin- 4′-methoxydaidzein) induced infertility in sheep *(93)*. Other species also had similar responses to isoflavones – these include quail *(94, 95)* and cheetahs *(96)*. Cats cannot make glucuronide conjugates and this may slow the metabolism and clearance of isoflavones, thereby enhancing their activity. Genistein was shown to antagonize estrogen binding to its receptors *(97, 98)*, although the estimated binding constant was between 0.1 and 1 μM. An appreciation of the importance of ER and isoflavone action came from the discovery of ERβ *(99)*, which binds genistein at low nM levels, concentrations relevant to physiological concentrations. However, ERβ, unlike ERα, is regarded by some as mediating protective mechanisms. Daidzein is a weaker estrogen than genistein, whereas coumestrol (a phytoestrogen in *Alfa alfa*) is much stronger *(100)*. However, the daidzein metabolite equol (Fig. 2) is a strong estrogen agonist. Equol has an asymmetric C_3 carbon atom. It is found in vivo as the *S*-isomer and has an ERβ binding constant of 0.73 nM. In contrast, the *R*-isomer has a binding constant of 15.4 nM *(101)*. As for genistein, both *R*- and *S*-equol are somewhat weaker ligands for ERα *(101)*. It is worth noting that all the daidzein metabolites that involve reduction of the heterocyclic ring have an asymmetric C_3 carbon atom – whether their *R*- and *S*-isomers have differential biological activities is yet to be determined.

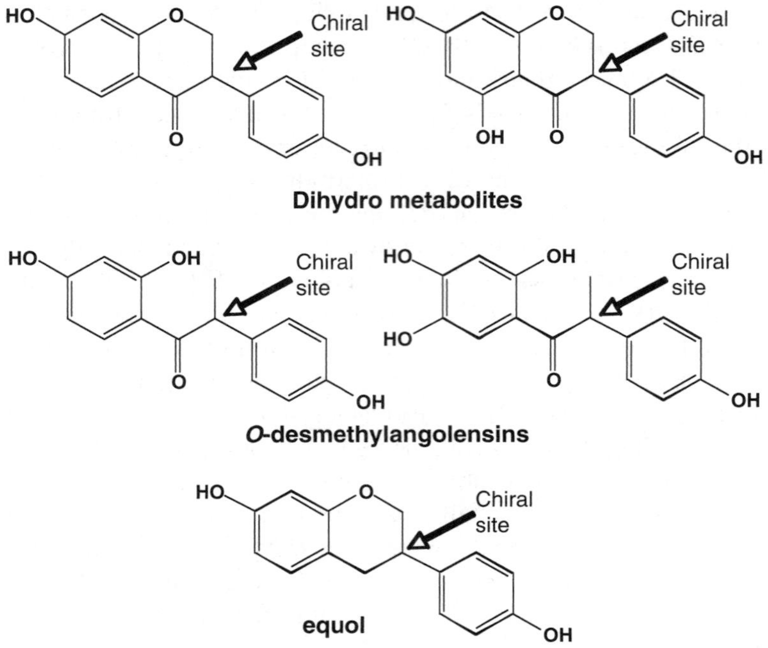

Fig. 2. Metabolites of daidzein and genistein. Note that each of the metabolites has an optically active carbon atom (marked with an *arrow*).

10. AROMATASE

The effect of genistein on blocking the aromatase inhibitor letrozole in nude mice *(82)* is in contrast to some, but not all, in vitro and cell culture studies of the action of genistein on aromatase. Early in vitro studies suggested that genistein and other isoflavones were inhibitors of aromatase *(102, 103)*. However, genistein (1 μM) increased aromatase activity in colon cancer epithelial cells *(104)* and human adrenocortical carcinoma cells *(105)*. This suggests that genistein upregulates the expression of aromatase more than it inhibits its enzymatic action. Another aspect of this issue is the effect of genistein on the synthesis of 17β-estradiol. In isolated ovarian follicles, genistein lowered testosterone, but had no effect on 17β-estradiol *(106)*. In MCF-7 cells, genistein (10 μM) inhibited aromatase and 17β-hydroxysteroid dehydrogenase *(107)*. Genistein inhibited 3β- and 17β-hydroxysteroid dehydrogenases in luteinized granulosa cells *(108)*, albeit at concentrations >10 μM *(109)*.

However, the response of aromatase to genistein may depend on the animal model or specific cell type used. Rats administered genistein have lowered testicular aromatase activity *(110)*. In contrast, in glial cells expressing three distinct ERs and a zebrafish aromatase gene, genistein upregulated aromatase expression *(111)*. Timing of the assessment of up- or downregulation aromatase mRNA expression or protein levels may also be a factor *(112)*. Combinations of isoflavones and other phytoestrogens may both increase/decrease aromatase expression *(111, 112)* and decrease aromatase activity

(113). Regulation of how much genistein reaches target cells may determine whether the overall effect of genistein is stimulatory or inhibitory. In the brain, the amount of genistein is predicted to be low. Accordingly, genistein has been shown to stimulate protein synthesis in ovariectomized rats *(114)*. It is not known whether this is a direct estrogenic effect, due to its stimulation of aromatase activity. Stimulation of brain protein synthesis by isoflavones may have important quality-of-life issues above and beyond cancer risk–benefit considerations.

11. ANDROGEN-DEPENDENT CARCINOGENESIS

Prostate-specific androgen (PSA) is under the regulation of the androgen receptor (AR). Genistein lowers PSA secretion in AR+ve LNCaP human prostate cancer cells through androgen-dependent and -independent mechanisms *(115)*. Interestingly, it did so at concentrations less than 1 μM.

12. PROTEIN TYROSINE KINASE INHIBITION

Besides the estrogen-like effects of genistein and other isoflavones, their mostly widely described effect is as protein tyrosine kinase (PTK) inhibitors *(49)*. However, their inhibitor constants are in the μM range. Many investigators observing isoflavone-induced changes in phosphotyrosine labeling of proteins in cells assume that the isoflavone effect is on direct PTK inhibition. However, they should also consider an indirect effect such as reduction in the amount of the protein. Nonetheless, there are tissues where μM amounts of isoflavones exist – in the small intestine (estimated to be up to 60 μM for a 50 mg daily dose – 185 μmol in 3–5 l of fluid), in urine in the bladder (up to 30 μM) *(116)*, in breast nipple aspirate (1–10 μM) *(117, 118)*, and in prostatic fluid (1–20 μM) *(119, 120)*. These higher concentrations may not only impact PTK inhibition but also other mechanisms reviewed in this chapter.

13. CELL-CYCLE REGULATION

Inhibitory effects of isoflavones on the cell cycle have been known for over 30 years, beginning with rotenone (Fig. 3) *(121)*. Genistein causes cell-cycle arrest at the G_0/G_1 transition *(122)* (Fig. 4) and at the G_2/M transition *(123)* (Fig. 5). It decreases cyclin B, which forms complexes with cell-cycle-dependent kinases CDK4 and CDK2 *(123)*. Genistein also increases proteins that inhibit the progress of the cell cycle (p21^{WAF1}, p27^{KIP1}, and p16^{INK4a}) *(121, 124–127)*. Interestingly, genistein's effect on cell-cycle arrest by upregulation of p21^{WAF1} may depend on ERβ; silencing of ERβ blocked the effect of genistein *(128)*. In addition, epigenetic mechanisms may play a part by reversal of hypermethylation of p16^{INK4a} *(129)* or by chromatin remodeling *(130)*. In addition, genistein downregulates Mdm2, which removes phosphorylated p53 from the nucleus *(131)*. Finally, genistein increases Myt-1 and reduces the phosphorylation of Wee-1, protein kinases that transcriptionally repress cyclin B1 *(132)*.

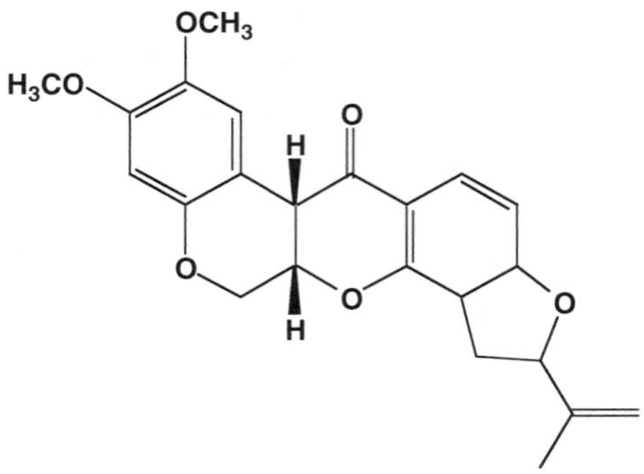

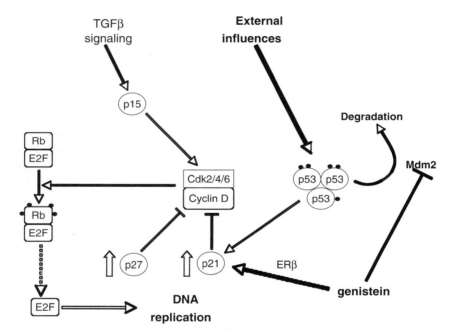

Fig. 3. Chemical structure of retonone, an isoflavone from *Lonchocarpus nicouz.*

Fig. 4. The G₁/S checkpoint in cell-cycle regulation. Cyclin D forms a complex with the cyclin-dependent kinases (cdk) that phosphorylates the retinoblastoma protein (Rb) that is complexed with the transcription factor E2F. Phosphorylation of Rb releases E2F to initiate DNA synthesis. The activity of the cyclin D/cdk (2, 4) complex is downregulated by p21 and p27. These two proteins are upregulated by genistein. p21 upregulation by genistein may be dependent on ERβ. Phosphorylated p53 also blocks cyclin D/cdk (2, 4) activity – this is reversed by removal of p53 from the nucleus by Mdm2. Genistein also reduces Mdm2 function.

14. SIGNALING PATHWAYS

Genistein was originally cast as an inhibitor of the epidermal growth factor pathway *(49)*. However, it is also a regulator of NF-κB (Fig. 6), mitogen-activated protein

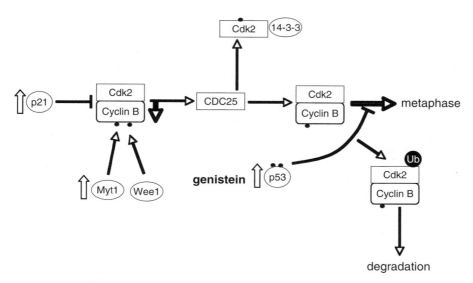

Fig. 5. The G2/M checkpoint in cell-cycle regulation. The cdk2/cyclin B complex is dephosphory-lated by CDC25 to initiate the metaphase. Genistein blocks cdc2/cyclin B via its upregulation of p21, promotes phosphorylation of cdck2/cyclin B by Myt1 and Wee1, and by upregulating p53 blocks cdk2/cyclin B.

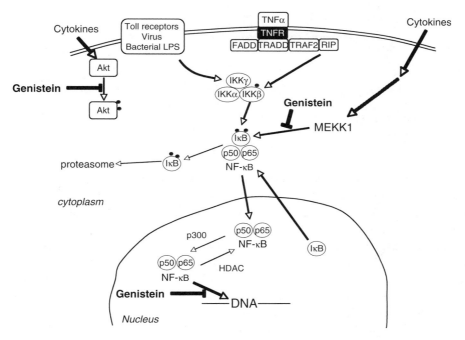

Fig. 6. The NF-κB pathway. Cytokines and TNFα lead to phosphorylation of IKKβ. IκB dissociates from the NF-κB (the p50/p65 complex) which then moves into the nucleus. NF-κB is acetylated by p300 (Creb) – this is reversed by histone deacetylase.

kinases (MAPKs or ERKs) (Fig. 7), p53, and AR pathways. Genistein blocks binding of NF-κB to DNA and reduces phosphorylation of IκB *(133)*, possibly by the mitogen-activated kinase kinase 1 (MEKK1) *(52)*. Epidermal growth factor is a regulator of Akt phosphorylation (at Ser473) and this is inhibited by genistein. Since Akt also regulates the NF-κB pathway, genistein may have a dual role, acting on both Akt and NF-κB *(134)*. Genistein also inhibits Akt-GSK-3β signaling *(135)*. Upstream of NF-κB are the MAP kinase pathways. Genistein inhibits activation of p38 MAPK by TGF-β in prostate epithelial cells *(136)* and ERK1/2 *(137)*.

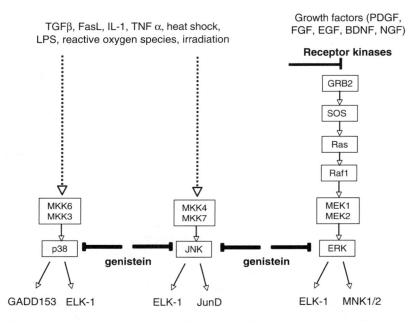

Fig. 7. MAP kinase regulation. Genistein inhibits the tyrosine kinase activities of the growth factors such as PDGF, EGF, FGF, BDNF, and NGF. It also inhibits the downstream kinases p38, JNK and ERK1/2.

Genistein has roles as antioxidant. It reacts in a direct manner with reactive oxygen species and related oxidants such as peroxynitrite and hypochlorous acid in vitro *(138)* and in a phorbol ester-driven oxidative burst both in DMSO-differentiated HL-60 cells *(139)* and in freshly isolated polymorphonuclear cells *(140)* to form nitrated and chlorinated isoflavones. Chlorinated isoflavones are stronger antioxidants in models of LDL oxidation *(139)*. Genistein also inhibited tumor necrosis factor alpha (TNFα)-induced adhesion of fluorescently labeled neutrophils to the vascular wall *(141)*. Importantly, this only occurred under conditions of shear stress and is PPAR-γ dependent *(142)*. Interestingly, the position of chlorine substitution of daidzein either enhanced (3'-chlorination) or inhibited (6- or 8-chlorination) PPAR-γ-dependent effects *(142)*. In addition to the direct effects, genistein also increased the cytosolic accumulation and nuclear translocation of the transcription factor, Nrf1 and Nrf2 *(143)*, that mediate the response to oxidative stress. It downregulates cyclooxygenase-2 expression *(144)* and inhibits phosphorylation of the transcription factors STAT-3 and STAT-5 *(145)*. It activates insulin-like growth factor 1-receptor signaling at low (<4 μM) concentrations *(146)* and inhibits at high concentrations (>25 μM) *(147)*.

15. APOPTOSIS

Genistein initiates apoptosis of cancer cells when used at higher concentrations. Apoptosis can occur for cells that enter the cell cycle. Proteins associated with regulation of apoptosis are listed in Table 1. These include the Bcl-2 family (anti-apoptotic, Bcl-x_L, Bcl-2; pro-apoptotic, Bax, Bak and Bad), as well as caspases and endoplasmic reticulum stress-relevant regulators. In human hepatoma cells, genistein downregulates Bcl-2 and Bcl-x_L, and upregulates Bax and activates caspases *(148)* (Fig. 8). It has been suggested that apoptosis can occur at *dietary* levels of phytochemicals *(149)*. However, the investigators used genistein, its aglucone, at 2.5 μM which is not physiological since most of the circulating genistein is present as its β-glucuronide with <5% as the aglucone. A much more interesting experiment would be to examine the effect of a combination of different phytochemicals (diindolylmethane, EGCG, genistein, and indole-3-carbinol) all at realistic *physiological* concentrations to determine whether they act additively or synergistically. It is also important to note that in all cell culture experiments the

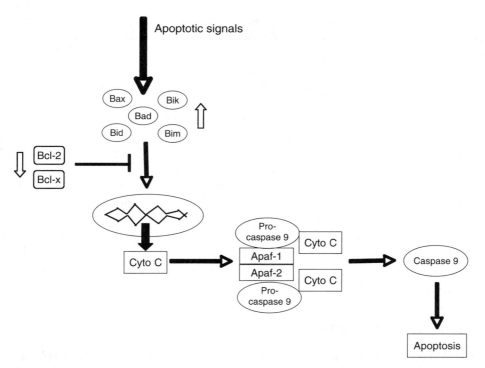

Fig. 8. Apoptosis regulation. A variety of influences can initiate apoptosis via upregulation of Bad, Bax, Bid, Bik and Bim – genistein does this, too. Genistein also downregulates the anti-apoptotic proteins Bcl-2 and Bcl-x. Cytochrome c released from mitochondria binds to the apoptosome and converts pro-caspase 9 to caspase 9. The latter then drives apoptosis.

long-term effect of the agents should be studied since apoptosis may increase with time as the phytochemicals disrupt the organization of the tumor cell.

16. METASTASIS

A limitation of most of the primary cancer chemoprevention models is that the tumors that appear do not exhibit metastasis, yet it is metastasis that leads to premature death, not the tumor per se. Therefore, it is the role of the isoflavones on preventing metastatic growth and tissue distribution of cancer cells that is most relevant to cancer mortality. Using MDA-MB-435 breast cancer cells expressing a GFP construct, Vantghem et al. *(150)* implanted them under the mammary fat pad of female nude mice and left them to grow for 5 weeks. They were resected and the animals placed on a control diet and one supplemented with genistein. After a further 5 weeks, the lungs were assessed. Genistein reduced by 10-fold the metastatic burden in the lung *(150)*. More research using this approach needs to be carried out using ER-positive cells and with other common isoflavones.

Genistein (100 and 250 ppm in the diet) also inhibits lung metastasis in a model of prostate cancer in nude mice created by implantation of PC3-M cells *(90)*. Genistein-mediated inhibition of activation of focal adhesion kinase (FAK) and of the p38 mitogen-activated protein kinase (MAPK)-heat shock protein 27 (HSP27) pathway has been shown to regulate PCa cell detachment and invasion effects, respectively. Additional benefits are associated with the combination of radiotherapy and genistein treatment *(91)*.

17. EPIGENETIC PHENOMENA

Genistein promotes DNA demethylation, "uncovering" the tumor suppressor GSTP1 in MDA-MB-468 cells *(151)*. Other epigenetic effects of genistein were observed in prostate cancer cells where it was shown to activate demethylation and acetylation of histone3-K9 at the PTEN and the CYLD promoter, while acetylation of histone 3-K9 at the p53 and the FOXO3a promoter occurred through reduction of endogenous SIRT1 activity *(152)*. Other effects of genistein on histone acetylation have been reported; genistein increased acetylated histones 3, 4, and H3/K4 at the p21 and p16 transcription start sites in prostate cancer cells *(130)*. Furthermore, genistein treatment increased the expression of histone acetyl transferases that function in transcriptional activation. As noted earlier, genistein also reduced the hypermethylation of p16^{INK4a} in prostate cancer cells *(129)*.

18. TUMOR SUPPRESSOR PATHWAYS

The first result hinting that genistein impacted tumor suppression was the elevation of p53 in HeLa cells *(153)*. However, in melanoma cells overexpressing p53, the inhibitory effect of genistein on cell growth was lost *(154)*. Genistein induces the upregulation of p53 protein, phosphorylation of p53 at ser15, activation of the sequence-specific DNA-binding properties of p53, and phosphorylation of the hCds1/Chk2 protein kinase at threonine 68 *(155)*. Furthermore, genistein induces phosphorylation of ATM on ser1981 and phosphorylation of histone H2AX on ser139 *(156)*. Genistein increases p53 expression in non-tumorigenic MCF-10F mammary epithelial cells *(157)*. However, the concentration (45 μM) was 3–4 orders of magnitude larger than would occur physiologically. Nonetheless, colonic cancer cells may be exposed to these concentrations; in HCT-116 cells genistein upregulated p53 *(158)*. Genistein elevated p53 protein levels in mouse dendritic cells, potentially affecting NF-κB signaling *(159)*.

There have been occasional reports on the effects of genistein on the tumor suppressors BRCA1/BRCA2 expression and protein levels in cells *(160, 161)*. However, when genistein is administered via the diet in the pre-pubertal period, it increases BRCA1 expression in the mammary gland *(162)*, consistent with lowered mammary tumorigenesis.

Genistein increases PTEN expression in the mammary gland of rats fed genistein (250 ppm in the diet) or soy protein isolate (216 ppm genistein and 160 ppm daidzein) from gestation day 4 *(163)*. The mammary glands of the female offspring were obtained 50 days after birth. PTEN expression was also upregulated by genistein in LNCaP and PC-3 prostate cancer cells *(164)*.

Genistein recently has been shown to increase the tumor suppressor EGR-1 and suppress the protooncogene MET at concentrations below 1 μM in normal breast epithelial cells (MCF-10F) *(165)*. This protein also binds to the transcription factor Sp1.

19. EXOSOME SIGNALING

A new area of research in cancer prevention is the role of tumor exosomes on immune tolerance. Exosomes arise from lysosomal processing of endosomes and are secreted by many cell types. They can fuse with other cells and thereby transfer proteins, RNA, and lipids from the tumor to natural killer (NK) cells. Exosomes from murine mammary tumor cells inhibit NK cell DNA synthesis when challenged with IL-2 *(166)*. Interestingly, when the polyphenol curcumin is incubated with the mammary tumor cells, the responsiveness of NK cells to IL-2 is restored *(167)*. This occurs significantly at 100 nM – certainly a concentration that can be achieved by dietary means. The reversal of the exosome effect was associated with curcumin-induced increased protein ubiquitination. This suggests that the proteins included in the exosomes and transferred to NK cells can be inactivated by dietary polyphenols. The role of isoflavones in regulating the exosome numbers secreted by cancer cells, their protein content, and posttranslational modifications remains to be pursued. These data suggest that isoflavones and other polyphenols play important roles in maintaining the immune surveillance against cancer and call into question the significance of results obtained with immunocompromised mouse models.

20. INTERACTIONS WITH OTHER PHYTOCHEMICALS

The systematic studies of most of NIH-sponsored research involve careful experimentation to determine the mechanism of action of single compounds. This approach, however, does not take into account the interaction between dietary components. When genistein was administered subcutaneously with the lignans enterodiol and enterolac-tone to OVEX nude mice with MCF-7 cell implants, tumor cell growth did not occur *(168)*. However, this combination also blocked beneficial effects of genistein on bone and caused uterine growth *(169)*. The combination of biochanin A, epigallocatechin-3-gallate (EGCG), and quercetin (administered subcutaneously) reduced the size of the tumor created by implantation of MCF-7 cells in nude mice *(85)*. Biochanin A in this combination was one-third of the dose when it was used on its own to demonstrate anti-tumor effects in this model. Since EGCG and quercetin had no significant effect when they were administered alone, the combination indicates that interactions occur for the effects of dietary components. In recent study, the effect of combining curcumin and genistein on the inhibition of pancreatic cancer cell growth was found to be synergistic *(170)*. Nonetheless, combinations aren't always beneficial. Although genistein signifi-cantly increases the oral bioavailability of EGCG in Min (–/–) mice, the animals have increased intestinal tumors *(171)*.

21. OMICS AND MECHANISMS OF ACTION

Microarray analysis (transcriptomics). Most mechanistic studies are carried out with the intent to test-specific hypotheses. This is the classical approach and it doesn't dis-tinguish whether the effects of the isoflavones are direct or indirect. In contrast, the implementation of reproducible DNA microarray analysis, particularly, over the past 5–6 years has allowed a broader appreciation of how isoflavones influence gene expression in cells and tissues. However, to do this, careful control of the experimental design to avoid systematic error is needed and sufficient numbers of replicates must be used *(172, 173)*. Also, the concept of "significance" is often limited to simple fold-change criteria. However, fold changes are only part of a Student *t* test – the *t* statistic contains not only the difference between means of two groups but also a function of the pooled variance. The more reproducible are microarray results (analytical and biological replicates), the smaller the fold changes that are significant. Indeed, for some factors such as PTEN, even a small change can be critical leading to either cell proliferation or apoptosis *(174)*.

A second issue is the *false discovery rate* (FDR). In simple experiments where one variable is being examined, we accept that a *P* value derived from the calculated *t* test that is less than 0.05 indicates that the null hypothesis can be rejected. As the number of variables increases, the *P* value has to be lowered. The Bonferroni correction (0.05/*n*) where *n* = number of variables, is very harsh *(175)*. Therefore, we must consider less stringent alternatives. One way is to plot a histogram of the *P* values – under the null hypothesis, the expected *P* values are uniformly distributed between 0 and 1. Therefore, a distribution showing an excess of expected genes as the *P* values approach 0 is evi-dence that some of the genes are true positives (Fig. 9). For instance, with an array with 5,000 genes that give measurable signals, the null hypothesis predicts that there will be 250 with *P* values <0.05. If we observe 377 genes that changed, then we can predict that 127 are true and 250 are false (however, we do not know which is which). The FDR is 67%. Only a few of the studies summarized in Table 2 take these issues into account.

Microarray analysis has been carried out using bladder *(176)*, breast *(177–181)*, endometrial *(182)*, lung *(183)*, pancreatic *(184)*, and prostate cancer cell lines

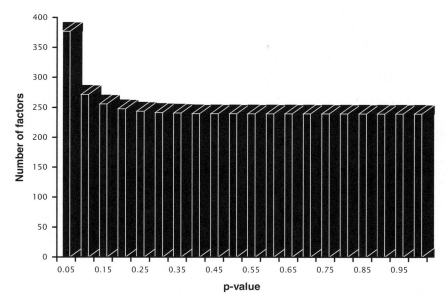

Fig. 9. Distribution of *P* values. Under the null hypothesis, the observed *P* values of a high dimensional system (e.g., a microarray) are distributed evenly between 0 and 1. This means that 5% of the measured factors will have *P* values <0.05. In this example of a 5,000 factor array, the expected number for *P* <0.05 under the null hypothesis is 250. However, 377 factors had *P* values <0.05. This represents an excess of 127 factors. So, 250 are false and 127 are true, although all 377 will look similar. Independent validation is necessary to define which is which.

(185–195). In many studies, genome-wide arrays were used *(179–181, 184, 187, 188, 190–192, 194, 195)*, whereas selective oligonucleotide arrays were used in the other cases *(176–178, 183, 185, 186, 189, 193)*. The major pathways or specific genes reported in these studies are summarized in Table 2. For the most part, the mechanisms associated with these changes in gene expression are consistent with the phenotypic changes observed in previous studies, i.e., for ER-positive cells, low concentrations (below 5 μM) of genistein leads to cell proliferation, whereas higher concentrations (10 μM and greater) cause cell-cycle inhibition and apoptosis. Genes that underwent changes in expression were mostly those expected to be associated with these biological events. Shioda et al. *(179)* stressed the importance of testing physiologically meaningful concentrations. However, these investigators used 3 μM genistein, which is not physiologic. The lowest concentration of genistein in any of these studies was 0.5 μM *(183)*, which exceeds the physiologic concentrations in blood.

The bladder is an exception to this generalism because of the much higher concentrations in urine. If the intake of isoflavones is 50 mg/day, this is approximately 150–180 μmol. If we assume 40% of the isoflavones are excreted in the urine per day and the 24-h urine volume is 2 l, the urine concentration of isoflavones will be 30–36 μM. Of course, it's not known exactly what isoflavone concentrations the bladder cells are exposed to, but they may substantially exceed other tissues.

Table 2
Impact of Genistein on Principal Changes in Gene Expression in Cultured Cancer Cells

Cell type	Concentration (μM)	Microarray type	Gene changes	References
Bladder TCCSUP	50	Custom array (884 selected cancer genes)	25 genes altered; divided into seven classes; most were upregulated; two were downregulated (NDR and DD1T3); egr-1 and c-fos; signal transduction; cell-cycle pathways	Chen et al. (*176*)
Breast MCF-7	50/100		Hsp105 upregulated; serum response factor, ERα, disabled homolog 2, and recombination activation gene 1	Chen et al. (*177*)
MCF-7	10	EstrArray (172 estrogen-responsive genes)	108 genes were upregulated and 64 downregulated; genistein was highly correlated ($R = 0.93$) with the effects of estradiol	Ise et al. (*178*)
MCF-7	3, 10	Human Genome U133A microarray (22,283 genes)	1,675 genes were informative; gene profile for genistein at 3 μM was closely related to that for 30 nM 17β-estradiol; cell-cycle pathway genes were upregulated, as were pathways in purine and pyrimidine synthesis and steroid biosynthesis; UCP-1 was upregulated (mitochondrial biogenesis)	Shioda et al. (*179*)

Cell line	Concentration	Microarray	Results	Reference
HCC1395	50	Human 1A (v2) microarray (18,716 genes)	397 genes had >2-fold change; 154 upregulated and 243 downregulated; MMP-2, MMP-7 and CXCL12 downregulated (activators of metastasis and invasion); upregulated TFPI-2, ATF3, DNMT1 and MTCBP-1 (inhibitors of metastasis and invasion)	Lee et al. (180)
MCF-7	1, 5, 25	Human Genome U133A Microarray	At 1 μM there was a pattern of increased mitogenic activity; significance cutoff ($P < 0.001$ and 1.5-fold change); 207, 232, and 245 genes changed at 1, 5, and 25 μM, respectively; CKS1B and CKS2 upregulated (associated with proliferation) at low concentration; pattern of apoptosis and decreased proliferation at the high concentrations, but conflicting results at low concentrations; ERα lowered, as were NCOA2 and NCOA3; AKR1C1 and AKR1C3 upregulated; Jun and Jun D upregulated as were the estrogen-responsive genes GREB1, EGR3, CXCL12; BIK and IL-1R1 were downregulated	Lavigne et al. (181)

(Continued)

Table 2
(Continued)

Cell type	Concentration (μM)	Microarray type	Gene changes	References
Endometrial Ishikawa	0.5, 5, 50, and 500	Custom cDNA Array (9,381 Unique cDNAs – Unigene build 144)	Overall, 667 genes changed (> or < 1.5-fold with 10% SEM); at 5 μM, 87 downregulated and 8 upregulated, and only 2 [1 up– (dual-specific phosphatase) and 1 downregulated (Trf)] at 0.5 μM; pathway analysis At 5 μM revealed that genes associated with Ras signaling, MAPK signaling, transcription, cell-cycle, cell proliferation, and cell migration were all down; upregulated genes included M-phase phosphoprotein 9, protein kinase Cα, ATP synthase, mitochondrial F1 complex $\sum$ subunit, steroidogenic acute regulatory protein, Cockayne syndrome 1	Konstantakopoulos et al. (*182*)
Lung carcinoma SPC-A-1	20	Oligo GEArray Human Apoptosis Microarray Human U133A	20 genes (out of 122) changed > two-fold; Bcl-2, TNF ligand and its receptor – apoptosis	Zou et al. (*183*)
Pancreatic Panc-1	10		47 genes significantly changed; egr-1 and IL-8 upregulated; EGFR, AKT2, CYP1B1, NELL2, SCD, DNA ligase III, and Rad were downregulated	Bai et al. (*184*)

Prostate LNCaP	36	Prostate-specific custom array (3,500 sequences)	870 genes examined; using a 2-fold cutoff, 29 genes were downregulated and 11 genes were upregulated; downregulated genes associated with transcription, translation, signal transduction, cell adhesion, ubiquitination, and mitochondrial functions; upregulated genes associated with transcription, signal transduction, and cell cytoskeletal structure	Rice et al. (*185*)
LNCaP PC-3	100	IntelliGene™ Cancer CHIP (557 genes)	Survivin, DNA topoisomerase II, CDC6, MAPK are downregulated; four genes upregulated (glutathione peroxidase; Ras homolog family, member D; aldolase A and quiescin Q6)	Suzuki et al. (*186*)
PC-3	5, 15, 30, and 50	Human genome U95 microarray (12,558 gene probes)	832 genes changed >2-fold; 774 downregulated, 58 upregulated; classes: cell growth, cell cycle, apoptosis, cell signaling transduction, angiogenesis, tumor cell invasion, and metastasis; TGFβ, VEGF and thrombospondin downregulated	Li and Sarkar (*187*, Li and Sarkar *188*)

(Continued)

Table 2
(Continued)

Cell type	Concentration (μM)	Microarray type	Gene changes	References
DU-145	50	Custom array (~6,000 genes)	Decreased NK-κB, PIM-2, defender against cell death 1	Ayala et al. (189)
LNCaP	1, 5, 25	Human genome U133A array (54,613 gene probes)	Concentration-dependent changes (8, 21 and 108 > 2-fold upregulated, and 22, 15, and 243 downregulated); downregulation of androgen upregulated androgen-responsive genes and upregulation of androgen down regulated androgen-responsive genes and five genes upregulated by both genistein and androgens; regulation of cell-cycle regulated genes consistent with cell-cycle inhibition; IGFR1 downregulation at 1 μM; two PPARisα-responsive (MEI and FACL2) genes upregulated at 5 and 25 μM	Takahashi et al. (190)
PC-3	30 with kinesin spindle protein inhibitor SB715992	Human Genome U133A Array (54,613 gene probes)	Cell proliferation, cell cycle, cell signaling, and apoptosis genes downregulated	Davis et al. (191)

Cell line	Concentration	Array	Results	Reference
PC-3	30–50	Human genome U95, U133A MMP-9 arrays	Upregulated osteoprotegrin, RANKL; downregulated	Li et al. (192)
PC-3 DU-145	28 μM	Human Focus Array (~8,500 genes)	For PC-3 cells, 78 genes were downregulated >50% and 82 two-fold upregulated; for DU-145 cells, 120 genes were downregulated and 25 were two-fold upregulated; lowered uPA and uPAR transcription; some MMPs and integrin subunits downregulated	Skogseth et al. (193)
LNCaP	1, 5, 25	Human genome U133A array	$P < 0.01$, > or < 1.5-fold change; genistein caused 3, 34 and 484 changes at 1, 5, and 25 μM; at 1 μM equol altered 14 genes and daidzein 29 genes; pathway analysis revealed significant effects of equol on many stages of cell-cycle control, nuclear division and cell proliferation; Daidzein's effects were much lower and were concentrated on cellular metabolism; common effects on androgen-responsive, IGF-1 pathway and MAP kinase-related pathways	Takahashi et al. (194)

(Continued)

Table 2
(Continued)

Cell type	Concentration (μM)	Microarray type	Gene changes	References
LNCaP	35 plus norepinephrine	Human genome U133A v2 array (54,675 probes)	Caused 201 genes to change in expression at $P < 0.002$; CDKN1A and WHSC2 upregulated; ATAD2, BUB3, BUB1B, CDC6, CENPE, CKS1B, DKFZP76E1312, DLG7, EIF5A, FEN1, FOXM1, KIAA1794, KIF20A, KIF2C, KIF4A, KNTC2, MCM4, MCM7, NUSAP1, POLD3, PRC1, PRIM1, SLC30A5, SMC2, SPBC24, TTK, UBE2S, UBE2T, UHRF1ZWINT downregulated	Mori et al. (195)

What is not often considered is that genistein circulating in the blood, and thereby able to reach tissues, is mostly conjugated with glucuronic acid, with only a small fraction in the aglucone (unconjugated) form. In this respect, genistein (and other isoflavones and their metabolites) is similar to 17β-estradiol. Only a small fraction of 17β-estradiol is unconjugated and available for tissue uptake *(196)*. Nonetheless, this fraction still has biological and biochemical activity. There is a substantial difference in genistein bioactivity between oral (dietary or by gavage) and peripheral intake (i.e., via a patch or subcutaneous injection) of estrogens *(197)*. For oral intake, the blood level of unconjugated genistein rarely exceeds 100 nM. Most of the toxicological data have been reported using experimental designs where genistein is administered by injection. Under these conditions of administration, unconjugated genistein concentrations can exceed 1 μM.

It is therefore more meaningful to examine microarray data from cells that are subject to cancer risk in vivo. Naciff et al. compared the dose responsive effects of 17α-ethinylestradiol, bisphenol A, and genistein on gene expression in the uterus of ovariectomized rats *(198)*. Genistein lowered the expression of more genes than it upregulated and behaved differently from 17α-ethinylestradiol and bisphenol A. Microarray analysis of gene expression in PC-3 bone tumors in SCID mice treated with genistein revealed that there were changes in cell growth, apoptosis, and metastasis, with a confirmed fall in MMP-9 *(199)*. Subsequent experiments indicated that genistein could augment the benefit of the anti-cancer drug docetaxel *(200)*. Another effect was the changes in gene expression caused by a soy isoflavone concentrate in wild-type and Nrf2 (–/–) mice, a factor that is associated with chemoprevention of prostate cancer *(201)*. Analysis was carried out on an Affymetrix mouse genome 430 2.0 array containing >45,101 probe sets; 1,438 genes were upregulated >2-fold and 1,338 were downregulated, covering a wide range of pathways. Gene classification revealed that they consisted of effects on electron transport, phase II metabolizing enzymes, cell growth and differentiation, apoptosis, cell cycle, transcription factors, transport, mRNA processing, and carbohydrate homeostasis.

22. PROTEOMICS

It is argued by many that gene expression is only one part of the – Omics strategy *(202)*. Gene transcripts have to be converted to proteins to fulfill their roles biologically and biochemically. Accordingly, techniques in protein chemistry at the global level have been developed using gel-based and gel-free workflows. The gel-free approach has been used extensively – it is based on the protease-driven hydrolysis of all the proteins present in a sample and then a two-dimensional separation of the resulting peptides based on their charge and hydrophobicity prior to tandem mass spectrometry *(203)*. The results from this approach were impressive, but were tempered by the realization that overfitting of the MSMS spectra had occurred. Investigators now use reverse or random databases to minimize false discovery of protein identification *(204)*. Also the initial definitions of what a gene is (in 2000) and hence what the predicted/expected proteins are undergoing change as the ENCODE project expands from the initial 1% survey of the humane genome *(205)*.

A further consideration is what happens to a protein once its formed by translation of the mRNA message. Many proteins have N-terminal signaling peptides that are removed once the protein is "in place" in the cell. Most proteins undergo extensive posttranslational modification (PTM). It is estimated that on average, PTM occur every 8–12 amino acid residues in proteins *(206)*. These can be important biochemically/functionally – e.g., phosphorylation, glycosylation, methylation, acetylation, myristoylation, nitrosylation, ubiquitinylation, sumoylation – as well as being the result of oxidative stress, e.g., oxidation, nitration, and reaction with electrophilic lipids and lipid aldehydes. Finally, many proteins are broken down into smaller parts, either intentionally like chromogranin in the brain *(207)* or as the result of the activation of metalloproteinases as part of the metastatic process. Therefore, there is a strong need to determine the actual protein forms in the system under study.

A better approach is to separate the proteins first. Biochemists have developed protein separation methods over the past 80–90 years. The challenge for present day investigators is how to scale these methods so as to be able to observe as many of the proteins of interest as possible while at the same time integrating the methods with mass spectrometry. A popular method is the use of 2D-isoelectric focusing/SDS-polyacrylamide gel electrophoresis *(208)*. Its advantage is that it can spread the separation of 500–800 proteins out over the 2D-gel. Proteins are separated not just by apparent molecular weight, but also by their isoelectric points. Importantly, every spot observed on the 2D-gel is a real protein, whether or not it is predicted by current interpretations of the human or other genomes. Many proteins form strings across the gel – those that give essentially flat lines (no measurable change in molecular weight) are often proteins undergoing phosphorylation or acetylation. Those strings that are at an angle (with increasing molecular weights) can be proteins in different stages of glycosylation. Limitations of 2D-gels are membrane proteins that are insoluble in the IEF buffer (7 M urea/2 M thiourea) and the reproducibility of the mobility of each spot. The latter issue has been largely overcome by the use of covalently attached pH gradients on plastic strips for the IEF first stage of analysis *(209)*. The introduction of fluorescent dyes (Cy dyes) that react with lysine and cysteine groups has further helped. This methodology enables control and treatment samples to be separately "colored" by individual Cy dyes and then the samples mixed prior to 2D-electrophoresis *(210)*. Changes in protein amount are determined by measuring the ratio of the two fluorescent tags for each protein spot.

Proteins insoluble in IEF buffers can usually be resolved by standard 1D-single concentration or gradient gel SDS-polyacrylamide electrophoresis *(211)*. The gel is cut into many fractions from low-to-high molecular weights. Since SDS denatures proteins, this is a particularly suitable method for effectively digesting proteins with proteases. The resulting peptides are analyzed by nanoLC-tandem mass spectrometry. The advantage of this Gel-LC method is that all the peptides for the particular molecular weight form of the protein are present in each fraction.

Proteins also form complexes that are essential for their function. Another 2D-electrophoresis method (2D-blue native or clear native electrophoresis) enables resolution of the intact protein complexes in the first dimension, followed by in-gel reduction with dithiothreitol and resolution of the proteins orthogonally using a gradient SDS-PAGE gel method *(212–214)*.

Using the 2D-gel approach, investigators have both examined mammary glands at different stages of development. In the former a potential pathway representing genistein-dependent protein differences in mammary gland tissue has been postulated *(215)*. GTP cyclohydrolase 1 was one of six proteins whose abundance was changed by genistein. It was significantly upregulated in day 21 animals injected with 500 µg genistein on days 16, 18, and 20 postpartum. This is the rate-limiting enzyme for the synthesis of tetrahydrobiopterin, a necessary cofactor for catecholamine synthesis and nitric oxide production *(216)*. Downstream of this enzyme, tyrosine hydroxylase was upregulated and this continued to day 50. This was proposed to reduce VEGFR2 and thereby alter angiogenesis and hence establishment of the mammary cancer. Importantly, these changes occurred in the epithelial cell layer lining the ducts in the mammary gland.

Kim et al. *(217)* demonstrated that approximately 25% of the mammary gland proteins detected on 2D-IEF/SDS-PAGE gel in day 21 and 50 day rats (at weaning and at maximum sensitivity to carcinogen) underwent statistically different changes in abundance and in mobility. Sixty-five of these proteins were identified by matrix-assisted laser desorption ionization – time of flight mass spectrometry (MALDI-MS) and confirmed by nanoLC-tandem mass spectrometry. Future studies are being directed at the modulating effects of polyphenols (genistein, resveratrol, and epigallocatechin-3-gallate) on these proteins with the goal of identifying the critical targets and mechanisms therein that alter the susceptibility of the mammary gland to cancer.

23. CONCLUSIONS

Isoflavones have structural similarities to physiologic estrogens. The soy isoflavone genistein in cellular and pre-clinical animal models has been shown to have estrogen-like effects, causing some concern about its safety. However, genistein and other common isoflavones have many other demonstrable mechanisms that may offset the estrogen-like effects, albeit that most occur at higher concentrations/doses. Also, there are many cancers that do not express estrogen receptors where genistein and combinations of isoflavones prevent tumorigenesis or existing tumor cell growth.

ACKNOWLEDGMENTS

Support for the UAB Center for Nutrient-Gene Interaction in Cancer Prevention is provided by a grant-in-aid (U54 CA100949, S. Barnes, PI) from the National Cancer Institute. Support for research on botanicals and dietary supplements at the Purdue University-University of Alabama at Birmingham Botanical Center for Age-related Disease is provided by a grant (P50 AT00477, Connie M. Weaver, PI) from the National Center for Complementary and Alternative Medicine and the NIH Office of Dietary Supplements. Acknowledgments are also given to colleagues in UAB Center for Nutrient-Gene Interaction (Drs. David Allison, Michael Crowley, Clinton Grubbs, Helen Kim, Coral Lamartiniere, Sreelatha Meleth and Grier Page), former graduate students, now Drs. Brenda Boersma and Tracy D'Alessandro, and colleagues in the UAB Center for Free Radical Biology (Drs. Victor Darley-Usmar and Dr. Rakesh Patel) for their contributions to the body of work performed on isoflavones.

REFERENCES

1. Barnes, S., Kim, H., Darley-Usmar, V., Patel, R., Xu, J., Boersma, B., and Luo, M. (2000) Beyond ER alpha and ER beta: Estrogen receptor binding is only part of the isoflavone story. *J Nutr* **130**, 656–7S.
2. Barnes, S., Prasain, J., D'Alessandro, T., Wang, C.C., Zhang, H.G., and Kim, H. (2006) In: Heber D., Blackburn G.L., Go V.L.W., and Milner J., eds. Nutritional Oncology. 559–71, San Diego, CA: Academic Press.
3. Steele, C.L., Gijzen, M., Qutob, D., and Dixon, R.A. (1999) Molecular characterization of the enzyme catalyzing the aryl migration reaction of isoflavonoid biosynthesis in soybean. *Arch Biochem Biophys* **367**, 146–50.
4. Barnes, S., Kirk, M., and Coward, L. (1994) Isoflavones and their conjugates in soy foods: Extraction conditions and analysis by HPLC-mass spectrometry. *J Agric Food Chem* **42**, 2466–74.
5. Prasain, J.K., Jones, K., Brissie, N., Moore, D.R., II, Wyss, J.M., and Barnes, S. (2004) Identification of puerarin and its metabolites in rats by liquid chromatography-tandem mass spectrometry. *J Agric Food Chem* **52**, 3708–12.
6. Talla, E., Njamen, D., Mbafor, J.T., Fomum, Z.T., Kamanyi, A., Mbanya, J.C., Giner, R.M., Recio, M.C., Máñez, S., and Ríos, J.L. (2003) Warangalone, the isoflavonoid anti-inflammatory principle of Erythrina addisoniae stem bark. *J Nat Prod* **66**, 891–93.
7. Milligan, S.R., Kalita, J.C., Pocock, V., Van De Kauter, V., Stevens, J.F., Deinzer, M.L., Rong, H., and De Keukeleire, D. (2000) The endocrine activities of 8-prenylnaringenin and related hop (*Humulus lupulus L.*) flavonoids. *J Clin Endocrinol Metab* **85**, 4912–15.
8. Walter, E.D. (1941) Genistin (an isoflavone glucoside) and its aglucone, genistein from soybean. *J Am Oil Chem Soc* **63**, 3273–76.
9. Adlercreutz, H., and Mazur, W. (1997) Phyto-oestrogens and Western diseases. *Ann Med* **29**, 95–120.
10. Horn-Ross, P.L., Barnes, S., Lee, M., Coward, L., Mandel, E., Koo, J., John, E.M., and Smith, M. (2000) Assessing phytoestrogen exposure in epidemiologic studies: Development of a database (United States). *Cancer Causes Contr* **11**, 289–98.
11. Price, K.R., and Fenwick, G.R. (1985) Naturally occurring oestrogens in foods—a review. *Food Addit Contam* **2**, 73–106.
12. Keung, W.M., and Vallee, B.L. (1998) Kudzu root: An ancient chinese source of modern antidipsotropic agents. *Phytochem* **47**, 499–506.
13. Reynolds, B.D., Blackmon, W.J., Wickremesinhe, E., Wells, M.H., and Constantin, R.J. (1990) Domestication of *Apios americana*. In: J. Janick, and J.E. Simon eds. Advances in new crops. 436–42, Portland, OR: Timber Press.
14. Barnes, S., Wang, C.C., Kirk, M., Smith-Johnson, M., Coward, L., Barnes, N.C., Vance, G., and Boersma, B. (2002) HPLC-mass spectrometry of isoflavonoids in soy and the American groundnut, *Apios americana*. *Adv Exp Med Biol* **505**, 77–88.
15. Nagata, C., Takatsuka, N., and Shimizu, H. (2002) Soy and Fish Oil Intake and Mortality in a Japanese Community. *Am J Epidemiol* **156**, 824–31.
16. Frankenfeld, C.L., Patterson, R.E., Kalhorn, T.F., Skor, H.E., Howald, W.N., and Lampe, J.W. (2002) Validation of a soy food frequency questionnaire with plasma concentrations of isoflavones in US adults. *J Am Diet Assoc* **102**, 1407–13.
17. Otero-Raviña, F., Grigorian-Shamagian, L., Blanco Rodríguez, R., Gómez Vázquez, J.L., Fernández Villaverde, J.M., and González-Juanatey, J.R. and Grupo Barbanza (2007) Changes in lipid profile after regular intake of canned fish. The influence of addition of isoflavones, omega-3 fatty acids and fitosterols. *Med Clin (Barc)* **129**, 81–85.
18. Coward, L., Barnes, N.C., Setchell, K.D.R., and Barnes, S. (1993) The antitumor isoflavones, genistein and daidzein, in soybean foods of American and Asian diets. *J Agric Food Chem* **41**, 1961–67.
19. Day, A.J., Cañada, F.J., Díaz, J.C., Kroon, P.A., Mclauchlan, R., Faulds, C.B., Plumb, G.W., Morgan, M.R., and Williamson, G. (2000) Dietary flavonoid and isoflavone glycosides are hydrolysed by the lactase site of lactase phlorizin hydrolase. *FEBS Lett* **468**, 166–70.
20. Sfakianos, J., Coward, L., Kirk, M., and Barnes, S. (1997) Intestinal uptake and biliary excretion of the isoflavone genistein in rats. *J Nutr* **127**, 1260–68.

21. Coldham, N.G., Howells, L.C., Santi, A., Montesissa, C., Langlais, C., King, L.J., Macpherson, D.D., and Sauer, M.J. (1999) Biotransformation of genistein in the rat: Elucidation of metabolite structure by product ion mass fragmentology. *J Steroid Biochem Mol Biol* **70**, 169–84.

22. Loo, G. (2003) Redox-sensitive mechanisms of phytochemical-mediated inhibition of cancer cell proliferation. *J Nutr Biochem* **14**, 64–73.

23. Surh, Y.J. (2003) Cancer chemoprevention with dietary phytochemicals. *Nat Rev Cancer* **3**, 768–80.

24. Tsuda, H., Ohshima, Y., Nomoto, H., Fujita, K., Matsuda, E., Iigo, M., Takasuka, N., and Moore, M.A. (2004) Cancer prevention by natural compounds. *Drug Metab Pharmacokinet* **19**, 245–63.

25. Surh, Y.J., Na, H.K., and Lee, S.S. (2004) Transcription factors and mitogen-activated protein kinases as molecular targets for chemoprevention with anti-inflammatory phytochemicals. *Biofactors* **21**, 103–08.

26. Liu, R.H. (2004) Potential synergy of phytochemicals in cancer prevention: Mechanism of action. *J Nutr* **134**, 3479S–3485S.

27. Surh, Y.J., Kundu, J.K., Na, H.K., and Lee, J.S. (2005) Redox-sensitive transcription factors as prime targets for chemoprevention with anti-inflammatory and antioxidative phytochemicals. *J Nutr* **135**, 2993S–3001S.

28. Ferguson, L.R., and Philpott, M. (2007) Cancer prevention by dietary bioactive components that target the immune response. *Curr Cancer Drug Targets* **7**, 459–64.

29. Nishino, H., Satomi, Y., Tokuda, H., and Masuda, M. (2007) Cancer control by phytochemicals. *Curr Pharm Des* **13**, 3394–99.

30. Kundu, J.K., and Surh, Y.J. (2008) Cancer chemopreventive and therapeutic potential of resveratrol: Mechanistic perspectives. *Cancer Lett* **269**, 243–61.

31. Aggarwal, B.B., Kunnumakkara, A.B., Harikumar, K.B., Tharakan, S.T., Sung, B., and Anand, P. (2008) Potential of spice-derived phytochemicals for cancer prevention. *Planta Med* **74**, 1560–69.

32. Kim, H., Peterson, T.G., and Barnes, S. (1998) Mechanisms of action of the soy isoflavone genistein: Emerging role for its effects via transforming growth factor beta signaling pathways. *Am J Clin Nutr* **68**, 1418S–1425S.

33. Polkowski, K., and Mazurek, A.P. (2000) Biological properties of genistein. A review of *in vitro* and in vivo data. *Acta Pol Pharm* **57**, 135–55.

34. Lamartiniere, C.A., Cotroneo, M.S., Fritz, W.A., Wang, J., Mentor-Marcel, R., and Elgavish, A. (2002) Genistein chemoprevention: Timing and mechanisms of action in murine mammary and prostate. *J Nutr* **132**, 552S–558S.

35. Magee, P.J., and Rowland, I.R. (2004) Phyto-oestrogens, their mechanism of action: Current evidence for a role in breast and prostate cancer. *Br J Nutr* **91**, 513–31.

36. Cross, H.S., Kállay, E., Lechner, D., Gerdenitsch, W., Adlercreutz, H., and Armbrecht, H.J. (2004) Phytoestrogens and vitamin D metabolism: A new concept for the prevention and therapy of colorectal, prostate, and mammary carcinomas. *J Nutr* **134**, 1207S–1212S.

37. Ravindranath, M.H., Muthugounder, S., Presser, N., and Viswanathan, S. (2004) Anticancer therapeutic potential of soy isoflavone, genistein. *Adv Exp Med Biol* **546**, 121–65.

38. Holzbeierlein, J.M., McIntosh, J., and Thrasher, J.B. (2005) The role of soy phytoestrogens in prostate cancer. *Curr Opin Urol* **15**, 17–22.

39. Bektic, J., Guggenberger, R., Eder, I.E., Pelzer, A.E., Berger, A.P., Bartsch, G., and Klocker, H. (2005) Molecular effects of the isoflavonoid genistein in prostate cancer. *Clin Prostate Cancer* **4**, 124–29.

40. Messina, M., Kucuk, O., and Lampe, J.W. (2006) An overview of the health effects of isoflavones with an emphasis on prostate cancer risk and prostate-specific antigen levels. *J AOAC Int* **89**, 1121–34.

41. Xiao, C.W., Wood, C., and Gilani, G.S. (2006) Nuclear receptors: Potential biomarkers for assessing physiological functions of soy proteins and phytoestrogens. *J AOAC Int* **89**, 1207–14.

42. Goetzl, M.A., Van Veldhuizen, P.J., and Thrasher, J.B. (2007) Effects of soy phytoestrogens on the prostate. *Prostate Cancer Prostatic Dis* **10**, 216–23.

43. Power, K.A., and Thompson, L.U. (2007) Can the combination of flaxseed and its lignans with soy and its isoflavones reduce the growth stimulatory effect of soy and its isoflavones on established breast cancer? *Mol Nutr Food Res* **51**, 845–56.

44. Rahman, I., Biswas, S.K., and Kirkham, P.A. (2006) Regulation of inflammation and redox signaling by dietary polyphenols. *Biochem Pharmacol* **72**, 1439–52.

45. Krishnan, V., Heath, H., and Bryant, H.U. (2000) Mechanism of action of estrogens and selective estrogen receptor modulators. *Vitam Horm* **60**, 123–47.

46. Moutsatsou, P. (2007) The spectrum of phytoestrogens in nature: Our knowledge is expanding. *Hormones (Athens)* **6**, 173–93.

47. Okura, A., Arakawa, H., Oka, H., Yoshinari, T., and Monden, Y. (1988) Effect of genistein on topoisomerase activity and on the growth of [Val 12]Ha-ras-transformed NIH 3T3 cells. *Biochem Biophys Res Commun* **157**, 183–89.

48. Scholar, E.M., and Toews, M.L. (1994) Inhibition of invasion of murine mammary carcinoma cells by the tyrosine kinase inhibitor genistein. *Cancer Lett* **87**, 159–62.

49. Akiyama, T., Ishida, J., Nakagawa, S., Ogawara, H., Watanabe, S., Itoh, N., Shibuya, M., and Fukami, Y. (1987) Genistein, a specific inhibitor of tyrosine-specific protein kinases. *J Biol Chem* **262**, 5592–95.

50. Shelnutt, S.R., Cimino, C.O., Wiggins, P.A., Ronis, M.J., and Badger, T.M. (2002) Pharmacokinetics of the glucuronide and sulfate conjugates of genistein and daidzein in men and women after consumption of a soy beverage. *Am J Clin Nutr* **76**, 588–94.

51. Kuiper, G.G., Lemmen, J.G., Carlsson, B., Corton, J.C., Safe, S.H., van der Saag, P.T., van der Burg, B., and Gustafsson, J.A. (1998) Interaction of estrogenic chemicals and phytoestrogens with estrogen receptor beta. *Endocrinology* **139**, 4252–63.

52. Banerjee, S., Li, Y., Wang, Z., and Sarkar, F.H. (2008) Multi-targeted therapy of cancer by genistein. *Cancer Lett* **269**, 226–42.

53. Katanoda, K., and Qiu, D. (2007) Comparison of Time Trends in Female Breast Cancer Incidence (1973–1997) in East Asia, Europe and USA, from Cancer Incidence in Five Continents, Vols IV–VIII. *Jpn J Clin Oncol* **37**, 638–639.

54. Hsing, A.W., Tsao, L., and Devesa, S.S. (2000) International trends and patterns of prostate cancer incidence and mortality. *Int J Cancer* **85**, 60–67.

55. Qiu, D., and Tanaka, S. (2006) International comparisons of cumulative risk of stomach cancer, from cancer incidence in five continents Vol. VIII. *Jpn J Clin Oncol* **36**, 123–4.

56. Howson, C.P., Hiyama, T., and Wynder, E.L. (1986) The decline in gastric cancer: Epidemiology of an unplanned triumph. *Epidemiol Rev* **8**, 1–26.

57. Shimizu, H., Ross, R.K., Bernstein, L., Yatani, R., Henderson, B.E., and Mack, T.M. (1991) Cancers of the prostate and breast among Japanese and white immigrants in Los Angeles County. *Br J Cancer* **63**, 963–66.

58. Brawer, M.K. (2005) Prostatic intraepithelial neoplasia: An overview. *Rev Urol* **7**(Suppl 3), S11–S18.

59. Stemmermann, G.N. (1991) The pathology of breast cancer in Japanese women compared to other ethnic groups: A review. *Breast Cancer Res Treat* **18**, S67–S72.

60. Chia, K.S., Reilly, M., Tan, C.S., Lee, J., Pawitan, Y., Adami, H.O., Hall, P., and Mow, B. (2005) Profound changes in breast cancer incidence may reflect changes into a Westernized lifestyle: A comparative population-based study in Singapore and Sweden. *Int J Cancer* **113**, 302–06.

61. Qin, L.Q., Xu, J.Y., Wang, P.Y., and Hoshi, K. (2006) Soyfood intake in the prevention of breast cancer risk in women: A meta-analysis of observational epidemiological studies. *J Nutr Sci Vitaminol (Tokyo)* **52**, 428–36.

62. Wu, A.H., Yu, M.C., Tseng, C.C., and Pike, M.C. (2008) Epidemiology of soy exposures and breast cancer risk. *Br J Cancer* **98**, 9–14.

63. Shu, X.O., Jin, F., Dai, Q., Wen, W., Potter, J.D., Kushi, L.H., Ruan, Z., Gao, Y.T., and Zheng, W. (2001) Soyfood intake during adolescence and subsequent risk of breast cancer among Chinese women. *Cancer Epidemiol Biomarkers Prev* **10**, 483–88.

64. Messina, M., and Wood, C.E. (2008) Soy isoflavones, estrogen therapy, and breast cancer risk: Analysis and commentary. *Nutrition J* **17**, 7.

65. Troll, W., Wiesner, R., Shellabarger, C.J., Holtzman, S., and Stone, J.P. (1980) Soybean diet lowers breast tumor incidence in irradiated rats. *Carcinogenesis* **1**, 469–72.

66. Barnes, S., Grubbs, C., Setchell, K.D.R., and Carlson, J. (1990) Soybeans inhibit mammary tumors in models of breast cancer. *Prog Clin Biol Res* **347**, 239–53.

67. Simmen, R.C., Eason, R.R., Till, S.R., Chatman, L., Jr, Velarde, M.C., Geng, Y., Korourian, S., and Badger, T.M. (2005) Inhibition of NMU-induced mammary tumorigenesis by dietary soy. *Cancer Lett* **224**, 45–52.
68. Lamartiniere, C.A., Moore, J., Holland, M., and Barnes, S. (1995) Genistein and chemoprevention of breast cancer. *Proc Soc Exp Biol Med* **208**, 120–23.
69. Murrill, W.B., Brown, N.M., Zhang, J.-X., Manzolillo, P.A., Barnes, S., and Lamartiniere, C.A. (1996) Prepubertal genistein exposure suppresses mammary cancer and enhances gland differentiation in rats. *Carcinogenesis* **17**, 1451–57.
70. Fritz, W.A., Coward, L., Wang, J., and Lamartiniere, C.A. (1998) Dietary genistein: Perinatal mammary cancer prevention, bioavailability and toxicity testing in the rat. *Carcinogenesis* **19**, 2151–58.
71. Hilakivi-Clarke, L., Onojafe, I., Raygada, M., Cho, E., Skaar, T., Russo, I., and Clarke, R. (1999) Prepubertal exposure to zearalenone or genistein reduces mammary tumorigenesis. *Br J Cancer* **80**, 1682–88.
72. Mishra, P., Kale, R.K., and Kar, A. (2008) Chemoprevention of mammary tumorigenesis and chemomodulation of the antioxidative enzymes and peroxidative damage in prepubertal Sprague Dawley rats by Biochanin A. *Mol Cell Biochem* **312**, 1–9.
73. Lamartiniere, C.A., Cotroneo, M.S., Fritz, W.A., Wang, J., Mentor-Marcel, R., and Elgavish, A. (2002) Genistein chemoprevention: Timing and mechanisms of action in murine mammary and prostate. *J Nutr* **132**, 552S–558S.
74. Kim, H., Hall, P., Smith, M., Kirk, M., Prasain, J.K., Barnes, S., and Grubbs, C. (2004) Chemoprevention by grape seed extract and genistein in carcinogen-induced mammary cancer in rats is diet-dependent. *J Nutr* **134**, 3445S–52S.
75. Constantinou, A.I., Lantvit, D., Hawthorne, M., Xu, X., van Breemen, R.B., and Pezzuto, J.M. (2001) Chemopreventive effects of soy protein and purified soy isoflavones on DMBA-induced mammary tumors in female Sprague-Dawley rats. *Nutr Cancer* **41**, 75–81.
76. Hsieh, C.Y., Santell, R.C., Haslam, S.Z., and Helferich, W.G. (1998) Estrogenic effects of genistein on the growth of estrogen receptor-positive human breast cancer (MCF-7) cells *in vitro* and *in vivo*. *Cancer Res* **58**, 3833–38.
77. Allred, C.D., Allred, K.F., Ju, Y.H., Goeppinger, T.S., Doerge, D.R., and Helferich, W.G. (2004) Soy processing influences growth of estrogen-dependent breast cancer tumors. *Carcinogenesis* **25**, 1649–57.
78. Messina, M., and Barnes, S. (1991) Workshop report from the Division of Cancer Etiology, National Cancer Institute, National Institutes of Health. The role of soy products in reducing risks of certain cancers. *J Natil Cancer Inst* **83**, 541–46.
79. Ju, Y.H., Fultz, J., Allred, K.F., Doerge, D.R., and Helferich, W.G. (2006) Effects of dietary daidzein and its metabolite, equol, at physiological concentrations on the growth of estrogen-dependent human breast cancer (MCF-7) tumors implanted in ovariectomized athymic mice. *Carcinogenesis* **27**, 856–63.
80. Ju, Y.H., Allred, K.F., Allred, C.D., and Helferich, W.G. (2006) Genistein stimulates growth of human breast cancer cells in a novel, postmenopausal animal model, with low plasma estradiol concentrations. *Carcinogenesis* **27**, 1292–99.
81. Ju, Y.H., Doerge, D.R., Allred, K.F., Allred, C.D., and Helferich, W.G. (2002) Dietary genistein negates the inhibitory effect of tamoxifen on growth of estrogen-dependent human breast cancer (MCF-7) cells implanted in athymic mice. *Cancer Res* **62**, 2474–77.
82. Ju, Y.H., Doerge, D.R., Woodling, K.A., Hartman, J.A., Kwak, J., and Helferich, W.G. (2008) Dietary Genistein Negates the Inhibitory Effect of Letrozole On The Growth Of Aromatase-expressing Estrogen-Dependent Human Breast Cancer Cells (MCF-7Ca) *In Vivo*. *Carcinogenesis* **29**, 2162–68.
83. Shao, Z.M., Wu, J., Shen, Z.Z., and Barsky, S.H. (1998) Genistein exerts multiple suppressive effects on human breast carcinoma cells. *Cancer Res* **58**, 4851–57.
84. Constantinou, A.I., Krygier, A.E., and Mehta, R.R. (1998) Genistein induces maturation of cultured human breast cancer cells and prevents tumor growth in nude mice. *Am J Clin Nutr* **68**, 1426S–1430S.
85. Moon, Y.J., Shin, B.S., An, G., and Morris, M.E. (2008) Biochanin A inhibits breast cancer tumor growth in a murine xenograft model. *Pharm Res* **25**, 2158–63.

86. Santell, R.C., Kieu, N., and Helferich, W.G. (2000) Genistein inhibits growth of estrogen-independent human breast cancer cells in culture but not in athymic mice. *J Nutr* **130**, 1665–69.

87. Hillman, G.G., Wang, Y., Che, M., Raffoul, J.J., Yudelev, M., Kucuk, O., and Sarkar, F.H. (2007) Progression of renal cell carcinoma is inhibited by genistein and radiation in an orthotopic model. *BMC Cancer* **9**(7), 4.

88. Singh, A.V., Franke, A.A., Blackburn, G.L., and Zhou, J.R. (2006) Soy phytochemicals prevent orthotopic growth and metastasis of bladder cancer in mice by alterations of cancer cell proliferation and apoptosis and tumor angiogenesis. *Cancer Res* **66**, 1851–58.

89. Büchler, P., Gukovskaya, A.S., Mouria, M., Büchler, M.C., Büchler, M.W., Friess, H., Pandol, S.J., Reber, H.A., and Hines, O.J. (2003) Prevention of metastatic pancreatic cancer growth in vivo by induction of apoptosis with genistein, a naturally occurring isoflavonoid. *Pancreas* **26**, 264–73.

90. Lakshman, M., Xu, L., Ananthanarayanan, V., Cooper, J., Takimoto, C.H., Helenowski, I., Pelling, J.C., and Bergan, R.C. (2008) Dietary genistein inhibits metastasis of human prostate cancer in mice. *Cancer Res* **68**, 2024–32.

91. Raffoul, J.J., Banerjee, S., Che, M., Knoll, Z.E., Doerge, D.R., Abrams, J., Kucuk, O., Sarkar, F.H., and Hillman, G.G. (2007) Soy isoflavones enhance radiotherapy in a metastatic prostate cancer model. *Int J Cancer* **120**, 2491–98.

92. Wang, Y., Raffoul, J.J., Che, M., Doerge, D.R., Joiner, M.C., Kucuk, O., Sarkar, F.H., and Hillman, G.G. (2006) Prostate cancer treatment is enhanced by genistein *in vitro* and in vivo in a syngeneic orthotopic tumor model. *Radiat Res* **166**, 73–80.

93. Lightfoot, R.J., Smith, J.F., Cumming, I.A., Marshall, T., Wroth, R.H., and Hearnshaw, H. (1974) Infertility in ewes caused by prolonged grazing on oestrogenic pastures: Oestrus, fertilization and cervical mucus. *Aust J Biol Sci* **27**, 409–14.

94. Leopold, A.S., Erwin, M., Oh, J., and Browning, B. (1976) Phytoestrogens: Adverse effects on reproduction in California quail. *Science* **191**, 98–100.

95. Wilhelms, K.W., Scanes, C.G., and Anderson, L.L. (2006) Lack of estrogenic or antiestrogenic actions of soy isoflavones in an avian model: The Japanese quail. *Poult Sci* **85**, 1885–89.

96. Setchell, K.D., Gosselin, S.J., Welsh, M.B., Johnston, J.O., Balistreri, W.F., Kramer, L.W., Dresser, B.L., and Tarr, M.J. (1987) Dietary estrogens–a probable cause of infertility and liver disease in captive cheetahs. *Gastroenterology* **93**, 225–33.

97. Martin, P.M., Horwitz, K.B., Ryan, D.S., and McGuire, W.L. (1978) Phytoestrogen interaction with estrogen receptors in human breast cancer cells. *Endocrinology* **103**, 1860–67.

98. Mathieson, R.A., and Kitts, W.D. (1980) Binding of phyto-oestrogen and oestradiol-17 beta by cytoplasmic receptors in the pituitary gland and hypothalamus of the ewe. *J Endocrinol* **85**, 317–25.

99. Kuiper, G.G., Enmark, E., Pelto-Huikko, M., Nilsson, S., and Gustafsson, J.A. (1996) Cloning of a novel receptor expressed in rat prostate and ovary. *Proc Natl Acad Sci U S A* **93**, 5925–30.

100. Kuiper, G.G., Carlsson, B., Grandien, K., Enmark, E., Häggblad, J., Nilsson, S., and Gustafsson, J.A. (1997) Comparison of the ligand binding specificity and transcript tissue distribution of estrogen receptors alpha and beta. *Endocrinology* **138**, 863–70.

101. Setchell, K.D., Clerici, C., Lephart, E.D., Cole, S.J., Heenan, C., Castellani, D., Wolfe, B.E., Nechemias-Zimmer, L., Brown, N.M., Lund, T.D., Handa, R.J., and Heubi, J.E. (2005) S-equol, a potent ligand for estrogen receptor beta, is the exclusive enantiomeric form of the soy isoflavone metabolite produced by human intestinal bacterial flora. *Am J Clin Nutr* **81**, 1072–79.

102. Pelissero, C., Lenczowski, M.J., Chinzi, D., Davail-Cuisset, B., Sumpter, J.P., and Fostier, A. (1996) Effects of flavonoids on aromatase activity, an *in vitro* study. *J Steroid Biochem Mol Biol* **57**, 215–23.

103. Kao, Y.C., Zhou, C., Sherman, M., Laughton, C.A., and Chen, S. (1998) Molecular basis of the inhibition of human aromatase (estrogen synthetase) by flavone and isoflavone phytoestrogens: A site-directed mutagenesis study. *Environ Health Perspect* **106**, 85–92.

104. Fiorelli, G., Picariello, L., Martineti, V., Tonelli, F., and Brandi, M.L. (1999) Estrogen synthesis in human colon cancer epithelial cells. *J Steroid Biochem Mol Biol* **71**, 223–30.

105. Sanderson, J.T., Hordijk, J., Denison, M.S., Springsteel, M.F., Nantz, M.H., and van den Berg, M. (2004) Induction and inhibition of aromatase (CYP19) activity by natural and synthetic flavonoid compounds in H295R human adrenocortical carcinoma cells. *Toxicol Sci* **82**, 70–79.

106. Myllymäki, S., Haavisto, T., Vainio, M., Toppari, J., and Paranko, J. (2005) *In vitro* effects of diethyl-stilbestrol, genistein, 4-tert-butylphenol, and 4-tert-octylphenol on steroidogenic activity of isolated immature rat ovarian follicles. *Toxicol Appl Pharmacol* **204**, 69–80.

107. Brooks, J.D., and Thompson, L.U. (2005) Mammalian lignans and genistein decrease the activities of aromatase and 17beta-hydroxysteroid dehydrogenase in MCF-7 cells. *J Steroid Biochem Mol Biol* **94**, 461–67.

108. Whitehead, S.A., Cross, J.E., Burden, C., and Lacey, M. (2002) Acute and chronic effects of genistein, tyrphostin and lavendustin A on steroid synthesis in luteinized human granulosa cells. *Hum Reprod* **17**, 589–94.

109. Lacey, M., Bohday, J., Fonseka, S.M., Ullah, A.I., and Whitehead, S.A. (2005) Dose-response effects of phytoestrogens on the activity and expression of 3beta-hydroxysteroid dehydrogenase and aromatase in human granulosa-luteal cells. *J Steroid Biochem Mol Biol* **96**, 279–86.

110. Fritz, W.A., Cotroneo, M.S., Wang, J., Eltoum, I.E., and Lamartiniere, C.A. (2003) Dietary diethyl-stilbestrol but not genistein adversely affects rat testicular development. *J Nutr* **133**, 2287–93.

111. Le Page, Y., Scholze, M., Kah, O., and Pakdel, F. (2006) Assessment of xenoestrogens using three distinct estrogen receptors and the zebrafish brain aromatase gene in a highly responsive glial cell system. *Environ Health Perspect* **114**, 752–58.

112. Rice, S., Mason, H.D., and Whitehead, S.A. (2006) Phytoestrogens and their low dose combinations inhibit mRNA expression and activity of aromatase in human granulosa-luteal cells. *J Steroid Biochem Mol Biol* **101**, 216–25.

113. van Meeuwen, J.A., Korthagen, N., de Jong, P.C., Piersma, A.H., and van den Berg, M. (2007) (Anti)estrogenic effects of phytochemicals on human primary mammary fibroblasts, MCF-7 cells and their co-culture. *Toxicol Appl Pharmacol* **221**, 372–83.

114. Lyou, S., Kawano, S., Yamada, T., Okuyama, S., Terashima, T., Hayase, K., and Yokogoshi, H. (2008) Role of estrogen receptors and aromatase on brain protein synthesis rates in ovariectomized female rats fed genistein. *Nutr Neurosci* **11**, 155–60.

115. Davis, J.N., Muqim, N., Bhuiyan, M., Kucuk, O., Pienta, K.J., and Sarkar, F.H. (2000) Inhibition of prostate specific antigen expression by genistein in prostate cancer cells. *Int J Oncol* **16**, 1091–97.

116. Maubach, J., Bracke, M.E., Heyerick, A., Depypere, H.T., Serreyn, R.F., Mareel, M.M., and De Keukeleire, D. (2003) Quantitation of soy-derived phytoestrogens in human breast tissue and biological fluids by high-performance liquid chromatography. *J Chromatogr B Analyt Technol Biomed Life Sci* **784**, 137–44.

117. Petrakis, N.L., Barnes, S., King, E.B., Lowenstein, J., Wiencke, J., Lee, M.M., Miike, R., Kirk, M., and Coward, L. (1996) Stimulatory influence of soy protein isolate on breast secretion in pre- and post-menopausal women. *Cancer Epidemiol Biomarkers Prev* **5**, 785–94.

118. Maskarinec, G., Hebshi, S., Custer, L., and Franke, A.A. (2008) The relation of soy intake and isoflavone levels in nipple aspirate fluid. *Eur J Cancer Prev* **17**, 67–70.

119. Hedlund, T.E., Maroni, P.D., Ferucci, P.G., Dayton, R., Barnes, S., Jones, K., Moore, R., Ogden, L.G., Wähälä, K., Sackett, H.M., and Gray, K.J. (2005) Long-term dietary habits affect soy isoflavone metabolism and accumulation in prostatic fluid in caucasian men. *J Nutr* **135**, 1400–06.

120. Hedlund, T.E., van Bokhoven, A., Johannes, W.U., Nordeen, S.K., and Ogden, L.G. (2006) Prostatic fluid concentrations of isoflavonoids in soy consumers are sufficient to inhibit growth of benign and malignant prostatic epithelial cells *in vitro*. *Prostate* **66**, 557–66.

121. Löffer, M., and Schneider, F. (1982) Further characterization of the growth inhibitory effect of rotenone on *in vitro* cultured Ehrlich ascites tumour cells. *Mol Cell Biochem* **48**, 77–90.

122. Kuzumaki, T., Kobayashi, T., and Ishikawa, K. (1998) Genistein induces p21(Cip1/WAF1) expression and blocks the G1 to S phase transition in mouse fibroblast and melanoma cells, Biochem. *Biophys Res Commun* **251**, 291–95.

123. Pagliacci, M.C., Smacchia, M., Migliorati, G., Grignani, F., Riccardi, C., and Nicoletti, I. (1994) Growth-inhibitory effects of the natural phyto-oestrogen genistein in MCF-7 human breast cancer cells, Eur. *J Cancer* **30A**, 1675–82.

124. Davis, J.N., Singh, B., Bhuiyan, M., and Sarkar, F.H. (1998) Genistein-induced upregulation of p21WAF1, downregulation of cyclin B, and induction of apoptosis in prostate cancer cells, Nutr. *Cancer* **32**, 123–31.

125. Choi, Y.H., Zhang, L., Lee, W.H., and Park, K.Y. (1998) Genistein-induced G2/M arrest is associated with the inhibition of cyclin B1 and the induction of p21 in human breast carcinoma cells. *Int J Oncol* **13**, 391–96.

126. Shen, J.C., Klein, R.D., Wei, Q., Guan, Y., Contois, J.H., Wang, T.T., Chang, S., and Hursting, S.D. (2000) Low-dose genistein induces cyclin-dependent kinase inhibitors and G(1) cell-cycle arrest in human prostate cancer cells. *Mol Carcinog* **29**, 92–102.

127. Frey, R.S., Li, J., and Singletary, K.W. (2001) Effects of genistein on cell proliferation and cell cycle arrest in nonneoplastic human mammary epithelial cells: Involvement of Cdc2, p21(waf/cip1), p27(kip1), and Cdc25C expression. *Biochem Pharmacol* **61**, 979–89.

128. Matsumura, K., Tanaka, T., Kawashima, H., and Nakatani, T. (2008) Involvement of the estrogen receptor beta in genistein-induced expression of p21(waf1/cip1) in PC-3 prostate cancer cells. *Anticancer Res* **28**, 709–14.

129. Fang, M.Z., Chen, D., Sun, Y., Jin, Z., Christman, J.K., and Yang, C.S. (2005) Reversal of hypermethylation and reactivation of p16INK4a, RARbeta, and MGMT genes by genistein and other isoflavones from soy. *Clin Cancer Res* **11**, 7033–41.

130. Majid, S., Kikuno, N., Nelles, J., Noonan, E., Tanaka, Y., Kawamoto, K., Hirata, H., Li, L.C., Zhao, H., Okino, S.T., Place, R.F., Pookot, D., and Dahiya, R. (2008) Genistein induces the p21WAF1/CIP1 and p16INK4a tumor suppressor genes in prostate cancer cells by epigenetic mechanisms involving active chromatin modification. *Cancer Res* **68**, 2736–44.

131. Li, M., Zhang, Z., Hill, D.L., Chen, X., Wang, H., and Zhang, R. (2005) Genistein, a dietary isoflavone, down-regulates the MDM2 oncogene at both transcriptional and posttranslational levels. *Cancer Res* **65**, 8200–08.

132. El Touny, L.H. (2006) Banerjee PP Identification of both Myt-1 and Wee-1 as necessary mediators of the p21-independent inactivation of the cdc-2/cyclin B1 complex and growth inhibition of TRAMP cancer cells by genistein. *Prostate* **66**, 1542–55.

133. Natarajan, K., Manna, S.K., Chaturvedi, M.M., and Aggarwal, B.B. (1998) Protein tyrosine kinase inhibitors block tumor necrosis factor-induced activation of nuclear factor-kappaB, degradation of IkappaBalpha, nuclear translocation of p65, and subsequent gene expression. *Arch Biochem Biophys* **352**, 59–70.

134. Li, Y., and Sarkar, F.H. (2002) Inhibition of nuclear factor kappaB activation in PC3 cells by genistein is mediated via Akt signaling pathway. *Clin Cancer Res* **8**, 2369–77.

135. El Touny, L.H., and Banerjee, P.P. (2007) Akt GSK-3 pathway as a target in genistein-induced inhibition of TRAMP prostate cancer progression toward a poorly differentiated phenotype. *Carcinogenesis* **28**, 1710–17.

136. Huang, X., Chen, S., Xu, L., Liu, Y., Deb, D.K., Platanias, L.C., and Bergan, R.C. (2005) Genistein inhibits p38 MAP kinase activation, matrix metalloproteinase type 2, and cell invasion in human prostate epithelial cells. *Cancer Res* **65**, 3470–78.

137. Lee, M.W., Bach, J.H., Lee, H.J., Lee, D.Y., Joo, W.S., Kim, Y.S., Park, S.C., Kim, K.Y., Lee, W.B., and Kim, S.S. (2005) The activation of ERK1/2 via a tyrosine kinase pathway attenuates trail-induced apoptosis in HeLa cells. *Cancer Invest* **23**, 586–92.

138. Boersma, B.J., Patel, R.P., Kirk, M., Darley-Usmar, V.M., and Barnes, S. (1999) Chlorination and Nitration of Soy Isoflavones. *Arch Biochem Biophys* **368**, 265–75.

139. Boersma, B.J., D'Alessandro, T., Benton, M.R., Kirk, M., Wilson, L.S., Prasain, J., Botting, N.P., Barnes, S., Darley-Usmar, V.M., and Patel, R.P. (2003) Neutrophil myeloperoxidase chlorinates soy isoflavones and enhances their antioxidant properties. *Free Rad Biol Med* **35**, 1417–30.

140. D'Alessandro, T., Prasain, J., Botting, N.P., Moore, R., Darley-Usmar, V.M., Patel, R.P., and Barnes, S. (2003) Polyphenols, inflammatory response, and cancer prevention: Chlorination of isoflavones by human neutrophils. *J Nutr* **133**, 3773S–3777S.

141. Chacko, B.K., Chandler, R.T., Mundhekar, A., Pruitt, H.M., Kucik, D.F., Kevil, C.G., Barnes, S., and Patel, R.P. (2005) Revealing anti-inflammatory mechanisms of soy-isoflavones by flow: Modulation of leukocyte-endothelial cell interactions. *Am J Physiol* **289**, H908–H15.

142. Chacko, B.K., Chandler, R.T., D'Alessandro, T.L., Mundhekar, A., Khoo, N.K., Botting, N., Barnes, S., and Patel, R.P. (2007) Anti-inflammatory effects of isoflavones are dependent on flow and human endothelial cell PPARγ. *J Nutr* **137**, 351–56.

143. Hernandez-Montes, E., Pollard, S.E., Vauzour, D., Jofre-Montseny, L., Rota, C., Rimbach, G., Weinberg, P.D., and Spencer, J.P. (2006) Activation of glutathione peroxidase via Nrf1 mediates genistein's protection against oxidative endothelial cell injury, Biochem. *Biophys Res Commun* **346**, 851–59.

144. Lau, T.Y., and Leung, L.K. (2006) Soya isoflavones suppress phorbol 12-myristate 13-acetate-induced COX-2 expression in MCF-7 cells. *Br J Nutr* **96**, 169–76.

145. Li, H.C., and Zhang, G.Y. (2003) Activation of STAT3 induced by cerebral ischemia in rat hippocampus and its possible mechanisms. *Sheng Li Xue Bao* **55**, 311–16.

146. Chen, W.F., Gao, Q.G., and Wong, M.S. (2007) Mechanism involved in genistein activation of insulin-like growth factor 1 receptor expression in human breast cancer cells. *Br J Nutr* **98**, 1120–25.

147. Kim, E.J., Shin, H.K., and Park, J.H. (2005) Genistein inhibits insulin-like growth factor-I receptor signaling in HT-29 human colon cancer cells: A possible mechanism of the growth inhibitory effect of genistein. *J Med Food* **8**, 431–38.

148. Su, S.J., Chow, N.H., Kung, M.L., Hung, T.C., and Chang, K.L. (2003) Effects of soy isoflavones on apoptosis induction and G2-M arrest in human hepatoma cells involvement of caspase-3 activation, Bcl-2 and Bcl-XL downregulation, and Cdc2 kinase activity. *Nutr Cancer* **45**, 113–23.

149. Moiseeva, E.P., Almeida, G.M., Jones, G.D., and Manson, M.M. (2007) Extended treatment with physiologic concentrations of dietary phytochemicals results in altered gene expression, reduced growth, and apoptosis of cancer cells. *Mol Cancer Ther* **6**, 3071–79.

150. Vantyghem, S.A., Wilson, S.M., Postenka, C.O., Al-Katib, W., Tuck, A.B., and Chambers, A.F. (2005) Dietary genistein reduces metastasis in a postsurgical orthotopic breast cancer model. *Cancer Res* **65**, 3396–403.

151. King-Batoon, A., Leszczynska, J.M., and Klein, C.B. (2008) Modulation of gene methylation by genistein or lycopene in breast cancer cells. *Environ Mol Mutagen* **49**, 36–45.

152. Kikuno, N., Shiina, H., Urakami, S., Kawamoto, K., Hirata, H., Tanaka, Y., Majid, S., Igawa, M., and Dahiya, R. (2008) Genistein mediated histone acetylation and demethylation activates tumor suppressor genes in prostate cancer cells. *Int J Cancer* **123**, 552–60.

153. Chen, Z.P., and Yeung, D.C. (1996) Regulation of p53 expression in HeLa cells. *Biochem Mol Biol Int* **38**, 607–16.

154. Rauth, S., Kichina, J., and Green, A. (1997) Inhibition of growth and induction of differentiation of metastatic melanoma cells *in vitro* by genistein: Chemosensitivity is regulated by cellular p53. *Br J Cancer* **75**, 1559–66.

155. Ye, R., Bodero, A., Zhou, B.B., Khanna, K.K., Lavin, M.F., and Lees-Miller, S.P. (2001) The plant isoflavenoid genistein activates p53 and Chk2 in an ATM-dependent manner. *J Biol Chem* **276**, 4828–33.

156. Ye, R., Goodarzi, A.A., Kurz, E.U., Saito, S., Higashimoto, Y., Lavin, M.F., Appella, E., Anderson, C.W., and Lees-Miller, S.P. (2004) The isoflavonoids genistein and quercetin activate different stress signaling pathways as shown by analysis of site-specific phosphorylation of ATM, p53 and histone H2AX. *DNA Repair (Amst)* **3**, 235–44.

157. Frey, R.S., Li, J., and Singletary, K.W. (2001) Effects of genistein on cell proliferation and cell cycle arrest in nonneoplastic human mammary epithelial cells: Involvement of Cdc2, p21(waf/cip1), p27(kip1), and Cdc25C expression. *Biochem Pharmacol* **61**, 979–89.

158. Wilson, L.C., Baek, S.J., Call, A., and Eling, T.E. (2003) Nonsteroidal anti-inflammatory drug-activated gene (NAG-1) is induced by genistein through the expression of p53 in colorectal cancer cells. *Int J Cancer* **105**, 747–53.

159. Dijsselbloem, N., Goriely, S., Albarani, V., Gerlo, S., Francoz, S., Marine, J.C., Goldman, M., Haegeman, G., and Vanden Berghe, W. (2007) A critical role for p53 in the control of NF-kappaB-dependent gene expression in TLR4-stimulated dendritic cells exposed to genistein. *J Immunol* **178**, 5048–57.

160. Vissac-Sabatier, C., Bignon, Y.J., and Bernard-Gallon, D.J. (2003) Effects of the phytoestrogens genistein and daidzein on BRCA2 tumor suppressor gene expression in breast cell lines. *Nutr Cancer* **45**, 247–55.

161. Vissac-Sabatier, C., Coxam, V., Déchelotte, P., Picherit, C., Horcajada, M.N., Davicco, M.J., Lebecque, P., Bignon, Y.J., and Bernard-Gallon, D. (2003) Phytoestrogen-rich diets modulate expression of Brca1 and Brca2 tumor suppressor genes in mammary glands of female Wistar rats. *Cancer Res* **63**, 6607–12.

162. Cabanes, A., Wang, M., Olivo, S., DeAssis, S., Gustafsson, J.A., Khan, G., and Hilakivi-Clarke, L. (2004) Prepubertal estradiol and genistein exposures up-regulate BRCA1 mRNA and reduce mammary tumorigenesis. *Carcinogenesis* **25**, 741–48.

163. Dave, B., Eason, R.R., Till, S.R., Geng, Y., Velarde, M.C., Badger, T.M., and Simmen, R.C. (2005) The soy isoflavone genistein promotes apoptosis in mammary epithelial cells by inducing the tumor suppressor PTEN. *Carcinogenesis* **26**, 1793–803.

164. Cao, F., Jin, T.Y., and Zhou, Y.F. (2006) Inhibitory effect of isoflavones on prostate cancer cells and PTEN gene. *Biomed Environ Sci* **19**, 35–41.

165. Singletary, K., and Ellington, A. (2006) Genistein suppresses proliferation and MET oncogene expression and induces EGR-1 tumor suppressor expression in immortalized human breast epithelial cells. *Anticancer Res* **26**, 1039–48.

166. Liu, C., Yu, S., Zinn, K., Wang, J., Zhang, L., Jia, Y., Kappes, J.C., Barnes, S., Kimberly, R.P., Grizzle, W.E., and Zhang, H.G. (2006) Murine mammary carcinoma exosomes promote tumor growth by suppression of NK cell function. *J Immunol* **176**, 1375–85.

167. Zhang, H.G., Kim, H., Liu, C., Yu, S., Wang, J., Grizzle, W.E., Kimberly, R.P., and Barnes, S. (2007) Curcumin reverses breast tumor exosomes mediated immune suppression of NK cell tumor cytotoxicity. *Biochim Biophys Acta* **1773**, 1116–23.

168. Power, K.A., Saarinen, N.M., Chen, J.M., and Thompson, L.U. (2006) Mammalian lignans enterolactone and enterodiol, alone and in combination with the isoflavone genistein, do not promote the growth of MCF-7 xenografts in ovariectomized athymic nude mice. *Int J Cancer* **118**, 1316–20.

169. Power, K.A., Ward, W.E., Chen, J.M., Saarinen, N.M., and Thompson, L.U. (2006) Genistein alone and in combination with the mammalian lignans enterolactone and enterodiol induce estrogenic effects on bone and uterus in a postmenopausal breast cancer mouse model. *Bone* **39**, 117–24.

170. Wang, Z., Desmoulin, S., Banerjee, S., Kong, D., Li, Y., Deraniyagala, R.L., Abbruzzese, J., and Sarkar, F.H. (2008) Synergistic effects of multiple natural products in pancreatic cancer cells. *Life Sci* **83**, 293–300.

171. Lambert, J.D., Kwon, S.J., Ju, J., Bose, M., Lee, M.J., Hong, J., Hao, X., and Yang, C.S. (2008) Effect of genistein on the bioavailability and intestinal cancer chemopreventive activity of (-)-epigallocatechin-3-gallate. *Carcinogenesis* **29**, 2019–24.

172. Barnes, S., Allison, D.B., Page, G.P., Carpenter, M., Gadbury, G.L., Meleth, S, Horn-Ross, P., Kim, H., Lamartiniere, C.A., and Grubbs, C.J. (2006) Genistein and polyphenols in the study of cancer prevention: Chemistry, biology, statistics, and experimental design. In: Kaput J., and Rodrigues R. eds. Discovering the Path to Personalized Nutrition. 1st ed., 55–62, New York: Wiley & Sons.

173. Zakharkin, S.O., Kim, K., Mehta, T., Chen, L., Barnes, S., Scheirer, K.E., Parrish, R.S., Allison, D.B., and Page, G.P. (2005) Sources of variation in Affymetrix microarray experiments. *BMC Bioinformatics* **6**, 214.

174. Trotman, L.C., Niki, M., Dotan, Z.A., Koutcher, J.A., Di Cristofano, A., Xiao, A., Khoo, A.S., Roy-Burman, P., Greenberg, N.M., Van Dyk, T., Carlos Cordon-Cardo, C., and Pandolfi, P.P. (2003) Pten Dose Dictates Cancer Progression in the Prostate. *PLoS Biology* **1**, 385–96.

175. Bonferroni, C.E. (1935) Il calcolo delle assicurazioni su gruppi di teste. In: *Studi in Onore del Professore Salvatore Ortu Carboni*. 13–60, Rome: Italy.

176. Chen, C.C., Shieh, B., Jin, Y.T., Liau, Y.E., Huang, C.H., Liou, J.T., Wu, L.W., Huang, W., Young, K.C., Lai, M.D., Liu, H.S., and Li, C. (2001) Microarray profiling of gene expression patterns in bladder tumor cells treated with genistein. *J Biomed Sci* **8**, 214–22.

177. Chen, W.F., Huang, M.H., Tzang, C.H., Yang, M., and Wong, M.S. (2003) Inhibitory actions of genistein in human breast cancer (MCF-7) cells. *Biochim Biophys Acta* **1638**, 187–96.

178. Ise, R., Han, D., Takahasi, Y., Teresaka, S., Inoue, A., Tanji, M., and Kiyama, R. (2005) Expression profiling of the estrogen responsive genes in response to phytoestrogens using a customized DNA microarray. *FEBS Lttr* **579**, 1732–40.

179. Shioda, T., Chesnes, J., Coser, K.R., Zou, L., Hur, J., Dean, K.L., Sonnenschein, C., Soto, A.M., and Isselbacher, K.J. (2006 Aug 8) Importance of dosage standardization for interpreting transcriptomal signature profiles: Evidence from studies of xenoestrogens. *Proc Natl Acad Sci U S A* **103**, 12033–38.

180. Lee, W.Y., Huang, S.C., Tzeng, C.C., Chang, T.L., and Hsu, K.F. (2007) Alterations of metastasis-related genes identified using an oligonucleotide microarray of genistein-treated HCC1395 breast cancer cells. *Nutr Cancer* **58**, 239–46.

181. Lavigne, J.A., Takahashi, Y., Chandramouli, G.V., Liu, H., Perkins, S.N., Hursting, S.D., and Wang, T.T. (2008) Concentration-dependent effects of genistein on global gene expression in MCF-7 breast cancer cells: An oligo microarray study. *Breast Cancer Res Treat* **110**, 85–98.

182. Konstantakopoulos, N., Montgomery, K.G., Chamberlain, N., Quinn, M.A., Baker, M.S., Rice, G.E., Georgiou, H.M., and Campbell, I.G. (2006) Changes in gene expressions elicited by physiological concentrations of genistein on human endometrial cancer cells. *Mol Carcinog* **45**, 752–63.

183. Zou, H., Zhan, S., and Cao, K. (2008) Apoptotic activity of genistein on human lung adenocarcinoma SPC-A-1 cells and preliminary exploration of its mechanisms using microarray. *Biomed Pharmacother* **62**, 583–89.

184. Bai, J., Sata, N., Nagai, H., Wada, T., Yoshida, K., Mano, H., Sata, F., and Kishi, R. (2004) Genistein-induced changes in gene expression in Panc 1 cells at physiological concentrations of genistein. *Pancreas* **29**, 93–98.

185. Rice, L., Samedi, V.G., Medrano, T.A., Sweeney, C.A., Baker, H.V., Stenstrom, A., Furman, J., and Shiverick, K.T. (2002) Mechanisms of the growth inhibitory effects of the isoflavonoid biochanin A on LNCaP cells and xenografts. *Prostate* **52**, 201–12.

186. Suzuki, K., Koike, H., Matsui, H., Ono, Y., Hasumi, M., Nakazato, H., Okugi, H., Sekine, Y., Oki, K., Ito, K., Yamamoto, T., Fukabori, Y., Kurokawa, K., and Yamanaka, H. (2002) Genistein, a soy isoflavone, induces glutathione peroxidase in the human prostate cancer cell lines LNCaP and PC-3. *Int J Cancer* **99**, 846–52.

187. Li, Y., and Sarkar, F.H. (2002) Down-regulation of invasion and angiogenesis-related genes identified by cDNA microarray analysis of PC3 prostate cancer cells treated with genistein. *Cancer Lett* **186**, 157–64.

188. Li, Y., and Sarkar, F.H. (2002) Gene expression profiles of genistein-treated PC3 prostate cancer cells. *J Nutr* **132**, 3623–31.

189. Ayala, G.E., Dai, H., Ittmann, M., Li, R., Powell, M., Frolov, A., Wheeler, T.M., Thompson, T.C., and Rowley, D. (2004) Growth and survival mechanisms associated with perineural invasion in prostate cancer. *Cancer Res* **64**, 6082–90.

190. Takahashi, Y., Lavigne, J.A., Hursting, S.D., Chandramouli, G.V., Perkins, S.N., Barrett, J.C., and Wang, T.T. (2004) Using DNA microarray analyses to elucidate the effects of genistein in androgen-responsive prostate cancer cells: Identification of novel targets. *Mol Carcinog* **41**, 108–19.

191. Davis, D.A., Sarkar, S.H., Hussain, M., Li, Y., and Sarkar, F.H. (2006) Increased therapeutic potential of an experimental anti-mitotic inhibitor SB715992 by genistein in PC-3 human prostate cancer cell line. *BMC Cancer* **6**, 22.

192. Li, Y., Kucuk, O., Hussain, M., Abrams, J., Cher, M.L., and Sarkar, F.H. (2006) Antitumor and antimetastatic activities of docetaxel are enhanced by genistein through regulation of osteoprotegerin/receptor activator of nuclear factor-kappaB (RANK)/RANK ligand/MMP-9 signaling in prostate cancer. *Cancer Res* **66**, 4816–25.

193. Skogseth, H., Follestad, T., Larsson, E., and Halgunset, J. (2006) Transcription levels of invasion-related genes in prostate cancer cells are modified by inhibitors of tyrosine kinase. *APMIS* **114**, 364–71.

194. Takahashi, Y., Lavigne, J.A., Hursting, S.D., Chandramouli, G.V., Perkins, S.N., Kim, Y.S., and Wang, T.T. (2006) Molecular signatures of soy-derived phytochemicals in androgen-responsive prostate cancer cells: A comparison study using DNA microarray. *Mol Carcinog* **45**, 943–56.

195. Mori, R., Xiong, S., Wang, Q., Tarabolous, C., Shimada, H., Panteris, E., Danenbehrg, K.D., Danenberg, P.V., and Pinski, J.K. (2009) Gene profiling and pathway analysis of neuroendocrine transdifferentiated prostate cancer cells. *Prostate* **69**, 12–23.

196. Willcox, D.L., McColm, S.C., Arthur, P.G., and Yovich, J.L. (1983) The application of rate dialysis to the determination of free steroids in plasma. *Anal Biochem* **135**, 304–11.

197. Menon, D.V., and Vongpatanasin, W. (2006) Effects of transdermal estrogen replacement therapy on cardiovascular risk factors. *Treat Endocrinol* **5**, 37–51.

198. Naciff, J.M., Jump, M.L., Torontali, S.M., Carr, G.J., Tiesman, J.P., Overmann, G.J., and Daston, G.P. (2002) Gene expression profile induced by 17alpha-ethynyl estradiol, bisphenol A, and genistein in the developing female reproductive system of the rat. *Toxicol Sci* **68**, 184–99.

199. Li, Y., Che, M., Bhagat, S., Ellis, K.L., Kucuk, O., Doerge, D.R., Abrams, J., Cher, M.L., and Sarkar, F.H. (2004) Regulation of gene expression and inhibition of experimental prostate cancer bone metastasis by dietary genistein. *Neoplasia* **6**, 354–63.
200. Li, Y., Kucuk, O., Hussain, M., Abrams, J., Cher, M.L., and Sarkar, F.H. (2006) Antitumor and antimetastatic activities of docetaxel are enhanced by genistein through regulation of osteoprotegerin/receptor activator of nuclear factor-kappaB (RANK)/RANK ligand/MMP-9 signaling in prostate cancer. *Cancer Res* **66**, 4816–25.
201. Barve, A., Khor, T.O., Nair, S., Lin, W., Yu, S., Jain, M.R., Chan, J.Y., and Kong, A.N. (2008) Pharmacogenomic profile of soy isoflavone concentrate in the prostate of Nrf2 deficient and wild-type mice. *J Pharm Sci* **97**, 4528–45.
202. Hochstrasser, D. (2008) Should the Human Proteome Project Be Gene- or Protein-centric? *J Proteome Res* **7**, 5071.
203. Washburn, M.P., Wolters, D., and Yates, J.R., 3rd. (2001) Large-scale analysis of the yeast proteome by multidimensional protein identification technology. *Nat Biotechnol* **19**, 242–47.
204. Resing, K.A., Meyer-Arendt, K., Mendoza, A.M., Aveline-Wolf, L.D., Jonscher, K.R., Pierce, K.G., Old, W.M., Cheung, H.T., Russell, S., Wattawa, J.L., Goehle, G.R., Knight, R.D., and Ahn, N.G. (2004) Improving reproducibility and sensitivity in identifying human proteins by shotgun proteomics. *Anal Chem* **76**, 3556–68.
205. Denoeud, F., Kapranov, P., Ucla, C., Frankish, A., Castelo, R., Drenkow, J., Lagarde, J., Alioto, T., Manzano, C., Chrast, J., Dike, S., Wyss, C., Henrichsen, C.N., Holroyd, N., Dickson, M.C., Taylor, R., Hance, Z., Foissac, S., Myers, R.M., Rogers, J., Hubbard, T., Harrow, J., Guigo, R., Gingeras, T.R., Antonarakis, S.E., and Reymond, A. (2007) Prominent use of distal 5′ transcription start sites and discovery of a large number of additional exons in ENCODE regions. *Genome Res* **17**, 746–59.
206. Nielsen, M.L., Savitski, M.M., and Zubarev, R.A. (2006) Extent of modifications in human proteome samples and their effect on dynamic range of analysis in shotgun proteomics. *Mol Cell Proteomics* **5**, 2384–91.
207. Taupenot, L., Harper, K.L., and O'Connor, D.T. (2003) The chromogranin-secretogranin family. *N Engl J Med* **348**, 1134–49.
208. O'Farrell, P.H. (1975) High resolution two-dimensional electrophoresis of proteins. *J Biol Chem* **250**, 4007–21.
209. Kim, H., Page, G.P., and Barnes, S. (2004) Proteomics and mass spectrometry in nutrition research. *Nutrition* **20**, 155–65.
210. Unlü, M., Morgan, M.E., and Minden, J.S. (1997) Difference gel electrophoresis: A single gel method for detecting changes in protein extracts. *Electrophoresis* **18**, 2071–77.
211. Laemmli, U.K. (1970) Cleavage of structural proteins during the assembly of the head of bacteriophage T4. *Nature* **227**, 680–85.
212. Schägger, H., and von Jagow, G. (1991) Blue native electrophoresis for isolation of membrane protein complexes in enzymatically active form. *Anal Biochem* **199**, 223–31.
213. Brookes, P.S., Pinner, A., Ramachandran, A., Coward, L., Barnes, S., Kim, H., and Darley-Usmar, V.M. (2002) High throughput 2D blue-native electrophoresis – a tool for functional proteomics of mitochondria and signaling complexes. *Proteomics* **2**, 969–77.
214. Wittig, I., Karas, M., and Schägger, H. (2007) High resolution clear native electrophoresis for in-gel functional assays and fluorescence studies of membrane protein complexes. *Mol Cell Proteomics* **6**, 1215–25.
215. Rowell, C., Carpenter, D.M., and Lamartiniere, C.A. (2005) Chemoprevention of breast cancer, proteomic discovery of genistein action in the rat mammary gland. *J Nutr* **135**, 2953S–2959S.
216. Nomura, T., Tazawa, M., Ohtsuki, M., Sumi-Ichinose, C., Hagino, Y., Ota, A., Nakashima, A., Mori, K., Sugimoto, T., Ueno, O., Nozawa, Y., Ichinose, H., and Nagatsu, T. (1998) Enzymes related to catecholamine biosynthesis in Tetrahymena pyriformis. Presence of GTP cyclohydrolase I. *Comp Biochem Physiol B Biochem Mol Biol* **120**, 753–60.
217. Kim, H., Cope, M., Herring, R., Robinson, G., Wilson, L., Page, G.P., and Barnes, S. (2008) 2D difference gel electrophoresis of pre-pubertal and pubertal rat mammary gland proteomes. *J Proteome Res* **7**, 4638–50.

28 The Anticarcinogenic Properties of Culinary Herbs and Spices

Guy H. Johnson and Lyssa Balick

Key Points

1. In vitro and epidemiological studies have demonstrated a potential link between chronic inflammation and cancer. Herbs and spices intake, especially in therapeutic dosages, may help decrease inflammation.
2. Important mechanisms in cancer prevention include attenuation of free radical formation, removal of radicals before damage occurs, repair of oxidative damage, elimination of damaged molecules, and the prevention of mutations. Many culinary herbs and spices, for example, rosemary, oregano, cinnamon, basil, cloves, are inherently high in antioxidant activity measured in vitro.
3. Several spices, or their active ingredients, have been evaluated for their anticancer potential using intact animal models. Spices and herbs have been shown to prevent or delay carcinogenesis in multiple organ sites.
4. Some spices and herbs have been shown to inhibit carcinogenesis by altering detoxifying enzymes. Mechanistic studies have found that garlic can prevent tumor initiation and promotion by altering the ratios of phase I and phase II liver enzymes.
5. There are emerging data in several areas to suggest that a variety of culinary herbs and spices reduce the risk of cancer. However, there is very little evidence from human studies in this area. In addition, human data on dose–response and biochemical mechanism are largely unavailable. Better designed epidemiological and intervention studies are clearly needed in this area.

Key Words: Herbs; spices; cancer prevention

1. INTRODUCTION

Cancer is one of the leading global causes of death in the world *(1)*. The purpose of this chapter is to review scientific evidence on the possibility that components of culinary spices and herbs (Fig. 1) help prevent or mitigate this constellation of diseases. Abundant anecdotal information documents the historical use of herbs and spices for their health benefits. Papyri from Ancient Egypt in 1555 BCE classified coriander, fennel, juniper, cumin, garlic, and thyme as health-promoting spices. As early as 460–377 BCE, Hippocrates recorded medicinal uses for over 300 herbs and spices (including

From: *Nutrition and Health: Bioactive Compounds and Cancer*
Edited by: J.A. Milner, D.F. Romagnolo, DOI 10.1007/978-1-60761-627-6_28,
© Springer Science+Business Media, LLC 2010

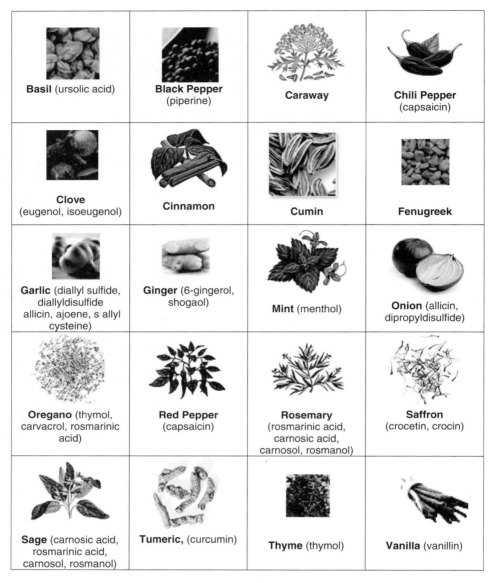

Fig. 1. Selected spices and herbs (and phytochemicals) with chemopreventive properties.

garlic, cinnamon, and rosemary) in Ancient Greece and Rome. Roughly 500 years later, Theophrastus, a Greek physician and botanist, published information on the health benefits of over 600 herbs. Cumin, turmeric, and other seed plants were used several 1,000 years ago as part of ancient Indian medical practices and this use has endured to the present *(2, 3)*. Worldwide, 80% of indigenous populations use plant- and herb-based medicines as their primary source of health care *(4)*.

Western medicine is rooted in plant-based medicine. The United States used plants as the primary source of medicine from the time of the Mayflower (1620) until after World

War I (1930) *(4)*. Many modern drugs such as aspirin from willow bark and morphine from the opium poppy are based on herbal sources. Researchers and pharmaceutical companies continue to investigate components in spices and herbs for their ability to prevent and/or treat cancer and other diseases *(3, 5)*.

The use of spices, herbs, and other alternative practices for the treatment/prevention of cancer and other diseases is increasing. Spending on alternative therapies in the United States increased by 45% to an estimated $27 billion between 1990 and 1997 (Table 1). Similar trends occurred in Australia, Germany, the United Kingdom, and Spain *(6, 7, 8)*. Aggarwal and Shishodia *(9)* have concluded that bioactive compounds from herbs and spices may be found to be efficacious for both the prevention and the treatment of different forms of cancer. The areas of most intense investigation are discussed briefly below.

Table 1
Spice Production in Tons and Cancer Rates in Selected Countries, 2000[a]

	Spice production, in tons	*Cancer rates, all sites but skin, male[b]*	*Cancer rates, all sites but skin, female[c]*
India	2,255,800	72.4	88.8
China	584,871	199.7	72.5
United States	6,120	536.8	458.8

[a]Production data from 2000 faostat.fao.org, taken from http://www.foodmarketexchange. com/datacenter/product/herb/herb/detail/dc_pi_hs_herb0406.htm. Cancer data from the World Health Organization GLOBOCAN 2002, which approximates canccer rates from around 2000 (but could be earlier).
[b]Crude rate per 100,000 males.
[c]Crude rate per 100,000 females.

2. THERAPEUTIC PROPERTIES OF HERBS AND SPICES

2.1. Anti-inflammatory Properties

In vitro and epidemiological studies have demonstrated a potential link between chronic inflammation and cancer *(10)*. Herb and spice intake, especially in therapeutic dosages, may help decrease inflammation. Studies with animal models and in vitro experiments have shown that sage, black cumin, and cinnamon can suppress or reduce various biomarkers of inflammation *(9, 11, 3)*. Some human experimental studies have shown that ginger and turmeric inhibit the inflammatory process. In addition, limited epidemiological evidence has suggested that populations that consume foods rich in specific polyphenols (such as ginger) have lower incidences of inflammatory diseases including cancer *(3)*.

Several molecular targets involved in the inflammatory process are currently being investigated for their effects on cancer. These targets include nuclear factor-kappa B (NF-kB), signal transducer and activator of transcription 3 (STAT3), v-akt murine thymoma viral oncogene (Akt), B-cell CLL/lymphoma 2 (Bcl-2), apoptosis regulator Bcl-X (Bcl-XL), caspases, poly (ADP-ribose) polymerase (PARP), IkappaB kinase (IKK), epidermal growth factor receptor (EGFR), human epidermal growth factor receptor 2 (HER2), Jun N-terminal kinase (JNK), mitogen-activated protein kinase (MAPK), cyclooxygenase 2 (COX2), and 5-lipoxygenase (5-LOX).

In vitro and animal studies have shown that spices and herbs such as ginger, garlic, and fenugreek (or bioactive substances in these foods including curcumin from turmeric and capsaicin from red pepper) affect one or more inflammatory processes. Preliminary research is also being conducted in humans with curcumin and garlic. These spices are being studied in therapeutic dosages and in combination with other cancer medications. This research has the potential to lead to targeted interventions in cancer prevention and/or treatment (9, 12).

2.2. Antioxidant Properties

Important mechanisms in cancer prevention include attenuation of free radical formation, removal of radicals before damage occurs, repair of oxidative damage, elimination of damaged molecules, and the prevention of mutations (13, 14, 15). Many culinary herbs and spices (e.g., rosemary, oregano, cinnamon, basil, cloves) are inherently high in antioxidant activity measured in vitro (16). Curcumin is also a potent antioxidant with free radical scavenging ability several times higher than that of vitamin E (13).

Antioxidants in foods may work in combination to produce synergistic effects. Flavonoid-rich plant foods contain many different antioxidant compounds (17, 18). For example, the antioxidant values measured by the oxygen radical absorbance capacity (ORAC) assay of some salad vegetables increased when spices and herbs were added to salad dressing (17, 19).

Studies in animal models have suggested that selected spices and herbs have antioxidant activity in vivo (13). Limited information on the ability of antioxidants in culinary herbs and spices to promote health in humans is available and more research on the bioavailability and protective mechanisms of spices and herbs is needed to assess their potential preventative and/or therapeutic benefits (9).

2.3. Effects on Tumor Cells in Culture

Tumorigenesis is a multi-step process that can become activated through environmental agents such as cigarette smoke, stress, oxidation, or numerous inflammatory compounds (20). In vitro studies with spices and herbs have demonstrated inhibitory effects on tumor cells. Curcumin has been shown to decrease tumor growth by interfering with NF-kB and other factors such as i-NOS and COX-1 activity (21, 22, 23). Capsaicin, cinnamon, ginger, and caraway have also been shown to inhibit animal and/or human tumor cells in vitro, and several cell culture studies have observed a decrease in NF-kB concentration when herbs/spices were added to the medium (21, 24, 25, 26, 27, 28). Oil from garlic and onion was shown to prevent tumor growth in several cell culture studies (21, 23), and Belman (29) reported that there was a dose–response for onion but not for garlic.

2.4. Effects on Cancer Initiation, Promotion, and Progression in Intact Animals

Several spices (or their active ingredients) have been evaluated for their anticancer potential using intact animal models. Spices and herbs have been shown to prevent or delay carcinogenesis in multiple organ sites. Saffron extracts (e.g., crocin and crocetin) have been shown to inhibit and/or delay the formation of skin and colon cancer in mice and rats. Curcumin has been shown to help prevent skin, stomach, colon, breast, and liver cancers in mice, while ginger and capsaicin (the pungent component in hot peppers) have been shown to help prevent cancer promotion and tumor formation in animals *(13, 30)*.

2.5. Effects on Specific Detoxifying Enzymes

Some spices and herbs have been shown to inhibit carcinogenesis by altering detoxifying enzymes. Mechanistic studies have found that garlic can prevent tumor initiation and promotion by altering the ratios of phase I and phase II liver enzymes *(21, 31, 32)*. An in vitro study by Gerhauser et al. *(23)* demonstrated that curcumin and active compounds in garlic were among the most powerful plant compounds examined on their ability to affect the detoxification process. In addition, cancer-induced mice fed rosemary had increases in liver detoxification enzymes *(33, 34)*.

2.6. Effects on Bacterial Infections

Culinary spices and herbs are well known for their anti-bacterial properties and anecdotal information shows that these foods have been used around the world to prevent bacterial infection and disease *(3)*. In vitro studies have demonstrated that cinnamon, clove, ginger, thyme, oregano, garlic, and turmeric have anti-bacterial properties *(30, 35, 36, 33)*. In addition, bacterial strains subjected to repeated exposure to herbs and spices do not develop resistance as often happens with repeated exposure to synthetic antibiotics *(33)*. Population studies have linked *Helicobacter pylori* infections to some types of cancers. Furthermore, in vitro and animal studies have shown that garlic and onion can prevent *H. pylori* growth *(37)* under some conditions. However, human intervention studies have not consistently replicated this finding *(38, 32, 39)*.

2.7. Human Observational and Population Studies

The amount of spice consumed in the diet varies dramatically according to geographic location. There is currently no system to measure worldwide spice intake. However, the Food and Agricultural Organization (FAO) tracks spices produced by country. The data presented in Table 1 show that India and China were the top producers of spices in 2000 while the United States produced much smaller amounts. Interestingly, the highest spice producing countries tend to have the lowest overall cancer rates *(40)*. Nevertheless, the significance of these crude estimates with respect to public health is unknown because they do not account for factors such as income, environmental factors, and accuracy of data collection.

Several population-based studies have noted that the incidence of colon, gastrointestinal, breast, and other cancers in Southeast Asia are much lower than in western countries. This observation is consistent with the hypothesis that common spices such as garlic, curry, and chili play a role in reducing cancer incidence (20, 2, 22). Other observational studies have shown that garlic intake is associated with lower incidence of colorectal, esophageal, breast, and/or ovarian cancer in the United States, Australia, Europe, and China (41, 42, 39).

2.8. *Human Intervention Studies with Cancer Patients or Healthy Subjects*

Controlled intervention studies designed to test the effect of spices or spice extracts on cancer in humans are limited (13). Published data indicate that extracts from curcumin and garlic are well tolerated in large doses (43). However, the long-term effects of these spices have not been documented (44). Many spices have a high antioxidant activity in vitro. However, there are very few data on bioavailability in humans. For example, Sharma et al. (45) reported that curcumin, or its metabolites, at doses of 36–180 mg for up to 29 days were not detected in blood or urine of 15 advanced colorectal cancer patients aged 41–72 living in the United Kingdom. In a subsequent study, Sharma et al. (46) found that metabolites of curcumin were detectable for up to 1 h in blood and urine of three patients with advanced colorectal cancer who took 3,600 mg of this compound. In addition, Cheng et al. (47) found that metabolites of curcumin were detectable in blood and urine for almost 12 h (peak 1–2 h, all doses) in 24 patients who ingested 4,000–8,000 mg/day for 3 months. The fact that a compound is not detected in large amounts in biological tissues does not necessarily mean it lacks bioactivity. Such compounds may be metabolized quickly to more efficacious compounds in the tissues or converted more slowly to beneficial compounds by intestinal bacteria (45, 31).

Garlic supplementation in animals has prompted lower rates of gastric and other cancers and in vitro and animal studies suggest that garlic can reduce *H. pylori* infection. However, long-term garlic supplementation has not reduced cancer rates or *H. pylori* infections on a consistent basis (48, 13, 38).

In vitro studies have demonstrated that ginger has anti-inflammatory properties (e.g., reduced COX2 activity in platelets), but this effect has not been replicated in humans (13). However, several studies have shown that ginger can prevent and/or reduce the side effects of cancer chemotherapy in humans (49).

Several clinical trials are underway to investigate the efficacy of curcumin in cancer patients. A variety of treatments ranging from large doses of curcumin to curcumin combined with other cancer medications are being investigated. Other spices, herbs, and extracts being studied include garlic for breast and stomach cancer, ginger for cancer nausea, and capsaicin for cancer pain (clinicaltrials.gov).

3. RESEARCH ON SELECTED SPICES AND SPICE EXTRACTS

Many spices, spice extracts, and herbs have the potential to prevent or mitigate the effects of cancer. However, curcumin (from turmeric) and garlic have been researched the most extensively. A synopsis of this research is provided below.

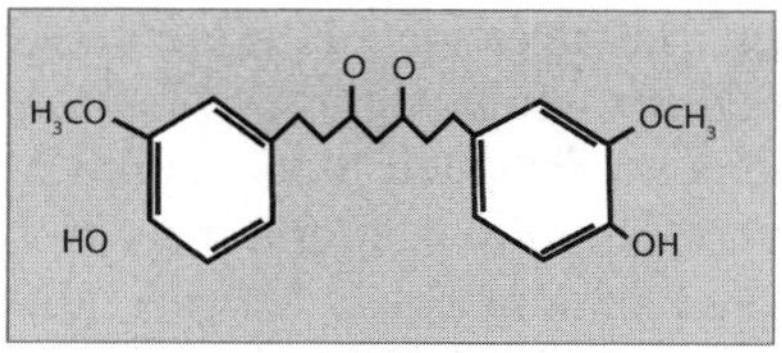

Structure of curcumin (diferuloylmethane)

Fig. 2. Structure of curcumin deferuloylmethane. Reproduced with copyright permission by Jagetia and Aggarwal *(50)*.

3.1. Curcumin

Curcumin (Fig. 2) is an active compound in turmeric and contributes to the yellow color found in such foods as curries and yellow mustard. Curcumin has been used in Ayruvedic medicine for at least 5,000 years. This compound has been used by people in India to treat various ailments (e.g., gastrointestinal disorders, liver disorders, aches, pains, wounds, sprains) for centuries with no known side effects *(152)*. Aggarwal *(152)* has concluded that numerous lines of evidence suggest that curcumin could help prevent or mitigate the effects of skin, oral, stomach, intestinal, colon, mammary, breast, liver, prostate, blood, bone marrow, brain, gastrointestinal, head and neck, pancreatic, esophageal, lung, and ovarian cancers.

3.1.1. Anti-inflammatory/Antioxidant Properties

Both animal and in vitro studies have shown that curcumin acts as an anti-inflammatory compound by inhibiting the COX-2, LOX, NADPH oxidase (NOX), and inductible nitric oxide synthase (i-NOS) pathways. COX-2 and NOX are often involved in tumors and malignant tissues and LOX and i-NOS are associated with different types of human cancers *(51, 52, 53)*. Both in vitro and animal studies have demonstrated the effect of turmeric, curcumin, and/or curcumin analogues on the inhibition of these enzymes *(152)*.

Interleukin 6 (IL-6), a biomarker associated with inflammation, induces STAT3 activity, which has been detected in head and neck squamous cell carcinoma, leukemias, lymphomas, and multiple myeloma *(54, 55)*. Bharti et al. *(54)* demonstrated that curcumin was able to inhibit STAT3 activity in vitro.

Curcumin also inhibits NF-kB, which affects cancer and many other diseases. NF-kB mediates inflammation and plays a pivotal role in controlling cell proliferation, oncogenesis, and cell transformation *(51)*. Ingested or topically applied curcumin has been shown to inhibit NF-kB in several in vitro cancer lines and animal studies *(152, 52)*. Additionally, the role of curcumin and NF-kB is currently being investigated in a clinical trial at the MD Anderson Cancer Center in multiple myeloma patients *(151, 56)*. Preliminary results, which have not yet been published, suggest that 2–12 g of curcumin/day greatly decreased the amount of NF-kB in some patients after 24 weeks. However, this result was not seen in all patients *(56)*.

A separate phase II clinical trial investigated the effect of curcumin (8 g for 8 weeks or more) on NF-kB (as well as other biological effects of curcumin) in 25 pancreatic cancer patients *(12)*. Of 19 patients who provided blood samples, there was a nonsignificant ($p < 0.10$) decline in NF-kB concentrations after 8 days of treatment *(12)*.

Curcumin is also considered an antioxidant because it helps inhibit free radical production and oxidative damage *(51, 57, 58)*. In vitro studies have shown that curcumin can induce heme oxygenase-1 (HO-1) and protect endothelial cells against oxidative stress *(59)*.

Curcumin is a potent scavenger of reactive oxygen species (ROS) including superoxide anion, 9 hydroxyl radical, singlet oxygen, and peroxynitrite *(59, 58)*. Both in vitro and animal studies have demonstrated that curcumin can protect lipids, hemoglobin, and/or DNA against oxidative degradation. Curcumin has also been shown to inhibit ROS-generating enzymes as well as cyclooxygenase (COX) and lipoxygenase (LOX) activity in mouse epidermis *(59, 57)*. A few in vitro studies have shown that curcumin can increase the production of ROS *(57, 58)* under certain conditions. Interestingly, ROS increases are related to mechanisms of curcumin-induced apoptosis, which are dependent on increasing ROS *(57, 58)*.

3.1.2. EFFECTS OF CURCUMIN ON TUMOR CELLS IN CULTURE

Curcumin works to prevent tumor growth in cell cultures by several mechanisms. It has been shown to inhibit angiogenesis (an obligatory process for tumor growth) in several experiments *(60)*. Zhang et al. *(61)* found that curcumin suppressed COX-2 activity and reduced tumor size in different calf, mouse, rabbit, and other animal cultures. A separate study found that curcumin inhibited tumor growth in human colorectal cancer cells *(51)*. Curcumin has also been shown to suppress or delay tumor growth by inhibiting i-NOS and LOX activity in several animal and human cancer lines. This compound has been shown to help inhibit the tumor suppressor gene, p53, in some cancer lines *(55)*. Curcumin has also been shown to induce apoptosis and suppress the growth of several T-cell leukemia cell lines in a dose-dependent manner *(57, 62)*.

NF-kB activation has been observed in many cancer cell lines, and the inhibition of NF-kB has resulted in a decrease in cancer and tumor cells *(55)*. Curcumin has been shown to decrease the amount of NF-kB and the size and growth rate of tumors in both animal and human tissue cultures. Curcumin has also been shown to inhibit the production of tumor necrosis factor (TNF) in both animal and human cells. TNF suppression is linked to the inhibition of NF-kB production *(51)*.

Activator protein-1 (AP1) is another transcription factor that has been closely linked with the proliferation and transformation of tumor cells. The activation of this factor is closely related to that of NF-kB. Curcumin has been shown to inhibit the tumor growth and the activation of AP-I in different cell lines *(55, 63)*.

Several studies have suggested that the anticancer effects of curcumin analogues may be even more potent than that of the parent compound. For example, several analogs were up to 10 times more effective than natural curcumin in inhibiting tumor growth in over 60 different human tumor cell lines. Analogues were well tolerated with little toxicity *(52)*.

3.1.3. EFFECTS OF CURCUMIN ON CANCER INITIATION, PROMOTION, OR PROGRESSION IN INTACT ANIMALS

Curcumin has been tested extensively in animals. Several studies have demonstrated that topically applied curcumin can inhibit tumor formation on mouse skin. Ingestion of curcumin decreased the number and/or size of skin, liver, colorectal, oral, and stomach tumors in animal models. Curcumin also decreased cancer-related weight loss and the amount of adenocarcinoma at different cancer sites (e.g., stomach, colon, and liver) *(64)*

Angiogenesis is involved in the conversion of premalignant to malignant cells and occurs in breast, prostate, liver, ovarian, and other tumors. Animal and in vitro studies have demonstrated that curcumin affects angiogenesis through the downregulation of transcription factors (e.g., NF-kB), proangiogenic factors [e.g., vascular endothelial growth factor (VEGF), COX-2], and inhibition of cell motility, cellular adhesion molecules, endothelial cell migration, invasion, and extracellular proteolysis *(60)*. Several studies have demonstrated the antiangiogenic effects of curcumin in mice *(64)*. For example, Yoysungnoen et al. *(65)* examined neocapillary formation in liver cells and found lower capillary density in tumors of mice who received 3,000 mg/kg of curcumin compared to controls.

Curcumin has been tested in animal models with malignant tumors *(64)*. For example, Ohashi et al. *(66)* found that 100–200 mg/kg of curcumin given to mice daily for 20 days suppressed intrahepatic metastasis in a dose-dependent manner compared to controls (although tumor growth was not affected).

Several xenograph experiments have demonstrated the ability of curcumin to inhibit cancer initiation, promotion, or progression. Shanker et al. *(67)* found that curcumin inhibited tumor growth, metastasis, and angiogenesis in mice who were implanted with prostate cancer cells. Kunnumakkara et al. *(68)* demonstrated that curcumin decreased tumor size, inhibited apoptosis, and suppressed NF-kB activity in pancreatic cancer using mouse xenograph experiments. Aggarwal *(30)* and Bachmeier et al. *(69)* found that mice implanted with human breast cancer cells had decreased metastasis to the lung, and suppressed NF-KB, COX 2, and matrix metalloproteinase (MMP) activity compared to controls. Li et al. *(70)* observed that curcumin reduced the expression of double minute (MDM2) oncogene in mice who received prostate cancer xenographs. MDM2 is dependent on the p53 gene and is currently being investigated for new cancer therapy treatment *(70)*. Hong et al. *(71)* reported that curcumin decreased pancreatic tumor size and inhibited MMP activity in mice with implanted prostate cancer cells. Curcumin also suppressed tumor growth and/or density in mice with xenographed head and neck and liver tumors *(72, 65)*.

Curcumin has been shown to increase immune response in both in vitro and animal models *(57, 73, 50)*. Specific effects of curcumin on the immune system are presented in Fig. 3.

Animal studies include research by Antony et al. *(74)* who reported that mice fed curcumin had higher plaque-forming cells (PFCs), bone marrow cells, and white blood cell counts compared to control animals. Yasni et al. *(75)* found that mice fed turmeric for 3–5 weeks had increased T lymphocytes throughout the experimental period *(73)*. Immune effects may play an important role in cancer prevention as well as in cancer treatment *(50)*.

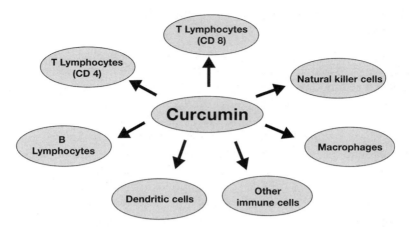

Regulation of various immune cells by curcumin (diferuloylmethane)

Fig. 3. Regulation of immune cells by curcumin (deferuloylmethane). Reproduced with copyright permission by Jagetia and Aggarwal *(50)*.

Some reports have suggested that curcumin can protect animals against radiation. Rats who received curcumin had lower levels of lung toxicity, liver and lipid peroxidation, and chromosomal damage compared to controls *(76)*. Some protection from radiation has been observed in humans. However, the evidence is not yet conclusive *(152)*.

3.1.4. EFFECTS OF CURCUMIN ON SPECIFIC DETOXIFYING ENZYMES

Modulation of enzymes involved in the activation and detoxification of carcinogens is one function of chemopreventive agents including curcumin *(64)*. Phase I enzymes such as cytochrome P450 (CYP) convert compounds (e.g., tetrachloromethane and aflatoxin B1) to toxic-reactive metabolites. Turmeric, curcumin, and curcumin analogues have inhibited CYP enzymes in vitro *(64, 77)*. Sharma et al. *(77)* concluded that understanding these metabolic effects can also help determine potential drug interactions in clinical use.

Curcumin has been shown to increase the activity of several phase II detoxifying enzymes. Separate studies found that feeding mice 1–2% of the diet as curcumin increased the activity of glutathione-S-transferase (GST), glutathione (GSH), DP-glucuronosyltransferase (UGT), and/or quinone reductase activity in the liver, kidney, intestine, and/or prostate compared to controls *(64, 59, 78, 79, 80, 81)*. Surh and Chun *(64)* have shown that curcumin can disrupt the Nrf2–Keap1 complex which is associated with an increase in the expression of detoxifying enzymes [e.g., heme oxygenase- 159 (HO-159)]. This study also demonstrated increased activity of glutamate–cysteine ligase (GCL) gene expression, which in turn increases phase II enzyme activity. Curcumin has also been shown to induce HO-1 activity in human hepatocytes, vascular endothelial cells, and renal proximal tubule cells *(64)*.

Curcumin has also been shown to inhibit the activity of procarcinogen benzo[a]pyrene (B[a]P) which is present in the detoxification process. For example, curcumin has been shown to decrease the levels of phase I enzymes, activate B[a]P in the liver, and increase the levels of phase II enzymes, which are involved in the detoxification of metabolites derived from B[a]P *(57)*.

3.1.5. EFFECTS OF CURCUMIN ON BACTERIAL INFECTIONS

Curcumin has been shown to affect infection with bacterial strains (e.g., *H. pylori*) in vitro *(82, 2)*. Both Münzenmaier et al. *(83)* and Foryst-Ludwig et al. *(84)* showed that curcumin also downregulated NF-kB and IL-8 in vitro. These compounds are induced by several *H. pylori* strains. There is currently no conclusive evidence that treatment with curcumin has an effect on *H. pylori* infection in humans *(2)*. Di Mario et al. *(85)* administered curcumin in combination with *N*-acetylcysteine, pantoprazole, and lactoferrin to 25 Italian males and females with functional dyspepsia and a positive *H. pylori* infection for 7 days. Only 3 of 25 patients (12%) were cured of this infection after 2 months. However, significant decreases occurred for both reported severity of symptoms ($p < 0.001$) and serum pepsinogens [sPGI ($p < 0.02$), sPGII ($p < 0.001$)] at day 7 and after 2 months of treatment.

3.1.6. HUMAN OBSERVATIONAL STUDIES ON CURCUMIN

As mentioned in the introduction, populations differ in both their dietary intake of spices and herbs and their rates of cancer morbidity and mortality. Worldwide, those populations who consume the most spices tend to have the lowest cancer rates. Curcumin has been consumed for centuries in Asian countries without any observed toxicity *(86)*. According to Menon and Sudheer *(51)*, "more than one billion people consume curcumin regularly in their diets." Eigner and Scholz *(87)* reported that in parts of Asia, people consume up to 1.5 g of turmeric/day. Mohandas and Desai *(88)* attribute the low incidence of bowel cancers in India at least partially to the high amounts of curcumin (from turmeric) in the diet. However, there is a lack of detailed information as to how the turmeric is consumed, prepared, or combined with other foods and/or spices. More epidemiologic data are needed to better understand the possible associations between intake of turmeric and curcumin and cancer incidence *(88)*.

3.1.7. HUMAN INTERVENTION STUDIES WITH CURCUMIN ON CANCER PATIENTS OR HEALTHY SUBJECTS

Considerable research has demonstrated that curcumin has the potential to prevent and delay cancer. However, the effectiveness of this compound has not been systematically examined in multicenter, randomized, double-blind, placebo-controlled clinical trials *(152)*. The most comprehensive studies on curcumin have been conducted on safety. For example, curcumin was found to have no toxic side effects in humans in dosages from 8 to 12 g/day *(50)*.

A limited number of case studies, pilot studies, and/or phase I/II trials have been conducted with curcumin. Most of these studies have employed cancer patients. Sixty-two

patients with external cancerous lesions who used a topical ointment made from curcumin and turmeric reported some symptomatic relief (either reduced itching, dryness,
or smell). In addition, 10% of these subjects reported reduced tumor size. However,
these findings must be interpreted with caution because this experiment had no control
group and the data were self-reported *(89, 64)*.

Polasa et al. *(90)* gave 1.5 g/day of turmeric to 16 smokers for 30 days and reported
that urinary excretion of mutagens was significantly reduced ($p < 001$). Six smokers who
did not receive turmeric had no changes in urinary mutagens after 30 days.

A pilot study in the United Kingdom *(45)* gave 15 patients with advanced colorectal
cancer 36–180 mg/day of curcumin extracts for up to 4 months. All doses of the extracts
were well tolerated. As noted earlier, curcumin and its metabolites were not detected
in blood or urine, but they were recovered from feces. One-third of the patients in this
study experienced stable disease for 2–4 months, and one additional patient exhibited
decreased amounts of a tumor marker (carcino-embryonic antigen). A subsequent phase
I clinical trial *(46)* provided curcumin supplementation with 0.45–3.6 g/day for up to
4 months to 15 patients diagnosed with progressive advanced colorectal cancer. There
was little toxicity with the exception of mild diarrhea. Curcumin and its sulfate metabolites were detected in plasma and urine, but only for 1 h in three patients who consumed 3.6 g/day of curcumin. The consumption of curcumin inhibited prostaglandin E2
(PGE2) production. Two of the 15 patients experienced radiologically stable conditions
for 4 months after the treatment with curcumin *(46)*.

A phase I clinical trial in Taiwan *(47)* examined the effects of curcumin supplementation in 25 patients with high-risk or premalignant lesions of the bladder, skin,
cervix, stomach, or oral mucosa. Patients took curcumin for 3 months in increasing
doses from 500 to 12,000 mg/day. Skin biopsy was performed immediately before
and after curcumin supplementation. Patients tolerated curcumin supplementation up
to 8,000 mg/day. Blood serum levels peaked 1–2 h after ingestion; after 12 h, concentrations usually declined to baseline. Improvement in lesions was seen in 7 of the
25 patients. One patient did not complete the study and two of the patients developed
malignancies despite curcumin use *(47)*.

Dhillon et al. *(12)* conducted a phase II clinical trial to investigate the biological
effects of curcumin in 25 American male and female patients (mean age $= 65$) with
advanced pancreatic cancer. Patients received 8 g curcumin daily until disease progression (restaging was done every 8 weeks). Nineteen of the 25 patients who were enrolled
completed the 8-week trial and were evaluated. No toxicity was observed in any of
the patients. Significant reductions in COX-2 ($p < 0.03$) and STAT3 ($p < 0.009$) were
observed after curcumin treatment. In addition, NF-kB levels declined, but not significantly ($p < 0.10$). Of the two patients with clinical biological activity, one had stabilized
disease for over 18 months and the second one had a transitory regression in tumor
size (73%) and decreased levels of all cytokines (e.g., IL-6, IL-8, IL-10, IL-1, NF-kB,
COX-2).

A concern regarding clinical trials with curcumin is the apparent low bioavailability of this compound *(31)*. As mentioned above, even at high doses (e.g.,
400–8,000 mg/day), curcumin is not detectable in blood after 12 h. Efficient first-pass

metabolism or alteration of curcumin in the gut may explain the apparent poor systemic availability of this compound when taken orally *(31)*. However, as noted previously, the fact that a compound is not detected in large amounts in biological tissues does not necessarily mean it is not bioactive. Such compounds may be metabolized quickly to other efficacious compounds, or modification by bacteria in the intestinal tract may prompt conversion to beneficial compounds that are subsequently absorbed *(45, 31)*.

Curcumin bioavailability in humans may be enhanced by the use of synergistic compounds. For example, Shoba et al. *(91)* found that 10 male healthy human volunteers from India who ingested 20 mg of piperine (from black pepper) in combination with 2,000 mg of curcumin had greatly enhanced (2,000%) curcumin bioavailability *(31)*.

Several clinical trials from pilot phase to phase III trials are underway to investigate the efficacy of curcumin in cancer patients (clinicaltrials.gov). A variety of treatments ranging from large doses of curcumin to curcumin combined with other cancer medications are being investigated.

3.2. Garlic

Garlic (classified as both a spice and a vegetable) belongs to the Allium class of plants along with onions, chives, leeks, and scallions. Garlic was used to treat tumors over 3,500 years ago in Ancient Egypt *(49)* and is used today as a spice for foods worldwide and as a dietary supplement in western countries *(92)*.

Garlic contains many potentially bioactive compounds including arginine, oligosaccharides, flavonoids, and selenium, all of which may be beneficial to health *(93, 94)*. This spice also contains many organosulfur compounds (OCS), which may have a role in cancer prevention *(95, 32, 96)* (Fig. 4). These substances include water-soluble allicin, alliin, *S*-allyl cysteine (SAC), *S*-allyl mercaptocysteine (SAMC), and oil-soluble diallyl sulfide (DAS), diallyl disulfide (DADS), and diallyl trisulfide (DATS) (Fig. 5). Other organosulfur compounds that have been examined include aged garlic extract (AGE), garlic powder, garlic oil, garlic homogenate, and raw garlic. Some of the active compounds in garlic are presented in Fig. 3.

3.2.1. LIMITATIONS OF GARLIC RESEARCH

There are more than 2,000 scientific publications on the chemistry and biological effects of garlic. However, studies do not always identify the type and/or form (e.g., extract) of garlic employed *(37)*. In addition, many studies do not use a chemically standardized product, although this approach tends to be in use in more recent experiments. The composition of garlic depends on the source, age, storage conditions, type of processing, and method of consumption *(37, 32, 98, 99, 96, 100)*. The amount and composition of organosulfur compounds differ among strains of garlic, and this variability is exacerbated by the volatile and reactive nature of these compounds *(37, 32, 96)*.

Cancer-related garlic research is far from conclusive. Nevertheless, there is considerable evidence that garlic and its active compounds play a role in cancer prevention and/or progression. This research is summarized below.

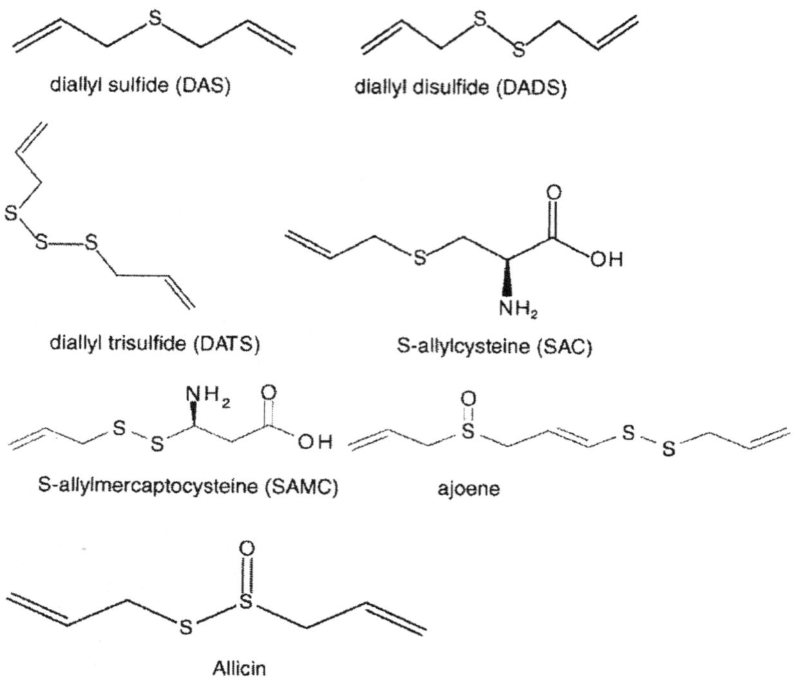

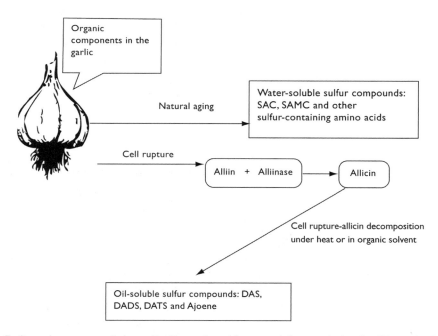

Fig. 4. Chemical structures of garlic compounds. Reproduced by copyright permission by Wu et al. *(97).*

Fig. 5. Organic compounds in garlic. Reproduced by copyright permission by Wu et al. *(97).*

3.2.2. ANTI-INFLAMMATORY/ANTIOXIDANT PROPERTIES OF GARLIC

The antioxidant and anti-inflammatory activity of garlic is seen in a variety of forms *(95)*. Garlic and its active compounds consistently exhibit good antioxidant activity, scavenge free radicals, and induce the activity of several antioxidant enzymes including glutathione peroxidase, GST, and superoxide dismutase *(101, 95, 32, 100, 92)*.

Garlic OSC have been reported to exhibit good antioxidant activity *(95, 32)*. For example, Prasad et al. *(104)* found that when mice were given either low (250 mg/animal) or high (500 mg/animal) amounts of the organosulfur compound DAS, levels of testosterone-induced oxidative stress were lower and levels of antioxidant enzymes were higher compared to controls. DADS can also inhibit lipid peroxidation in the liver in vitro *(105)*. Organosulfur compounds, SAC and SAMC (major compounds in aged garlic extract), have been shown to exhibit free radical scavenging activity in in vitro experiments *(100)*.

Garlic has been shown to lower ROS formation through the inhibition of myeloperoxidase (MPO). This enzyme can prompt activation of mutagens (e.g., tobacco smoke) and environmental pollutants *(32)* and lead to the generation of ROS. Gedik et al. *(106)* found that administration of aqueous garlic extract for 28 days reduced oxidative damage (decreased MPO activity) in rats with biliary obstruction as compared to controls. Sener et al. *(107)* reported that rats given aqueous garlic extract exhibited decreased MPO activity and oxidative damage induced by thermal stress as compared to controls.

Moreover, garlic has the ability to decrease the inflammatory response *(32)*. For example, garlic has been shown to decrease both leukocyte helper cells and inflammatory cytokine production in vitro *(32)*. Lang et al. *(108)* found that allicin inhibited inflammatory biomarkers such as interleukin 1 beta (IL-1β), interleukin 8 (IL-8), and interferon-gamma-inducible protein 10 (IP-10). In addition, Dirsch and Vollmar *(109)* demonstrated that ajoene, a component of crushed garlic, inhibited COX-2 activity in vitro.

3.2.3. EFFECTS OF GARLIC ON TUMOR CELLS IN CULTURE

Garlic and its active compounds have been shown to suppress the proliferation of cancer cells in culture. Antitumorigenic effects have been demonstrated for many types of cancers including mammary, colon, lung, skin, and prostate tumor cell lines in both animal models and humans *(49, 97)*. Generally, the effect on apoptosis was both dose and time dependent *(97)*.

As early as 1958, Weisberger found that selenium compounds and allium enzymes in garlic could suppress the growth of mouse and rat tumor cells in culture. Wesiberger also found that these compounds suppressed tumor growth when they were injected into intact animals. Chu et al. *(110)* found that SAC and SAMC suppressed cancer cell proliferation in the prostate as well as restore E-cadherin expression. Chu et al. *(110)* also found that SAC and SAMC restored E-cadherin in other human cancer cell lines including ovarian, nasopharyngeal, and esophageal. Some researchers have concluded that inactivation of E-cadherin is a key component in cancer development and that garlic derivatives may play a role in cancer prevention through the activation of this factor *(95, 110)*.

Some evidence suggests that garlic compounds can modify cell division by blocking cells within the G1, S, or G2/M phases *(105, 97, 98)*. In vitro data suggest that OSC (such as DADS, SAMC, and DAS) can contribute to cell arrest in the G2/M phase of the cell cycle *(105, 98)*, but this mechanism has not yet been consistently demonstrated in human or animal models *(32, 105)*.

DADS, DAS, and DATS have been shown to inhibit p53 activity and increase the number of apoptotic cancer cells in several cell lines *(99, 98)*. DAS and DADS have also been shown to increase the concentration of BCL2-associated X protein (BAX) and/or decrease levels of B-cell CLL/lymphoma 2 (Bcl-2) in vitro, which correlate to inhibition and promotion of the p53 gene, respectively *(98, 99)*.

NF-kB activation has been observed in many cancer cell lines and the inhibition of NF-kB has resulted in a decrease in cancer and tumor cells *(55)*. The organosulfur compound SAC has been shown to inhibit NF-kB activation in several in vitro experiments *(100)*. Overall, the mechanisms by which garlic may inhibit tumor growth are not well understood *(32, 97)*. However, it has been hypothesized that both the water-soluble and oil-soluble OSC in garlic may work together to facilitate transport through the lipid bilayer of the cell membrane *(97)*. Compounds with high biological activity (e.g., DADS, SAMC, DAS) seem to have a high number of sulfur atoms, which could potentially increase GSH production *(97, 101, 102, 103)*.

A few in vitro studies have been conducted to assess the toxicity of garlic compounds but Wu et al. *(97)* have concluded that more research is needed to assess their long-term safety.

3.2.4. EFFECTS OF GARLIC ON CANCER INITIATION, PROMOTION, AND PROGRESSION IN INTACT ANIMALS

Garlic and its active compounds have been shown to inhibit carcinogenesis at multiple sites in animals treated with a variety of carcinogens *(49, 32)*. Cancer chemoprevention by garlic and its active compounds has been demonstrated at the initiation, promotion, and progression stages in intact animals *(111)*. The ability of garlic to suppress cancer at various stages does not appear to be species, tissue, or carcinogen dependent *(112, 99)*. The organosulfur compound, DAS, has been shown to prevent the initiation and progression of cancer in several animal models. For example, Singh and Shukla *(113)* found that 250 μg of DAS applied to Swiss albino mice 3 times/week for 32 weeks decreased the incidence of skin tumors in mice compared to untreated controls. Anti-tumor properties of DAS on mouse skin carcinogenesis have also been observed in several other studies *(105)*. Shukla et al. *(114)* found that mice injected daily with 250 μg of DAS for 7 days and then implanted with ascites tumor cells had a 67% higher chance of survival than untreated controls after 8 weeks. Arunkumar et al. *(115, 116)* found that DAS inhibited cancer induction in the rat prostate. DAS and other organosulfur compounds have also provided protection from mammary gland, lung, colon, esophageal, colon, skin, and stomach cancers in rats and mice *(49, 97)*.

Other compounds from garlic have been shown to prevent or delay cancer in intact animals. As mentioned above, Weisberger and Pensky *(117)* found suppressed ascites tumor cell growth (both size and number) in intact Swiss Albino mice given the selenium garlic compound S-ethyl L-cysteine sulfoxide treated with alliinase. There was no significant effect on tumor growth or number when the compounds were administered to the mice separately.

AGE has been shown to demonstrate a number of chemopreventative and tumor growth effects in animal models *(118, 119)*. For example, AGE and its constituents were shown to inhibit the development of chemically induced tumors in the bladder, mammary gland, colon, esophagus, lung, skin, and stomach of rodents *(118)*. Lamm and Riggs *(119)* found that oral AGE added to drinking water (5, 50, and 500 mg/100 ml) inhibited bladder tumor growth in a dose-dependent manner in mice. AGE and its constituents may inhibit carcinogen activation, enhance detoxification of phase I and phase II enzymes, and provide protection from carcinogens *(118, 119)*. However, AGE may also be toxic when injected into mice at high doses *(119)*.

Some studies have compared the effects of garlic and/or bioactive garlic compounds on the development of cancer in intact animals. Schaffer et al. *(120)* studied the effects of dietary garlic powder (20 g/kg) or selenium garlic compounds including SAC and DADS (57 μMol/kg) on the occurrence of mammary tumors in rats. Tumor incidence was reduced by 76, 41, and 53% after 23 days in rats fed garlic, SAC, and DADS, respectively, compared to controls. Analogous data for total tumor number were reduced 81, 35, and 65%, respectively.

3.2.5. EFFECTS OF GARLIC ON SPECIFIC DETOXIFYING ENZYMES

Phase I detoxification reactions usually involve the cytochrome P450 (Cyp 450) system, which can act on a wide variety of chemical carcinogens, drugs, and environmental toxins *(121)*. Garlic and its active compounds appear to modify both phase I and phase II detoxification activities. OSC with at least one allyl (but not methyl) group including DAS, DAD, AMTS, and whole garlic appear to have the strongest effect in this system, although considerable variability has been observed among these compounds *(121, 98, 122)*.

The ability of garlic and its active compounds to modify phase I enzymes, specifically Cyp P450 activity, is specific. Several Cyp P450 enzymes (e.g., Cyp 1A1, 1A2, 3A4, 2B1, 2B4, 2E1) are increased by various allyl organosulfur components while others are downregulated *(123, 32)*. For example, Wargovich *(121)* demonstrated that the CYP mechanism (CYP2E1) was shut down within 24 h in the liver of rats given 50 mg/kg orally of either DAS or allylmethylsulfide (both oil-soluble compounds). This effect was not seen in experiments with water-soluble garlic compounds. In addition, Chen et al. *(124)* observed that garlic oil was able to inhibit Cyp P4502B1 in a dose-dependent manner when given to rats 3 times/week for 6 weeks.

Dalvi *(125)* found that rats given a single dose of DAS (500 mg/kg), but not 50 mg/kg, experienced decreased levels of cytochrome P-450, aminopyrine N-demethylase, and aniline hydroxylase after 24 h with no liver damage.

Garlic and its active compounds can also facilitate detoxification of carcinogens through upregulation of Phase II-conjugating enzymes (e.g., GST, epoxide hydrolase, quinone reductase, and UDP-glucuronosyltransferase) *(123, 105, 98)*. It appears that different OSC have different effects on phase II detoxification *(123)*. Chen et al. *(124)*

observed that garlic oil administered to rats for 6 weeks increased GST in a dose-dependent manner. In addition, highly purified forms of allylsulfides (e.g., DAS, DADS, DATS) administered to rats at a concentration of 10 or 100 μmol/kg body weight for 14 consecutive days caused an increase in the activities of several phase II enzymes including GST, quinone reductase, and glutathione peroxidase *(126, 105)*.

Sumiyoshi and Wargovich *(122)* compared the effectiveness of lipid- and water-soluble OSC in mice prior to ip injection of the carcinogen 1,2-dimethylhydrazine (DMII). Administration of DAS and SAC (200 mg/kg) significantly inhibited colonic nuclear damage in mice by 47 and 36%, respectively ($p < 0.05$). The number and incidence of colonic tumors were also significantly inhibited by this compound ($p < 0.05$). Sumiyoshi hypothesized that OSC containing allyl groups can stimulate GST activity in both the liver and colon, which could potentially facilitate detoxification and cancer prevention. This conclusion has been suggested by subsequent studies *(121)* and whole garlic as well as other allyl group garlic compounds (e.g., DAS, DAD, AMTS) have been shown to increase the amounts of phase II detoxification enzymes *(121, 98)*.

3.2.6. EFFECTS OF GARLIC ON BACTERIAL INFECTIONS

Garlic oil and OSC compounds have been shown to strongly inhibit the bacterial growth of *H. pylori* in vitro and in a few animal models. However, studies in humans have mostly shown no correlation between the *H. pylori* infection and the use of garlic *(99, 38, 127, 128)*. You et al. *(38)* conducted a large ($n = 3365$) randomized, placebo-controlled factorial design trial among subjects (aged 35–64) living in Linqu County, Shandong Province, China. The subjects were randomized to receive a one-time antibiotic treatment for *H. pylori* infection and/or 7.3 years oral supplementation with a vitamin preparation and/or a garlic preparation. The outcome measure was prevalence of advanced precancerous gastric lesions. Two-week antibiotic treatment significantly decreased the prevalence of both gastric cancer lesions and gastric cancer incidence after 7.3 years ($p < 0.05$). However, vitamin and garlic supplementations did not have an effect compared to controls.

Fani et al. *(127)* conducted a clinical trial among 75 male and female Iranian patients (mean age 37.5 years) with nonulcer chronic dyspepsia and positive *H. pylori* status. The subjects received 15 g of garlic and 20 mg of antibiotic (omeprazole) daily for 2 weeks. Seventy-seven patients with duodenal ulcer (mean age 37.4 years) and positive *H. pylori* status served as the control group and received quadruple antibiotic therapy (omeprazole 20 mg BID, amoxicillin 1 g BID, bismuth subitrate 2 tablet TID, metronida-zole 500 mg BID) for 2 weeks. The response rate to treatment (demonstrated by a negative *H. pylori* test) was much lower in the garlic (12%) vs. the control group (90.9%; $p < 0.001$). Treatment with multi antibiotics was about seven times more effective than treatment with a single antibiotic and garlic. Two additional clinical trials *(128)* that assessed the effect of garlic on the inhibition of *H. pylori* reported no effect.

Garlic in vitro also exhibits a broad antibiotic spectrum against a variety of gram-positive and gram-negative bacteria *(37)*. Specifically, garlic has inhibited growth of the genera *Aerobacter, Aeromonas, Bacillus, Citrella, Citrobacter, Clostridium, Enterobacter, Escherichia, Klebsiella, Lactobacillus, Leuconostoc, Micrococcus, Mycobacterium, Proteus, Providencia, Pseudomonas, Salmonella, Serratia, Shigella,*

Staphylococcus, *Streptococcus*, and *Vibrio* in vitro *(37)*. Similar to turmeric, garlic appears not to display resistance to antibiotics *(37)*.

3.2.7. HUMAN OBSERVATIONAL STUDIES ON GARLIC

The association between garlic intake and cancer risk has been demonstrated in several epidemiological studies for different types of cancers (e.g., colon, gastrointestinal). One of the first epidemiological studies *(129)* with garlic assessed a potential association with stomach cancer in China. In two Chinese provinces, a 10-fold difference in the death rate from this cancer correlated with garlic consumption of 20 g/day in the low-risk area and <1 g/day in the high-risk area *(129)*

Fleischauer and Arab *(130)* conducted a meta analysis on garlic consumption and cancer risk based on 19 case–control studies. It was concluded that although the analysis had some limitations (e.g., low study power, lack of variability in garlic consumption, poor adjustment for potential cofounders), there is suggestive evidence of a protective association between garlic consumption and cancer incidence. A separate meta analysis by Fleischauer et al. *(131)* concluded that those populations who consumed the most garlic (any consumption to about 9–10 cloves/week, average 28.8 g) had reduced risk of colon and stomach cancers compared to those who consumed no or low amounts of garlic (no consumption to about 1 clove/week, average 3.5 g).

The European Prospective Investigation into Cancer and Nutrition (EPIC) is an ongoing population study of dietary consumption and cancer risk among 519,978 subjects (366,521 women and 153,457 men) most aged 35–70 years. A recent analysis of food intake *(132)* suggested that consumption of onion and garlic reduced the risk of intestinal and stomach cancers, but it was probably not associated with cancer of the lung, prostate, colon, or breast.

A prospective cohort study in the United States *(133)* obtained data on food intake (including garlic) in 1986 for 41,837 women aged 55–69 years using a 127-item food frequency questionnaire. Garlic showed the strongest inverse association with colon cancer incidence after 5 years of follow-up using data from the state health registry of Iowa (p <0.10). One or more servings of garlic (fresh or powdered) per week was associated with a 35% lower risk of cancers anywhere in the colon, while a 50% lower risk was found for cancer of the distal colon *(133)*.

Devrim and Durak *(95)* concluded that there is suggestive evidence of a protective association between garlic intake and prostate cancer based on a review of several case–control and population-based studies. However, the results of these studies are not entirely consistent. Hsing et al. *(134)* investigated the relationship between consumption of allium-containing vegetables (including garlic) and the risk of prostate cancer in 238 subjects with confirmed prostate cancer and 471 apparently healthy controls (Chinese males, aged 16 and older). Men with the highest intake of garlic exhibited reduced incidence of prostate cancer. The risk of prostate cancer was independent of body size, intake of other foods, or total calorie intake and was more pronounced for men with localized than advanced prostate cancer. A case–control study in England also found that garlic intake (either in food or supplement form) was associated with reduced risk of prostate cancer among British men aged 75 or less *(135)*.

Chan et al. *(136)* examined food consumption in 532 pancreatic cancer cases and 1,701 age- and sex-matched controls in the San Francisco bay area. Those subjects that consumed the highest amount of onions and garlic had 54% lower incidence of pancreatic cancer compared to those in the lowest consumption category. However, the study did not distinguish between garlic and onion consumption. Therefore, it was not possible to attribute this association to garlic per se.

A case–control study *(137)* showed that garlic and onion consumption was significantly linked to reduced breast cancer incidence (diagnosed between 1986 and 1989) among 345 patients in France (*p* for trend <0.000001). However, this study did not examine the amount of garlic consumed or distinguish between consumption of garlic and onion.

3.2.8. HUMAN INTERVENTION STUDIES WITH GARLIC ON CANCER PATIENTS OR HEALTHY SUBJECTS

The results of intervention studies on the effect of garlic (or garlic compounds) supplementation on cancer are inconsistent. Milner *(32)* hypothesized that there is a variable response to the intake of garlic and other allium vegetables among individuals. Factors responsible for this variability include genetic background (nutrigenetic effects), DNA methylation and histone regulation (nutritional epigenomic effects), ability to induce or repress gene expression patterns (nutritional transcriptomics effects), occurrence and activity of specific proteins (nutriproteomic effects), and/or dose and temporal changes in cellular small-molecular-weight compounds (metabolomics effects). Further research is needed to better predict who will respond to garlic and/or other allium foods *(32)*.

Durak et al. *(138)* administered Turkish men (27 subjects with benign prostate hyperplasia (BPH) and nine patients with prostate cancer) 1 ml/kg of aqueous garlic extract/day for 1 month. The BPH group had a lower prostate mass and both groups had decreased urinary frequency and stronger urinary output at the end of the study compared to baseline (*p* <0.01). The cancer group also experienced decreased PSA concentrations as a result of garlic supplementation (*p* <0.01).

Tanaka et al. *(139)* conducted a double-blind clinical trial among 51 Japanese patients (aged 40–79) with colorectal adenomas. The experimental group received a high dose of aged garlic extract (AGE) (2.4 ml/day) and the control group received a low dose of this substance (0.16 ml/day). Each subject took three capsules a day for 12 months. Those in the high dosage group had fewer and smaller adenomas at 6 and 12 month evaluations compared to controls (*p* <0.04).

Ishikawa et al. *(140)* conducted a double-blind trial among 50 Japanese cancer patients with inoperable cancer of the liver, pancreas, or colon. Subjects received either aged garlic extract (500 mg/day) or a placebo for 6 months. The garlic treatment significantly increased both the number of natural killer (NK) cells (*p* <0.05) and NK cell activity (*p* <0.01) compared to controls. There was no difference between the two groups in self-reported quality of life.

Li et al. *(141)* conducted a double-blind intervention study on over 5,000 Chinese men and women (aged 35–74) who were at high risk of gastric cancer. The intervention group took 200 mg of synthetic garlic and 100 µg of selenium/day for 1 month of the year between 1989 and 1991. There was a significant (no *p*-value provided) 22% decrease in gastric cancer morbidity and a 47% decrease in gastric cancer incidence after 5 years in the male treatment group compared to controls. No effect was found among females.

As noted previously, several clinical trials have examined the effect of garlic supplementation on gastric cancer associated with *H. pylori* infection *(38, 127, 128)*. However, the results of these studies were either negative or inconclusive.

Several clinical trials with garlic are currently in progress. These studies include the effects of garlic supplementation in combination with prescription medication on breast cancer, and garlic supplementation in patients with lymphoma (clinicaltrials.gov).

3.3. Other Culinary Spices and Herbs

Curcumin and garlic have been the most extensively studied spices for their potential ability to inhibit and/or prevent cancer. Nevertheless, many other culinary spices and herbs have been investigated to a lesser extent. The most information is available for saffron, ginger, and capsaicin, and a summary of this research is presented below.

3.3.1. SAFFRON

Saffron (*Crocus sativus*) extracts have been shown to inhibit skin, colon, and soft tissue tumors in several in vitro and animal experiments *(13, 142, 143)*. A dose response inhibitory effect on tumor growth has been observed in some in vitro experiments *(144)*. Saffron has also been shown to decrease the mean number of tumors and tumor growth rate and to extend lifespan in some animal models *(143)*. Saffron exhibits low toxicity (Schmidt) and high oral doses have been administered to animals (20.7 g/kg) without toxic effects *(143)*.

Crocetin, an extract of saffron (Fig. 6), has been found to have a dose-dependent effect on inhibiting DNA and RNA synthesis in tumor cells in vitro *(13, 145)*. Crocin, another saffron extract, has been shown to demonstrate an antitumor effect in female, but not male, rats, suggesting this effect may be hormone dependent *(13, 143, 145)*.

The mechanism(s) of saffron's anticarcinogenic effect have not been determined *(13, 143)*. Some hypotheses include inhibition of free radical formation, inhibition of DNA/RNA synthesis, inhibition of cell proliferation, induction of apoptosis, inhibition of different cellular pathways, and/or changes in phase I/phase II detoxification enzymes *(143, 144)*. Findings of in vitro and animal studies have not been verified in human clinical trials. More evidence is clearly needed before the potential effects of saffron on cancer prevention may be clarified *(143, 13)*.

3.3.2. GINGER

Ginger and some of its components (e.g., gingerol, shoagaol) (Fig. 7) have been shown to exhibit strong antioxidant and anti-inflammatory activity in both in vitro and in animal models *(15)*. For example, 6-gingerol inhibited angiogenesis and caused cell

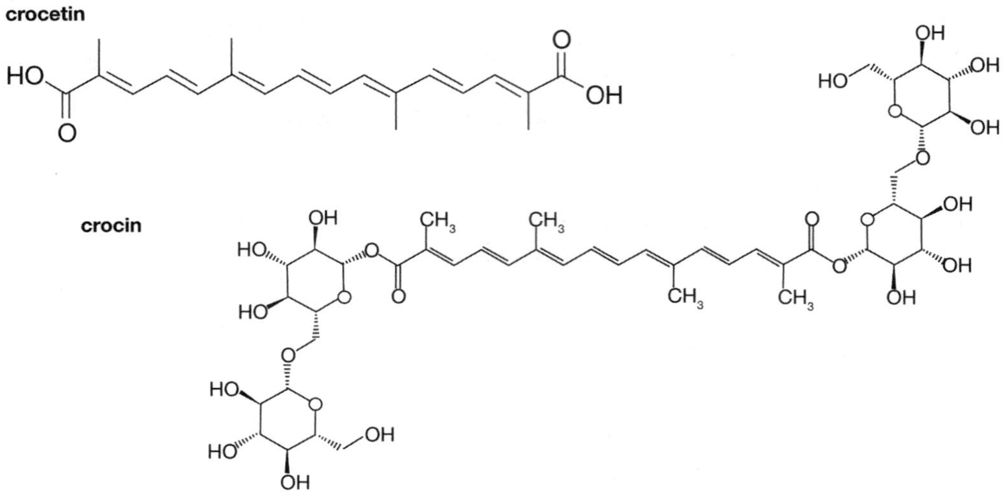

crocetin

crocin

Fig. 6. Chemical structures of saffron compounds.

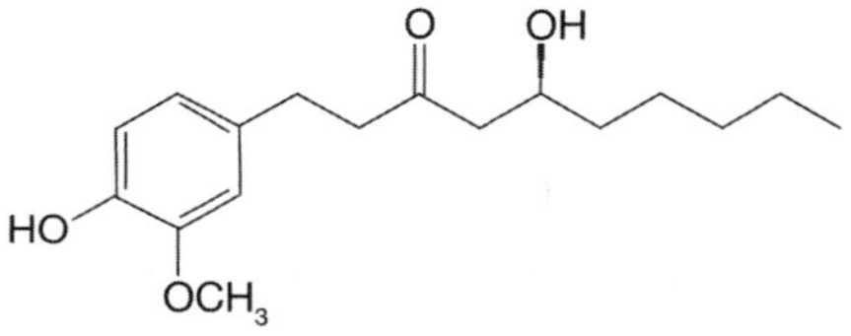

6-gingerol 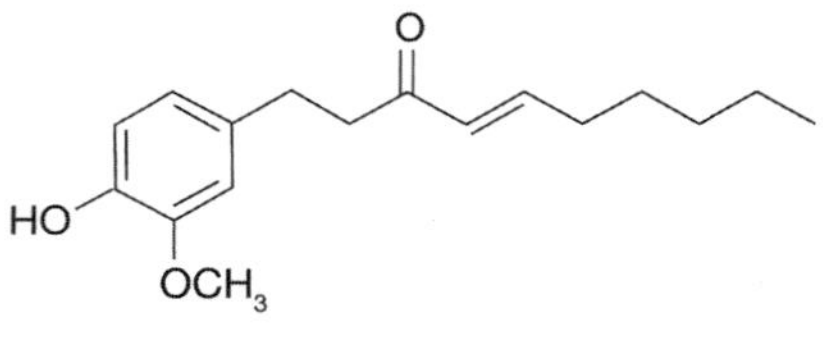   **6-shogaol**

Fig. 7. Chemical structures of ginger compounds.

cycle arrest in human endothelial cells *(60)*. 6-Gingerol has also been shown to inhibit the production of inflammatory enzymes such as nitric oxide synthase (NOS) in several in vitro experiments *(60)*.

Ginger and its active compounds have been shown to inhibit skin, colon, breast, and gastrointestinal tumors in animal models, prevent metastasis in murine skin cancer cells, and induce apoptosis in in vitro experiments *(15, 60)*. Some experiments have found that ginger compounds in vitro have induced apoptosis in a dose-dependent manner *(60)*. Mechanisms that have been observed in in vitro experiments include inhibition of Epstein Barr virus, decreased Bcl-2 expression, inhibition of NF-kB, and inhibition of free radical production *(60)*.

There is also emerging evidence that ginger may reduce nausea in chemotherapy patients *(60)*. Several clinical trials are underway to confirm this observation and to determine the most effective dose (clinicaltrials.gov).

3.3.3. CAPSAICIN

Capsaicin (Fig. 8) has been investigated in several studies for its chemopreventive properties. This substance has been shown to prevent oxidative damage or lipid perox-

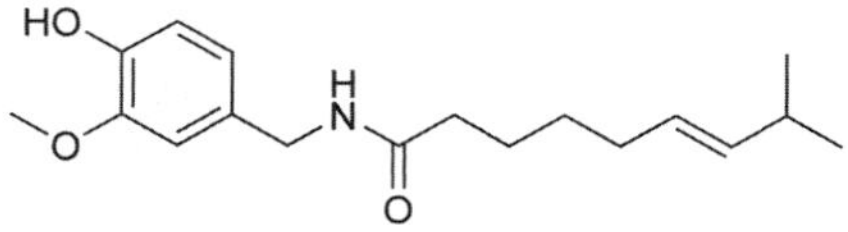

Fig. 8. Chemical structure of capsaicin.

idation in various organs of experimental animals and to have anti-inflammatory properties in both in vitro and animal experiments (Surh, 1998). Capsaicin has been shown to activate AP-1, inhibit tumor formation and cytochrome P-450 expression in some animal models *(146, 147)*, and to inhibit NF-kB production in several cancer cell lines *(146)*.

Capsaicin has shown promise in reducing pain in both animal and human models *(147)*. A clinical trial is currently underway to investigate whether capsaicin can decrease pain in head and neck cancer (clinical trials.gov).

Results of some studies in both human and animal models suggest that capsaicin is a potential carcinogen, especially in high dosages. However, there is a much larger body of data suggesting the compound has chemopreventive and chemoprotective effects *(146, 147)*. The World Cancer Research Fund (WCRF) and the American Institute for Cancer Research (AICR) have noted that this evidence based solely on case–control studies is inconsistent and concluded "there is limited evidence suggesting that [dietary] capsaicin is associated with an increased risk of stomach cancer" *(148)*. However, these data are likely confounded by other risk factors such socioeconomic status, the availability of refrigeration, and contamination with *H. pylori (148, 149)*. Further research is needed to determine the long-term health effects of capsaicin in humans *(149, 150)*.

4. CONCLUSIONS

There are emerging data in several areas to suggest that a variety of culinary herbs and spices reduce the risk of cancer. However, there is very little evidence from human studies in this area. In addition, human data on dose–response and biochemical mechanisms are largely unavailable. More well-designed epidemiological and intervention studies in this area are clearly needed. Reliable estimates of the quantities of spices and herbs consumed by free-living population are not available because the amounts of these ingredients present in foods made at home or purchased from manufacturers are largely undocumented. A very crude estimate of usage in the United States can be obtained from data on the inventory and production of herbs and spices collected by the US Department of Agriculture. Similar inventory data are available in other countries including Australia and Greece *(3)*. Nevertheless, this lack of intake data has severely limited the amount and quality of observational data that are available.

Curcumin shows the most evidence of chemoprevention among bioactive compounds in spices. However, more data are needed, especially from randomized, placebo-controlled long-term clinical trials, before definitive conclusions can be made *(152)*. Additionally, research on curcumin is needed to determine what types (e.g., dietary or supplement) and dosages should be used for optimal bioavailability and efficacy *(64, 152)*.

Potential interactions of culinary spices and herbs and/or supplements with other food components also need more research *(32)*. Both observational and experimental data suggest that the bioactive compounds in spices and herbs can have a synergistic relationship with other bioactive substances, either from other spices or foods, to enhance their chemopreventive effects *(152, 32)*. For example, Shoba et al. *(91)* found that 10 healthy men volunteers from India who ingested 20 mg of piperine from black pepper in combination with 2,000 mg of curcumin had greatly enhanced (2,000%) curcumin bioavailability. In addition, hamster studies have shown that the administration of a combination of tomato and garlic resulted in a much greater suppression of tumor incidence and number and better detoxification (e.g., decreased Phase I and increased Phase II enzyme activity) than when these compounds were administered separately *(32)*. Nevertheless, very little data on the effect of combining bioactive food components on the prevention and treatment of cancer are currently available *(32)*.

More experimental data are needed on the optimal doses of spices and herbs necessary for chemoprevention. For example, the effective dose of the garlic organosulfur compound DAS in animals ranges from 50 to 400 mg/kg/day, which is equivalent to 3.5–28 g/day of DAS in a 150 lbs human subject *(99)*. Epidemiologic studies have found that garlic consumed in much lower doses of 18.3 g/week (about 4–5 cloves) is inversely associated with several types of cancers in humans *(99)*.

Finally, herbs and spices are natural substances and there is great variability in the amount, chemical composition, and activity of the bioactive compounds they contain. Growing conditions, storage, transport, preparation, and part of the plant used are some of the factors that may affect the structure and amount of bioactive compounds present in spices and herbs *(32, 37)*. It is important that researchers publish detailed information on the cultivar, source, and other information about the materials used.

For thousands of years, people have consumed culinary spices and herbs for both pleasure and medicinal purposes. However, rigorous scientific evidence to support this practice is only now becoming available. These data are encouraging and suggest that future studies in humans are warranted to determine the potential for spices and herbs to serve as inexpensive and effective agents to help prevent and/or manage cancer.

REFERENCES

1. Abdullaev, F.I. (2002 Jan) Cancer chemopreventive and tumoricidal properties of saffron (Crocus sativus L.). *Exp Biol Med (Maywood)* **227**(1), 20–25.
2. Sinha, R., Anderson, D.E., McDonald, S.S., and Greenwald, P. (2003 Jul–Sep) Cancer risk and diet in India. *J Postgrad Med* **49**(3), 222–28.
3. Tapsell, L.C., Hemphill, I., Cobiac, L., Patch, C.S., Sullivan, D.R., Fenech, M., Roodenrys, S., Keogh, J.B., Clifton, P.M., Williams, P.G., Fazio, V.A., and Inge, K.E. (2006 Aug 21) Health benefits of herbs and spices: The past, the present, the future. *Med J Aust* **185**(4 Suppl), S4–S24.
4. Mahady, G.B. (2001 Mar) Global harmonization of herbal health claims. *J Nutr* **131**(3s), 1120S–3S.
5. Vickers, A., and Zollman, C. (1999 Oct 16) ABC of complementary medicine: Herbal medicine. *BMJ* **319**(7216), 1050–53.

6. Eisenberg, D., Kessler, R.C., Foster, C., Norlock, F.E., Calkins, D.R., and Delbanco, T.L. (1993) Unconventional medicine in the United States: Prevalence, cost and patterns of use. *N Engl J Med* **328**, 246–52.

7. Tascilar, M., de Jong, F.A., Verweij, J., and Mathijssen, R.H. (2006 Jul–Aug) Complementary and alternative medicine during cancer treatment: Beyond innocence. *Oncologist* **11**(7), 732–41.

8. Ritchie, M.R. (2007 Nov) Use of herbal supplements and nutritional supplements in the UK: what do we know about their pattern of usage? *Proc Nutr Soc* **66**(4), 479–82.

9. Aggarwal, B.B., and Shishodia, S. (2006 May 14) Molecular targets of dietary agents for prevention and therapy of cancer. *Biochem Pharmacol* **71**(10), 1397–421.

10. Maeda, S., and Omata, M. (2008 May) Inflammation and cancer: Role of nuclear factor-kappaB activation. *Cancer Sci* **99**(5), 836–42.

11. Kim, D.H., Kim, C.H., Kim, M.S., Kim, J.Y., Jung, K.J., Chung, J.H., An, W.G., Lee, J.W., Yu, B.P., and Chung, H.Y. (2007 Oct) Suppression of age-related inflammatory NF-kappaB activation by cinnamaldehyde. *Biogerontology* **8**(5), 545–54.

12. Dhillon, N., Aggarwal, B.B., Newman, R.A., Wolff, R.A., Kunnumakkara, A.B., Abbruzzese, J.L., Ng, C.S., Badmaev, V., and Kurzrock, R. (2008 Jul 15) Phase II Trial of Curcumin in Patients with Advanced Pancreatic Cancer. *Clin Cancer Res* **14**(14), 4491–99.

13. Lampe, J.W. (2003 Sep) Spicing up a vegetarian diet: Chemopreventive effects of phytochemicals. *Am J Clin Nutr* **78**(3 Suppl), 579S–583S.

14. Kwon, K.B., Park, B.H., and Ryu, D.G. (2007 Feb) Chemotherapy through mitochondrial apoptosis using nutritional supplements and herbs: A brief overview. *J Bioenerg Biomembr* **39**(1), 31–34.

15. Surh, Y.J. (2002 Aug) Anti-tumor promoting potential of selected spice ingredients with antioxidative and anti-inflammatory activities: A short review. *Food Chem Toxicol* **40**(8), 1091–97.

16. Halvorsen, B.L., Carlsen, M.H., Phillips, K.M., Bohn, S.K., Holte, K., Jacobs, D.R., Jr, and Blomhoff, R. (2006 Jul) Content of redox-active compounds (ie, antioxidants) in foods consumed in the United States. *Am J Clin Nutr* **84**(1), 95–135.

17. Baghurst, K.. Herbs and spices: An integral part of the daily diet. Position paper, November 2006. National Centre of Excellence in Functional Foods, Australia.

18. Liu, R.H. (2004 Dec) Potential synergy of phytochemicals in cancer prevention: Mechanism of action. *J Nutr* **134**(12 Suppl), 3479S–3485S.

19. Ninfali, P., Mea, G., Giorgini, S., Rocchi, M., and Bacchiocca, M. (2005 Feb) Antioxidant capacity of vegetables, spices and dressings relevant to nutrition. *Br J Nutr* **93**(2), 257–66.

20. Dorai, T., and Aggarwal, B.B. (2004 Nov 25) Role of chemopreventive agents in cancer therapy. *Cancer Lett* **215**(2), 129–40.

21. Lee, B.M., and Park, K.K. (2003 Feb–Mar) Beneficial and adverse effects of chemopreventive agents. *Mutat Res* **523–524**, 265.

22. Sarkar, F.H., and Li, Y. (2004 Nov 2) Cell signaling pathways altered by natural chemopreventive agents. *Mutat Res* **555**(1–2), 53–64.

23. Gerhäuser, C., Klimo, K., Heiss, E., Neumann, I., Gamal-Eldeen, A., Knauft, J., Liu, G.Y., Sitthimonchai, S., and Frank, N. (2003 Feb–Mar) Mechanism-based in vitro screening of potential cancer chemopreventive agents. *Mutat Res* **523–524**, 163–72.

24. Modly, C.E., Das, M., Don, P.S., Marcelo, C.L., Mukhtar, H., and Bickers, D.R. (1986 Jul–Aug) Capsaicin as an in vitro inhibitor of benzo(a)pyrene metabolism and its DNA binding in human and murine keratinocytes. *Drug Metab Dispos* **14**(4), 413–16.

25. Rhode, J., Fogoros, S., Zick, S., Wahl, H., Griffith, K.A., Huang, J., and Liu, J.R. (2007 Dec 20) Ginger inhibits cell growth and modulates angiogenic factors in ovarian cancer cells. *BMC Complement Altern Med* **7**, 44.

26. Manju V, Nalini N. (2006 Oct) Effect of ginger on bacterial enzymes in 1,2-dimethylhydrazine induced experimental colon carcinogenesis. *Eur J Cancer Prev* **15**(5), 377–83.

27. Deeptha, K., Kamaleeswari, M., Sengottuvelan, M., and Nalini, N. (2006 Nov) Dose dependent inhibitory effect of dietary caraway on 1,2-dimethylhydrazine induced colonic aberrant crypt foci and bacterial enzyme activity in rats. *Invest New Drugs* **24**(6), 479–88.

28. Liao, B.C., Hsieh, C.W., Liu, Y.C., Tzeng, T.T., Sun, Y.W., and Wung, B.S. (2008 Jun 1) Cinnamaldehyde inhibits the tumor necrosis factor-alpha-induced expression of cell adhesion molecules in endothelial cells by suppressing NF-kappaB activation: Effects upon IkappaB and Nrf2. *Toxicol Appl Pharmacol* **229**(2), 161–71.

29. Belman, S. (1983) Onion and garlic oils inhibit tumor promotion. *Carcinogenesis* **4**, 1063–65.

30. Aggarwal, B.B., Shishodia, S., Takada, Y., Banerjee, S., Newman, R.A., Bueso-Ramos, C.E., and Price, J.E. (2005 Oct 15) Curcumin suppresses the paclitaxel-induced nuclear factor-kappaB pathway in breast cancer cells and inhibits lung metastasis of human breast cancer in nude mice. *Clin Cancer Res* **11**(20), 7490–98.

31. Sharma, R.A., Steward, W.P., and Gescher, A.J. (2007) Pharmacokinetics and pharmacodynamics of curcumin. *Adv Exp Med Biol* **595**, 453–70.

32. Milner, J.A. (2006 Mar) Preclinical perspectives on garlic and cancer. *J Nutr* **136**(3 Suppl), 827S–831S.

33. Lai, P.K., and Roy, J. (2004 Jun) Antimicrobial and chemopreventive properties of herbs and spices. *Curr Med Chem* **11**(11), 1451–60.

34. Singletary, K.W. (1996 Feb 27) Rosemary extract and carnosol stimulate rat liver glutathione-S-transferase and quinone reductase activities. *Cancer Lett* **100**(1–2), 139–44.

35. Araújo, C.C., and Leon, L.L. (2001 Jul) Biological activities of Curcuma longa L. *Mem Inst Oswaldo Cruz* **96**(5), 723–28.

36. Chaieb, K., Hajlaoui, H., Zmantar, T., Kahla-Nakbi, A.B., Rouabhia, M., Mahdouani, K., and Bakhrouf, A. (2007 Jun) The chemical composition and biological activity of clove essential oil, Eugenia caryophyllata (Syzigium aromaticum L. Myrtaceae): a short review. *Phytother Res* **21**(6), 501–06.

37. Sivam, G.P. (2001 Mar) Protection against Helicobacter pylori and other bacterial infections by garlic. *J Nutr* **131**(3s), 1106S–8S.

38. You, W.C., Brown, L.M., Zhang, L., Li, J.Y., Jin, M.L., Chang, Y.S., Ma, J.L., Pan, K.F., Liu, W.D., Hu, Y., Crystal-Mansour, S., Pee, D., Blot, W.J., Fraumeni, J.F., Jr., Xu, G.W., and Gail, M.H. (2006 July 19) Randomized double-blind factorial trial of three treatments to reduce the prevalence of precancerous gastric lesions. *J Natl Cancer Inst* **98**(14), 974–83.

39. Ngo, S.N., Williams, D.B., Cobiac, L., and Head, R.J. (2007 Oct) Does garlic reduce risk of colorectal cancer? A systematic review. *J Nutr* **137**(10), 2264–69.

40. Ferlay, J., Bray, F., and Pisani, P. Parkin D.M. Globocan. (2004) Cancer Incidence, Mortality and Prevalence Worldwide IARC CancerBase No. 5. version 2.0. 2004, Lyon: IARC*Press*.

41. Galeone, C., Pelucchi, C., Levi, F., Negri, E., Franceschi, S., Talamini, R., Giacosa, A., and La Vecchia, C. (2006 Nov) Onion and garlic use and human cancer. *Am J Clin Nutr* **84**(5), 1027–32.

42. Millen, A.E., Subar, A.F., Graubard, B.I., Peters, U., Hayes, R.B., Weissfeld, J.L., and Yokochi, L.A. (2007 Dec) Ziegler RG; PLCO Cancer Screening Trial Project Team. Fruit and vegetable intake and prevalence of colorectal adenoma in a cancer screening trial. *Am J Clin Nutr* **86**(6), 1754–64.

43. Anand, P., Kunnumakkara, A.B., Newman, R.A., and Aggarwal, B.B. (2007 Nov–Dec) Bioavailability of curcumin: Problems and promises. *Mol Pharm* **4**(6), 807–18.

44. Verschoyle, R.D., Steward, W.P., and Gescher, A.J. (2007) Putative cancer chemopreventive agents of dietary origin-how safe are they? *Nutr Cancer* **59**(2), 152–62.

45. Sharma, R.A., McLelland, H.R., Hill, K.A., Ireson, C.R., Euden, S.A., Manson, M.M., Pirmohamed, M., Marnett, L.J., Gescher, A.J., and Steward, W.P. (2001 Jul) Pharmacodynamic and pharmacokinetic study of oral Curcuma extract in patients with colorectal cancer. *Clin Cancer Res* **7**(7), 1894–900.

46. Sharma, R.A., Euden, S.A., Platton, S.L., Cooke, D.N., Shafayat, A., Hewitt, H.R., Marczylo, T.H., Morgan, B., Hemingway, D., Plummer, S.M., Pirmohamed, M., Gescher, A.J., and Steward, W.P. (2004 Oct 15) Phase I clinical trial of oral curcumin: Biomarkers of systemic activity and compliance. *Clin Cancer Res* **10**(20), 6847–54.

47. Cheng, A.L., Hsu, C.H., Lin, J.K., Hsu, M.M., Ho, Y.F., Shen, T.S., Ko, J.Y., Lin, J.T., Lin, B.R., Ming-Shiang, W., Yu, H.S., Jee, S.H., Chen, G.S., Chen, T.M., Chen, C.A., Lai, M.K., Pu, Y.S., Pan,

M.H., Wang, Y.J., Tsai, C.C., and Hsieh, C.Y. (2001 Jul-Aug) Phase I clinical trial of curcumin, a chemopreventive agent, in patients with high-risk or pre-malignant lesions. *Anticancer Res* **21**(4B), 2895–900.

48. Pittler, M.H., and Ernst, E. (2007 Nov) Clinical effectiveness of garlic (Allium sativum). *Mol Nutr Food Res* **51**(11), 1382–85.

49. Shukla, Y., and Kalra, N. (2007 Mar 18) Cancer chemoprevention with garlic and its constituents. *Cancer Lett* **247**(2), 167–81.

50. Jagetia, G.C., and Aggarwal, B.B. (2007 Jan) "Spicing up" of the immune system by curcumin. *J Clin Immunol* **27**(1), 19–35 Epub 2007 Jan 9.

51. Menon, V.P., and Sudheer, A.R. (2007) Antioxidant and anti-inflammatory properties of curcumin. *Adv Exp Med Biol* **595**, 105–25.

52. Mosley, C.A., Liotta, D.C., and Snyder, J.P. (2007) Highly active anticancer curcumin analogues. *Adv Exp Med Biol* **595**, 77–103.

53. Murakami, A., Ohigashi, H., and Targeting, N.O.X. (2007 Dec 1) INOS and COX-2 in inflammatory cells: Chemoprevention using food phytochemicals. *Int J Cancer* **121**(11), 2357–63.

54. Bharti, A.C., Donato, N., and Aggarwal, B.B. (2003 Oct 1) Curcumin (diferuloylmethane) inhibits constitutive and IL-6-inducible STAT3 phosphorylation in human multiple myeloma cells. *J Immunol* **171**(7), 3863–71.

55. Shishodia, S., Singh, T., and Chaturvedi, M.M. (2007) Modulation of transcription factors by curcumin. *Adv Exp Med Biol* **595**, 127–48.

56. Vadhan-Raj, S., Weber, D.M., Wang, M., Giralt, S.A., Thomas, S.K., Alexanian, R., Zhou, X., Patel, P., Bueso-Ramos, C.E., Newman, R.A., and Aggarwal, B.B. Curcumin downregulates NF-kB and related genes in patients with multiple myeloma: Results of a phase I/II study. *ASH Annu Meet Abstr* **110** Abstract 1177.

57. Kuttan, G., Kumar, K.B., Guruvayoorappan, C., and Kuttan, R. (2007) Antitumor, anti-invasion, and antimetastatic effects of curcumin. *Adv Exp Med Biol* **595**, 173–84.

58. Karunagaran, D., Joseph, J., and Kumar, T.R. (2007) Cell growth regulation. *Adv Exp Med Biol* **595**, 245–68.

59. Lin, J.K. (2007) Molecular targets of curcumin. *Adv Exp Med Biol* **595**, 227–43.

60. Bhandarkar, S.S., and Arbiser, J.L. (2007) Curcumin as an inhibitor of angiogenesis. *Adv Exp Med Biol* **595**, 185–95.

61. Zhang, F., Altorki, N.K., Mestre, J.R., Subbaramaiah, K., and Dannenberg, A.J. (1999 Mar) Curcumin inhibits cyclooxygenase-2 transcription in bile acid- and phorbol ester-treated human gastrointestinal epithelial cells. Carcinogenesis 20(3):445–51.

62. Hussain, A.R., Al-Rasheed, M., Manogaran, P.S., Al-Hussein, K.A., Platanias, L.C., Al Kuraya, K., and Uddin, S. (2006 Feb) Curcumin induces apoptosis via inhibition of PI3′-kinase/AKT pathway in acute T cell leukemias. *Apoptosis* **11**(2), 245–54.

63. Singh, S., and Khar, A. (2006 May) Biological effects of curcumin and its role in cancer chemoprevention and therapy. *Anticancer Agents Med Chem* **6**(3), 259–70.

64. Surh, Y.J., and Chun, K.S. (2007) Cancer chemopreventive effects of curcumin. *Adv Exp Med Biol* **595**, 149–72.

65. Yoysungnoen, P., Wirachwong, P., Bhattarakosol, P., Niimi, H., and Patumraj, S. (2005) Antiangiogenic activity of curcumin in hepatocellular carcinoma cells implanted nude mice. *Clin Hemorheol Microcirc* **33**(2), 127–35.

66. Ohashi, Y., Tsuchiya, Y., Koizumi, K., Sakurai, H., and Saiki, I. (2003) Prevention of intrahepatic metastasis by curcumin in an orthotopic implantation model. *Oncology* **65**(3), 250–58.

67. Shankar, S., Ganapathy, S., Chen, Q., and Srivastava, R.K. (2008 Jan) Curcumin sensitizes TRAIL-resistant xenografts: Molecular mechanisms of apoptosis, metastasis and angiogenesis. *Mol Cancer* **29**(7), 16.

68. Kunnumakkara, A.B., Guha, S., Krishnan, S., Diagaradjane, P., Gelovani, J., and Aggarwal, B.B. (2007 Apr 15) Curcumin potentiates antitumor activity of gemcitabine in an orthotopic model of pancreatic cancer through suppression of proliferation, angiogenesis, and inhibition of nuclear factor-kappaB-regulated gene products. *Cancer Res* **67**(8), 3853–61.

69. Bachmeier, B., Nerlich, A.G., Iancu, C.M., Cilli, M., Schleicher, E., Vené, R., Dell'Eva, R., Jochum, M., Albini, A., and Pfeffer, U. (2007) The chemopreventive polyphenol Curcumin prevents hematogenous breast cancer metastases in immunodeficient mice. *Cell Physiol Biochem* **19**(1–4), 137–52.

70. Li, M., Zhang, Z., Hill, D.L., Wang, H., and Zhang, R. (2007 Mar 1) Curcumin, a dietary component, has anticancer, chemosensitization, and radiosensitization effects by down-regulating the MDM2 oncogene through the PI3K/mTOR/ETS2 pathway. *Cancer Res* **67**(5), 1988–96.

71. Hong, J.H., Ahn, K.S., Bae, E., Jeon, S.S., and Choi, H.Y. (2006) The effects of curcumin on the invasiveness of prostate cancer in vitro and in vivo. *Prostate Cancer Prostatic Dis* **9**(2), 147–52.

72. LoTempio, M.M., Veena, M.S., Steele, H.L., Ramamurthy, B., Ramalingam, T.S., Cohen, A.N., Chakrabarti, R., Srivatsan, E.S., and Wang, M.B. (2005 Oct 1) Curcumin suppresses growth of head and neck squamous cell carcinoma. *Clin Cancer Res* **11**(19 Pt 1), 6994–7002.

73. Gautam, S.C., Gao, X., and Dulchavsky, S. (2007) Immunomodulation by curcumin. *Adv Exp Med Biol* **595**, 321–41.

74. Antony, S., Kuttan, R., and Kuttan, G. (1999 Sep–Dec) Immunomodulatory activity of curcumin. *Immunol Invest* **28**(5–6), 291–303.

75. Yasni, S., Yoshiie, K., Oda, H., Sugano, M., and Imaizumi, K. (1993 Aug) Dietary Curcuma xanthorrhiza Roxb. increases mitogenic responses of splenic lymphocytes in rats, and alters populations of the lymphocytes in mice. *J Nutr Sci Vitaminol (Tokyo)* **39**(4), 345–54.

76. Garg, A.K., Buchholz, T.A., and Aggarwal, B.B. (2005 Nov–Dec) Chemosensitization and radiosensitization of tumors by plant polyphenols. *Antioxid Redox Signal* **7**(11–12), 1630–47.

77. Sharma, R.A., Gescher, A.J., and Steward, W.P. (2005 Sep) Curcumin: The story so far. *Eur J Cancer* **41**(13), 1955–68.

78. Singh, S.V., Hu, X., Srivastava, S.K., Singh, M., Xia, H., Orchard, J.L., and Zaren, H.A. (1998) Mechanism of inhibition of benzo[a]pyrene-induced forestomach cancer in mice by dietary curcumin. *Carcinogenesis* **19**, 1357–60.

79. Iqbal, M., Sharma, S.D., Okazaki, Y., Fujisawa, M., and Okada, S. (2003 Jan) Dietary supplementation of curcumin enhances antioxidant and phase II metabolizing enzymes in ddY male mice: Possible role in protection against chemical carcinogenesis and toxicity. *Pharmacol Toxicol* **92**(1), 33–38.

80. Jones, S.B., and Brooks, J.D. (2006 Mar 15) Modest induction of phase 2 enzyme activity in the F-344 rat prostate. *BMC Cancer* **6**, 62.

81. Van der Logt, E.M., Roelofs, H.M., van Lieshout, E.M., Nagengast, F.M., and Peters, W.H. (2004 Mar-Apr) Effects of dietary anticarcinogens and nonsteroidal anti-inflammatory drugs on rat gastrointestinal UDP-glucuronosyltransferases. *Anticancer Res* **24**(2B), 843–49.

82. Mahady, G.B., Pendland, S.L., Yun, G., and Lu, Z.Z. (2002 Nov–Dec) Turmeric (Curcuma longa) and curcumin inhibit the growth of Helicobacter pylori, a group 1 carcinogen. *Anticancer Res* **22**(6C), 4179–81.

83. Münzenmaier, A., Lange, C., Glocker, E., Covacci, A., Moran, A., Bereswill, S., Baeuerle, P.A., Kist, M., and Pahl, H.L. (1997 Dec 15) A secreted/shed product of Helicobacter pylori activates transcription factor nuclear factor-kappa B. *J Immunol* **159**(12), 6140–47.

84. Foryst-Ludwig, A., Neumann, M., Schneider-Brachert, W., and Naumann, M. (2004 Apr 16) Curcumin blocks NF-kappaB and the motogenic response in Helicobacter pylori-infected epithelial cells. *Biochem Biophys Res Commun* **316**(4), 1065–72.

85. Di Mario, F., Cavallaro, L.G., Nouvenne, A., Stefani, N., Cavestro, G.M., Iori, V., Maino, M., Comparato, G., Fanigliulo, L., Morana, E., Pilotto, A., Martelli, L., Martelli, M., Leandro, G., and Franzè, A. (2007 Jun) A curcumin-based 1-week triple therapy for eradication of Helicobacter pylori infection: Something to learn from failure? *Helicobacter* **12**(3), 238–43.

86. Maheshwari, R.K., Singh, A.K., Gaddipati, J., and Srimal, R.C. (2006 Mar 27) Multiple biological activities of curcumin: A short review. *Life Sci* **78**(18), 2081–87.

87. Eigner, D., and Scholz, D. (1999 Oct) Ferula asa-foetida and Curcuma longa in traditional medical treatment and diet in Nepal. *J Ethnopharmacol* **67**(1), 1–6.

88. Mohandas, K.M., and Desai, D.C. (1999 Jul–Sep) Epidemiology of digestive tract cancers in India. V. Large and small bowel. *Indian J Gastroenterol* **18**(3), 118–21.

89. Kuttan, R., Sudheeran, P.C., and Josph, C.D. (1987 Feb 28) Turmeric and curcumin as topical agents in cancer therapy. *Tumori* **73**(1), 29–31.
90. Polasa, K., Raghuram, T.C., Krishna, T.P., and Krishnaswamy, K. (1992 Mar) Effect of turmeric on urinary mutagens in smokers. *Mutagenesis* **7**(2), 107–09.
91. Shoba, G., Joy, D., Joseph, T., Majeed, M., Rajendran, R., and Srinivas, P.S. (1998 May) Influence of piperine on the pharmacokinetics of curcumin in animals and human volunteers. *Planta Med* **64**(4), 353–56.
92. Banerjee, S.K., Mukherjee, P.K., and Maulik, S.K. (2003 Feb) Garlic as an antioxidant: The good, the bad and the ugly. *Phytother Res* **17**(2), 97–106. Review.
93. http://www.cancer.gov/cancertopics/factsheet/Prevention/garlic-and-cancer-prevention.
94. Milner, J.A. (1996) Garlic: Its anticarcinogenic and antitumorigenic properties. *Nutr Rev* **54**, S82–S86.
95. Devrim, E., and Durak, I. (2007 Nov) Is garlic a promising food for benign prostatic hyperplasia and prostate cancer? *Mol Nutr Food Res* **51**(11), 1319–23.
96. Milner, J.A. (2001 Mar) A historical perspective on garlic and cancer. *J Nutr* **131**(3s), 1027S–31S.
97. Wu, X., Kassie, F., and Mersch-Sundermann, V. (2005 Mar) Induction of apoptosis in tumor cells by naturally occurring sulfur-containing compounds. *Mutat Res* **589**(2), 81–102.
98. Thomson, M., and Ali, M. (2003 Feb) Garlic [Allium sativum]: a review of its potential use as an anti-cancer agent. *Curr Cancer Drug Targets* **3**(1), 67–81.
99. Bianchini, F., and Vainio, H. (2001 Sep) Allium vegetables and organosulfur compounds: Do they help prevent cancer? *Environ Health Perspect* **109**(9), 893–902.
100. Amagase, H. (2006 Mar) Clarifying the real bioactive constituents of garlic. *J Nutr* **136**(3 Suppl), 716S–725S.
101. Kris-Etherton, P.M., Hecker, K.D., Bonanome, A., Coval, S.M., Binkoski, A.E., Hilpert, K.F., Griel, A.E., and Etherton, T.D. (2002 Dec 30) Bioactive compounds in foods: Their role in the prevention of cardiovascular disease and cancer. *Am J Med* **113**(Suppl 9B), 71S–88S.
102. Khanum, F., Anilakumar, K.R., and Viswanathan, K.R. (2004) Anticarcinogenic properties of garlic: A review. *Crit Rev Food Sci Nutr* **44**(6), 479–88.
103. Maurya, A.K., and Singh, S.V. (1991 May 1) Differential induction of glutathione transferase isoenzymes of mice stomach by diallyl sulfide, a naturally occurring anticarcinogen. *Cancer Lett* **57**(2), 121–29.
104. Prasad, S., Kalra, N., and Shukla, Y. (2006) Modulatory effects of diallyl sulfide against testosterone-induced oxidative stress in Swiss albino mice. *Asian J Androl* **8**, 719–23.
105. Sengupta, A., Ghosh, S., and Bhattacharjee, S. (2004 Jul–Sep) Allium vegetables in cancer prevention: An overview. *Asian Pac J Cancer Prev* **5**(3), 237–45.
106. Gedik, N., Kabasakal, L., Sehirli, O., Ercan, F., Sirvanci, S., Keyer-Uysal, M., and Sener, G. (2005 Apr 15) Long-term administration of aqueous garlic extract (AGE) alleviates liver fibrosis and oxidative damage induced by biliary obstruction in rats. *Life Sci* **76**(22), 2593–606.
107. Sener, G., Satýroğlu, H., Ozer Sehirli, A., and Kaçmaz, A. (2003 May 23) Protective effect of aqueous garlic extract against oxidative organ damage in a rat model of thermal injury. *Life Sci* **73**(1), 81–91.
108. Lang, A., Lahav, M., Sakhnini, E., Barshack, I., Fidder, H.H., Avidan, B., Bardan, E., Hershkoviz, R., Bar-Meir, S., and Chowers, Y. (2004 Oct) Allicin inhibits spontaneous and TNF-alpha induced secretion of proinflammatory cytokines and chemokines from intestinal epithelial cells. *Clin Nutr* **23**(5), 1199–208.
109. Dirsch, V.B., and Vollmar, A.M. (2001) Ajoene, a Natural Product with Non-Steroidal Anti-Inflammatory Drug (NSAID)-Like Properties? Biochem. *Pharmacol* **61**, 587–93.
110. Chu, Q., Ling, M.T., Feng, H., Cheung, H.W., Tsao, S.W., Wang, X., and Wong, Y.C. (2006 Nov) A novel anticancer effect of garlic derivatives: Inhibition of cancer cell invasion through restoration of E-cadherin expression. *Carcinogenesis* **27**(11), 2180–89.
111. Ross, S.A., Finley, J.W., and Milner, J.A. (2006 Mar) Allyl sulfur compounds from garlic modulate aberrant crypt formation. *J Nutr* **136**(3 Suppl), 852S–4S.
112. El-Bayoumy, K., Sinha, R., Pinto, J.T., and Rivlin, R.S. (2006 Mar) Cancer chemoprevention by garlic and garlic-containing sulfur and selenium compounds. *J Nutr* **136**(3 Suppl), 864S–869S.

113. Singh, A., and Shukla, Y. (1998 Sep) Antitumor activity of diallyl sulfide in two-stage mouse skin model of carcinogenesis. *Biomed Environ Sci* **11**(3), 258–63.
114. Shukla, Y., Arora, A., and Singh, A. (2002 Mar) Antitumorigenic potential of diallyl sulfide in Ehrlich ascites tumor bearing mice. *Biomed Environ Sci* **15**(1), 41–47.
115. Arunkumar, A., Vijayababu, M.R., Venkataraman, P., Senthilkumar, K., and Arunakaran, J. (2006) Chemoprevention of rat prostate carcinogenesis by diallyl disulfide, an organosulfur compound of garlic. *Biol Pharm Bull* **29**, 375–79.
116. Arunkumar, A., Vijayababu, M.R., Gunadharini, N., Krishnamoorthy, G., and Arunakaran, J. (2007 Jun 18) Induction of apoptosis and histone hyperacetylation by diallyl disulfide in prostate cancer cell line PC-3. *Cancer Lett* **251**(1), 59–67.
117. Weisberger, A.S., and Pensky, J. (1958 Dec) Tumor inhibition by a sulfhydryl-blocking agent related to an active principle of garlic (Allium sativum). *Cancer Res* **18**(11), 1301–08.
118. Kyo, E., Uda, N., Kasuga, S., and Itakura, Y. (2001 Mar) Immunomodulatory effects of aged garlic extract. *J Nutr* **131**(3s), 1075S–9S.
119. Lamm, D.L., and Riggs, D.R. (2000 Feb) The potential application of Allium sativum (garlic) for the treatment of bladder cancer. *Urol Clin North Am* **27**(1), 157–62.
120. Schaffer, E.M., Liu, J.Z., Green, J., Dangler, C.A., and Milner, J.A. (1996 Apr 19) Garlic and associated allyl sulfur components inhibit N-methyl-N-nitrosourea induced rat mammary carcinogenesis. *Cancer Lett* **102**(1–2), 199–204.
121. Wargovich, M.J. (2006 Mar) Diallylsulfide and allylmethylsulfide are uniquely effective among organosulfur compounds in inhibiting CYP2E1 protein in animal models. *J Nutr* **136**(3 Suppl), 832S–834S.
122. Sumiyoshi, H., and Wargovich, M.J. (1990 Aug 15) Chemoprevention of 1,2- dimethylhydrazine-induced colon cancer in mice by naturally occurring organosulfur compounds. *Cancer Res* **50**(16), 5084–87.
123. Pinto, J.T., Krasnikov, B.F., and Cooper, A.J. (2006 Mar) Redox-sensitive proteins are potential targets of garlic-derived mercaptocysteine derivatives. *J Nutr* **136**(3 Suppl), 835S–841S.
124. Chen, H.W., Yang, J.J., Tsai, C.W., Wu, J.J., Sheen, L.Y., Ou, C.C., and Lii, C.K. (2001 May) Dietary fat and garlic oil independently regulate hepatic cytochrome p(450) 2B1 and the placental form of glutathione S-transferase expression in rats. *J Nutr* **131**(5), 1438–43.
125. Dalvi, R.R. (1992 May) Alterations in hepatic phase I and phase II biotransformation enzymes by garlic oil in rats. *Toxicol Lett* **60**(3), 299–305.
126. Fukao, T., Hosono, T., Misawa, S., Seki, T., and Ariga, T. (2004 May) The effects of allyl sulfides on the induction of phase II detoxification enzymes and liver injury by carbon tetrachloride. *Food Chem Toxicol* **42**(5), 743–49.
127. Fani, A., Fani, I., Delavar, M., Fani, P., Eshrati, B., and Elahi, M. (2007 May–Jun) Combined garlic-omeprazole versus standard quadruple therapy for eradication of Helicobacter pylori infection. *Indian J Gastroenterol* **26**(3), 145–6.
128. Martin, K.W., and Ernst, E. (2003 Feb) Herbal medicines for treatment of bacterial infections: A review of controlled clinical trials. *J Antimicrob Chemother* **51**(2), 241–46 Review.
129. Mei, X., Wang, M.C., Xu, H.X., Pan, X.Y., Gao, C.Y., Han, N., and Fu, M.Y. (1982) Garlic and gastric cancer – the effect of garlic on nitrite and nitrate in gastric juice. *Acta Nutr Sin* **4**, 53–56.
130. Fleischauer, A.T., and Arab, L. (2001 Mar) Garlic and cancer: A critical review of the epidemiologic literature. *J Nutr* **131**(3s), 032S–40S.
131. Fleischauer, A.T., Poole, C., and Arab, L. (2000 Oct) Garlic consumption and cancer prevention: Meta-analyses of colorectal and stomach cancers. *Am J Clin Nutr* **72**(4), 1047–52.
132. Gonzalez, C.A., and Riboli, E. (2006) Diet and cancer prevention: Where we are, where we are going. *Nutr Cancer* **56**(2), 225–31.
133. Steinmetz, K.A., Kushi, L.H., Bostick, R.M., Folsom, A.R., and Potter, J.D. (1994 Jan 1) Vegetables, fruit, and colon cancer in the Iowa Women's Health Study. *Am J Epidemiol* **139**(1), 1–15.
134. Hsing, A.W., Chokkalingam, A.P., Gao, Y.T., Madigan, M.P., Deng, J., Gridley, G., and Fraumeni, J.F., Jr. (2002 Nov 6) Allium vegetables and risk of prostate cancer: A population-based study. *J Natl Cancer Inst* **94**(21), 1648–51.

135. Key, T.J., Silcocks, P.B., Davey, G.K., Appleby, P.N., and Bishop, D.T. (1997) A case-control study of diet and prostate cancer. *Br J Cancer* **76**(5), 678–87.

136. Chan, J.M., Wang, F., and Holly, E.A. (2005 Sep) Vegetable and fruit intake and pancreatic cancer in a population-based case-control study in the San Francisco bay area. *Cancer Epidemiol Biomarkers Prev* **14**(9), 2093–97.

137. Challier, B., Perarnau, J.M., and Viel, J.F. (1998 Dec) Garlic, onion and cereal fibre as protective factors for breast cancer: A French case-control study. *Eur J Epidemiol* **14**(8), 737–47.

138. Durak, I., Yilmaz, E., Devrim, E., Perk, H., and Kamaz, M. (2003) Consumption of aqueous garlic extract leads to significant improvement in patients with benign prostate hyperplasia and prostate cancer. *Nutr Res* **23**, 199–204.

139. Tanaka, S., Haruma, K., Yoshihara, M., Kajiyama, G., Kira, K., Amagase, H., and Chayama, K. (2006 Mar) Aged garlic extract has potential suppressive effect on colorectal adenomas in humans. *J Nutr* **136**(3 Suppl), 821S–6S.

140. Ishikawa, H., Saeki, T., Otani, T., Suzuki, T., Shimozuma, K., Nishino, H., Fukuda, S., and Morimoto, K. (2006 Mar) Aged garlic extract prevents a decline of NK cell number and activity in patients with advanced cancer. *J Nutr* **136**(3 Suppl), 816S–820S.

141. Li, H., Li, H.Q., Wang, Y., Xu, H.X., Fan, W.T., Wang, M.L., Sun, P.H., and Xie, X.Y. (2004 Aug) An intervention study to prevent gastric cancer by micro-selenium and large dose of allitridum. *Chin Med J (Engl)* **117**(8), 1155–60.

142. Schmidt, M., Betti, G., and Hensel, A. (2007) Saffron in phytotherapy: Pharmacology and clinical uses. *Wien Med Wochenschr* **157**(13–14), 315–19.

143. Abdullaev, F.I., and Espinosa-Aguirre, J.J. (2004) Biomedical properties of saffron and its potential use in cancer therapy and chemoprevention trials. *Cancer Detect Prev* **28**(6), 426–32.

144. Nair, S.C., Kurumboor, S.K., and Hasegawa, J.H. (1995 Winter) Saffron chemoprevention in biology and medicine: A review. *Cancer Biother* **10**(4), 257–64.

145. Giaccio, M. (2004) Crocetin from saffron: An active component of an ancient spice. *Crit Rev Food Sci Nutr* **44**(3), 155–72.

146. Surh, Y.J., Lee, E., and Lee, J.M. (1998 June 18) Chemoprotective properties of some pungent ingredients present in red pepper and ginger. *Mutat Res* **402**(1–2), 259–67.

147. Yun, T.K. (1999) Update from Asia. Asian studies on cancer chemoprevention. *Ann N Y Acad Sci* **889**, 157–92.

148. Marmot, M., Atinmo, T., Byers, T., Chen, J., Hirohata, T., Jackson, A., James, W.P.T., Kolonel, L.N., Kumanyika, S., Leitzmann, C., Mann, J., Powers, H.J., Reddy, K.S., Riboli, E., Rivera, J.A., Schatzkin, A., Seidell, J.C., Shuker, D.E., Uauy, R., Willett, W., and Zeisel, S.H. (2007) Food, nutrition, physical activity, and the prevention of cancer: A global perspective. Research report. WCRF/AICR Expert Report. American Institute for Cancer Research, Washington, DC.

149. Surh, Y.J., and Lee, S.S. (1996 Mar) Capsaicin in hot chili pepper: Carcinogen, co-carcinogen or anticarcinogen? *Food Chem Toxicol* **34**(3), 313–16.

150. Surh, Y.J., and Lee, S.S. (1995) Capsaicin, a double-edged sword: Toxicity, metabolism, and chemopreventive potential. *Life Sci* **56**(22), 1845–55.

151. Aggarwal, B. Personal communication, Jul 11, 2007.

152. Aggarwal, B.B., Sundaram, C., Malani, N., and Ichikawa, H. (2007) Curcumin: The Indian solid gold. *Adv Exp Med Biol* **595**, 1–75.

29 Cancer Prevention with Berries: Role of Anthocyanins

Gary D. Stoner, Li-Shu Wang, Christine Sardo, Nancy Zikri, Stephen S. Hecht, and Susan R. Mallery

Key Points

1. Berries have been part of the human diet for many centuries. They are a rich source of known chemopreventive agents including provitamin A carotenoids, C, E, and folate, calcium and selenium, simple and complex phenols, and phytosterols.
2. It has been found that freeze-dried berries can inhibit cancer development in the esophagus, colon, oral cavity, and mammary gland of rodents. Studies suggest that the most active inhibitory compounds in berries are the anthocyanins, the most abundant flavonoids in berries.
3. Berries function to inhibit carcinogenesis by reducing the growth rate of premalignant cells, inhibiting angiogenesis and inflammation, and stimulating apoptosis, cell differentiation, and cell adhesion. Molecular studies indicate that berries exhibit a genome-wide effect on the expression of genes associated with these different cellular functions.
4. The ability of berries to prevent cancer is likely due to the localized absorption of berry compounds into target tissues. Topical treatment of oral dysplastic lesions with a black raspberry gel for a period of 6 weeks resulted in a reduction in histological grade and restoration of loss of heterozygosity (LOH) in about 50% of the lesions. Consumption of black raspberry powder (60 g/day) in a slurry of water for only 2–4 weeks reduced the Ki-67 cell proliferation index in colon tumors taken at surgery from cancer patients.
5. The protective effects of berries on cancer development at specific sites in animals are impressive; however, there is little evidence that berry consumption leads to significant side effects either in animals or in humans. It seems reasonable to suggest that berries be part of the daily diet, and that in individuals at high risk, the daily consumption of several grams of berry powder could well elicit protection.

Key Words: Berries; cancer chemoprevention; anthocyanins; esophagus; colon; oral cavity; molecular mechanisms

From: *Nutrition and Health: Bioactive Compounds and Cancer*
Edited by: J.A. Milner, D.F. Romagnolo, DOI 10.1007/978-1-60761-627-6_29,
© Springer Science+Business Media, LLC 2010

1. INTRODUCTION

1.1. Rationale for the Use of Berries in Cancer Prevention

Wild berries have been a part of the human diet for many centuries *(1)*. Their major use is for nutrition, although some varieties have been used for medicinal purposes. The most important commercial varieties of berries include members of the *Vaccinium* genus (blueberry, lingonberry, cranberry, bilberry), *Rubus* genus (blackberry, red raspberry, black raspberry, cloudberry), *Fragaria* genus (strawberry), and the *Sambucus* genus (elderberry, red elderberry). These berries contain a vast array of phytochemicals, many of which are of potential importance for human health. Phytochemicals are non-nutritive compounds, produced mainly by secondary metabolism, that protect the plant from UV light, predators, and parasites, regulate chemical pathways, and provide flavor and color to the berry. Perhaps the most interesting phytochemicals in berries are the polyphenols, which impart to berries much of their antioxidant potential *(2)*. The polyphenols can be divided into phenolic acids, which consist of an aromatic ring structure with at least one hydroxyl group, and the flavonoids, which are more complex molecules *(1)*. The phenolic acids represent about 30% of the daily intake of polyphenols in humans and the flavonoids about 70%. There are several groups of flavonoids, including the anthocyanidins, flavanols, flavonols, isoflavones, flavones, and flavonones. These groups differ in the number and distribution of hydroxyl groups on the basic chemical structure. More complete descriptions of the classes of phytochemicals in berries, including the flavonoids, are found in recent reviews by Seeram *(3)* and from our laboratory *(4, 5)*.

The anthocyanins are among the most abundant flavonoids in berries *(3)*. They are responsible for the color of berries; thus, the darker berries such as black raspberries, blueberries, blackberries, and black currents have the highest levels of anthocyanins. The anthocyanins occur in berries and other foodstuffs as glycosides, having glucose, galactose, rhamnose, xylose, or arabinose attached to an aglycone nucleus *(3)*. The deglycosylated or aglycone forms of anthocyanins are known as anthocyanidins. The six most common anthocyanidin skeletons are cyanidin, pelarogonidin, malvidin, petunidin, delphinidin, and peonidin (Fig. 1). The sugar components of anthocyanins are usually conjugated to the anthocyanidin skeleton via the C3 hydroxyl group in ring C. Several hundred anthocyanins are known in nature, varying in the basic anthocyanidin skeleton and the extent and position to which the glycosides are attached to the skeleton. Of potential importance to human health is the relatively high concentration of anthocyanins in the diet. The daily intake of anthocyanins in the United States is estimated to be about 200 mg, whereas the intake of other dietary flavonoids such as quercetin, genistein, and apigenin is about 25 mg/day *(4)*. Epidemiologic studies suggest that the consumption of anthocyanins lowers the risk of cancer, cardiovascular disease, diabetes, and arthritis, in part, due to their potent antioxidant and anti-inflammatory activities *(5)*.

In the mid-1980s, our laboratory was evaluating the ability of the naturally occurring polyphenol, ellagic acid to inhibit *N*-nitrosomethylbenzylamine (NMBA)-induced cancer in the rodent esophagus when administered in the diet *(6)*. While conducting

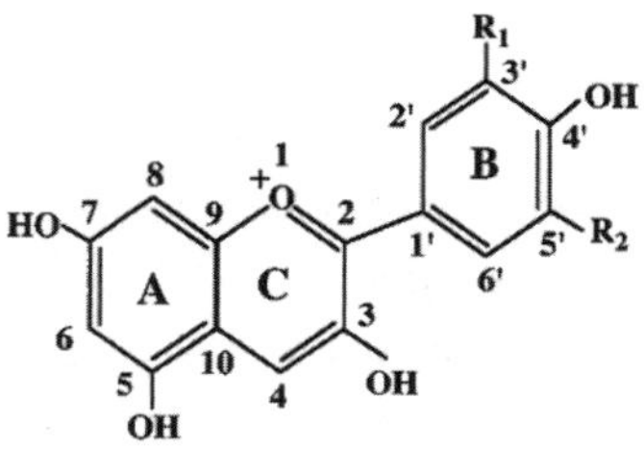

Name	R1	R2
Delphinidin	OH	OH
Petunidin	OCH$_3$	H
Cyanidin	OH	H
Pelargonidin	H	H
Peonidin	OCH$_3$	H
Malvidin	OCH$_3$	OCH$_3$

Fig. 1. Chemical structure of anthocyanidins. Adapted from *(5)*.

studies with ellagic acid, we decided to identify foods in which it might be found. We extracted ellagic acid from a series of lyophilized fruits and found high concentrations (630–1,500 mg/kg dry weight) in black raspberries (BRB), blackberries, red raspberries, strawberries, and cranberries *(7)*. Interestingly, the ellagic acid was far more abundant in the seed and pulp of the berries; very little was detected in the juice. Because berries are composed of 85–90% water (juice), we reasoned that the removal of water from the berries by freeze-drying would result in about a 10-fold concentration of the ellagic acid, and that one might prevent cancer in rodents and humans using freeze-dried berry powder containing "enriched" levels of ellagic acid. In the present report, we summarize investigations of the ability of freeze-dried berry powders and berry extracts to inhibit chemically induced cancer in rodents and provide evidence that the preventive effects of the berries are not due solely to their content of ellagic acid. In fact, recent data suggest that the anthocyanins in berries may be the most important determinants of their cancer-preventive effects *(8)*. We also summarize known cellular and molecular mechanisms by which berries and their component anthocyanins elicit cancer-preventive effects in vivo. Because of the extensive amount of available data, the reader is referred to recent reviews from our laboratory and others for discussions of the effects of berry extracts and berry anthocyanins on normal and tumor cells in vitro *(4, 5)*. We also discuss the results of epidemiological studies to determine whether berry consumption is protective against cancer in humans. Finally, we discuss results of completed and ongoing clinical trials of berries as chemopreventive agents for colon, oral, and esophagus cancer in humans.

2. PREVENTION OF CANCER IN ANIMALS WITH BERRY POWDERS AND ANTHOCYANINS

2.1. Preparation of Freeze-Dried Berry Powders

Most investigations of the cancer-inhibitory effects of freeze-dried berries in animals have been conducted with black raspberries (BRB) obtained from a single farm in Ohio. The rationale for the choice of BRB for study is their high content of anthocyanins and ellagic acid and their high antioxidant potential relative to most other berry types *(9)*. The rationale for obtaining berries from a single farm stems from observations that the contents of ellagic acid and anthocyanins in BRB obtained from 12 different farms in Ohio during a single year can vary as much as two to threefold *(10)*. The BRB are picked mechanically, washed with water, and placed in a −20°C freezer on the farm within 2–4 h of the time of picking. They are then shipped frozen to Van Drunen Farms (Momence, IL) where they are freeze-dried and ground into a powder. For animal studies, both the seed and pulp of the berries are ground into a powder. Berry powders are packaged in double polyethylene bags, placed in carton boxes, and shipped frozen to the Ohio State University Innovation Centre where they remain frozen until used in experimental studies. Each batch of freeze-dried BRB powder is analyzed routinely for content of certain vitamins, minerals, carotenoids, simple phenols, and phytosterols by Covance Laboratories, Inc. (Madison, WI); for ellagic and chlorogenic acids by Brunswick Laboratories (Norton, MA); and for anthocyanin content in the laboratory of Dr. Steven Schwartz, Department of Food Science and Technology, Ohio State University. Table 1 shows the contents of these berry components in BRB obtained from crop year 2006. In general, with the exception of vitamin C, which degrades while berries are frozen, the components measured in freeze-dried berries remain relatively stable for at least 1 year when the berry powder is stored at −20°C. BRB powders are also tested for content of pesticides, herbicides, and fungicides. These agents are usually undetectable or present at no effect levels as defined by the US Environmental Protection Agency.

2.2. Evaluation of Freeze-Dried BRB Powder for Cancer Prevention in Animals

Dietary freeze-dried BRB powder has been demonstrated to inhibit carcinogen-induced cancer in the esophagus and colon of F-344 rats, and in the cheek pouch of Syrian golden hamsters, as well as spontaneous tumors of the small intestine in APC Min mice *(11–13)* (Table 2). Most investigations have been conducted using the F-344 rat model of esophageal squamous cell carcinoma in which tumors have been induced with the carcinogen, NMBA *(14)*. Historically, BRB have been administered in the diet at 5 and 10% either before, during, and after treatment of the rats with NMBA (complete carcinogenesis protocol; Fig. 2a) or only after NMBA treatment (post-initiation protocol; Fig. 2b) to evaluate the anti-initiation and anti-promotion/progression effects of the berries *(4)*. At the end of the bioassay (25–30 weeks), the incidence, multiplicity, and size of esophageal tumors are determined. Typically, the BRB diets have not been effective in reducing esophageal tumor incidence or size in NMBA-treated animals. However, they have reduced the number of tumors per esophagus, i.e., the tumor

Table 1

Levels of Nutrients and Potential Chemopreventive Agents in Freeze-Dried Black Raspberries[a]

Components	mg/100 g
Minerals	
Calcium	188.00
Copper	0.75
Iron	4.80
Magnesium	171.00
Manganese	3.56
Phosphorus	209.00
Potassium	1570.00
Selenium	<5.00
Zinc	2.16
Vitamins	
A from carotene	132.00
Ascorbic acid	6.60
α-Carotene	<0.03
β-Carotene	<0.07
α-Tocopherol	10.40
β-Tocopherol	3.51
γ-Tocopherol	11.20
Folate	0.14
Sterols	
β-Sitosterol	110.00
Campesterol	5.50
Stigmasterol	1.00
Cholesterol	<1.00
Simple phenols	
Ellagic acid	447.00
Ferulic acid	47.10
P-Coumaric acid	6.92
Chlorogenic acid	0.14
Quercetin	36.50
Anthocyanins (complex phenols)	
Cyanidin-3-O-glucoside	278.50
Cyanidin-3-O-sambubioside	56.00
Cyanidin-3-O-rutinoside	1790.00
Cyanidin-3-O-xylosylrutinoside	853.50

[a]Components reported in mg/100 g sample, except selenium level reported in μg/100 g and vitamin A in IU. Data from crop year 2006.

Table 2
Effects of 5 and 10% Black Raspberry Diets on Tumor Development in Rodents[a]

Species	Organ	Carcinogen[b]	Inhibition of tumor multiplicity (%)
Rat	Esophagus	NMBA	38–61
Rat	Colon	AOM	42–71
Hamster	Cheek pouch	DMBA	~40
Mouse (Min)[c]	Small intestine	Spontaneous	~50

[a]Adapted from Stoner et al. (4, 40).
[b]NMBA, N-nitrosomethylbenzylamine; AOM, azoxymethane; DMBA, 7,12-dimethylbenz[a]anthracene.
[c]Unpublished data.

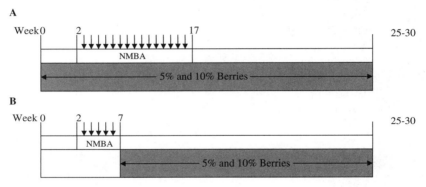

Fig. 2. Experimental protocols for the complete carcinogenesis bioassay (**a**) and the anti-promotion/progression bioassay (**b**). In (**a**), rats are treated with NMBA (0.25 mg/kg bw) once per week for 15 weeks, and berry diet is administered 2 weeks prior to and during NMBA treatment and until the end of the bioassay (25–30 weeks) (11, 40). In (**b**), rats are treated with NMBA (0.25 mg/kg bw) three times/week for 5 weeks and then placed on berry diets until the end of the bioassay (11, 40).

multiplicity (11). BRB are generally more effective in the complete carcinogenesis protocol (Fig. 2a) than when given in the diet only after treatment of the animals with NMBA, i.e., post-initiation. Undoubtedly, the reason for this is that BRB diets have been shown to affect initiation events by influencing the metabolism of NMBA, leading to reduced levels of O^6-methylguanine (O^6-MeGua) adducts in esophageal DNA (11). This undoubtedly results in reduced mutagenesis in key genes involved in esophageal tumor development. One such gene is the *H*-ras oncogene, which is mutationally activated in about 5–10% of early dysplastic lesions in NMBA-treated esophagus and in nearly 100% of NMBA-induced esophageal tumors (15). These results suggest that dysplastic foci containing cells with *H*-ras mutations are the ones that progress on to form tumors. DNA microarray studies have shown that dietary BRB influence the expression levels of specific esophageal cytochrome P450 enzymes and liver phase II enzymes.

Nevertheless, it is not known whether these enzymes are involved in the metabolic activation and/or detoxification of NMBA *(16)*.

Recent data suggest that the efficacy of BRB treatment in the post-initiation protocol (Fig. 2b) is influenced markedly by two factors: (a) the timing of initial treatment with dietary BRB following NMBA exposure and (b) the duration of BRB treatment. In general, the berries are most effective (about 70% inhibition of tumor multiplicity) when added to the diet within 1 week after treatment of the rats with NMBA (week 8) and when maintained in the diet until the end of the 25- to 30-week bioassay (Fig. 3). They are less effective when added to the diet at week 8 and then removed from the diet at week 17. This result suggests that the inhibitory effect of the berries is not permanent and that continued treatment is required to prevent tumor development. The berries were even less effective when their addition to the diet after NMBA treatment was delayed until week 17, suggesting that they are less effective in preventing the progression of more advanced preneoplastic lesions than less advanced lesions. Finally, even when added to the diet at a concentration as high as 20%, the berries were ineffective in regressing already developed tumors, suggesting that they have little, if any, therapeutic value in the rodent esophagus *(17)*.

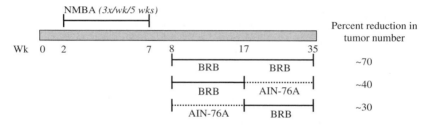

Fig. 3. Effects of 5% black raspberry diet on NMBA-induced rat esophageal tumorigenesis. BRB, black raspberries; AIN-76A, control diet contains no known chemopreventive components. Adapted from *(8)*.

Dietary BRB were also found to inhibit azoxymethane (AOM)-induced colon carcinogenesis in rats when given in a post-initiation protocol (Table 2) *(12)*. When administered at 2.5, 5.0, and 10% of the diet, BRB reduced the total tumor (adenoma + adenocarcinoma) multiplicity by 42, 45, and 71%, respectively, relative to AOM controls. In addition, the levels of urinary 8-hydroxy-2′-deoxyguanosine (8-OHdG) in AOM-treated rats fed 2.5, 5, and 10% BRB diets were reduced by 73, 81, and 83%, respectively (Fig. 4). These results suggest that the berries markedly reduced oxidative DNA damage in AOM-exposed rats.

Inhibition of cancer in the Syrian golden hamster cheek pouch by the dietary administration of BRB was demonstrated by Casto et al. (Table 2) *(13)*. Tumors were induced by painting the cheek pouches of hamsters with 7,12-dimethylbenz(a)anthracene (DMBA). Hamsters were fed either 5 or 10% BRB prior to and after treatment with DMBA. Interestingly, treatment with 5% BRB caused a significant ($P < 0.05$) reduction in tumor multiplicity but the reduction with 10% berries was not significant. BRB reduced the levels of DNA adducts in DMBA-treated pouch tissues as determined by ^{32}P-post-labeling techniques.

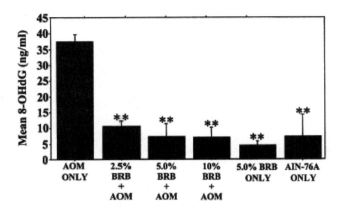

Fig. 4. Effect of 2.5, 5, and 10% black raspberry diets on urinary 8-OH-dGua levels in AOM-treated rats. BRB, black raspberries; AOM, azoxymethane; AIN-76A, control diet contains no known chemopreventive components. Adapted from *(12)*.

In a recent report, dietary berries and ellagic acid were found to diminish estrogen-mediated mammary tumorigenesis in ACI rats (Table 3) *(18)*. Female ACI rats were fed either control diet or diets supplemented with either powdered blueberries or BRB at 2.5% w/w each or ellagic acid at 400 ppm. After 2 weeks, the rats received implants of 17β-estradiol for a period of 24 weeks. Although none of the treatments influenced tumor incidence at 24 weeks, tumor volume and multiplicity were reduced significantly by berries. Compared with controls, ellagic acid reduced the tumor volume by 75% and multiplicity by 44%. BRB diminished tumor volume by >69% and tumor multiplicity by 37%. Blueberries produced a 40% reduction in tumor volume, but had no effect on tumor multiplicity. Although the reason(s) for the reduction in estrogen-mediated mammary tumorigenesis by ellagic acid and the berry diets were not determined, it is possible that these agents influence the metabolism of estradiol in the liver such that

Table 3
Effects of Black Raspberry, Blueberry, and Ellagic Acid Diets on Tumor Indices in ACI Rats Treated with 17β-Estradiol[a]

	Mammary tumor	
Treatment	*Volume (mm³)*	*Multiplicity*
Control diet	685 ± 240	7.9 ± 1.3
BB diet	409 ± 73	8.2 ± 1.0
BRB diet	211 ± 69[b]	4.7 ± 0.7
Ellagic acid diet	168 ± 34[b]	4.5 ± 0.5[b]

[a]BRB, black raspberries; BB, blueberries. Data adapted from Aiyer et al. *(18)*.
[b]Values are statistically different from animals fed control diet (*P* < 0.05).

less hormone reaches the mammary gland. It is also possible that ellagic acid and other berry compounds may bind to estrogen receptors, thus, competitively inhibiting the pro-carcinogenic effects of estrogen.

2.3. Evaluation of Other Berry Types for Prevention of Cancer in Animals

Strawberry, blackberry, and blueberry powders have also been tested for their ability to prevent NMBA tumorigenesis in the rat esophagus when added at 5 and 10% of the diet (Table 4) *(19)*. The sources of these berries and their conversion into powders have been described in detail *(19–21)*. Strawberries and blackberries were nearly as effective in preventing tumors as BRB. However, blueberries were inactive. Both straw-berries and blackberries reduced the formation of NMBA-induced O^6-MeGua adducts in esophageal DNA, whereas blueberries had no effect on adduct formation (data not shown). The reason(s) for the inactivity of blueberries is unknown. Unlike the other three berry types, blueberries have only very low levels of ellagitannins *(7)*. In addition, blueberry anthocyanins have a delphinidin skeleton whereas the anthocyanins in BRB and blackberries have a cyanidin skeleton and those in strawberries have both pelaro-gonidin and cyanidin skeletons *(1)*. These differences in chemical composition may be responsible for the different biological activities of the berry types. A second bioassay

Table 4

Effects of Freeze-Dried Strawberries, Blackberries, and Blueberries on NMBA-Induced Rat Esophageal Tumorigenesis when Administered in the Diet Before, During, and After NMBA Treatment (Complete Prevention Protocol)[a]

Treatment	Rats (n)	Tumor incidence (% inhibition)	Tumor multiplicity (% inhibition)
Vehicle control	15	0	0.0
10% STRW	15	0	0.0
NMBA control	15	100	4.1 ± 0.2
NMBA + 5% STRW	15	100	$3.1 \pm 1.0 \ (24)^{b}$
NMBA + 10% STRW	15	80 (20)	$1.8 \pm 1.4 \ (56)^{b}$
Vehicle control	10	0	0.0
10% BLB	10	0	0.0
NMBA control	17	82	2.8 ± 0.6
NMBA + 5% BLB	20	75 (8)	$1.5 \pm 0.4 \ (46)^{b}$
NMBA + 10% BLB	18	70 (15)	$2.3 \pm 0.5 \ (18)$
Vehicle control	10	0	0.0
10% BB	10	0	0.0
NMBA control	24	91	2.2 ± 0.3
NMBA + 5% BB	24	92 (0)	$2.5 \pm 0.3 \ (0)^{b}$
NMBA + 10% BB	23	96 (0)	$2.6 \pm 0.3 \ (0)$

[a]Abbreviations are as follows: STRW, strawberries; BLB, blackberries; BB, blueberries; NMBA, *N*-nitrosomethylbenzylamine.

[b]Statistically significant relative to NMBA controls ($P < 0.05$). STRW data are taken from *(20)*. BLB data are from *(19)* and BB data are from *(21)*.

using blueberries is currently being utilized to confirm the previous results and further determine the basis for the inactivity of blueberries.

Chemoprevention of lung cancer has proven to be difficult, both in rodents and in humans. Thus, it is perhaps not surprising that a diet containing 10% freeze-dried strawberries was ineffective in reducing lung tumors in mice that were induced either by 4-(methylnitrosamino)-1-(3-pyridyl)-1-butanone (NNK) or benzo(a)pyrene (B(a)P) (22). In this study, strain A/J mice were administered the strawberry diet beginning 1 week before initial carcinogen treatment and throughout the study. NNK and B(a)P were administered i.p. over a 2-week period beginning at week 2 of the bioassay. At 24 weeks, there were no differences in lung tumor incidence or multiplicity in any of the groups. Successes in reducing carcinogen-induced cancers in the oral cavity, esophagus, and colon, where berry components come into direct contact with the tissues, and the failure to inhibit lung tumors in mice suggest that the active components in berries fail to reach the lung in sufficient amounts to elicit protection. This conclusion is supported by studies documenting that the anthocyanins and ellagitannins from berry juices are poorly absorbed in rodents and their plasma levels decline rapidly (23). However, the protective effects of dietary BRB powder against estrogen-mediated mammary cancer in rats suggest that sufficient amounts of protective compounds reach the mammary gland through systemic delivery. Thus, the protective effects of dietary berry powders appear to be organ and site dependent.

2.4. Studies to Identify the Anthocyanins as Active Inhibitory Components in Berries

To identify the active chemopreventive constituents of black raspberries, we have used bioactivity-guided fractionation. Initially, we extracted freeze-dried BRB with organic solvents and water and tested these extract fractions for their ability to inhibit chemically induced transformation of Syrian hamster embryo (SHE) cells (24). Of five extract fractions tested, an alcohol extract of BRB was found to be the most effective in inhibiting cell transformation. These same extract fractions were evaluated by Huang et al. (25) for their effects on transactivation of activated protein-1 (AP-1) and nuclear factor-κB (NF-κB) induced by the carcinogen, benzo(a)pyrene diol-epoxide (BPDE), in mouse epidermal cells. Again, the alcohol extract was found to be the most effective in down-regulating AP-1 and NF-κB activities, and its effects were mediated via inhibition of mitogen-activated protein kinase (MAPK) activation and inhibitory subunit κB phosphorylation, respectively. Subsequent studies utilizing cultured human oral and colon cancer cells, and rat esophageal epithelial cells of differing tumorigenic potential, confirmed that an alcohol extract of BRB was the most effective of several extracts tested in inhibiting cell proliferation and in stimulating apoptosis and cell differentiation (26–28).

The alcohol extract was then fractionated by high-performance liquid chromatography (HPLC) to yield several bioactive subfractions (29). These subfractions were tested individually for their ability to down-regulate AP-1 and NF-κB activities in mouse epidermal cells and, interestingly, the major constituents of the most active subfractions were three of the four anthocyanins in BRB, i.e., cyanidin-3-*O*-glucoside, cyanidin-3-*O*-rutinoside, and cyanidin 3-*O*-(2^G-xylosylrutinoside) (29). Thus, these in vitro results suggested that the anthocyanins in BRB account for at least some of their chemopreventive activity.

In a follow-up study, we extended the in vitro observations and determined whether the anthocyanins in BRB are among the most active chemopreventive components in vivo. F-344 rats were fed diets containing either (a) 5% whole BRB powder, (b) an anthocyanin-rich fraction, (c) an alcohol/H_2O-soluble extract, (d) an alcohol-insoluble (residue) fraction, (e) a hexane extract, and (f) a sugar fraction before, during, and after treatment with NMBA *(8)*. The scheme for the preparation of these different extracts/fractions is given in Fig. 5. The anthocyanin fraction and the alcohol/H_2O-soluble extract each contained the same amount of anthocyanins (~3.8 μmol/g diet) as were present in the diet containing 5% whole BRB powder. The residue fraction contained less than 0.02 μmol anthocyanins/g of diet, and the hexane extract and the sugar fraction had only trace quantities of anthocyanins. The results of these studies are shown in Fig. 6a, b. The anthocyanin treatments (diet groups a–c) were about equally effective in reducing NMBA tumorigenesis (multiplicity and size) in the esophagus confirming that the anthocyanins in BRB have chemopreventive potential in vivo. Interestingly, the organic-insoluble (residue) fraction (d) was also effective, suggesting that components other than the anthocyanins may be chemopreventive. Our preliminary analysis of this fraction indicates that it contains a number of ellagitannins. As expected, the hexane and sugar fractions were inactive, presumably because they contained only trace quantities of anthocyanins and other bioactives. Our conclusion from these studies is that the anthocyanins in BRB are important for their cancer-inhibitory effects. The ellagitannins

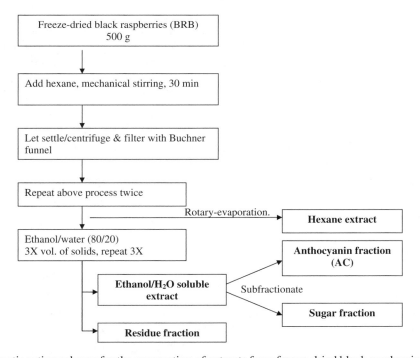

Fig. 5. Fractionation scheme for the preparation of extracts from freeze-dried black raspberries (BRB).

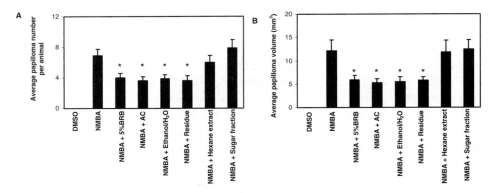

Fig. 6. Effect of diets containing BRB or BRB residues/fractions on papilloma development in NMBA-treated rat esophagus. Rats treated with NMBA + 5% BRB, NMBA + anthocyanin fraction (AC), NMBA + ethanol/H$_2$O soluble extract (ethanol/H$_2$O), and NMBA + residue fraction (residue) had fewer papillomas (**a**) and smaller papilloma volume (**b**) than rats treated with NMBA only. Bars represent mean ± SD, $n = 15$. The symbol (*) indicates significantly lower ($P < 0.05$) than rats treated with NMBA only.

may also prove to be important. The role of vitamins, minerals, and phytosterols in BRB as chemopreventive agents may be important, but it does not appear to be as important as that of the anthocyanins and ellagitannins.

Other laboratories have provided evidence for the chemopreventive activity of berry anthocyanins in vivo. Lala et al. *(30)* reported that diets containing anthocyanin-rich extracts from bilberry, chokeberry, or grape reduced the number of aberrant crypt foci (ACF) in the colon of rats treated with AOM. Colonic cell proliferation was reduced significantly ($P < 0.05$) in rats fed bilberry and chokeberry anthocyanins, and cyclooxygenase-2 (COX-2) mRNA expression was reduced in the colon of rats fed bilberry and grape anthocyanins. Cooke et al. *(31)* found that the adenoma numbers in the intestinal mucosa of Apc (*Min*) mice fed diets containing an anthocyanin mixture from bilberry, or pure cyanidin-3-glucoside (C3G), were reduced by 45% ($P < 0.05$) and 30% ($P < 0.05$), respectively. Anthocyanins were found in plasma and in quantifiable levels in the intestinal mucosa and urine of the mice. Both studies concluded that anthocyanins should be further developed as potential chemopreventive agents for human colon cancer.

2.5. Cellular and Molecular Mechanisms for the Chemopreventive Effects of BRB

Most experimental studies of the cellular and molecular mechanisms by which freeze-dried berries exhibit chemopreventive efficacy in vivo have been conducted using BRB and the NMBA model of rat esophageal carcinogenesis. Initial studies were conducted using esophageal tissues taken from rats at several time points following their treatment with NMBA (i.e., post-initiation). Whole esophagus (representing a mixture of normal, hyperplastic, and dysplastic epithelium) and esophageal papillomas taken from rats treated with NMBA only or with NMBA + 5 or 10% dietary BRB were used for study. Gene expression in these tissues was measured using quantitative immunohisto-chemistry and real-time PCR.

BRB diets were initially shown to inhibit the growth rate of preneoplastic cells in NMBA-treated esophagus as determined by reduced nuclear staining of proliferating cell nuclear antigen (PCNA) *(11)*. This was later found to correlate with reduced mRNA and protein expression levels of c-Jun, a component of activator protein-1 (AP-1), and reduced immunostaining for ERK 1/2, a mitogen-activated protein kinase, both associated with cellular proliferation *(8, 32)*. In another study, BRB were found to inhibit angiogenesis in NMBA-treated esophagus as indicated by reduced microvessel density and decreased mRNA expression levels of vascular endothelial growth factor-1 (VEGF-1) *(33)*. BRB diets were also shown to inhibit mRNA and protein expression levels of the pro-inflammatory enzymes, COX-2 and inducible nitric oxide synthase (iNOS), which correlated with reduced levels of prostaglandin E_2 (PGE_2)and nitrite/nitrate, respectively, in NMBA-treated esophagus *(32)*. Increased PGE_2 levels in tissues can lead to increased proliferation, inflammation, angiogenesis, and metastasis and to reduced apoptosis *(32)*. More recently, BRB diets were shown to stimulate apoptosis in NMBA-treated preneoplastic esophagus and in esophageal papillomas as determined by staining for apoptotic cells using TUNEL and by demonstrating reduced mRNA and protein expression levels of Bcl-2 and increased mRNA and protein expression levels of Bax *(8)*. In this same study, BRB were shown by immunohistochemistry to reduce the protein expression levels of additional genes in preneoplastic tissues and in papillomas including NF-κb and hypoxia-inhibitory factor-1α (HIF-1α), genes associated with multiple cellular functions including inflammation and angiogenesis. These studies using quantitative immunohistochemistry and real-time PCR have demonstrated, therefore, the ability of freeze-dried BRB to influence the expression of genes associated with cellular proliferation, apoptosis, angiogenesis, and inflammation as summarized in Table 5.

A recent investigation used DNA microarray to further assess the effects of a 5% BRB diet on genes associated with rat esophageal carcinogenesis *(16)*. In this study, the effects of the berry diet on early events in esophageal carcinogenesis were determined by feeding 5- to 6-week-old rats with 5% BRB for a period of 3 weeks. During the third week of berry feeding, each rat received three subcutaneous injections of NMBA (0.5 mg/kg) and 24 h after the last injection, their esophagi were removed for histopathological evaluation and molecular analysis. NMBA treatment led to profound changes in the epithelium including inflammation, increased basal cell proliferation, and evidence of significant toxicity. These epithelial changes were much less pronounced in NMBA-treated rats fed 5% BRB. Nearly 2,300 esophageal genes were dysregulated by the NMBA treatment, and 462 of these were restored to near-normal levels of expression with BRB. These restored genes were associated with multiple cellular functions including cell cycle, proliferation, apoptosis, angiogenesis, cell to cell communication, cell adhesion, inflammation, oxidative stress, carcinogen metabolism, etc., indicating that the active components in BRB elicit a genome-wide effect in modulating genes involved in the early events of esophageal toxicity and carcinogenesis. Perhaps, this is not surprising in view of the large number of chemopreventive agents in berries that most

Table 5
Cellular Functions and Associated Genes Affected by BRB in NMBA-Treated Rat Esophagus

Function	Genes/events	References
Cell proliferation	↓ PCNA, Ki-67	Kresty et al. (11)
	↓ AP-1 (c-Jun)	Chen et al. (32)
	↓ COX-2, PGE$_2$	Chen et al. (32)
	↓ Erk1/2	Wang et al. (8)
Apoptosis	↑ TUNEL	Wang et al. (8)
	↓ Bcl-2	Wang et al. (8)
	↑ Bax	Wang et al. (8)
	↓ Caspase-3	Zikri et al. (28)
Inflammation	↓ COX-2, PGE$_2$	Chen et al. (32)
	↓ iNOS, nitrite/nitrate	Chen et al. (32)
	↓ NF-κB	Wang et al. (8)
	↓ CD45 (leukocyte common antigen)	Wang et al. (8)
Angiogenesis	↓ VEGF-1	Chen et al. (33)
	↓ HIF-1α	Wang et al. (8)
	↓ Microvessel density	Chen et al. (33)

likely act on different signaling pathways. In contrast, the treatment of control (non-NMBA treated) rats with the 5% BRB diet for 3 weeks led to changes in the expression levels of only 36 genes in the esophagus (34). For the most part, these genes were not associated with cancer development in the rat esophagus or in other tissues.

3. EPIDEMIOLOGICAL STUDIES

There have been relatively few epidemiological studies to assess the potential cancer-preventive effects of berries in humans. One study of 1,271 Massachusetts residents reported a reduced relative risk of cancer death (RR = 0.3) among subjects who consumed less than one serving of strawberries per week (35). The actual amount of strawberries consumed was not reported. Another study examined the effect of fruit and vegetable consumption, including strawberries and blueberries, on the incidence of colon and rectal cancers in the Nurses' Health Study (88,764 women) and the Health Professionals' Follow-up Study (47,325 men) and concluded that the frequent consumption of all fruits and vegetables examined did not confer protection from colon or rectal cancer (36). A weak inverse association was found between colorectal adenoma growth and fruit and berry consumption in Norway. However, the types and amounts of berries consumed were not discussed (37). Fruit intake, including berries, does not appear to be related to risk of prostate cancer and, if anything, may be associated with a slightly elevated risk (38). A major difficulty in making definitive conclusions regarding the relationship between the intake of berry and risk for human cancer is that of separating berry consumption from that of other fruits in epidemiological studies. In addition, the seasonal use of many berry types during the year compromises the acquisition of accurate consumption data. Probably, the most extensive database on berry consumption by humans as a function of age, gender, berry type, and geographic location resides in Finland *(39)*. To date, however, there do not appear to be any studies relating berry use in Finland to cancer occurrence or outcome.

4. INTERVENTION STUDIES IN HUMANS

There have been relatively few clinical trials to evaluate the potential anticancer effects of berries. Some of the available data in humans were derived from pharmacokinetic studies of the absorption, distribution, metabolism, and excretion of berry compounds, obtained either from foodstuffs or as purified compounds. An extensive summary of these studies was provided by Seeram *(3)*. To our knowledge, all other data have been derived from studies in our laboratories, including a phase I clinical trial of the safety/tolerability of BRB and limited phase IB trials to evaluate the ability of BRB powder, administered in different formulations, to modulate biomarkers of neoplastic progression in Barrett's esophagus, colon polyps, colon adenocarcinomas, and oral dysplasia. The results from our studies have been summarized recently in two reviews *(4–40)* and will be discussed only briefly here.

4.1. Phase I Clinical Trial of BRB

We conducted a phase I trial in 11 subjects to determine the safety/tolerability of BRB and to measure anthocyanins and ellagic acid in plasma and urine *(41)*. Subjects were fed 45 g (equivalent to a 5% berry diet in animals) of BRB powder as a slurry in water daily for 7 days. Blood and urine samples were collected prior to and after berry treatment. The berries were found to be well tolerated. The only clinical observation was a low incidence of mild or moderate constipation in 4 of the 11 subjects. Maximum concentrations of anthocyanins and ellagic acid in plasma occurred at 1–2 h, and maximum quantities in urine appeared from within 4 h. The uptake of the anthocyanins into plasma was reflective of their relative concentrations in black raspberry powder with cyanidin-3-rutinoside > cyanidin-3-xylosylrutinoside > cyanidin-3-glucoside = cyanidin-3-sambubioside. Overall, the uptake of ellagic acid and the anthocyanins was less than 1% of the administered dose. Thus, as is the case with many other phenolic compounds, the anthocyanins and ellagic acid have limited bioavailability in humans.

4.2. Effects of BRB Powder on Biomarkers of Neoplastic Progression in Colon, Oral Cavity, and Esophagus

Several investigations concerning the effects of berry powders on cancer development in the human colon, oral cavity, and esophagus are either ongoing or have been completed. A brief discussion of the results of these studies is provided based on cancer type.

Colon cancer: Based upon positive results of the inhibitory effects of BRB on colon tumor development in rodents *(12)*, we initiated a study in 30 subjects with colorectal cancer to determine if the oral administration of BRB would modulate biomarkers of colon cancer development. Biopsies of normal and tumor tissues were collected at baseline. Subjects consumed 20 g of freeze-dried BRB powder, as a slurry in water, three times a day (60 g total), until their scheduled surgery date, usually within 2–4 weeks. Post-treatment biopsy specimens of normal and tumor tissues were collected during the surgery. Pre-and post-treatment specimens from 30 patients were analyzed for the effects of BRB on cell proliferation using Ki-67, apoptosis by TUNEL, and angiogenesis by staining for CD105. Because the Wnt pathway is altered in about 70% of sporadic colon cancers, we examined, by immunohistochemistry, the nuclear staining of β-catenin, membrane and cytoplasmic staining of E-cadherin, and the protein expression levels of c-Myc and cyclin D1. Although there was a trend for changes in the expression of all biomarkers in tumors relative to that seen in normal colon, only the reduction in Ki-67 cell proliferation rates in both normal and, to a larger extent, tumor tissues was significant (Table 6). Nevertheless, we were encouraged by the fact that biomarkers of tumor development in human colon were modulated by such short-term treatment with BRB. In addition, the recovery of berry anthocyanins from normal colon tissue specimens from BRB-treated patients indicated that the anthocyanins were absorbed locally into colon tissue.

Oral cancer: Studies have been undertaken to determine if BRB might exert a protective effect on the development of oral cancer in humans. A preliminary phase I study evaluated the utility of a mucoadhesive gel for the localized delivery of berry anthocyanins to human oral mucosa *(42)*. Gels containing 5 and 10% BRB powder were formulated to insure the stability of the anthocyanins. Maximum stability of these compounds in the gel was observed at pH 3.5 and at a temperature of 4°C. When the gel was applied topically to the oral mucosa of normal subjects, the anthocyanins were found to be readily absorbed into the tissue as evidenced by detectable blood levels within 5 min after gel application. In addition, all four anthocyanins in black raspberries were found to penetrate into explant tissues of oral mucosa, in vitro, with the greatest penetration being from the 10% berry gel. Based upon these results, the effects of topical application of the 10% BRB gel to oral intraepithelial neoplastic (IEN) lesions in 17 patients and normal tissues in 10 patients, 4×/day for 6 weeks, were evaluated *(43)*. None of the 27 participants developed toxicities associated with gel treatment. Histologic regression of the intraepithelial neoplasia (IEN) lesions was observed in a subset of patients as well as a statistically significant reduction in loss of heterozygosity (LOH) at three tumor-suppressor gene (*INK4a/ARF, p53, FHIT*) loci. Gene expression studies revealed that the berry gel reduced the expression of COX-2 and iNOS in dysplastic lesions and uniformly suppressed genes associated with RNA processing, growth factor recycling, and inhibition of apoptosis *(44)*. The authors concluded that further evaluation of BRB gels for chemoprevention of oral IEN lesions is warranted.

Barrett's esophagus: Barrett's esophagus is the only recognized precursor lesion to esophageal adenocarcinoma, a cancer that has increased dramatically in incidence throughout the Western world over the last three decades *(45)*. A study was undertaken to determine if the oral administration of BRB powder would influence parameters

Table 6
Summary of the Effects of BRB Dietary Intervention (60 g/day) on Modulation of Biomarkers in Human Normal and Cancerous Colon Tissue

	Normal				Tumor			
	Pre-trt (mean ± SE)	Post-trt (mean ± SE)	Difference (mean ± SE)	P value	Pre-trt (mean ± SE)	Post-trt (mean ± SE)	Difference (mean ± SE)	P value
Ki-67	11.30 ± 1.41	8.00 ± 1.07	-3.30 ± 1.23	0.016*	55.20 ± 2.81	49.12 ± 2.28	-6.08 ± 1.83	0.005[a]
TUNEL	0.58 ± 0.10	1.08 ± 0.33	0.50 ± 0.33	0.16	4.49 ± 0.95	6.64 ± 1.17	2.15 ± 1.20	0.14
CD105	2.55 ± 0.39	1.69 ± −0.29	-0.86 ± 0.48	0.10	6.66 ± 1.59	4.14 ± 0.77	-2.52 ± 1.70	0.12
β-Catenin	0.016 ± 0.003	0.018 ± 0.002	0.003 ± 0.002	0.14	0.054 ± 0.006	0.044 ± 0.007	-0.011 ± 0.008	0.06
E-Cadherin	0.17 ± 0.02	0.17 ± 0.02	-0.01 ± 0.03	0.84	0.15 ± 0.02	0.12 ± 0.02	-0.04 ± 0.02	0.10
C-myc	0.19 ± 0.03	0.17 ± 0.03	-0.02 ± 0.02	0.05	0.22 ± 0.03	0.19 ± 0.03	-0.02 ± 0.04	0.28
Cyclin-D1	20.84 ± 2.37	24.48 ± 2.74	3.65 ± 2.14	0.19	38.62 ± 2.80	38.64 ± 2.81	0.02 ± 2.21	0.91

[a]Statistically significant by Wilcoxon signed rank test. Unpublished data.

associated with the progression of Barrett's lesions *(46)*. Twenty Barrett's patients consumed 32 or 45 g (female and male, respectively) of BRB powder daily, as a slurry in water for 26 weeks. Biopsies of Barrett's lesions were taken before and after berry treatment for biomarker analysis. Based upon interim results from 10 of the 20 patients, berry treatment did not result in a reduction in segment length of Barrett's lesions at 26 weeks. Urine was collected from each subject at baseline and at weeks 12 and 26 of the study and evaluated for the oxidative damage biomarkers 8-hydroxy-deoxyguanosine (8-OHdG) and 8-epi-prostaglandin F2α (8-Iso-PGF2). Levels of urinary 8-Iso-PGF2 were significantly reduced, but there was no significant change in mean levels of urinary 8-OHdG. The authors concluded that the daily consumption of freeze-dried black raspberries promotes reductions in the urinary excretion of two biomarkers of oxidative stress, 8-Iso-PGF2, and to a lesser more variable extent, 8-OHdG, among patients with Barrett's esophagus. A concern from this study is that the transit time of the BRB slurry across the esophagus, when consumed orally, is very rapid and may not permit sufficient localized absorption of berry compounds into Barrett's lesions to be effective.

5. TISSUE SPECIFICITY

Animal studies demonstrating the effectiveness of berry powders to prevent cancer in the oral cavity, esophagus, and colon, but not in the lung, suggest that the localized absorption of berry compounds is critical for chemopreventive efficacy. This was further confirmed in humans by the observation that berry compounds are effective when absorbed locally by target tissues (e.g., the oral cavity and colon) in sufficient concentrations to demonstrate efficacy. In that regard, it seems likely that the inability of oral BRB powder to exhibit any effects on Barrett's esophageal lesions was related to insufficient absorption of berry compounds into these lesions. Thus, in order to protect against esophageal adenocarcinoma development in humans, it seems necessary to develop delivery systems that enhance the uptake of berry compounds into Barrett's lesions. The same is probably true for protection against the development of esophageal squamous cell carcinoma from dysplastic lesions and for protection in internal organs such as the liver and lung.

6. CONCLUSIONS AND RECOMMENDATIONS FOR INTAKE/DIETARY CHANGES

It is difficult to make specific recommendations for the dietary uptake of berries for cancer prevention for the following reasons: (a) epidemiological data on the relationship between berry consumption and the prevention of cancer in humans are insufficient and do not provide guidelines as to desirable daily intakes of any berry type; (b) experimental data indicate that berry consumption may be protective against the development of cancer at some sites in humans. However, these studies are preliminary and require verification; (c) the quantity of berries required on a routine basis to prevent the development of cancer at a specific organ site is likely to vary significantly from one individual to another and from one risk group to another. For example, one might expect that a higher intake of berries would be required to induce regression of a polyp in the colon than would be needed to prevent initial polyp development. Nevertheless, the protective effects of berries on cancer development at specific sites in animals are impressive and, to date, there is little evidence that berry consumption leads to significant side effects either in animals or in humans. Thus, it seems reasonable to suggest that berries be part of the daily diet, and that in individuals at high risk, the daily consumption of several grams of berry powder could well elicit protection.

REFERENCES

1. deBoer, J.D. (2005) Berries and their role in human health. In: A Survey of Research into the Health Benefits of Berries. 1–103, Victoria, BC, Canada: DeBoer Consulting.
2. Leonard, S.S., Cutler, D., Ding, M., Vallyathan, V., Castronova, V., and Shi, X. (2002) Antioxidant properties of fruit and vegetable juices: More to the story than ascorbic acid. *Ann Clin Lab Sci* **32**, 193–2.
3. Seeram, N.P. (2006) Berries. In: Heber D., Blackburn G., Go V. and Milner J. eds. Nutritional Oncology. 615–28, Amsterdam: Elsevier, Inc, Chapter 37.
4. Stoner, G.D., Wang, L.-S., and Casto, B.C. (2008) Laboratory and clinical studies of cancer chemoprevention by antioxidants in berries. *Carcinogenesis* **29**, 1665–74.
5. Wang, L.-S., and Stoner, G.D. (2008) Anthocyanins and their role in cancer prevention. *Cancer Lett* **269**, 281–90.
6. Mandal, S., and Stoner, G.D. (1990) Inhibition of *N*-nitrosobenzylmethylamine-induced esophageal tumorigenesis in rats by ellagic acid. *Carcinogenesis* **11**, 55–61.
7. Daniel, E.M., Krupnick, A.S., Heur, Y.-H., Blinzler, J.A., Nims, R.W., and Stoner, G.D. (1989) Extraction, stability, and quantitation of ellagic acid in various fruits and nuts. *J Food Comp Anal* **2**, 338–49.
8. Wang, L.-S., Hecht, S., Carmella, S., Yu, N., Larue, B., Henry, C., McIntyre, C., Rocha, C., Lechner, J.F., and Stoner, G.D. (2009) Anthocyanins in black raspberries prevent esophageal tumors in rats. Cancer Prev Res **2**, 84–93.
9. Moyer, R.A., Hummer, K.E., Finn, C.E., Balz, F., and Wrolstad, R.E. (2002) Anthocyaninis, phenolics, and antioxidant capacity in diverse small fruits *Vaccinium, Rubus*, and *Ribes. J Agric Food Chem* **50**, 519–25.
10. Tulio, A.Z., Jr., Reese, R.N., Wyzgoski, F.J., Rinaldi, P.L., Fu, R., Scheerens, J.C., and Miller, A.R. (2008) Cyanidin 3-rutinoside and cyanidin 3-xylosylrutinoside as primary phenolic antioxidants in black raspberry. *J Agric Food Chem* **56**, 1880–8.
11. Kresty, L.A., Morse, M.A., Morgan, C., Carlton, P.S., Lu, J., Gupta, A., Blackwood, M., and Stoner, G.D. (2001) Chemoprevention of esophageal tumorigenesis by dietary administration of lyophilized black raspberries. *Cancer Res* **61**, 6112–8.
12. Harris, G.K., Gupta, A., Nines, R.G., Kresty, L.A., Habib, S.G., Frankel, W.L., LaPerle, K., Gallaher, D.D., Schwartz, S.J., and Stoner, G.D. (2002) Effects of lyophilized black raspberries on azoxymethane-induced colon cancer and 8-hydroxy-2ʹ-deoxyguanosine levels in the Fischer 344 rat. *Nutr Cancer* **40**, 125–33.
13. Casto, B.C., Kresty, L.A., Kraly, C.L., Pearl, D.K., Knobloch, T.J., Schut, H.A., Stoner, G.D., Mallery, S.R., and Weghorst, C.M. (2002) Chemoprevention of oral cancer by black raspberries. *Anticancer Res* **22**, 4005–16.
14. Stoner, G.D., Chen, T., and Wang, L.-S. (2007) Chemoprevention of esophageal squamous cell carcinoma. *Toxicol Appl Pharmacol* **224**, 337–49.
15. Wang, Y., You, M., Reynolds, S.H., Stoner, G.D., and Anderson, M.W. (1990) Mutational activation of the cellular Harvey *ras* oncogene in rat esophageal papillomas induced by methylbenzylnitrosamine. *Cancer Res* **50**, 1591–5.
16. Stoner, G.D., Dombkowski, A.A., Reen, R.K., Cukovic, D., Salagrama, S., Wang, L.-S., and Lechner, J.F. (2008) Carcinogen-altered genes in rat esophagus positively modulated to normal levels of expression by both phenethyl isothiocyanate and black raspberries. *Cancer Res* **68**, 6460–7.
17. Stoner, G.D., and Aziz, R.M. (2007) Prevention and therapy of squamous cell carcinoma of the rodent esophagus using freeze-dried black raspberries. *Acta Pharmacol Sin* **9**, 1422–8.

18. Aiyer, H.S., Srinivasan, C., and Gupta, R.C. (2008) Dietary berries and ellagic acid diminish estrogen-mediated mammary tumorigenesis in ACI rats. *Nutr Cancer* **60**, 227–34.

19. Stoner, G.D., Chen, T., Kresty, L.A., Aziz, R.M., Reinemann, T., and Nines, R.G. (2006) Protection against esophageal cancer in rodents with lyophilized berries: Potential mechanisms. *Nutr Cancer* **54**, 33–46.

20. Carlton, P.S., Kresty, L.A., Siglin, J.C., Morgan, C., Lu, J., and Stoner, G.D. (2001) Inhibition of *N*-nitrosomethylbenzylamine-induced tumorigenesis in the rat esophagus by dietary freeze-dried strawberries. *Carcinogenesis* **22**, 441–6.

21. Aziz, R.M., Nines, R., Rodrigo, K., Harris, K., Hudson, T., Gupta, A., Morse, M., Carlton, P., and Stoner, G.D. (2002) The effect of freeze-dried blueberries on N-nitrosomethylbenzylamine tumorigenesis in the rat esophagus. *Pharmaceutical Biology* **40**, 43–49.

22. Carlton, P.S., Kresty, L.A., and Stoner, G.D. (2000) Failure of dietary lyophilized strawberries to inhibit 4-(methylnitrosamino)-1-(3-pyridyl)-1-butanone-and benzo[a]pyrene-induced lung tumorigenesis in strain A/J mice. *Cancer Lett* **159**, 113–7.

23. Borges, G., Roowi, S., Rouanet, J.M., Duthie, G.G., Lean, M.E., and Crozier, A. (2007) The bioavailability of raspberry anthocyanins and ellagitannins in rats. *Mol Nutr Food Res* **6**, 714–25.

24. Xue, H., Aziz, R.M., Sun, N., Cassady, J.M., Kamendulis, L.M., Xu, Y., Stoner, G.D., and Klaunig, J.E. (2001) Inhibition of cellular transformation by berry extracts. *Carcinogenesis* **22**, 351–61.

25. Huang, C., Huang, Y., Li, J., Hu, W., Aziz, R., Tang, M.-S., Sun, N., Cassady, J., and Stoner, G.D. (2002) Inhibition of BPDE-induced transactivation of AP-1 and NFκB by black raspberry extracts. *Cancer Res* **62**, 6857–63.

26. Han, C., Ding, H., Casto, B., Stoner, G.D., and D'Ambrosio, S.M. (2005) Inhibition of the growth of premalignant and malignant human oral cell lines by extracts and components of black raspberries. *Nutr Cancer* **51**, 207–17.

27. Rodrigo, K., Rawal, Y., Renner, R.J., Schwartz, S.J., Tian, Q., Larson, P.E., and Mallery, S.R. (2006) Suppression of the tumorigenic phenotype in human oral squamous cell carcinoma cells by an ethanol extract derived from freeze-dried black raspberries. *Nutr Cancer* **54**, 58–68.

28. Zikri, N., Hecht, S.S., Schwartz, S., Tian, Q., Carmella, S., Lechner, J.F., and Stoner, G.D. (2009) Black raspberry components inhibit proliferation, induce apoptosis and modulate gene expression in rat esophageal epithelial cells. *Nutr and Cancer* **61**, 816–26.

29. Hecht, S.S., Huang, C., Stoner, G.D., Li, J., Kenney, P.M.J., Sturla, S.J., and Carmella, S.G. (2006) Identification of cyanidin glycosides as constituents of freeze-dried black raspberries which inhibit anti-benzo(a)pyrene-7,8-diol-9,10-epoxide induced NFκB and AP-1 activity. *Carcinogenesis* **27**, 1617–26.

30. Lala, G., Malik, M., Zhao, C., He, J., Kwon, T., Guisti, M.M., and Magnuson, B.A. (2006) Anthocyanin-rich extracts inhibit multiple biomarkers of colon cancer in rats. *Nutr Cancer* **54**, 84–93.

31. Cooke, D., Schwartz, M., Boocock, D., Winterhalter, P., Steward, W.P., Gescher, A.J., and Marczylo, T.H. (2006) Effect of cyanidin-3-glucoside and an anthocyanin mixture from bilberry on adenoma development in the ApcMin mouse model of intestinal carcinogenesis – relationship with tissue anthocyanin levels. *Int J Cancer* **119**, 2213–20.

32. Chen, T., Hwang, H., Rose, M.E., Nines, R.G., and Stoner, G.D. (2006) Chemopreventive properties of black raspberries in *N*-nitrosomethylbenzylamine-induced rat esophageal tumorigenesis: Downregulation of COX-2, iNOS and c-Jun. *Cancer Res* **66**, 2853–9.

33. Chen, T., Rose, M.E., Hwang, H., Nines, R.G., and Stoner, G.D. (2006) Black raspberries inhibit *N*-Nitrosomethylbenzylamine-induced angiogenesis in rat esophagus parallel to the suppression of COX-2 and iNOS. *Carcinogenesis* **27**, 2301–7.

34. Lechner, J.F., Reen, R.K., Dombkowski, A.A., Cukovic, D., Salagrama, S., Wang, L.-S., and Stoner, G.D. (2008) Effects of a black raspberry diet on gene expression in the rat esophagus. *Nutr and Cancer* **60**, 61–69.

35. Colditz, G.A., Branch, L.G., Lipnick, R.J., Willett, W.C., Rosner, B., Posner, B.M., and Hennekens, C.H. (1985) Increased green and yellow vegetable intake and lowered cancer deaths in an elderly population. *Am J Clin Nutr* **41**, 32–36.

36. Michels, K.B., Giovannucci, E., Joshipura, K.J., Rosner, B.A., Stampfer, M.J., Fuchs, C.S., Colditz, G.A., Speizer, F.E., and Willett, W.C. (2000) Prospective study of fruit and vegetable consumption and incidence of colon and rectal cancers. *J Natl Cancer Inst* **92**, 1740–52.

37. Almendingen, K., Hofstad, B., and Morten, H.V. (2004) Dietary habits and growth and recurrence of colorectal adenomas: Results from a three-year endoscopic follow-up study. *Nutr Cancer* **49**, 131–8.

38. Chan, J.M., and Giovannucci, E.L. (2001) Vegetables, fruits, associated micronutrients, and risk of prostate cancer. *Epid Rev* **23**, 82–86.

39. Kahkonen, M.P., Hopia, A.I., and Heinonen, M. (2001) Berry phenolics and their antioxidant activity. *J Agric Food Chem* **49**, 4076–82.

40. Stoner, G.D., Zikri, N., Wang, Li.-S., Chen, T., Hecht, S.S., Huang, C., Sardo, C., and Lechner, J.F. (2007) Cancer prevention with freeze-dried berries and berry components. *Seminars Cancer Biol* **17**, 403–10.

41. Stoner, G.D., Sardo, C., Apseloff, G., Mullet, D., Wargo, W., Pound, V., Singh, A., Sanders, J., Aziz, R., Casto, B., and Sun, X.L. (2005) Pharmacokinetics of anthocyanins and ellagic acid in healthy volunteers fed freeze-dried black raspberries daily for 7 days. *J Clin Pharmacol* **45**, 1153–64.

42. Mallery, S.R., Stoner, G.D., Larsen, P.E., Fields, H.W., Rodrigo, K.A., Schwartz, S.J., Tian, Q., Dai, J., and Mumper, R.J. (2007) Formulation and *in-vitro* and *in-vivo* evaluation of a mucoadhesive gel containing freeze dried black raspberries: Implications for oral cancer chemoprevention. *Pharmaceut Res* **24**, 728–37.

43. Shumway, B.S., Kresty, L.A., Larsen, P.E., Zwick, J.C., Lu, B., Fields, H.W., Mumper, R.J., Stoner, G.D., and Mallery, S.R. (2008) Effects of a topically applied bioadhesive berry gel on loss of heterozygosity indices in premalignant oral lesions. *Clin Cancer Res* **14**, 2412–30.

44. Mallery, S.R., Zwick, J.C., Pei, P., Tong, M., Larsen, P.E., Shumway, B.S., Lu, B., Fields, H.W., Mumper, R.J., and Stoner, G.D. (2008) Application of a bioadhesive black raspberry gel modulates gene expression and reduces cyclooxygenase 2 protein in human premalignant oral lesions. *Cancer Res* **68**, 4945–57.

45. Spechler, S. (2002) Barrett's esophagus. *N Engl J Med* **346**, 836–42.

46. Kresty, L.A., Frankel, W.L., Hammond, C.D., Baird, M.E., Mele, J.M., Stoner, G.D., and Fromkes, J.J. (2006) Transitioning from preclinical to clinical chemopreventive assessments of lyophilized black raspberries: Interim results show berries modulate markers of oxidative stress in Barrett's esophagus patients. *Nutr Cancer* **54**, 148–56.

30 Pomegranate

David Heber

Key Points

1. The pomegranate fruit has been used for medicinal purposes since ancient times, but extensive research on the bioactive substances in the pomegranate has potential applications in the chemoprevention of common forms of cancer.
2. Pomegranates have been shown to contain 124 different phytochemicals, and some of these act in concert to exert antioxidant and anti-inflammatory effects on cancer cells. Pomegranate juice made by squeezing whole fruit has the highest concentration of ellagitannins of any commonly consumed juice and contains the unique ellagitannin, punicalagin.
3. Punicalagin is the largest molecular weight polyphenol known. Pomegranate ellagitannins are not absorbed intact into the blood stream but are hydrolyzed to ellagic acid over several hours in the intestine. They are also metabolized by gut flora into urolithins which are conjugated in the liver and excreted in the urine. These urolithins are also bioactive and inhibit prostate cancer cell growth. Inhibition of nuclear factor kappa-B activation has been shown in prostate cancer cells and in human prostate cancer xenografts in mice. Inhibition of angiogenesis by inhibition of HIF-1 alpha activation of VEGF has also been demonstrated in animals with xenografts.
4. In clinical studies, pomegranate juice administration led to a decrease in the rate of rise of prostate-specific antigen after primary treatment with surgery or radiation. Continued translational research on the chemopreventive potential of pomegranate ellagitannins is ongoing.

Key Words: Pomegranate; ellagitannins; prostate cancer; urolithins

1. INTRODUCTION

While it is widely accepted that eating a diet rich in fruits and vegetables may lead to a reduction in the risk of common forms of cancer and may be useful in cancer prevention, both basic and clinical evidences of benefits of particular classes of bioactive substances have been developed specifically for pomegranate juice and pomegranate juice extracts. Research on basic mechanisms of action in cell culture, animal model systems, and limited clinical research in prostate cancer patients has been carried out with pomegranate juice. Clinical studies demonstrated a marked reduction in the rate of increase of prostate-specific antigen (PSA), an important marker of prostate cancer

From: *Nutrition and Health: Bioactive Compounds and Cancer*
Edited by: J.A. Milner, D.F. Romagnolo, DOI 10.1007/978-1-60761-627-6_30,
© Springer Science+Business Media, LLC 2010

progression in men previously treated for prostate cancer. There has also been significant progress in defining the pharmacokinetics and metabolism of ellagitannins from pomegranate juice in humans.

2. BIOACTIVITY OF POMEGRANATE POLYPHENOLS AND METABOLITES

Ellagitannins (ETs) are a family of bioactive polyphenols from fruits and nuts such as pomegranates, black raspberries, raspberries, strawberries, walnuts, and almonds (1, 2). Squeezing whole pomegranate fruit (*Punica granatum* L.) yields the richest source of ellagitannins among fruit juices. This juice has been used for centuries in ancient cultures for medicinal purposes (3). Commercial pomegranate juice (PJ), which has recently become popular in the United States, has more potent antioxidant properties than other common fruit juices attributed to its high content of polyphenols. Emerging science has demonstrated anti-cancer effects with the most impressive data so far in prostate cancer. However, the inhibition of sub-cellular pathways of inflammation triggered by nuclear factor kappa-B (NF-κB), angiogenesis under hypoxic conditions triggered by hypoxia-inducible factor-1 alpha (HIF-1α), and cellular proliferation along with stimulation of apoptosis suggests that ellagitannins through multiple pathways may find utility as a dietary agent for the prevention and treatment of many common forms of cancer.

The most abundant polyphenols in PJ are ellagitannins (ETs), which are hydrolyzable tannins that release ellagic acid (EA) on hydrolysis (4) and following metabolism by gut flora form urolithins such as urolithin A (see Fig. 1). Punicalagin is unique to pomegranate and is part of a family of ellagitannins which include the minor tannins called punicalin and gallagic acid (structures not shown). All these ellagitannins have in common the ability to be hydrolyzed to ellagic acid resulting in a prolonged release into the blood of ellagic acid.

Among the pomegranate ETs, punicalagin, which is the largest polyphenol known with a molecular weight of greater than 1,000, has been reported to be responsible for over half of the juice's potent antioxidant activity (4). Punicalagin is most abundant in the fruit husk as opposed to the juicy seeds called arils found within the fruit. It is by pressing the whole fruit during processing that ellagitannins are extracted into PJ in significant quantities, reaching levels of >2 g/l juice (4). PJ also contains other polyphenols such as anthocyanins (cyanidin, delphinidin, and pelargonidin glycosides) and flavonols (quercetin, kaempferol, and luteolin glycosides) (4). In all some 124 phytochemicals have been identified in the pomegranate (5).

Following metabolism by gut flora, urolithins A and B are formed and conjugated in the liver prior to excretion in the urine over 12–56 h after a single administration of 8 oz of pomegranate juice. These urolithins circulate in the blood as well and can reach many of the target organs where the effects of pomegranate ellagitannins are noted.

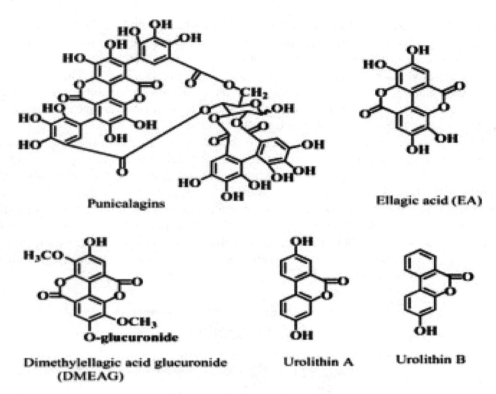

Punicalagins

Ellagic acid (EA)

O-glucuronide

Dimethylellagic acid glucuronide
(DMEAG)

Urolithin A

Urolithin B

Fig. 1. Chemical structures of punicalagin isomers, the major ET present in pomegranate juice and its metabolites, dimethylellagic acid glucuronide, ellagic acid, and urolithins A and B.

3. CANCER PREVENTIVE POTENTIAL OF POMEGRANATE POLYPHENOLS

Results from studies in cells, animals, and humans clearly point to the importance of following ellagitannin metabolites as markers of PJ intake and studying them in detail to explain the effects of PJ on inhibition of prostate cancer cell growth in vitro and in SCID mice with orthotopically transplanted human prostate cancer cells.

Our group and others have also shown that pomegranate fruit extract and its purified ETs inhibit the proliferation of human cancer cells and modulate inflammatory subcellular signaling pathways and apoptosis (6–8).

Based on the observation that a pomegranate fruit extract inhibited prostate cancer growth in athymic nude mice, some authors have proposed that anthocyanins are responsible for the inhibition observed (9). However, these studies did not identify the metabolites that might be responsible for this activity, and it is unlikely that anthocyanins account for the unique profile of activities observed with pomegranate juice and pomegranate extracts. In fact, ETs have previously been shown to exhibit in vitro and in vivo anticarcinogenic properties such as induction of cell-cycle arrest and apoptosis, as well as the inhibition of tumor formation and growth in animals *(10)*. Therefore, it is unnecessary to invoke the idea that the anthocyanins are required for the health benefits observed in cancer models and in the human intervention studies to date.

Inflammation is a hallmark of prostate cancer and is universally found in prostate tissue at the time of prostatectomy. Inflammation has also been implicated in colon cancer, breast cancer, and other common forms of cancer. In fact, proliferative inflammatory atrophy may be a precursor to PIN and prostate cancer *(11)*.

Multiple molecular targets are related to the inflammatory pathway in prostate and other types of cancer cells (see Fig. 2). Inflammatory cells are found in prostate tissue at the time of prostatectomy and expression of NF-κB is increased in more advanced lesions. In fact, nuclear localization of NF-κB is a risk factor for prostate cancer recurrence following prostatectomy *(12)*. In other cancers as well this transcription factor has been found to be central. It is fair to say that without this transcription factor, you cannot have inflammation. Whether this is the only pathway mediating the effects of ellagitannins is unknown and it is entirely possible that other interacting pathways reviewed below may well be involved.

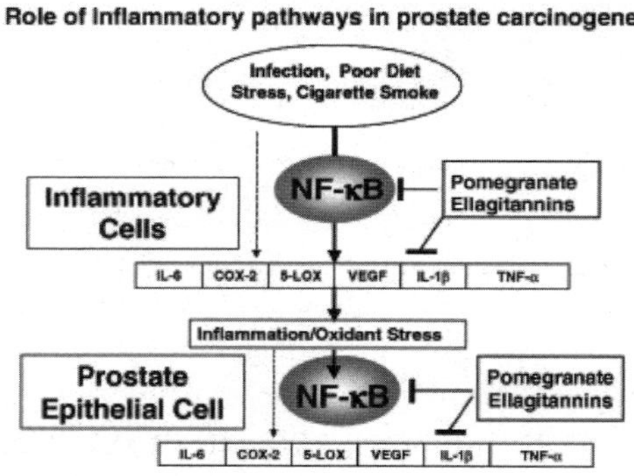

Fig. 2. NF-κB activation in inflammatory cells can lead to oxidant stress and inflammation in prostate epithelial cells. Constitutive activation of NF-κB is then found in prostate cancer cells and may be the result of the interaction of inflammatory stromal cells and epithelial cells.

NF-κB activation leads to immune activation, inflammation, and cell proliferation *(13, 14)*. NF-κB can also upregulate the transcription of genes that produce collagenases, cell adhesion molecules, and inflammatory cytokines including TNFα, IL-1, 2, 6, and 8 *(15–17)*. NF-κB regulates genes involved in the immune and inflammatory responses, as well as cell-cycle control and cell death in response to pro-inflammatory cytokines such as IL-1 and TNFα *(18, 19)*. NF-κB is also associated with the transcription of genes involved in cell survival such as Bcl_x and inhibitors of apoptosis.

Constitutive activation of NF-κB has been identified in prostate cancers *(20)*. Interestingly, the genes coding for the NF-κB proteins p52 and p65 have been mapped to sites of frequent rearrangement and amplification which give rise to many cancers. PC-3 and DU145 prostate cancer cell lines and prostate carcinoma xenografts have demonstrated constitutive NF-κB activity through constitutive activation of the IκB kinase α (IKKα) protein complex *(21–23)*.

Activation of NF-κB also regulates a number of downstream genes including cyclooxygenase-2 (COX-2). COX-2 is the key enzyme regulating the production of prostaglandins, central mediators of inflammation. The expression of cyclooxygenase-2 is induced by several extracellular signals including pro-inflammatory and growth-promoting stimuli. Expression of cyclooxygenase-2 mRNA is regulated by several transcription factors including the cyclic-AMP response element binding protein (CREB), NF-κB, and the CCAAT-enhancer binding protein (C/EBP). Cyclooxygenase-2 is also affected post-transcriptionally, at the level of mRNA stability. Inflammatory cells such as macrophages and mast cells release angiogenic factors and cytokines such as TNFα, IL-1, and VEGF *(24)* which signal cell growth and proliferation.

ETs and their hydrolysis product, ellagic acid (EA), inhibit prostate cancer cell growth through cell-cycle arrest and stimulation of apoptosis *(10, 25, 26)*. In addition, they inhibit the activation of inflammatory pathways including but not limited to the NF-κB pathway. Inhibition of angiogenesis has also been demonstrated both in vitro and in vivo for prostate cancer. The universal nature of these mechanisms in common forms of cancer suggests that pomegranate ellagitannins which have been tested in both prostate and colon cancer cells by our group may also be useful dietary agents for the prevention and treatment of other forms of cancer such as breast cancer.

4. MECHANISTIC INSIGHTS FROM CELL CULTURE AND ANIMAL STUDIES

In cell culture, combinations of ellagitannins are more potent than any single compound *(27–30)*. They have activity in combination against both prostate and colon cancer cells. While punicalagin is the most active of the ellagitannins, it is possible to design experiments which demonstrate the additional effects of the other phytochemicals found in pomegranate juice.

Overall, the significance of these in vitro findings is in doubt since only ellagic acid is found in the circulation after ingestion of pomegranate juice along with urolithins. The latter are formed by gut bacteria and recirculated through the liver prior to excretion in the urine. Urolithins also inhibit the growth of both androgen-dependent and androgen-independent prostate cancer cell lines, with IC_{50} values lower than EA. Future studies to evaluate the mechanistic basis for the anti-proliferative effects of urolithins are required. On the basis of current knowledge of polyphenol bioavailability, the IC_{50} values that we observed in the in vitro anti-proliferative assays far exceeded physiologically achievable levels.

Angiogenesis is critical to tumor growth and is stimulated by tissue hypoxia due to poor oxygen delivery. In turn, cellular hypoxia leads to angiogenesis via the induction of hypoxia-inducible factor-1alpha (HIF-1alpha) and vascular endothelial growth factor (VEGF) at a cellular level. Pomegranate juice and extracts, which are rich sources of ellagitannins, have been shown to have chemopreventive potential against prostate cancer, but there have been no studies on the effects of an ellagitannin-rich pomegranate extract on angiogenesis. Human prostate cancer cells (LNCaP) and human umbilical vein endothelial cells (HUVEC) were incubated with a pomegranate extract standardized to ellagitannin content (POMx), under normoxic and hypoxic conditions in vitro.

POMx inhibited the proliferation of LNCaP and HUVEC cells significantly under both normoxic and hypoxic conditions. HIF-1 alpha and VEGF protein levels were also reduced by POMx under hypoxic conditions *(30)*.

Recently there have been a number of reports on anti-proliferative, pro-apoptotic, and antiangiogenic activities by pomegranate polyphenols, as well as inhibition of NF-κβ activity and xenograft growth *(6, 25, 26)*. In a recent study from our group (Sartippour et al.) human prostate cancer cells (LAPC4) were injected subcutaneously into severe combined immunodeficient (SCID) mice and the effects of oral administration of POMx on tumor growth, microvessel density, and HIF-1alpha and VEGF expression were determined after 4 weeks of treatment. POMx decreased prostate cancer xenograft size, tumor vessel density, VEGF peptide levels, and HIF-1alpha expression after 4 weeks of treatment in SCID mice *(30)*. These results demonstrate that an ellagitannin-rich pomegranate extract can inhibit tumor-associated angiogenesis as one of several potential mechanisms for slowing the growth of prostate cancer in chemopreventive applications. Further studies in humans are needed to confirm that angiogenesis can be inhibited by an ellagitannin-rich pomegranate extract administered orally as a dietary supplement.

5. EVIDENCE OF BIOACTIVITY FROM HUMAN CLINICAL STUDIES

A clinical study in men with rising PSA after surgery or radiotherapy was begun in January, 2003. Eligible patients had a detectable PSA greater than 0.2 ng/ml and less than 5 ng/ml, and a Gleason score of 7 or less. Patients were treated with 8 oz of pomegranate juice daily (wonderful variety, 570 mg total polyphenol gallic acid equivalents). Interim results were published in 2007 *(31)* and showed a significant increase in mean PSA doubling time following treatment, from 15 months at baseline to 54 months post-treatment ($p < 0.001$). The PSA doubling time is a predictor of survival in prostate cancer patients with recurrent disease. The study was amended to allow patients to continue treatment and to undergo evaluation in 3 month intervals until disease progression. In an ex vivo mitogenic bioassay, serum obtained from these PJ-treated patients who were given 8 oz of PJ daily for 2 years also inhibited proliferation and stimulated apoptosis of LNCaP prostate cancer cells in vitro. Future studies have been designed to determine if EA, urolithins, and related metabolites in patient sera are responsible for these anti-proliferative and pro-apoptotic effects.

6. DETAILED STUDIES OF BIOAVAILABILITY AND METABOLISM

Since bioavailability of phytochemicals is critical to their bioactivity, this was studied in 18 volunteers to quantitate the plasma appearance and disappearance rates of EA hydrolyzed from ET's in administered PJ *(32)*. In addition, it was demonstrated that the absorbed EA hydrolyzed from PJ punicalagin is converted to dimethylellagic acid glucuronide in plasma and urine on the day of administration of PJ *(32, 33)*. Urolithins derived from EA appeared in human urine after the disappearance of DMEAG about 12 h after juice administration.

Additional bioavailability data on DMEAG and urolithins were obtained in mice in support of our planned studies of PJ effects on orthotopically transplanted LNCaP cells in SCID mice *(34)*. Studies in rats and in humans have shown that ETs are hydrolyzed in the gut to EA and that EA is metabolized by the colon microflora to form the urolithins A and B. Urolithins can be absorbed into the enterohepatic circulation and excreted in urine and feces *(35–37)*. EA and urolithins can accumulate in the intestine and prostate *(34, 38)*. ET's, EA, and urolithin-A exhibit cancer chemopreventive activities in various cell and animal models. Oral administration of PE to wild-type mice led to increased plasma levels of EA, but EA was not detected in the prostate gland. On the other hand, intraperitoneal administration of PE led to 10-fold higher EA levels in the plasma and detectable and higher EA levels in the prostate, intestine, and colon relative to other organ systems. The detectable EA levels in prostate tissue following intraperitoneal but not oral administration were likely due to higher plasma levels attained after intraperitoneal administration.

Intraperitoneal and oral administration of synthesized UA led to uptake of UA and it conjugates in prostate tissue, and UA levels were higher in prostate, colon, and intestinal tissues relative to other organs. It is unclear why pomegranate ET metabolites localize at higher levels in prostate, colon, and intestinal tissues relative to the other organs studied. Importantly, the predilection of bioactive pomegranate ET metabolites to localize in prostate tissue, combined with clinical data demonstrating the anti-cancer effects of PJ, suggests the potential for pomegranate products to play a role in prostate cancer chemoprevention. Whether urolithins in human prostate tissue can be used as a biomarker following long-term administration of PJ or PE remains to be determined.

7. CONCLUSIONS

The ellagitannins found in pomegranate fruit are very potent antioxidants exceeding the in vitro antioxidant potency of other common refrigerated juices *(39)*. While there are limited treatment options for prostate cancer patients who have undergone primary therapy such as radical prostatectomy with curative intent but have progressive elevation of their PSA, PJ given daily for 2 years to 40 prostate cancer patients with rising PSA provides evidence for the possible utilization of a non-toxic option for prevention or delay of prostate carcinogenesis. It is remarkable that 85% of patients responded to PJ in this study. Both in vitro and in vivo investigations in prostate cancer models of the molecular mechanisms that may account for these PJ effects have been explored.

However, while researchers tend to focus on the idea of a single pathway, it is evident that pomegranate ellagitannins like other phytochemicals work through multiple targeted pathways. Nonetheless, evidence that NF-κB activation is associated with heightened proliferation, increased neo-angiogenesis, and resistance to apoptosis suggests that the anti-tumor action of PJ polyphenols is significantly mediated through their NF-κB inhibitory effects. This hypothesis is given added support by the recent implication of NF-κB as an independent risk factor for PSA rise (i.e., biochemical recurrence) after prostatectomy. Studies of the effects of pomegranate juice and dietary supplements made from pomegranate extract in patients prior to prostatectomy and after biochemical recurrence with rising PSA are ongoing and should provide further information on the prostate cancer preventive and treatment potential of the juice made from this ancient fruit. Additional studies in other forms of cancer including colon cancer and breast cancer may reveal additional potentials for pomegranate juice in cancer chemoprevention.

REFERENCES

1. Clifford, M.N., and Scalbert, A. (2000) Ellagitannins-nature, occurrence and dietary burden. *J Sci Food Agric* **80**, 1118–25.
2. Amakura, Y., Okada, M., Sumiko, T., and Tonogai, Y. (2000) High-performance liquid chromatographic determination with photodiode array detection of ellagic acid in fresh and processed fruits. *J Chromatogr A* **896**, 87–93.
3. Longtin, R. (2003) The pomegranate: Nature's power fruit? *J Natl Cancer Inst* **95**, 346–8.
4. Gil, M.I., Tomas-Barberan, F.A., Hess-Pierce, B., Holcroft, D.M., and Kader, A.A. (2000) Antioxidant activity of pomegranate juice and its relationship with phenolic composition and processing. *J Agric Food Chem* **48**, 4581–9.
5. Seeram, N.P., Schulman, R.N., and Heber, D. (2006) Pomegranates: Ancient Roots to Modern Medicine. Boca Raton, Florida: CRC Press.
6. Afaq, F., Saleem, M., Krueger, C.G., Reed, J.D., and Mukhtar, H. (2005) Anthocyanin- and hydrolysable tannin-rich pomegranate fruit extract modulates MAPK and NF-κB pathways and inhibits skin tumorigenesis in CD-1 mice. *Int J Cancer* **113**, 423–33.
7. Seeram, N.P., Adams, L.S., Henning, S.M., Niu, Y., Zhang, Y., Nair, M.G., and Heber, D. (2005) In vitro antiproliferative, apoptotic and antioxidant activities of punicalagin, ellagic acid and a total pomegranate tannin extract are enhanced in combination with other polyphenols as found in pomegranate juice. *J Nutr Biochem* **16**, 360–7.
8. Adams, L.S., Seeram, N.P., Aggarwal, B.B., Takada, Y., Sand, D., and Heber, D. (2006) Pomegranate juice, total pomegranate tannins and punicalagin suppress inflammatory cell signaling in colon cancer cells. *J Agric Food Chem* **54**, 980–5.
9. Malik, A., Afaq, F., Sarfaraz, S., Adhami, V.M., Syed, D.N., and Mukhtar, H. (2005) Pomegranate fruit juice for chemoprevention and chemotherapy of prostate cancer. *Proc Natl Acad Sci USA* **102**, 14813–8.
10. Castonguay, A., Gali, H.U., Perchellet, E.M., Gao, X.M., Boukharta, M., Jalbert, G. et al. (1997) Antitumorigenic and antipromoting activities of ellagic acid, ellagitannins and ligomeric anthocyanin and procyanidin. *Int J Oncol* **10**, 367–73.
11. De Marzo, A.M., Meeker, A.K., Zha, S., Luo, J., Nakayama, M., and Platz, E.A. (2003) Human prostate cancer precursors and pathobiology. *Urology* **62**, 55–62.
12. Fradet, L., Bégin, L.R., Karakiewicz, P., Masson, A.M., and Saad, F. (2004) Nuclear factor-kappaB nuclear localization is predictive of biochemical recurrence in patients with positive margin prostate cancer. *Clin Cancer Res* **10**, 8460–4.
13. Biswas, D.K., Curz, A.P., Gansberger, E., and Pardee, A.B. (2000) Epidermal growth factor-induced nuclear factor kappa B activation: A major pathway of cell-cycle progression in estrogen-receptor negative breast cancer cells. *Proc Natl Acad Sci USA* **97**, 8542–7.
14. Kim, D.W., Sovak, M.A., and Zanieski, G. (2000) Activation of NF-kappaB/Rel occurs early during neoplastic transformation of mammary cells. *Carcinogenesis* **21**, 871–9.
15. Conner, E.M., and Grisham, M.B. (1996) Inflammation, free radicals and antioxidants. *Nutrition* **12**, 274–7.
16. Allison, A.C. (1997) Antioxidant drug targeting. *Adv Pharmacol* **38**, 273–91.
17. Winyard, P.G., and Blake, D.R. (1997) Antioxidants, redox-regulated transcription factors and inflammation. *Adv Pharmacol* **38**, 403–21.
18. Mayo, M.W., and Baldwin, A.S. (2000) The transcription factor NF-kappaB: Control of oncogenesis and cancer therapy resistance. *Biochim Biophys Acta* **1470**, M55–M62.
19. Rayet, B., and Gelinas, C. (1999) Aberrant rel/nfκb genes and activity in human cancer. *Oncogene* **18**, 6938–45.

20. Domingo-Domenech, J., Mellado, B., Ferrer, B., Truan, D., Codony-Servat, B., Sauleda, S. et al. (2005) Activation of nuclear factor-kappaB in human prostate carcinogenesis and association to biochemical relapse. *Br J Cancer* **93**, 1285–94.

21. Palayoor, S.T., Youmell, M.Y., Claderwood, S.K., Coleman, C.N., and Price, B.D. (1999) Constitutive activation of IkB kinase a and NFκB in prostate cancer cells is inhibited by ibuprofen. *Oncogene* **18**, 7389–94.

22. Gasparian, A.V., Yao, Y.J., Kowalczyk, D., Lyakh, L.A., Karseladze, A., Slaga, T.J. et al. (2002) The role of IKK in sonctitutive activation of NF-kappaB in pancreatic carcinoma cells. *J Cell Sci* **155**, 141–51.

23. Suh, J., Payvandi, F., Edelstein, L., Amenta, P., Zong, W., Gelinas, C. et al. (2002) Mechanisms of constitutive NFκB activation in human prostate cancer cells. *Prostate* **52**, 183–200.

24. O'Byrne, K.J., and Dalgleish, A.G. (2001) Chronic immune activation and inflammation as the cause of malignancy. *Br J Cancer* **85**, 473–83.

25. Lansky, E.P., Jiang, W., Mo, H., Bravo, L., Froom, P., Yu, W., Harris, N.M., Neeman, I., and Campbell, M.J. (2005) Possible synergistic prostate cancer suppression by anatomically discrete pomegranate fractions. *Invest New Drugs* **23**, 11–20.

26. Albrecht, M., Jiang, W., Kumi-Diaka, J. et al. (2004) Pomegranate extracts potently suppress proliferation, xenograft growth, and invasion of human prostate cancer cells. *J Med Food* **7**, 274–83.

27. Losso, J.N., Bansode, R.R., Trappey, A., Bawadi, A.A., and Truax, R. (2004) In vitro anti-proliferative activities of ellagic acid. *J Nutr Biochem* **15**, 672–8.

28. Narayanan, B.A., Geoffroy, O., Willingham, M.C., Re, G.G., and Nixon, D.W. (1999) p53/p21(WAF1/CIP1) expression and its possible role in G1 arrest and apoptosis in ellagic acid treated cancer cells. *Cancer Lett* **136**, 215–21.

29. Seeram, N.P., Adams, L.S., Henning, S.M., Niu, Y., Zhang, Y., Nair, M.G., and Heber, D. (2005) In vitro antiproliferative, apoptotic and antioxidant activities of punicalagin, ellagic acid and a total pomegranate tannin extract are enhanced in combination with other polyphenols as found in pomegranate juice. *J Nutr Biochem* **16**, 360–7.

30. Sartippour, M.R., Seeram, N.P., Rao, J.Y., Moro, A., Harris, D.M., Henning, S.M., and Heber, D. (2008) Ellagitannin-rich pomegranate extract inhibits angiogenesis in prostate cancer in vitro and in vivo. *Int J Oncol* **32**, 475–80.

31. Pantuck, A.J., Leppert, J.T., Zomorodian, N., Aronson, W., Hong, J., Barnard, R.J., Seeram, N.P., Liker, H., Wang, H., Elashoff, R., Heber, D., Aviram, M., Ignarro, L., and Belldegrun, A. (2006) Phase II study of pomegranate juice for men with rising prostate-specific antigen following surgery or radiation for prostate cancer. *Clin Cancer Res* **12**, 4018–26.

32. Seeram, N.P., Lee, R., and Heber, D. (2004) Bioavailability of ellagic acid in human plasma after consumption of ellagitannins from pomegranate (*Punica granatum* L.) juice. *Clin Chim Acta* **348**, 63–68.

33. Seeram, N.P., Henning, S.M., Zhang, Y., Suchard, M., Li, Z., and Heber, D. (2006) Pomegranate juice ellagitannin metabolites are present in human plasma and some persist in urine for up to 48 hours. *J Nutr* **136**, 2481–5.

34. Seeram, N.P., Aronson, W.J., Zhang, Y., Henning, S.M., Moro, A., Lee, R.P., and Heber, D. (2007) Pomegranate ellagitannin-derived metabolites inhibit prostate cancer growth and localize to the mouse prostate gland. *J Agric Food Chem* **55**, 7732–7.

35. Cerdá, B., Llorach, R., Cerón, J.J., Espín, J.C., and Tomás-Barberán, F.A. (2003) Evaluation of the bioavailability and metabolism in the rat of punicalagin, an antioxidant polyphenol from pomegranate juice. *Eur J Nutr* **42**, 18–28.

36. Cerdá, B., Espín, J.C., Parra, S., Martínez, P., and Tomás-Barberán, F.A. (2004) The potent in vitro antioxidant ellagitannins from pomegranate juice are metabolised into bioavailable but poor antioxidant hydroxy-6H-dibenzopyran-6-one derivatives by the colonic microflora of healthy humans. *Eur J Nutr* **43**, 205–20.

37. Espín, J.C., González-Barrio, R., Cerdá, B., López-Bote, C., Rey, A.I., and Tomás-Barberán, F.A. (2007) Iberian pig as a model to clarify obscure points in the bioavailability and metabolism of ellagitannins in humans. *J Agric Food Chem* **55**, 10476–85.

38. Larrosa, M., Tomás-Barberán, F.A., and Espín, J.C. (2006) The dietary hydrolysable tannin punicalagin releases ellagic acid that induces apoptosis in human colon adenocarcinoma Caco-2 cells by using the mitochondrial pathway. *J Nutr Biochem* **17**, 611–25.
39. Seeram, N.P., Aviram, M., Zhang, Y., Henning, S.M., Feng, L., Dreher, M., and Heber, D. (2008) Comparison of antioxidant potency of commonly consumed polyphenol-rich beverages in the United States. *J Agric Food Chem* **56**, 1415–22.

31 Alcohol and Cancer: Biological Basis

Keith Singletary

Key Points

1. For decades, it has been well documented that alcohol intake increases risk for cancers of the upper aerodigestive tract (oral cavity, pharynx, larynx, and esophagus), especially at high levels of intake, as well as for breast, colon, and liver cancers.
2. Many types of cancer associations were observed for all types of alcoholic beverages, suggesting that ethanol is the main carcinogenic constituent of alcohol drinks.
3. Alcohol has multiple actions in modifying carcinogenesis, not only directly, such as disordering cell membranes, but also indirectly, such as a consequence of ethanol oxidation to acetaldehyde and other reactive intermediates.
4. The magnitude, specificity, and variability of ethanol's actions can depend on the dose and duration of exposure and on specific biochemical and molecular characteristics of the tissues to which ethanol comes in contact.
5. The possible mechanisms underlying alcohol's carcinogenicity include the causation of DNA damage by alcohol's metabolic product acetaldehyde, alcohol's effect in increasing estrogen levels, alcohol being a solvent for carcinogens, alcohol-induced generation of reactive oxygen species, alcohol-associated alterations in nutritional status, and deleterious effects of alcohol on the host immune system.

Key Words: Alcohol; ethanol; acetaldehyde; carcinogen; oxidative stress; hormones; cancer

1. INTRODUCTION

For decades, it has been well documented that alcohol intake increases the risk for cancers of the upper aerodigestive tract (oral cavity, pharynx, larynx, and esophagus), especially at high levels of intake *(1–4)*. For instance, as early as 1977, alcohol intake was identified as a risk factor for breast cancer and resulted in numerous subsequent epidemiological reports supporting the role of alcohol in breast cancer causation *(5, 6)*. In fact, alcohol's interrelationship with breast cancer was listed as 1 of the top 10 greatest recent discoveries in nutrition *(7)*. Thus, alcohol consumption can augment to varying degrees carcinogenesis at several organ sites including those in

From: *Nutrition and Health: Bioactive Compounds and Cancer*
Edited by: J.A. Milner, D.F. Romagnolo, DOI 10.1007/978-1-60761-627-6_31,
© Springer Science+Business Media, LLC 2010

the upper aerodigestive tract, liver, colon, and breast. The epidemiological evidence for the role of alcohol in these and other cancers has recently been reviewed in depth *(5)* and will not be discussed at length in this chapter. The evidence that alcohol enhances cancer risk is strongest for tumors of the upper aerodigestive tract (UADT), colon (particularly in men), and the female breast *(5, 6, 8–10)*. There is also strong evidence that alcohol intake is an independent risk factor for liver cancer, especially as a consequence of cirrhosis *(4)*. Collectively, data from various animal models provide supportive evidence that ethanol can increase cancer when provided alone (liver, head, neck, fore-stomach, and breast) and when co-administered with known carcinogens *(2, 11–14)*. In these carcinogen-induced animal tumor models, ethanol has been observed to be a stimulator of both the initiation and the post-initiation stages of experimental carcinogenesis *(15–28)*. In light of the total evidence, the IARC has concluded that there is "sufficient evidence" of ethanol's carcinogenicity in animals *(2, 11)*. Likewise based on findings of epidemiological studies and preclinical mechanistic data, the IARC indicates that alcohol drinking is "carcinogenic to humans" *(2, 11)*. In general, these cancer associations were observed for all types of alcoholic beverages, suggesting that ethanol is the main carcinogenic constituent of alcohol drinks. It also should be kept in mind that many of these alcohol–cancer associations are most prominent at high levels of alcohol consumption. The biological basis for this enhancing effect of alcohol intake on these various cancers remains an area of active scientific inquiry, especially the extent to which other dietary and lifestyle factors and genetic predisposition can modify the impact of alcohol on cancer risk *(29)*. This chapter, therefore, will focus on providing insights into potential mechanisms of action whereby alcohol stimulates cancer development and highlighting areas for future investigation.

It is readily apparent that alcohol has multiple actions in modifying carcinogenesis, not only directly, such as disordering cell membranes, but also indirectly, such as a consequence of ethanol oxidation to acetaldehyde and other reactive intermediates *(2, 4, 16, 29–31)*. The magnitude, specificity, and variability in ethanol's actions can depend on the dose and duration of exposure and on specific biochemical and molecular characteristics of the target tissues. A recent summary of possible mechanisms underlying alcohol's carcinogenicity provides strong evidence that acetaldehyde causes DNA damage and alcohol increases estrogen levels; moderate evidence that alcohol is a solvent for carcinogens, generates reactive oxygen species (ROS), and alters folate status; and weak evidence that alcohol causes cancer by reducing host defenses and causing nutritional deficiencies *(2)*.

The literature may use various terms to describe units of alcohol consumption. Generally in the United States, an alcoholic drink is recognized to contain about 14 g of ethanol which translates to approximately 1.5 oz (44 ml) of liquor, a 5 oz (148 ml) glass of wine, or a 12 oz (355 ml) glass of beer. For purposes of this overview, high alcohol intake is considered ≥3 drinks/day. Furthermore, the term alcohol will be used interchangeably with the word ethanol, the major biologically active constituent of alcoholic beverages.

2. ETHANOL METABOLISM: ACETALDEHYDE AND OXIDATIVE STRESS

Ingested ethanol is absorbed predominantly in the stomach and duodenum and is eliminated from the body by several metabolic processes. The liver is the main site of ethanol metabolism, although it may occur in other tissues. Individual variability in absorption, distribution, and elimination of ethanol is affected by genetic and environmental factors, which cumulatively can contribute to differences in the clinical consequences, harmful effects, and cancer risks associated with chronic ethanol consumption *(4, 32–35)*.

There are three metabolic pathways for the oxidation of ethanol to its primary product acetaldehyde (Fig. 1), a known carcinogen *(36)*. Peroxisomal catalase-mediated metabolism to acetaldehyde is considered a minor pathway. A second oxidative pathway involving microsomal cytochrome P4502E1 (CYP2E1)-catalyzed conversion of ethanol to acetaldehyde may have particular importance in metabolizing ethanol in non-liver tissues, especially those lacking appreciable alcohol dehydrogenase (ADH) activity. CYP2E1-dependent ethanol oxidation (Km = 8–10 mM) plays a greater role in ethanol elimination following consumption of large amounts of alcohol that subsequently result in elevated blood alcohol content. Reactive oxygen species (ROS) such as hydroxyl radicals, superoxide anions, and hydroxyethyl radicals are also a by-product of cytochrome P450 catalysis and can contribute to cancer-promoting tissue damage. By far the major contributor to ethanol oxidation to acetaldehyde is cytosolic ADH (Km of liver

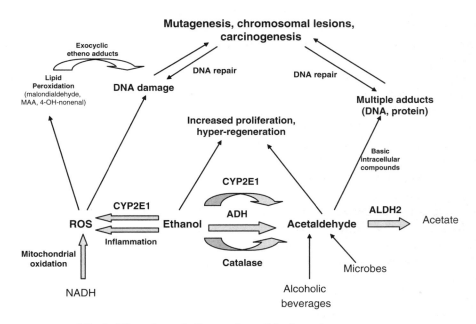

Fig. 1. Ethanol metabolism and possible damaging outcomes.

ADH = 0.2–2.0 mM). Acetaldehyde is subsequently converted to acetate *(37)* through a reaction catalyzed primarily by mitochondrial acetaldehyde dehydrogenase 2 (ALDH2). To a smaller extent acetaldehyde may also be detoxified in the liver by CYP2E1, which is referred to as the microsomal acetaldehyde oxidizing system *(38)*. Acetate ultimately can be oxidized to CO_2 or metabolized to acetyl-CoA. Allelic variation in ADH and ALDH2 enzymes, as discussed below, may have considerable impact on risk for several alcohol-related cancers. Particularly, individuals with elevated acetaldehyde levels following drinking due to increased formation and/or impaired elimination exhibit higher rates of alcohol-related cancers and other problems. There also are nonoxidative pathways of ethanol metabolism to phosphatidyl ethanol (catalyzed by phospholipase D) and fatty acid ethyl esters that, to date, make only a small contribution to ethanol's impact on carcinogenesis *(36)*.

Acetaldehyde, the primary oxidative metabolite of ethanol, is considered to be an important mediator of ethanol's cancer-promoting actions, particularly in the upper aerodigestive tract (UADT) and colon *(39–41)*. Actually, exposure of tissues to acetaldehyde may come from several sources. First, alcoholic beverages, especially whiskey and beer, may contain high levels of acetaldehyde *(4)*. Second, as discussed above, acetaldehyde can be formed from ethanol by ADH in a variety of tissues such as liver, UADT mucosa, colon, and the parotid glands. An under-appreciated third source of acetaldehyde results from microbial metabolism of ethanol in the oral cavity and the colon *(4, 42)*. Salivary acetaldehyde concentrations measured after ethanol intake have been detected at levels many-fold higher than those in corresponding blood samples, a response that can be ameliorated by using an antibiotic rinse prior to consuming alcohol *(43)*. In alcoholics it has been also noted that smoking and poor oral hygiene can further increase acetaldehyde levels *(44)*. Likewise, in the colon, high acetaldehyde levels may be a consequence of microbial oxidation of ethanol *(45)*. Depending on the organ, *Neisseria* species, *Streptococcus* (viridans group), *Rothia* species, and the yeast *Candida albicans* are micro-organisms identified as being potential participants in this conversion *(46, 47)*. High levels of acetaldehyde in the oral cavity also may be explained by the fact that the ALDH activity of microbes and oral mucosa is low. Dissimilarities in relative activities of ADH and ALDH have been observed at several sites along the GI tract. For example, Yin et al. *(48, 49)* reported that esophageal ADH activity was 4-fold higher than ADH activity in the gastric mucosa, whereas esophageal ALDH activity was 20% stomach ALDH activity. This would then account for selective tissue accumulation of acetaldehyde during alcohol ingestion. Of interest, alcohol consumers with the less active aldehyde dehydrogenase enzyme encoded by the ALDH2*2 allele exhibited 2–3-fold higher concentrations of acetaldehyde in the mouth compared to those with normal ALDH2, and salivary acetaldehyde concentrations 9-fold higher than blood levels *(50)*. Tissue accumulation and toxicity of acetaldehyde also may be a concern in other sites beyond the UADT. Recently, it was reported that acute oral administration of ethanol to female rats (0.6 g–6.3 g/kg body weight) resulted in prolonged accumulation of acetaldehyde in mammary tissue to levels higher than those measured in blood *(51)*. These researchers also have suggested that, at least in mammary tissue, xanthine oxidoreductase and CYP2E1 may be additional enzymes contributing to steady-state acetaldehyde levels *(52–54)*.

Acetaldehyde is considered by the International Agency for Research on Cancer (IARC) as a human carcinogen, and is classified as an animal carcinogen, too. In rodents acetaldehyde inhalation leads to nasal and laryngeal cancers and its consumption leads to hyperproliferation and inflammation of UADT mucosa *(2)*. In humans, those populations having allelic variants that lead to higher tissue exposure to acetaldehyde have higher cancer risks *(4, 50, 55)*.

Acetaldehyde's action as a carcinogen is due, in part, to its genotoxicity and the consequent generation of genetic abnormalities *(56–59)*. Both stable and unstable adducts can be formed not only with specific amino acid residues of proteins but also with nucleic acids (such as that formed by reaction with deoxyguanosine, N2-ethyl-dG). Covalent DNA adduct formation is considered to be a critical initiating event in the process of chemically induced cancer. This DNA adduct and acetaldehyde can be detected in human urine, although the extent of its mutagenicity in cancer target tissues is not well characterized *(60, 61)*. In Aldh2–/– mice, having minimal capacity to metabolize away acetaldehyde, consumption of ethanol led to higher covalent binding of ethanol metabolites to DNA in several organs compared to Aldh 2+/+ mice with normal acetaldehyde oxidizing capacity *(62)*. In human alcohol abusers, white blood cell (WBC) acetaldehyde–DNA adducts may reach levels 7-fold greater than those in non-consumers *(63)*. Habitual or moderate drinkers with polymorphisms in alcohol metabolizing enzymes that lead to elevated circulating acetaldehyde have significantly higher frequencies of sister chromatid exchanges and micronuclei frequency in peripheral lymphocytes, an established biomarker of genomic instability *(64–67)*. DNA–acetaldehyde adducts can be formed in a dose-dependent manner even at low concentrations that are relatively nontoxic to human buccal epithelial cells *(57)*. Moreover, acetaldehyde in combination with other biological molecules (such as polyamines) that accumulate in tissues damaged by ethanol exposure may generate other forms of stable DNA damage such as crotonaldehyde–DNA and N2-propano-dG–DNA adducts that can lead to particularly damaging DNA–DNA and DNA–protein cross-links *(56)*. Again, habitual drinkers with polymorphisms leading to inactive forms of ALDH2 evidence a greater frequency of chromosomal aberrations and other evidence of genetic damage in blood samples *(68)*. What may compound this carcinogenic and genotoxic action of acetaldehyde is that it also may bind to and compromise the function of cellular proteins involved in DNA synthesis and repair, in maintaining normal DNA cytosine methylation and in mounting antioxidant defenses *(69–71)*. Furthermore, ethanol metabolism may disrupt critical intracellular signaling events that contribute to maintaining genomic stability *(72, 73)*. Recently, for example, ethanol-treated hepatic cells exhibited more highly acetylated microtubules, presumably due to acetaldehyde, that substantially disrupted microtubule integrity *(74)*. Acetaldehyde–protein adducts and malondialdehyde adducts (generated from lipid peroxidation) also may stimulate an immune response and induce inflammatory processes particularly in certain types of liver cells, all of which can further exacerbate local tissue damage and elevate disease risk *(58, 75–77)*. Acetaldehyde may contribute to precancerous lesion formation, as has been reported in the colon (accelerated crypt cell formation, polyp formation, and hyper-regeneration) and in the oral cavity (leukoplakia) *(78–81)*.

There is another consequence of ethanol metabolism that may be important in contributing to cancer particularly in the liver and that is the generation of oxidative stress *(32, 58, 82–85)*. ROS may be produced by multiple pathways that are triggered following consumption of ethanol (Fig. 1). For example, ethanol oxidation via P4502E1 and oxidation in the mitochondria of NADH (that is generated by ADH as ethanol is oxidized) produce ROS. Ethanol-associated inflammation also can produce ROS. Besides contributing to liver cirrhosis and cancer, ROS generation may also be associated with extrahepatic cancers. For example, ethanol-induced oxidative stress and acetaldehyde formation have been detected in rat mammary tissue that was accompanied by ultracellular aberrations in epithelial cell structure *(52, 54)*. The magnitude of ROS generated depends on the amounts of ethanol consumed as well as the individual's genotype encoding for ethanol metabolizing enzymes. Whatever the source of increased ROS, the consequences can include increased direct DNA damage (such as formation of 8-oxo-dG) or indirect DNA damage following ROS-induced lipid peroxidation. Lipid peroxidation produces malondialdehyde, 4-OH nonenal, and other metabolites, all of which subsequently can form adducts and modify cellular proteins *(75, 86)*. In fact, exocyclic etheno adducts, generated by reaction of DNA bases with lipid peroxidation products such as trans-4-hydroxy-2-nonenal, can be detected in the urine of alcoholics with fatty liver. There are other damaging cellular consequences of ROS formation. For example, in mouse liver the oxidation of cytosolic proteins, such as those participating in stress responses, intermediary metabolism, and antioxidant defense, leads to increased protein degradation *(87)*. This may certainly create cellular dysfunction and susceptibility to toxic agents that are contributors to cancer development. Moreover, oxidative stress may contribute to redox imbalance and disturbances in signaling cascades within liver cells, such as those described for mitogen-activated protein (MAP) kinases, NFkappaB, and AP-1 *(88)*. The extent to which these ROS-induced processes of protein degradation and signaling disruption occur in tissues other than the liver deserves further study and is likely to depend on the dose of ethanol.

Lastly, exposure of tissues to ethanol-generated ROS and acetaldehyde can lead to enhanced cell proliferation and damage-induced hyper-regeneration *(81)*, at least in the gastrointestinal tract. Such consequences of acetaldehyde and ROS formation combined with their genotoxic effects and their impairment of cellular repair capacities likely contribute to a tissue environment conducive to cancer promotion.

3. ALCOHOL AND CARCINOGEN BIOACTIVATION

Direct exposure of tissues to ethanol such as occurs in the UADT may lead to solvent effects of ethanol on membranes that may enhance the bioavailability of tobacco-related and other carcinogens. Carcinogens and xenobiotics normally can be metabolized and detoxified to excretable forms by numerous enzymes *(84, 89)*. However, in numerous tissues ethanol may stimulate carcinogenesis by inducing enzymes involved in carcinogen bioactivation *(84, 89–93)*. Specifically, ethanol may induce enzymes that metabolically activate inert procarcinogens to DNA-reactive intermediates. Decades ago it was discovered that chronic exposure of the liver to ethanol resulted in increased activity of the cytochrome P450s of the microsomal ethanol oxidizing system, especially CYP2E1

(84). There is substantial human variability in CYP2E1 induction but, nonetheless, its induction can increase the metabolic activation of such carcinogens as hydrazines and nitrosamines *(94)*. Likewise, induction of CYP3A4 and possibly CYP1A2 by ethanol increases activation of such procarcinogens as aflatoxin and heterocyclic amines such as 2-amino-1-methyl-6-phenylimidazo[4,5-*b*]pyridine (PhIP), which in animals are know to cause tumor formation in several tissues *(90, 91)*. The induction of CYP 3A4 activity was due to multiple mechanisms including stabilization of mRNA and protein *(91)*. It is of interest to note that exposure of human breast epithelial cells to ethanol and acetaldehyde increased adduct formation by the polycyclic aromatic hydrocarbon benzo[a]pyrene (BP, 95). This occurred at physiologically relevant concentrations of ethanol and acetaldehyde, and in part, was the result of an ethanol-induced decrease in expression of the phase II detoxification enzyme glutathione-*S*-transferase π. Furthermore, this effect of ethanol on these human breast epithelial cells led to formation of 8-oxo-dG adducts and the inhibition of the BP–DNA adduct removal *(96)*. These data suggest, therefore, that ethanol may impact the steady-state levels of DNA-reactive metabolites by affecting both activation and detoxification of suspected carcinogens. With regard to the latter, ethanol-induced CYP2E1 metabolism may not only stimulate carcinogen bioactivation but also stimulate the release of ROS that in turn could deplete the cell of reduced glutathione and other thiol substrates that are important for carcinogen detoxification pathways *(32, 82, 84)*.

Another consequence and concern related to ethanol-induced enzyme activity, specifically for CYP3A4 is that sex hormone metabolite profiles may be altered. CYP3A4 is the most abundant enzyme in human liver and, due to its role in steroid hormone interconversions, may play a role in breast and prostate carcinogenesis *(97)*.

It should be noted that the consequences of ethanol-associated induction of carcinogen and hormone metabolizing enzymes are complex and depend in large part on the structure of the carcinogen as well as whether ethanol exposure is acute or chronic. In contrast to the stimulating effects of chronic ethanol consumption, acute ethanol exposure may inhibit the metabolism of drugs and carcinogens *(84)*. For those enzymes capable of reacting with ethanol (and/or acetaldehyde) following acute alcohol dosing, the reaction with ethanol can occur at the expense of another substrate, such as a carcinogen, leading to competitive inhibition of carcinogen bioactivation. In mice, for example, concomitant dosing with alcohol and the lung carcinogen *N*-nitrosodimethylamine (NDMA) actually resulted in competitive inhibition of NDMA metabolism in the liver, which led to enhanced exposure of the lungs to NDMA in the circulation and subsequently to increased lung tumorigenesis *(98)*.

4. ALCOHOL AND GENE INTERACTIONS

The primary enzymes catalyzing alcohol metabolism are ADH and ALDH. There is considerable ethnic variation in the distribution of these forms and their biological characteristics. Augmented formation of acetaldehyde and/or its deficient detoxification can lead to elevated tissue exposure and resultant deleterious consequences. Thus, variant alleles encoding ADH and ALDH2 enzymes can play particularly important roles in determining peak blood acetaldehyde and ROS concentrations that can ultimately impact the magnitude of acetaldehyde- and ROS-mediated damage to cellular macro-molecules *(4, 33, 34)*. Several examples of these polymorphisms and their impact on risk of certain cancers will be illustrated. A more detailed description of the genetics of alcohol metabolism can be found in the review by Edenberg *(34)*.

ADH polymorphisms. There are seven ADH enzymes encoded on genes in chromosome 4q that are capable of oxidizing ethanol. Polymorphic forms of at least two genes have been studied for their impacts on alcohol drinking and cancer risk. The polymorphisms of ADH1B and ADH1C are ADH1B*1, ADH1B*2, ADH1C*1, and ADH1C*2. ADH1B genes encode β subunits and ADH1C genes encode γ subunits of ADH that are capable of forming homo- or heterodimers *(33)*. ADH1B*2 exhibits considerably more (about 40-fold) activity compared to the reference allele ADH1B*1 (Fig. 2). The frequency of ADH1B*2 allele is higher in Asians and less prevalent in individuals of Caucasian and African descent. Those East Asian heavy drinkers heterozygous for the ADH1B alleles (ADH1B*1/2) are reported to have higher levels of ethanol persisting in the blood for longer periods as compared to those homozygous for the ADH1B*2 allele *(99)*. Furthermore, acetaldehyde levels in saliva of ADH1B*1 carriers were higher than in their corresponding blood samples and were about 30-fold higher than salivary levels in those ADH1B*2 carriers. The higher salivary acetaldehyde levels in the ADH1B*1 carriers were associated with considerable oral micro-organism overgrowth. The less active ADH1B*1 form is associated with the higher risk for UADT cancer in East Asian drinkers and also may confer higher risk in Central Europeans as well *(4, 55, 99–102)*. Its presence has a dramatic multiplicative effect on those consuming both alcohol and tobacco *(103)*, and there also appears to be significant gene–gene interaction with ALDH2 *(55)*.

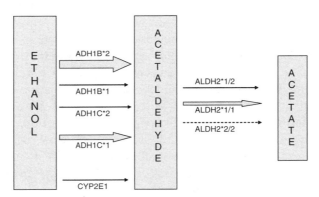

Fig. 2. Polymorphisms in alcohol and aldehyde dehydrogenases that may influence the alcohol–cancer relationship.

Among Western populations, ADH1C is a rate-limiting factor in acetaldehyde metabolism *(55)*. The ADH1C*1 form has been estimated to have about 2.5-fold the activity in metabolizing ethanol compared to the reference ADH1C*2. In this regard, it has been reported that individuals homozygous for ADH1C*1 have nearly twice the salivary acetaldehyde concentration following alcohol intake compared to heterozygous populations *(104)*. The prevalence of the ADH1C*1 is more consistently associated with increased risk for cancers of the head, neck, and esophagus for populations consuming high amounts of ethanol (>40 g/day). On the other hand, at low levels of ethanol consumption, evidence for this relationship is inconsistent *(4, 105)*. Similarly, the relationship of ADH1C*1 to alcohol and colon cancer is inconsistent *(4)*. On the other hand, a majority of studies of alcohol and breast cancer that include examination of the role of ADH polymorphisms report findings that ADH1C*1 homozygosity increases risk *(4, 106, 107)*.

As far as other ethanol oxidizing enzymes are concerned, no associations between cytochrome P4502E1 and liver and esophageal cancers have been reported *(4)*.

ALDH polymorphisms. Two main ALDH enzymes metabolize acetaldehyde to acetate, the cytosolic ALDH1 and mitochondrial ALDH2 *(33, 34)* (Fig. 2). The low Km homotetrameric mitochondrial ALDH2*1 is most active in metabolizing acetaldehyde. The variant of ALDH2 that codes for a nearly inactive form of ALDH2 is ALDH2*2. This inactive allele is much more common in Chinese, Japanese, and Koreans compared to those of European or African descent and is responsible for the acetaldehyde-induced alcohol flushing reaction that usually mitigates high alcohol consumption *(33, 34)*. Those that are heterozygous or homozygous for ALDH2*2 exhibit nearly undetectable acetaldehyde metabolizing activity. This explains why alcohol-consuming populations, homozygous or heterozygous for the inactive allele, have about 18-fold and 5-fold higher concentrations of peak blood and saliva acetaldehyde, respectively, compared to those with ALDH2*1/1 *(108)*. Moreover, those with the ALDH2*1/2 genotype who consume moderate doses of alcohol exhibit salivary acetaldehyde levels 2–3-fold higher than those levels measured in individuals with the ALDH2*1/1 genotype *(109)*. This is consistent with the observation that those males with low-activity ALDH2 alleles who consume high amounts of alcohol have greater than a 10-fold elevation in oral, throat, laryngeal, and esophageal cancer risks *(55, 101, 102, 110)*. A particularly compelling demonstration of the impact of ALDH genetics on cancer risk was reported in a case–control study of Japanese men by Yokoyama et al. *(101)*. These investigators observed that light-to-moderate drinkers with inactive ALDH2 evidenced a 5–10-fold increase in esophageal cancer risk compared to those with the active allele. Of note, they detected that the risk for light drinkers with the inactive allele was comparable to the risk for moderate drinkers with the active allele. Likewise, risk for moderate drinkers with the inactive allele was similar to heavy drinkers with the active allele. Furthermore, those with the inactive allele were at increased risk for a second tumor. Much less information has been gathered regarding increased cancer risks in women harboring these inactive alleles, and current observations suggest that male–female disparities do exist among lifestyle-associated risk factors for UADT cancers *(55)*. There is also disturbing evidence that alcohol consumption is increasing for those Japanese with the ALDH2*2 polymorphism, a group previously thought to be protected from alcoholism (due to aversive effects of the flushing response to drinking) and consequent high UADT cancer risk *(34)*. It has been reported that low vegetable and fruit intake also contributed to higher UADT risk among high alcohol consumers *(101, 102, 111)*.

Other polymorphisms. Polymorphisms for glutathine-*S*-transferase (GST), a phase II enzyme involved in carcinogen detoxification, have been studied. Women who are drinking alcohol and null for GSTM1 or GSTT1 have been reported to have either increased breast cancer risk or have had increased levels of carcinogen–DNA adducts detected in their breast tissue *(112–114)*. This relationship deserves further clarification. No association of GSTM1 genotype and lifestyle factors with esophageal cancer in Japanese was reported *(101)*. Data regarding alcohol intake and cancer risk in those with polymorphisms for the CYP2E1 gene, genes encoding enzymes for folate metabolism, and for DNA repair genes are inconclusive *(2, 115, 116)*. There is some evidence that CYP2E1 expression may interact with certain ADH and ALDH alleles in modifying an alcohol–cancer interaction *(81, 117)*. Also related to this topic, it will be informative to confirm in multiple cancer target tissues how loss of tumor suppressor gene function (such as p53) exacerbates the carcinogenic effects of alcohol in mice *(118)*.

5. ALCOHOL, HORMONES, AND GROWTH FACTORS

Alcohol intake, particularly at high levels, impairs normal functioning of most endocrine systems and can affect the hormone sensitivity of endocrine target tissues *(119, 120)*. The magnitude and direction of change in hormone levels depends on numerous factors including the specific hormonal system, target tissue, gender, lifestyle factors, age, and alcohol drinking pattern. Epidemiological, clinical, and preclinical studies point to several ways by which ethanol may affect the hormonal environment of normal and neoplastic cells, especially as it relates to estrogen and breast cancer *(16, 30, 31)* (Fig. 3). This is especially important, since it is considered that lifetime exposure to estrogens directly contributes to breast cancer risk *(121)*. Circulating estrogens in women may be generated from ovarian synthesis or from peripheral conversion (aromatization) of other steroid substrates such as testosterone, androstenedione, and hydroepiandrosterone sulfate. Alcohol-associated changes in the hormonal milieu have been observed in both premenopausal and postmenopausal women. For example, in a cross-sectional study of premenopausal women, alcoholic beverage intake was associated with significantly higher levels of estradiol, androstenedione, and testosterone averaged throughout the menstrual cycle, as well as higher progesterone levels during the luteal phase *(122)*. The literature collectively suggests that there is a positive association between chronic and acute ethanol intake and circulating estrogens *(123–131)*. The effect of alcohol may also include derangements of menstrual cycle and reproductive hormone function. The relationship between alcohol intake and levels of androgens and progesterone appears to be less consistent. In postmenopausal women, observational studies are inconsistent *(132–134)*, although in a recent large cross-sectional study, a significant positive relationship between alcohol drinking and sex steroids in the blood of both pre- and postmenopausal women was detected *(123)*. Of particular interest are reports that postmenopausal women who consume alcohol and use exogenous estrogen have substantial elevations in serum estradiol concentrations *(128, 133)*, although a recent large study found no significant interactions *(123)*. It is likely that the impact of ethanol on circulating estrogens is, in part, a result of decreased metabolic clearance and/or increased production *(119, 120, 133)*. This cancer-promoting environment due to higher estrogen exposure may be further exacerbated by the fact that blood levels of acetaldehyde are significantly increased during the peak estradiol phase of the menstrual cycle of women who drink and for those female alcohol consumers using synthetic

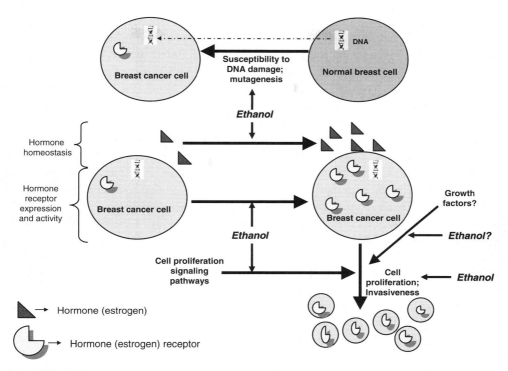

Fig. 3. Potential actions of ethanol in stimulating hormone-responsive breast cancer.

estrogens *(135)*. The interaction of alcohol and oral estradiol needs to be more carefully characterized for their combined impact on circulating estrogen and ultimately cancer risk *(134)*.

As with other cancers, genetic variability may contribute to this hormonal mechanism of alcohol and breast cancer. Coutelle et al. *(136)* reported that those women with the ADH1C*1 allele consuming small amounts of alcohol (0.225 g ethanol/kg body weight) exhibited both an increase (27–38%) in circulating estradiol levels and an increase (1.8-fold) in breast cancer risk. In another study, however, ADH1C genotype was not found to influence the relationship between alcohol and breast cancer *(137)*.

An additional hormone-related issue to consider is that there is some evidence in cell cultures that ethanol exposure may stimulate androgen aromatization in breast cancer cells *(138, 139)*.

The effect of a hormone on a target cell is in large part determined by binding of the hormone ligand to its cognate receptor. Therefore, it is important to consider how alcohol may affect hormone receptor expression or ligand–receptor dynamics. For example, a well-characterized response of some cells to estradiol binding to the estrogen receptor-alpha (ERα) is upregulation of a number of estrogen-responsive genes including that for the progesterone receptor (PR). Therefore, ethanol intake may stimulate cancer cell proliferation not only by increasing circulating levels of estrogens but also by increasing cancer cell hormone receptor expression and hormone responsiveness. The association of alcohol intake with specific steroid hormone receptor tumor subtypes in breast cancer has been the subject of numerous investigations with inconsistent results. Recently, a meta-analysis of such epidemiological studies found support for a positive relationship between alcohol drinking and the development of all ER-expressing (ER+) tumors, including ER+PR+ and ER+PR− tumors *(140)*. The mechanisms responsible for this finding are unknown, but, in light of the observation that both PR+ and PR− subtypes of tumors were increased, biological explanations would need to include both classical ER-mediated estrogenic modes of action as well as hormone-independent pathways.

Cell culture experiments point to the capacity of ethanol to increase the content of ER in human breast cancer cells *(138, 141)*. These changes in ER content were associated with an increase in cancer cell proliferation particularly in ER+ cells *(141)*. Moreover, treatment of breast cancer cells in culture with ethanol-induced ligand-independent activation of the ERα that in part involved signaling by cyclic AMP and protein kinase A pathways *(142)*. Fan et al. *(143)* reported an ethanol-induced downregulation of the tumor suppressor BRCA1 along with an upregulation of ERα expression and transcriptional activity in human breast cancer cells in vitro. Others have also reported a decreased BRCA1 expression that occurred along with decreased expression of proteins maintaining tissue organization, such as E-cadherin and α- and β-catenin *(144, 145)*. These findings are consistent with other studies using a variety of cancer cell lines, which show that ethanol exposure can affect cell adhesion and substantially enhance invasiveness. This action of ethanol was due in part to its action on a number of biological intermediates including vascular endothelial growth factor (VEGF), matrix metalloproteinases, NFkappaB, transforming growth factor-beta (TGFβ), and ErbB2/Her2 *(146–152)*. Taken together, these data suggest that breast and other neoplasms may be affected by ethanol in multiple ways leading to increased exposure to estrogens and other hormones, to heightened sensitivity to hormonal stimulation, and to aberrations in hormone-associated signaling cascades. Thus, ethanol may have a variety of actions that could lead to greater tumor development, including increased tumor cell proliferation, suppression of tumor suppressor gene-mediated genomic stability, and stimulation of tumor invasiveness and metastases. These in vitro observations warrant confirmation in appropriate animal models.

Alcohol drinking may affect carcinogenesis by mechanisms other than those involving sex steroid hormone levels and responsiveness. For example, insulin-like growth factor-1 (IGF-1) is a peptide hormone that exhibits multiple actions in regulating cell proliferation and apoptosis, largely mediated through the IGF-1 receptor *(153, 154)*. IGF-1 bound to its binding proteins (BP), predominantly IGFBP-3, makes IGF-1 unavailable for binding to its receptor. Thus, the expression of IGF-1 and its BP contributes to regulation of breast cancer proliferation. There is evidence that increasing blood concentrations of IGF-1 are associated with increased risk not only for pre and postmenopausal breast cancer but also for prostate and colorectal cancers *(155, 156)*. It has been suggested that the promotion of breast cancer by alcohol also may be a consequence of perturbations in growth factor dynamics *(157, 158)*. Both controlled and cross-sectional studies in women have examined the relationship of alcohol to circulating IGF-1 levels and some to IGFBP status, but the results are mixed *(159–162)*. Cell culture and animal studies have reported inconsistent effects of ethanol on IGF-1 levels, cell division, and intracellular signaling pathways. Some of these inconsistent findings may be due to variability in ethanol doses used and tissue-specific differences in responses to ethanol *(163–171)*. Because of the importance of IGF-I in chronic disease risk, the dose–response relationship and the factors contributing to variability in IGF-I and IGFBP responses to alcohol drinking need to be better characterized, particularly for breast cancer. Furthermore, the effects of ethanol on other growth factor and hormonal systems as well as diverse signaling pathways that can influence numerous cancers, such as AMPK, PPAR, and G-proteins, deserve more attention *(172–178)*.

In regard to other hormones, there is inconsistent evidence linking circulating prolactin levels with breast cancer risk. In humans, it is unclear how alcohol intake affects this relationship. In preclinical studies, ethanol influenced prolactin homeostasis and in a short-term feeding study alcohol intake (0.4 g/kg body weight) increased blood concentrations of prolactin *(179–181)*. Characterizing the effects of alcohol on prolactin status is important since locally produced prolactin and stimulation of the prolactin receptor in mammary tissue can affect breast carcinogenesis *(182)*.

A phenomenon related to the alcohol–breast cancer interaction is that alcohol intake is associated with the development of high-risk breast characteristics (mammographic parenchymal or fibroglandular densities) that are influenced by sex hormones and growth factors. The number of breast parenchymal cells and the integrity of the surrounding collagen matrix are reflected in the amount of radiologically dense breast tissue. Mammographic percent density has been identified as a strong and independent risk factor for breast cancer *(183, 184)*. In fact, women with mammographic densities occupying over 60–70% of the breast have 4–6 times higher risk for breast cancer than those women with breast densities occupying <10% of the breast. These dense patterns are associated with atypical hyperplasia, carcinoma in situ, with atypical cytology of nipple aspirates, and may be the consequence of enhanced mitogenesis and mutagenesis in the breast *(183–185)*. Estrogens and growth factors are associated with the prevalence of these breast structures as are dietary factors *(183, 186–189)*, such as alcohol consumption. In regard to alcohol intake, most but not all investigations report a positive association between alcohol drinking and the percentage of the breast occupied by mammographic densities *(189–198)*. These human data are supported by preclinical experiments in rodents. In the rat mammary gland of young, virgin females, immature terminal end bud (TEB) structures are highly susceptible to carcinogen-induced DNA damage and tumorigenesis. With ageing, TEB mature into more differentiated alveolar bud (AVB) structures that are less sensitive to carcinogen-induced damage. Compared to control rats, it was observed that the intake of ethanol by young, virgin female rats was associated with an increased ratio of TEB to AVB structures, a change indicative of less differentiation and maturation of the TEB to AVB *(199, 200)*. This action was associated with a small decrease in estradiol and more marked suppression of circulating progesterone levels *(199)*. These changes would suggest that ethanol-fed rats would have greater mammary gland susceptibility to carcinogen-induced tumorigenesis. This contention is supported by other studies in which female rats consuming ethanol exhibited enhanced initiation of chemically induced breast carcinogenesis *(16)*. The molecular mechanisms responsible for these effects of ethanol on maturation and differentiation of breast structures and, potentially, on development of preneoplastic breast lesions warrants further scrutiny.

6. OTHER BIOLOGICAL ACTIONS/INTERACTIONS

There are additional actions of alcohol that have been identified as potential mediators of its procarcinogenic influence. For example, alcohol drinking, especially at high levels, may affect the risk of cancer by compromising the status and function of nutrients that participate in maintenance of normal cell proliferation, differentiation, and routine functions. Evidence from preclinical studies suggest that ethanol compromises the bioavailability of dietary folate and interferes with folate-mediated methionine synthesis *(201–205)*. Thus, low folate intake along with exposure to ethanol and/or acetaldehyde could lead to inhibition of important methylation reactions catalyzed by *S*-adenosylmethionine, and consequently affect DNA repair processes, DNA stability, and the epigenetic control of gene expression through hypomethyation of DNA. This alcohol–folate interaction may in part explain epidemiological observations that ethanol consumption and low dietary folate increase risk for several cancers *(115, 201, 206–214)*, although the results are not entirely consistent. The interrelationships among alcohol, one-carbon metabolism, and carcinogenesis are complex and depend not only on folate status but also on the activity of other dietary factors such as vitamins B12, B6, and riboflavin, and the lipotropes choline and betaine *(206, 215)*. Alcohol consumption also has been associated with changes in the status of nutrients and biologically active dietary constituents such as beta-carotene, lutein, zeaxanthin, and vitamins A, B12, C, and alpha-tocopherol *(216–221)*. Taken together these findings suggest that alcohol intake, especially at high levels, may contribute to increased cancer risks by disrupting the disposition or biological functions of cancer preventive dietary factors. Thus, considerable additional research is needed to better understand the overall impact of alcohol on these dietary constituents and their molecular/epigenetic consequences before a public health recommendation on alcohol, vitamin nutrition, and cancer can be made.

Alcohol has distinctly different effects on the immune system depending on dose and frequency of exposure. A biphasic influence has been reported in that high doses of alcohol result in broad suppression of immune system activities that are associated with greater susceptibility to infectious diseases. On the other hand, moderate intake appears to have a beneficial effect on the immune system and inflammatory processes when compared to heavy drinkers and abstainers *(222–227)*. Based on observations from numerous preclinical studies, the deleterious effects of alcohol exposure on immunity are due to its actions in compromising humoral competence of the host, delaying activation of adaptive immunity, and altering inflammatory cytokine responses and neuroendocrine functions, to name a few *(228–235)*. Some of these actions may be due to ethanol-induced generation of ROS or lipid peroxidation products *(236, 237)*. However, there are fewer studies that have characterized the interplay of alcohol and immunity in affecting the development at several sites. Some studies indicate that ethanol intake by mice can suppress host resistance to metastatic spread of implanted tumors (especially melanomas) in rodents, in part due to the effect of alcohol in decreasing natural killer (NK) cell activity and compromising associated signaling pathways *(237–249)*. This aspect of alcohol's impact on cancer deserves further attention in both preclinical and clinical studies.

7. CONCLUSIONS AND FUTURE RESEARCH OPPORTUNITIES

Overall, there is clearly a need for better characterization of individual risk factors affecting the alcohol–cancer relationship so that prevention and early detection strategies can be enhanced. Some of these issues are especially important in situations where an alcohol-associated cancer risk may be modest in a general population, but greater in subgroups with biological characteristics that make them at substantially higher risk for cancers due to alcohol intake. Several research questions still need to be addressed:

What is the dose–response relationship between alcoholic beverage intake or ethanol exposure and the mechanisms associated with cancer promotion? Increased cancer risk is most evident at high intakes of ethanol, but what is the magnitude of the effect at lower levels of ethanol exposure? Furthermore, particularly in extrahepatic and nonUADT tissues, the local concentrations of ethanol, acetaldehyde, and other reactive metabolites (e.g., ROS) need to be better quantified, since these local metabolite levels may be considerably different in quality and quantity compared to those in the circulation.

What are other contributors to genetic variability in alcohol-associated cancer risks? Attention has been given to ADH and ALDH polymorphisms as modifiers of the alcohol–cancer relationship. Yet, further insights into the impact of gene variants for enzymes involved in one-carbon metabolism, in DNA methylation, in DNA repair, and in phase I and II metabolism of hormones and xenobiotics are warranted. For example, the interactive effects of methyl group diet, alcohol intake, and specific MTHFR polymorphisms need to be better understood *(215)*. Related to this is the issue as to whether and with what magnitude other lifestyle factors modify the alcohol–gene–cancer interaction.

What is the impact of ethanol intake on endocrine-related and growth factor-associated signaling pathways? And how might subtle changes in immune system efficacy affect susceptibility to cancer? The dose-, gender-, and cancer-specific differences in the influence of ethanol on these signaling pathways, physiological control of cell growth and differentiation, and even immune surveillance should be better characterized. This hormone and growth factor issue is likely to be of particular importance for breast cancer, but may have implications for other cancers as well.

REFERENCES

1. Poschl, G., and Seitz, H. (2004) Alcohol and cancer. *Alcohol Alcohol* **39**, 155–65.
2. Boffetta, P., and Hashibe, M. (2006) Alcohol and cancer. *Lancet* **7**, 149–56.
3. Seitz, H., and Becker, P. (2007) Alcohol metabolism and cancer risk. *Alcohol Res Health* **30**, 38–47.
4. Seitz, H., and Stickel, F. (2007) Molecular mechanisms of alcohol-mediated carcinogenesis. *Nat Rev Cancer* **7**, 599–612.
5. World Cancer Research Fund/American Institute for Cancer Research. (2007) Food Nutrition Physical Activity and the Prevention of Cancer: A Global Perspective World. Washington DC: American Institute for Cancer Research.
6. World Health Organization/International Agency for Research on Cancer. (2007) Carcinogenicity of alcoholic beverages. *Lancet Oncol* **8**, 292–293.
7. Katan, M., Boekschoten, M., Connor, W., Mensink, R., Serdell, J., Vessby, B., and Willett, W. (2009) Which are the greatest recent discovering and the greatest future challenges in nutrition? *Eur J Clin Nutr* **63**, 2–10.

8. Tjonneland, A., Christensen, J., Olsen, A. et al. (2007) Alcohol intake and breast cancer risk: The European Prospective Investigation into Cancer and Nutrition (EPIC). *Cancer Causes Control* **18**, 361–73.

9. Franke, A., Teyssen, S., and Singer, H. (2005) Alcohol-related diseases of the esophagus and stomach. *Dig Dis* **23**, 204–13.

10. Riedel, F., Goessler, U., and Hormann, K. (2005) Alcohol-related diseases of the mouth and throat. *Dig Dis* **23**, 195–203.

11. IARC. Preamble to the IARC monographs on the evaluation of carcinogenic risks to humans. http://monographs.iarc.fr/ENG/Preamble/CurrentPreamble.pdf

12. US National Toxicology Program. Toxicology and carcinogenesis studies of urethane and ethanol. NTP Technical Report No. 510.

13. Soffritti, M., Belpoggi, F., Cevolani, D. et al. (2002) Results of long term experimental studies on the carcinogenicity of methyl alcohol and ethyl alcohol in rats. *Ann NY Acad Sci* **982**, 46–69.

14. Watabiki, T., Okii, Y., Tokiyasu, T. et al. (2000) Long term ethanol consumption in mice causes mammary tumors in females and liver fibrosis in males. *Alcohol Clin Exp Res* **24**, 117S–125S.

15. Freedman, A., and Shklar, G. (1978) Alcohol and hamster buccal pouch carcinogenesis. *Oral Surg Oral Med Oral Pathol* **46**, 794–805.

16. Singletary, K., and Gapstur, S. (2001) Alcohol and breast cancer: Review of epidemiologic and experimental evidence and potential mechanisms. *JAMA* **286**, 2143–51.

17. Castonguay, A., Rivenson, A., Trushin, A. et al. (1984) Effects of chronic ethanol consumption on the metabolism and carcinogenicity of N'-nitrosonornicotine in F344 rats. *Cancer Res* **44**, 2285–90.

18. Anderson, L., Carter, J., Logsdon, D., Driver, C., and Kovatch, R. (1992) Characterization of ethanol's enhancement of tumorigenesis by N-nitrosodimethylamine in mice. *Carcinogenesis* **13**, 2107–11.

19. Tanaka, T., Nishikawa, A., Iwata, H. et al. (1989) Enhancing effect of ethanol on aflatoxin B1-induced hepatocarcinogenesis in male ACI/N rats. *Jpn J Cancer Res* **80**, 526–30.

20. Yamagiwa, K., Mizumoto, R., Higashi, S. et al. (1994) Alcohol ingestion enhances hepatocarcinogenesis induced by synthetic estrogen and progestin in the rat. *Cancer Detect Prev* **18**, 103–14.

21. Shikata, N., Singh, Y., Senzaki, H., Shirai, K., Watanabe, T., and Tsubura, A. (1996) Effect of ethanol on esophageal cell proliferation and the development of N-methyl-N'-nitro-N-nitrosoguanidine induced-esophageal carcinoma in shrews. *J Cancer Res Clin Oncol* **122**, 613–8.

22. Maier, H., Tisch, M., Schneeberg, E., and Born, A. (1999) An association of chronic alcohol consumption with morphological alterations of the laryngeal mucosa in rats. *Eur Arch Otorhinolaryngeal* **256**, 247–9.

23. Hakkak, R., Korourian, S., Ronis, M., and Badger, T. (1996) Effects of ethanol and diet treatment on azoxymethane-induced liver and gastrointestinal neoplasia of male rats. *Cancer Lett* **107**, 257–64.

24. Singletary, K. (1997) Ethanol and experimental breast cancer: A review. *Alcohol Clin Exp Res* **21**, 334–9.

25. Tatsuta, M., Iishi, H., Baba, M. et al. (1997) Enhancement by ethyl alcohol of experimental hepatocarcinogenesis induced by N-nitrosomorpholine. *Int J Cancer* **71**, 1045–8.

26. Roy, H., Gulizia, J., Karolski, W., Ratashak, A., Sorrell, M., and Tuma, D. (2002) Ethanol promotes intestinal tumorigenesis in the MIN mouse. *Cancer Epidemiol Biomark Prev* **11**, 1499–502.

27. Tsutsumi, M., George, J., Ishizawa, K., Fukumura, A., and Takase, S. (2006) Effect of chronic dietary ethanol in the promotion of N-nitrosomethylbenzylamine-induced esophageal carcinogenesis in rats. *J Gastroenterol Hepatol* **21**, 805–13.

28. Stevens, M. (1979) Synergistic effect of alcohol on epidermoid carcinogenesis in the larynx. *Otolaryngol Head Neck Surg* **87**, 751–6.

29. Poschl, G., Stickel, F., Wang, X., and seitz, H. (2004) Alcohol and cancer; genetic and nutritional aspects. *Proc Nutr Soc* **63**, 65–71.

30. Dumitrescu, R., and Shields, P. (2005) The etiology of alcohol-induced breast cancer. *Alcohol* **35**, 213–25.

31. Purohit, V., Khalsa, J., and Serrano, J. (2005) Mechanisms of alcohol-associated cancers: Introduction and summary of symposium. *Alcohol* **35**, 155–60.

32. Koop, D. (2006) Alcohol metabolism's damaging effects on the cell. *Alcohol Res Health* **29**, 274–80.

33. Hurley, T., Edenberg, H., and Li, T. (2002) The pharmacogenomics of alcoholism. In: Pharmacogenomics: The Search for Individualized Therapies. 417–441, Weinheim, Germany: Wiley-VCH.

34. Edenberg, H. (2007) The genetics of alcohol metabolism. *Alcohol Res Health* **30**, 5–13.

35. Baun, R., Straif, K., Gresse, Y., Secretan, B., Elghissassi, F., Bouvard, V., Altieri, A., and Cogliano, V. (2007) Carcinogenicity of alcoholic beverages. *Lancet* **8**, 292–293.

36. Zakhari, S. (2006) Overview: How is alcohol metabolized by the body? *Alcohol Res Health* **29**, 245–54.

37. Deitrich, R., Petersen, D., and Vasiliou, V. (2007) Removal of acetaldehyde from the body. *Novartis Found Symp* **285**, 23–40.

38. Kunitoh, S., Imaoka, S., Hiroi, T., Yabusaki, Y., Monna, T., and Funae, Y. (1997) Acetaldehyde as well as ethanol is metabolized by human CYP2E1. *J Pharmacol ExpTher* **280**, 527–32.

39. Salaspuro, M. (2007) Interrelationship between alcohol, smoking, acetaldehyde and cancer. *Novartis Found Symp* **285**, 80–89.

40. Seitz, H., and Homann, N. (2007) The role of acetaldehyde in alcohol-associated cancer of the gastrointestinal tract. *Novartis Found Symp* **258**, 110–9.

41. Seitz, H., and Meier, P. (2007) The role of acetaldehyde in upper digestive tract cancer in alcoholics. *Transl Res* **149**, 293–7.

42. Kurkivuori, J., Salaspuro, V., Kaihovaara, P. et al. (2007) Acetaldehyde production from ethanol by oral streptococci. *Oral Oncol* **43**, 181–6.

43. Homann, N., Jousimies-Somer, H., Jokelainen, K., Heine, R., and Salaspuro, M. (1997) High acetaldehyde levels in saliva after ethanol consumption: Methodologic aspects and pathologic implications. *Carcinogenesis* **18**, 1739–43.

44. Homann, N., Tillonen, J., Meurman, J., Rintamaki, H., Lindqvist, C., Rautio, M. et al. (2000) Increased salivary acetaldehyde levels in heavy drinkers and smokers: A microbiological approach to oral cavity cancer. *Carcinogenesis* **21**, 663–8.

45. Homann, N., Tillonen, J., and Salaspuro, M. (2000) Microbially produced acetaldehyde from ethanol may increase the risk of colon cancer via folate deficiency. *Int J Cancer* **86**, 169–73.

46. Väkeväinen, S., Tilloren, J., Blom, M., Jousimies-Somer, H., and Salaspuro, M. (2001) Acetaldehyde production and other ADH-related characteristics of aerobic bacteria isolated from hypochloric human stomach. *Alcoh Clin Exp Res* **25**, 421–6.

47. Salaspuro, M. (2003) Acetaldehyde, microbes and cancer. *Crit Rev Clin Lab Sci* **40**, 183–208.

48. Yin, S., Chou, F., Chao, S. et al. (1993) Alcohol and acetaldehyde dehydrogenases in human esophagus: Comparison with the stomach enzyme activities. *Alcohol Clin Exp Res* **17**, 376–81.

49. Yin, S., Liao, C., Wu, C. et al. (1997) Human stomach alcohol and aldehyde dehydrogenase: Comparison of expression pattern and activities in the alimentary tract. *Gastroenterol* **112**, 766–75.

50. Srivastava, S., and Salaspuro, M. (2000) High salivary acetaldehyde after a moderate dose of alcohol in ALDH2-deficient subjects: Strong evidence for the local carcinogenic action of acetaldehyde. *Alcohol Clin Exp Res* **24**, 873–7.

51. Castro, G., Delgado-deLayno, A., Fanelli, S., Maciel, M., Diaz-Gomez, M., and Castro, J. (2007) Acetaldehyde accumulation in rat mammary tissue after an acute treatment with alcohol. *J Appl Toxicol* **28**, 315–21.

52. Castro, G., Delgado-deLayno, A., Costantini, M., and Castro, J. (2001) Cytosolic xanthine oxidoreductase-mediated bioactivation of ethanol to acetaldehyde and free radicals in rat breast tissue: Its potential role in alcohol-promoted mammary cancer. *Toxicol* **160**, 11–18.

53. Castro, G., Delgado-deLayno, A., Costantini, M., and castro, J. (2003) Rat breast microsomal biotransformation of ethanol to acetaldehyde but not free radicals: Its potential role in the association between alcohol drinking and breast tumor promotion. *Teratog Carcinog Mutagen* **23**(Suppl 1), 61–70.

54. Castro, G., DeCastro, C., Maciel, M. et al. (2006) Ethanol-induced oxidative stress and acetaldehyde formation in rat mammary tissue: Potential factors involved in alcohol drinking promotion of breast cancer. *Toxicol* **219**, 208–19.

55. Yokoyama, A., and Omori, T. (2003) Genetic polymorphisms of alcohol and aldehyde dehydrogenases and risk for esophageal and head and neck cancers. *Jpn J Clin Oncol* **33**, 111–21.

56. Brooks, P., and Theravathu, J. (2005) DNA adducts from acetaldehyde: Implications for alcohol-related carcinogenesis. *Alcohol* **35**, 187–93.

57. Vaca, C., Nilsson, J., Fang, J., and Grafström, R. (1998) Formation of DNA adducts in human buccal epithelial cells exposed to acetaldehyde and methylglyoxal in vitro. *Chem Biol Inter* **108**, 197–208.

58. Tuma, D., and Casey, C. (2003) Dangerous byproducts of alcohol breakdown: Focus on adducts. *Alcohol Res Health* **27**, 285–90.

59. Matter, B., Guza, R., Zhao, J., Li, Z., Jones, R., and Tretyakova, N. (2007) Sequence distribution of acetaldehyde-derived N2-ethyl-dG adducts along duplex DNA. *Chem Res Toxicol* **20**, 1379–87.

60. Brooks, P., and Theruvathu, J. (2006) Acetaldehyde-DNA adducts: Implications for molecular mechanisms of alcohol-related carcinogenesis. In: Cho, C., Purohit, V. eds. Alcohol Tobacco and Cancer. 78–96, Basel: Karger.

61. Yamada, Y., Imai, T., Ishizak, M., and Honda, R. (2006) ALDH2 and CYP2E1 genotypes, urinary acetaldehyde excretion and the health consequences of moderate alcohol consumers. *J Hum Genet* **51**, 104–11.

62. Ogawa, M., Oyama, T., Isse, T. et al. (2007) A comparison of covalent binding of ethanol metabolites to DNA according to Aldh2 genotype. *Toxicol Lett* **168**, 148–54.

63. Fang, J., and Vaca, C. (1997) Detection of DNA adducts of acetaldehyde in peripheral white blood cells of alcohol abusers. *Carcinogenesis* **18**, 627–32.

64. Ishikawa, H., Ishikawa, T., Yamamoto, H., Fukao, A., and Yokoyama, K. (2007) Genotoxic effects of alcohol in human peripheral lymphocytes modulated by ADH1B and ALDH2 gene polymorphisms. *Mutat Res* **615**, 134–42.

65. Ishikawa, H., Miyatsu, Y., Kurihara, K., and Yokoyama, K. (2006) Gene environmental interactions between alcohol drinking behavior and ALDH2 and CYP2E1 polymorphisms and their impact on micronuclei frequency in human lymphocytes. *Mutat Res* **594**, 1–9.

66. Morimoto, K., and Takeshita, T. (1996) Low Km aldehyde dehydrogenase (ALDH2) polymorphism, alcohol drinking behavior, and chromosome alterations in peripheral lymphocytes. *Environ Health Perspect* **104**, 563–7.

67. Ishikawa, H., Yamamoto, H., Tian, Y., Kawano, M., Yamauchi, T., and Yokoyama, K. (2003) Effects of ALDH2 gene polymorphisms and alcohol drinking behavior on micronuclei frequency in non-smokers. *Mutat Res* **541**, 71–80.

68. Matsuda, T., Yabushita, H., Kanaly, R., Shibutani, S., and Yokoyama, A. (2006) Increased DNA damage in ALDH2-deficient alcoholics. *Chem Res Toxicol* **19**, 1374–8.

69. Garro, A., Espina, N., McBeth, D., Wang, S., and Wu-Wang, C. (1992) Effects of alcohol consumption on DNA methylation reactions and gene expression: Implications for increased cancer risk. *Eur J Cancer Prev* **1**(Suppl 3), 19–23.

70. Wilson, D., Tentler, J., Carney, J., Wislon, T., and Kelley, M. (1994) Acute ethanol exposure suppresses the repair of O6-methylguanine DNA lesions in castrated adult male rats. *Alcohol Clin Exp Res* **18**, 1267–71.

71. Brooks, P. (1997) DNA damage, DNA repair, and alcohol toxicity—a review. *Alcohol Clin Exp Res* **21**, 1073–82.

72. Aroor, A., and Shukla, S. (2004) MAP kinase signaling in diverse effects of ethanol. *Life Sci* **74**, 2339–64.

73. Shukla, S., Lee, Y., Park, P., and Aroor, A. (2007) Acetaldehyde alters MAP kinase signaling and epigenetic histone modifications in hepatocytes. *Novartis Found Symp* **285**, 217–24.

74. Kannarkat, G., Tuma, D., and Tuma, P. (2006) Microtubules are more stable and more highly acetylated in ethanol-treated hepatic cells. *J Hepatol* **44**, 963–70.

75. Worrall, S., DeJersey, J., Shanley, B., and Wilce, P. (1990) Antibodies against acetaldehyde-modified epitopes: Presence in alcoholic, non-alcoholic liver disease and control subjects. *Alcohol Alcohol* **25**, 509–17.

76. Tuma, D., Thiele, G., Xu, D. et al. (1996) Acetaldehyde and malondialdehyde react together to generate distinct protein adducts in the liver during long term ethanol administration. *Hepatol* **23**, 872–80.

77. Thiele, G., Klassen, I., and Tuma, D. (2008) Formation and immunological properties of aldehyde-derived protein adducts following alcohol consumption. *Meth Mol Biol* **447**, 235–57.

78. Warnakulasuriya, S., Parkkila, S., Nagao, T. et al. (2008) Demonstration of ethanol-induced protein adducts in oral leukoplakia (pre-cancer) and cancer. *J Oral Pathol Med* **37**, 157–65.

79. Petti, S., and Scully, C. (2006) Association between different alcoholic beverages and leukoplakia among non- to moderate-drinking adults: A matched case-control study. *Eur J Cancer* **42**, 512–27.

80. Bardou, M., Montembault, S., Giraud, V., Balian, A., Borotto, E., Houdayer, C., Capron, F., Chaput, J., and Naveau, S. (2002) Excessive alcohol consumption favours high risk polyp or colorectal cancer occurrence among patients with adenomas: A case-control study. *Gut* **50**, 38–42.

81. Simanowski, U., Stickel, F., Maier, H., Gartner, U., and Seitz, H. (1995) Effect of alcohol on gastrointestinal tract cell regeneration as a possible mechanism in alcohol-associated carcinogenesis. *Alcohol* **12**, 111–5.

82. Wu, D., and Cederbaum, A. (2003) Alcohol, oxidative stress and free radical damage. *Alcohol Res Health* **27**, 277–84.

83. Kim, Y., Eom, S., Ogawa, T. et al. (2007) Ethanol-induced oxidative DNA damage and CYP2E1 expression in liver tissue of Aldh2 knockout mice. *J Occup Health* **49**, 363–9.

84. Lieber, C. (2004) The discovery of the microsomal ethanol oxidizing system and its physiologic and pathologic role. *Drug Metab Rev* **36**, 511–29.

85. Bartsch, H., and Nair, J. (2005) Accumulation of lipid peroxidation-derived DNA lesions: Potential lead markers for chemoprevention of inflammation-driven malignancies. *Mutat Res* **591**, 34–44.

86. Arteel, G. (2008) Alcohol-induced oxidative stress in the liver: In vivo measurements. *Method Mol Biol* **447**, 185–97.

87. Kim, B., Hood, B., Aragon, R. et al. (2006) Increased oxidation and degradation of cytosolic proteins in alcohol-exposed mouse liver and hepatoma cells. *Proteomics* **6**, 1250–60.

88. Zima, T., and Kalousova, M. (2005) Oxidative stress and signal transduction pathways in alcoholic liver disease. *Alcohol Clin Exp Res* **29**(Suppl 11), 110S–115S.

89. Djordjevic, D., Nikolic, J., and Stefanovic, V. (1998) Ethanol interactions with other cytochrome P450 substrates including drugs, xenobiotics and carcinogens. *Pathol Biol (Paris)* **46**, 760–70.

90. Hamitouche, S., Poupon, J., Dreano, Y., Amet, Y., and Lucas, D. (2006) Ethanol oxidation into acetaldehyde by 16 recombinant human cytochrome P450 isoforms: Role of CYP2C isoforms in human liver microsomes. *Toxicol Lett* **167**, 221–30.

91. Feierman, D., Melinkov, Z., and Nanji, A. (2003) Induction of CYP3A by ethanol in multiple in vitro and in vivo models. *Alcohol Clin Exp Res* **27**, 981–8.

92. Chabra, S., Souliotis, V., Krytopoulos, S., and Anderson, L. (1996) Nitrosamines, alcohol, and gastrointestinal tract cancer: Recent epidemiology and experimentation. *In Vivo* **10**, 265–84.

93. Seitz, H., and Osswald, B. (1992) Effect of alcohol on procarcinogen bioactivation. In: Watson, R. ed. Alcohol and Cancer. 55–72, Boca Raton, FLO: CRC Press.

94. Mori, Y., Koide, A., Kobayashi, Y., Morimura, K., Kaneko, M., and Fukushima, S. (2002) Effect of ethanol treatment on metabolic activation and detoxification of esophagus carcinogenic N-nitrosoamines in rat liver. *Mutagenesis* **17**, 251–6.

95. Barnes, S., Singletary, K., and Frey, R. (2000) Ethanol and acetaldehyde enhance benzo[a[pyrene-DNA adduct formation in human mammary epithelial cells. *Carcinogenesis* **21**, 2123–8.

96. Singletary, K., Barnes, S., and VanBreemen, R. (2004) Ethanol inhibits benzo[a]pyrene-DNA adduct removal and increases 8-oxo-deoxyguanosine formation in human mammary epithelial cells. *Cancer Lett* **203**, 139–44.

97. Keshava, C., McNanlies, E., and Weston, A. (2004) CYP3A4 polymorphisms—potential risk factors for breast and prostate cancers: A HuGE review. *Am J Epidemiol* **160**, 825–41.

98. Anderson, L. (1988) Increased numbers of N-nitrosodimethylamine-initiated lung tumors in mice by chronic co-administration of ethanol. *Carcinogenesis* **9**, 1717–9.

99. Yokoyama, A., Tsutsumi, F., Imazeki, H., Suwa, Y., Nakamura, C., and Yokoyama, T. (2007) Contribution of the alcohol dehydrogenase 1B genotype and oral microorganisms to high salivary acetaldehyde concentrations in Japanese alcoholic men. *Int J Cancer* **121**, 1047–54.

100. Hashike, M., Boffetta, P., Zaridze, D., Shangina, O., Szeszema-Dabrowska, N., Mates, D., Janout, V., Fabianova, E., Bencko, V., Moullan, N., Chabrier, A., Hung, R.,, Hall, J., Canzian, F., and Brennan, P. (2006) Evidence for an important role of the alcohol and aldehyde-metabolizing genes in cancers of the upper aerodigestive tract. *Cancer Epidemiol Biomark Prev* **15**, 696–703.

101. 101.Yokoyama, A., Kato, H., Yokoyama, T., Tsujinaka, T., Muto, M., Omori, T., Haneda, T., Kumagai, Y., Ioaki, H., Yokoyama, M., Watanabe, H., Fukuda, H., and Yoshimizu, H. (2002) Genetic polymorphisms of alcohol and aldehyde dehydrogenases and glutathione-S-transferase M1 and drinking, smoking, and diet in Japanese men with esophageal squamous cell carcinoma. *Carcinogenesis* **23**, 1851–9.

102. Asakage, T., Yokoyama, A., Haneda, T., Yamazaki, M., Muto, M., Yokoyama, T., Kato, H., Igahi, H., Tsujinaka, T., Kumagar, Y., Yokoyama, M., Omori, T., and Watanabe, H. (2007) Genetic polymorphisms of alcohol and aldehyde dehydrogenases, and drinking, smoking and diet in Japanese men with oral and pharyngeal squamous cell carcinoma. *Carcinogenesis* **28**, 865–74.

103. Lee, C., Lee, J., Wu, D. et al. (2008) Carcinogenic impact of ADH1B and ALDH2 genes on squamous cell carcinoma risk of the esophagus with regard to the consumption of alcohol, tobacco and betel quid. *Int J Cancer* **122**, 1347–56.

104. Visapaa, J., Gotte, K., Benesova, M., Homann, N., Conradt, C. et al. (2004) Increased cancer risk in heavy drinkers with the alcohol dehydrogenase 3*1 allele possibly due to salivary acetaldehyde. *Gut* **53**, 871–6.

105. Terry, M., Gammon, M., Zhang, F., Vaughan, T., Chow, W., Risch, H., Schoenberg, J., Mayne, S., Stanford, J., West, A., Rotterdam, H., Blot, W., Fraumeni, J., and Santella, R. (2007) Alcohol dehydrogenase 3 and risk of esophageal and gastric adenocarcinoma. *Cancer Causes Control* **18**, 1039–46.

106. Freudenheim, J., Ambrosone, C., Moysich, K., Vena, J., Graham, S., Marshall, J., Muti, P., Laughlin, R., Nemoto, T., Harty, L., Crits, G., Chan, G., Chan, A., and Shields, P. (1999) Alcohol dehydrogenase 3 genotype modification of the association of alcohol consumption with breast cancer risk. *Cancer Causes Control* **10**, 369–77.

107. Terry, M., Gammon, M., Zhang, F., Knight, J., Wang, Q., Britton, J., Teitelbaum, S., Neugat, A., and Santella, R. (2006) ADH3 genotype, alcohol intake and breast cancer risk. *Carcinogenesis* **27**, 840–47.

108. Enomoto, N., Takase, S., Yasuhara, M., and Takada, A. (1991) Acetaldehyde metabolism in different aldehyde dehydrogenase-2 genotypes. *Alcohol Clin Exp Res* **15**, 141–4.

109. Väkeväinen, S., Tilloren, J., Agarwal, D., Srivastava, N., and Salaspuro, M. (2000) High salivary acetaldehyde after a moderate dose of alcohol in ALDH2-deficient subjects: Strong evidence for the local carcinogenic action of acetaldehyde. *Alcoh Clin Exp Res* **24**, 873–7.

110. Hiraki, A., Matsuo, K., Wakai, K., Suzuki, T., Hasegawa, Y., and Tajima, K. (2007) Gene-gene and gene-environmental interactions between alcohol drinking habit and polymorphisms in alcohol-metabolizing enzyme genes and risk of head and neck cancers in. *Japan Cancer Sci* **98**, 1087–91.

111. Boccia, S., Cadoni, G., Sayed-Tabatabaei, F. et al. (2008) CYP1A1, CYP2E1, GSTT1, EPHX1 exons 3 and 4, and NAT2 polymorphisms, smoking, consumption of alcohol and fruit and vegetables and risk of head and neck cancer. *J Cancer Res Clin Oncol* **134**, 93–100.

112. Park, S., Yoo, K., Lee, S. et al. (2000) Alcohol consumption, glutathione-S-transferase M1 and T1 genetic polymorphisms and breast cancer risk. *Pharmacogen* **10**, 301–9.

113. Zheng, T., Holford, T., Zahm, S. et al. (2003) Glutathione-S-transferase M1 and T1 genetic polymorphisms, alcohol consumption and breast cancer risk. *Br J Cancer* **88**, 58–62.

114. Rundle, A., Tang, D., Mooney, L., Grumet, S., and Perera, F. (2003) The interaction between alcohol consumption and GSTM1 genotype on polycyclic aromatic hydrocarbon-DNA adduct levels in breast tissue. *Cancer Epidemiol Biomark Prev* **12**, 911–4.

115. Giovanucci, E., Chen, J., Smith-Warner, S. et al. (2003) Methylenetetrahydrofolate reductase, alcohol dehydrogenase, diet and risk for colorectal adenomas. *Cancer Epidemiol Biomark Prev* **12**, 970–9.

116. Hansen, R., Sorenson, M., Tjonneland, A. et al. (2008) A haplotype of polymorphisms in ASE-1, RAI and ERCC1 and the effects of tobacco smoking and alcohol consumption on risk of colorectal cancer: A Danish prospective case-cohort study. *BMC Cancer* **20**, 54.

117. Guo, Y., Wang, Q., Liu, Y., Chen, H., Qi, Z., and Guo, Q. (2008) Genetic polymorphisms in cytochrome P450 2E1, alcohol and aldehyde dehydrogenases and the risk of esophageal squamous cell carcinoma in Gansu Chinese males. *World J Gastroenterol* **14**, 1444–9.

118. Pani, G., Fusco, S., Colavitti, R. et al. (2004) Abrogation of hepatocyte apoptosis and early appearance of liver dysplasia in ethanol-fed p53-deficient mice. *Biochem Biophys Res Commun* **325**, 97–100.

119. Ronis, M., Wands, J., Badger, T., DeLa Monte, S., Lang, C., and Calissendorff, J. (2007) Alcohol-induced disruption of endocrine signaling. *Alcohol Clin Exp Res* **31**, 1269–85.

120. Emanuele, N., and Emanuele, M. (1997) The endocrine system: Alcohol alters critical hormone balance. *Alcohol Health Res World* **21**, 53–80.

121. Key, T., and Verasala, P. (1999) Endogenous hormones and the etiology of breast cancer. *Breast Cancer Res* **1**, 18–21.

122. Garcia-Closas, M., Herbstman, J., Schiffman, M., Glass, A., and Dorgan, J. (2002) Relationship between serum hormone concentrations, reproductive history, alcohol consumption and genetic polymorphisms in pre-menopausal women. *Int J Cancer* **102**, 172–8.

123. Rinaldi, S., Peeters, P., Bezemer, J. et al. (2006) Relationship of alcohol intake and sex steroid concentrations in blood of pre- and post-menopausal women: The European Prospective Investigation into Cancer and Nutrition. *Cancer Causes Control* **17**, 1033–43.

124. Maskarinec, G., Morimoto, Y., Takata, Y., Murphy, S., and Stanczyk, F. (2006) Alcohol and dietary fibre intakes affect circulating sex hormones among premenopausal women. *Publ Health Nutr* **9**, 875–81.

125. Reichman, M., Judd, J., Longcope, C. et al. (1993) Effects of alcohol consumption on plasma and urinary hormone concentrations in premenopausal women. *J Natl Cancer Inst* **85**, 722–7.

126. Mendelson, J., Mello, N., Teoh, S., and Ellingboe, J. (1989) Alcohol effects on luteinizing hormone releasing hormone-stimulated anterior pituitary and gonadal hormones in women. *J Pharmacol Exp Ther* **250**, 2902–9.

127. Mendelson, J., Mello, N., Cristofaro, P. et al. (1987) Alcohol effects on naloxone-stimulated luteinizing hormone, prolactin, and estradiol in women. *J Stud Alcohol* **48**, 287–94.

128. Ginsberg, E. (1999) Estrogen, alcohol, and breast cancer risk. *J Ster Biochem Mol Biol* **69**, 299–306.

129. Dorgan, J., Reichamn, M., Judd, J. et al. (1994) The relation of reported alcohol ingestion to plasma levels of estrogens and androgens in premenopausal women (Maryland, United states). *Cancer Causes Control* **5**, 53–60.

130. Mendelson, J., Lukas, S., Mello, N., Amass, L., Ellingboe, J., and Skupny, A. (1988) Acute alcohol effects on plasma estradiol levels in women. *Psychopharmacol* **94**, 464–7.

131. Mendelson, J., and Mello, N. (1988) Chronic alcohol effects on anterior pituitary and ovarian hormones in healthy women. *J Pharmacol Exp Ther* **245**, 407–12.

132. Dorgan, J., Baer, D., Albert, D. et al. (2001) Serum hormones and the alcohol-breast cancer association in postmenopausal women. *J Natl Cancer Inst* **93**, 710–5.

133. Ginsburg, E., Mello, N., Mendelson, J. et al. (1996) Effects of alcohol ingestion on estrogens in postmenopausal women. *JAMA* **276**, 1747–51.

134. Nielsen, N., and Gronback, M. (2008) Interactions between intakes of alcohol and postmenopausal hormones on risk of breast cancer. *Int J Cancer* **122**, 1109–13.

135. Eriksson, P., Fukunaga, T., Sarkola, T., Lindholm, H., and Ahola, L. (1996) Estrogen-related acetaldehyde elevation in women during alcohol intoxication. *Alcohol Clin Exp Res* **20**, 1192–5.

136. Coutelle, C., Hohn, B., Benesova, M., Oneta, C., Quattrochi, P., Roth, H., Schmidt-Gayk, H., Schneeweis, A., Bastert, G., and Seitz, H. (2004) Rick factors in alcohol associated breast cancer: Alcohol dehydrogenase polymorphism and estrogens. *Int J Cancer* **25**, 1127–32.

137. Hines, L., Hankinson, S., Smith-Warner, S. et al. (2000) A prospective study of the effect of alcohol consumption and ADH3 genotype on plasma steroid hormone levels and breast cancer risk. *Cancer Epidemiol Biomark Prev* **9**, 1099–105.

138. Etique, N., Chandard, D., Chesnel, A., Merlin, J., Flament, S., and BGrillier-Vuissoz, I. (2004) Ethanol stimulates proliferation, ERalpha and aromatase expression in MCF-7 human breast cancer cells. *Int J Mol Med* **13**, 149–55.

139. Purohit, V. (2000) Can alcohol promote aromatization of androgens to estrogens? *Alcohol* **22**, 123–7.

140. Suzuki, R., Orsini, N., Mignone, L., Saji, S., and Wolk, A. (2008) Alcohol intake and risk of breast cancer defined by estrogen and progesterone receptor status: A meta-analysis of epidemiological studies. *Int J Cancer* **122**, 1832–41.

141. Frey, R., Singletary, K., and Yan, W. (2001) Effect of ethanol on proliferation and estrogen receptor α expression in human breast cancer cells. *Cancer Lett* **165**, 131–7.

142. Etique, N., Flament, S., Lecomte, J., and Grillier-Vuissoz, I. (2007) Ethanol-induced ligand-independent activation of ER-alpha mediated by cyclicAMP/PKA signaling pathway: An in vitro study on MCF-7 breast cancer cells. *Int J Oncol* **31**, 1509–18.

143. Fan, S., Meng, Q., Gao, B. et al. (2000) Alcohol stimulates estrogen receptor signaling in human breast cancer cell lines. *Cancer Res* **60**, 5635–9.

144. Meng, Q., Gao, B., Goldberg, I., Rosen, E., and Fan, S. (2000) Stimulation of cell invasion and migration by alcohol in breast cancer cells. *Biochem Biophys Res Comm* **273**, 448–53.

145. Luo, J., and Miller, M. (2000) Ethanol enhances erb B-mediated invasion of human breast cancer cells in culture. *Br Cancer Res Treat* **63**, 61–69.

146. Miller, M., Mooney, S., and Middletown, F. (2006) Transforming growth factor-beta 1 and ethanol affect transcription and translation of genes and proteins for cell adhesion molecules in B104 neuroblastoma cells. *J Neurochem* **97**, 1182–90.

147. Luo, J. (2006) Role of matrix metalloproteinase-2 in ethanol-induced invasion by breast cancer cells. *J Gastroenterol Hepatol* **21**(Suppl 3), S65–S68.

148. Ke, Z., Lin, M., Fan, Z. et al. (2006) MMP-2 mediates ethanol-induced invasion of mammary epithelial cells over-expressing ErbB2. *Int J Cancer* **119**, 8–16.

149. Aye, M., Ma, C., Lin, H., Bower, K., Wiggins, R., and Luo, J. (2004) Ethanol-induced in vitro invasion of breast cancer cells: The contribution of MMP-2 by fibroblasts. *Int J Cancer* **112**, 738–46.

150. Gu, J., Bailey, A., Sartin, A., Makey, I., and Brady, A. (2005) Ethanol stimulate tumor progression and expression of vascular endothelial growth factor in chick embryos. *Cancer* **103**, 422–31.

151. Tan, W., Bailey, A., Shparago, M. et al. (2007) Chronic alcohol consumption stimulates VEGF expression, tumor angiogenesis, and progression of melanoma in mice. *Cancer Biol Ther* **6**, 1211–7.

152. Hsiang, C., Wu, S., Chen, J. et al. (2007) Acetaldehyde induces matrix metalloproteinase-3 gene expression via nuclear factor-kappaB and activator protein-1 signaling pathways in human hepatocellular carcinoma cells: Association with the invasive potential. *Toxicol Lett* **171**, 78–86.

153. Westley, B., Clayton, S., Daws, M., Molloy, C. and May, F. (1998) Interactions between oestrogen and insulin-like growth factor signaling pathways in the control of breast epithelial cell proliferation. *Biochem Soc Symp* **63**, 35–44.

154. Yu, H., and Rohan, T. (2000) Role of insulin-like growth factor family in cancer development and progression. *J Natl Cancer Inst* **92**, 1472–89.

155. Frasca, F., Pandini, G., Sciacca, L. et al. (2008) The role of insulin-like growth factors and IGF-1 receptors in cancer and other diseases. *Arch Physiol Biochem* **114**, 23–37.

156. Pollak, M. (2007) Insulin-like growth factor-regulated signaling and cancer development. *Recent Rev Cancer Res* **174**, 49–53.

157. Stoll, B. (1999) Alcohol intake and late-stage promotion of breast cancer. *Eur J Cancer* **35**, 1653–8.

158. Yu, H., and Berkel, J. (1999) Do insulin-like growth factors mediate the effect of ethanol on breast cancer? *Med Hypoth* **52**, 491–6.

159. Dees, W., Hiney, S., and Srivastava, V. (1998) Alcohol's effects on female puberty: The role of insulin-like growth factor. *Alcoh Health Res World* **22**, 165–69.

160. Lavigne, J., Baer, D., Wimbrozo, H., Albert, P., Brown, E., Judd, J., Campbell, W., Giffen, C., Dorgan, J., Hartman, T., Barrett, J., Hursting, S., and Taylor, P. (2005) Effects of alcohol on insulin-like growth factor 1 and insulin-like growth factor binding protein 3 in postmenopausal women. *Am J Clin Nutr* **81**, 503–7.

161. Lavigne, J., Wimbrozo, H., Clevidence, B., Alberts, P., Reichman, M., Campbell, W., Barrett, J., Hursting, S., Judd, J., and Taylor, P. (2004) Effects of alcohol and menstrual cycle on insulin-like growth factor-1 and insulin-like growth factor binding protein 3. *Cancer Epidemiol Biomarkers Prev* **13**, 2264–7.

162. DeLellis, K., Rinaldi, S., Kaaks, R., Kolonel, L., Henderson, B., and LeMarchand, L. (2004) Dietary and lifestyle correlates of plasma insulin-like growth factor-1 (IGF-1) and IGF binding protein-3 (IGFBP-3): The multiethnic cohort. *Cancer Epidemiol Biomark Prev* **13**, 1444–51.

163. Srivastava, V., Hiney, J., Mattison, J., Bartke, A., and Dees, W. (2007) The alcohol-induced suppression of ovarian insulin-like growth factor-1 gene transcription is independent of growth hormone and its receptor. *Alcohol Clin Exp Res* **31**, 880–6.

164. Srivastava, V., Hiney, J., Mattison, J., Bartjke, A., and Dees, W. (2007) The alcohol-induced suppression of ovarian insulin-like growth factor-1 gene transcription is independent of growth hormone and its receptor. *Alcohol Clin Exp Res* **31**, 880–6.

165. Magne, L., Blanc, E., Marchand, A., Fafournoux, P., Barouki, R., Rouach, H., and Garlatti, M. (2007) Stabilization of IGFBP-1 mRNA by ethanol in hepatoma cells involves the JNK pathway. *J Hepatol* **47**, 691–8.

166. Lee, S., Alam, R., Ho, C. et al. (2007) Involvement of p42/44 MAPK in the effects of ethanol on secretion of insulin-like growth factor (IGF)-1 and insulin-like growth factor binding protein (IGFBP)-1 in primary cultured rat hepatocytes. *Int J Neurosci* **117**, 187–201.

167. Tomono, M., and Kiss, Z. (1995) Ethanol enhances the stimulatory effect of insulin and insulin-like growth factor-1 on DNA synthesis in NIH 3T3 fibroblasts. *Biochem Biophys Res Comm* **208**, 63–67.

168. Lang, C., Fan, J., Lipton, B., Potter, B., and McDonough, K. (1998) Modulation of the insulin like growth factor system by chronic ethanol feeding. *Alcohol Clin Exp Res* **22**, 823–9.

169. Srivastava, V., Hiney, J., Nuberg, C., and Dees, W. (1995) Effect of ethanol on the synthesis of insulin-like growth factor-1 (IGF-1) and IGF-1 receptor in late prepubertal rats: A correlation with serum IGF-1. *Alcoh Clin Exp Res* **19**, 1467–73.

170. Seller, A., Ross, B., Green, J., and Rubin, R. (2000) Differential effects of ethanol on insulin-like growth factor-1 receptor signaling. *Alcohol Clin Exp Res* **24**, 140–8.

171. Smith, D., Yang, H., Scheff, A., Ploch, S., and Schalch, D. (1992) Ethanol-fed Sprague Dawley rats maintain normal levels of insulin-like growth factor-1. *J Nutr* **122**, 220–33.

172. Sarkar, D., and Boyadjieva, N. (2007) Ethanol alters production and secretion of estrogen-regulated growth factors that control prolactin-secreting tumors in the pituitary. *Alcohol Clin Exp Res* **31**, 2101–5.

173. Chaturvedi, K., and Sarkar, D. (2008) Alteration in G proteins and prolactin levels in pituitary after ethanol and estrogen treatment. *Alcohol Clin Exp Res* **32**, 806–13.

174. You, M., Matsumoto, M., Pacold, C., Cho, W., and Crabb, D. (2004) The role of AMP-activated protein kinase in the action of ethanol in the liver. *Gastroenterol* **127**, 1798–808.

175. Venkata, M., Aung, C., Cabot, P., Monteith, G., and Roberts-Thomson, S. (2008) PPARalpha and PPARbeta are differentially affected by ethanol and the ethanol metabolite acetaldehyde in the MCF-7 breast cancer cell line. *Toxicol Sci* **102**, 120–8.

176. Hallak, H., and Rubin, R. (2004) Ethanol inhibits palmitoylation of G protein G alpha (s). *J Neurochem* **89**, 919–27.

177. Hoek, J., and Kholodenko, B. (1998) The intracellular signaling network as a target of ethanol. *Alcohol Clin Exp Res* **22**, 224S–230S.

178. Castaneda, F., Rosin-Steiner, S., and Jung, K. (2006) Functional genomics analysis of low concentrations of ethanol in human hepatocellular carcinoma (HepG2) cells: Role of genes involved in transcriptional and translational processes. *Int J Med Sci* **4**, 28–35.

179. Diaz, I., Cano, P., Jimenez-Ortega, V., Nova, E., Romeo, J., Marcos, A., and Esquifino, A. (2007) Effects of moderate consumption of distilled and fermented alcohol on some aspects of neuroimmunomodulation. *Neuromodul* **14**, 200–5.

180. Jimenez-Ortega, V., Cardinali, D., Fernandez-Mateos, P., Reyes-Toso, C., and Esquifino, A. (2006) Effect of ethanol on 24-h hormonal changes in prolactin release mechanisms in growing male rats. *Endocrine* **30**, 269–78.

181. Menella, J., and Pepino, M. (2006) Short-term effects of alcohol consumption on the hormonal milieu and mood states in nulliparous women. *Alcohol* **38**, 29–36.

182. Wennbo, H., and Tornell, J. (2000) The role of prolactin and growth hormone in breast cancer. *Oncogene* **19**, 1072–6.

183. Boyd, N., Martin, L., Yaffe, M., and Minkin, S. (2006) Mammographic density: A hormonally responsive factor for breast cancer. *J Br Menopause Soc* **12**, 186–93.

184. Boyd, N., Lockwood, G., Byng, J., Tritchler, D., and Yaffe, M. (1998) Mammographic densities and breast cancer risk. *Cancer Epidemiol Biomark Prev* **7**, 1133–44.

185. Lee, M., Petraikis, N., Wrensch, M., King, E., Miike, R., and Sickles, E. (1994) Association of abnormal nipple aspirate cytology and mammographic pattern and density. *Cancer Epidemiol Biomark Prev* **3**, 33–36.

186. DosSantos-Silva, I., Johnson, N., DeStavola, B. et al. (2006) The insulin like growth factor system and mammographic features in premenopausal and postmenopausal women. *Cancer Epidemiol Biomark Prev* **15**, 449–55.

187. Byrne, C., Colditz, G., Willett, W., Speizer, F., Pollak, M., and Hankinson, S. (2000) Plasma insulin-like growth factor (IGF) 1, IGF-binding protein 3, and mammographic density. *Cancer Res* **60**, 3744–8.

188. Tamimi, R., Cox, D., Kraft, P. et al. (2007) Common genetic variation in IGF-1, IGFBP-1 and IGFBP-3 in relation to mammographic density: A cross-sectional study. *Breast Cancer Res* **9**, R18.

189. Johansson, H., Gandini, S., Bonanni, B. et al. (2008) Relationships between circulating hormone levels, mammographic percent density and breast cancer risk factors in postmenopausal women. *Breast Cancer Res Treat* **108**, 57–67.

190. Keleman, L., Pankratz, V., Sellers, T. et al. (2008) Age-specific trends in mammographic density: The Minnesota Breast Cancer Family Study. *Am J Epidemiol* **167**, 1027–36.

191. Maskarinec, G., Takata, Y., Pagano, I., Lurie, G., Wilkens, L., and Kolonel, L. (2006) Alcohol consumption and mammographic density in multiethnic population. *Int J Cancer* **118**, 2579–83.

192. Funkhouser, E., Waterbor, J., Cole, P., and Rubin, E. (1993) Mammographic patterns and breast cancer risk factors among women having elective screening. *South Med J* **86**, 177–80.

193. Herrinton, L., Saftlas, A., Stanford, J., Brinton, L., and Wolfe, J. (1993) Do alcohol intake and mammographic densities interact in regard to the risk for breast cancer? *Cancer* **71**, 3029–35.

194. Vachon, C., Kuni, C., Anderson, K., Anderson, V., and Sellers, T. (2000) Association of mammographically defined percent breast density with epidemiologic risk factors for breast cancer (United States). *Cancer Causes Control* **11**, 653–62.

195. Sala, E., Warren, R., Duffy, S., Welch, A., Luben, R., and Day, N. (2000) High risk mammographic parenchymal patterns and diet: A case-control study. *Br J Cancer* **83**, 121–6.

196. Brisson, J., Verrault, R., Morrison, A., Tennina, S., and Meyer, F. (1989) Diet, mammographic features of breast tissue, and breast cancer risk. *Am J Epidemiol* **130**, 14–24.

197. Berube, S., Diorio, C., Verhoek-Oftedahl, W., and Brisson, J. (2004) Vitamin D, calcium and mammographic breast densities. *Cancer Epidemiol Biomark Prev* **13**, 1466–72.

198. Boyd, N., Connelly, P., Bung, J. et al. (1995) Plasma lipids, lipoproteins, and mammographic densities. *Cancer Epidemiol Biomark Prev* **4**, 727–33.

199. Singletary, K., and McNary, M. (1992) Effect of moderate ethanol consumption on mammary gland structural development and DNA synthesis in the female rat. *Alcohol* **9**, 95–101.

200. Singletary, K., and McNary, M. (1994) Influence of ethanol intake on mammary gland morphology and cell proliferation in normal and carcinogen-treated rats. *Alcohol Clin Exp Res* **18**, 1261–6.

201. Mason, J., and Choi, S. (2005) Effects of alcohol on folate metabolism: Implications for carcinogenesis. *Alcohol* **35**, 235–41.

202. Schalinske, K., and Nieman, K. (2005) Disruption of methyl group metabolism by ethanol. *Nutr Rev* **63**, 387–91.

203. Halsted, C., Villaneuva, J., Devlin, A., and Chandler, C. (2002) Metabolic interactions of alcohol and folate. *J Nutr* **132**, 2367S–2372S.

204. Anonymous. (1994) Folate, alcohol, methionine, and colon cancer risk: Is there a unifying theme? *Nut Rev* **52**, 18–20.

205. Stempak, J., Sohn, K., Chiang, E., Shane, B., and Kim, Y. (2005) Cell and stage of transformation-specific effects of folate deficiency on methionine cycle intermediates and DNA methylation in an in vitro model. *Carcinogenesis* **26**, 981–90.

206. Ziegler, R. (2007) One-carbon metabolism, colorectal carcinogenesis, chemoprevention – with caution. *J Natl Cancer Inst* **99**, 1214–1215.

207. Zhang, S., Hankinson, S., Hunter, D., Giovanucci, E., Colditz, G., and Willett, W. (2005) Folate intake and risk of breast cancer characterized by hormone receptor status. *Cancer Epidemiol Biomark Prev* **14**, 2004–8.

208. Cui, Y., Page, D., Chlebowski, R., Beresford, S., Hendrix, S., Lane, D., and Rohan, T. (2007) Alcohol and folate consumption and the risk of benign proliferative disorders of the breast. *Int J Cancer* **121**, 1346–51.

209. Cho, E., Holmes, M., Hankinson, S., and Willett, W. (2007) Nutrients involved in one-carbon metabolism and risk of breast cancer among premenopausal women Cancer. *Epidemiol Biomark Prev* **16**, 2787–90.

210. Sellers, T., Vierkant, R., Cerhan, J. et al. (2002) Interaction of dietary folate intake, alcohol, and risk of hormone-receptor-defined breast cancer in a prospective study of postmenopausal women. *Cancer Epidemiol Biomark Prev* **11**, 1104–7.

211. Sellers, T., Kushi, L., Cerhan, J. et al. (2001) Dietary folate, alcohol, and risk of breast cancer in a prospective study of postmenopausal women. *Epidemiol* **12**, 420–8.

212. Stolzenberg-Solomon, R., Chang, S., Leitzmann, M. et al. (2006) Folate intake, alcohol use and post-menopausal breast cancer risk in the Prostate, Lung, Colorectal and Ovarian Cancer Screening Trial. *Am J Clin Nutr* **83**, 895–904.

213. Feigelson, H., Jonas, C., Robertson, A., McCullough, M., Thun, M., and Calle, E. (2003) Alcohol, folate, methionine, and risk of incident breast cancer in the American Cancer Society Cancer prevention Study II Nutrition Cohort. *Cancer Epidemiol Biomark Prev* **12**, 161–4.

214. Boyaparti, S., Bostick, R., McGlynn, K. et al. (2004) Folate intake, MTHFR C677T polymorphism, alcohol consumption, and risk for sporadic colorectal adenoma (United States). *Cancer Causes Control* **15**, 493–501.

215. Kim, D. (2007) The interactive effect of methyl-group diet and polymorphisms of methylenetetrahydrofolate reductase on the risk of colorectal cancer. *Mutat Res* **622**, 14–18.

216. Wang, X. (2005) Alcohol, vitamin A and cancer. *Alcohol* **35**, 251–8.

217. Larsson, S., Giovanucci, E., and Wolk, A. (2007) Folate and risk of breast cancer: A meta-analysis. *J Natl Cancer Inst* **99**, 64–76.

218. Drewnowski, A., Rock, C., Henderson, S. et al. (1997) Serum beta-carotene and vitamin C as biomarkers of vegetable and fruit intakes in a community-based sample of French adults. *Am J Clin Nutr* **65**, 1796–802.

219. Forman, M., Beecher, G., Lanza, E. et al. (1995) Effect of alcohol consumption on plasma carotenoid concentrations in pre-menopausal women: A controlled dietary study. *Am J Clin Nutr* **62**, 131–5.

220. Laufer, E., Hartman, T., Baer, D. et al. (2004) Effects of moderate alcohol consumption on folate and vitamin B12 status in postmenopausal women. *Eur J Clin Nutr* **58**, 1518–24.

221. Hartman, T., Baer, D., Graham, L. et al. (2005) Moderate alcohol consumption and levels of antioxidant vitamins and isoprostane in postmenopausal women. *Eur J Clin Nutr* **59**, 161–8.

222. Romeo, J., Warnberg, J., Nova, E., Diaz, L., Gomez-Martinez, S., and Marcos, A. (2007) Moderate alcohol consumption and the immune system: A review. *Br J Nutr* **98**(Suppl 1), S111–S15.

223. Diaz, L., Montero, A., Gonzalez-Gross, M., Vallejo, A., Romeo, J., and Marcos, A. (2002) Influence of alcohol consumption on immunological status: A review. *Eur J Clin Nutr* **56**(Suppl 3), S50–S53.

224. Goral, J., Karavitis, J., and Kovacs, E. (2008) Exposure-dependent effects of ethanol on the innate immune system. *Alcohol* **42**, 237–47.

225. Brown, L., Cook, R., Jerrells, T. et al. (2006) Acute and chronic alcohol abuse modulate immunity. *Alcohol Clin Exp Res* **30**, 1624–31.

226. Pruett, S., Yan, Y., and Wu, W. (1994) A brief review of immunomodulation by acute administration of ethanol: Involvement of neuroendocrine pathways. *Alcohol Alcohol* **2**(Suppl), 431–7.

227. Waldschmidt, T., Cook, R., and Kovacs, E. (2006) Alcohol and inflammation and immune responses: Summary of the 2005 Alcohol and Immunity Research Interest Group (AIRIG) meeting. *Alcohol* **38**, 121–5.

228. Verma, S., Alexander, C., Carlson, M., Tygrett, L., and Waldschmidt, T. (2008) B-cell studies in chronic ethanol mice. *Meth Mol Biol* **447**, 295–323.

229. Jerrells, T., Slukvin, I., Sibley, D., and Fuseler, J. (1994) Increased susceptibility of experimental animals to infectious organisms as a consequence of ethanol consumption. *Alcohol Alcohol* **2**(Suppl), 425–30.

230. Szabo, G. (1999) Consequences of alcohol consumption on host defense. *Alcohol Alcohol* **34**, 830–41.

231. Bhattacharya, Ra.nd, and Shuhart, M. (2003) Hepatitis C and alcohol: Interactions, outcomes and implications. *J Clin Gastroenterol* **36**, 242–52.

232. Ness, K., Fan, J., Wilke, W., Coleman, R., Cook, R., and Schlueter, A. (2008) Chronic ethanol consumption decreases murine Langerhans cell numbers and delays migration of Langerhans cells as well as dermal dendritic cells. *Alcohol Clin Exp Res* **32**, 657–68.

233. Singal, A., and Anand, B. (2007) Mechanisms of synergy between alcohol and hepatitis C. *J Clin Gastroenterol* **41**, 761–72.

234. Chen, C.P., Boyadjieva, N.I., Advis, J.P., and Sarkar, D.K. (2006) Ethanol suppression of the hypothalamic proopiomelanocortin level and the splenic NK cell cytolytic activity is associated with a reduction in the expression of proinflammatory cytokines but not anti-inflammatory cytokines in neuroendocrine and immune cells. *Alcohol Clin Exp Res* **30**, 1925–32.

235. McVicker, B., Tuma, D., Kharbanda, K., Kubik, J., and Casey, C. (2007) Effect of chronic ethanol administration on the in vitro production of proinflammatory cytokines by rat Kupffer cells in the presence of apoptotic cells. *Alcohol Clin Exp Res* **31**, 122–9.

236. Osna, N., White, R., Todero, S. et al. (2007) Ethanol-induced oxidative stress suppresses generation of peptides for antigen presentation by hepatoma cells. *Hepatol* **45**, 53–61.

237. Watson, R., Odeleye, O., Eskelson, C., and Mufti, S. (1992) Alcohol stimulation of lipid peroxidation and esophageal tumor growth in mice immunocompromised by retrovirus infection. *Alcohol* **9**, 495–500.

238. Mufti, S., Darban, H., and Watson, R. (1989) Alcohol, cancer and immunomodulation. *Crit Rev Oncol Hematol* **9**, 243–61.

239. Taylor, A., Ben-Eliyahu, S., Yirmiya, R., Chang, M., Norman, D., and Chiapelli, F. (1993) Actions of alcohol on immunity and neoplasia in fetal alcohol exposed and adult rats. *Alcohol Alcohol* **2**(Suppl), 69–74.

240. Wu, W., and Pruett, S. (1999) Ethanol decreases host resistance to pulmonary metastases in a mouse model: Role of natural killer cells and ethanol-induced stress response. *Int J Cancer* **82**, 886–92.

241. Ben-Eliyahu, S., Page, G., Yirmaya, R., and Taylor, A. (1996) Acute alcohol intoxication suppresses natural killer cell activity and promotes tumor metastasis. *Nat Med* **2**, 457–60.

242. Hebert, P., and Pruett, S. (2003) Ethanol decreases natural killer cell activation but only minimally affects anatomical distribution after administration of polyinosinic: Polycytidylic acid; role in resistance to B16F10 melanoma. *Alcohol Clin Exp Res* **27**, 1622–31.

243. Blank, S., and Meadows, G. (1996) Ethanol modulates metastatic potential of B16BL6 melanoma and host responses. *Alcohol Clin Exp Res* **20**, 624–8.

244. Spitzer, J., Nunez, N., Meadows, S., Gallucci, R., Blank, S., and Meadows, G. (2000) The modulation of B16BL6 melanoma metastasis is not directly mediated by cytolytic activity of natural killer cells in alcohol-consuming mice. *Alcohol Clin Exp Res* **24**, 837–44.

245. Zhou, J., and Meadows, G. (2003) Alcohol consumption decreases IL-2-induced NF-kappaB activity in enriched NK cells from C57BL/6 mice. *Toxicol Sci* **73**, 72–79.

246. Meadows, G., Wallendal, M., Kosugi, A., Wunderlich, J., and Singer, D. (1992) Ethanol induces marked changes in lymphocyte populations and natural killer cell activity in mice. *Alcohol Clin Exp Res* **16**, 474–9.

247. Yirmaya, R., Ben-Eliyahu, S., Gale, R., Shavit, Y., Liebeskind, J., and Taylor, A. (1992) Ethanol increases tumor progression in rats: Possible involvement of natural killer cells. *Brain Behav Immun* **6**, 74–86.

248. Zhang, H., and Meadows, G. (2008) Chronic alcohol consumption perturbs the balance between thymus-derived and bone marrow-derived natural killer cells in the spleen. *J Leukoc Biol* **83**, 41–47.

249. Boyadjieva, N., Meadows, G., and Sarkar, D. (1999) Effects of ethanol consumption on the beta-endorphin levels and natural killer cell activity in rats. *Ann NY Acad Sci* **885**, 383–6.

32 Aryl Hydrocarbon Receptor-Mediated Carcinogenesis and Modulation by Dietary Xenobiotic and Natural Ligands

Donato F. Romagnolo, Stephanie C. Degner, and Ornella Selmin

Key Points

1. The aryl hydrocarbon receptor (AhR) is a ligand-activated transcription factor of the helix-loop-helix/PAS family. Many compounds interact with the AhR including xenobiotic ("xeno" = foreign) polycyclic aromatic hydrocarbons (PAH) and dioxins, endogenous ligands, and natural bioactive compounds. The activation of the AhR leads to increased expression of Phase I enzymes at xenobiotic responsive elements (XRE) and production of chemically reactive species known to induce cancer. Conversely, activation of the AhR leads to decreased expression of the tumor-suppressor genes *p16* and *BRCA-1*.
2. Data from both animal and human studies suggest that the persistent activation of the AhR may be a risk factor and promote various types of cancer. In particular, PAH appear to preferentially induce mammary tumors in preclinical models. Natural modulators of the AhR include the phytoalexin resveratrol, the indole compounds indole-3-carbinol (I3C) and its condensation product 3,3′-diindolylmethane (DIM), several flavonoids, and catechins.
3. Data from cell culture and animal studies suggest that at relatively low concentration (∼10 μM), DIM may exert antagonistic protective effects, whereas at higher levels (∼100 μM), it may exert agonistic effects and activate the expression of P450. Animal studies reported that the compound I3C may also promote tumor development. The therapeutic properties of these compounds may be influenced by various factors including cell context, timing of exposure, concentration, and relative binding affinity for the AhR.
4. Both the bioavailability and pharmacokinetics of AhR ligands from phytochemicals may influence the therapeutic values of preventative strategies based on AhR antagonists.
5. Although further investigations are necessary to assess the potential benefits of AhR-based strategies against cancer, it is suggested that several phytochemicals may exert protective effects and reduce the risk of toxicity and cancer through competitive transformation of the AhR.

Key Words: Aromatic hydrocarbon receptor; xenobiotics; resveratrol; indole-3-carbinol (I3C); 3,3′-diindolylmethane (DIM); cancer prevention

From: *Nutrition and Health: Bioactive Compounds and Cancer*
Edited by: J.A. Milner, D.F. Romagnolo, DOI 10.1007/978-1-60761-627-6_32,
© Springer Science+Business Media, LLC 2010

1. INTRODUCTION

The aryl hydrocarbon receptor (AhR) is a ligand-activated transcription factor of the helix-loop-helix/PAS family which comprises hypoxia-inducible factor-1α (HIF1α), PAS, and SIM *(1)*. Many compounds interact with the AhR including xenobiotics, endogenous ligands, and natural bioactive compounds (Table 1). In the absence of exogenous ligands, the AhR is found in the cytoplasm associated to a number of chaperone proteins including Hsp90, XAP2, and p23. This complex stabilizes the AhR in the cytoplasm and protects it from degradation. The binding of ligands to the AhR induces the displacement of XAP2 and allows migration of the liganded AhR to the nucleus where it associates with the aryl hydrocarbon receptor nuclear translocator (ARNT), of which three different isoforms have been identified (ARNT-1, ARNT-2, and ARNT-3). Upon nuclear release of the Hsp90 protein, the AhR/ARNT heterocomplex binds to specific DNA core sequences termed xenobiotic or dioxin-responsive elements (XRE = 5'-GCGTG-3') (Fig. 1).

Table 1
Xenobiotic, Endogenous, and Natural AhR Ligands

Class	Examples	Sources
Exogenous xenobiotic AhR ligands		
Halogenated aromatic hydrocarbons (HAHs)	2,3,7,8-Tetrachlorodibenzo-*p*-dioxin Dibenzofurans Azo(xy)benzenes, Naphthalenes	Contamination from industrial processes including chlorine bleaching in paper manufacturing and waste incineration, dietary exposure from fatty foods such as milk, fish, and meat
Polychlorinated biphenyls (PCBs)	3,3',4,4'-Tetrachlorobiphenyl (tetraCB), 3,3',4,4',5-pentaCB, 3,3',4,4',5,5'-hexaCB	Transformer oils, capacitors, heat exchangers, hydraulic fluids, flame retardants, adhesives; dietary exposure from meat, liver, milk, and eggs
Polyaromatic hydrocarbons (PAHs)	Benzo(a)pyrene Benzanthracenes Benzoflavones 3-Methylcholanthrene	Products of combustion found in smoke exhaust, chimney soot, and charbroiled foods; other dietary sources include cereals, oils, fats, some fruits, and vegetables
Phthalates	Butyl phthalate (BBP) Dibutyl phthalate (DBP)	Perfumes, cosmetics, lotions, nail polish, lacquers, and varnishes, present in indoor air and dust, found in a variety of foods, milk, breast milk

Phenols	Bisphenol A (BPA) 4-*n*-Nonylphenol (nNP)	Polycarbonate plastic, detected in drinking water, canned meats, vegetables, fruit, and infant formula Additive in some plastics, soaps, cosmetics, paints, herbicides, pesticides
Candidate endogenous AhR ligands		
Indigoids	Indigo Indirubin	
Heme metabolites	Bilirubin Biliverdin	Degradation of heme
Arachidonic acid metabolites	Prostaglandin G2 Lipoxin A4	Produced from cyclooxygenase and lipoxygenase pathways
Tryptophan metabolites	Tryptamine Indole acetic acid (IAA)	
Tryptophan photoproducts	6-Formylindolo[3,2-*b*]carbazole (FICZ) 6,12-Diformylindolo[3,2-*b*]carbazole (dFICZ)	Produced from UV irradiation of tryptophan in the skin
Natural dietary AhR ligands		
Indoles	Indole-3-carbinol (I3C) Indolo[3,2-*b*]carbazole (ICZ) 3,3′-Diindolylmethane (DIM)	Cruciferous vegetables such as broccoli, brussels sprouts, cabbage, cauliflower, collard greens, kale, radish, rutabaga, and turnip
Polyphenolic curcuminoid	Curcumin	Found in turmeric, a spice obtained from rhizomes of *Curcuma longa*
Polyphenolic stilbene	Resveratrol	Grapes, wine, peanuts, soy, and some berries
Flavonoids	Quercetin, kaempferol, chrysin, galangin, baicalein, genistein, daidzein, apigenin	In a variety of fruits and vegetables including apples, onions, kale, broccoli, berries, teas

Data presented in Table 1 were compiled from Amakura *(103)*, Ciolino *(127)*, Phillips *(140)*, Safe *(85)*, Zhang *(96)*, Denison *(97)*, Krüger *(86)*, La Rocca *(141)*, Moon *(142)*, Nguyen *(143)*, Sathyanarayana *(144)*, and Willhite *(145)*.

The *CYP1A1* gene has been used extensively as a sentinel marker of exposure to environmental ligands of the AhR and to investigate the regulation of Phase I enzymes in detoxification *(2, 3)*. The binding of the dioxin prototype 2,3,7,8 tetrachlorodibenzo-*p*-dioxin (TCDD) to the AhR triggers the recruitment of the AhR/ARNT complex to XREs located in the enhancer region of CYP1A1 inducing changes in chromatin

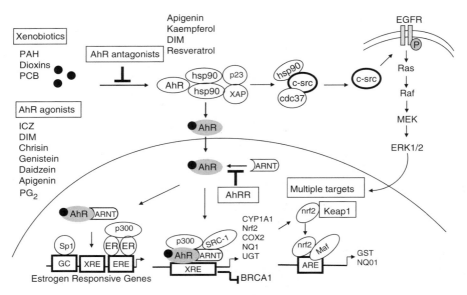

Fig. 1. Effects of xenobiotics, natural ligands, and endogenous compounds on activation of the AhR pathway. Upon binding to ligands, the AhR translocates to the nucleus where it activates (CYP1A1, Nrf2, COX-2, NQO1, UGT) or represses (BRCA-1) transcription of target genes at xenobiotic responsive elements (XRE) or through interaction with transcription factors bound to their cognate elements (Sp, AP-1, ERE). The activation of Nrf2 leads to parallel activation of Phase II enzymes by Nrf2/Maf transcription complexes at antioxidant responsive elements (ARE). The activation of the AhR leads to parallel phosphorylation of the epidermal growth factor receptor (EGFR) by the cytosolic factor c-src and downstream activation of the MAPK pathways and related targets. These events are triggered by various ligands of the AhR including xenobiotic PAH, dioxins, and PCB as well as endogenous ligands (PG2). Natural compounds may exert agonistic or antagonistic effects based on concentrations, timing of exposure, and cell context. Details are in the text.

organization and DNA bending. These conformational changes facilitate the interaction with a series of transcription cofactors, including p/CIP, p300, and GTFs, which in turn interact with NF-1 and TBP proteins bound to CAAT and TATA boxes, respectively. The coordinate recruitment of these factors leads to activation of Pol II-mediated transcription *(4)*.

Several studies have also documented that the AhR may regulate expression through non-XRE-mediated mechanisms. For example, the AhR binds directly to cofactors that possess histone acetyl transferase (HAT) activity including SRC-1 and CBP or to transcription factors bound to their cognate response elements such as Sp1 and the estrogen receptor (ER). Through these mechanisms the AhR may sequester or tether transcription factors thus influencing transcription of target genes *(5)*.

1.1. Activation of Phase I and II Enzymes by AhR

Specific genes that harbor XRE sequences in their promoter include members of the cytochrome P450 family of Phase I metabolizing enzymes such as *CYP1A1*, *CYP1B1*, and *CYP1A2* and the Phase II detoxification NAD(P)H:quinone oxidoreductase1 (*NQO1*) and UDP-glucuronosyltransferase-1A6 (*UGT1A6*) genes *(6)*. The activation of Phase I enzymes leads to the production of chemically reactive species, which are modified to inactive products by Phase II enzymes. For example, benzo[a]pyrene (B[a]P), a prototype polycyclic aromatic hydrocarbon (PAH) found in tobacco smoke and grilled foods activates the expression of CYP1A1, which in turn participates in the biotransformation of B[a]P to the highly mutagenic diol-epoxide 7r,8t-dihydroxy-9t,10-epoxy-7,8,9,10-tetrahydrobenzo[a]pyrene (BPDE) *(7)*. Phase II enzymes such as glutathione *S*-transferase (GST) inactivate BPDE through enzymatic conjugation. The activation of the AhR by TCDD also induces transcription of Phase I (CYP1A, CYP1A2, and CYP1B1) and Phase II (UGT and GST, NQO1) enzymes *(8, 9)*. However, unlike PAHs, TCDD is resistant to metabolic breakdown and this property is responsible for its accumulation in the food chain and fatty tissue. A possible consequence of TCDD accumulation in tissue (half-life $\sim$8–10 years) may be the persistent activation of the AhR increasing the likelihood for tumor development *(10)*.

The expression of Phase II enzymes is linked to the transcription activity of the AhR, which directly stimulates transcription of the nuclear factor erythroid 2-related factor-2 (Nrf2) through the AhR/XRE pathway *(11)*. The Nrf2 protein is localized in its inactive form to the cytoplasm bound to a Keap1 complex. However, both the accumulation of AhR/CYP1A1-generated reactive oxygen species and electrophiles *(12)* and thiol modification of Keap1 cysteine residues by isothiocyanate compounds induce the release of Nrf2 from the Keap1 complex. The released Nrf2 forms a heterodimer with Maf proteins (MafF, MafG, MafK) activating the transcription of GST and NQO1 genes at antioxidant responsive elements (ARE = 5′-A/GTGAC/GNNNGCA/G-3′) (Fig. 1). Whereas the ARE is found in many Phase II genes, the XRE is found in both Phase I and Phase II genes.

The fact that the AhR can control directly or indirectly the expression of Phase I and II enzymes provides an integrated system of detoxification against potential carcinogens. Therefore, the dietary intake of bioactive compounds that couple inhibition of Phase I and activation of Phase II enzymes may have beneficial effects against AhR-mediated carcinogens *(11)*.

1.2. Endogenous Role for the AhR

In addition to acting as a sensor of exposure to xenobiotics and natural ligands, the AhR may modulate the effects of endogenous ligands (Table 1) *(13)*. Several eicosanoid molecules, in particular 5,6 dihydroxy-eicosatetraenoic acid isomers (5,6-DiHETEs) and prostaglandin-2 (PG$_2$), are activators of the AhR. The cross-talk between eicosanoid and AhR-mediated pathways may have important implications in inflammation and cancer. Using human pulmonary microvascular endothelial cells under conditions of hypoxia, Zhang and Walker *(14)* showed constitutive elevation of CYP1A1 mRNA, which was dependent on expression of the AhR in the absence of exogenous ligands. Moreover, Baba et al. *(15)* demonstrated that the AhR played a central role in female reproduction by regulating the expression of the ovarian P450 aromatase, Cyp19, an enzyme involved in estrogen synthesis. These studies indicated that the AhR directly regulated the expression of the *CyP19* gene through physical interaction with the nuclear orphan receptor Ad4BP/SF-1, thus providing a mechanism through which the AhR may influence estrogen levels.

1.3. Cross-Talk Between AhR- and ER-Regulated Pathways

Mechanisms through which the AhR interferes with the physiological actions of steroid hormones, in particular estrogen, have been extensively reviewed (16). The ligand-activated AhR alters transcriptional activation by the ER through binding to XREs located in proximity to estrogen receptor elements (ERE) (5). The occupancy of XRE by the AhR heterocomplex and the direct interaction with the AhR have been shown to disrupt the formation of ER/SP-1 and ER/AP-1 DNA complexes and compete for limited cofactors (e.g., NF-1) (Fig. 1). The activation of the AhR by exogenous ligands can rapidly reduce ER protein levels through proteasomal degradation (17). Reducing the nuclear levels of ERα protein or its transcriptional activity may lower the expression of the progesterone receptor (PR). In turn, reduced PR levels may hamper the actions of progesterone on endometrial differentiation during the secretory phase and favor the development of endometrial pathologies (18, 19).

The liganded AhR activates ERα signaling in the absence of estrogen. Two possible mechanisms have been described. First, the binding of ligands to the AhR induces the release of c-src from a cytosolic complex that comprises hsp90 and cdc37 (20). The released c-src activates several protein kinases leading to phosphorylation and activation of the ERα. Second, in the absence of estrogen, the AhR/ARNT complex interacts with the nuclear ERα and the cofactor p300/CBP activating the expression of ER responsive genes. Conversely, in the presence of estrogen, the activated AhR inhibits transcription of estrogen-responsive genes (21). Recent studies suggested that the ability of the AhR to activate the ER in the absence of estrogens was limited to PAH including 3-methylcholanthrene (3-MC) and B[a]P, whereas no proestrogenic effects were seen in the presence of TCDD. Moreover, TCDD exerted antiestrogenic effects due to preferential reduction of ERβ activity (22). Therefore, the activation of the AhR can lead to induction or inhibition of estrogen-regulated genes depending on type of AhR ligand, cell context, and involvement of specific (ER/Sp1 or ER/AP-1) transcription complexes.

1.4. AhR Cross-Talk with EGFR Pathways

The epidermal growth factor receptor (EGFR) family is involved in the regulation of cell proliferation, differentiation, and embryonic development by controlling several downstream signaling transduction cascades, principally MAPK, Akt, and JNK pathways (23). Increased expression of EGFR has been described in most human epithelial cancers. Administration of EGF induces effects similar to those caused by dioxin intoxication including fatty liver, lack of palatal fusion, and skin tumors.

The AhR-induced release of c-src from the hsp90/cdc37/c-src complex has been proposed as a mechanism of activation of the EGFR pathway (Fig. 1). The c-src translocates to the plasma membrane and phosphorylates the EGFR, which in turn activates MAPK/ERK1/2 signal transduction leading to transcriptional activation of genes involved in inflammation including cyclooxygenase-2 (COX-2) (24). It has also been suggested that activation of the AhR may increase the levels of cAMP, which in turn activates PKA-mediated phosphorylation of EGFR and CREB proteins *(25)*. Under normoxic conditions, EGFR signaling activated by the phosphoinositide 3-kinase/Akt pathway leading to increased expression of HIF-1α. The HIF-1α stimulates the expression of genes necessary for cell survival and inhibition of apoptosis under hypoxic conditions *(26)*. Thus, cross-talk between AhR and EGFR/HIF-1α pathways may be important in cancer since activation of the EGFR and hypoxia in tumors are conditions that increase resistance to apoptosis.

1.5. AhR-Mediated Effects on Cell Cycle Checkpoints

Several observations point to an inhibitory role of the AhR in regulation of cell cycle progression through the G1 phase *(27)*. The Rb protein is functionally inactivated in its hyperphosphorylated form. Two models have been proposed for AhR-mediated cell cycle arrest through pRb. In the first model, the AhR forms a quaternary structure comprising hypophosphorylated "active" pRb, E2F, and DP. The latter is an E2F-binding partner in transactivation. The direct binding of the AhR/pRb complex to E2F represses transcription of genes necessary for cell cycle progression including cyclin E. The second model suggests that suppression of cell cycle progression by AhR ligands results from interaction between pRb and the liganded AhR, where pRb is functioning as a coactivator bound to the AhR. The heterocomplex comprising pRb, AhR, and ARNT activates at XRE the expression of p27 *(28)*. Both mechanisms seem to coexist and block cdk2 activity thus preventing pRb inactivation.

The AhR-mediated cell cycle arrest and stimulation of p27 expression are in contrast with the evidence TCDD is one of the most potent tumor promoters in animal model systems *(29)*. In keeping with this notion, TCDD has been shown to repress expression of the cell cycle checkpoints p53 and p16 through hypermethylation of the p16 and p53 promoter regions *(30)*. This silencing effect was dependent on the concomitant expression of the AhR. Also, activation of the AhR by the dioxin TCDD induced expression of *c-fos* and *c-jun* proto-oncogenes and a large increase in transcription factor AP-1 *(31)*. Moreover, the recruitment of the activated AhR to XRE has been shown to repress the expression of the *BRCA-1* gene *(32)*, while increasing transcription of the proinflammatory gene, COX-2 *(33, 34)*. The lack of functional cdk inhibitors p16 and p53, combined with mysregulation of DNA repair linked to BRCA-1 and increased COX-2 expression, is a recognized hallmark of many human cancers. These cumulative observations have led to the conclusion TCDD may accelerate the rate at which DNA-damaged cells convert to a neoplastic phenotype through a yin-yang mechanism: under normal conditions of exposure to DNA-damaging agents the AhR would function as a transient checkpoint. However, under conditions of persistent exposure to AhR ligands or severe DNA damage caused by AhR ligands (e.g., PAH) the binding of the AhR to E2F-1 may block its apoptotic properties leading to proliferation. This yin-yang mechanism may explain, at least in part, how activation of the AhR pathway contributes to tumorigenesis *(29)*.

Expression levels of the AhR protein may influence this mechanism and alter cell cycle regulation. For example, the constitutive overexpression of the AhR resulted in promotion of hepatocarcinogenesis in mice that were treated with a single injection of the hepatocarcinogen *N*-nitrosodiethylamine *(35)*. Moreover, constitutively active AhR was reported to upregulate CYP1B1 before tumor formation in a rat model of mammary tumorigenesis *(36)*. Furthermore, higher binding affinity of AhR ligands may reduce the rate of proteosomal degradation of the AhR increasing the activity of the AhR/ARNT heterocomplex at target promoter elements and the activation of growth factor pathways.

2. AHR-MEDIATED CARCINOGENESIS

2.1. Animal Models

The use of AhR knockout models has provided insights into the role of the AhR in normal physiology and carcinogenesis. AhR knockout mice exhibit reduced viability, lower fertility, and impaired liver development *(37)*. AhR-null mice had reduced basal and inducible CYP1A1 expression *(38)*, and were resistant to malignancies induced by PAHs and dioxins. Reduced B[a]P-induced mutagenesis and genotoxicity in AhR knockout mice was attributed to impaired CYP1A1 expression and metabolism of B[*a*]P to reactive intermediates *(39)*. In the absence of exogenous ligands, AhR-null mice with transgenic adenocarcinoma of the mouse prostate (TRAMP) displayed increased frequency of prostate tumors compared to AhR wild-type TRAMP mice *(40)*, implying the AhR may function as a tumor suppressor.

Results of animal studies suggested that the exposure to PAH may be a risk factor in the etiology of mammary tumors. For example, DMBA, a prototypical PAH and ligand of the AhR, preferentially induced mammary cancers in rats *(41)* and mice *(42)*. The DMBA-induced rat and mouse mammary tumors expressed higher levels of AhR protein *(43)*. In female rats treated with DMBA, levels of *CYP1B1*, but not CYP1A1 mRNA, were elevated in mammary tumors *(44)*. CYP1B1 is a 17β-estradiol-hydroxylase that catalyzes the production of 4-hydroxyestradiol (4HE), a known mammary carcinogen *(45)*. The incidence of DMBA-induced rat mammary tumors was reduced by cotreatment with the AhR ligands 6-methyl-1,3,8-trichlorodibenzofuran (6-MCDF) and 8-methyl-1,3,6-trichlorodibenzofuran (8-MCDF) *(43)*. The preventive properties of these compounds were related to their weak agonist activity for the AhR. The ability of dioxins to induce tumors differed between males and females. The treatment with TCDD induced hepatocelullar carcinogenesis in female, but not male, Sprague-Dawley rats implying the existence of cross-talk between AhR and ovarian steroid-regulated pathways *(46)*.

2.2. In Utero Exposure to AhR Ligands

In transplacental carcinogenesis studies, AhR ligands administered to mothers increased the incidence of cancer in offsprings *(47)*. To examine the role of AhR polymorphisms on susceptibility to transplacental carcinogenesis, 3-MC and DMBA were administered to either AhR responsive or AhR non-responsive pregnant mice during gestation *(48)*. Offsprings that were AhR responsive had greater incidence of lung and liver tumors compared to AhR non-responsive littermates. In a mouse model, the in utero exposure to the PAH compounds, dibenzo[a,l]pyrene (DB[a,l]P), induced aggressive T-cell lymphoblastic lymphoma and lung tumors in offsprings *(49)*. Compared to exposure after 3 weeks of nursing, the in utero exposure to DB[a,l]P resulted in greater lung tumor multiplicity in offsprings *(50)*. In a rat mammary cancer model, prenatal exposure to TCDD altered mammary gland differentiation and increased the susceptibility of female offsprings to DMBA-induced mammary tumors *(51)*.

2.3. Human Studies

The AhR is expressed in a wide variety of normal human tissues. Basal expression for both AhR and ARNT was detected in liver, heart, spleen, testis, and at higher levels in the lung and kidney *(52)*. However, there appears to be a large inter-individual variation between AhR and ARNT mRNA expression levels in liver and lungs. In another study, levels of AhR mRNA were relatively lower in normal pancreatic tissue, intermediate in 60% of chronic pancreatitis samples (9/15), and expressed at higher levels in 93% (14/15) of pancreatic cancer samples *(53)*. Increased AhR expression was also observed in about 50% (49/107) of human lung adenocarcinomas. The increased levels of AhR were associated with increased expression of CYP1A1 in smoking adenocarcinoma patients *(54)*. Studies examining AhR expression in bronchiolar epithelial cells reported increased expression of the AhR in neoplastic cells, especially adenocarcinoma samples *(55)*.

The expression of ARNT2, a homolog of ARNT, was found in 75.2% of breast tumor tissue compared to only 17.6% in normal tissue and was associated with favorable disease outcome for patients *(56)*. Many of the tumors expressing ARNT2 were also ER-positive. In human primary acute lymphoblastic leukemia tumors, the *AhR* gene was methylated in 33% of cases, suggesting the AhR could be a tumor suppressor *(57)*. In addition, studies have suggested that AhR polymorphisms influence individual susceptibility to colon cancer following exposure to AhR-carcinogens *(58–61)*.

The AhR repressor (AhRR) protein negatively regulates the AhR pathway through competitive binding to ARNT reducing the recruitment of the AhR/ARNT heterocomplex to XREs harbored in promoters of various genes. In normal human tissues, AhRR mRNA expression was detected in human liver, breast, colon, kidney, lung, bladder, uterus, testis, ovary, and adrenal gland tissues *(62)*. Conversely, the expression of AHRR was downregulated in tumors of the colon, breast, lung, stomach, and ovary. Furthermore, hypermethylation of the AHRR promoter was observed in the majority of colon, ovarian, prostate, and cervical cancers *(63)*. These observations suggested the reduced expression of AhRR may be a predisposing factor in tumorigenesis.

Breast tissues from breast cancer patients showed a disproportionate presence of PAH:DNA adducts suggesting there exists an important link between exposure to AhR ligands and risk of breast cancer *(64)*.

3. HUMAN EXPOSURE TO AhR XENOBIOTICS

3.1. PAH

Through diet, environmental pollution, and cigarette smoke, humans are exposed to a complex mixture of xenobiotics and ligands of the AhR including PAHs, dioxins, dioxin-like polychlorinated biphenylenes (PCB), and bisphenols. The relative binding affinity of these compounds for the AhR influences the transcriptional activity of the

Table 2
Binding Affinity of TCDD and Various PAH for the AhR

Selected AhR ligand	EC50 AhR-binding values
High affinity	
TCDD	1.0×10^{-8} M
3-Methylcholanthrene	2.8×10^{-8} M
Intermediate affinity	
Dimethylbenzo[a]anthracene	3.2×10^{-7} M
Benzo[a]pyrene	3.6×10^{-7} M
Low affinity	
Benzo[e]pyrene	1.0×10^{-4} M

Data in Table 2 were obtained from Piskorska-Pliszczynska *(146)*.

AhR (Table 2). Of the many PAHs present in the environment, B[a]P is considered a prototype and classic DNA-damaging agent and mammary carcinogen *(65, 66)*. The daily average ingestion of B[a]P from food sources is estimated to be ~2.2 μg/day *(67, 68)* with a median intake level of ~ 3 μg/day *(69, 70)*. The concentration of B[a]P in foods is influenced by geographical location and industrial environment *(71, 72)*. Common dietary sources of B[a]P are well-cooked meats, cereals, oils, and fats *(73)*.

3.2. Dioxins

An important class of environmental contaminants found in foods is halogenated hydrocarbons, of which TCDD is the prototype *(74, 75)*. TCDD was classified as a Group 1 human carcinogen by the International Agency for Cancer Research (IARC) *(10, 76)*. Dioxins found in the environment originate from waste incinerators, chlorine bleaching in pulp and paper manufacturing, and the production of some pesticides, herbicides, and fungicides *(77)*. It is estimated that approximately 90% of human exposure to dioxins is from dietary ingestion from fish, meat, and dairy products *(78, 79)*. The average daily intake of TCDD toxic equivalents (TEqs) per adult in the US is estimated to range from 0.3 to 3.0 pg/kg body weight *(80)*.

Population studies detected the accumulation of TCDD in breast milk *(81, 82)*, suggesting this agent may accumulate in breast tissue at levels sufficient to induce mammary neoplasia. The mean dietary dioxin and dioxin-like PCB intake estimates for adults in the USA were the highest in a study that compared the risk of exposure in several industrialized countries *(83)*. Increased incidence of breast cancer has been reported in human populations residing in industrialized areas for which high levels of dioxins were found in air, soil, drinking water, and cow's milk *(84)*.

3.3. PCB and Bisphenols

Many PCB, found in insulators, flame retardants, and adhesives, are chemically stable and environmentally ubiquitous *(85)*. Phthalates and phenols found in plastic that modulate AhR activity include bisphenol A (BPA), 4-*n*-nonylphenol (nNP), benzyl butyl phthalate (BBP), 4-chloro-3-methylphenol (CMP), 2,4-dichlorophenol (DCP), resorcinol, bis(2-ethylhexyl) phthalate (DEHP), diisodecyl phthalate (DIDP), and dibutyl phthalate (DBP) *(86)*. The exposure to PCB and bisphenols during gestation and through breast milk may increase cancer risk *(87–89)*.

4. SYNTHETIC MODULATORS OF THE AHR

4.1. α-Naphthoflavone and 3′-Methoxy-4′-Nitroflavone

Compounds that have antagonistic activities may prevent the formation of the AhR/ARNT heterocomplex. For example, the synthetic compound 3′-methoxy-4′-nitroflavone (3M4NF) has been characterized as a "pure" antagonist of the AhR by blocking the translocation of the AhR to the nucleus *(90)*. A second mechanism of action of AhR antagonists is the formation of an AhR/ARNT heterocomplex that binds DNA but is less active at the transcriptional level *(91)*. For example, the synthetic compound ANF was reported to antagonize the TCDD-induced binding of AhR/ARNT complexes to XRE by forming an inactive complex with the AhR *(92)*. The ANF has been categorized as a "partial" antagonist by directly competing for binding sites of the cytosolic AhR *(93, 94)*. Studies documented that the cotreatment with ANF reversed in a dose-dependent fashion the repressive effects of B[a]P on BRCA-1 expression, while preventing the activation of CYP1A1 *(95)*. These cumulative observations provide important experimental clues for the development of dietary strategies based on natural modulators of the AhR *(96, 97)*.

5. NATURAL LIGANDS OF THE AhR

5.1. Resveratrol

The compound *resveratrol* (3,5,4′-trihydroxystilbene) (RES) is a phytoalexin found in grapes, wine, berries, peanuts, and soy *(98)*. RES has multiple anticancer effects including induction of cell cycle arrest and apoptosis *(99, 100)*. Studies have documented that RES inhibited carcinogen-induced preneoplastic lesions in the murine mammary gland *(101)* as well as tumorigenesis in the mouse-skin model *(102)*. Resveratrol has been shown to antagonize TCDD-induced AhR activity as measured by a AhR bioassay *(103, 104)*. Interestingly, RES has a similar molecular size and planar structure to TCDD. In human mammary epithelial cells, RES inhibited TCDD-induced AhR-binding activity and expression of CYP1A1 and CYP1B1 *(105)*. RES can also act as a phytoestrogen and it is a partial agonist for the ER *(106)*. It induced mRNA levels of BRCA-1 in a panel of breast tumor cell lines *(107)*.

5.2. Indoles

The consumption of cruciferous vegetables is believed to protect against several types of cancer through the action of glucosinolates *(108)*. Upon metabolic breakdown, glucosinolates generate several compounds including isothiocyanates, thiocyanates, nitriles, cyanoepithioalkanes, and indoles. Indoles include indol-3-carbinol (I3C), which is produced during crushing of plant tissue. In the acidic environment of the stomach,

I3C condenses to generate 3,3'-diindolylmethane (DIM) and indolo[3,2-b]carbazole (ICZ) *(97, 109)*. The metabolite ICZ (K_d = 1.9 × 10^{-10} M) is a potent activator of the AhR whereas DIM (K_d = 9 × 10^{-8} M) and I3C (K_d = 2.7 × 10^{-5} M) are weaker ligands *(4, 110, 111)*. The relative binding affinity of ICZ approximates that of the dioxin compound TCDD (K_d = 7.1 × 10^{-12} M).

The consumption of 25 g of Brassica vegetables generates intake levels of I3C in excess of 700 μg/day *(110)*. Other estimates suggest that human consumption of 100 g of Brussels sprouts may generate plasma levels of I3C ranging from 10 to 50 μM *(112)*. Several studies have shown that I3C has chemopreventive properties against chemically-induced and spontaneous tumors *(113–116)*. Experimental evidence indicated I3C reduced the formation of colonic aberrant crypt foci and DNA adduct formation in rat models of colon carcinogenesis *(117)*. In MCF-7 and MDA-MB-468 breast cancer cell lines, the treatment with I3C resulted in the dose-dependent accumulation of BRCA-1, a nuclear factor required in DNA repair *(118)*. The ability of I3C to modulate the cancer process appeared to be influenced by the timing of exposure. For example, when administered before a carcinogen, I3C acted to protect cancer initiation, whereas when administered after a carcinogen, I3C promoted carcinogenesis *(113, 119)*. Moreover, I3C has been shown to promote development of colonic lesions in a rat model *(120)* and enhance uterine carcinogenesis *(121)*. The latter effect was attributed primarily to induction of CYP1B1-dependent 4HE activity. The enzyme CYP1B1 catalyzes the metabolism of estradiol to the catechol 4HE. The latter is a strong ligand of the ER and stimulates uterine and mammary tumor development. These data suggest that I3C may exert protective effects in normal cells, whereas it may enhance growth of existing lesions.

Pharmacokinetic studies indicated that DIM is the predominant I3C-derived metabolic product *(122)*. These results likely explain why the treatment with DIM (5 mg/kg body weight) was more effective than IC3 in reducing the formation of mammary tumors induced by the carcinogen and AhR ligand, DMBA. At concentrations ranging from 10 to 50 μM, the condensation product DIM induced the formation of the nuclear AhR heterocomplex, but it did not influence basal CYP1A1 expression. At concentrations ranging from 10 to 50 μM, DIM repressed estrogen-induced expression in MCF-7 cells *(123, 124)*. In contrast, concentrations of 100 μM DIM induced CYP1A1 expression to a degree similar to that observed for 1 nM TCDD *(123)*. These data suggest that at relatively low levels of exposure, DIM may exert protective effects and interfere with the activity of the AhR, whereas at higher concentrations (>50 μM) DIM may favor transformation of the AhR and activation of P450s *(117)*. Therefore, through diet it may be advantageous to achieve human plasma concentrations of DIM (∼10 μM) sufficient to exert antagonistic effects against the AhR, while preventing activation of P450s. The short-term bioavailability of DIM (4–12 h) suggests that daily intake of Brassica vegetables or repeated dosing may be necessary to reach target micromolar levels of DIM in human plasma *(125)*. Through the AhR-mediated activation of Nrf2 expression, indoles and isothiocyanates may exert synergistic effects and inducing Phase II enzymes such as GST *(6, 126)*.

5.3. Flavonoids

The total dietary intake of flavonoids from plants has been estimated to be ~1 g/day. Several flavonoids that have been investigated for their antagonistic and agonistic actions on the AhR include kaempferol, quercitin, and apigenin. Although these compounds are structurally related, hydroxyl substitutions seem to influence their binding affinity for the AhR (Table 3). Compared to kaempferol and apigenin, quercitin possesses an extra OH group on the B-ring, which may increase its binding affinity for the AhR. Results of AhR-binding affinity studies varied and were influenced by cell type, time of exposure, and concentration of flavonoids used. Kaempferol at concentrations ranging from 1 to 10 µM did not induce CYP1A1 expression in MCF-7 breast cancer cells *(127)*. These results suggested that kaempferol did not exhibit significant AhR agonist activity. However, in human hepatoma H2pG2 cells at concentrations ~10 µM or higher kaempferol acted as an AhR antagonist by interacting with the AhR-ligand binding site and preventing TCDD-induced CYP1A1 expression *(128)*. In MCF-7 cells,

Table 3
Antagonistic IC50 of α-Naphthoflavone and Natural Ligands of the AhR

Compound	IC 50 against TCDD
α-Naphthoflavone	0.39×10^{-6}
Flavones	
Apigenin	3.2×10^{-6}
Luteolin	6.5×10^{-6}
Flavonols	
Galangin	0.2×10^{-6}
Kaempferol	2.1×10^{-6}
Quercetin	1.5×10^{-6}
Flavanones	
Naringenin	6.7×10^{-6}
Isoflavones	
Daidzein	$>5.0 \times 10^{-5}$
Genistein	$>5.0 \times 10^{-5}$
Catechins	
(-)-Epigallocatechin gallate	3.5×10^{-5}
(-)-Epicatechin gallate	8.0×10^{-5}
(-)-Epigallocatechin	$>2.0 \times 10^{-4}$
Indoles	
3,3′-diindolylmethane	5.0×10^{-5}
Indol-3-carbinol	2.3×10^{-3}
Phytoalexins	
Resveratrol	1.9×10^{-6}

Data were obtained from Amakura et al. *(103)*, Jellinck et al. *(111)*, and Ashida et al. *(130)*.

both kaempferol and quercitin at doses ranging from 1 to 10 µM exerted antagonistic activity and inhibited TCDD-induced XRE-promoter activity *(96)*. In human hepatoma HepG2 cells, apigenin (at least 10 µM) exhibited antagonistic activities *(128)*.

5.4. Cathechins

Catechins represent ∼15–30% of dry weight of green tea although composition of green tea extracts can be highly variable. The major catechins present in tea are catechin (-)-epigallocatechin-3-gallate (EGCG), (-)epigallocatechin (EGC), (-)-epicatechin-3-gallate (ECG), and (-)-epicathenic (EC). Results of studies that measured the effects of these compounds on AhR activity have been discordant. Dietary levels of EGCG (∼1–2 µM) were found to suppress transformation of the AhR by TCDD *(129)* and CYP1A1 expression *(130, 131)*. These concentrations approximated those measured in human serum (4.4 µM) following supplementation with 525 mg EGCG *(132)*. However, in other studies higher concentrations of green tea extracts (25–50 µM) *(133)* or EGCG and EGC (∼50 µM) *(134)* were required to antagonize the activation of the AhR by TCDD.

6. CONCLUSIONS

The AhR has a promiscuous ligand-binding site that interacts with many dietary xenobiotic and natural compounds *(97)*. The daily intake of natural compounds has been estimated to be higher than the reported exposures to dioxins and dioxin-like PCBs. For example, potatoes, cruciferous vegetables, breads, hamburgers, grapefruit juice *(135)*, fruits, and herbs *(136)* have been shown to contain agonists of the AhR. The activation of the AhR has been reported to directly induce at XRE the expression of COX-2 *(33, 34)* which converts arachidonic acid to prostaglandins. Prostaglandin-2 and 12-R-HETE have been shown to activate the AhR *(97, 137)*. Therefore, chemopreventative approaches targeted to the AhR should take into account the contribution of both dietary natural and endogenously occurring AhR agonists *(128)*.

In designing preventative strategies based on AhR modulators it may be important to consider whether these compounds exert tissue-specific effects, the influence of concentration and timing of exposure, the relative binding affinity for the AhR, and whether AhR ligands present in physiological mixtures exert additive cancer preventing or promoting effects (Fig. 1). For example, human studies have reported AhR-related induction of the P450 enzyme CYP1A2 following intake of cruciferous vegetables *(138)*. Moreover, animal studies showed that the Brassica-derived compound, I3C, promoted tumor development *(139)*. Whereas these results could be related to use of supraphysiological concentrations, it is possible that several ligands administered as part of a diet may reach levels sufficient to activate the AhR pathway. Therefore, both the bioavailability and pharmacokinetics of AhR ligands from phytochemicals may influence the therapeutic values of preventative strategies based on AhR antagonists. Although further investigations are necessary to assess the potential benefits of AhR-based strategies against cancer, it is suggested that several vegetable bioactive compounds may exert protective effects and reduce the risk of toxicity and cancer through competitive transformation of the AhR.

ACKNOWLEDGMENTS

This research has been supported by grants from the Arizona Biomedical Research Commission (100116, 8015), the Susan G. Komen Breast Cancer Foundation (BCTR0707643), the US Department Breast Cancer Research Program (DAMD17-00-1-0130), the National Institute of Environmental Health Sciences, National Institutes of Health (ES009966), and Training Grant in Toxicology and Toxicogenomics (T32 ES-07091-24).

REFERENCES

1. Perdew, G.H. (2008) Ah receptor binding to its cognate response element is required for dioxin-mediated toxicity. *Toxicol Sci* **106**, 301–03.
2. Hankinson, O. (2005) Role of coactivators in transcriptional activation by the aryl hydrocarbon receptor. *Arch Biochem Biophys* **433**, 379–86.
3. Matthews, J., Wihlén, B., Thomsen, J., and Gustafsson, J.A. (2005) Aryl hydrocarbon receptor-mediated transcription: Ligand-dependent recruitment of estrogen receptor alpha to 2,3,7,8-tetrachlorodibenzo-p-dioxin-responsive promoters. *Mol Cell Biol* **25**, 5317–28.
4. Hestermann, E.V., and Brown, M. (2003) Agonist and chemopreventative ligands induce differential transcriptional cofactor recruitment by aryl hydrocarbon receptor. *Mol Cell Biol* **23**, 7920–25.
5. Safe, S. (2001) Molecular biology of the Ah receptor and its role in carcinogenesis. *Toxicol Lett* **120**, 1–7.
6. Hayes, J.D., Kelleher, M.O., and Eggleston, I.M. (2008) The cancer chemopreventive actions of phytochemicals derived from glucosinolates. *Eur J Nutr* **47**, 73–88.
7. Ruddon, R. (1995) Cancer Biology. 3rd ed., New York: Oxford University Press.
8. Hankinson, O. (1995) The aryl hydrocarbon receptor complex. *Annu Rev Pharmacol Toxicol* **35**, 307–40.
9. Hahn, M.E. (2002) Aryl hydrocarbon receptors: Diversity and evolution. *Chem Biol Interact* **141**, 131–60.
10. Steenland, K., Bertazzi, P., Baccarelli, A., and Kogevinas, M. (2004) Dioxin revisited: Developments since the 1997 IARC classification of dioxin as a human carcinogen. *Environ Health Perspect* **112**, 1265–68.
11. Miao, W., Hu, L., Scrivens, P.J., and Batist, G. (2005) Transcriptional regulation of NF-E2 p45-related factor (NRF2) expression by the aryl hydrocarbon receptor-xenobiotic response element signaling pathway: Direct cross-talk between phase I and II drug-metabolizing enzymes. *J Biol Chem* **280**, 20340–48.
12. Köhle, C., and Bock, K.W. (2006) Activation of coupled Ah receptor and Nrf2 gene batteries by dietary phytochemicals in relation to chemoprevention. *Biochem Pharmacol* **72**, 795–805.
13. Nebert, D.W., and Karp, C.L. (2008) Endogenous functions of the Aryl hydrocarbon receptor: Intersection of cytochromeP450 (CYP1)-metabolized eicosanoids and AHR biology. *J Biol Chem*, Aug 18 [Epub ahead of print] PMID: 18713746.
14. Zhang, N., and Walker, M.K. (2007) Crosstalk between the aryl hydrocarbon receptor and hypoxia on the constitutive expression of cytochrome P4501A1 mRNA. *Cardiovasc Toxicol* **7**, 282–90.
15. Baba, T., Mimura, J., Nakamura, N., Harada, N., Yamamoto, M., Morohashi, K., and Fujii-Kuriyama, Y. (2005) Intrinsic function of the aryl hydrocarbon (dioxin) receptor as a key factor in female Reproduction. *Mol Cell Biol* **22**, 10040–51.
16. Pocar, P., Fischer, B., Klonisch, T., and Hombach-Klonisch, S. (2005) Molecular interactions of the aryl hydrocarbon receptor and its biological and toxicological relevance for reproduction. *Reproduction* **129**, 379–89.

17. Wormke, M., Stoner, M., Saville, B., and Safe, S. (2000) Crosstalk between estrogen receptor alpha and the aryl hydrocarbon receptor in breast cancer cells involves unidirectional activation of proteasomes. *FEBS Lett* **478**, 109–12.

18. Fujimoto, J., Sakaguchi, H., Aoki, I., Khatun, S., Toyoki, H., and Tamaya, T. (2000) Steroid receptors and metastatic potential in endometrial cancers. *J Steroid Biochem Mol Biol* **75**, 209–12.

19. Fujimoto, J., Sakaguchi, H., Aoki, I., Toyoki, H., and Tamaya, T. (2002) Clinical implications of the expression of estrogen receptor-alpha and -beta in primary and metastatic lesions of uterine endometrial cancers. *Oncology* **62**, 269–77.

20. Park, S., Dong, B., and Matsumura, F. (2007) Rapid activation of c-Src kinase by dioxin is mediated by the Cdc37-HSP90 complex as part of Ah receptor signaling in MCF10A cells. *Biochemistry* **46**, 899–908.

21. Ohtake, F., Takeyama, K., Matsumoto, T. et al. (2003) Modulation of oestrogen receptor signalling by association with the activated dioxin receptor. *Nature* **423**, 545–50.

22. Rüegg, J., Swedenborg, E., Wahlström, D. et al. (2008) The transcription factor aryl hydrocarbon receptor nuclear translocator functions as an estrogen receptor beta-selective coactivator, and its recruitment to alternative pathways mediates antiestrogenic effects of dioxin. *Mol Endocrinol* **2**, 304–16.

23. Haarmann-Stemmann, T., Bothe, H., and Abel, J. (2008) Growth factors, cytokines and their receptors as downstream targets of arylhydrocarbon receptor (AhR) signaling pathways. *Biochem Pharmacol*, Sep 20. [Epub ahead of print] PMID: 18848820.

24. Fritsche, E., Schafer, C., Calles, C. et al. (2007) Lightening up the UV response by identification of the arylhydrocarbon receptor as a cytoplasmatic target for ultraviolet B radiation. *Proc Natl Acad Sci U S A* **104**, 8851–56.

25. Johansson, C.C., Yndestad, A., Enserink, J.M. et al. (2004) The epidermal growth factor-like growth factor amphiregulin is strongly induced by the adenosine 30,50-onophosphate pathway in various cell types. *Endocrinology* **145**, 5177–84.

26. Peng, X.H., Karna, P., Cao, Z., Jiang, B.H., Zhou, M., and Yang, L. (2006) Cross-talk between epidermal growth factor receptor and hypoxia-inducible factor-1alpha signal pathways increases resistance to apoptosis by up-regulating survivin gene expression. *J Biol Chem* **281**, 25903–14.

27. Puga, A., Barnes, S.J., Dalton, T.P., Chang, C., Knudsen, E.S., and Maier, M.A. (2000) Aromatic hydrocarbon receptor interaction with the retinoblastoma protein potentiates repression of E2F-dependent transcription and cell cycle arrest. *J Biol Chem* **275**, 2943–50.

28. Huang, G., and Elferink, C.J. (2005) Multiple mechanisms are involved in Ah receptor-mediated cell cycle arrest. *Mol Pharmacol* **67**, 88–96.

29. Marlowe, J.L., and Puga, A. (2005) Aryl hydrocarbon receptor, cell cycle regulation, toxicity, and tumorigenesis. *J Cell Biochem* **96**, 1174–84.

30. Ray, S.S., and Swanson, H.I. (2004) Dioxin-induced immortalization of normal human keratinocytes and silencing of p53 and p16INK4a. *J Biol Chem* **279**, 27187–93.

31. Puga, A., Nebert, D.W., and Carrier, F. (1992) Dioxin induces expression of c-fos and c-jun proto-oncogenes and a large increase in transcription factor AP-1. *DNA Cell Biol* **11**, 269–81.

32. Hockings, J.K., Degner, S.C., Morgan, S.S., Kemp, M.Q., and Romagnolo, D.F. (2008) Involvement of a specificity proteins-binding element in regulation of basal and estrogen-induced transcription activity of the BRCA1 gene. *Breast Cancer Res* **10**, R29.

33. Degner, S.C., Kemp, M.Q., Hockings, J.K., and Romagnolo, D.F. (2007) Cyclooxygenase-2 promoter activation by the aromatic hydrocarbon receptor in breast cancer mcf-7 cells: Repressive effects of conjugated linoleic acid. *Nutr Cancer* **59**, 248–57.

34. Degner, S.C., Papoutsis, A.J., Selmin, O., and Romagnolo, D.F. (2009) Targeting of aryl hydrocarbon receptor-mediated activation of COX-2 expression by the indole-3-carbinol metabolite 3,3′-diindolylmethane in breast cancer cells. *J Nutr* **139**, 26–32.

35. Moennikes, O., Loeppen, S., Buchmann, A. et al. (2004) A constitutively active dioxin/aryl hydrocarbon receptor promotes hepatocarcinogenesis in mice. *Cancer Res* **64**, 4707–10.

36. Yang, X., Solomon, S., Fraser, L.R. et al. (2008) Constitutive regulation of CYP1B1 by the aryl hydrocarbon receptor (AhR) in pre-malignant and malignant mammary tissue. *J Cell Biochem* **104**, 402–17.

37. Harstad, E.B., Guite, C.A., Thomae, T.L., and Bradfield, C.A. (2006) Liver deformation in Ahr-null mice: Evidence for aberrant hepatic perfusion in early development. *Mol Pharmacol* **69**, 1534–41.

38. Fernandez-Salguero, P., Pineau, T., Hilbert, D.M. et al. (1995) Immune system impairment and hepatic fibrosis in mice lacking the dioxin-binding Ah receptor. *Science* **268**, 722–26.

39. Shimizu, Y., Nakatsuru, Y., Ichinose, M. et al. (2000) Benzo[a]pyrene carcinogenicity is lost in mice lacking the aryl hydrocarbon receptor. *Proc Natl Acad Sci U S A* **97**, 779–82.

40. Fritz, W.A., Lin, T.M., and Peterson, R.E. (2008) The aryl hydrocarbon receptor (AhR) inhibits vanadate-induced vascular endothelial growth factor (VEGF) production in TRAMP prostates. *Carcinogenesis* **29**, 1077–82.

41. Papaconstantinou, A.D., Shanmugam, I., Shan, L. et al. (2006) Gene expression profiling in the mammary gland of rats treated with 7,12-dimethylbenz[a]anthracene. *Int J Cancer* **118**, 17–24.

42. Currier, N., Solomon, S.E., Demicco, E.G. et al. (2005) Oncogenic signaling pathways activated in DMBA-induced mouse mammary tumors. *Toxicol Pathol* **33**, 726–37.

43. McDougal, A., Wilson, C., and Safe, S. (1997) Inhibition of 7,12-dimethylbenz[a]anthracene-induced rat mammary tumor growth by aryl hydrocarbon receptor agonists. *Cancer Lett* **120**, 53–63.

44. Trombino, A.F., Near, R.I., Matulka, R.A. et al. (2000) Expression of the aryl hydrocarbon receptor/transcription factor (AhR) and AhR-regulated CYP1 gene transcripts in a rat model of mammary tumorigenesis. *Breast Cancer Res Treat* **63**, 117–31.

45. Liehr, J.G., and Ricci, M.J. (1996) 4-Hydroxylation of estrogens as marker of human mammary tumors. *Proc Natl Acad Sci U S A* **93**, 3294–96.

46. Kociba, R.J., Keyes, D.G., Beyer, J.E. et al. (1978) Results of a two-year chronic toxicity and oncogenicity study of 2,3,7,8-tetrachlorodibenzo-p-dioxin in rats. *Toxicol Appl Pharmacol* **46**, 279–303.

47. Nebert, D.W. (1989) The Ah locus: Genetic differences in toxicity, cancer, mutation, and birth defects. *Crit Rev Toxicol* **20**, 153–74.

48. Anderson, L.M., Ruskie, S., Carter, J., Pittinger, S., Kovatch, R.M., and Riggs, C.W. (1995) Fetal mouse susceptibility to transplacental carcinogenesis: Differential influence of Ah receptor phenotype on effects of 3-methylcholanthrene, 12-dimethylbenz[a]anthracene, and benzo[a]pyrene. *Pharmacogenetics* **5**, 364–72.

49. Yu, Z., Loehr, C.V., Fischer, K.A. et al. (2006) In utero exposure of mice to dibenzo[a,l]pyrene produces lymphoma in offspring: Role of the aryl hydrocarbon receptor. *Cancer Res* **66**, 755–62.

50. Castro, D.J., Löhr, C.V., Fischer, K.A., Pereira, C.B., and Williams, D.E. (2008) Lymphoma and lung cancer in offspring born to pregnant mice dosed with dibenzo[a,l]pyrene: The importance of in utero vs. lactational exposure. *Toxicol Appl Pharmacol*, Sep 24. [Epub ahead of print].

51. Jenkins, S., Rowell, C., Wang, J., and Lamartiniere, C.A. (2007) Prenatal TCDD exposure predisposes for mammary cancer in rats. *Reprod Toxicol* **23**, 391–96.

52. Hayashi, S., Watanabe, J., Nakachi, K., Eguchi, H., Gotoh, O., and Kawajiri, K. (1994) Interindividual difference in expression of human Ah receptor and related P450 genes. *Carcinogenesis* **15**, 801–06.

53. Koliopanos, A., Kleeff, J., Xiao, Y. et al. (2002) Increased arylhydrocarbon receptor expression offers a potential therapeutic target for pancreatic cancer. *Oncogene* **21**, 6059–70.

54. Chang, J.T., Chang, H., Chen, P.H., Lin, S.L., and Lin, P. (2007) Requirement of aryl hydrocarbon receptor overexpression for CYP1B1 up-regulation and cell growth in human lung adenocarcinomas. *Clin Cancer Res* **13**, 38–45.

55. Lin, P., Chang, H., Tsai, W.T. et al. (2003) Overexpression of aryl hydrocarbon receptor in human lung carcinomas. *Toxicol Pathol* **31**, 22–30.

56. Martinez, V., Kennedy, S., Doolan, P. et al. (2008) Drug metabolism-related genes as potential biomarkers: Analysis of expression in normal and tumour breast tissue. *Breast Cancer Res Treat* **110**, 521–30.

57. Mulero-Navarro, S., Carvajal-Gonzalez, J.M., Herranz, M. et al. (2006) The dioxin receptor is silenced by promoter hypermethylation in human acute lymphoblastic leukemia through inhibition of Sp1 binding. *Carcinogenesis* **27**, 1099–104.

58. Shin, A., Shrubsole, M.J., Rice, J.M. et al. (2008) Meat intake, heterocyclic amine exposure, and metabolizing enzyme polymorphisms in relation to colorectal polyp risk. *Cancer Epidemiol Biomarkers Prev* **17**, 320–29.

59. Bin, P., Leng, S., Cheng, J. et al. (2008) Association of aryl hydrocarbon receptor gene polymorphisms and urinary 1-hydroxypyrene in polycyclic aromatic hydrocarbon-exposed workers. *Cancer Epidemiol Biomarkers Prev* **17**, 1702–08.

60. Kim, J.H., Kim, H., Lee, K.Y. et al. (2007) Aryl hydrocarbon receptor gene polymorphisms affect lung cancer risk. *Lung Cancer* **56**, 9–15.

61. Chen, D., Tian, T., Wang, H. et al. (2008) Association of human aryl hydrocarbon receptor gene polymorphisms with risk of lung cancer among cigarette smokers in a Chinese population. *Pharmacogenet Genomics*, Sep 24. [Epub ahead of print].

62. Tsuchiya, Y., Nakajima, M., Itoh, S., Iwanari, M., and Yokoi, T. (2003) Expression of aryl hydrocarbon receptor repressor in normal human tissues and inducibility by polycyclic aromatic hydrocarbons in human tumor-derived cell lines. *Toxicol Sci* **72**, 253–59.

63. Zudaire, E., Cuesta, N., Murty, V. et al. (2008) The aryl hydrocarbon receptor repressor is a putative tumor suppressor gene in multiple human cancers. *J Clin Invest* **118**, 640–50.

64. Schlezinger, J.J., Liu, D., Farago, M., Seldin, D.C., Belguise, K., Sonenshein, G.E., and Sherr, D.H. (2006) A role for the aryl hydrocarbon receptor in mammary gland tumorigenesis. *Biol Chem* **387**, 1175–87.

65. Russo, J., Tahin, Q., Lareef, M.H., Hu, Y.-F., and Russo, I.H. (2002) Neoplastic transformation of human breast epithelial cells by estrogens and chemical carcinogens. *Environ Mol Mutagen* **39**, 254–63.

66. Hecht, S.S. (2002) Tobacco smoke carcinogens and breast cancer. *Environ Mol Mutagen* **39**, 119–26.

67. Hattemer-Frey, H.A., and Travis, C.C. (1991) Benzo-a-pyrene: Environmental partitioning and human exposure. *Toxicol Ind Health* **7**, 141–57.

68. Burchiel, S.W., and Luster, M.I. (2001) Signaling by environmental polycyclic aromatic hydrocarbons in human lymphocytes. *Clin Immunol* **98**, 2–10.

69. Menzie, C.A., Potocki, B.B., and Santodonato, J. (1992) Exposure to carcinogenic PAHs in the environment. *Environ Sci Technol* **26**, 1278–84.

70. Lodovici, M., Dolara, P., Casalini, C., Ciappellano, S., and Testolin, G. (1995) Polycyclic aromatic hydrocarbon contamination in the Italian diet. *Food Addit Contam* **12**, 703–13.

71. Jakszyn, P., Agudo, A., Ibáñez, R. et al. (2004) Development of a food database of nitrosamines, heterocyclic amines, and polycyclic aromatic hydrocarbons. *J Nutr* **134**, 2011–14.

72. Sram, R.J., and Binkova, B. (2000) Molecular epidemiology studies on occupational and environmental exposure to mutagens and carcinogens. *Environ Health Perspect* **108**(suppl 1), 451–60.

73. Ibáñez, R., Agudo, A., Berenguer, A. et al. (2005) Dietary intake of polycyclic aromatic hydrocarbons in a Spanish population. *J Food Prot* **68**, 2190–95.

74. Huff, J., Lucier, G., and Tritscher, A. (1994) Carcinogenicity of TCDD: Experimental, mechanistic, and epidemiologic evidence. *Annu Rev Pharmacol Toxicol* **34**, 343–72.

75. Hahn, M.E. (2002) Aryl hydrocarbon receptors: Diversity and evolution. *Chem Biol Interact* **141**, 131–60.

76. Kogevinas, M. (2001) Human health effects of dioxins: Cancer, reproductive and endocrine system effects. *Hum Reprod Update* **7**, 331–39.

77. Gilpin, R.K., Wagel, D.J., and Solch, J.G. (2003) Production, distribution, and fate of polychlorinated dibenzo-*p*-dioxins, dibenzofurans, and related organohalogens in the environment. In: Schecter, A. and Gasiewicz, T.A., eds. *Dioxins and Health*. Hoboken, NJ: Wiley, 89–136.

78. Fries, G.F. (1995) A review of the significance of animal food products as potential pathways of human exposures to dioxins. *J Anim Sci* **73**, 1639–50.

79. Liem, A.K., Furst, P., and Rappe, C. (2000) Exposure of populations to dioxins and related compounds. *Food Addit Contam* **17**, 241–59.

80. Schecter, G., Frank, S., Riedel, K., Meger-Kossien, I., and Renner, T. (2000) Biomonitoring of exposure to polycyclic aromatic hydrocarbons of nonoccupationally exposed person. *Cancer Epidemiol Biomarkers Prev* **9**, 373–80.

81. Hooper, K., Petreas, M.X., Chuvakova, T. et al. (1998) Analysis of breast milk to assess exposure to chlorinated contaminants in Kazakstan: High levels of 2,3,7,8-tetrachlorodibenzo-p-dioxin (TCDD) in agricultural villages of southern Kazakstan. *Environ Health Perspect* **106**, 797–806.

82. Weiss, J., Papke, O., Bignert, A. et al. (2003) Concentrations of dioxin and other organochlorines (PCBs, DDTs, HCHs) in human milk from Seveso, Milan and a Lombardian rural area in Italy: A study performed 25 years after the heavy dioxin exposure in Seveso. *Acta Paediatr* **92**, 467–72.

83. Fattore, E., Fanelli, R., Turrini, A., and di Domenico, A. (2006) Current dietary exposure to polychlorodibenzo-p-dioxins, polychlorodibenzofurans, and dioxin-like polychlorobiphenyls in Italy. *Mol Nutr Food Res* **50**, 915–21.

84. Revich, B., Aksel, E., Ushakova, T. et al. (2001) Dioxin exposure and public health in Chapaevsk, Russia. *Chemosphere* **43**, 951–66.

85. Safe, S. (1993) Toxicology, structure-function relationship, and human and environmental health impacts of polychlorinated biphenyls: Progress and problems. *Environ Health Perspect* **100**, 259–68.

86. Krüger, T., Long, M., and Bonefeld-Jørgensen, E.C. (2008) Plastic components affect the activation of the aryl hydrocarbon and the androgen receptor. *Toxicology* **246**, 112–23.

87. Arisawa, K., Takeda, H., and Mikasa, H. (2005) Background exposure to PCDDs/PCDFs/PCBs and its potential health effects: A review of epidemiologic studies. *J Med Invest* **52**, 10–21.

88. Thundiyil, J.G., Solomon, G.M., and Miller, M.D. (2007) Transgenerational exposures: Persistent chemical pollutants in the environment and breast milk. *Pediatr Clin North Am* **54**, 81–101.

89. Solomon, G.M., and Weiss, P.M. (2002) Chemical contaminants in breast milk: Time trends and regional variability. *Environ Health Perspect* **110**, A339–A47.

90. Lu, Y.F., Santostefano, M., Cunningham, B.D., Threadgill, M.D., and Safe, S. (1995) Identification of 3′-methoxy-4′-nitroflavone as a pure aryl hydrocarbon (Ah) receptor antagonist and evidence for more than one form of the nuclear Ah receptor in MCF-7 human breast cancer cells. *Arch Biochem Biophys* **316**, 470–77.

91. Gasiewicz, T.A., Kende, A.S., Rucci, G., Whitney, B., and Willey, J.J. (1996) Analysis of structural requirements for Ah receptor antagonist activity: Ellipticines, flavones, and related compounds. *Biochem Pharmacol* **52**, 1787–803.

92. Gasiewicz, T.A., Henry, E.C., and Collins, L.L. (2008) Expression and activity of aryl hydrocarbon receptors in development and cancer. *Crit Rev Eukaryot Gene Expr* **18**, 279–321.

93. Merchant, M., Arellano, L., and Safe, S. (1990) The mechanism of action of alpha- naphthoflavone as an inhibitor of 2,3,7,8-tetrachlorodibenzo-p-dioxin-induced CYP1A1 gene expression. *Arch Biochem Biophys* **281**, 84–89.

94. Wilhelmsson, A., Whitelaw, M.L., Gustafsson, J.A., and Poellinger, L. (1994) Agonistic and antagonistic effects of a-naphthoflavone on dioxin receptor function: Role of the basic region helix-loop-helix dioxin receptor partner factor. *Arnt J Biol Chem* **269**, 19028–33.

95. Jeffy, B.D., Chen, E.J., Gudas, J.M., and Romagnolo, D.F. (2000) Disruption of cell cycle kinetics by benzo[a]pyrene: Inverse expression patterns of BRCA-1 and p53 in MCF-7 cells arrested in S and G2. *Neoplasia* **2**, 460–70.

96. Zhang, S., Qin, C., and Safe, S.H. (2003) Flavonoids as aryl hydrocarbon receptor agonists/antagonists: Effects of structure and cell context. *Environ Health Perspect* **111**, 1877–82.

97. Denison, M.S., and Nagy, S.R. (2003) Activation of the aryl hydrocarbon receptor by structurally diverse exogenousand endogenous chemicals. *Annu Rev Pharmacol Toxicol* **43**, 309–34.

98. Park, E.J., and Pezzuto, J.M. (2002) Botanicals in cancer chemoprevention. *Cancer Metastasis Rev* **21**, 231–55.

99. Bode, A.M., and Dong, Z. (2004) Targeting signal transduction pathways by chemopreventive agents. *Mutat Res* **555**, 33–51.

100. Signorell, P., and Ghidoni, R. (2005) Resveratrol as an anticancer nutrient: Molecular basis, open questions and promises. *J Nutr Biochem* **16**, 449–66.

101. Banerjee, S., Bueso-Ramos, C., and Aggarwal, B.B. (2002) Suppression of 7,12 dimethyl-lbenz(a)anthracene-induced mammary carcinogenesis in rats by resveratrol: Role of nuclear factor-kappaB, cyclooxygenase 2, and matrix metalloprotease 9. *Cancer Res* **62**, 4945–54.

102. Jang, M., Cai, L., and Udeani, G.O. (1997) Cancer chemopreventive activity of resveratrol, a natural product derived from grapes. *Science* **275**, 218–20.

103. Amakura, Y., Tsutsumi, T., Sasaki, K., Yoshida, T., and Maitani, T. (2003) Screening of the inhibitory effect of vegetable constituents on the aryl hydrocarbon receptor-mediated activity induced by 2,3,7,8-tetrachlorodibenzo-p-dioxin. *Biol Pharm Bull* **26**, 1754–60.

104. de Medina, P., Casper, R., Savouret, J.F., and Poirot, M. (2005) Synthesis and biological properties of new stilbene derivatives of resveratrol as new selective aryl hydrocarbon modulators. *J Med Chem* **48**, 287–91.

105. Chen, Y., Tseng, S.H., Lai, H.S., and Chen, W.J. (2004) Resveratrol-induced cellular apoptosis and cell cycle arrest in neuroblastoma cells and antitumor effects on neuroblastoma in mice. *Surgery* **36**, 57–66.

106. Gehm, B.D., McAndrews, J.M., Chien, P.Y., and Jameson, J.L. (1997) Resveratrol, a polyphenolic compound found in grapes and wine, is an agonist for the estrogen receptor. *Proc Natl Acad Sci U S A* **94**, 14138–43.

107. Fustier, P., Le Corre, L., Chalabi, N., Vissac-Sabatier, C., Communal, Y., Bignon, Y.J., and Bernard-Gallon, D.J. (2003) Resveratrol increases BRCA1 and BRCA2 mRNA expression in breast tumour cell lines. *Br J Cancer* **89**, 168–72.

108. Kim, Y.S., and Milner, J.A. (2005) Targets for indole-3-carbinol in cancer prevention. *J Nutr Biochem* **16**, 65–73.

109. Wortelboer, H.M., van der Linden, E.C., de Kruif, C.A. et al. (1992) Effects of indole-3-carbinol on biotransformation enzymes in the rat: In vivo changes in liver and small intestinal mucosa in comparison with primary hepatocyte cultures. *Food Chem Toxicol* **30**, 589–99.

110. Bjeldanes, L.F., Kim, J.Y., Grose, K.R., Bartholomew, J.C., and Bradfield, C.A. (1991) Aromatic hydrocarbon responsiveness-receptor agonists generated from indole-3-carbinol in vitro and in vivo: Comparisons with 2,3,7,8-tetrachlorodibenzo-p-dioxin. *Proc Natl Acad Sci USA* **88**, 9543–47.

111. Jellinck, P.H., Forkert, P.G., Riddick, D.S., Okey, A.B., Michnovicz, J.J., and Bradlow, H.L. (1993) Ah receptor binding properties of indole carbinols and induction of hepatic estradiol hydroxylation. *Biochem Pharmacol* **45**, 1129–36.

112. Fenwick, G.R., Heaney, R.K., and Mullin, W.J. (1983) Glucosinolates and their breakdown products in food and food plants. *Crit Rev Food Sci Nutr* **18**, 123–201.

113. Wattenberg, L.W., and Loub, W.D. (1978) Inhibition of polycyclic aromatic hydrocarbon-induced neoplasia by naturally occurring indoles. *Cancer Res* **38**, 1410–13.

114. Fong, A.T., Hendricks, J.D., Dashwood, R.H., Van Winkle, S., Lee, B.C., and Bailey, G.S. (1988) Modulation of diethylnitrosamine-induced hepatocarcinogenesis and O6-ethylguanine formation in rainbow trout by indole-3-carbinol, beta naphthoflavone, and Aroclor 1254. *Toxicol Appl Pharmacol* **96**, 93–100.

115. Bradlow, H.L., Michnovicz, J., Telang, N.T., and Osborne, M.P. (1991) Effects of dietary indole-3-carbinol on estradiol metabolism and spontaneous mammary tumors in mice. *Carcinogenesis* **12**, 1571–74.

116. Bradlow, H.L. (2008) Indole-3-carbinol as a chemoprotective agent in breast and prostate cancer. *In Vivo* **22**, 441–45.

117. Xu, M., Schut, H.A., Bjeldanes, L.F., Williams, D.E., Bailey, G.S., and Dashwood, R.H. (1997) Inhibition of 2-amino-3-methylimidazo[4,5-f]quinoline-DNA adducts by indole-3-carbinol: Dose-response studies in the rat colon. *Carcinogenesis* **18**, 2149–53.

118. Meng, Q., Yuan, F., Goldberg, I.D., Rosen, E.M., Auborn, K., and Fan, S. (2000) Indole-3-carbinol is a negative regulator of estrogen receptor-alpha signaling in human tumor cells. *J Nutr* **130**, 2927–31.

119. Bailey, G.S., Hendricks, J.D., Shelton, D.W., Nixon, J.E., and Pawlowski, N.E. (1987) Enhancement of carcinogenesis by the natural anticarcinogen indole-3-carbinol. *J Natl Cancer Inst* **78**, 931–34.

120. Exon, J.H., Henningsen, G.M., Osborne, C.A., and Koller, L.D. (1984) Toxicologic, pathologic, and immunotoxic effects of 2,4-dichlorophenol in rats. *J Toxicol Environ Health* **14**, 723–30.

121. Yoshida, M., Katashima, S., Ando, J. et al. (2004) Dietary indole-3-carbinol promotes endometrial adenocarcinoma development in rats initiated with N-ethyl-N'-nitro-N-nitrosoguanidine, with induction of cytochrome P450s in the liver and consequent modulation of estrogen metabolism. *Carcinogenesis* **25**, 2257–64.

122. Reed, G.A., Arneson, D.W., Putnam, W.C. et al. (2006) Single-dose and multiple-dose administration of indole-3-carbinol to women: Pharmacokinetics based on 3,3'-diindolylmethane. *Cancer Epidemiol Biomarkers Prev* **15**, 477–81.

123. Chen, I., McDougal, A., Wang, F., and Safe, S. (1998) Aryl hydrocarbon receptor-mediated antiestrogenic and antitumorigenic activity of diindolylmethane. *Carcinogenesis* **19**, 1631–39.

124. Grubbs, C.J., Steele, V.E., Casebolt, T. et al. (1995) Chemoprevention of chemically-induced mammary carcinogenesis by indole-3-carbinol. *Anticancer Res* **15**, 709–16.

125. Reed, G.A., Sunega, J.M., Sullivan, D.K. et al. (2008) Single-dose pharmacokinetics and tolerability of absorption-enhanced 3,3'-diindolylmethane in healthy subjects. *Cancer Epidemiol Biomarkers Prev* **17**, 2619–24.

126. Bonnesen, C., Eggleston, I.M., and Hayes, J.D. (2001) Dietary indoles and isothiocyanates that are generated from cruciferous vegetables can both stimulate apoptosis and confer protection against DNA damage in human colon cell lines. *Cancer Res* **61**, 6120–30.

127. Ciolino, H.P., Daschner, P.J., and Yeh, G.C. (1999) Dietary flavonols quercetin and kaempferol are ligands of the aryl hydrocarbon receptor that affect CYP1A1 transcription differentially. *Biochem J* **340**, 715–22.

128. Puppala, D., Gairola, C.G., and Swanson, H.I. (2007) Identification of kaempferol as an inhibitor of cigarette smoke-induced activation of the aryl hydrocarbon receptor and cell transformation. *Carcinogenesis* **28**, 639–47.

129. Fukuda, I., Sakane, I., Yabushita, Y. et al. (2004) Pigments in green tea leaves (Camellia sinensis) suppress transformation of the aryl hydrocarbon receptor induced by dioxin. *J Agric Food Chem* **52**, 2499–506.

130. Ashida, H., Fukuda, I., Yamashita, T., and Kanazawa, K. (2000) Flavones and flavonols at dietary levels inhibit a transformation of aryl hydrocarbon receptor induced by dioxin. *FEBS Lett* **476**, 213–17.

131. Williams, S.N., Shih, H., Guenette, D.K. et al. (2000) Comparative studies on the effects of green tea extracts and individual tea catechins on human CYP1A gene expression. *Chem Biol Interact* **128**, 211–29.

132. Nakagawa, K., Okuda, S., and Miyazawa, T. (1997) Dose-dependent incorporation of tea catechins, (-)-epigallocatechin-3-gallate and (-)-epigallocatechin, into human plasma. *Biosci Biotechnol Biochem* **61**, 1981–85.

133. Amakura, Y., Tsutsumi, T., Nakamura, M. et al. (2002) Preliminary screening of the inhibitory effect of food extracts on activation of the aryl hydrocarbon receptor induced by 2,3,7,8-tetrachlorodibenzo-p-dioxin. *Biol Pharm Bull* **25**, 272–74.

134. Palermo, C.M., Hernando, J.I., Dertinger, S.D., Kende, A.S., and Gasiewicz, T.A. (2003) Identification of potential aryl hydrocarbon receptor antagonists in green tea. *Chem Res Toxicol* **16**, 865–72.

135. De Waard, W.J., Aarts, J.M., Peijnenburg, A.C., De Kok, T.M., Van Schooten, F.J., and Hoogenboom, L.A. (2008) Ah receptor agonist activity in frequently consumed food items. *Food Addit Contam Part A Chem Anal Control Expo Risk Assess* **25**, 779–87.

136. Connor, K.T., Harris, M.A., Edwards, M. et al. (2008) AH receptor agonist activity in human blood measure with a cell-based bioassay: Evidence for naturally occurring AH receptor ligands in vivo. *J Expo Sci Environ Epidemiol* **18**, 369–80.

137. Chiaro, C.R., Patel, R.D., and Perdew, G.H. (2008) 12(R)-HETE, an Arachidonic Acid Derivative, is an Activator of the Aryl Hydrocarbon (Ah) Receptor. *Mol Pharmacol*, Sep **8**. [Epub ahead of print] PMID: 18779363.

138. Kall, M.A., Vang, O., and Clausen, J. (1996) Effects of dietary broccoli on human in vivo drug metabolizing enzymes: Evaluation of caffeine, oestrone and chlorzoxazone metabolism. *Carcinogenesis* **17**, 793–99.

139. Dashwood, R.H. (1998) Indole-3-carbinol: Anticarcinogen or tumor promoter in brassica vegetables? *Chem Biol Interact* **110**, 1–5.
140. Phillips, D.H. (1999) Polycyclic aromatic hydrocarbons in the diet. *Mutat Res* **443**, 139–47.
141. La Rocca, C., and Mantovani, A. (2006) From environment to food: The case of PCB. *Ann Ist Super Sanita* **42**, 410–16.
142. Moon, Y.J., Wang, X., and Morris, M.E. (2006) Dietary flavonoids: Effects on xenobiotic and carcinogen metabolism. *Toxicol In Vitro* **20**, 187–210.
143. Nguyen, L.P., and Bradfield, C.A. (2008) The search for endogenous activators of the aryl hydrocarbon receptor. *Chem Res Toxicol* **21**, 102–16.
144. Sathyanarayana, S. (2008) Phthalates and children's health. *Curr Probl Pediatr Adolesc Health Care* **38**, 34–49.
145. Willhite, C.C., Ball, G.L., and McLellan, C.J. (2008) Derivation of a bisphenol A oral reference dose (RfD) and drinking-water equivalent concentration. *J Toxicol Environ Health B Crit Rev* **11**, 69–146.
146. Piskorska-Pliszczynska, J., Keys, B., Safe, S., and Newman, M.S. (1986) The cytosolic receptor binding affinities and AHH induction potencies of 29 polynuclear aromatic hydrocarbons. *Toxicol Lett* **34**, 67–74.

33 Opportunities and Challenges for Communicating Food and Health Relationships to American Consumers

Susan Borra, Wendy Reinhardt Kapsak, and Elizabeth Rahavi

Key Points

1. Health and nutrition advice from the United States (U.S.) government and many health associations and nutrition experts emphasizes the need for Americans to include more healthful foods in their diets. Yet, despite the wealth of sound nutrition advice available to consumers, obesity and many other chronic diseases still plague a staggering number of Americans.
2. What type of information will provide the motivation consumers need to improve their lifestyles to avoid chronic diseases like obesity, heart disease, or cancer? As the science of food and nutrition continues to evolve, communication strategies that consider consumer perceptions are imperative. Health professionals, educators, and journalists can help change consumer behaviors by first understanding their attitudes, awareness, and interest in foods and beverages that may provide added health benefits.
3. This chapter provides a detailed discussion of consumer research that was fielded to gauge Americans' attitudes toward food and health, including attitudes toward foods and food components with added health and wellness benefits. With information that considers the consumer perspective, food and nutrition communicators can better relate with consumers and guide them to make informed and healthful food choices that maintain good health and minimize disease risk.

Key Words: Functional foods; food components; health benefits; communication

1. INTRODUCTION

Health and nutrition advice from the United States (U.S.) government and many health associations and nutrition experts emphasizes the need for Americans to include more healthful foods in their diets. Yet, despite the wealth of sound nutrition advice available to consumers, obesity and many other diet-related chronic diseases still plague a staggering number of Americans. What type of information will provide the motivation

From: *Nutrition and Health: Bioactive Compounds and Cancer*
Edited by: J.A. Milner, D.F. Romagnolo, DOI 10.1007/978-1-60761-627-6_33,
© Springer Science+Business Media, LLC 2010

consumers need to improve their lifestyles to avoid chronic diseases like obesity, heart disease, or cancer?

As the science of food and nutrition continues to evolve, communication strategies that consider consumer perceptions are imperative. Health professionals, educators, and journalists can help change consumer behaviors by first understanding their attitudes, awareness, and interest in foods and beverages that may provide added health benefits. This chapter provides a detailed discussion of two consumer research surveys that were fielded to gauge Americans' attitudes toward food and health, including attitudes toward foods and food components with added health and wellness benefits.

In 2009, the International Food Information Council (IFIC) commissioned its sixth survey to study Americans' awareness and attitudes toward "functional foods" – foods and beverages that provide benefits beyond basic nutrition. Functional foods include a wide variety of foods and food components believed to improve overall health and well-being, reduce the risk of specific diseases, or minimize the effects of other health concerns. Examples can include fruits and vegetables, whole grains, fortified or enhanced foods and beverages, and some dietary supplements.

Results from IFIC's 2009 *Functional Foods/Foods for Health Survey*, conducted every 2–3 years since 1998, provide ongoing consumer insights into the interests and beliefs about foods and food components and their roles in reducing the risk of disease and promoting health and wellness *(1)*. The research was designed to:

- measure and track changes in consumer awareness and interest in functional foods and food components;
- explore how awareness levels and maturity of food/benefit pairs impact behavior and perceptions; and
- gauge consumer awareness and attitudes toward using individual genetic information to make nutrition and diet-related recommendations.

This chapter also includes some key findings from the IFIC Foundation *Food & Health Survey*, a survey conducted in early 2009 to explore consumer attitudes toward food, nutrition, and health *(2)*. A segment of this survey also explored consumer perceptions of and interest in added benefits offered by foods and beverages. With information that considers the consumer perspective, food and nutrition communicators can better relate with consumers and guide them to make informed and healthful food choices that maintain good health and minimize disease risk.

2. METHODOLOGY

2.1. IFIC Functional Foods/Foods for Health Survey

IFIC commissioned Cogent Research of Cambridge, MA, to conduct a quantitative study of American consumers' attitudes, awareness, and interest in functional foods. Between May 11 and 20, 2009, 1,000 adults, 18 years and older, were randomly selected to participate in a 20-min web-based survey. Questions were either open-ended or participants were prompted and asked to rate specific responses. Data were weighted by education, age, and ethnicity to allow the findings to be representative of the American population.

This chapter predominately reports on key findings from this web-based quantitative survey and offers perspectives on the trends and evolution of consumer attitudes and awareness to help enhance understanding of consumer behaviors specifically related to foods and food components for added health and wellness benefits.

Note: When consumers were asked questions about "food," it was defined as "everything people eat, including fruits, vegetables, grains, meats, dairy, as well as beverages, herbs, spices, and dietary supplements."

2.2. IFIC Foundation Food & Health Survey

The *2009 IFIC Foundation Food & Health Survey*, also highlighted in this chapter, is designed to provide ongoing consumer insights into how consumers view their own diets, their efforts to improve them, and their understanding of the components of their diets. The 2009 survey builds upon the data released in the 2006, 2007, and 2008 *Food & Health Survey*, which included questions to evaluate consumers' knowledge and attitudes toward overall diet, physical activity, weight, nutrients, and food safety. New questions were added in 2009 to explore consumers' interests in certain functional components when making good and beverage selections for themselves and, if applicable, their children.

This chapter includes a few key findings from the 2009 *Food & Health Survey,* which offer additional perspectives and insights into findings from the *IFIC 2009 Consumer Attitudes Toward Functional Foods/Foods for Health* consumer research.

3. RESEARCH FINDINGS

3.1. General Attitudes Toward Health

Findings from the IFIC Foundation *Food & Health Survey* reveal that although the majority of Americans (81%) rate their health status as "excellent," "very good," or "good," significantly fewer (58%) say they are "somewhat" or "extremely satisfied" with their health status. This gap indicates that some Americans who consider themselves to be healthy also perceive room for improvement.

The IFIC *Functional Foods/Food for Health Survey* shows that the majority (66%) of U.S. consumers remain confident that they have a "great amount" of control over their own health. U.S. consumers who believe they have a "great amount" of control over their own health include those who also believe that "food and nutrition" play a "great role" in maintaining or improving overall health (73 vs. 53% who believe it plays a "moderate role" and 26% who believe it plays "no or a limited role"); consumers who are single (72 vs. 57% of those who are married); females (70 vs. 62% males); and consumers who state their overall health is "excellent" (86%) or "good" (66%) vs. 46% of those who report their health as "fair" or "poor".

Consistent with previous surveys, consumers overwhelmingly believe food and nutrition play the greatest role in maintaining or improving health (72%), more so than exercise (62%) or family history (39%). Americans who are most likely to cite the role of "food and nutrition" in improving health as "great" are consumers who state that their overall health is "excellent" (82%) or "good" (78%) vs. 68% of those who state their health is "fair" or "poor"; supplement users (78 vs. 62% of non-users); and those who are the primary household shopper (75 vs. 57% who are not the primary household shopper). Americans' belief that family health history plays a "moderate" to "great role" in maintaining and improving health (87%) has remained fairly stable since 2005 (90%), but reflects an overall increase compared to previous years (82% in 2002, 80% in 2000, and 85% in 1998).

Heart-related and circulatory conditions, including general heart health, blood pressure, stroke, and high cholesterol, remain top health concerns of consumers. Almost half (48%) of all Americans cite heart disease as their top health concern, which is a significant decrease from 2007 (53%) and 2005 (54%). This decline may be the result of significantly fewer Americans reporting concern about cholesterol (9%) compared to 2007 (13%). Consistent with 2007, the number of consumers mentioning weight as a top health concern remains higher (31%) than cancer (24%). Interestingly, while the number of Americans mentioning weight as a top health concern (31%) remains consistent with 2007 (33%) 2005 (34%), this percentage has doubled since 2000 (14%). Females are more likely to mention weight as a top health concern (36 vs. 25% males). Diabetes remains as the fourth largest health concern (17%). Although other health issues continue to be consistently less of a concern, nutrition/diet has increased in concern compared to previous years (16 in 2009 and 2007 vs. 7% in 2005 and 12% in 2002) (Fig. 1).

In previous Surveys, consumers were asked to report specific dietary changes they have made over the past year to improve or maintain their overall health. These changes were categorized as either additions or reductions to the diet. Americans continue to

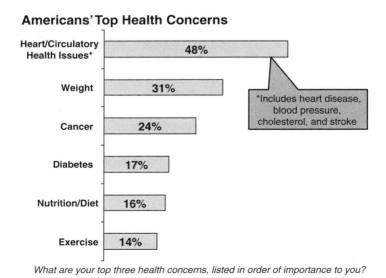

What are your top three health concerns, listed in order of importance to you?
(Unaided, Multiple Responses) (n=1005)

Fig. 1. Americans' top health concerns *(1)*.

focus on removing foods or food components from the diet with about half of consumers reporting changes that involve reductions, including trying to consume less fat, reducing calorie intake, and eating less sugar. In contrast, only about one in four consumers report changes that involve adding more healthful foods to the diet, including eating more vegetables, fruits, and grains, getting more fiber, and drinking more water. *Food & Health* data indicates that Americans generally make changes to their diet in an effort to improve overall well-being (64%) and to lose weight (61%).

The vast majority (89%) of consumers agree that certain foods have health benefits that go beyond basic nutrition and may reduce the risk of disease or other health concerns. Consumers most likely to "strongly agree" that certain foods have health benefits beyond basic nutrition are those who report that their healthy status is "excellent" (71 vs. 51% "good" and 44% "fair" or "poor"); dietary supplement users (58 vs. 44% nonusers); those with a college education (60 vs. 49% of those who have a high school degree or less and 53% of those who have some college); and those who are single (56 vs. 47% of those who are married).

Overall, consumers believe in very specific benefits offered by certain foods and beverages. These include improving heart health (85%), improving physical energy or stamina (82%), maintaining overall health and wellness (82%), improving digestive health (81%), improving immune system function (80%), providing higher levels of satiety (73%), and reducing the risk of getting specific diseases (73%), among others. In line with this finding, more than 85% of all Americans say they are currently consuming or would be interested in consuming foods or beverages for these added benefits, as well as others.

3.2. Awareness and Interest in Functional Foods/Foods for Health

Similar to 2007 and 2005, 9 out of 10 Americans are able, on an unaided basis, to name a specific food or component and its associated health benefit. This represents a steady and significant increase compared to 84% in 2002, 82% in 2000, and 77% in 1998. On an unaided basis, the top "functional foods" named by consumers in the 2009 *Functional Foods/Foods for Health* quantitative survey were

1. fruits and vegetables;
2. fish, fish oil, seafood;
3. dairy (including milk and yogurt);
4. meat and poultry;
5. herbs/spices;
6. fiber
7. tea and green tea;
8. nuts;
9. whole grains and other grains;
10. water;
11. cereal;
12. oats/oat bran/oatmeal; and
13. vitamins/supplements.

Seven out of ten (71%) consumers name fruits and vegetables as foods that provide benefits beyond basic nutrition, either generically or specifically, which has significantly increased from 2007 (66%). Significantly more Americans mention fruits (48%) compared to 2007 (37%) while slightly fewer mention vegetables (40% in 2009 vs. 44% in 2007).

When asked about the type of health benefit associated with the named foods, consumers' reported food/health associations are dominated by their top health concerns of heart disease, weight maintenance, and cancer. Most Americans report (unaided) food/health associations for reduced risk of cardiovascular disease (34%) followed by digestive health (19%); vitamin deficiency (19%); general health (18%); bone health (14%); reduced risk of cancer (11%); eye health (11%); immune health (9%); and weight maintenance (6%). More specifically, on an unaided basis, Americans associate fish/fish oil/seafood, oats/oat bran, garlic, cereal, and whole grains with benefits related to cardiovascular disease. For cancer, Americans associate broccoli, tomatoes, other fruits, and green, leafy vegetables. The top foods/food components that consumers associate with weight maintenance include green tea and vegetables. Other top food/food component and health benefit associations include dairy for bones and osteoporosis, carrots for eye health, and fiber and whole grains for intestinal health.

In the 2007 IFIC *Functional Foods/Foods for Health Survey*, consumers were asked to consider a specific health concern and name a food or food component believed to reduce the risk of that disease or condition. Overall, awareness of the associations between specific foods and reduced risk of health concerns grew stronger. Compared to previous years, significantly more Americans are able to name a specific food or food component associated with menopause, aging, breast cancer, high blood pressure, colon cancer, eye disease, mental performance, diabetes, and weight management/maintaining a healthy weight.

The following foods and food components were mentioned by consumers as potentially reducing the risk of certain cancers: milk, broccoli, green, leafy vegetables, and soy for reducing the risk of breast cancer; tomatoes and saw palmetto for the reducing the risk of prostate cancer; and fiber, whole grains, green leafy vegetables, broccoli, water, and bran for reducing the risk of colon cancer.

Americans remain highly interested in learning more about foods and food components to improve health and decrease risk for disease. This high level of interest – 43% are "very interested" and another 41% are "somewhat interested" – has remained unchanged over previous years. Americans who are more likely to be "very interested" in learning more about functional foods are those who report their health as "excellent" (57 vs. 51% of those who consider their health to be "very good," 40% "good," and 37% "fair" or "poor"); dietary supplement users (52 vs. 28% non-users); those who are single (52 vs. 31% of those who are married); and females (49 vs. 37% males).

3.3. Consumption Behaviors and Awareness of Food/Health Benefit Pairs

Consumers were then asked, on an aided basis, whether they are aware of specific food components, their corresponding food sources, and associated health benefits. With the exception of a few associations, awareness increased significantly since 2007. The dominant food/health associations continue to be those related to bone health (e.g., calcium and vitamin D), cardiovascular disease (e.g., omega-3 fats, fiber, and whole grains), cancer, and benefits associated with fiber (e.g., digestive health and reduced risk of heart disease and cancer).

With regard to cancer, awareness of "soy protein/soy found, for example, in soy-based products such as meat alternatives, nutritional bars, and beverages, such as soymilk, for reduced risk of cancer" significantly increased (55%) from 2007 (47%). Awareness of "fiber, found, for example, in vegetables, fruits, and some breads and cereals, for reduced risk of cancer" remained stable (78%). Awareness of "antioxidants, found for example in fruits and vegetables, dark chocolate, and certain teas, for protection against free radical damage implicated in aging and various chronic diseases" and "lycopene, found for example in processed tomato products, such as tomato sauce, for the reduced risk of cancer" also increased (81 vs. 72% in 2007 and 61 vs. 49% in 2007, respectively).

Additional specific food/health associations that have increased in terms of consumers' awareness since 2007 include: calcium and vitamin D for the promotion of both health (93 vs. 89% and 90 vs. 81%, respectively); whole grains and B vitamins for reduced risk of heart disease (83 vs. 72% and 78 vs. 61%, respectively); potassium for reduced risk of high blood pressure and stroke (78 vs. 64%); (monounsaturated fats for reduced risk of heart disease (73 vs. 63%); probiotics for maintaining a healthy digestive system (72 vs. 58%); omega-3 fatty acids for cognitive development, especially in children (72 vs. 53%), folate or folic acid for reduced risk of heart disease (70 vs. 55%) among several others.

The functional foods or food components already being consumed by Americans parallel their awareness of food associations. When prompted with specific food or food component and health benefit pairs, consumers report they are already eating specific foods or components related to some of their top health concerns, including cardiovascular disease, weight management, cancer, and benefits related to bone health. Of those who are aware of various associations, roughly 25–60% of all Americans are currently consuming specific foods/food components for related health benefits. The foods or components that Americans are most likely to be eating for a specified health condition are calcium, found for example in dairy foods such as milk, cheese, or yogurt or in calcium-fortified foods or beverages, for the promotion of bone health" (58%); "vitamin D, found for example in fortified foods and beverages, for the promotion of bone health" (56%); "fiber, found for example in vegetables, fruits, and some fortified foods such as breads and cereals, for a reduced risk of heart disease" and ". . .for digestive health" (both at 56%); "protein, found, for example, in meat, dairy, beans, nuts, soy, and some fortified foods and beverages, for maintaining optimal health" (56%); and "antioxidants, found for example in fruits and vegetables, whole grains, dark chocolate, coffee, and certain teas, for protection against free radical damage implicated in aging and various chronic diseases" (54%). Fiber is the food component most likely to be eaten by Americans for the reduced risk of cancer (54%).

In addition, 35–60% of consumers report they are "very likely" to begin eating specific food components or nutrients for health benefits. Generally, Americans who are more likely to consume foods and beverages for a specific benefit are those who believe they have a "great amount" of control over their health; those who report being in "excellent" health; are dietary supplement users; are single; and are 55 years and older compared to those 54 years and younger. In addition, food/health associations with lower levels of awareness tend to be those involving lesser health concerns, such as cognitive development, eye health, oral health, or lesser known food components, such as lutein, lycopene, prebiotic fiber, plant sterols, and xylitol. Similarly, food components less likely to be consumed for health benefits also tend to be lesser known, such as probiotics, prebiotic fiber, plant sterols, xylitol, and soy protein.

3.4. Communication and Sources of Information on Health and Nutrition

The mass media continue to be Americans' top source of information on health and nutrition (unaided). Similar to 2007, nearly three-quarters of Americans name the news media (70%), especially electronic media outlets such as the Internet (54%) and television news (25%), as their top source of information about health and nutrition. Roughly a third of all consumers name medical sources (34%), including physicians (31%), as a top source of information on health and nutrition. However, this reflects a significant decrease from 2005 (44% medical sources with 43% physicians).

Although Americans may look to the media for information on health and nutrition, they do not consider this to be the most credible source. Similar to 2007, many consumers (36%) name medical sources such as physicians, nutritionists, and dietitians as the most believable providers of information on the health benefits of food or food components (unaided). However, the mass media remain a credible source among nearly a quarter of all consumers (27%), and this has remained consistent over the years (24% in 2007, 23% in 2005 and 2002, 22% in 2000, and 29% in 1998). (Fig. 2).

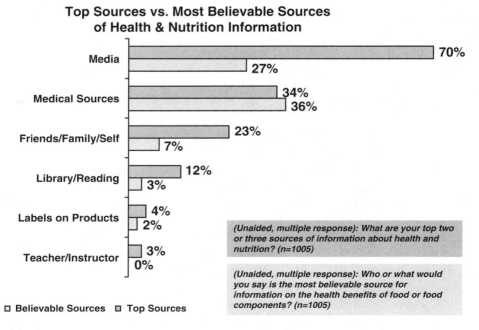

Fig. 2. Top sources vs. most believable sources of health and nutrition information *(1)*.

Americans most likely to mention medical sources among their top sources of information are those who perceive "food and nutrition" as playing a "great" (36%) or "moderate" (33%) role in maintaining or improving their overall health vs. 15% of those who believe that it plays a "small" or "no role."

When asked to rate specific sources of information that impact their decision to try a food or food component with added benefits, Americans continue to rate health professionals as the most influential (83% cite either a "moderate" or "great extent"). Dietitians (71%); health associations (68%); and fitness experts (57%) were also mentioned as very influential. Compared to 2007, significantly fewer Americans named health associations (68% vs. 73% in 2007); TV news programs (48% vs. 54%); magazines (44% vs. 53%); newspapers (38% vs. 44%); government officials (32% vs. 40%); and radio news programs (28% vs. 36%) as influential sources of information.

3.5. Nutrigenomics/"Personalized Nutrition"

In 2005, questions were added to the *IFIC Functional Foods/Foods for Health Survey* regarding the concept of nutrigenomics; this line of questioning was also included in the 2007 and 2009 surveys. Consumers were asked how much they have heard or read about using individual genetic information to provide personalized nutrition or diet-related recommendations. Results indicate that awareness is similar to 2007. Approximately half of Americans report knowing "a little bit" about this practice (46%). The percentage of Americans in 2009 knowing "a lot" or "a fair amount" about this practice (24%) remained stable since 2007 (25%), however, this is elevated from when the question was first asked in 2005 (18%). Those who are most likely to know "a lot" or about this concept include consumers who consider their health status to be "excellent" (23% vs. 4% reporting "very good," 3% reporting "good," and 3% in "fair" or "poor" health); consumers who take dietary supplements (6% vs. 3% of non- users); and those who are single (7% vs. 3% who are married). (Fig. 3).

The majority of Americans (78%) expressed favorability toward the concept of using genetic information to provide personalized nutrition and/or diet recommendations. However, it appears that favorability may have softened as significantly less people say that they are "very favorable" toward this concept (26% vs. 32% in 2007 and 29% in 2005) and significantly more saying that they are "somewhat favorable" (52% vs. 47% in 2007 and 42% in 2005). Americans most likely to have a "very favorable" opinion toward personalized nutrition are consumers who consider themselves to be in "excellent" health (42% vs. 27% "very good," 22% "good," and 26% "fair" or "poor") and believe "food and nutrition" play a "great" role in overall health (29% vs. 18% who believe it plays a "moderate" role and 6% who say it plays "limited" or "no" role). In 2007, when asked why they are favorable toward nutrigenomics, "maintaining health and preventing disease" remains the primary reason cited by 18% of Americans (Fig. 4). This question was not repeated in 2009.

More than three-quarters (78%) of Americans are interested in learning more about the use of genetic information to provide nutrition and/or diet-related recommendations to optimize health and reduce the risk of diseases to which they are genetically predisposed (vs. 77% in 2007 and 70% in 2005). About a third remain "very interested" (32

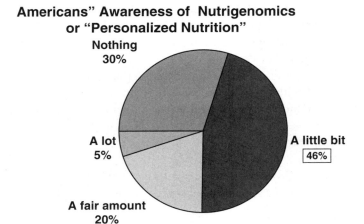

Americans" Awareness of Nutrigenomics or "Personalized Nutrition"

Recent advances in science are making it possible to look at an individual's genetic information (i.e. DNA) to determine a wide range of things about that person's current or future health. Genetic information can be used to provide people with important nutrition and/or diet-related recommendations in order to optimize overall health and reduce the risk of diseases to which they are genetically predisposed. How much, if at all, have you heard or read about this area? (n=1005)

Fig. 3. Americans' awareness of nutrigenomics or "personalized nutrition" *(1)*.

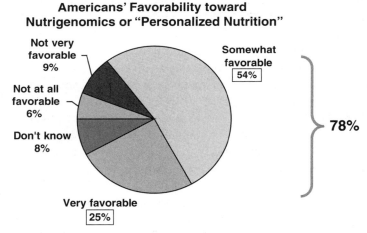

Americans' Favorability toward Nutrigenomics or "Personalized Nutrition"

In general, how favorable are you toward the idea of using genetic information to provide people with nutrition and/or diet-related recommendations? (n=1005)

Fig. 4. Americans' favorability toward nutrigenomics or "personalized nutrition" *(1)*.

vs. 31% in 2007 and 28% in 2005). Those who are "somewhat interested" remained stable compared to 2007 (47% vs. 45% in 2007 and 41% in 2005). Fewer Americans are "not very" or "not at all interested" (17% vs. 19% in 2007 and 23% in 2005). Those most likely to be "very interested" in learning more about nutrigenomics or "personalized nutrition" are consumers who believe food and nutrition play a "great" (31%) or "moderate role" (16%) in maintaining or improving overall health (vs. 17% "limited or no role"); consumers who believe that they have a "great" amount of control over their health (35% vs. 26% who say they have "moderate" control and 17% who say they have "small" or "no" control over their health); those who report their health status to be "excellent" (49% vs. 35% "very good," 29% "good," and 28% "fair" or "poor"); dietary supplement users (37% vs. 22% non-users); consumers with children under the ages of 18 living at home (37% vs. 30% without children at home); and primary household shoppers (37% vs. 23% of those who are not the primary shopper).

In 2007, we asked questions about terminology with respect to this emerging science. American consumers overwhelmingly continue to prefer the terms "personalized nutrition" (76%) and "individualized nutrition" (73%) rather than "nutrigenetics" (50%) or "nutritional genomics" (40%) to describe the practice of using genetic information to develop personalized diet and health recommendations. Compared to 2005, slightly fewer consumers say that medical sources, including physicians, nutritionists, dietitians, and other medical professionals, are the most believable information resource on genetics as it relates to diet and nutrition (33 vs. 37% in 2005). According to our 2009 survey, physicians continue to be the most believable source, although this has decreased (21 vs. 28% in 2005). Similar to 2005, very few cite dietitians (4 vs. 2% in 2005) and nutritionists (3% in both 2005 and 2007) as the most believable source. Other sources cited by less than 10% of consumers include news media, medical journals/books, government agency/U.S. Surgeon General, and friends and family.

4. CONCLUSIONS

This research confirms many of IFIC's earlier findings about foods and beverages that provide added benefits and reveals some new trends in consumers' attitudes, beliefs, and behaviors about food and health. Americans continue to have a high level of awareness and interest in "functional foods," or foods and food components with added benefits, and how a personalized nutrition plan that incorporates these foods can help optimize health and reduce the risk of disease. The vast majority of Americans believe that they have some control over their health, with food and nutrition identified as playing a great role in improving or maintaining health, followed by exercise and family history. Heart disease, weight, and cancer continue to be the top health concerns of Americans, while diabetes and nutrition/diet follow as other important health concerns.

Americans are increasingly aware of specific health benefits associated with various foods and food components. Accordingly, consumers are most aware of food/health benefit associations related to their greatest health concerns of cardiovascular disease, weight maintenance, and cancer, as well as those that have been well established and promoted over time, such as calcium for bone health. Still, newer food associations have entered the minds of some Americans, including health benefits related to probiotics and soy/soy protein. However, as in past surveys, consumers more easily identify whole foods that are generic in nature and fall into a wide spectrum of non-descript categories such as "vegetables," "fruits," or "dairy foods." In some respects it is not surprising that consumers more readily mention certain foods or food categories that contain healthful components rather than the components themselves. For example, consumers may identify fish, fish oil, certain nuts, and flax as being "good" for their hearts and other conditions, but they may not be able to articulate that omega-3 fatty acids are the healthful component that they all have in common. Cross-promotion of foods containing specific components can be helpful and may contribute to increased consumer awareness and consumption over time.

The emerging science of nutrigenomics – preferentially called "personalized nutrition" by most consumers – was explored again after being introduced in the survey in 2005. Americans are increasingly open to the concept of genetic information being used to provide personalized nutrition recommendations. This survey found that Americans report a greater knowledge of this new development, and they are interested in learning more.

Results from the *2009 IFIC Foundation Food & Health Survey* indicate that about two-thirds of Americans are making changes to improve the healthfulness of their diet. The majority of Americans who report that they are consuming certain foods and food components for health benefits are doing so for benefits related to bone health, cardiovascular disease, and cancer. Still, even more consumers are willing to begin eating specific foods and food components for these and other health benefits.

The majority of Americans believe in the concept that certain foods and food components have specific benefits, such as decreasing the risk of certain diseases or improving health attributes such as immune health, and their interest in learning more about foods and their relationships with specific health benefits remains strong. The findings from this research suggest that today's consumers are primed for information and messages about foods and food components that provide benefits beyond basic nutrition and how to incorporate them into their diet. Many are already attempting to make changes to improve the healthfulness of their diets in an effort to reduce risk of disease, yet still more can be done to increase their knowledge about the benefits of specific foods and food components and their consumption.

In 2002, IFIC completed quantitative research with Americans to better understand how to build effective health messages *(3)*. Four factors, time, level of awareness, belief in efficacy, and relevance of the health concern or issue, play an important role in determining where to start a conversation about food and health.

This earlier research conducted by IFIC revealed that the longer the length of time a person had been exposed to information related to a diet and health relationship, the more likely they were to be aware of the benefits certain foods can provide in reducing the risk of disease. For example, the message "calcium builds strong bones" has been touted by many different and trusted information sources for many years, and through this quantitative research, IFIC found that Americans are very aware of this diet and health pairing. The same is not necessarily true for more recent diet and health pairings such as lycopene and a reduced risk of prostate cancer.

Level of awareness is the second factor in effective health messaging. Of those who had heard something about a diet and health pair, those who had heard "a lot" were more likely to believe in the efficacy of the association. Efficacy is the belief that a certain food can, in fact, provide a specific health benefit.

Belief in efficacy – the third factor in building effective health messages – increases with time and level of awareness. Efficacy is a challenging concept for many consumers to grasp because the benefits of food or food components on their health status are usually not an effect that is easily seen or felt immediately. Rather, it can take decades before the effects of eating well seem to "pay off." IFIC's research in this area revealed that if a person believes that a food can provide a specific health benefit then they are more likely to be consuming that food for that benefit.

Finally, it is also important to consider the individual themselves and their perception of the particular health concern or issue. One of the most common barriers cited for not increasing the consumption of foods that provide benefits is that the associated disease or health issue is "not a concern" or the individual perceives they are "not at risk."

Effective health messaging is the key to motivating people to take health into their own hands. Messages that provide the appropriate information for the individual's level of knowledge and help them to set actionable goals regarding foods that are relevant to their lifestyle and health conditions will likely be successful. One size does not fit all.

Collectively, this body of publicly available consumer research provided by IFIC and the IFIC Foundation indicates that there is a window of opportunity for nutrition and health professionals to communicate the potential health benefits of foods and food components and how they may be associated with the practice of "personalized nutrition." Both the media and health professionals are looked upon as sources of credible and influential information related to the role of food in health and disease. Health professionals, researchers, educators, and journalists can seize this opportunity to deliver more personalized nutrition messages that help consumers enjoy health-promoting foods as part of an overall healthful lifestyle.

4.1. Guidelines for Communicating the Emerging Science of Dietary Components for Health

Americans acquire health and nutrition information from numerous sources *(4)*. With more and more information coming from mass media, it is important for everyone in the communication chain to provide consistent and scientifically accurate information. To aid in this process, the IFIC Foundation partnered with the Institute of Food Technologists (IFT) to develop the *Guidelines for Communicating the Emerging Science of Dietary Components for Health*. These *Guidelines* include a checklist for communicators to help enhance the public's understanding of foods, food components, and dietary supplements and their role in a healthful lifestyle.

Communicators, ranging from health professionals, educators, scientists, scientific journal editors, government officials, and journalists, should consider these points when translating how the latest research about food and nutrition could change what's on the public's plate:

- Serve up plain talk about food and health.
- State that scientific research is evolutionary, not revolutionary.
- Carefully craft communications.
- Make messages meaningful.
- Cite study specifics.
- Point out the peer-review process as a key measure of a study's objectivity.
- Consider the full facts when assessing a study's objectivity.

For more information on the *Guidelines*, visit http://www.foodinsight.org/Resources/ Detail.aspx?topic=Guidelines_for_Communicating_the_Emerging_Science_of_Dietary _Components_for_Health.

5. ADDITIONAL RESOURCES

1. International Food Information Council Foundation. (2001) *IFIC Review: How to Understand and Interpret Food and Health-Related Scientific Studies.* September 2001. http://www.foodinsight.org/linkclick.aspx?fileticket=d8IZK7B4MGY%3d&tabid=93. Accessed February 25, 2010.
2. International Food Information Council Foundation. (2007) Understanding and effectively communicating food and nutrition science: Leading consumers to better health. *IFIC Foundation Continuing Professional Education Module.* November 2007. http://foodinsight.staging.r2integrated.com/Resources/Detail.aspx?topic=Understanding _and_Effectively_Communicating_Food_and_Nutrition_Science_Leading_Consumers_ to_Better_Health_CPE_Program. Accessed February 25, 2010.
3. International Food Information Council Foundation. (2008) *Tools for Effective Communication: Beginning a New Conversation with Consumers.* http://www. ific.org/tools/intro.cfm. Accessed on December 8, 2008.
4. Borra, S., Kelly, L., Tuttle, M., and Neville, K. (2001) Developing actionable dietary guidance messages: Dietary fat as a case study. *J Am Diet Assoc.* 101, 678–84.
5. US Department of Health and Human Services, National Institutes of Health, National Cancer Institute. (2001) Making Health Communication Programs Work, Bethesda, MD.

REFERENCES

1. International Food Information Council. (2009) *Functional Foods/Foods for Health Consumer Trending Survey Executive Summary.* August 2009. http://www.foodinsight.org/Resources/Detail.aspx? topic=2009_Functional_Foods_Foods_For_Health_Consumer_Trending_Survey_Executive_Summary. Accessed on February 25, 2010.
2. International Food Information Council Foundation. (2009) *Food & Health Survey.* May 2009. http://www.foodinsight.org/Resources/Detail.aspx?topic=2009_Food_Health_Survey_Consumer_ Attitudes_toward_Food_Nutrition_and_Health. Accessed on February 25, 2010.
3. International Food Information Council. (2002) *Functional Foods: Attitudinal Research.* August 2002. http://www.foodinsight.org/Resources/Detail.aspx?topic=2002_Functional_Foods_Attitudinal_ Research. Accessed on February 25, 2010.
4. International Food Information Council Foundation, Institute of Food Technologists. (2005) *Guidelines for Communicating the Emerging Science of Dietary Components for Health.* March 2005. http://www.foodinsight.org/Resources/Detail.aspx?topic=Guidelines_for_Communicating_the_ Emerging_Science_of_Dietary_Components_for_Health . Accessed on February 25, 2010.

Subject Index

Note: The letters 'f' and 't' following the locators refer to figures and tables respectively.

A

AARP Diet and Health Study cohort, 220
Aberrant crypt foci (ACF), 171, 184–185, 188t,
    369–370, 372, 401–402, 429, 541, 580,
    615–617, 714, 772
Acrodermatitis enteropathica (AE), 501
ACS, *see* American Cancer Society (ACS)
Activating transcription factor (ATF), 30, 56, 129,
    265
Activator protein-1 (AP-1), 129–135
    activation suppressed by EGCG, 130–131
        activation of Fyn, 130
        H-*Ras*-activated AP-1 pathway, 130–131
        inhibitory effects, 131
        MAP kinase/AP-1 signaling pathway,
            inhibits, 130
        Ras pathway, 130
    cell transformation, 129
    EGCG, 129
    flavonol compounds
        kaempferol/quercetin/myricetin, *see*
            Flavonol compounds
    [6]-gingerol modulates AP-1 activation, *see*
        [6]-gingerol
    inhibited by black tea theaflavins, 131
        anticancer activity, 131
        polyphenols, 131
        UVB-induced AP-1 activation, inhibitors,
            131
    inhibited by xanthine 70, caffeine analogue,
        132–133
        anticancer drugs, 132
        effects of caffeine, 132
        oral administration, 132
        proliferation of cells, 132

and resveratrol, *see* Resveratrol
transcription factors, 129
    ATF and MAF protein families, 129
    Fos family, 129
    Jun protein family, 129
in tumor promotion, 129f
Acute myeloid leukemia (AML), 479, 626
Acute phase response, 155, 436
AE, *see* Acrodermatitis enteropathica (AE)
Aged garlic extract (AGE), 569, 571, 579, 683,
    685, 687, 690
AHR-mediated carcinogenesis, 768–769
    animal models, 768
    human studies
        AhR repressor (AhRR) protein, 769
        utero exposure to AhR ligands, 768–769
AICR, *see* American Institute for Cancer Research
    (AICR)
2007 AICR/WCRF
    report, 547
    Second Expert Report on Food, Nutrition,
        Physical Activity, and the Prevention of
        Cancer, 28
Ajoene, 568t, 569, 572, 575–579, 672f, 685
Alcohol and cancer
    alcohol and carcinogen bioactivation, 740–741
    alcohol and gene interactions, 741–744
        ADH1C, rate-limiting factor, 742
        ADH polymorphisms, 742–743, 742f
        ALDH polymorphisms, 743
        other polymorphisms, 743–744
        polymorphisms in alcohol and aldehyde
            dehydrogenases, 742f
    alcohol, hormones, and growth factors, 744–747
        alcohol–breast cancer interaction, 747
        biological intermediates, 746

From: *Nutrition and Health: Bioactive Compounds and Cancer*
Edited by: J.A. Milner, D.F. Romagnolo, DOI 10.1007/978-1-60761-627-6,
© Springer Science+Business Media, LLC 2010

About the Editors

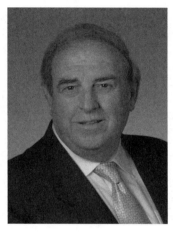

John Milner, Ph.D., is chief of the Nutritional Science Research Group, Division of Cancer Prevention, National Cancer Institute. From 1989 to 2000, he was head of and a professor in the Department of Nutrition at The Pennsylvania State University, where he also served as director of the Graduate Program in Nutrition. Before joining Penn State, he was a faculty member for 13 years in the Food Science Department and in the Division of Nutritional Sciences at the University of Illinois, Urbana-Champaign. While at the University of Illinois he served as the director of the Division of Nutritional Sciences and as an assistant director of the Agricultural Experiment Station.

Dr. Milner earned a Ph.D. from Cornell University in nutrition, with a minor in biochemistry and physiology and a B.S. in Animal Sciences from Oklahoma State University. Dr. Milner is a member of several professional organizations, including the American Society for Nutrition, American Association of Cancer Research, American Chemical Society's Food and Chemistry Division, the Institute of Food Technology and the International Society of Nutrigenetics/Nutrigenomics. He is a fellow in the American Association for the Advancement of Science and an honorary member of the American Dietetic Association.

He has served in an advisory capacity as a member of the US Department of Agriculture's Human Nutrition Board of Scientific Counselors, Joint USDA/HHS Dietary Guidelines Committee, and for the Food, Nutrition and Safety Committee within the International Life Sciences Institute (ILSI). Dr. Milner has served as president of the American Society for Nutrition (formerly the American Institute of Nutrition) and has testified before the Subcommittee on Appropriations in Washington, DC and the Presidential Commission on Dietary Supplement Labels in Baltimore, Maryland. He has served as a member of the National Academy of Sciences Committee on Military Nutrition Research, the US Olympic Committee Dietary Guidelines Task Force, the External Advisory Board for the Pennington Biomedical Research Center, as a member and vice-chair for the Counsel of Experts of United States Pharmacopoeia Committee on Bioavailability and Nutrient Absorption, a member of the External Advisory Board for the European Commission SeaFood Plus initiative, and as the chair of the World Cancer Research Fund/American Institute for Cancer Research Mechanisms Working Group. He is currently a member of the Global Board of Trustees for ILSI, liaison to the International Food Information Council (IFIC), member of the Danone Institute's International

Functional Foods and Health Claims Knowledge Center Committee, a member of the Board for the McCormick Science Institute, and a member of the Mushroom Research Board. In 2008 he received the David A. Kritchevsky Career Achievement Award in Nutrition from the American Society for Nutrition.

Dr. Milner has published more than 200 book chapters, monographs, and journal articles. He serves on the editorial boards for *Cancer Prevention Research*, *Food and Nutrition Research*, *Nutrition and Cancer*, *Nutrfood*, *Journal of Nutritional Biochemistry*, *Journal of Alternative and Complementary Medicine*, *Journal of Ovarian Research*, *and The Journal of Medical Foods*. In his current position he promotes research that deals with the physiological importance of dietary bioactive compounds as modifiers of cancer risk and tumor behavior. Much of his own current research focuses on the anticancer properties of garlic and associated allyl sulfur compounds. In addition to presentations about nutrition and genomics he has been invited to speak about garlic and health, selenium nutriture, antioxidants and health, functional foods and health promotion, and nutrition for cancer prevention.

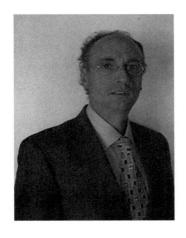

Donato F. Romagnolo, Ph.D., is professor of Nutritional and Cancer Biology at The University of Arizona. Dr. Romagnolo is a member of the Arizona Cancer and The Toxicology Centers, The BIO5 Institute, and the Southwest Environmental Health Sciences Center at The University of Arizona. He is currently a member of the Executive Committees for the Graduate Program in Nutritional Sciences, the Cancer Biology Graduate Program, The Training Grant in Cancer Biology, The Training Grant in Toxicology and Toxicogenomis, and served as member for the Advisory Board and chair of the Environmental Gene Expression Group of the Southwest Environmental Health Sciences Center, and chair for the Research Frontiers in Nutritional Sciences Conference, Department of Nutritional Sciences, at The University of Arizona. Dr. Romagnolo is instructor for undergraduate Nutritional Biology and graduate Metabolic Integration at The University of Arizona.

Dr. Romagnolo earned a M.S. and a Ph.D. from Virginia Polytechnic Institute and State University, and a B.S. from The University of Padua, Padua, Italy. He was a postdoctoral fellow at the National Institutes of Environmental Health Sciences, National Institutes of Health. Dr. Romagnolo is a member of several professional organizations, including the American Society for Nutrition, American Association of Cancer Research, and the American Association for the Advancement of Science.

He has published book chapters, monographs, and original research in cancer and nutrition scientific journals including *Cancer Research, The Journal of Nutrition, Nutrition and Cancer, Breast Cancer Research, Molecular Carcinogenesis, Environmental and Molecular Mutagenesis, Neoplasia, and Experimental Biology and Medicine.* Dr. Romagnolo has been a member of scientific review panels and received research funding from the National Institutes of Health, The US Department Breast Cancer Research Program, the Susan G. Komen Breast Cancer Foundation, and the Arizona Biomedical Research Commission. Dr. Romagnolo is currently a member of the RIS Gene Expression Group of the American Society of Nutrition.

In his current position he promotes research that deals with the role of dietary xenobiotics and natural bioactive compounds as epigenetic regulators of expression of genes involved in cancer and inflammation. Current research focuses primarily on the role of ligands of the aromatic hydrocarbon receptor on epigenetic regulation of the breast cancer tumor suppressor (BRCA1) and proinflammatory (COX-2) genes.

About the Series Editor

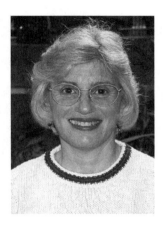

Dr. Adrianne Bendich is clinical director, Medical Affairs at GlaxoSmithKline (GSK) Consumer Healthcare where she is responsible for leading the innovation and medical programs in support of many well-known brands including TUMS and Os-Cal. Dr. Bendich had primary responsibility for GSK's support for the Women's Health Initiative (WHI) intervention study. Prior to joining GSK, Dr. Bendich was at Roche Vitamins Inc. and was involved with the groundbreaking clinical studies showing that folic acid-containing multivitamins significantly reduced major classes of birth defects. Dr. Bendich has co-authored over 100 major clinical research studies in the area of preventive nutrition. Dr. Bendich is recognized as a leading authority on antioxidants, nutrition and immunity and pregnancy outcomes, vitamin safety and the cost-effectiveness of vitamin/mineral supplementation.

Dr. Bendich is the editor of nine books including "Preventive Nutrition: The Comprehensive Guide for Health Professionals" co-edited with Dr. Richard Deckelbaum and is Series Editor of "Nutrition and Health" for Humana Press with 29 published volumes including "Probiotics in Pediatric Medicine" edited by Dr. Sonia Michail and Dr. Philip Sherman; " Handbook of Nutrition and Pregnancy" edited by Dr. Carol Lammi-Keefe, Dr. Sarah Couch, and Dr. Elliot Philipson; "Nutrition and Rheumatic Disease" edited by Dr. Laura Coleman; " Nutrition and Kidney Disease" edited by Dr. Laura Byham-Grey, Dr. Jerrilynn Burrowes, and Dr. Glenn Chertow; "Nutrition and Health in Developing Countries" edited by Dr. Richard Semba and Dr. Martin Bloem; "Calcium in Human Health" edited by Dr. Robert Heaney and Dr. Connie Weaver; and "Nutrition and Bone Health" edited by Dr. Michael Holick and Dr. Bess Dawson-Hughes.

Dr. Bendich served as associate editor for "*Nutrition*" the International Journal; served on the Editorial Board of the *Journal of Women's Health and Gender-based Medicine* and was a member of the board of directors of the American College of Nutrition.

Dr. Bendich was the recipient of the Roche Research Award, is a *Tribute to Women and Industry* Awardee, and was a recipient of the Burroughs Wellcome Visiting Professorship in Basic Medical Sciences, 2000–2001. In 2008, Dr. Bendich was given the Council for Responsible Nutrition (CRN) Apple Award in recognition of her many contributions to the scientific understanding of dietary supplements. Dr. Bendich holds academic appointments as adjunct professor in the Department of Preventive Medicine and Community Health at UMDNJ and has an adjunct appointment at the Institute of Nutrition, Columbia University P&S, and is an adjunct research professor, Rutgers University, Newark Campus. She is listed in Who's Who in American Women.

Printed in the United States of America